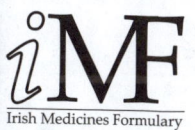

iMF
Irish Medicines Formulary

August 2017

CW01500480

Contents

1
2
3
4
5
6
7
8
9
10
11
12
13
14
15
16

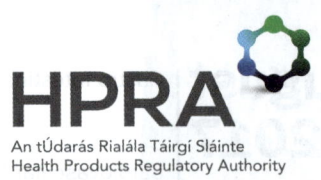

DOMPERIDONE-CONTAINING MEDICINES: REMINDER OF THE RISK OF CARDIAC ADVERSE REACTIONS-RESTRICTED INDICATION, CONTRAINDICATIONS AND REDUCED DOSE AND DURATION OF USE

In 2014 a European-wide review recommended restrictions on the use of domperidone-containing medicines following an evaluation of the benefits and risks of domperidone. This review was triggered due to concerns regarding cardiac adverse effects associated with domperidone use.

After evaluation of available evidence on the efficacy and safety of domperidone from various sources (non-clinical and clinical, published and unpublished), the review confirmed that there was a small increased risk of serious cardiac adverse effects associated with the use of domperidone, including QT prolongation, torsades de pointes, ventricular arrhythmia and sudden cardiac arrest. This risk was higher in patients > 60 years, adults taking daily oral doses of >30 mg and those concomitantly taking QT prolonging medicines or CYP3A4 inhibitors. The review concluded that the benefit-risk profile remains positive in the treatment of nausea and vomiting, when there is adherence to the risk minimisation measures set out in the product information.

Domperidone should be used at the lowest effective dose for the shortest possible duration (not exceeding 1 week). The maximum recommended dose of domperidone in adults is 10 mg orally up to 3 times daily or 30 mg twice daily as suppositories. The recommended dose of domperidone for children is 0.25mg/kg bodyweight up to 3 times daily orally (oral suspensions should be given in adapted graduated oral syringes).

Domperidone is contraindicated in patients with moderate or severe hepatic impairment, conditions where cardiac conduction is, or could be, impaired, and in patients with underlying cardiac disease. Co-administration with QT prolonging medicines or potent CYP3A4 inhibitors is also contraindicated.

Healthcare Professionals are reminded of the following advice to support the safe and appropriate use of domperidone:

Reminder of restricted indication

• The use of domperidone is restricted to the relief of symptoms of nausea and vomiting.

Reminder of contraindications

Domperidone should not be used in:

• patients with conditions where cardiac conduction is, or could be, impaired,

• patients with underlying cardiac diseases such as congestive heart failure,

• patients receiving other medications known to prolong QT interval or potent CYP3A4 inhibitors, and

• patients with moderate to severe hepatic impairment.

Reminder of the restrictions on dose
Oral formulations

- For adults and adolescents over 12 years of age and weighing 35kg or more, the recommended maximum dose in 24 hours is 30mg (dose interval: 10mg up to three times a day)

- In children under 12 years of age and weighing less than 35kg, the recommended maximum dose in 24 hours is 0.75mg/kg body weight (dose interval: 0.25mg/kg body weight up to three times a day).

- In order to accurately measure doses to paediatric patients, oral suspensions should be given using an adapted graduated oral syringe.

Reminder of the restrictions on dose
Suppository formulation

- Suppositories should only be used in adults and adolescents weighing 35kg or more, the recommended maximum daily dose in 24 hours is 60mg (dose interval: 30mg twice a day).

- Note: there are currently no suppository formulations of domperidone authorised in Ireland.

Reminder of the duration of treatment

- Domperidone should be used at the lowest effective dose for the shortest possible duration.

- The maximum treatment duration should not usually exceed one week.

- Patients currently receiving long-term treatment with domperidone should be reassessed at a routine appointment to advise on treatment continuation, dose change, or cessation.

Key Message

Domperidone is associated with a small increased risk of serious cardiac adverse effects. HCPs are reminded of the following risk minimisation measures:

Therapeutic Indications: Use of domperidone is restricted to the relief of symptoms of nausea and vomiting.

Contraindications: Domperidone is contraindicated in patients who have known existing prolongation of cardiac conduction intervals, particularly QTc, in patients with significant electrolyte disturbances or underlying cardiac diseases such as congestive heart failure, in patients who are concomitantly taking QT-prolonging drugs or potent CYP3A4 inhibitors (regardless of their QT prolonging effects) and in patients who have moderate or severe hepatic impairment.

Dose and duration of use: HCPs should adhere to the dose and duration of use for adults, adolescents and children recommended in the Summary of Product Characteristics. Patients >60 years of age should consult a Healthcare Professional before taking domperidone. Domperidone should be used at the lowest effective dose for the shortest duration necessary. The maximum treatment period should not usually exceed one week.

*Products currently authorised in Ireland include Motilium and Domerid. Further details are available at www.hpra.ie

---

This information is supplied by the Health Products Regulatory Authority (HPRA) for use in the IMF. However, the HPRA is independent and impartial to any other information contained in this formulary.

iii

Guide to using IMF

Information in IMF is presented in a consistent format for maximum clarity and ease of use. This page explains the format and the type of information contained under each heading.

7

Chapter Name and Number
e.g. Ophthalmology

7.1 - Glaucoma

Class Effects
Information included is common to ALL members of this broad therapeutic area or drug class and includes: **Indications, Contraindications (CI), Drug Interactions, Special Precautions (SP), Use in Pregnancy and Lactation, Adverse Drug Reactions (ADR).**

7.1.1 - Topical Beta-Blockers

In This Chapter: *Molecules included in this chapter are named either by their International Non-Proprietary Name (INN) or British Approved Name (BAN) (adrenaline).*

Class Effects
Information included is common to ALL members of this **specific** therapeutic area or drug class under the same headings as the broad therapeutic area above.

Molecule (INN or BAN)

ATC Code: The Anatomical Therapeutic Chemical (ATC) classification system, WHO Collaborating Centre for Drug Statistics Methodology.

Sport: Guidelines in accordance with the World Anti-Doping Code published by WADA (World Anti-Doping Agency). They are not a substitute for consultation of the full Anti-Doping Code and expert professional opinion. Restrictions may relate to use in certain sports or use under certain circumstances. The ultimate responsibility lies with the athlete.

Driving: Guidelines according to the licensed Summary of Product Characteristics (SPC) and/or the DRUID project (Driving Under the Influence of Drugs, Alcohol and Medicines). This information does not take into account co-administered medicinals or alcohol intake.

Indications: Additional or different indications to those listed under Class Effects. May pertain to a specific brand listed below.

Dose: Adult: Adult dosing information for all brands/formulations listed below.

Dose: Adult, Elderly: Dosing is listed under this heading if there are no dose modifications required for elderly patients.

Elderly: Specific dose modifications and/or precautions required for the elderly.

Renal Impairment: Specific dose modifications and/or precautions required.

Hepatic Impairment: As for Renal above.

Child: Specific dosing for children according to the Irish license for each brand. If there is no Child dosing specified the product is NOT for use in children. Always check Class Effects above.

CI: Additional or different contraindications to those listed under Class Effects. May pertain to a specific brand listed below.

Interactions: Effect of Other Drugs on the Drug (molecule listed above): *Effect on the drug listed above is first (always in italics):* Followed by the drugs where co-admin is contraindicated, not recommended or where a specific action needs to be taken.

Effect of the Drug (molecule listed above) on Other Drugs: Drugs which are affected are always listed first. *They are followed by the effect that the drug (listed above) has on other drugs (effect always in italics).*

SP: Additional or different special precautions to those listed under Class Effects. May pertain to a specific brand listed below.

Pregnancy, Lactation: Information in addition to Class Effects above; whether the drug can be used or if there are any special precautions. Any statement applies to both pregnancy and lactation unless specified.

ADR: Additional or different ADRs to those listed under Class Effects. May pertain to a specific brand listed below. Where the information is available the frequency and/or seriousness of the ADRs are highlighted. ADRs from post-marketing surveillance are not included.

Notes: The prescriber is directed to the Class Effects above or to other sections of the publication in the case of combination products.

Interchangeability: Highlights the brands listed below deemed interchangeable by the Health Products Regulatory Authority (HPRA).

Reference Price: Lists the reference price as published by the HSE.

Following the prescribing information for the molecule above, all brands licensed and marketed in Ireland are listed. Where the innovator brand still exists, it is listed first followed by the generic equivalents in alphabetical order.

Brand Name *(Pharmaceutical Company)* Dispensing Status. Reimbursement Status.
Price, strength-pack size, Euro price. If reimbursed (GMS, HT, DTS), the reimbursed price is published. If not reimbursed, the trade price is published. Where companies do not provide pricing information, products are listed as 'Price, not published by company'. If the price to wholesaler (PTW) is supplied for these products, the Euro price is published and clarified (PTW).
Type of formulation, active ingredient(s) (always in italics), followed by a description of the formulation(s). *Noteworthy excipients (always in italics) (see Appendix for list of noteworthy excipients).*
Store: Specific storage requirements.
Notes: Any additional information pertaining to brand above. Full Prescribing Information for brands available at www.hpra.ie.

Content in IMF

IMF is provided as a decision support resource and is not a substitute for professional opinion or the manufacturer's Full Prescribing Information **(FPI)**. Users are strongly advised to consult the Summary of Product Characteristics (SPC) for the manufacturer's **FPI** available from the Health Products Regulatory Authority (HPRA) website, www.hpra.ie.

Prices listed in IMF are for comparative purposes only. For reimbursed products, the reimbursed price is published; reimbursement may be under the General Medical Services Scheme (GMS), the High Tech Scheme (HT) or the Dental Treatment Service Scheme (DTS). For products that are not reimbursed, the trade price or price to wholesaler (PTW) is published.

Product-related information is based on SPC information sourced from the HPRA and updates supplied by pharmaceutical companies. Pricing information is based on information supplied by individual pharmaceutical companies and published GMS and High Tech updates. All information contained in IMF is deemed accurate at the time of going to press.

While every effort is made to ensure information included is accurate and up to date, the publisher, contributors, advisors, manufacturers, marketing authorisation (MA) holders, designer and printer of IMF do not accept any liability for errors or omissions.

No part of IMF may be reproduced in any form without the written permission of the publisher. Please address editorial queries to formulary@meridianireland.com.

Copies of **IMF** can be purchased online at www.imfmedia.ie or by telephoning +353-1-8390073 or e-mailing sales@meridianireland.com.

IMF is updated twice yearly and the latest edition should always be used in practice.

Symbols Used in IMF

Dispensing Status:
A: Product subject to prescription which may not be renewed.
B: Product subject to prescription which may be renewed.
C: Product subject to restricted prescription
OTC Product not subject to prescription i.e. available over the counter (may be available for general sale in supermarket or only in pharmacy).
CD: A drug controlled under the Misuse of Drugs Act and amendments.
For more information regarding Legal Category or Dispensing Status of Medicines, see www.hpra.ie

Reimbursement Status:
A number of pharmaceutical reimbursement schemes operate in Ireland including:
GMS: Reimbursed in full by the Primary Care Reimbursement Service (PCRS) under the General Medical Services Scheme (GMS). This applies to eligible medicines supplied to patients entitled to a Medical Card.

HT: High Tech Scheme – applicable to certain medicines prescribed in hospitals using a specific prescription form.

D: Reimbursed under the Dental Treatment Service Scheme (DTS) for eligible medicines supplied to patients entitled to a medical card. D* is used when only certain strength(s) or pack size(s) are reimbursed.

HOS: Products usually used in a hospital setting.

HSEi: Specifically for vaccines supplied by the HSE. See www.immunisation.ie

(Adult): Adult Vaccines
(Child): Primary Childhood Vaccines
(Restricted): Restricted Vaccines (require authorisation)
(Used): Vaccines used by the HSE

Medicines Subject to Additional Monitoring Requirements
▼ This medicinal product is subject to additional monitoring. This symbol (inverted black triangle) will be used in all EU member states to identify medicines under additional monitoring and will appear in the product information. In IMF the inverted black triangle will appear next to the brand name of the product. Further information on additional monitoring is available from www.hpra.ie and www.ema.europa.eu

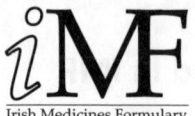

Irish Medicines Formulary

August 2017

Changes Since Edition 21

New Chemical Entities, New Combinations (existing chemical entities)

Apremilast 4.4.1 Drugs Suppressing Rheumatic Disease Process
Brivaracetam 3.1.6 Miscellaneous Antiepileptics
Cobicistat 9.3.2 Protease Inhibitors (HIV)
Everolimus 13.2.1 Immunosuppressants
Naltrexone, Bupropion 16.2 Obesity
Nintedanib (Oncology) 13.1.6 Protein Kinase Inhibitors
Nintedanib (IPF) 2.2.4 PAH, Idiopathic Pulmonary Fibrosis (IPF)
Trifluridine, Tipiracil 13.1.3 Antimetabolites

New Generic Equivalents

48 new generic equivalents/formulations

Discontinued Products, Presentations, Packs

Alomide 0.1% Eye Drops
Atrovent UDVs (250mcg, 500mcg)
Aulin Topical Gel
Betoptic Eye Drops 0.5%, Single Dose 0.25%
Bravelle Parenteral 75 IU
Camcolit 400mg
Carbamazepine Essential Supps (formerly Tegretol)
Clonamox (range)
Emadine Eye Drops
Esomeprazole Mylan 20mg, 40mg
Laxose Oral Soln (300mL-pack only)
Maxidex Eye Ointment
Maxitrol 0.1% Eye Ointment
Mefac 250mg (500-pack only)
MOXIVIG 0.5% Eye Drops
Mysoline (1000-pack only)
Myzaar 50mg, 100mg
Nitrocine Parenteral 1mg/mL
Norvir Oral Soln 80mg/mL
Pabal Parenteral 100mcg/mL
Pantoprazole TEVA Parenteral 40mg

Parlodel 2.5mg (100-pack only)
Persantin Retard 200mg
Pioglitazone Rowex 15mg, 30mg, 45mg
Prapexin 0.088mg, 0.18mg Standard/R
Prindavam 4/1.25mg
Protizole 20mg, 40mg
Provera 5mg (100-pack only)
Rabeprazole (Gerard) 10mg, 20mg
Rabiclon 10mg, 20mg
Rapilysin Parenteral
Regurin 20mg
Romep 20mg (7-pack only)
Setinin XL Tablets
Slow K 600mg
Sonata 5mg, 10mg
Tradol Effervescent 50mg (50-pack only)
Tradol Parenteral 50mg/mL (1mL-pack only)
Vedixal XL Prolonged/R 37.5mg (7-pack only)
ViraferonPeg Parenteral
Zeffix Oral Soln
Zytiga (250mg-strength only)

Editor:
Arlene Cock-Wall

Publisher:
Meridian Ireland

Medical Advisor:
Dr John Gilbert, GP

Managing Editor:
Brian Wall

49 Castlerosse View
Baldoyle
Dublin 13
D13 K0V9
Ireland
E-mail: formulary@meridianireland.com
www.imfmedia.ie
Developed, designed and printed in Ireland

1

Gastro-Intestinal Drugs

1.1 - Dyspepsia, GORD

Class Effects
Metallic salts, simethicone and compound alginates are used first-line for symptomatic relief of hyperacidity (heartburn, dyspepsia, indigestion, flatulence) and gastro-oesophageal reflux (GORD) (acid regurgitation, heartburn, indigestion). Some ARE indicated for use during pregnancy; unless specified, use only with medical advice.

CI: Hypersensitivity to any member of the class.
SP: Many of these products are available without prescription. If symptoms persist, advise patient to seek medical advice; do not exceed recommended dose.

1.1.1 - Metallic Salts

In This Chapter: *Metallic salts (aluminium, calcium, magnesium) of (hydroxides, carbonates, bicarbonates).*

Class Effects
Interactions: Effect of Metallic Salts (Antacids) on Other Drugs: ACEIs, analgesics, tetracyclines, fluoroquinolones, azole antifungals, vitamins, H2-antagonists, digoxin, iron salts, neuroleptics, thyroxin, penicillamine, beta-blockers (atenolol, metoprolol, propranolol), cefdinir, cefpodoxime, glucocorticoids, chloroquine, bisphosphonates, cyclines, diflunisal, ethambutol, sodium fluoride, indomethacin, isoniazid, lincosamides, neuroleptic phenothiazines: *Decreased absorption due to altered gastric pH or formation of complexes (admin 2 hours apart; 4 hours for fluoroquinolones).* Drugs where excretion is urinary pH sensitive (aspirin): *Increased or decreased excretion.* Lithium: *Reduced plasma levels.* Quinidine: *Increased plasma levels.* Polystyrene sulfonate (Kayexalate): *Caution, reduced effectiveness of the resin.*
SP: *Aluminium,* may be involved in porphyrin metabolism abnormalities; caution, porphyriacs on haemodialysis. May lead to phosphate depletion syndrome especially with low phosphate diet (malnutrition). With renal impairment, plasma aluminium and magnesium levels increase; long-term exposure to high doses may lead to encephalopathy,

dementia, microcytic anaemia or worsening dialysis-induced osteomalacia. Constipating. Aluminium hydroxide is not well absorbed from the GI tract; systemic effects rare but can occur at high doses or prolonged use.
Magnesium, CNS depression (with renal impairment or failure). Laxative effect.
Calcium, constipating, may delay gastric emptying; Ca/Mg mixture avoids lower GI effects.
Sodium bicarbonate, rebound hyperacidity if taken in excess.
Pregnancy, Lactation: First trimester, not recommended; some products ARE indicated for treatment of heartburn of pregnancy. Use calcium carbonate containing products for shortest duration.
Notes: See Class Effects 1.1 Dyspepsia, GORD.

Aluminium, Magnesium (GI)
ATC Code: A02AD01. **Sport:** Permitted.
Driving: Unlikely to impair.
Indications: Symptoms of dyspepsia.
Dose: Adult, Elderly: 5-10mL taken 20-60 minutes after meals and at night.
Renal Impairment: Failure, contraindicated.
CI: Severely debilitated.
SP: NOTE: Sodium content. Prolonged use or at high doses may result in increased bone resorption, hypercalciuria, osteomalacia in patients with low phosphorus diet or infants under 2 years.
Pregnancy, Lactation: Pregnancy if considered essential. Lactation, considered compatible.
ADR: *Uncommon,* diarrhoea, constipation.
Notes: See 1.1.1 Metallic Salts.

    Maalox Suspension 200/175 *(SANOFI)* OTC. GMS.
    Price, (500mL) €2.49.
    Oral susp, aluminium/magnesium (hydroxide) 175/200. White viscous aqueous; peppermint odour, taste. *Sorbitol, sodium 1.59mg/5mL.* **Store:** Below 25 deg C.

1.1.2 - Compound Alginates

In This Chapter: *Alginates (and metallic salts).*

Class Effects
Alginic acid reacts with gastric acid to form a viscous foamy gel, floating on top of gastric contents helping to prevent reflux.
CI: Hypersensitivity to any member of the class.
Notes: See Class Effects 1.1.1 Metallic Salts.

Alginates
ATC Code: A02BX13. **Sport:** Permitted.
Driving: Not applicable.
Indications: Gastric regurgitation (infants). GORD, hiatus hernia (infants, young children).
Dose: Adult, Elderly: Not for use.
Child: *Infants* (age 1-2 years), under 4.5kg, 1 sachet; over 4.5kg, 2 sachets. *Admin, breast fed,* add 5mL cooled boiled water to powder in a glass, mix immediately to smooth paste; add another 10mL of water and mix; give after each feed using spoon or feeding bottle. *Bottle fed,* mix contents of sachet(s) immediately into minimum 115mL (for 1 sachet) or 225mL (for 2 sachets) of each feed in the bottle; shake well. Not for use in premature infants, children under 1 year (except with medical supervision), children over 2 years. Admin max. 6 times in 24 hours.
Renal Impairment: Contraindicated (high sodium content, hypernatraemia risk).
CI: Use only with healthcare professional recommendation. Intestinal obstruction, established diarrhoea; excessive water loss (fever, diarrhoea, vomiting, high room temperature); gastroenteritis (requiring rehydration with fluid replacement).
Interactions: Effect of Other Drugs on Alginates: *Co-admin not recommended:* Thickening agents, infant milk

1.2 Antispasmodics

preparations containing thickening agents (risk of over-thickening stomach content).

SP: Hypernatraemia (admin oral fluids, monitor electrolytes). Abnormal stool consistency (diarrhoea, constipation); investigate changes in bowel habit.

ADR: Altered stool consistency (constipation, diarrhoea).

Notes: See 1.1.2 Compound Alginates.

> **Gaviscon Infant Sachets** *(R/Benckiser)* OTC.
> *Price,* (30) €3.03 (PTW).
> *Sachet,* magnesium 87.5mg/sodium alginate 225mg per dose. Off-white powder for oral susp. *Sodium 21mg/dose.* **Store:** Below 30 deg C.

Alginates, Metallic Salts

ATC Code: A02BX13. **Sport:** Permitted.
Driving: Unlikely to impair.

Indications: GORD and symptoms; including during pregnancy.

Dose: Adult, Elderly: *Gaviscon Advance,* chew 1-2 tabs thoroughly OR take 5-10mL after meals and at bedtime; no improvement after 7 days, review. *Gaviscon Susp, Acidex,* age over 12 years, 10-20mL after meals and at bedtime.

Child: *Gaviscon Advance,* under 12 years only on medical advice. *Acidex, Gaviscon Suspension,* age 6-12 years, 5-10mL after meals and at night; *Gaviscon Suspension,* admin only with medical advice.

Renal Impairment: Caution, highly salt-restricted diet.

SP: Avoid large amounts of milk, milk products. Hypercalcaemia, nephrocalcinosis, recurrent calcium-containing renal calculi, caution (calcium content). Signs of appendicitis or inflamed bowel, not recommended. Not for admin within 1-2 hours of other oral medicines.

Pregnancy, Lactation: Can be used if clinically needed.

Notes: See 1.1.2 Compound Alginates.

> **Gaviscon Advance** *(R/Benckiser)* OTC. GMS.
> *Price,* tabs (60) €4.37. Susp (500mL) €7.68.
> *Chew tab,* sodium alginate, potassium bicarbonate 500/100mg. Off-white (cream) round flat; peppermint (odour, flavour). Marked with logo; GA500 on reverse. *Sodium 103mg,* aspartame. **Store:** Below 30 deg C; original pack.
> *Oral susp,* as above 100/20mg per 1mL. Off-white viscous. *Sodium 106mg,* potassium 78mg per 10mL, parabens.
> **Gaviscon Suspension** *(R/Benckiser)* OTC. GMS.
> *Price,* (500mL) €3.53.
> *Oral susp,* calcium carbonate 160mg, sodium (bicarbonate 267mg, alginate 500mg) per 10mL. Opaque viscous pink; fennel-odour. *Sodium 141mg/10mL,* parabens. **Store:** Below 30 deg C; do not refrigerate.
> **Acidex Oral Suspension** *(Pinewood)* OTC. GMS.
> *Price,* (200mL) €1.83. (500mL) €2.92.
> *Oral susp,* calcium carbonate 160mg, sodium (bicarbonate 267mg, alginate 500mg) per 10mL. Pink aniseed-flavour. *Sodium 141mg/10mL,* parabens.

1.2 - Antispasmodics

In This Chapter: *Alverine, hyoscine, mebeverine, peppermint oil.*

Class Effects

Mebeverine is also used in combination in laxative preparations. Hyoscine hydrobromide, is also used in the prevention of motion sickness; available without prescription, brand *Kwells.*

CI: Hypersensitivity to any member of the class.

Notes: See Class Effects 1.5.2 Bulk Forming Laxatives (mebeverine combinations).

Alverine

ATC Code: A03AX08. **Sport:** Permitted.
Driving: Dizziness.

Indications: GI smooth muscle spasm (IBS, diverticular disease of colon).

Dose: Adult, Elderly: 60-120mg 1-3 times daily.

Child: Under 12 years, not recommended.

CI: Paralytic ileus, intestinal obstruction.

SP: Seek medical advice if (older than 40 years, passed blood from bowel, feeling sick or vomiting, lost appetite or weight, pale or feeling tired, severe constipation, fever, recently travelled abroad, vaginal bleeding or discharge, difficulty or pain passing urine, may be pregnant).

Pregnancy, Lactation: Not recommended.

ADR: *Incidence not known,* nausea, headache, dizziness, itching, rash, allergic reaction, anaphylaxis, dyspnoea, jaundice, abnormal LFTs.

Notes: See 1.2 Antispasmodics.

> **Spasmonal 60mg, Forte 120mg** *(Meda)* B. GMS.
> *Price,* 60mg (100) €13.87. 120mg (60) €16.64.
> *Capsule,* alverine citrate. Opaque blue/grey. Marked SP/strength.

Hyoscine Butylbromide

ATC Code: A03BB01. **Sport:** Permitted.
Driving: Accommodation disorder, dizziness.

Indications: *Buscopan Rx,* spasm relief (GI, GU tract). *Buscopan Parenteral,* acute spasm (renal, biliary colic), radiology to reduce pain or spasm. *Buscopan (OTC),* spasm relief (GI), symptomatic relief (IBS).

Dose: Adult, Elderly: ORAL, *Buscopan Rx,* 20mg 4-times daily swallowed whole with water. *Buscopan (OTC),* GI spasm, as for Rx above; IBS, 10mg up to 3-times daily; increase as for Rx above. *Admin,* swallow whole with water. PARENTERAL, initially 20mg (IM or slow IV); repeat after 30 minutes if required; max. 100mg/day. Endoscopy, may need to repeat dose more frequently.

Child: ORAL, *Buscopan Rx,* age 6-12 years, 10mg 3-times daily; under 6 years, not recommended. *Admin,* swallow whole with water. *Buscopan (OTC),* under 12 years, not recommended.

CI: *Both formulations,* myasthenia gravis, megacolon, narrow angle glaucoma. *Parenteral,* tachycardia, prostatic enlargement with urinary retention, mechanical stenoses (region of GI tract), paralytic ileus. IM route, haematoma risk if treated with anticoagulants.

Interactions: Effect of Other Drugs on Hyoscine Butylbromide: *Mutual diminished effect with co-admin:* Dopamine antagonists (metoclopramide).

Effect of Hyoscine Butylbromide on Other Drugs: TCADs, antihistamines, quinidine, amantadine, antipsychotics (phenothiazines, butyrophenones), disopyramide, other anticholinergics (tiotropium, ipratropium, atropine-like compounds): *Anticholinergic effect intensified.* Beta-adrenergics: *Tachycardic effects enhanced.*

SP: Investigate severe, unexplained abdominal pain or symptoms of fever, nausea, vomiting, bowel changes, abdominal tenderness, decreased BP, fainting, blood in stools. Can cause tachycardia, hypotension, anaphylaxis, caution (cardiac failure, coronary heart disease, cardiac arrhythmia, hypertension, cardiac surgery). Intestinal or urinary outlet obstruction, pyrexia, untreated narrow angle glaucoma, caution (anticholinergic complications).

Pregnancy, Lactation: Avoid (oral); not recommended (parenteral).

ADR: Oral, *uncommon,* skin reactions, tachycardia, dry mouth, constipation, dyshidrosis. Parenteral, *common,* accommodation disorders, tachycardia, dizziness, dry mouth. Injection site pain (especially IM route).

Notes: See 1.2 Antispasmodics.

> **Buscopan Rx 10mg** *(SANOFI)* B. GMS.
> *Price,* (56) €1.31.
> *Tablet,* hyoscine butylbromide. White round s/c. *Sucrose.* **Store:** Below 30 deg C; original pack.
> **Buscopan 10mg** *(SANOFI)* OTC.
> *Price,* not published by company.
> *Tablet,* hyoscine butylbromide. White round s/c. *Sucrose.* **Store:** Below 30 deg C; original pack; protect (light).
> **Buscopan Parenteral** *(SANOFI)* A. GMS.
> *Price,* 20mg (10) €2.56.
> *Injection,* hyoscine butylbromide 20mg/1mL. Colourless (almost) clear soln. **Store:** Below 30 deg C in outer carton.

2

Mebeverine

ATC Code: A03AA04. **Sport:** Permitted.
Driving: Unlikely to impair.
Indications: Irritable bowel syndrome (IBS) (GI spasm).
Dose: Adult, Elderly: 1 tab 3-times daily, 20 minutes before meals.
Child: Under 10 years, not recommended.
SP: Exclude organic diseases of bowel, malignancy.
Pregnancy, Lactation: Not recommended.
ADR: *Very rarely*, urticaria, angioedema, facial oedema, exanthema/rash.
Notes: See 1.2 Antispasmodics.

Colofac 135mg *(BGP)* B. GMS.
Price, (100) €5.23.
Tablet, mebeverine HCl. White round s/c. *Lactose, sucrose.*

Peppermint Oil

Sport: Permitted.
Driving: Unlikely to impair.
Indications: IBS (discomfort, abdominal colic, distension).
Dose: Adult, Elderly: Initially 1 cap 3-times daily 30-60 minutes before food; titrate to 2 caps 3-times daily if discomfort severe. Do not break/chew or take immediately after food.
Child: Under 15 years, not recommended.
CI: Hypersensitivity (menthol, peanut, soya).
Interactions: Effect of Other Drugs on Peppermint Oil: *Co-admin not recommended*: Antacids.
SP: Max. 2-3 months per course.
Pregnancy, Lactation: If benefit outweighs risk.
ADR: *Frequency unknown*, hypersensitivity, burning sensation of mucosa, anorectal discomfort, dyspepsia, gastro-oesophageal reflux, nausea, vomiting.
Notes: See 1.2 Antispasmodics.

Colpermin 187mg *(McNeil)* OTC. GMS.
Price, (100) €14.86.
Capsule, peppermint oil. Hard gelatin blue/dark blue (blue band) containing oily mixture g/r, e/c; peppermint odour. *Arachis oil.*

1.3 - Ulcer Management

Class Effects
The principle drug classes used in the treatment and prophylaxis GI ulceration include H2-antagonists, proton pump inhibitors (PPIs) and prostaglandin analogues. Cytoprotectants are also used.
CI: Hypersensitivity to any member of the class.
SP: Decreased gastric acidity may increase gastric counts of bacteria normally present in GI tract. Acid-reducing drugs may lead to slightly increased risk of Salmonella and/or Campylobacter GI infections.

1.3.1 - H2-Antagonists

In This Chapter: *Cimetidine, nizatidine, ranitidine.*

Class Effects
H2-antagonists block the histamine receptors (H2-receptors) on parietal cells.
CI: Use in children, under 12 years, unless otherwise specified; over 12 years, as for Adult.
Interactions: Effect of H2-Antagonists on Other Drugs: Bioavailability affected for drugs requiring acidic gastric pH for absorption: *Absorption reduced (ketoconazole, atazanavir, delavirdine, gefitinib)* or *increased (triazolam, midazolam, glipizide).*
SP: May mask symptoms and allow transient healing of gastric ulcer; caution, patients in middle age or with new or recently changed dyspeptic symptoms; exclude malignancy (symptoms may be masked). *Infection*, including increased infectious complications in severely injured patients; increased risk of community-acquired pneumonia in current users (elderly, chronic lung disease,

diabetes, immunocompromised). *Regular supervision*, patients with history of peptic ulcer, especially elderly, those taking NSAIDs or on long-term maintenance. *Porphyriacs*, avoid as may precipitate acute attack.
Pregnancy, Lactation: Only if considered essential and benefit outweighs risk.
Notes: See Class Effects 1.3 Ulcer Management.

Cimetidine

ATC Code: A02BA01. **Sport:** Permitted.
Driving: Unlikely to impair.
Indications: Duodenal and benign gastric ulceration, stomal ulcer, reflux oesophagitis, other conditions requiring reduced gastric acid secretion, Zollinger-Ellison syndrome. Long-term maintenance of benign peptic ulcer, NSAID-associated.
Dose: Adult, Elderly: *Ulceration*, duodenal, benign gastric ulcers, 800mg as single dose at bedtime OR 200mg 3-times daily and 400mg at bedtime OR 400mg 4-times daily and at bedtime.
Reflux oesophagitis, 400mg 4-times daily and at bedtime (4-8 weeks).
Zollinger-Ellison Syndrome, 400mg 4-times daily (or higher dose).
Prophylaxis, haemorrhage from 'stress' ulceration, up to max. 2.4g daily in divided doses (200-400mg every 4-6 hours by oral, nasogastric or parenteral routes; direct IV injection max. 200mg).
Acid aspiration (Mendelson's Syndrome), 400mg as single dose 90-120 minutes before general anaesthesia induction or start of labour; if risk persists, 400mg (parenteral if appropriate) 4-hourly to max. 2.4g/day.
Pancreatic insufficiency, Pancreatic Enzyme Supplement Protection, 800-1600mg/day in 4 divided doses, 60-90 minutes before meals; max. by any route 2.4g/day.
Child: Over 2 years, 25-30mg/kg/day in divided doses, oral or parenteral.
Renal Impairment: CrCl (mL/min) below 15, 200mg twice daily; 15-30, 200mg 3-times daily; 30-50, 200mg 4-times daily. Removed by haemodialysis.
Interactions: Effect of Other Drugs on Cimetidine: *Effect potentiated*: Drugs or illness reducing blood count.
Effect of Cimetidine on Other Drugs: Oral anticoagulants, phenytoin, theophylline, IV lidocaine: *Reduce dose.*
ADR: *Common*, headache, dizziness, diarrhoea, rash, myalgia, fatigue.
Notes: See 1.3.1 H2-Antagonists.

Cimeldine 400mg *(Clonmel)* B. GMS.
Price, (60) €11.35.
Tablet, cimetidine. Pale-green oblong f/c. Marked with logo 275.

Nizatidine

ATC Code: A02BA04. **Sport:** Permitted.
Driving: Unlikely to impair.
Indications: Ulceration, duodenal, benign gastric, NSAID-associated. Prevention of duodenal ulcer recurrence.
Dose: Adult, Elderly: 300mg/day as single dose (evening) OR 150mg twice daily. Prophylaxis, 150mg (evening).
Renal Impairment: *Dose 300mg/day*, CrCl (mL/min) 20-50, 150mg in evening; below 20, 150mg alternate days. *Dose 150mg/day*, CrCl (mL/min) 20-50, 150mg alternate days; below 20, 150mg every third day.
Interactions: Effect of Other Drugs on Nizatidine: *Absorption reduced (up to 20%)*: Charcoal.
Effect of Nizatidine on Other Drugs: High dose salicylates: Absorption Increased.
ADR: Sweating, urticaria.
Notes: See 1.3.1 H2-Antagonists.

Axid 150mg, 300mg *(Flynn)* B. GMS.
Price, (30) 150mg, €11.75. 300mg, €16.70.
Capsule, nizatidine. Hard contains off-white granular powder. 150mg: Pale/dark-yellow. Marked Flynn 3144. 300mg: Pale-yellow/brown. Marked Flynn 3145.

Ranitidine

ATC Code: A02BA02. **Sport:** Permitted.
Driving: Caution, dizziness, headache, confusion, hallucination.
Indications: *Oral, parenteral,* duodenal and gastric ulcer including associated with NSAIDs. Prevention, of NSAID (including aspirin) associated duodenal ulcer. Treatment, post-operative ulcer, reflux oesophagitis, Zollinger-Ellison's Syndrome, other conditions where gastric acid reduction is beneficial. *Parenteral,* prophylaxis, duodenal ulcer including NSAID-associated, acid aspiration (Mendelson's Syndrome), stress lesions of upper GI tract, recurrent upper GI tract haemorrhage. *Children,* short-term treatment, peptic ulcer, GORD including reflux oesophagitis, symptomatic GORD relief, parenteral (age 6 months to 18 years), oral (age 3-18 years).
Dose: Adult, Elderly: Age 12 years and over: ORAL, *ulcer* (duodenal, gastric, NSAID-associated), 300mg as single dose at night OR 150mg twice daily; increase to 300mg twice daily if needed; maintenance, 150-300mg at night. Prophylaxis, duodenal ulcer, 150mg at night; NSAID-associated ulcer, 150mg twice daily (with NSAID).
Reflux oesophagitis, 300mg/day as single dose or 150mg twice daily; moderate or severe, 150mg 4-times daily OR 300mg twice daily. Long-term relapse prevention, 150mg twice daily.
Zollinger-Ellison Syndrome, 150mg 3-4 times daily; increase to 300mg 4-times daily if needed; max. 6g/day.
Obstetrics, 150mg at start of labour, then 150mg 6-hourly.
PARENTERAL (age 12 years and over), 50mg slow IV (over 2 minutes) 6-8 hourly OR 25mg/hour intermittent IV infusion for 2 hours repeated 6-8 hourly OR 50mg IM 6-8 hourly.
Prophylaxis, upper GI haemorrhage from stress ulceration, initially 50mg by slow IV, then continuous IV infusion 0.125-0.25mg/kg/hour; when oral suitable, 150mg tabs twice daily.
Acid aspiration (Mendelson's Syndrome), 50mg IM or slow IV over 1 minute, 45-60 minutes before induction of anaesthesia.
Child: ORAL (age 3-11 years, over 30kg): Peptic ulcer, 4-8mg/kg/day*; max. 300mg/day. GORD, 5-10mg/kg/day*; max. 600mg/day. *(in 2 divided doses).
PARENTERAL (age 6 months to 11 years): Acute, ulcer/GORD, 2-2.5mg/kg; max. 50mg by slow IV infusion over 10 minutes or continuous IV infusion with loading dose 0.45mg/kg then 0.15mg/kg/hour. Stress ulceration, prophylaxis, 1mg/kg; max. 50mg every 6-8 hours OR 125-250mcg/kg/hour by continuous IV infusion. Neonates (under 1 month), limited data. Age 12 years and over, as for Adult above.
Renal Impairment: CrCl (mL/min) below 50 (30*), oral 150mg/day (or 25mg parenterally). *Brand *Gertac.*
Interactions: Effect of Other Drugs on Ranitidine: *Decreased absorption:* Antacids, sucralfate (high doses of 2g) (allow 2-hour dose interval).
Effect of Ranitidine on Other Drugs: Procainamide, N-acetylprocainamide: *Reduced excretion, plasma levels increased.* Coumarins (warfarin): *Altered prothrombin time, monitor.*
SP: Asystole, bradycardia risk with rapid IV admin; do not exceed recommended admin rate or dose.
ADR: *Uncommon,* abdominal pain, constipation, nausea.
Notes: See 1.3.1 H2-Antagonists.
Interchangeability: Same strengths of all ranitidine f/c, effervescent tabs and oral soln listed below are deemed interchangeable.

Zantac 150mg, 300mg, Effervescent, Syrup *(GSK)* B. GMS.
Price, 150mg (60) €11.18. 300mg (30) €10.30. Eff 150mg (30) €8.00. Syrup (300mL) €19.22.
Tablet, ranitidine HCl. White f/c. 150mg: Round. Marked GXEC2. 300mg: Cap-shaped. Marked GXEC3.

Effervescent tablet, as above 150mg. White (pale-yellow) round; dissolves in water to give clear orange/grapefruit flavoured soln. Marked GSLHK. *Aspartame, sorbitol, sodium 328mg/tab.*
Oral syrup, as above 150mg/10mL. Clear colourless (pale-yellow) liquid; mint odour. *Ethanol, sorbitol, parabens.*
Zantac Parenteral 50mg/2mL *(GSK)* A.
Price, (5) €3.54 (PTW).
Injection, ranitidine HCl. Clear colourless (pale-yellow) aqueous soln. *Sodium 1.3mg, potassium 0.6mg per amp.*
Gertac 150mg, 300mg *(Gerard)* B. GMS.
Price, 150mg (60) €10.95. 300mg (30) €10.10.
Tablet, ranitidine HCl. White (beige) f/c. Marked G. 150mg: Marked 00 over 30. 300mg: Cap-shaped. Marked 0031.
Ranitic 150mg, 300mg *(Rowex)* B. GMS.
Price, 150mg (60) €10.95. 300mg (30) €10.10.
Tablet, ranitidine HCl. White scored (facilitates breaking) f/c. 150mg: Round. 300mg: Oblong. *Lactose.*
Ranitidine (Accord) Effervescent 150mg *(Accord)* B. GMS.
Price, (30) €7.56.
Effervescent tablet, ranitidine HCl. Light-orange round flat; peppermint odour. *Sodium 533mg/tab; Sunset Yellow.*
Ranitidine Oral Soln *(Rosemont)* B. GMS.
Price, (300mL) €11.38.
Oral soln, ranitidine HCl equiv. to ranitidine 150mg/10mL. Straw-coloured; mint odour. *Ethanol, sorbitol.* **Store:** Below 25 deg C.
Ranopine 150mg, 300mg *(Pinewood)* B. GMS.
Price, 150mg (60) €10.95. 300mg (30) €10.10.
Tablet, ranitidine HCl. White (off-white) f/c. Marked RAN/strength. 150mg: Round. 300mg: Cap-shaped.

1.3.2 - Proton Pump Inhibitors

In This Chapter: *Esomeprazole, lansoprazole, omeprazole, pantoprazole, rabeprazole.*

Class Effects

Proton pump inhibitors (PPIs) are specific inhibitors of the acid pump in parietal cells.
CI: Use in children unless otherwise specified.
Interactions: Effect of Other Drugs on PPIs: *Discourage co-admin (omeprazole, esomeprazole):* Clopidogrel.
Effect of PPIs on Other Drugs: Atazanavir (significantly reduced bioavailability): *Co-admin contraindicated.* Drug absorption pH dependent e.g. nelfinavir (reduced bioavailability): *Increased or decreased absorption.* Ketoconazole, itraconazole, posaconazole, vitamin B12 (cyanocobalamin), erlotinib: *Decreased absorption.* Digoxin: *Monitor plasma levels.* Warfarin: *Monitor prothrombin time, INR.* Methotrexate: *Elevated and prolonged serum levels especially at high dose (methotrexate 300mg); possible toxicity.* Tacrolimus: *Serum levels increased.*
SP: Exclude (gastric, oesophageal) malignancy prior to initiating. Use with antibiotics to eradicate *H. pylori.* May increase counts of bacteria normally present in upper GI tract; slightly increased GI infection risk (Salmonella, Campylobacter; in hospitalised patients possibly *Clostridium difficile*) (not all PPIs).
Class effects include severe hypomagnesaemia (long-term use). Increased fracture risk of hip, wrist, spine (especially elderly, risk factors present). Increased Chromogranin A (CgA) may interfere with investigations for neuroendocrine tumours (discontinue 5 days before CgA measurement). Subacute cutaneous lupus erythematosus (SCLE); if lesions occur (especially sun exposed skin), if accompanied by arthralgia, consider discontinuing PPI.
Pregnancy, Lactation: Unless otherwise stated, use only if considered essential (benefit outweighs risk). Some PPIs do pass into breast milk; levels deemed low enough not to affect the breastfed infant.
ADR: *Oral, common,* headache, constipation, diarrhoea, nausea, vomiting, abdominal pain (uncommon with pantoprazole). *Parenteral,* injection-site reactions.
Notes: See Class Effects 1.3 Ulcer Management and 1.3.1 H2-Antagonists.

Esomeprazole

ATC Code: A02BC05. **Sport:** Permitted.
Driving: Unlikely to impair.

Indications: *Oral*, GORD, peptic ulcer relapse, NSAID-associated ulcer (gastric, duodenal), Zollinger Ellison Syndrome, prolonged treatment after IV induced prevention of peptic ulcer re-bleeding, *H. pylori* eradication (with antibacterials) in *H. pylori*-associated duodenal ulcer. Adolescents from 12 years, GORD, *H. pylori*-associated duodenal ulcer. *Parenteral*, gastric antisecretory treatment (GORD in adults, children 1-18 years; NSAID-associated gastric or duodenal ulcers; prevention of re-bleeding following therapeutic endoscopy for acute bleeding gastric or duodenal ulcers).

Dose: Adult, Elderly: ORAL, *GORD, erosive reflux oesophagitis*, 40mg once daily. Relapse prevention, symptomatic treatment, 20mg once daily ('on-demand' CAN be used).

H. pylori eradication, esomeprazole 20mg + amoxicillin 1g + clarithromycin 500mg, all twice daily for 7 days.

NSAID-associated ulceration, gastric ulcer healing, gastric or duodenal ulcer prevention, 20mg once daily ('on-demand' NOT recommended).

Re-bleeding after IV-induced prevention, 40mg once daily.

Zollinger Ellison Syndrome, 40mg twice daily; range 80-160mg/day. *Admin*, swallow tabs whole with liquid; do not chew or crush.

PARENTERAL, *gastric antisecretory treatment*, 20-40mg once daily by IV injection over 3 minutes OR IV infusion over 10-30 minutes.

Bleeding ulcers, 80mg as bolus infusion over 30 minutes, then 8mg/hour as continuous IV infusion over 72 hours; follow with oral acid-suppression 40mg once daily (4 weeks).

Child: ORAL, GORD, age 12 years and over, as for Adult above. *H. pylori* eradication, above 40kg, as for Adult; 30-40kg, esomeprazole 20mg + amoxicillin 750mg + clarithromycin 7.5mg/kg body weight, all twice daily for 7 days.

PARENTERAL, *gastric antisecretory treatment, erosive oesophagitis*, age 1-11 years, under 20kg, 10mg/day; 20kg and over, 10-20mg/day; age 12-18 years, 40mg/day. *GORD* symptomatic treatment, age 1-11 years, 10mg/day; age 12-18 years, 20mg/day. All dosed once daily.

Renal Impairment: Severe, caution.

Hepatic Impairment: Severe, max. 20mg/day. *Parenteral*, bleeding ulcer treatment, initially 80mg bolus infusion then 4mg/hour for 72 hours.

CI: Substituted benzimidazole hypersensitivity.

Interactions: Effect of Other Drugs on Esomeprazole: *Co-admin contraindicated*: Nelfinavir (reduced nelfinavir exposure); atazanavir. *Co-admin not recommended*: Atazanavir (reduced atazanavir exposure; if unavoidable, increase atazanavir to 400mg + ritonavir 100mg; max. esomeprazole 20mg). *Co-admin avoid*: Clopidogrel. *Plasma levels increased*: Voriconazole (severe hepatic impairment, consider dose adjustment). *Plasma levels decreased*: CYP2C19 or CYP3A4 inducers, rifampicin, St John's Wort.

Effect of Esomeprazole on Other Drugs: CYP2C19 metabolised drugs (diazepam, citalopram, imipramine, clomipramine, phenytoin, cilostazol): *CYP2C19 inhibited; increased plasma levels (reduce dose); effect may be more pronounced with parenteral high dose regimen.* Warfarin, coumarins: *Elevated INR, monitor.* Cisapride: *Increased AUC, prolonged elimination half-life (t1/2).*

SP: 'On-demand' treatment, monitor for symptom change; caution CYP2C19-associated interactions.

ADR: Summary, *most common*, headache, abdominal pain, diarrhoea, nausea, flatulence.

Notes: See 1.3.2 Proton Pump Inhibitors. See Omeprazole below.

Interchangeability: Same strengths of all brands of esomeprazole gastro-resistant (g/r) caps/tabs listed below are deemed interchangeable.

Reference Price: (28) 20mg, €3.64. 40mg, €6.44.

Nexium 20mg, 40mg *(AstraZeneca)* B. GMS.
Price, 20mg (7) €3.33; (14) €6.65; (28) €13.31. 40mg (7) €3.55 (28) €14.21.
Tablet (g/r), esomeprazole magnesium trihydrate. Oblong f/c. Marked strength; logo on reverse. 20mg: Light-pink. 40mg: Pink. *Sucrose*. **Store:** Below 30 deg C; original pack.

Nexium Parenteral 40mg *(AstraZeneca)* A. HOS.
Price, (1) €6.28 (PTW).
Injection or infusion, esomeprazole (as sodium salt). White (off-white) porous cake or powder for soln. *Sodium 1mmoL/vial*. **Store:** Below 30 deg C; protect from light; normal indoor light (max. 24 hours).

Emazole 20mg, 40mg *(Rowex)* B. GMS.
Price, (28) see reference price above.
Tablet (g/r), esomeprazole. Oval f/c. 20mg: Light-pink. 40mg: Pink scored (divisible into equal halves). *Sucrose*.

Esomeprazole Actavis 20mg, 40mg *(Accord)* B. GMS.
Price, (28) see reference price above.
Capsule (g/r), esomeprazole magnesium dihydrate. Hard opaque. Marked with strength. 20mg: Yellow/white. 40mg: Yellow.

Esomeprazole Krka 20mg, 40mg *(Krka)* B. GMS.
Price, (28) see reference price above.
Capsule (g/r), esomeprazole. Hard; contain white (almost) pellets. 20mg: Slightly-pink. 40mg: Off-pink. *Sucrose*.

Esomeprazole TEVA 20mg, 40mg *(TEVA)* B. GMS.
Price, (28) see reference price above.
Tablet (g/r), esomeprazole magnesium. Brick-red round f/c. Marked with strength. *Sucrose, lactose*.

Nepramel 20mg, 40mg *(Clonmel)* B. GMS.
Price, (28) see reference price above.
Capsule (g/r), esomeprazole magnesium dihydrate. Opaque. Contains off-white (greyish) spherical microgranules. Marked with strength. 20mg: Yellow/white. 40mg: Yellow/yellow. *Sucrose, benzoate*.

Nexazole 20mg, 40mg *(Pinewood)* B. GMS.
Price, (28) see reference price above.
Capsule (g/r), esomeprazole magnesium dihydrate. Slightly pink. Contains white (almost) pellets. *Sucrose*.

Lansoprazole

ATC Code: A02BC03. **Sport:** Permitted.
Driving: Unlikely to impair.

Indications: Duodenal and benign gastric ulcer, reflux oesophagitis (RO), GORD, Zollinger-Ellison syndrome, *H. pylori* eradication (with antibiotics), NSAID-associated benign gastric and duodenal ulcers.

Dose: Adult: *Ulcer* (duodenal, gastric, NSAID-associated), RO, GORD, 30mg/day; maintenance, 15-30mg/day. Gastric and duodenal ulcer, RO prophylaxis, 15mg/day; increase to 30mg/day if needed.

Zollinger-Ellison Syndrome, initially 60mg/day; increase if needed; 120mg/day or more admin in 2 divided doses; max. 180mg/day. *Admin*, oral once daily (morning); swallow tabs whole with water or dissolve orodispersible tabs on tongue; 30 minutes before food; do not crush or chew.

H. pylori eradication, lansoprazole 30mg + clarithromycin 250-500mg + (amoxicillin 1g OR metronidazole 400-500mg) OR lansoprazole 30mg + amoxicillin 1g + metronidazole 400-500mg; all twice daily for 7 days.

Elderly: Max. 30mg/day.

Child: Not recommended; under 1 year, avoid.

Hepatic Impairment: Moderate to severe, reduce dose by 50%.

Interactions: Effect of Other Drugs on Lansoprazole: *Co-admin caution*: Phenytoin, carbamazepine, theophylline, warfarin. *Bioavailability reduced*: Antacids, sucralfate (allow 1-hour dosing interval).

ADR: *Common*, headache, dizziness, vomiting, nausea, diarrhoea, stomach ache, constipation, flatulence, dry mouth or throat, fundic gland polyps (benign), increased liver enzymes, urticaria, itching, rash, fatigue. See Notes below.

Notes: See 1.3.2 Proton Pump Inhibitors.

Interchangeability: Same strengths of all brands of lansoprazole gastro-resistant (g/r) caps/orodispersible tabs listed below are deemed interchangeable.

Reference Price: (28) 15mg, €3.08. 30mg, €4.76.

1.3.2 Proton Pump Inhibitors

Zoton FasTab 15mg, 30mg *(Pfizer)* B. GMS.
Price, 15mg (28) €6.90. 30mg (14) €7.44; (28) €13.72.
OroDisp tablet, lansoprazole. White (yellowish white) round flat speckled. Contains orange (dark brown) granules g/r. Marked with strength. Strawberry flavoured. *Aspartame, lactose*. **Store:** Below 25 deg C; original pack.

Lansoprazole Actavis 15mg, 30mg *(Accord)* B. GMS.
Price, (28) see reference price above.
Capsule, lansoprazole. Hard opaque g/r; contains white (almost) spherical microgranules. 15mg: Yellow. 30mg: White. *Sucrose*.

Lansoprazole Krka 15mg, 30mg *(Krka)* B. GMS.
Price, (28) see reference price above.
Capsule, lansoprazole. Hard g/r; contain white (light-brown or lightly-pink) e/c pellets. 15mg: White/red-brownish. 30mg: White. *Sucrose*.

Lansoprazole Pinewood 15mg, 30mg *(Pinewood)* B. GMS.
Price, (28) see reference price above.
Capsule, lansoprazole. Hard opaque g/r; contain white (almost) spherical granules. 15mg: Yellow. 30mg: White. *Sucrose*.

Lansoprazole TEVA OroDisp 15mg, 30mg *(TEVA)* B. GMS.
Price, (28) see reference price above.
OroDisp tablet, as above. White (off-white) flat round; contain white (greyish) g/r granules. Marked with strength. *Lactose, aspartame, sucrose*.

Lansoprazole TEVA Pharma 15mg, 30mg *(TEVA)* B. GMS.
Price, (28) see reference price above.
Capsule, lansoprazole. Hard opaque white/white g/r; contains beige micropellets. Marked L and strength. *Sucrose*.

Lanzol 15mg, 30mg *(Rowex)* B. GMS.
Price, (28) see reference price above.
Capsule, lansoprazole. Opaque hard gelatin g/r; contains pellets e/c. 15mg: Yellow. 30mg: White. *Sucrose*. **Store:** Below 25 deg C; original pack to protect (moisture).

Razolager 15mg, 30mg *(Gerard)* B. GMS.
Price, (28) see reference price above.
Capsule, lansoprazole. Hard g/r; contains white (almost) microgranules. 15mg: Yellow. 30mg: White. *Sucrose*. **Store:** Below 25 deg C.

Zomel 15mg, 30mg *(Clonmel)* B. GMS.
Price, (28) see reference price above.
Capsule, lansoprazole. Hard opaque. 15mg: Yellow. 30mg: White. *Sucrose*.

Omeprazole

ATC Code: A02BC01. **Sport:** Permitted.
Driving: Not likely to affect; dizziness, visual disturbances reported.
Indications: Oesophageal reflux disease, treatment and prevention of relapse of duodenal and gastric ulcer, NSAID-associated ulcer, *H. pylori* eradication (with antibiotics), prophylaxis of acid aspiration, Zollinger-Ellison syndrome. *Children* over (1 year, 10kg), reflux oesophagitis, symptomatic GORD treatment; over 4 years, treatment of *H. pylori*-associated duodenal ulcer (with antibiotics).
Dose: Adult, Elderly: *Oesophageal reflux* disease, usually 20mg/day; range 10-20mg/day, up to 40mg/day; long-term management of healed reflux oesophagitis, 20-40mg once daily. *Acid reflux*, 10mg/day; increase to 20mg if symptoms return.
Ulcer, duodenal, gastric, usually 20mg/day; if needed increase to 40mg/day; maintenance, relapse prevention, as for acid reflux ulcer. Those at risk for recurrence (under 60 years, symptoms persisting for more than 1 year, smokers), or severe reflux oesophagitis or poorly responsive gastric ulcer, 20mg/day; titrate to 40mg/day if needed. *NSAID-associated* ulcer, 20mg/day.
H. pylori eradication, *triple therapy*, omeprazole 20mg + clarithromycin 250mg + metronidazole 400mg (tinidazole) OR omeprazole 20mg + amoxicillin 1g + clarithromycin 500mg, all twice daily for 7 days; *dual therapy*, omeprazole 20mg + amoxicillin 1g, both twice daily for 14 days OR omeprazole 40mg once daily + clarithromycin 500mg both 3-times daily for 14 days.
Prophylaxis, acid aspiration, 40mg evening before surgery, then 40mg 2-6 hours before surgery.
Zollinger-Ellison Syndrome, initially 60mg; range 20-120mg/day; dose above 80mg, admin in 2 divided doses.
Admin, swallow all g/r tabs/caps whole, do not crush or chew; on empty stomach before food. Food delays absorption; does not tend to change bioavailability.
Child: Severe reflux oesophagitis, over 2 years, refractory to conventional treatment, 10-20kg (10mg/day); over 20kg (20mg/day). Children 2-6 years, tab may be dispersed.

Under 2 years, limited data, infants, no data. *Losec Mups*, over 1 year, 10-20kg, 10mg/day; max. 20mg/day; age 2 years and over (above 20kg), 20mg/day; max. 40mg/day if needed. *Admin*, once daily.
Losec Mups, H. pylori eradication, over 4 years, all admin twice daily for 7 days; weight (15kg-30kg), omeprazole 10mg + amoxicillin 25mg/kg + clarithromycin 7.5mg/kg; (30kg-40kg), omeprazole 20mg + amoxicillin 750mg + clarithromycin 7.5mg/kg; (over 40kg), omeprazole 20mg + amoxicillin 1g + clarithromycin 500mg.
Hepatic Impairment: Oral, max. 20mg/day.
CI: Substituted benzimidazole hypersensitivity.
Interactions: Effect of Other Drugs on Omeprazole: Co-admin contraindicated: Atazanavir, nelfinavir. *Mutually increased plasma levels*: Clarithromycin. *Plasma levels decreased*: St John's Wort. *Plasma levels increased*: Voriconazole.
Effect of Omeprazole on Other Drugs: Erythromycin, clarithromycin, roxithromycin: *Absorption increased*. Diazepam, phenytoin; warfarin and other Vitamin K antagonists (monitor INR, consider dose reduction); hexobarbital, citalopram, imipramine, clomipramine, tacrolimus, cilostazol: *Plasma levels increased*. Disulfiram: *Hepatic metabolism inhibited*. Ciclosporin: *Possible increased plasma levels, monitor*. Digoxin: *Increased bioavailability*. Atazanavir, ritonavir: *Plasma levels decreased*.
SP: Some children with chronic illnesses may require long-term treatment although not recommended.
Pregnancy, Lactation: Pregnancy, can be used. Lactation, is excreted in breast milk; unlikely to affect child at therapeutic doses.
ADR: *Common*, flatulence. See Notes below.
Notes: See 1.3.2 Proton Pump Inhibitors.
Interchangeability: Same strengths of all brands of omeprazole gastro-resistant (g/r) caps/tabs listed below are deemed interchangeable.
Reference Price: 10mg (28) €3.36; (30) €3.60. 20mg (28) €2.80; (30) €3.00. 40mg (14) €2.80; (28) €5.60; (30) €6.00

Losec Mups 10mg, 20mg, 40mg *(AstraZeneca)* B. GMS.
Price, 10mg (28), €7.55. 20mg (7), €4.45; (28), €14.21. 40mg (14), €14.19.
Tablet (g/r), omeprazole magnesium. Oblong f/c; contains e/c coated pellets. Marked with logo; strength on reverse. 10mg: Light-pink. 20mg: Pink. 40mg: Dark red-brown. *Sucrose*. **Store:** Below 25 deg C.

Losamel 20mg *(Clonmel)* B. GMS.
Price, (30) see reference price above.
Tablet (g/r), omeprazole. Light-grey. *Lactose*.

Omeprazole Actavis 10mg, 20mg, 40mg *(Accord)* B. GMS.
Price, (28) 10mg, 20mg, (14) 40mg, see reference price above.
Capsule (g/r), omeprazole. Hard gelatin opaque; contains cream-white spherical microgranules. 10mg, 20mg: Yellow. 40mg: Blue/white. *Sucrose*.

Omeprazole Bluefish Tablets *(Bluefish)* B. GMS.
Price, (28) 10mg, (14) 40mg, see reference price above.
Capsule (g/r), omeprazole 10mg, 40mg. Opaque; contains white (beige) granules. Marked 0 and strength. 10mg: Red/orange. 40mg: Blue/orange. *Sucrose*.

Omeprazole Mylan 10mg, 20mg, 40mg *(Gerard)* B. GMS.
Price, (28) 10mg, 20mg, (14) 40mg, see reference price above.
Capsule (g/r), omeprazole. Hard opaque. Marked Mylan, OM and strength. 10mg: Light-pink/white. 20mg: Dark-pink/white. 40mg: Dark-pink. *Sucrose; tartrazine, Allura red (20mg)*, Sunset Yellow *(40mg)*. **Store:** Below 25 deg C; original pack/tightly closed to protect (moisture).

Omeprazole Pinewood 20mg *(Pinewood)* B. GMS.
Price, (28) see reference price above.
Capsule (g/r), omeprazole. Opaque yellow; contains white (cream/white) e/c microgranules. *Sucrose*.

Omeprazole TEVA 10mg, 20mg, 40mg *(TEVA)* B. GMS.
Price, (28) 10mg, 20mg, (14) 40mg, see reference price above.
Capsule (g/r), omeprazole. Contains white (off-white) micropellets. Marked 0 and strength. 10mg: Orange/red. 20mg, 40mg: Orange/blue. *Sucrose*.

Romep 10mg, 20mg, 40mg *(Rowex)* B. GMS.
Price, (28) 10mg, 20mg, (14) 40mg, see reference price above.
Capsule (g/r), omeprazole. Contains white (beige) coated pellets (granules). Marked OME/strength. 10mg: Light-brown. 20mg: White. 40mg: White/light brown. *Lactose*.

Pantoprazole

ATC Code: A02BC02. **Sport:** Permitted.
Driving: Dizziness, visual disturbances.
Indications: *Oral,* (20mg strength), GORD, reflux oesophagitis (RO), mild reflux disease, NSAID-associated ulceration, prevention of gastro-duodenal ulcers; (40mg strength), moderate/severe RO, ulcer (duodenal, gastric), Zollinger-Ellison syndrome, other pathological hypersecretory conditions, *H. pylori* eradication. *Parenteral,* as for oral (40mg), excluding *H. pylori* eradication, and other pathological hypersecretory conditions.

Dose: Adult: ORAL, (20mg strength), mild reflux, 20mg/day; when relief achieved, 20mg/day 'on-demand' to control reoccurrence. GORD, RO, 20mg/day; relapse, increase to 40mg/day; after healing reduce to 20mg/day. NSAID-associated ulceration, 20mg/day. ORAL (40mg strength), moderate/severe RO, ulcer (duodenal, gastric), 40mg/day; no response, increase to 80mg/day. *H. pylori* eradication, pantoprazole 40mg + amoxicillin 1g + clarithromycin 500mg OR pantoprazole 40mg + metronidazole 400mg (or tinidazole 500mg) + clarithromycin 250mg OR pantoprazole 40mg + amoxicillin 1g + metronidazole 400mg (or tinidazole 500mg); all twice daily for 7 days.
Zollinger-Ellison Syndrome, 80mg/day; titrate up or down as needed; temporary increases above 160mg/day possible. *Admin,* do not crush or chew g/r tabs; swallow whole with liquid 1 hour before food.
PARENTERAL, ulcer (duodenal, gastric), RO (moderate, severe), 40mg/day IV over 2-15 minutes. Zollinger-Ellison Syndrome, initially 80mg/day as for oral. If rapid acid control required, initially 160mg IV. Switch to oral soonest.

Elderly: Over 65 years, max. 40mg/day.

Child: Over 12 years, as for Adult; under 12 years (oral) or under 18 years (parenteral), not recommended.

Renal Impairment: As for Elderly above.

Hepatic Impairment: Severe, max. 20mg/day OR 40mg every other day; monitor liver enzymes; if elevated discontinue. 40mg must not be used in *H. pylori* eradication combination treatment.

Interactions: Effect of Pantoprazole on Other Drugs: Vitamin B12 (cyanocobalamin), ketoconazole: *Reduced absorption.* Coumarins (warfarin): *Monitor prothrombin time/INR.*

SP: GI complications with use in prevention of NSAID-associated ulceration, assess risk (age, over 65 years, gastric or duodenal ulcer, upper GI bleeding).

Pregnancy, Lactation: Pregnancy, avoid. Lactation, stop drug or stop breastfeeding.

ADR: *Common,* fundic gland polyps (benign).

Notes: See 1.3.2 Proton Pump Inhibitors.

Interchangeability: Same strengths of all brands of pantoprazole gastro-resistant (g/r) tabs listed below are deemed interchangeable.

Reference Price: 20mg (28) €2.52; (30) €2.70. 40mg (28) €3.08; (30) €3.30.

Protium 20mg, 40mg *(Takeda)* B. GMS.
Price, (28) 20mg, €3.08; 40mg, €3.36.
Tablet (g/r), pantoprazole sodium sesquihydrate. Yellow oval. 20mg: f/c. Marked P20. 40mg: e/c. Marked P40. *Mannitol.* **Store:** No special conditions.
Protium Parenteral 40mg *(Takeda)* A. HOS.
Price, (5) €29.90 (PTW).
Injection, pantoprazole sodium. White (almost) powder for soln. **Store:** Below 25 deg C; protect (light).
Nolpaza 20mg, 40mg *(Krka)* B. GMS.
Price, (28) see reference price above.
Tablet (g/r), pantoprazole sodium sesquihydrate. Light brownish-yellow oval. *Sorbitol.* **Store:** Original pack to protect (moisture).
Pantium 20mg, 40mg *(Clonmel)* B. GMS.
Price, (28) see reference price above.
Tablet (g/r), pantoprazole sodium sesquihydrate. Yellow oval. *Maltitol.* **Store:** Below 25 deg C.
Pantoflux 20mg, 40mg *(Accord)* B. GMS.
Price, (28) see reference price above.
Tablet (g/r), pantoprazole sodium sesquihydrate. Elliptical. 20mg:

Light-yellow. 40mg: Dark-yellow. *Mannitol.* **Store:** No special conditions.
Pantoprazole Bluefish 20mg, 40mg *(Bluefish)* B. GMS.
Price, (30) see reference price above.
Tablet (g/r), pantoprazole sodium sesquihydrate. Yellow oval concave smooth. **Store:** Below 30 deg C.
Pantoprazole Mylan 20mg, 40mg *(Gerard)* B. GMS.
Price, (28) see reference price above.
Tablet (g/r), pantoprazole sodium sesquihydrate. Dark-yellow f/c. 20mg: Marked PS2. 40mg: Marked PS4. **Store:** No special conditions (blister); tightly closed (bottles).
Pantoprazole TEVA Pharma 20mg, 40mg *(TEVA)* B. GMS.
Price, (28) see reference price above.
Tablet (g/r), pantoprazole sodium sesquihydrate. Yellow oval f/c. **Store:** Below 30 deg C.
Pantoprazole Rowex 20mg, 40mg *(Rowex)* B. GMS.
Price, (28) see reference price above.
Tablet (g/r), pantoprazole sodium sesquihydrate. Yellow oval. Marked with strength. *Ponceau 4R.* **Store:** No special conditions.
Zolepant 20mg, 40mg *(Pinewood)* B. GMS.
Price, (28) see reference price above.
Tablet (g/r), pantoprazole sodium sesquihydrate. Light-brownish-yellow. *Mannitol, sorbitol.* **Store:** Original pack to protect (moisture).

Rabeprazole

ATC Code: A02BC04. **Sport:** Permitted.
Driving: Caution.
Indications: Duodenal, benign gastric ulcer, GORD (symptomatic, long-term management), Zollinger-Ellison Syndrome, *H. pylori* eradication.

Dose: Adult, Elderly: *Ulcer (active),* duodenal, benign gastric, 20mg/day. *Zollinger-Ellison* Syndrome, initially 60mg/day; titrate to 60mg twice daily if needed.
GORD, 20mg/day; symptomatic, 10mg/day, then 10mg/day as 'on-demand' therapy; maintenance, 10-20mg/day.
H. pylori eradication, 20mg rabeprazole + 500mg clarithromycin + 1g amoxicillin all twice daily (7 days).
Admin, oral once daily (morning); swallow tabs whole; do not crush or chew.

Hepatic Impairment: Severe, caution.

CI: Substituted benzimidazole hypersensitivity.

SP: Reduced Vitamin B absorption risk.

Pregnancy, Lactation: Contraindicated.

ADR: *Common,* infection, insomnia, headache, dizziness, cough, pharyngitis, rhinitis, diarrhoea, vomiting, nausea, abdominal pain, flatulence, fundic gland polyps (benign), pain (non-specific), back pain, asthenia, flu-like illness. See Notes below.

Notes: See 1.3.2 Proton Pump Inhibitors.

Interchangeability: Same strengths of all brands of rabeprazole gastro-resistant (g/r) tabs listed below are deemed interchangeable.

Reference Price: 10mg (28) €4.76; (30) €5.10. 20mg (28) €6.44; (30) €6.90.

Pariet 10mg, 20mg *(Janssen-Cilag)* B. GMS.
Price, (28) see reference price above.
Tablet (g/r), rabeprazole sodium. f/c. 10mg. Pink. Marked E 241. 20mg: Yellow. Marked E243. *Mannitol.* **Store:** Below 25 deg C; do not refrigerate.
Rabeprazole Actavis 10mg, 20mg *(Accord)* B. GMS.
Price, (28) see reference price above.
Tablet, rabeprazole sodium. Elliptical g/r coated. 10mg: Pink. 20mg: Yellow. **Store:** Below 25 deg C; original pack to protect (moisture).
Rabeprazole Clonmel 10mg, 20mg *(Clonmel)* B. GMS.
Price, (28) see reference price above.
Tablet, rabeprazole sodium. Round g/r. 10mg: Pink. 20mg: Yellow. **Store:** Below 25 deg C.
Rabeprazole Krka 10mg, 20mg *(Krka)* B. GMS.
Price, (28) see reference price above.
Tablet, rabeprazole sodium. Round g/r. 10mg: Orange-pink. 20mg: Brownish-yellow. **Store:** Below 30 deg C; original pack to protect (moisture, light).
Rabeprazole (Rowex) 10mg, 20mg *(Rowex)* B. GMS.
Price, (28) see reference price above.
Tablet, rabeprazole sodium. Round g/r, f/c. 10mg: Pink. 20mg: Yellow. *Mannitol.* **Store:** Below 25 deg C; original pack.

1.3.3 Prostaglandin Analogues

1.3.3 - Prostaglandin Analogues

In This Chapter: *Misoprostol.*

Class Effects
Misoprostol, an analogue of prostaglandin E1 (PGE1), promotes peptic ulcer healing and symptomatic relief.

Misoprostol

ATC Code: A02BB01. **Sport:** Permitted.
Driving: Caution, dizziness.

Indications: Short-term management, duodenal and gastric ulcer. Management and prophylaxis, NSAID-associated peptic ulcer.

Dose: Adult, Elderly: *Ulcer,* duodenal, gastric, NSAID-induced, 800mcg/day in 2-4 divided doses (breakfast and/or each main meal and bedtime). *Prophylaxis,* NSAID-induced peptic ulcer, 200mcg 2-4 times daily.

Child: Not evaluated.

Interactions: Effect of Other Drugs on Misoprostol: *Co-admin avoid:* Magnesium-containing antacids may worsen misoprostol-induced diarrhoea.

SP: Not for use in pre-menopausal women unless NSAID therapy is required and there is a high risk of complications from NSAID-induced ulcer (see Pregnancy below). Caution, where hypotension might cause severe complications (cerebrovascular disease, CAD, severe PVD including hypertension), conditions predisposing to diarrhoea (inflammatory bowel disease) or where dehydration is potentially dangerous.

Pregnancy, Lactation: Pregnancy, contraindicated (increases uterine tone and contractions, may cause expulsion of products of conception). Exclude pregnancy before initiation; ensure adequate contraception. Lactation, not for use; excretion of misoprostol could cause diarrhoea in infant.

ADR: *Very common,* diarrhoea, rash. *Common,* dizziness, headache, abdominal pain, constipation, dyspepsia, flatulence, nausea, vomiting.

Notes: See 1.3 Ulcer Management.

Cytotec 200mcg *(Pfizer)* A. GMS.
Price, (60) €14.57. (112) €26.83.
Tablet, misoprostol. White (off-white) flat hexagonal scored. Marked Searle over 1461. *Hydrogenated castor oil.* **Store:** Below 30 deg C; original pack.

1.3.4 - Chelates, Complexes

In This Chapter: *Sucralfate.*

Class Effects
Sucralfate is non-systemic; only minimally absorbed from GI tract. It exerts a generalised cytoprotective effect by preventing GI mucosal injury.

Sucralfate

ATC Code: A02BX02. **Sport:** Permitted.
Driving: Dizziness, drowsiness.

Indications: Duodenal and gastric ulcer, chronic gastritis (tabs, susp). Prophylaxis, GI haemorrhage from stress ulceration in the seriously ill (susp).

Dose: Adult, Elderly: *Ulceration,* 2g twice daily in morning and at bedtime OR 1g 4-times daily, 1 hour before meals and at bedtime; max. 8g/day. Tabs may be dispersed in 10-15mL water for ease of admin. *Stress ulceration prophylaxis,* 1g 6-times daily; max. 8g/day. Take antacids half an hour before or after *Antepsin* tabs/susp. *Elderly,* use lowest effective dose.

Child: Under 14 years, no dose recommendation. Monitor aluminium, phosphate, calcium, alkaline phosphatase.

Renal Impairment: Severe or chronic, extreme caution (increased aluminium absorption). Dialysis, not recommended.

Interactions: Effect of Other Drugs on Sucralfate: *Co-admin not recommended:* Citrates (may increase

aluminium blood levels). *Co-admin, enhanced aluminium absorption/toxicity:* Other aluminium-containing drugs.

Effect of Sucralfate on Other Drugs: Tetracyclines, ciprofloxacin, norfloxacin, ketoconazole, sulpiride, digoxin, warfarin, phenytoin, theophylline, levothyroxine, quinidine, H2-antagonists: *Bioavailability reduced, allow 2-hour dosing interval; where bioavailability is critical, admin separately.* Enteral feeds by nasogastric tube: *Separate admin by 1 hour (bezoar formation).*

SP: Bezoar formation (insoluble mass within gastric lumen), usually with underlying predisposing conditions (delayed gastric emptying, receiving concomitant enteral feeding). Caution, admin to severely ill. Aspiration may occur with tabs in patients with swallowing difficulty.

Pregnancy, Lactation: Pregnancy, only if clearly necessary. Lactation, caution; not known if excreted in human milk.

ADR: *Common,* constipation.

Notes: See 1.3 Ulcer Management.

Antepsin 1g, Oral Susp 1g/5mL *(Chugai)* B. GMS.
Price, tabs (50) susp (250mL) €7.73.
Tablet, sucralfate. White oblong scored (facilitates breaking). *Oral susp,* as above. White (off-white) viscous; aniseed odour. *Parabens.*

1.4 - Anti-Diarrhoeals

Class Effects
Acute diarrhoea, treatment is symptomatic; drugs affecting gastric motility may be used adjunctive to rehydration (fluids, electrolytes). Chronic diarrhoea, treatment is usually of underlying causative disorder. Colestyramine is also used for relief of diarrhoea associated with ileal resection, Crohn's disease, vagotomy and diabetic vagal neuropathy and management of radiation-induced diarrhoea.

CI: Hypersensitivity to any member of the class.

SP: Correct dehydration, electrolyte imbalance before commencing treatment.

Notes: See 2.3.1 Anion Exchange Resins (colestyramine).

1.4.1 - Drugs Affecting Gastric Motility

In This Chapter: *Co-phenotrope, loperamide.*

Class Effects
Co-phenotrope (diphenoxylate, atropine combination); diphenoxylate, a synthetic opioid derivative, has selective effects on GI smooth muscle; at therapeutic doses it is devoid of 'morphine type subjective effects'. Atropine is included in the formulation as an anti-abusing agent.

Indications: Acute diarrhoea, adjunctive with rehydration. Symptomatic diarrhoea associated with chronic inflammatory bowel disease (Crohn's disease, ulcerative colitis). Post-surgical diarrhoea including ileostomy. *Loperamide* is used to control intractable diarrhoea in children under specialist supervision.

CI: Acute ulcerative colitis.

SP: Diphenoxylate should be avoided in patients with antibiotic-associated colitis or diarrhoea associated with entero-toxin-producing bacteria.

Pregnancy, Lactation: Pregnancy, lactation not recommended.

Notes: See 1.4 Anti-Diarrhoeals.

Diphenoxylate, Atropine (co-phenotrope)

ATC Code: A07DA01, A03BA01. **Sport:** Permitted.
Driving: Caution.

Dose: Adult, Elderly: Initially 4 tabs, then 2 tabs 6-hourly until diarrhoea controlled.

Child: Not recommended.

CI: Jaundice, intestinal obstruction, acute ulcerative colitis, pseudo-membranous colitis.

Interactions: Effect of Co-Phenotrope on Other Drugs: CNS depressants (ALCOHOL, barbiturates, tranquilisers), other anticholinergics: *Effect enhanced.* MAOIs: CNS excitation or depression, hyper- or hypotension; avoid co-admin for 14 days after MAOI cessation. Levodopa, ketoconazole: Absorption reduced by antimuscarinics. Bethanecol/carbachol, galantamine, donepezil, neostigmine/pyridostigmine, pilocarpine: Muscarinic effects antagonised. Domperidone, metoclopramide, cisapride: Effects antagonised by opioid analgesics.

SP: Advanced hepato-renal disease, abnormal liver function, caution. Increased susceptibility to atropine in Down's syndrome. At high doses (40-60mg) typical opioid effects are produced, see Notes below.

ADR: CNS and GI disturbances, hypersensitivity reactions, anticholinergic effects.

Notes: See 1.4.1 Drugs Affecting Gastric Motility. See also 4.2.2 Opioid Analgesics.

> **Lomotil Tabs** (Concordia) B. GMS.
> Price, (100) €12.44.
> Tablet, diphenoxylate HCl 2.5mg, atropine sulfate 0.025mg. White. Marked GS10. Sucrose, sorbitol.

Loperamide

ATC Code: A07DA03. **Sport:** Permitted.
Driving: Tiredness, dizziness, drowsiness.

Dose: Adult, Elderly: Acute diarrhoea, initially 2-4mg, then 2mg 3-times daily or after each episode of diarrhoea; max. 10mg/day. Chronic diarrhoea, initially 4-8mg/day in divided doses; maintenance admin twice daily.

Child: Acute diarrhoea, age 9-12 years, as for Adult above. Age 4-8 years, max. 4mg/day in divided doses. Under 4 years, contraindicated.

Hepatic Impairment: Caution, CNS toxicity.

CI: Bacterial enterocolitis (Salmonella, Shigella, Campylobacter), pseudomembranous colitis (antibiotic-associated), acute dysentery. Conditions where inhibition of peristalsis is to be avoided. Discontinue if constipation, abdominal distension or ileus develop.

SP: Consider specific therapy (anti-infectives), particularly if treatment is needed for more than 3 days. Severe acute attacks of ulcerative colitis, avoid; less severe attacks, caution. Abuse/misuse of loperamide as an opioid substitute reported with opioid addiction.

ADR: Common, headache, constipation, nausea, flatulence.

Notes: See 1.4.1 Drugs Affecting Gastric Motility.

> **Imodium 2mg** (McNeil) B. GMS.
> Price, 2mg (60) €5.52.
> Capsule, loperamide HCl 2mg. Hard gelatin opaque green/dark-grey; contains white powder. Lactose.

1.4.2 - Rehydration, Fluids, Electrolytes

In This Chapter: Electrolytes, glucose.

Class Effects

Oral rehydration therapy embraces 4 aspects i.e. electrolyte correction (usually sodium and potassium chloride); bicarbonate (sodium bicarbonate or citrate) to address metabolic acidosis; water to replace fluid loss; carbohydrate to facilitate absorption of both fluid and electrolytes (usually glucose).

CI: Hypersensitivity to any member of the class.

SP: Hypernatraemia. Inadequate replacement.

Pregnancy, Lactation: Pregnancy, lactation, use only with medical supervision.

Electrolytes, Glucose (oral)

ATC Code: A07CA91. **Sport:** Permitted.
Driving: Unlikely to impair.

Indications: Oral management, dehydration and electrolyte imbalance associated with acute watery diarrhoea, including gastro-enteritis.

Dose: Adult, Elderly: Contents of 1-2 sachets after every loose motion; reconstitute in 200mL boiled and cooled water.

Child: Children, contents of 1 sachet after every loose motion; reconstitute and substitute in equivalent volume

as feeds (1-1.5 times usual feed volume); under 12 months, only on medical advice.

Notes: See 1.4.2 Rehydration, Fluids, Electrolytes.

> **Dioralyte** (SANOFI) OTC. GMS.
> Price, sachets (20) €5.05.
> Oral soln, sodium chloride 0.47g, potassium chloride 0.3g, disodium hydrogen citrate 0.53g, glucose 3.56g per sachet. White homogeneous granular powder (neutral, flavoured). **Store:** Below 25 deg C; reconstituted soln in refrigerator (max. 24 hours).

Electrolytes, Glucose (parenteral)

ATC Code: B05BB02. **Sport:** Permitted.
Driving: No special advice.

Indications: Prevention and treatment, potassium, sodium and chloride depletion due to loss of GI fluid, chronic laxative abuse, malabsorption syndromes, mucous secreting villous adenoma of small intestine, renal salt-losing conditions especially where energy source required.

Dose: Adult, Elderly: Hypokalaemia, prevention and mild potassium deficiency, up to 50mmoL/day IV; severe hypokalaemia, up to 20mmoL potassium in 500mL IV over 2-3 hours with ECG control. Max. 2-3mmoL/kg/24 hours. Max. rate 10-40mmoL/hour to avoid hyperkalaemia. Peripheral infusion, potassium concentration to be below 60mmoL/L to avoid pain.
Carbohydrate and fluid depletion, 500mL to 3L IV per 24 hours.

Child: Carbohydrate and fluid depletion, body weight 0-10kg, 100mL/kg/24 hours; 10-20kg, 1000mL+(50mL/kg over 10kg) per 24 hours; 20kg, 1500mL + (20mL/kg over 20kg) per 24 hours. Hypokalaemia, as for Adult above.

Renal Impairment: Severe (with oliguria/anuria), contraindicated.

CI: Hyperchloraemia, hyperkalaemia, uncompensated HF, severe CHF, Addison's disease, fluid and sodium retention, acute ischaemic stroke, head trauma (first 24 hours), uncompensated diabetes, hyperosmolar coma, hyperglycaemia, hyperlactataemia, other glucose intolerances.

Interactions: Effect of Other Drugs on Electrolyte, Glucose Solutions: Co-admin caution: Potassium-sparing drugs (potassium-sparing diuretics, ACEIs, ciclosporin); potassium salts; corticosteroids (associated with sodium and water retention).

SP: Caution, cardiac disease, conditions predisposing to hyperkalaemia. Monitor regularly (clinical status, serum electrolytes, ECG) especially with cardiac or renal impairment. Diabetics, insulin may need adjustment. Glucose not for admin through same infusion equipment as whole blood as haemolysis and clumping can occur.

Pregnancy, Lactation: No special warnings or precautions reported.

ADR: Associated with admin technique (febrile response, injection-site reaction, local pain/reaction, vein irritation, venous thrombosis, phlebitis, extravasation, hypervolaemia). Anaphylactic reaction, hypersensitivity, chills, hyponatraemia.

Notes: See 1.4.2 Rehydration, Fluids, Electrolytes.

> **Potassium/Sodium, Glucose Parenteral** (Baxter) A.
> Price, not published by company.
> Infusion, potassium chloride 0.3%, sodium chloride 0.18%, glucose 4% w/v. Clear colourless soln. pH (3.5-5.5).

1.5 - Constipation, Laxatives

Class Effects

Laxatives promote defecation and have 2 main uses, treatment of constipation; bowel evacuation prior to diagnostic procedures. May be stimulant (contact), bulk-forming or osmotic laxatives or faecal softeners.

CI: Hypersensitivity to any member of the class.

SP: Prolonged use not usually recommended. Extended use may be necessary with severe chronic or resistant constipation secondary to multiple sclerosis or Parkinson's Disease or induced by regular constipating medications.

1.5.1 Stimulant Laxatives

1.5.1 - Stimulant Laxatives

In This Chapter: Bisacodyl, co-danthromer, glycerol and citrate combinations, pyridostigmine, senna.

Class Effects
These laxatives increase stool evacuation by increasing peristalsis in the intestine.

CI: Intestinal obstruction, ileus, acute abdominal conditions (appendicitis, acute inflammatory bowel disease), other abdominal conditions (undiagnosed or persistent, acute surgical), severe dehydration.

Interactions: Effect of Other Drugs on Stimulant Laxatives: Co-admin caution: Drugs affecting water or electrolyte balance (NSAIDs, drugs inducing SIADH including TCADs, SSRIs, antipsychotics, carbamazepine) or causing hypokalaemia (diuretics, corticosteroids, lithium, laxative over-use) or where hypokalaemia is a risk (cardiac glycosides).

Effect of Stimulant Laxatives on Other Drugs: Anti-epileptics, contraceptives, anti-diabetics, antibiotics: *Absorption may be modified.*

SP: *Caution*, recent GI surgery, inflammatory bowel disease. Monitor fluid, electrolytes in elderly, renal impairment, acute MI, unstable angina, debilitated, conditions causing dehydration. Haematochezia, generally mild/self-limiting. *Enema*, lubricate tip of nozzle with drop of contents to aid insertion.

Notes: See 1.5 Constipation, Laxatives.

Bisacodyl

ATC Code: A06AB02. **Sport:** Permitted.
Driving: Dizziness, syncope due to vasovagal response.
Indications: Colon evacuation in constipation or preparation for radiological investigation.

Dose: Adult, Elderly: *Constipation*, 1-2 tabs (5-10mg) daily before bedtime or insert 1 supp rectally (10mg) daily for immediate effect (10-30 minutes). *Diagnostic procedures*, 2 tabs (10mg) twice daily (morning, evening) and insert 1 supp rectally (10mg) following morning. *Admin*, swallow tabs whole with adequate water.
Child: Age 4-10 years, *constipation*, 1 tab (5mg) at bedtime or insert 1 supp rectally (5mg) daily for immediate effect (10-30 minutes); chronic or persistent constipation, use with medical supervision. *Diagnostic procedures*, 1 tab (5mg) in evening and insert 1 supp rectally (5mg) following morning. Age 10 years and older, as for Adult above.
Interactions: Effect of Other Drugs on Bisacodyl: *Resistance of tablet coating reduced*: Antacids, milk-products.
Pregnancy, Lactation: Pregnancy, avoid (especially first trimester). Lactation, use only if benefit outweighs risk.
ADR: *Common*, abdominal pain/cramps, nausea, diarrhoea.
Notes: See 1.5.1 Stimulant Laxatives.
Dulcolax Tablets, Supps (SANOFI) OTC.
Price, tabs 5mg (20) €2.37; (40) €4.31. (60) €5.13; (100) €6.24. Supps 5mg (5) €1.59. 10mg (10) €2.95. (20) €5.45.
Tablet, bisacodyl 5mg. Round yellow s/c e/c. *Lactose, sucrose*.
Store: Below 25 deg C in outer carton.
Supps, as above 5mg (Children), 10mg (Adult). Smooth white torpedo-shaped. **Store:** Below 25 deg C in outer carton.

Co-Danthromer

ATC Code: A06AB53. **Sport:** Permitted.
Driving: May cause unusual tiredness or weakness.
Indications: Prophylaxis and treatment, constipation in terminally ill.
Dose: Adult, Elderly: Admin 5-10mL at bedtime.
Child: Generally, avoid. If recommended, 2.5-5mL at bedtime.
Renal Impairment: Hypermagnesaemia may occur.
CI: Intestinal obstruction, appendicitis, inflamed bowel.
Interactions: Effect of Other Drugs on Co-Danthromer:

Stool softener laxative co-admin: May enhance dantron systemic absorption.
SP: Urine coloured red; avoid prolonged contact with skin e.g. incontinent patients (irritation, excoriation).
Pregnancy, Lactation: Contraindicated.
ADR: Temporary pink or red colouring of urine and peri-anal skin, superficial skin sloughing, tiredness, weakness, rash, abdominal cramp. See SP above.
Notes: See 1.5.1 Stimulant Laxatives.
Co-Danthromer 25/200 Susp *(Pinewood)* B. GMS.
Price, (300mL) 25/200mg, €45.90.
Oral susp, dantron, poloxamer 188 25/200mg (sugar-free). Yellow; peach flavour. *Sorbitol, propylene glycol, parabens, ethanol*.

Glycerol

ATC Code: A06AG04. **Sport:** Permitted.
Driving: No effect noted.
Indications: Treatment, constipation.
Dose: Adult, Elderly: Age 12 years and over, insert 1 supp (Adult Strength) moistening tip with water to aid insertion.
Child: Using appropriate formulation (Child, Infant), insert 1 supp moistening tip to aid insertion.
CI: Intestinal obstruction/blockage.
SP: Prolonged use not recommended. May interfere with glucose control in diabetics. If symptoms persist, consult medical advice.
Pregnancy, Lactation: No harmful effects. Avoid, first trimester.
ADR: Abdominal cramp.
Notes: See 1.5.1 Stimulant Laxatives.
Glycerol Supps Adult, Child, Infant *(Martindale)* OTC.
Price, not published by company.
Supp, glycerol 70% w/w. Adult 4g, child 2g, infant 1g. Amber-coloured.

Glycerol, Citrates (laxative)

ATC Code: A16AX09. A06AD11. **Sport:** Permitted.
Driving: Unlikely to impair.
Indications: Evacuation of colon in constipation, prior to surgical and diagnostic procedure and in obstetrics prior to delivery.
Dose: Adult, Elderly: Insert full length of nozzle into rectum and squeeze tube until total contents administered; severe, 2 tubes may be needed.
Child: As for Adult, insert nozzle half-length only. Under 3 years, not recommended.
CI: Inflammatory or ulcerative bowel disease, acute GI conditions.
SP: Diarrhoea and fluid loss with excessive use. Prolonged use, interference with absorption of some vitamins.
Pregnancy, Lactation: Use with medical supervision.
ADR: Slight cramp. Irritation of anal canal with prolonged use.
Notes: See 1.5.1 Stimulant Laxatives.
Micolette Micro-Enema *(Pinewood)* OTC.
Price, not published by company.
Rectal soln (enema), sodium citrate 450mg, sodium lauryl sulphoacetate 45mg, glycerol 625mg. Translucent gel-like soln. *Potassium sorbate*.

Pyridostigmine (GI)

ATC Code: N07AA02. **Sport:** Permitted.
Driving: Impaired visual acuity and ability to react.
Indications: Myasthenia gravis, paralytic ileus, post-operative urinary retention.
Dose: Adult, Elderly: *Myasthenia gravis*, 30-120mg at intervals throughout the day (usual duration of action is 3-4 hours in day; longer effect of 6 hours obtained with a dose before bed); max. range 5-20 tabs.
Paralytic ileus, usually 60-240mg/day.
Child: Under 6 years, initially 30mg; age 6-12 years, 60mg. Increase gradually in 15-30mg/day increments; max. range 30-360mg/day.
Paralytic ileus, usually 15-60mg/day.

Renal Impairment: Lower doses may be needed.
CI: GI or urinary obstruction.
Interactions: Effect of Other Drugs on Pyridostigmine: *Effect diminished*: Aminoglycosides, polymyxins, clindamycin, chloroquine, lithium, procainamide, propranolol, quinidine.
Effect of Pyridostigmine on Other Drugs: Non-depolarising muscle relaxants: *Effect antagonised.* Suxamethonium: *Effect Enhanced.*
SP: Extreme caution with obstructive respiratory diseases (bronchial asthma, COPD); caution, arrhythmias, recent coronary occlusion, hypotension, vagotonia, peptic ulcer, epilepsy, Parkinson's Disease, hyperthyroidism. At high doses of pyridostigmine, myasthenic patient may need atropine or other anticholinergics to counteract the muscarinic effects. NOTE: Possibility of cholinergic crisis (pyridostigmine overdose) and differentiate from myasthenic crisis (increased disease severity). After thymectomy, pyridostigmine requirement may be decreased.
Pregnancy, Lactation: Pregnancy, lactation, if benefit outweighs risk. Avoid excessive doses; monitor newborn.
ADR: *Muscarinic effects*, nausea, vomiting, diarrhoea, abdominal cramps, increased (peristaltic, bronchial) secretion, salivation, bradycardia, miosis; *nicotinic effects*, muscle spasms, fasciculation and muscular weakness.
Notes: See 1.5.1 Stimulant Laxatives.

Mestinon 60mg *(Meda)* B. GMS.
Price, (200) €58.15.
Tablet, pyridostigmine bromide. White (off white) round scored (divisible into equal halves). Marked V M60. *Lactose.*

Sennoside
ATC Code: A06AB06. **Sport:** Permitted.
Driving: None known.
Indications: Laxative in treatment of occasional constipation.
Dose: Adult, Elderly: Age 12 years and over, 2-4 tablets in 24 hours OR 10mL syrup. *Admin*, oral at NIGHT.
Child: *Tabs*, over 12 years as for Adult; under 12 years, not recommended.
Syrup, under 12 years, with medical advice; age 6-12 years, 5mL OR age 2-6 years 2.5mL in 24 hours. *Admin*, as single dose in MORNING.
SP: Prolonged use not recommended.
Pregnancy, Lactation: Not recommended.
ADR: *Unknown incidence*, hypersensitivity, urticaria, asthma, hypogammaglobulinaemia, hypokalaemia, cachexia, abdominal (pain, spasm), diarrhoea, GI mucosal pigmentation, pruritus, generalised exanthema, finger clubbing, tetany, hyper trophic osteoarthropathy, chromaturia.
Notes: See 1.5.1 Stimulant Laxatives.

Senokot 7.5mg Tabs, Syrup *(R/Benckiser)* OTC.
Price, not published by company.
Tablet, sennosides 7.5mg/tab (sennoside B). Round greenish-brown. Marked S. *Lactose.* **Store:** No special conditions.
Syrup, as above 7.5mg/5mL. Amber slightly viscous. **Store:** Below 25 deg C; do not freeze.

1.5.2 - Bulk Forming Laxatives

In This Chapter: *Ispaghula (and mebeverine combination), sterculia.*

Class Effects
These laxatives produce their effect by stimulating colonic motility (increased faecal volume) and reducing intraluminal recto-sigmoid pressure.
CI: Intestinal obstruction, colonic atony (senile mega-colon), reduced gut motility (natural, drug-induced), paralytic ileus.
Interactions: Effect of Bulk-Forming Laxatives on Other Drugs: Cardiac glycosides, coumarin derivatives, lithium, vitamins (B12), mineral (calcium, iron, zinc): *Delayed or*

reduced GI absorption. Medicinals inhibiting peristaltic movement (opioids): *Increase GI obstruction risk.*
SP: Do not admin in dry form. Maintain adequate fluid intake. Oesophageal obstruction is possible if not washed down with fluid. Preparations that swell in contact with fluid should not be taken immediately before bed or in recumbent position, especially elderly. Elderly or debilitated require medical supervision. Hypersensitivity reactions, discontinue.
Notes: See 1.5 Constipation, Laxatives.

Ispaghula Husk
ATC Code: A06AC01. **Sport:** Permitted.
Driving: Unlikely to impair.
Indications: Patients requiring high fibre regimen.
Dose: Adult, Elderly: Age 12 years and over, 1 sachet or 2x 5mL spoonfuls morning and evening, add 1 sachet or granules into glass of water (at least 150mL); drink as soon as effervescence subsides. Effect starts 12-24 hours later.
Child: Age 6-12 years, half to one level 5mL spoonful (depending on age, size), morning and evening. Under 6 years, as for 6-12 years, only when prescribed by a doctor. *Admin*, as for Adult above.
CI: Sudden changed bowel habit (more than 2 weeks), undiagnosed rectal bleeding and failure to defecate following laxative use, swallowing difficulty or throat problems. See Notes below.
SP: Ispaghula/psyllium husk contains potent allergens; avoid inhaling the powder to minimise sensitisation risk. No bowel movement after 3 days, consult doctor. Antidiabetic therapy may need adjustment.
Pregnancy, Lactation: Use can be considered.
ADR: Hypersensitivity with pruritus, bronchospasm and anaphylaxis; conjunctivitis, rhinitis, flatulence, abdominal distention, obstruction (intestinal, oesophageal), faecal impaction, skin rash.
Notes: See 1.5.2 Bulk Forming Laxatives.

Fybogel Citrus *(R/Benckiser)* OTC. GMS.
Price, (30) €2.68. (60) €5.35.
Sachet, ispaghula husk. Semi-transparent buff-coloured granules; orange odour. *Aspartame.*

Ispaghula Husk, Mebeverine
ATC Code: A06AC51. **Sport:** Permitted.
Driving: No or negligible effect.
Indications: Irritable bowel syndrome.
Dose: Adult, Elderly: Contents of 1 sachet morning and evening. A third dose may be taken before midday meal if needed. *Admin*, stir contents into glass of cold water (240mL); drink immediately; admin half hour before food; do not admin immediately before going to sleep. *Elderly, debilitated*, admin with medical supervision.
Child: Under 12 years, not recommended.
CI: See Notes below (ispaghula husk).
Interactions: Effect of Ispaghula, Mebeverine Combination on Other Drugs: Antihypertensives: *Dose adjustment.*
SP: Renal failure, potassium (supplements, -sparing diuretics); caution, hyperkalaemia.
Pregnancy, Lactation: Pregnancy, use if considered essential. Lactation, not recommended; mebeverine is excreted in human milk.
ADR: *Unknown incidence*, hypersensitivity, conjunctivitis, rhinitis, flatulence, abdominal distension, intestinal obstruction, faecal impaction, skin rash.
Notes: See Ispaghula Husk above. See 1.2 Antispasmodics (mebeverine).

Fybogel Mebeverine *(R/Benckiser)* OTC. GMS.
Price, (10) €3.15. (60) €18.93.
Granules (sachet), ispaghula 3.5g, mebeverine 135mg. Buff granules and orange spheroids for oral susp. *Potassium 2.5mmoL, sodium 2.57mmoL per dose; aspartame.* **Store:** Below 30 deg C; original pack.

1.5.3   Osmotic Laxatives

Sterculia

ATC Code: A06AC03. **Sport:** Permitted.
Driving: Unlikely to impair.

Indications: Constipation, including during pregnancy and lactation. Colostomy and ileostomy management. High Residue Diet management in diverticular disease of colon, other conditions requiring high fibre regimen. Initiation and maintenance of bowel action after rectal and anal surgery. Admin after ingestion of sharp foreign bodies to provide a coating and reduce possibility of intestinal damage during transit.

Dose: Adult, Elderly: Contents of 1-2 sachets or 1-2 heaped 5mL spoonfuls, once or twice daily after meals. *Admin*, with plenty of fluid; do not crush or chew granules.
Child: 6-12 years, half Adult dose or with medical advice.
SP: Ulcerative colitis, caution.
ADR: Oesophageal or intestinal obstruction, intestinal impaction, abdominal distention, flatulence.
Notes: See 1.5.2 Bulk Forming Laxatives.

Normacol 62% Granules *(Norgine)* OTC. GMS.
Price, (500g) €7.10. Sachets (60) €5.96.
Oral granules, sterculia. White irregular-shaped. *Sucrose, sodium hydrogen carbonate.*

1.5.3 - Osmotic Laxatives

In This Chapter: *Citrates, lactulose, macrogols, phosphates.*

Class Effects

Osmotic laxatives increase amount of water in large bowel, either by retaining fluid with which they were taken or by drawing fluid from body into bowel.
Notes: See 1.5 Constipation, Laxatives.

Citrates (laxative)

ATC Code: A06AD. **Sport:** Permitted.
Driving: No or negligible effect.

Indications: Laxative through faecal softening and lubricant properties. For evacuation of colon in constipation or prior to surgical and diagnostic procedure or in obstetrics prior to delivery.
Dose: Adult, Elderly: Contents of 1 micro-enema admin rectally as necessary. Lubricate nozzle tip with of contents to aid insertion.
Child: As for Adult; under 3 years, insert nozzle half of length.
SP: Prolonged use may lead to irritation of anal canal. Caution, large bowel inflammatory or ulcerative conditions, acute GI conditions. Seek medical advice if symptoms persist. Risk of intestinal necrosis with sorbitol and sodium polystyrene sulphonate (oral/rectal admin).
Pregnancy, Lactation: Only to be used as directed by physician at time of delivery.
ADR: No common reported adverse events.
Notes: See 1.5.3 Osmotic Laxatives.

Microlax Rectal Soln *(McNeil)* OTC.
Price, not published by company (5mL).
Rectal soln (enema), sodium citrate 450mg, sodium lauryl sulphoacetate 45mg. Colourless viscous liquid in micro-enema with elongated nozzle. *Sorbic acid.*

Lactulose

ATC Code: A06AD11. **Sport:** Permitted.
Driving: No or negligible effect.

Indications: Constipation. Hepatic encephalopathy, treatment and prevention of hepatic coma or precoma.
Dose: Adult, Elderly: *Constipation,* initially 15-45mL/day; maintenance, 15-30mL/day. *Hepatic encephalopathy,* initially 30-45mL 3-4 times daily. Adjust dose to produce 2-3 soft stools per day. *Admin*, diluted or undiluted; swallow immediately, do not hold in mouth; admin as single dose at same time each day (e.g. before breakfast) or in 2 divided doses. It may be 2-3 days before adequate effect occurs.

Child: *Duphalac, constipation,* (age 7-14 years), initially 15mL/day, maintenance 10-15mL/day; (age 1-6 years), initial and maintenance 5-10mL/day; (infants under 1 year), initial and maintenance, up to 5mL/day. *Admin*, see Adult above.
Laxose, constipation, 10-25mL/day for first 2-3 days; maintenance, 5-15mL/day.
CI: Galactosaemia, GI (obstruction, perforation or risk of).
Interactions: Effect of Lactulose on Other Drugs: Enteric coated mesalazine: *Lower stool pH may prevent mesalazine release.*
SP: Seek medical advice if there are painful abdominal symptoms before initiation, insufficient therapeutic effect after several days. Chronic use of unadjusted dose and misuse can lead to diarrhoea and disturbed electrolytes. Diabetics, dose in constipation should not be problematic; in hepatic encephalopathy, the higher dose may need consideration. Defecation reflex may be disturbed.
Pregnancy, Lactation: Pregnancy, can be used if considered necessary by physician. Lactation, can be used.
ADR: *Very common,* diarrhoea; *common,* flatulence, abdominal pain, nausea, vomiting.
Notes: See 1.5.3 Osmotic Laxatives.

Duphalac Oral Soln *(BGP)* OTC. GMS.
Price, 300mL, €1.23. 1L, €3.72.
Oral soln, lactulose 3.335g/5mL. Clear colourless (pale-brownish-yellow) viscous.

Laxose Oral Soln *(Pinewood)* OTC. GMS.
Price, 500mL, €4.07.
Oral soln, lactulose 3.335g/5mL. *Lactose, epilactose, galactose, tagatose, fructose.*

Macrogol, Electrolytes

ATC Code: A06AD65. **Sport:** Permitted.
Driving: Unlikely to impair; dizziness may occur.

Indications: GI lavage/bowel cleansing prior to (clinical procedures, diagnostic examination, surgery). Constipation, faecal impaction (adults, children). See Dose below.
Dose: Adult, Elderly: GI lavage, diagnostic procedures:
Klean-Prep, contents of 1 sachet dissolved in 1L water, usually 4L (4 sachets) admin at rate of 200-250mL over 10-15 minutes; until total volume consumed or rectal effluent clear. Admin night before or start 4 hours prior to procedure; admin via nasogastric tube at 20-30mL/min.
Moviprep, 1 sachet each (A + B) dissolved in 1L water; admin over 1-2 hours; repeat with second litre (1L evening before and 1L early morning on day of procedure OR 2L evening before procedure); recommend additional 1L clear fluid also be taken (water, clear soup, fruit juice without pulp, soft drinks, tea/coffee without milk). Allow 1 hour between end of fluid intake and start of colonoscopy; take no solid food from start of treatment until after procedure.
Chronic constipation *(Laxido, Macrolief, Molaxone, Movicol, Tevicon),* 1-3 sachets/day (divided doses); extended use, 1-2 sachets/day; max. 2 weeks. *Admin*, dissolve 1 sachet in 125mL water.
Faecal impaction *(Laxido, Macrolief, Molaxone, Movicol, Tevicon),* 8 sachets/day, admin within a 6-hour period for 3 days. *Admin*, dissolve 8 sachets in 1L of water. Impaired cardiovascular function, divide dose; max. 2 sachets in any 1 hour.
Child: *Laxido (Paed), Movicol (Paed), chronic constipation,* (age 2-6 years), 1 sachet/day; (7-11 years), 2 sachets/day; max. 4 sachets/day; (under 2 years), not recommended.
Faecal impaction, age 5-11 years, 4 sachets (day 1), then 6 sachets (day 2), then 8 sachets (day 3), then 10 sachets (day 4), then 12 sachets/day (days 5, 6 and 7); divided doses, admin within a 12-hour period. Under 5 years or impaired cardiovascular function, not recommended. Dissolve each sachet in 62.5mL water (quarter of a glass).
Laxido (adult), Macrolief, Tevicon, adolescents, as for Adult; under 12 years, not recommended.
Klean-Prep, Movicol (adult), Moviprep, under 18 years, not recommended.

Renal Impairment: *Laxido (Paed)*, faecal impaction (child) not recommended with impaired function.

CI: Intestinal perforation or obstruction, ileus, severe GI inflammatory disease (Crohn's disease, ulcerative colitis, toxic megacolon). Under 20kg, CHF (NYHA III/IV) *Klean-Prep.*

Interactions: Effect of Other Drugs on Macrogol, Electrolytes: *Co-admin not recommended*: Oral drugs with (narrow therapeutic index, short half-life); absorption reduced due to increased GI transit/decreased efficacy (antiepileptics); leave 1-hour dosing interval.

SP: Caution, impaired gag reflex, impaired consciousness, reflux oesophagitis, tendency to aspiration, regurgitation. Acute inflammatory bowel disease. Unconscious or semi-conscious, monitor (especially nasogastric route). Debilitated, fragile, poor health, renal impairment risk, fluid or electrolyte disturbances including decreased blood bicarbonate, hypercalcaemia, hypo- (phosphataemia, calcaemia, kalaemia, natraemia). Underlying renal impairment risk, use if benefit outweighs risk. Maintain adequate fluid intake (the fluid content of *Movicol* when re-constituted with water does not replace regular fluid intake).

Pregnancy, Lactation: Only if considered necessary. *Molaxole*, not recommended. *Movicol, Laxido Orange, Macrolief* can be used in pregnancy and lactation.

ADR: *Common, Klean-Prep, Moviprep*, nausea, abdominal distension/discomfort, flatulence; *Laxido Orange/Paed, Molaxole, Movicol, Macrolief*, reactions related to GI tract, due to expansion of contents of GI tract and increased motility; mild diarrhoea usually responds to dose reduction.

Notes: See 1.5.3 Osmotic Laxatives.

Klean-Prep *(Fannin)* B.
Price, (4) sachets, €7.28. Sachets + container, €7.89.
Oral soln, macrogol 3350 59g, sodium (sulfate anhydrous 5.685g, bicarbonate 1.685g, chloride 1.465g), potassium chloride 0.7425g per sachet. White granular powder for soln; vanilla flavour. *Aspartame.*

Laxido Orange, Laxido Paed Plain *(Galen)* B. GMS.
Price, sachets (20) €8.29; paediatric, €6.17.
Powder for oral soln (Orange), macrogol 3350 13.125g, sodium (chloride 350.7mg, bicarbonate 178.5mg), potassium chloride 46.6mg per sachet. White powder.
Paediatric powder for oral soln (Paed Plain), macrogol 3350 6.563g, sodium (chloride 175.4mg, hydrogen carbonate 89.3mg), potassium chloride 25.1mg. White powder.

Macrolief *(Rowex)* B. GMS.
Price, sachets (30) €7.50.
Powder for oral soln, macrogol 3350 13.125g, sodium (chloride 0.3507g, hydrogen carbonate 0.1785g), potassium chloride 0.0466g per sachet. White free-flowing powder. *Sorbitol; sodium 187mg, potassium 25mg per sachet.*

Molaxole *(Meda)* B. GMS.
Price, sachets (20) €7.02. (30) €8.91.
Oral soln, macrogol 3350 13.125g, sodium (chloride 350.7mg, bicarbonate 178.5mg), potassium chloride 46.6mg per sachet. White crystalline powder.

Movicol Sachet, Paed Plain *(Norgine)* B. GMS.
Price, sachets 13.8g (20) €7.07. (30) €10.62. Paed 6.9g (30) €7.71.
Oral soln, macrogol 3350 (13.125g) (paed 6.563g), sodium chloride (0.3507g) (paed 0.1754g), sodium bicarbonate (0.1785g) (paed 0.0893g), potassium chloride (0.0466g) (paed 0.0251g) per sachet. Free-flowing white (light-brown) powder.

Moviprep *(Norgine)* B.
Price, (4) sachets (A+B) €13.26.
Oral soln, macrogol 3350 100g, sodium (sulfate 7.5g, chloride 2.691g), potassium chloride 1.015g (A); ascorbic acid 4.7g, sodium ascorbate 5.9g (B) per sachet. Powder. *Aspartame (A).*

Tevicon 13.7g *(TEVA)* B. GMS.
Price, sachets (30) €9.98.
Oral soln, macrogol 3350 13.125g, sodium (chloride 350.7mg, hydrogen carbonate 178.5mg), potassium chloride 46.6mg per sachet. White powder. *Sodium 65mmoL/L of soln.*

1.5.4 - Opioid-Induced Constipation

In This Chapter: *Methylnaltrexone, naloxegol.*

Class Effects
Methylnaltrexone bromide and naloxegol act as peripherally-acting mu-opioid antagonists in the GI tract, without impacting on CNS opioid-mediated analgesic effects.

Methylnaltrexone
ATC Code: A06AH01. **Sport:** Permitted.
Driving: Dizziness.

Indications: Treatment, opioid-induced constipation in advanced illness (response to usual laxative therapy insufficient).

Dose: Adult, Elderly: Weight (38-61kg), admin 8mg; (62-114kg), admin 12mg as single dose every other day or at longer intervals if needed; 2 consecutive doses (24 hours apart) may be given only if no bowel movement on preceding day. Weight outside ranges above, 0.15mg/kg. *Admin*, by SC injection rotating sites; upper legs, abdomen, upper arms.

Child: Under 18 years, no data.

Renal Impairment: CrCl (mL/min) below 30 (weight 62-114kg) 8mg; outside this range, 0.075mg/kg. Dialysis, not recommended.

Hepatic Impairment: Severe, not recommended.

CI: Suspected mechanical GI obstruction, increased recurrent obstruction risk or acute surgical abdomen (potential for GI perforation).

SP: Severe persistent diarrhoea, discontinue. Bowel movement can have rapid onset (30-60 minutes). Only for use with palliative care in addition to usual laxatives in opioid-associated constipation. Colostomy, peritoneal catheter, active diverticular disease, faecal impaction, caution. GI perforation reported with conditions that may reduce structural wall integrity in GI tract e.g. peptic ulcer disease, pseudo obstruction (Ogilvie's syndrome), diverticular disease, infiltrative GI malignancies or peritoneal metastases. Opioid withdrawal symptoms reported.

Pregnancy, Lactation: Pregnancy, only if clearly necessary. Lactation, stop drug or stop breastfeeding.

ADR: Summary, *most common*, abdominal pain, nausea, flatulence, diarrhoea.

Notes: See 1.5 Constipation, Laxatives.

Relistor Parenteral 12mg/0.6mL *(SOBI)* A. GMS.
Price, (1) €32.24. (7) €224.81.
Injection, methylnaltrexone bromide. Sterile clear colourless (pale-yellow) soln; visible particle free. *Essentially sodium-free*. **Store:** Protect from light.

Naloxegol
ATC Code: A06AH03. **Sport:** Permitted.
Driving: No or negligible effect.

Indications: Opioid-induced constipation in adults (inadequate response to laxatives).

Dose: Adult, Elderly: Recommended 25mg/day. When initiating, halt laxative therapy until clinical effect determined. *CYP3A4 moderate inhibitor co-admin (diltiazem, verapamil)*: Initially 12.5mg/day; if tolerated, increase to 25mg/day. *Admin*, once daily in morning (to avoid bowel movements during the night) on empty stomach at least 30 minutes before first meal of day or 2 hours after. Swallowing difficulty, tablet can be crushed to a powder, mixed with half a glass of water (120mL) and drunk immediately; rinse glass with further 120mL and drink. Mixture can be admin through a nasogastric tube (CH 8 or greater); flush tube with water after admin.

Child: Under 18 years, safety/efficacy not established.

Renal Impairment: Moderate/severe, initially 12.5mg; discontinue if side effects impacting on tolerability occur. Increase to 25mg if tolerated. Mild, no adjustment.

Hepatic Impairment: Mild/moderate, no adjustment. Severe, not recommended.

CI: GI obstruction (or at increased risk of), underlying cancer with increased GI perforation risk e.g. GI or peritoneum malignancy, recurrent or advanced ovarian cancer, vascular endothelial growth factor (VEGF) inhibitor

13

1.5.5 Drugs Acting on Serotonin Receptors

treatment; severe ulcer disease, Crohn's disease, diverticulitis.

Interactions: Effect of Other Drugs on Naloxegol: *Co-admin contraindicated*: Strong CYP3A4 inhibitors (clarithromycin, ketoconazole, itraconazole, telithromycin, ritonavir, indinavir, saquinavir, grapefruit juice). *Co-admin caution*: Methadone. *Co-admin not recommended*: Strong CYP3A4 inducers.

SP: Blood-brain barrier integrity minimises naloxegol uptake to CNS; disruptions (primary brain malignancy, CNS metastases, other inflammatory conditions, active MS, advanced Alzheimer's disease), caution (risk/benefit). Severe abdominal pain and diarrhoea; consider lowering dose to 12.5mg. Opioid withdrawal syndrome reported; discontinue. Caution, MI (within 6 months), symptomatic CHF, overt cardiovascular disease, QT interval of 500 msec or above.

Pregnancy, Lactation: Not recommended.

ADR: Summary, *most common*, abdominal pain, diarrhoea, nausea, headache, flatulence.

Notes: See 1.5 Constipation, Laxatives.

▼ **Moventig 12.5mg, 25mg** *(KyowaKirin)* B. GMS.
Price, (30) 12.5mg, 25mg, €70.96.
Tablet, naloxegol oxalate. Oval mauve f/c. Marked nGL one side; strength on reverse.

1.5.5 - Drugs Acting on Serotonin Receptors

In This Chapter: *Prucalopride.*

Class Effects
Also called 5HT4-agonists.

Prucalopride

ATC Code: A03AE04. **Sport:** Permitted.
Driving: Minor influence, dizziness, fatigue.
Indications: Chronic constipation in adults (other laxatives not providing adequate relief).

Dose: Adult: 2mg once daily with or without food at any time of day; no effect after 4 weeks, reconsider benefit of continuing; exceeding 2mg/day not expected to increase efficacy; no data for use beyond 3 months.

Elderly: Over 65 years, initially 1mg; increase to 2mg if needed.

Child: Under 18 years, not recommended.

Renal Impairment: Severe, GFR (mL/min/1.73m2) below 30, 1mg once daily. Dialysis, contraindicated.

Hepatic Impairment: Severe, 1mg once daily; increase to 2mg if required and if tolerated (caution).

CI: Intestinal perforation or obstruction, severe GI inflammatory disease (Crohn's disease, ulcerative colitis, toxic megacolon). Dialysis.

Interactions: Effect of Other Drugs on Prucalopride: *Co-admin caution*: Drugs causing QTc prolongation. *Effects reduced*: Atropine-like substances.

Effect of Prucalopride on Other Drugs: Erythromycin: *Plasma levels increased*.

SP: Severe, unstable concomitant disease; arrhythmias, ischaemic cardiovascular disease, caution. Severe diarrhoea, oral contraceptive efficacy reduced.

Pregnancy, Lactation: Not recommended. Women of childbearing potential to ensure adequate contraception. Lactation, is excreted in breast milk.

ADR: Summary, *most frequent*, headache, GI symptoms (abdominal pain, nausea, diarrhoea).

Notes: See 1.5 Constipation, Laxatives.

Resolor 1mg, 2mg *(Shire)* B. GMS.
Price, (28) 1mg, €45.13. 2mg, €66.10.
Tablet, prucalopride succinate. Round f/c. Marked PRU and strength. 1mg: White (off-white). 2mg: Pink. *Lactose*.

1.6.1 - Corticosteroids (GI)

In This Chapter: *Budesonide, hydrocortisone, prednisolone.*

Class Effects
Sport: Use of corticosteroids in sport is described under systemic glucocorticoids. See Notes below.

Driving: See SP below (visual disturbances).

CI: Hypersensitivity to any member of the class. See Notes below (glucocorticoids).

Interactions: Effect of Other Drugs on Systemic Corticosteroids: *Co-admin not recommended*: Live vaccines. *Increased GI bleeding/ulceration risk*: Aspirin, NSAIDs. *Metabolism accelerated, reduced effect*: Rifamycins, carbamazepine, phenobarbital, phenytoin, primidone, aminoglutethimide, mifepristone. *Metabolism inhibited (plasma levels increased)*: Erythromycin, clarithromycin, ketoconazole, itraconazole. *Increased hypokalaemia risk (toxicity)*: Amphotericin (avoid co-admin), cardiac glycosides, bambuterol, fenoterol, formoterol, ritodrine, salbutamol, salmeterol, terbutaline, theophylline, carbenoxolone. *Plasma levels increased (prednisolone)*: Ritonavir, ciclosporin. *Plasma protein binding altered, increased exposure (prednisolone)*: Oestrogens, progestogens. *Increased systemic side-effect risk (avoid)*: CYP3A4 inhibitors (cobicistat).

Effect of Systemic Corticosteroids on Other Drugs: Salicylates: *Increased renal clearance; salicylate intoxication risk on steroid withdrawal*. Coumarins: *Effect enhanced, monitor INR*. Antidiabetics: *Hypoglycaemic effect antagonised*. Antihypertensives: *Hypotensive effect antagonised*. Methotrexate: *Increased haematological toxicity risk*. Diuretics: *Effect antagonised*. Acetazolamide, loop diuretics, thiazides: *Increased hypokalaemia risk*. Somatropin: *Growth promoting effect inhibited*.

SP: Caution, severe ulcerative disease, perforation risk. Systemic absorption may result in disturbances in hypothalamic-pituitary-adrenal (HPA) axis and reduced stress response (prolonged or excessive use). Topicals, systemic absorption may occur especially with local inflammation. Patients to carry treatment cards.

Visual disturbances with systemic and topical corticosteroid use, reported; consider ophthalmologist evaluation (cataract, glaucoma, rare diseases e.g. central serous chorioretinopathy). See Notes below.

Pregnancy, Lactation: Pregnancy, if benefit outweighs risk; avoid large amounts or prolonged use of topical steroids. Lactation, generally not recommended.

ADR: See Notes below (glucocorticoids).

Notes: Systemic effects, see Class Effects 11.1.1 Glucocorticoids.

Budesonide (GI) (systemic)

ATC Code: A07EA06. **Sport:** Prohibited (in-competition).
Driving: Unlikely to impair; see SP below.
Indications: *Caps, Granules*, mild to moderate Crohn's disease* (ileum and/or ascending colon). Microscopic colitis. Symptomatic relief, chronic diarrhoea with collagenous colitis, active collagenous colitis*. *Caps*, autoimmune hepatitis. *Rectal Foam*, treatment, ulcerative colitis (rectum, sigmoid colon). *Tabs*, mild to moderate active ulcerative colitis* (acetylsalicylic acid not sufficient). *(induction of remission).

Dose: Adult: *Budenofalk*, CAPS, Crohn's Disease, collagenous colitis, autoimmune hepatitis (remission induction), 3mg 3-times daily (9mg/day); autoimmune hepatitis (maintenance), 3mg twice daily (6mg/day); GRANULES, Crohn's disease, collagenous colitis, 1 sachet (9mg) once daily (morning, 30 minutes before breakfast). *Admin*, swallow caps/granules whole with plenty of water; do not crush or chew. RECTAL, insert 1 foam actuation daily, morning or evening.

Entocort CR, CAPS, active Crohn's Disease, microscopic colitis, 9mg/day (up to 8 weeks). *Admin*, once daily (morning). Swallow whole; do not crush or chew. Long-term use (prolong remission) or to replace prednisolone or prevent recurrence after surgery, 6mg/day.
Cortiment, TABS, ulcerative colitis, 9mg/day (morning) (up to 8 weeks); discontinue gradually.

Elderly: Limited data.

Child: *Budenofalk*, under 12 years, caps not recommended; age 12-18 years, no dose recommendation; under 18 years, granules not recommended. *Entocort CR, Cortiment*, under 18 years, not recommended.

Renal Impairment: Caution.

Hepatic Impairment: Increased systemic exposure, caution. Liver disease, without hepatic cirrhosis, 9mg/day was safe/well tolerated.

CI: Hepatic cirrhosis *(Budenofalk)*.

Interactions: Effect of Other Drugs on Budesonide: Plasma levels increased *(consider dose reduction)*: Ketoconazole, grapefruit juice *(co-admin not recommended)*. *Reduced absorption*: Colestyramine, antacids (admin 2 hours apart).

Effect of Budesonide on Other Drugs: Cardiac glycosides: *Action potentiated by hypokalaemia.*

SP: Lower systemic levels than oral glucocorticoids; caution, transfer from steroid therapy with higher systemic effect; monitor adrenocortical function; may unmask allergies (rhinitis, eczema). Autoimmune hepatitis, monitor transaminases.

ADR: *Common, Budenofalk*, Cushing's syndrome, dyspepsia, increased infection risk, hypokalaemia, muscle/joint pain, muscle weakness and twitching, osteoporosis, headache, depression, irritability, euphoria, allergic exanthema, petechiae, ecchymosis, delayed wound healing, contact dermatitis. *Entocort*, palpitations, Cushingoid features, blurred vision, dyspepsia, hypokalaemia, muscle cramp, behavioural changes (nervousness, insomnia, mood swings), menstrual disorders, skin reactions (urticaria, exanthema).

Notes: See Class Effects 1.6.1 Corticosteroids (GI). Systemic effects, see Class Effects 11.1.1 Glucocorticoids.

Budenofalk Caps, Granules, Rectal Foam *(Dr Falk)* B. GMS.
Price, caps 3mg (100) €85.28. Granules (sachets) 9mg (60) €164.32. Foam (1) €71.20.
Capsule, budesonide 3mg. Hard pink; contains granules g/r. *Lactose, sucrose.* **Store:** No special conditions.
Rectal foam (pressurised container), as above 2mg/1.2g dose. White (pale white) creamy firm. *Cetyl alcohol, propylene glycol.* **Store:** Do not refrigerate, freeze or expose to temperature above 50 deg C.
Granules (sachet), as above 9mg. White (off-white) granules g/r; lemon smell. *Sucrose, lactose, sorbitol.* **Store:** No special conditions.

Cortiment 9mg *(Ferring)* B. GMS.
Price, (30) €91.80.
Prolonged/R tablet, budesonide. White (off-white) f/c, g/r. Marked MX9. *Lactose.*

Entocort CR 3mg *(Tillotts)* B. GMS.
Price, (100) €90.59.
Prolonged/R capsule, budesonide. Hard gelatin opaque light-grey/pink g/r. Marked CIR 3mg. *Sucrose.* **Store:** Below 30 deg C; original pack.

Hydrocortisone (rectal)

ATC Code: A07EA02. **Sport:** Prohibited (in-competition).
Driving: Unlikely to impair.

Indications: Distal ulcerative colitis, procto-sigmoiditis, granular proctitis.

Dose: Adult, Elderly: 1 applicator-full inserted into rectum once or twice daily for 2-3 weeks, then every second day.

Child: As for Adult above.

CI: Obstruction, abscess, perforation, peritonitis, fresh intestinal anastomoses, extensive fistulae.

ADR: Irritation may occur. Prolonged extensive use may cause systemic effects.

Notes: See Class Effects 1.6.1 Corticosteroids (GI). Systemic effects, see Class Effects 11.1.1 Glucocorticoids.

Colifoam 10% Rectal Foam *(Meda)* A. GMS.
Price, (1) €9.12.
Rectal foam, hydrocortisone acetate 10% w/w (approx. 14 doses). White odourless. *Parabens, cetyl alcohol, propylene glycol.* **Store:** Below 25 deg C; do not refrigerate or freeze.

Prednisolone (rectal)

ATC Code: A07EA01. **Sport:** Prohibited (in-competition).
Driving: Unlikely to impair.

Indications: Treatment, proctitis, ulcerative colitis.

Dose: Adult, Elderly: Insert 1 metered dose rectally once or twice daily for 2 weeks; continue for another 2 weeks if response is good; discontinue at discretion of physician.

Child: Not recommended.

CI: Local infection may be masked with peritonitis, intestinal obstruction, bowel perforation. Not for use during disease remission,

Notes: See Class Effects 1.6.1 Corticosteroids (GI). Systemic effects, see Class Effects 11.1.1 Glucocorticoids.

Prednisolone Rectal Foam *(Essential Generics)* A. GMS.
Price, 14-dose (1) €73.07.
Rectal foam, prednisolone metasulphobenzoate sodium equiv. to prednisolone 20mg. White (pale-cream) metered-dose. *Cetostearyl alcohol, sorbic acid.*

1.6.2 - Aminosalicylates (GI)

In This Chapter: *Mesalazine, olsalazine, sulfasalazine.*

Class Effects

Aminosalicylates are anti-inflammatories used to treat inflammatory bowel disease and some types of arthritis.

CI: Hypersensitivity to any member of the class/salicylates.

Interactions: Effect of Aminosalicylates on Other Drugs: *Co-admin not recommended (possible increased Reye's syndrome risk)*: Varicella vaccine (allow 6-week interval before salicylate admin). *Increased renal toxicity*: Nephrotoxic agents (NSAIDs, azathioprine), monitor function.

Effect of Aminosalicylates on Other Drugs: Digoxin: *Absorption decreased by sulfasalazine (no data with mesalazine)*. Warfarin: *Altered INR.* Azathioprine, tioguanine, 6-mercaptopurine: *Increased immunosuppressive effect (caution, life-threatening infection; leucopenia, monitor haematology; use lowest dose).*

SP: Caution, sulfasalazine or sulfonamide hypersensitivity. Severe allergy, asthma. Severe life-threatening systemic hypersensitivity reactions (DRESS), serious skin reactions (exfoliative dermatitis, Steven's-Johnson syndrome, toxic epidermal necrolysis) reported. Unexplained bleeding, bruising, purpura, anaemia, fever, sore throat; investigate haematology; blood dyscrasias, discontinue immediately. Caution, liver impairment, mild/moderate renal impairment; monitor function (prior to initiation, during treatment).

Mesalazine

ATC Code: A07EC02. **Sport:** Permitted.
Driving: No or negligible effect.

Indications: *Asacolon* (tabs), mild acute ulcerative colitis (maintenance of remission, surgically induced remission of Crohn's Disease; (supps), proctitis, procto-sigmoiditis, adjunctive (adults). *Pentasa* (Prolonged/R tabs, granules in sachets), mild/moderate ulcerative colitis; (Prolonged/R tabs), Crohn's Disease; (rectal susp), active ulcerative colitis; (supps), ulcerative proctitis. *Salofalk*, (all oral and rectal formulations) treatment of acute episodes and maintenance of remission of ulcerative colitis, (tabs) Crohn's Disease. *Mezavant*, induction and maintenance of remission, mild to moderate active ulcerative colitis.

Dose: Adult: *Asacolon*, ulcerative colitis, remission induction, 2.4g (3 tabs)/day; titrate to 4g/day if needed; maintenance, 1.2-2.4g/day. Crohn's Disease, remission

15

1.6.2 Aminosalicylates (GI)

maintenance, 2.4g (3 tabs)/day OR 1 supp inserted rectally 3-times daily after defecation; severe, insert 1 supp morning and evening. Admin, in divided doses; swallow tabs whole with water; do not crush or chew; do not swallow supps.

Mezavant, remission induction, 2.4-4.8g/day; maintenance 2.4g/day. Admin, once daily with food; do not crush or chew tabs.

Pentasa ulcerative colitis active treatment, up to 4g/day once daily or 2-3 divided doses; maintenance, 2g once daily (tabs/sachets). Crohn's disease, active treatment and maintenance, up to 4g/day in 2 or 3 divided doses (oral) OR rectal (enema), 1g (100mL) at bedtime (2-3 weeks); (supps), acute 1 x1g supp twice daily (2-4 weeks); maintenance 1-2g daily. Admin, oral; do not chew; swallow tabs whole or wash granules down with water.

Salofalk, tabs, ulcerative colitis, 2x 250mg tabs 3-times daily; double if needed; max. 8-12 weeks; maintenance, 2 tabs 3-times daily. Granules, acute 1.5-3g/day preferably morning or 3 divided doses; remission maintenance, 0.5g 3-times daily (1.5g/day) OR 3g as single daily dose (morning); admin as for Pentasa Sachets. Supps, (250mg strength), acute, 2 x 250mg supps 3-times daily (double if needed); maintenance, 1 x 250mg supp 3-times daily; (1g strength), 1 x 1g supp once daily. Enema, 1 enema (60mL) before retiring; (foam), 2 administrations at bedtime.

Elderly: As for Adult unless severely impaired liver or renal function.

Child: Pentasa, age 6 years and older, (granules only), ulcerative colitis and Crohn's disease, initially 30-50mg/kg/day*; max. 75mg/kg/day (4g/day)*; maintenance, 15-30mg/kg/day*; max. 2g/day*. Weight under 40kg, half Adult dose; over 40kg, as for Adult above. Do not chew tabs or granules; tabs may be dispersed in 50mL cold water; wash down granules with water. Other formulations, limited data. Under 6 years, safety/efficacy not established. *(admin in divided doses).

Salofalk, granules, 250mg tabs (6 years and older), active disease and maintenance, 30-50mg/kg/day in divided doses; max. 75mg/kg/day (total not to exceed Adult dose). Usually, up to 40kg, half adult dose; over 40kg, as for Adult above. Supps, Enema, Rectal Foam, limited data.

Asacolon (6 years and older), active disease, initially 30-50mg/kg/day*; max. 4g/day; maintenance, 15-30mg/kg/day*; max. 2g/day. Weight under 40kg, half Adult dose; over 40kg, as for Adult above. *(admin in divided doses).

Mezavant, under 18 years, not recommended.

Renal Impairment: Severe, GFR (mL/min) below 30, contraindicated. Caution, raised blood urea, proteinuria.

Hepatic Impairment: Severe, contraindicated.

CI: Gastric, duodenal ulcer (Asacolon).

Interactions: Effect of Mesalazine on Other Drugs: Azathioprine, 6-mercaptopurine, tioguanine: Possible increased myelosuppressive effect, blood dyscrasias. Warfarin: May decrease anticoagulant effect.

SP: Acute intolerance, discontinue immediately. Determine urinary status, LFTs (ALT, AST) prior to and during treatment. Dehydration (restore normal electrolytes, fluid balance). Nephrotoxicity, cardiac hypersensitivity, do not reintroduce. Serious blood dyscrasias (rare). Empty shells of Asacolon tab coating may appear in stools. Adrenal function may be suppressed by budesonide; ACTH stimulation test for diagnosing pituitary insufficiency might show false results (low values).

Pregnancy, Lactation: Pregnancy, only if clearly indicated; crosses placental barrier; blood disorders reported in newborn (pancytopenia, leucopenia, thrombocytopenia, anaemia); renal failure. Underlying inflammatory bowel disorder may increase risk for adverse pregnancy outcome. Lactation, use only if benefit outweighs risk; excreted in breast milk. If diarrhoea develops in breast fed infants, stop breastfeeding.

ADR: Summary, Mezavant, most frequent, colitis (including ulcerative), abdominal pain, headache, abnormal LFTs, diarrhoea, nausea; Asacolon, reported, organ specific reactions (heart, lungs, liver, kidneys, pancreas, skin, subcutaneous tissue); Pentasa, most frequent, diarrhoea, nausea, abdominal pain, headache, vomiting, rash; hypersensitivity reactions, drug fever. Salofalk, rarely, headache, dizziness, myocarditis, pericarditis, abdominal pain, diarrhoea, flatulence, nausea, vomiting.

Notes: See Class Effects 1.6.2 Aminosalicylates (GI).

Asacolon 400mg, 800mg, Supps 500mg (Tillotts) B. GMS.
Price, tabs 400mg (100) €26.06. 800mg (90) €48.84. Supps 500mg (20) €11.21.
Tablet, mesalazine. Reddish-brown oblong g/r. Lactose.
Supps, as above. Light grey-brown torpedo-shaped. Lecithin.
Store: Below 25 deg C; do not refrigerate or freeze.
Mezavant XL 1200mg (Shire) B. GMS.
Price, (60) €61.95.
Prolonged/R tablet, mesalazine. Red-brown ellipsoid g/r, f/c. Marked S476.
Pentasa Prolonged/R Tabs, Sachets (Ferring) B. GMS.
Price, Prolonged/R tabs 500mg (100) €35.13. 1g (60) €43.75. Sachets 1g (50) €41.72. 2g (60) €97.50. 4g (30) €97.50.
Prolonged/R tablet, mesalazine 500mg, 1g. White-grey (pale white-brown) speckled. 500mg: Round scored. Marked 500mg; Pentasa on reverse. 1g: Oval. Marked Pentasa both sides.
Prolonged/R granules (sachets), as above 1g, 2g, 4g. White-grey (white-brown).
Pentasa Rectal Susp, Supps 1g (Ferring) B. GMS.
Price, enema (7) €26.77. Supps (28) €54.26.
Rectal susp, mesalazine 10mg/mL. White (slightly-yellow).
Supps, as above. White (tan) spotted oblong.
Salofalk Tabs, Granules (Dr Falk) B. GMS.
Price, tabs 250mg (100) €15.72. Granules 500mg (100) €36.93. 1g (50) €37.21. 1.5g (60) €56.49. 3g (60) €119.98.
Tablet, mesalazine 250mg. Yellow round g/r. Sodium 48mg/tab.
Prolonged/R oral granules, as above 500mg, 1g, 1.5g, 3g sachet. Greyish-white g/r stick-formed or round. Aspartame, sucrose.
Salofalk Enema 4g, Supps, Rectal Foam (Dr Falk) B. GMS.
Price, enema (7) €34.12. Supps (30) 250mg, €12.44. 1g, €44.43. Foam 1g, €34.07.
Rectal soln, mesalazine 4g/60mL. Cream-coloured; lubricated applicator. Benzoate, metabisulphite.
Supps, as above 250mg, 1g. Light-beige torpedo-shaped.
Rectal foam, as above 1g/actuation. White-greyish (slightly reddish-violet) creamy firm foam. Cetostearyl alcohol, propylene glycol, metabisulphite.

Olsalazine

ATC Code: A07EC03. Sport: Permitted.
Driving: Unlikely to impair.

Indications: Mild to moderate acute, long-term maintenance or remission of ulcerative colitis. Useful if sulfasalazine not tolerated.

Dose: Adult, Elderly: Acute, mild disease, initially 1g/day; titrate over 1 week to 3g/day if needed. Max. single dose 1g. Long-term maintenance of remission, 500mg twice daily. Admin, in divided doses, end of meal; empty stomach may cause loose stools or diarrhoea.

Child: Not recommended.

Renal Impairment: Severe, not recommended.

Pregnancy, Lactation: Pregnancy, if benefit outweighs risk. Lactation, may pass into breast milk; infant diarrhoea reported; use not recommended.

ADR: Common, headache, diarrhoea, nausea, rash, arthralgia.

Notes: See Class Effects 1.6.2 Aminosalicylates (GI).

Dipentum 250mg, 500mg (Atnahs) B. GMS.
Price, caps 250mg (112) €32.72. Tabs 500mg (60) €35.91.
Capsule, olsalazine sodium. Beige hard.
Tablet, as above. Yellow scored.

Sulfasalazine

ATC Code: A07EC01. Sport: Permitted.
Driving: Unlikely to impair.

Indications: Induction and maintenance of remission, ulcerative colitis, active Crohn's disease, rheumatoid arthritis. Rectal, treatment of proctocolitis, proctitis.

Dose: Adult, Elderly: ORAL, STANDARD/R, ulcerative colitis, Crohn's Disease, moderate to severe, 1-2g, 4-times daily (with steroids if needed); maintenance, reduce gradually to 2g/day. Rheumatoid arthritis, initially 0.5g/day; increase weekly by 0.5g as needed; max. 3g/day.

MODIFIED/R, rheumatoid arthritis, long-term treatment with NSAIDs, initially 1 tab/day; increase by 1 tab each week to 1 tab 4-times daily or 2 tabs 3-times daily.

RECTAL, 2 supps to be inserted after defecation morning and evening.

Child: Acute attack, relapse, 40-60mg/kg/day; maintenance 20-30mg/kg/day. Severe disease, oral and rectal routes may be used together. Dose adjusted according to body weight. Under 2 years, contraindicated.

Renal Impairment: Caution.

Hepatic Impairment: As for Renal above.

CI: Jaundice, porphyria.

Interactions: Effect of Other Drugs on Sulfasalazine: *Bone marrow suppression, leucopenia:* Azathioprine, thiopurine 6-mercaptopurine. *Increased GI adverse events (nausea):* Methotrexate in patients with rheumatoid arthritis.

Effect of Sulfasalazine on Other Drugs: Folic-acid antagonists, hypoglycaemics: *Increased effect.* Digoxin: *Reduced absorption; non-therapeutic serum levels.*

SP: Children with systemic onset juvenile RA, not recommended. Monitor haematology. Ensure adequate fluid intake to prevent crystalluria and kidney stone formation. G-6-PD deficiency, monitor for haemolytic anaemia; acute attacks precipitated in porphyriacs. Certain types of extended wear soft contact lenses may be permanently stained. Urinary normetanephrine measurement by liquid chromatography interference causing a false-positive test result.

Pregnancy, Lactation: Sulfonamides, pregnancy use only if clearly needed; folic acid deficiency may lead to neural tube defects in newborn. Lactation, caution especially premature infants or with glucose-6-phosphate dehydrogenase deficiency; reports of bloody stools or diarrhoea in breastfed infants.

ADR: *Very common,* gastric distress, nausea.

Notes: See Class Effects 1.6.2 Aminosalicylates (GI).

Salazopyrin 500mg, EN 500mg *(Pfizer)* B. GMS.
Price, 500mg (112), €10.16. EN, €11.23.
Tablet and g/r tablet (EN), sulfasalazine. Orange/yellow. Marked KPh. 500mg: Round. Marked 101. EN: Oval g/r. Marked 102.

1.6.3 - Drugs Affecting Immune Response (GI)

In This Chapter: *Infliximab, vedolizumab.*

Class Effects
Infliximab, a selective immunosuppressive, is used for number of rheumatoid conditions; also indicated for treatment of Crohn's Disease. See Notes below.

CI: Hypersensitivity to any member of the class.

Notes: See 4.4.1 Drugs Suppressing Rheumatic Disease Process and Infliximab.

Vedolizumab
ATC Code: L04AA33. **Sport:** Pending.
Driving: Minor influence; dizziness.
Indications: Treatment, ulcerative colitis, Crohn's disease (moderate to severely active), with inadequate or lost response or intolerant to (conventional therapy, TNF-alpha antagonist).

Dose: Adult, Elderly: *Ulcerative colitis,* 300mg by IV infusion over 30 minutes (weeks 0, 2, 6) then every 8 weeks; no benefit by week 10, carefully reconsider. Monitor during and after infusion.

Crohn's Disease, 300mg (weeks 0, 2, 6) as for ulcerative colitis above; no response, a dose at week 10 may be beneficial then every 8 weeks from week 14 in responding patients; no response by week 14, do not continue.

Patients with decreased response may benefit from 300mg every 4 weeks. *Re-treatment,* consider restarting with dosing every 4 weeks if therapy is interrupted.

Child: Age 0-17 years, safety and efficacy not established.

Renal Impairment: No dose recommendation.

Hepatic Impairment: No dose recommendation.

CI: Active severe infections (TB, sepsis, cytomegalovirus, listeriosis, opportunistic infections e.g. PML).

Interactions: Effect of Other Drugs on Vedolizumab: *Co-admin caution:* Live vaccines, especially live oral vaccines.

SP: Admin in setting equipped to manage acute hypersensitivity reactions (anaphylaxis). Observe during and for 2 hours after infusion (first 2 infusions) for acute hypersensitivity reactions; observe for 1 hour (subsequent infusions). Severe infusion reaction, discontinue immediately; mild or moderate, slow infusion rate or interrupt. Consider pre-treatment (antihistamine, hydrocortisone and/or paracetamol). Increased risk of opportunistic or GI infections, malignancy risk. Caution, previous natalizumab or rituximab treatment. Bring all immunisations up to date prior to initiation. Induction of remission in Crohn's disease may take up to 14 weeks. See Notes below.

Pregnancy, Lactation: Pregnancy, use only if benefit outweighs risk. Women of childbearing potential to ensure adequate contraception during and for 18 weeks after treatment. Lactation, stop breastfeeding or stop drug.

ADR: *Very common,* nasopharyngitis, headache, arthralgia.

▼ **Entyvio Parenteral 300mg** *(Takeda)* A.
Price, not published by company.
Infusion, vedolizumab 60mg/mL. Humanised IgG1 monoclonal antibody. White (off-white) cake/powder for conc for soln. **Store:** Refrigerate.

1.7 - Anal and Rectal Disorders

1.7.1 - Haemorrhoids, Anal Fissure

In This Chapter: *Glyceryl trinitrate.*

Class Effects
Many of these preparations have antiseptic, astringent and emollient properties providing symptomatic relief of discomfort associated with minor ano-rectal conditions. Many of these products are available without prescription as brands *Anusol* (cream, ointment, supps) and *Rowatanal* (cream).

CI: Hypersensitivity to any member of the class.

SP: Medical advice should be sought to determine cause of haemorrhoids; especially with rectal bleeding or blood in stools. Not for oral admin.

Glyceryl Trinitrate (rectal)
ATC Code: C05AE01. **Sport:** Permitted.
Driving: Caution.
Indications: Pain relief associated with chronic anal fissure.

Dose: Adult, Elderly: Apply 2.5cm strip of ointment to anal canal every 12 hours; max. 8 weeks.

Child: Under 18 years, not recommended.

Renal Impairment: Severe, caution.

Hepatic Impairment: As for Renal above.

Interactions: Effect of Other Drugs on Glyceryl Trinitrate: *Co-admin not recommended:* Nitric oxide donors (isosorbide dinitrate, amyl or butyl-nitrite). *Vasodilatory effect potentiated:* Acetyl cysteine. *Reduced therapeutic response:* Acetylsalicylic acid, NSAIDs.

Effect of Glyceryl Trinitrate on Other Drugs: Heparin: *Decreased efficacy; consider dose adjustment.* Alteplase: *Reduced thrombolytic activity.* Dihydroergotamine: *Plasma levels increased.*

SP: Increased haemorrhoidal bleeding, discontinue. Persistent anal pain, seek differential diagnosis.

Pregnancy, Lactation: Not recommended.

ADR: *Very common,* headache. *Common,* dizziness, nausea.

1.7.2 Haemorrhoidals, with Corticosteroids

Notes: See 1.7.1 Haemorrhoids, Anal Fissure. Additional information, see 2.2.3 Nitrates (glyceryl trinitrate).

Rectogesic Rectal Ointment *(KyowaKirin)* B. GMS.
Price, (30g) €46.49.
Ointment, glyceryl trinitrate 4mg/g. Off-white opaque. *Propylene glycol, lanolin.*

1.7.2 - Haemorrhoidals, with Corticosteroids

In This Chapter: *Corticosteroids include hydrocortisone, prednisolone, fluocortolone.*

Class Effects
Sport: Use of corticosteroids in sport is described under systemic glucocorticoids. See Notes below.

CI: Children, unless otherwise specified. TB, fungal, bacterial, viral lesions including herpes simplex, vaccinia, varicella. Hypersensitivity to any member of class.

SP: Use rectal formulations after bowel evacuation. If the condition is aggravated or if rectal bleeding occurs, seek medical advice. Local atrophy of skin, striae and superficial vascular dilatation may occur. Local skin reactions (contact dermatitis), sensitivity reactions. Systemic corticosteroid effects may occur (prolonged or excessive use) or with other corticosteroid co-admin (topical, oral). Superinfection, phaeochromocytoma crisis.

Pregnancy, Lactation: If benefit outweighs risk; under medical supervision.

ADR: Transient burning on application, especially if anoderm not intact. See SP above.

Notes: See Class Effects 1.7.1 Haemorrhoids, Anal Fissure and 1.6.1 Corticosteroids (GI). For systemic effects, see 11.1.1 Glucocorticoids.

Cinchocaine, Fluocortolone
ATC Code: C05AD04, C05AA08. **Sport:** Restricted.
Driving: Unlikely to impair.
Indications: Haemorrhoids, anal fissures and proctitis.
Dose: Adult, Elderly: Apply twice daily; on first day up to 4-times for faster relief.
Notes: See 1.7.2 Haemorrhoidals, with Corticosteroids.

Ultraproct Rectal Ointment *(Bayer)* B. GMS.
Price, (30g) €5.32.
Ointment, fluocortolone pivalate 0.92mg, fluocortolone caproate 0.95mg, cinchocaine HCl 5mg per 1g. Colourless (faintly yellow). *Castor oil.* **Store:** Below 25 deg C; replace cap tightly.

Cinchocaine, Hydrocortisone
ATC Code: C05AD04, AC5AA01. **Sport:** Restricted.
Driving: Unlikely to impair.
Indications: Pain, pruritus, inflammation associated with haemorrhoids, fissures, proctitis, perianal eczema, post ano-rectal surgery.
Dose: Adult, Elderly: Apply externally or by means of cannula into rectum, twice daily and after each bowel evacuation; duration 1 week.
Child: Under 3 years, avoid.
SP: Continuous treatment for more than 3 weeks (avoid under age 3 years; possibility of adrenocortical suppression and growth retardation).
ADR: Itching, pain or rash around back passage.
Notes: See 1.7.2 Haemorrhoidals, with Corticosteroids.

Proctosedyl Ointment *(SANOFI)* A. GMS.
Price, (30g) €8.23.
Ointment, hydrocortisone 5mg, cinchocaine HCl 5mg, aesculin 10mg, framycetin sulfate 10mg. Yellow-white translucent homogenous. *Wool fat.* **Store:** Below 25 deg C.

Cinchocaine, Prednisolone
ATC Code: C05AD04, C05AA04. **Sport:** Restricted.
Driving: Unlikely to impair.
Indications: Internal or external haemorrhoids, anal fissures, proctitis.

Dose: Adult, Elderly: Apply twice daily; 4 times daily for faster relief; max. use 1 week. Supps, insert 1 daily; severe, insert 1 supp 2-3 times daily on first day.
Notes: See 1.7.2 Haemorrhoidals, with Corticosteroids.

Scheriproct Rectal Ointment, Supps *(Bayer)* B. GMS.
Price, ointment (10g) €1.86. (30g) €4.24. Supps (12) €2.67.
Rectal ointment, prednisolone caproate equiv. to prednisolone 1.5mg, cinchocaine HCl 5mg. Colourless (faintly-yellow) homogenous translucent. *Castor oil.* **Store:** Below 25 deg C; replace cap tightly after use.
Supps, prednisolone caproate equiv. to prednisolone 1mg, cinchocaine HCl 1mg. White (yellowish). **Store:** Refrigerate.

Lidocaine, Hydrocortisone
ATC Code: C05AD01, AC5AA01. **Sport:** Restricted.
Driving: Unlikely to impair.
Indications: Anal and perianal conditions (pruritus, pain, inflammation) associated with haemorrhoids, anal fissures, loose stools.
Dose: Adult, Elderly: Age 14 years and over, spray once over affected area up to 3-times daily depending on severity.
Child: Under 14 years, use only with medical supervision.
CI: Not for use on broken or infected skin.
SP: Not for internal use, keep away from eyes, nose, mouth.
ADR: Lidocaine hypersensitivity.
Notes: See 1.7.2 Haemorrhoidals, with Corticosteroids and 14.2 Local Anaesthesia (lidocaine).

Perinal Spray *(Dermal)* B. GMS.
Price, (30mL) €7.85.
Cutaneous spray, hydrocortisone 0.2%, lidocaine HCl 1% w/w. Colourless (pale-yellow) soln.

Pramocaine (pramoxine), Hydrocortisone
ATC Code: C05AD07, AC5AA01. **Sport:** Prohibited (in-competition).
Driving: Unlikely to impair.
Indications: Itching, irritation, discomfort or pain associated with local, non-infective anal or perianal conditions; anorectal inflammation, fissures, pain and oedema (haemorrhoids, post-op), pruritus ani.
Dose: Adult, Elderly: 1 applicator-full per rectum, 2-3 times daily and after each bowel evacuation; max. 4 times daily.
CI: Ulcerations, fistulae or perforations.
Notes: See 1.7.2 Haemorrhoidals, with Corticosteroids.

Proctofoam HC *(Meda)* B. GMS.
Price, (24g) €6.08.
Rectal foam, hydrocortisone acetate 1%, pramocaine HCl 1% w/w. White aerosol. *Parabens, cetyl alcohol.* **Store:** Below 25 deg C; do not refrigerate. Pressurised container contains flammable propellant.

1.8 - Drugs Affecting GI Secretions

1.8.1 - Biliary Agents

In This Chapter: *Rowachol, ursodeoxycholic acid.*

Class Effects
These agents have a number of uses including gallstone dissolution.
CI: Hypersensitivity to any member of the class.

Rowachol
ATC Code: A05AX91. **Sport:** Permitted.
Driving: Unlikely to impair.
Indications: Management and dissolution of radiolucent gallstones in the functioning gall-bladder.
Dose: Adult, Elderly: 1-2 caps 3-times daily before meals.
Child: Age 6-14 years, 1 cap twice daily before meals.
Interactions: Effect of Other Drugs on Rowachol: *Caution:* Oral contraceptives, oral anticoagulants.
Pregnancy, Lactation: Only if considered essential by physician.
ADR: Slight taste of peppermint.

Notes: See 1.8.1 Biliary Agents.

Rowachol Capsules *(Rowa)* OTC. GMS.
Price, (50) €5.01.
Capsule, borneol 5mg, camphene 5mg, cineole 2mg, menthol 32mg, menthone 6mg, pinenes 17mg. Soft gelatine green g/r; contains greenish-yellow oral soln with strong aromatic odour. *Parabens*.

Ursodeoxycholic Acid (UDCA)

ATC Code: A05AA02. **Sport:** Permitted.
Driving: No or negligible effect.

Indications: Dissolution of cholesterol gallstones in functioning gall bladder. Primary biliary cirrhosis (stages I-III). Hepatobiliary disorders associated with cystic fibrosis (children age 1 month to 18 years).

Dose: Adult, Elderly: *Gallstone dissolution*, usually 10-12mg/kg/day (750mg) daily (evening at bedtime) with water. Do not crush or chew tabs.
Primary biliary cirrhosis, range 3-7 caps or 1.5-3.5 tabs (14 +/- 2mg per kg bodyweight) divided over day for first 3 months. When liver function parameters improve, admin once daily (evening).
Child: *Hepatobiliary disorders*, age 1 month to 18 years, 20mg/kg/day in 2-3 divided doses; increase to 30mg/kg/day if needed. Children up to 10kg, 20mg UDCA/kg/day using graduated syringe (not provided); 10kg and over, 20-25mg UDCA/kg/day using measuring cup.

CI: Acute inflammation (gall bladder, biliary tract), biliary tract occlusion (common bile duct, cystic duct), biliary colic, radio-opaque calcified gallstones, impaired contractility of gall bladder. Unsuccessful portoenterostomy or without recovery of good bile flow in children with biliary atresia (children with cystic fibrosis).

Interactions: Effect of Other Drugs on Ursodeoxycholic Acid: *Absorption/efficacy reduced*: Antacids containing aluminium hydroxide, colestyramine, colestipol. *Effect countered (gall stone dissolution)*: Oestrogenic hormones, cholesterol-lowering agent (clofibrate) (increased biliary lithiasis).
Effect of Ursodeoxycholic Acid on Other Drugs: Ciclosporin: *Increased absorption; monitor blood conc; consider dose adjustment. Absorption reduced (isolated cases)*. Nitrendipine: *Peak plasma conc reduced*. Dapsone: *Reduced therapeutic effect*.

SP: Monitor liver function parameters every 4 weeks during first 3 months; then every 3 months. Gallstone dissolution, visualise gall bladder (oral cholecystography) 6-10 months after beginning treatment; females should use effective non-hormonal contraception as hormonal contraceptives may increase biliary lithiasis. Advanced primary biliary cirrhosis, decompensation of hepatic cirrhosis observed. Diarrhoea, reduce dose; if persistent, discontinue.

Pregnancy, Lactation: Pregnancy, not for use unless clearly necessary; exclude pregnancy before initiating. Women of childbearing potential to ensure adequate contraception. Lactation, not recommended.

ADR: *Common*, diarrhoea, pasty stools.

Notes: See 1.8.1 Biliary Agents.

Ursofalk 250mg, 500mg, Susp *(Dr Falk)* B. GMS.
Price, (100) 250mg, €32.79. 500mg, €68.77. Susp 250mL, €31.37.
Capsule, ursodeoxycholic acid. White hard gelatin.
Tablet, as above. White oval f/c scored (divisible into equal halves).
Oral susp, as above 250mg/5mL. White with small air bubbles; lemon odour. *Sodium 11.39mg/5mL*.

1.8.2 - Bile Acid Sequestrants

In This Chapter: *Colestyramine*.

Class Effects
In addition to reduction of plasma cholesterol in hypercholesterolaemia, colestyramine is also indicated for relief of pruritus associated with (partial biliary obstruction, primary biliary cirrhosis), diarrhoea associated with (ileal

Bile Acid Sequestrants   1.8.2

resection, Crohn's disease, vagotomy, diabetic vagal neuropathy). Management, radiation-induced diarrhoea. See Notes below.

Notes: See 2.3.1 Anion Exchange Resins (colestyramine).

1.8.3 - Pancreatic Enzymes

In This Chapter: *Pancreatin*.

Class Effects
FIP units of protease, lipase and amylase activity are equivalent to Ph Eur Units.

CI: Hypersensitivity to porcine proteins or to any member of class.

SP: Oral medications not for admin during early stages of acute pancreatitis.

Pregnancy, Lactation: Only if clearly necessary; doses to provide adequate nutritional status only.

Pancreatin

ATC Code: A09AA02. **Sport:** Permitted.
Driving: Unlikely to impair.

Indications: Pancreatic exocrine (PE) insufficiency.

Dose: Adult, Elderly: *Creon 10000, 25000*, initially 1-2 (10000) caps or 1 (25000) cap with meals. If needed, increase by max. 2500 units of lipase/kg/meal (10000 units/kg/day). Higher doses, caution; especially young children (colonic damage reported in cystic fibrosis patients taking above 10000 units of lipase/kg/day).
Creon 40000, 1-2 caps with meals adjusting dose slowly; only to be used only if 40000 or more lipase units per meal/snack required; determine minimum effective dose using lower strengths; ensure adequate hydration.
Admin, during or immediately after a meal; swallow caps whole or open and mix granules with fluid or soft food and admin immediately or enteric coating may dissolve. Do not crush or chew; do not retain in mouth.
Child: *Creon For Children*, initially 100mg (5000 lipase units) of (g/r) granules (1 measure supplied in pack) admin with each feed or meal; titrate slowly if required; max. 10000 lipase units per day. *Admin*, young infants, mix granules with small amount of infant formula, expressed breast milk or fruit puree; give from a spoon directly before the feed; do not add to baby's bottle. Weaned infants, mix with acidic liquids or soft foods without chewing and admin immediately. See Adult above.

SP: High doses, strictures of ileo-caecum and large bowel reported; unusual abdominal symptoms, exclude colonic damage especially at high doses. Sourced from porcine pancreatic tissue.

Pregnancy, Lactation: Can be prescribed to pregnant women; can be used during breastfeeding.

ADR: *Very common*, abdominal pain. *Common*, nausea, vomiting, constipation, abdominal distention, diarrhoea.

Notes: See 1.8.3 Pancreatic Enzymes.

Creon, For Children *(BGP)* B. GMS.
Price, caps 10000U (100) €16.29; 25000U (50) €16.96; 40000U (100) €55.88. Children 5000U (20g) €23.82.
Capsule, (thousand U) 10, 25, 40, pancreatin. Hard gelatin g/r filled with g/r brown granules. 10000U: Lipase (L) 10000U (Ph Eur units), amylase (A) 8000U, protease (P) 600U equiv. to pancreatin 150mg. Brown/colourless. 25000: L 25000U, A 18000U, P 1000U equiv. to pancreatin 300mg. Orange/colourless. 40000: L 40000U, A 25000U, P 1600U. Brown/clear. *Cetyl alcohol*. **Store:** Below 25 deg C.
Oral granules (For Children), 5000U pancreatin. Lipase 5000U (Ph Eur Units), amylase 3600U, protease 200U equiv. to pancreatin 60.12mg. Round light-brown g/r. **Store:** Below 30 deg C; protect (moisture).

19

2

Cardiovascular Drugs

2.1 - Hypertension, Heart Failure

2.1.1 - Angiotensin Converting Enzyme Inhibitors (ACEIs) and Combinations

In This Chapter: *Benazepril, captopril, enalapril, lisinopril, perindopril (arginine, tert-butylamine, tosilate), quinapril, ramipril, trandolapril, zofenopril; combinations, captopril, enalapril, lisinopril, quinapril (hydrochlorothiazide), perindopril arginine (amlodipine, indapamide), perindopril tert-butylamine (indapamide), ramipril (piretanide, felodipine).*

Class Effects

Driving: Dizziness or fatigue may occur with initiation or change of antihypertensive (first-dose hypotension) and/or in combination with alcohol; caution until the effect of the drug is known.

Pharmacology: Angiotensin Converting Enzyme Inhibitors (ACEIs) are used in the treatment of high blood pressure (BP) and in congestive heart failure (CHF). Consider using ACEI combinations when there is insufficient control on monotherapy and patients have been stabilised on individual components.

CI: Hypersensitivity to any member of class (or combination). Use in children under 18 years unless otherwise specified. Aortic stenosis or outflow tract obstruction, renovascular disease. Angioedema (hereditary and/or idiopathic, or associated with ACEI admin). Severe renal impairment. Hyperkalaemia. See Interactions and Pregnancy below.
ACEI + Hydrochlorothiazide, anuria, severe renal impairment; hypersensitivity to sulfonamide-derivatives. Hydrochlorothiazide contraindicated with CrCl (mL/min) 30 or below (ineffective).
ACEI + Indapamide, sulfonamide hypersensitivity, severe impairment (renal, hepatic), hepatic encephalopathy, hypokalaemia (related to indapamide). Dialysis, untreated decompensated HF.
ACEI + Piretanide, dialysis, untreated decompensated HF, primary hyperaldosteronism, severe liver impairment, primary liver disease.
ACEI + Felodipine, unstable haemodynamic conditions (cardiovascular shock, untreated HF, acute MI, unstable angina pectoris, stroke), AV block II or III.

Interactions: Effect of Other Drugs on ACEIs: *Co-admin contraindicated:* Aliskiren (patients with diabetes mellitus or renal impairment GFR below 60mL/min/1.73m2). *Co-admin, limit to defined cases; close monitoring (renal function, potassium levels, BP):* AIIAs, ARBs, aliskiren (patients other than diabetics) (dual RAAS blockade). *Co-admin not recommended (hyperkalaemia):* Potassium-sparing diuretics (spironolactone, eplerenone, triamterene, amiloride); potassium supplements, immunosuppressants (ciclosporin, tacrolimus), indomethacin, heparin, epoetin, ketorolac, trimethoprim, co-trimoxazole (trimethoprim + sulfamethoxazole). *Co-admin caution:* Allopurinol. *Enhanced hypotensive effect:* ALCOHOL, alprostadil, general anaesthetics, antidepressants, anxiolytics, antipsychotics (chlorpromazine, phenothiazines), other antihypertensives (ACEIs, AIIAs, adrenergic neurone blockers, alpha-blockers, beta-blockers, calcium channel blockers, diuretics, vasodilators), dopaminergics (levodopa), muscle relaxants (baclofen), nitrates. *Reduced hypotensive effect:* NSAIDs (including aspirin at dose 3g/day or above), oestrogens, carbenoxolone, corticosteroids. *Increased renal impairment risk:* NSAIDs (including COX-2 inhibitors). *Increased angioedema risk:* mTOR inhibitors (temsirolimus, everolimus, sirolimus), DPP-4 inhibitors (vildagliptin), tissue plasminogen activators (tPA) (alteplase, reteplase, tenecteplase), racecadotril; caution (initiation); in case of angioedema, discontinue.

Hydrochlorothiazide Combinations: *Hypersensitivity:* Sulfonamides and derivatives. *Enhanced responsiveness:* Non-depolarising muscle relaxants (tubocurarine). *Reduced hydrochlorothiazide absorption:* Colestyramine, colestipol. *Increased urea:* Tetracyclines.

Indapamide Combinations: *Torsade de Pointes risk:* Non-antiarrhythmics (astemizole, erythromycin IV, halofantrine, pentamidine, terfenadine), antiarrhythmics Class Ia (quinidine, disopyramide), amiodarone, bretylium, sotalol. *Hypercalcaemia:* Calcium salts.
Piretanide Combinations: *Reduced hypotensive effect:* Sodium chloride, probenecid.
Felodipine, Amlodipine Combinations: *Caution:* Grapefruit juice.
Interactions: Effect of ACEIs on Other Drugs: Lithium: *Decreased renal clearance, lithium toxicity risk; co-admin not recommended.* Antidiabetics: *Increased hypoglycaemic effect.* Gold (sodium aurothiomalate) (parenteral): *Nitritoid reactions (vasodilatation, nausea, dizziness, hypotension).*
Piretanide Combinations: Adrenaline: *Reduced effect.* Muscle Relaxants: *Enhanced and/or prolonged effect.* Nephrotoxic and/or ototoxic antibiotics: *Increased toxicity.*
SP: Drugs affecting RAAS (ACEIs, AIIAs), hyperkalaemia is a risk, especially (elderly over 70 years, renal insufficiency,

diabetics, other potassium-sparing drugs, dehydration, acute cardiac decompensation, metabolic acidosis, worsening renal function, cellular lysis), see Interactions above. *Caution*, strongly activated RAAS (renovascular hypertension, salt and/or volume depletion, cardiac decompensation, CHF, severe hypertension). Dual RAAS blockade (ACE, AIIA, aliskiren), not recommended; increased adverse event risk (hypotension, hyperkalaemia, decreased renal function, renal failure). In HF, triple combination (ACEI, beta-blocker, ARB) shown no clinical benefit; triple combination (ACEI, mineralocorticoid receptor antagonist, ARB) not recommended (specialist supervision with frequent monitoring). ACEIs and AIIS co-admin not recommended with diabetic nephropathy. See Interactions above.

First-dose hypotension (pronounced); consider low initial dose. Diuretic co-admin, stop diuretic 2-3 days before ACEI (AIIA) or reduce ACEI (AIIA) dose. HF patients at high risk of hypotension, initiate with lower dose. Infants (especially newborns) more susceptible to haemodynamic effects; excessive, prolonged and unpredictable decreases in BP with complications (oliguria, seizures).

Clinically silent renovascular disease (PVD, generalised atherosclerosis), renal impairment, reduce dose, monitor. Collagen vascular disease, SLE, scleroderma, immunosuppressant therapy (agranulocytosis risk). High-flux dialysis membranes, LDL-apheresis with dextran sulfate adsorption, angio-oedema risk. Primary aldosteronism. Angioedema (face, extremities, lips, tongue, glottis, and/or larynx; may be fatal), discontinue immediately; incidence higher in black patients; may also be increased with mTOR inhibitor co-admin (sirolimus, everolimus, temsirolimus). Intestinal angioedema reported with ACEIs. ACEIs may be less effective in lowering BP in blacks (higher prevalence of low-renin states).

Desensitisation with hymenoptera venom (rarely, life-threatening anaphylactoid reactions). Stable CAD, with episode of unstable angina in first month, assess benefit/risk. Renal function RAAS dependant (severe CHF), ACEI may be associated with oliguria and/or progressive azotaemia, rarely acute renal failure. AIIAs have inhibitor effect on RAAS, may be associated with renal impairment. Left ventricular valvular and outflow tract obstruction (caution). Anaesthesia, hepatic impairment/cholestasis (especially prodrugs).

Combinations: *Hydrochlorothiazide*, hyperuricaemia/gout, altered insulin requirements, emergence of latent diabetes. Hydrochlorothiazide, a sulfonamide, can cause idiosyncratic acute transient myopia and acute angle-closure glaucoma; discontinue (risk factors e.g. sulfonamide or penicillin allergy). *Indapamide*, hepatic encephalopathy. *Piretanide*, gout, cerebrovascular disease, CHD. *Calcium Channel Blockers*, extrapyramidal syndrome.

Pregnancy, Lactation: *Pregnancy*, **first trimester**, **not recommended**, foetal exposure associated with increased cardiovascular malformations (atrial and/or ventricular septal defect, pulmonic stenosis, patent ductus arteriosus), CNS (microcephaly, spina bifida), kidney; **second and third trimesters, contra-indicated**, injury/death in developing foetus; prolonged ACEI/AIIA exposure induces human fetotoxicity (decreased renal function, oligohydramnios, skull ossification, retardation) and neonatal toxicity (renal failure, hypotension, hyperkalaemia). Monitor newborns of mothers taking ACEIs (hypotension, oliguria, hyperkalaemia). Use in women of child-bearing age, not recommended unless adequate contraception; do not use initiate during pregnancy; if pregnancy diagnosed, discontinue. Change patients planning pregnancy to an alternative. *Lactation*, not recommended, unless otherwise specified; if no suitable alternative, stop breastfeeding. Combinations, see Notes below.

ADR: Dual RAAS blockade (ACEIs, ARBs, aliskiren) associated with higher frequency of adverse events (hypotension, hyperkalaemia, decreased renal function including failure). Diuretic and/or calcium channel blocker combinations, see Notes below.

Notes: See 2.9.5 Thiazides (hydrochlorothiazide, indapamide) and 2.9.2 Loop Diuretics (piretanide) and 2.2.1 Calcium Channel Blockers (amlodipine, felodipine).

Benazepril

ATC Code: C09AA07. **Sport:** Permitted.
Driving: Caution (hypotension), see Notes below.
Indications: Hypertension. CHF, adjunctive. Chronic, progressive renal insufficiency/nephropathy.

Dose: Adult: *Hypertension*, initially 10mg/day; titrate at 1-2 week intervals to 20mg/day if needed; max. 40mg/day (1 or 2 divided doses). Diuretic co-admin, initially 5mg/day. *CHF*, initially 2.5mg/day; titrate after 2-4 weeks to 5mg/day if needed; titrate to 10mg/day, then 20mg/day. CHF with hypertension, initially 5mg/day.
Renal insufficiency, progressive chronic, 10mg/day (single dose once daily).

Elderly: *Hypertension*, initially 5mg/day; titrate to 10mg/day if required. Other indications, as for Adult.

Child: *Hypertension*, age 7-16 years (25kg or over and able to swallow tabs), 0.2mg/kg/day; max 10mg/day. Above 0.6mg/kg (or above 40mg/day), no data. *Admin*, once daily.

Renal Impairment: CrCl (mL/min) below 30, initially 5mg/day (hypertension) OR 2.5mg/day (CHF); titrate to 10mg/day if required. Children, GFR below 30, not recommended.

ADR: *Common*, palpitations, orthostatic symptoms, non-specific GI disorders, rash, flushing, pruritus, photosensitivity, urinary frequency, cough, respiratory tract symptoms, headache, dizziness, fatigue.

Notes: See 2.1.1 ACEIs.

> **Cibacen 5mg, 10mg** *(Meda)* B. GMS.
> *Price*, (28) 5mg, €10.08. 10mg, €13.44.
> *Tablet*, benazepril HCl. Scored f/c. Marked CG. 5mg: Light-yellow oval. Marked LV. 10mg: Dark-yellow. Marked HO. *Lactose*. **Store:** Below 25 deg C.

Captopril

ATC Code: C09AA01. **Sport:** Permitted.
Driving: Caution (hypotension), see Notes below.
Indications: Hypertension. CHF, adjunctive. Renal disease, renal complications of diabetes mellitus, glomerular diabetic nephropathy. Secondary prevention, post MI (clinically stable, with or without LVD).

Dose: Adult: *Hypertension*, initially 25-50mg/day; if needed titrate at 2-4 week intervals; max. 100-150mg/day or use combination. Strongly activated RAAS (hypovolaemia, renovascular hypertension, cardiac decompensation), initially, 6.25-12.5mg/day; gradually increase to 50mg-100mg daily.
CHF, initially, 6.25-12.5mg 2 or 3-times daily; maintenance 75-100mg/day; max. 150mg/day.
Post-MI, short-term, initiate soonest following appearance of signs/symptoms (stable haemodynamics). Initially 6.25mg, then 12.5mg after 2 hours, then 25mg after 12 hours; then from next day, 100mg/day in 2 divided doses for 4 weeks. Chronic, if not begun during first 24-hours, initiate between 3-16 days post-MI at 6.25mg, then 12.5mg 3-times daily for 2 days, then 25mg 3-times daily. Effective cardioprotection, 75-150mg/day in 2 or 3 doses.
Diabetic nephropathy, 75-100mg/day. Admin once or twice daily.

Elderly: *Hypertension*, initially 6.25mg twice daily.

Child: Safety/efficacy not fully established; use with close medical supervision. Initial dose about 0.3mg/kg body weight; where special precautions required (renal dysfunction, premature infants, newborns), initially 0.15mg/kg. Subsequent dosing, no further information available; adapt (dose/interval) according to response.

Renal Impairment: CrCl (mL/min) above 40, initially 25-50mg/day (max. 150mg/day); 21-40, initially 25mg/day (max. 100mg/day); 10-20, initially 12.5mg/day (max. 75mg/day); below 10, initially 6.25mg/day (max. 37.5mg/day). May be removed by haemodialysis; not adequately cleared by peritoneal dialysis.

ADR: *Common*, insomnia, dysgeusia, dizziness, dry irritating (non-productive) cough, dyspnoea, nausea, vomiting, epigastric discomfort, abdominal pain, diarrhoea, constipation, dry mouth, peptic ulcer, dyspepsia, pruritus with/without rash, rash, alopecia.

2.1.1 Angiotensin Converting Enzyme Inhibitors (ACEIs) and Combinations

Notes: See 2.1.1 ACEIs.

Capoten 25mg, 50mg *(BMS)* B. GMS.
Price, 25mg (28) €2.35. 50mg (28) €4.02. (56) €10.05.
Tablet, captopril. White. Marked with strength. 25mg: Square cross-scored (divisible into four equal doses). 50mg: Oval scored (divisible into two equal doses). *Lactose.*

Aceomel 12.5mg, 25mg, 50mg *(Clonmel)* B. GMS.
Price, (60) 12.5mg, €5.42. 25mg, €4.95. 50mg, €8.43.
Tablet, captopril. White flat round scored (divisible into equal halves). *Lactose.*

Captor 12.5mg, 25mg, 50mg *(Rowex)* B. GMS.
Price, 12.5mg (60) €5.43. 25mg (60) €4.95. 50mg (60) €8.43. 100, €14.05.
Tablet, captopril. White round scored (divisible into equal halves). *Lactose.*

Captopril, Hydrochlorothiazide

ATC Code: C09BA01. **Sport:** Prohibited.
Driving: Caution (hypotension), see Notes below.
Indications: Essential hypertension not controlled with monotherapy.
Dose: Adult, Elderly: Max. captopril/hydrochlorothiazide 50mg/25mg daily as single dose or 2 divided doses with or without food. *Elderly,* salt/volume depleted, diabetics, initially, 25mg/12.5mg.
Renal Impairment: CrCl (mL/min) 30-80, as for Elderly; below 30, contraindicated.
Notes: See 2.1.1 ACEIs.

Capozide *(BMS)* B. GMS.
Price, (30) €6.75.
Tablet, 50/25mg captopril/hydrochlorothiazide. White (off-white) scored (divisible into equal halves). Marked CH. *Lactose.*

Captor-HCT *(Rowex)* B. GMS.
Price, (30) 25/12.5mg, €5.84. 50/25mg, €6.62.
Tablet, 25/12.5mg, 50/25mg captopril/hydrochlorothiazide. White. Marked Cc. 25/12.5: Round scored (divisible into equal halves). 50/12.5: Octagonal scored (divisible into equal halves or quarters). *Lactose.*

Enalapril

ATC Code: C09AA02. **Sport:** Permitted.
Driving: Caution (hypotension), see Notes below.
Indications: Hypertension. CHF, adjunctive. Prophylaxis, CHF, symptomatic (asymptomatic LVD; ejection fraction 35% or less).
Dose: Adult: *Hypertension,* initially 5-20mg/day (mild, initially 5-10mg/day). Strongly activated RAAS, initially 5mg/day or less. Maintenance 20mg/day; max. 40mg/day.
CHF, asymptomatic LVD, week 1 (days 1-3), 2.5mg/day as single dose; (days 4-7), 5mg/day in 2 divided doses; week 2, 10mg/day, week 3 and 4, 20mg/day in 1-2 divided doses; max. 40mg/day in 2 divided doses. *Admin,* once daily in hypertension, with or without food.
Elderly: As for Renal below.
Child: Weight 20-50kg, initially, 2.5mg/day; max. 20mg/day. 50kg or more, initially 5mg; max. 40mg/day. Neonates, paediatrics (GFR below 30mL/min/1.73m2), not recommended.
Renal Impairment: CrCl (mL/min) 30-80, 5-10mg/day; 10-30, 2.5mg/day; 10 or less, 2.5mg on dialysis days (enalaprilat can be dialysed).
CI: Recent renal transplant.
Pregnancy, Lactation: Older infants, breastfeeding may be considered if treatment is necessary for mother and child observed for adverse effects.
ADR: *Very common,* headache, depression, blurred vision, dizziness, cough, nausea, asthenia.
Notes: See 2.1.1 ACEIs.

Innovace 2.5mg, 5mg, 10mg, 20mg *(MSD)* B. GMS.
Price, (28) 2.5mg, €3.91. 5mg, €3.84. 10mg, €5.39. 20mg, €6.40.
Tablet, enalapril maleate. 2.5mg: White round. Marked MSD 14. 5mg: White. Marked MSD 712. 10mg: Rust-red. Marked MSD 713. 5mg, 10mg: Rounded triangle-shaped scored. 20mg: Peach-coloured triangle-shaped scored. Marked MSD 714. *Lactose.*

Enap 5mg, 10mg, 20mg *(Rowex)* B. GMS.
Price, (30) 5mg, €3.93. 10mg, €5.66. 20mg, €6.72.
Tablet, enalapril maleate. Oblong scored (divisible into equal halves). Marked EN/strength. 5mg: White. 10mg: Red-brownish. 20mg: Light-orange. *Lactose.*

Enalapril, Hydrochlorothiazide

ATC Code: C09BA02. **Sport:** Prohibited.
Driving: Caution (hypotension), see Notes below.
Indications: Essential hypertension not controlled with monotherapy.
Dose: Adult, Elderly: 1 tab (20/12.5mg) daily; max. 2 tabs/day.
Renal Impairment: CrCl (mL/min) between 30-80, first titrate individual components; 30 or less, thiazides not appropriate.
Hepatic Impairment: Contraindicated.
CI: Hypertrophic cardiomyopathy. Acute hypertension, renal artery stenosis. CHF (fixed-combination); individual components may be used.
Notes: See 2.1.1 ACEIs.

Innozide *(MSD)* B. GMS.
Price, (28) €8.17.
Tablet, enalapril maleate/hydrochlorothiazide 20mg/12.5mg. Round fluted yellow scored. Marked MSD 718. *Lactose.*

Lisinopril

ATC Code: C09AA03. **Sport:** Permitted.
Driving: Caution (hypotension), see Notes below.
Indications: Hypertension. CHF, adjunctive. Renal disease, renal complications of diabetes mellitus, glomerular diabetic nephropathy. Secondary prevention, post MI (clinically stable, with or without LVD).
Dose: Adult: *Hypertension,* initially 10mg/day; maintenance 20mg/day. If needed titrate over 2-4 weeks; max. 80mg/day. Diuretic co-admin, initially 5mg/day. Renovascular hypertension, initially 2.5mg-5mg/day.
CHF, initially 2.5mg/day. Increase by max. 5-10mg at minimum 2 week intervals; max. 35mg/day.
Acute MI, commence within 24 hours of onset of symptoms. Initially 5mg, then 5mg after 24 hours, 10mg after 48 hours, then 10mg/day thereafter. Low systolic BP (120mmHg or less) or during first 3 days post-MI, 2.5mg/day. If hypotension occurs (systolic BP 100mmHg or less), maintenance 5mg/day (temporarily reduce to 2.5mg if needed).
Renal complications of diabetes mellitus, normotensive, initially 2.5-10mg/day; titrate to 20mg/day if required to achieve a reduction of microalbumin to below (20mcg/min or 30mg/day). Hypertensive, as for normotensive; objective sitting BP of 130/80mmHg. *Admin,* once daily with or without food.
Elderly: As for Renal or Adult (diuretic co-admin).
Child: Hypertension, age 6-16 years, weight 20kg to under 50kg, initially 2.5mg/day; max. 20mg/day. Weight 50kg and over, 5mg/day; max. 40mg/day. Admin once daily.
Renal Impairment: *Adult,* CrCl (mL/min) 10 or less, 2.5mg/day; 10-30, 2.5-5mg/day; 31-80, 5-10mg/day. If needed adjust dose and/or admin frequency; max. 40mg/day. Dialysable. *Child,* consider lower starting dose or increased dosing interval. Severe, not recommended.
CI: Cor pulmonale.
SP: Co-admin with tissue plasminogen activators (tPA) may increase angioedema risk.
ADR: *Common,* dizziness, headache, orthostatic effects (including hypotension), cough, diarrhoea, vomiting, renal dysfunction.
Notes: See 2.1.1 ACEIs.

Zestril 5mg, 10mg, 20mg *(AstraZeneca)* B. GMS.
Price, (28) 5mg, €3.94. 10mg, €4.86. 20mg, €5.58.
Tablet, lisinopril dihydrate. Round u/c. Marked with symbol and strength. 5mg: Pink scored (divisible into equal doses). 10mg: Pink. 20mg: Brownish-red.

Bellisin 10mg, 20mg *(Pharmadel)* B. GMS.
Price, (28) 10mg, €4.76. 20mg, €5.48.
Tablet, lisinopril dihydrate. Round scored u/c. Marked with strength. 10mg: Yellow. 20mg: Light peach. *Mannitol.*

Lestace 2.5mg, 5mg, 10mg, 20mg *(Accord)* B. GMS.
Price, (28) 2.5mg, €2.73. 5mg, €3.87. 10mg, €4.76. 20mg, €5.48.
Tablet, lisinopril dihydrate. Round. 2.5mg: Round. 5mg: Flat scored both sides. 10mg: Scored* light-pink. 20mg: Scored* pink. *Divisible into equal halves. *Mannitol.*

Angiotensin Converting Enzyme Inhibitors (ACEIs) and Combinations 2.1.1

Lisopress 2.5mg, 5mg, 10mg, 20mg *(GedeonRichter)* B. GMS.
Price, (28) 2.5mg, €2.73. 5mg, €3.87. 10mg, €4.76. 20mg, €5.48.
Tablet, lisinopril dihydrate. White. Marked with strength. 2.5mg: Round scored (facilitates breaking). 5mg: Round scored*. 10mg: Square scored*. 20mg: Pentagonal scored*. *Mannitol.* *(divisible into equal halves)
Lispril 5mg, 10mg, 20mg *(Rowex)* B. GMS.
Price, (30) 5mg, €4.14. 10mg, €5.11. 20mg, €5.86.
Tablet, lisinopril dihydrate. Round red mottled scored (divisible into equal doses).
Zesger 2.5mg, 5mg, 10mg, 20mg *(Gerard)* B. GMS.
Price, (28) 2.5mg, €2.73. 5mg, €3.87. 10mg, €4.76. 20mg, €5.48.
Tablet, lisinopril dihydrate. 2.5mg, 5mg: Round. 10mg: Square. 20mg: Pentagonal. White (almost) scored (divisible into equal doses). Marked with strength.
Zestan 2.5mg, 5mg, 10mg, 20mg *(Dexcel)* B. GMS.
Price, (28) 2.5mg, €2.73. 5mg, €3.87. 10mg, €4.76. 20mg, €5.48.
Tablet, lisinopril dihydrate. 2.5mg, 5mg: Scored both sides. 10mg, 20mg: Quadrisected. White. Marked with strength.

Lisinopril, Hydrochlorothiazide

ATC Code: C09BA03. **Sport:** Prohibited.
Driving: Caution (hypotension), see Notes below.
Indications: Essential hypertension not controlled with monotherapy.
Dose: Adult, Elderly: Initially, 1 tab/day (10/12.5 or 20/12.5); if required titrate after 2-4 weeks to 2 tabs/day; max. 40/25mg.
Renal Impairment: CrCl (mL/min) 30-80, not for initial therapy; first titrate individual components (initial lisinopril monotherapy 5-10mg); 30 or less, contraindicated.
ADR: *Common,* dizziness, headache, syncope, orthostatic effects, cough, diarrhoea, vomiting, renal dysfunction.
Notes: See 2.1.1 ACEIs.
Zestoretic Tablets *(AstraZeneca)* B. GMS.
Price, (28) €4.86.
Tablet, 10(20)/12.5mg lisinopril dihydrate/hydrochlorothiazide. Round u/c. 10mg: Peach. Marked Zt; 10 on reverse. 20mg: White scored (not intended to break tab). Marked 20 12.5. **Store:** Below 30 deg C; blister in outer carton to protect (light).
Lispril-Hydrochlorothiazide Tablets *(Rowex)* B. GMS.
Price, (30) 10/12.5mg, €5.10. 20/12.5mg, €5.86.
Tablet, 10(20)/12.5mg lisinopril/hydrochlorothiazide. Pink round scored.
Zesger Plus Tablets *(Gerard)* B. GMS.
Price, (28) €5.48.
Tablet, 20/12.5mg lisinopril dihydrate/hydrochlorothiazide. Pink round. Marked LHZ; 32.5 on reverse. **Store:** No special conditions.

Perindopril (arginine, tosilate)

ATC Code: C09AA04. **Sport:** Permitted.
Driving: Caution (hypotension), see Notes below.
Indications: Hypertension. Symptomatic CHF, adjunctive. Stable CAD, reduction of risk of cardiac events in patients with history of MI and/or revascularisation.
Dose: Adult: NOTE: Dosing is NOT the same for all perindopril salts.
Hypertension, initially 5mg/day; titrate to 10mg after 1 month if needed. Strongly activated RAAS, diuretic co-admin, initially 2.5mg under medical supervision.
CHF, initially 2.5mg/day; titrate to 5mg/day after 2 weeks*.
Stable CAD, reduction in cardiac events, initially 5mg once daily (2 weeks); titrate to 10mg/day*. *Admin,* once daily (morning) before food. Place OroDisp tabs on tongue for disintegration; swallow with saliva. *(if tolerated)
Elderly: *Hypertension,* initially 2.5mg/day; titrate to 5mg/day after 1 month then to 10mg if needed. CHF, as for Adult. *Stable CAD,* initially 2.5mg/day (week 1), then 5mg/day (week 2), then 10mg/day.
Renal Impairment: CrCl (mL/min) 30-60, initially 2.5mg/day; 15-30, 2.5mg every other day; below 15 (on haemodialysis), 2.5mg on dialysis day.
Interactions: Effect of Perindopril Arginine on Other Drugs: *Increased adverse effects (angioedema):* Estramustine.
ADR: *Common,* headache, dizziness, vertigo, paraesthesia, disturbed vision, tinnitus, hypotension, cough, dyspnoea, nausea, vomiting, abdominal pain, dysgeusia, dyspepsia,

diarrhoea, constipation, rash, pruritus, muscle cramp, asthenia.
Notes: See 2.1.1 ACEIs.
Interchangeability: Same strengths of all brands of perindopril (arginine, tosilate) f/c tabs and orodispersible tabs listed below are deemed interchangeable.
Reference Price: Perindopril arginine (30) 5mg, €5.18. 10mg, €8.46.
Coversyl Arginine Tablets, OroDisp *(Servier)* B. GMS.
Price, (30), see reference price above.
Tablet, perindopril arginine 5mg, 10mg. f/c. Marked with logo. 5mg: Light-green rod-shaped scored (divisible into equal halves). 10mg: Green round. Marked with heart. *Lactose.* **Store:** Tightly closed to protect (moisture).
OroDisp tablet, as above. White round. *Lactose, aspartame.* **Store:** As above.
Perindopril Tosilate TEVA 5mg, 10mg *(TEVA)* B. GMS.
Price, (30) see reference price above.
Tablet, perindopril tosilate. F/c. Marked T. 5mg: Light-green cap-shaped scored (divisible into equal halves). 10mg: Green round. Marked 10. *Lactose.*

Perindopril (arginine, tosilate), Amlodipine

ATC Code: C09BB04. **Sport:** Permitted.
Driving: Caution (hypotension), see Notes below.
Indications: Essential hypertension and/or stable coronary artery disease not controlled with components at same dose.
Dose: Adult, Elderly: 1 tab/day, morning before food. Fixed dose not suitable for initiation. *Elderly,* monitor creatinine and potassium.
Renal Impairment: CrCl (mL/min) below 60, not suitable, use individual components. Amlodipine cannot be dialysed.
Hepatic Impairment: Caution.
SP: Safety/efficacy of amlodipine in hypertensive crisis not established.
Notes: See 2.1.1 ACEIs.
Interchangeability: Same strengths of all brands of perindopril arginine/amlodipine tabs are deemed interchangeable (includes parallel imports; excludes perindopril tosilate).
Acerycal Tablets *(Servier)* B. GMS.
Price, (30) 5/5mg, €11.35. 5/10mg, €11.25. 10/5mg, €14.47. 10/10mg, €15.41.
Tablet, 5/5(10), 10/5(10) perindopril arginine/amlodipine besilate. White. Marked strength; logo on reverse. 5/5: Rod-shaped. 5/10: Square. 10/5: Triangular. 10/10: Round. *Lactose.*
Perindopril tosilate/Amlodipine TEVA *(TEVA)* B. GMS.
Price, (30) 5/5mg, €6.51. 5/10mg, €7.23. 10/5mg, €9.41. 10/10mg, €9.94.
Tablet, 5/5(10), 10/5(10) perindopril tosilate/amlodipine besilate. White. Marked strength. 5/5: Oval. 5/10: Square. 10/5 and 10/10: Round. *Lactose.*

Perindopril (arginine), Indapamide

ATC Code: C09BA04. **Sport:** Prohibited.
Driving: Caution (hypotension), see Notes below.
Indications: Essential hypertension not controlled with monotherapy.
Dose: Adult, Elderly: 1 tab/day, morning before food. *Elderly,* as for Renal below.
Renal Impairment: CrCl (mL/min) below 30, not recommended; 30-60, 1 tab/day.
ADR: *Most common,* (perindopril), dizziness, headache, paraesthesia, dysgeusia, visual impairment, vertigo, tinnitus, hypotension, cough, dyspnoea, abdominal pain, constipation, dyspepsia, diarrhoea, nausea, vomiting, pruritus, rash, muscle cramps and asthenia; (indapamide) hypersensitivity, rash.
Notes: See 2.1.1 ACEIs.
Interchangeability: Same strengths of all brands of perindopril arginine/indapamide and perindopril tosilate/indapamide tabs listed below and under Perindopril Tosilate, are deemed interchangeable.
Reference Price: (30) 2.5/0.625mg, €6.39. 5/1.25mg, €7.14.

2.1.1   Angiotensin Converting Enzyme Inhibitors (ACEIs) and Combinations

Coversyl Arginine Plus *(Servier)* B. GMS.
Price, (30) 2.5/0.625mg, 5/1.25mg, see reference price above. 10/2.5mg, €11.98.
Tablet, perindopril arginine/indapamide 2.5/0.625, 5/1.25mg, 10/2.5mg. White. 2.5/0.625 and 5/1.25: Rod-shaped. 10/2.5: Round. *Lactose.* **Store:** Protect (moisture).

Perindopril (arginine), Indapamide, Amlodipine

ATC Code: C09BX01. **Sport:** Prohibited.
Driving: Caution (hypotension), see Notes below.
Indications: Essential hypertension not controlled with monotherapy.
Dose: Adult, Elderly: 1 tab per day as single dose in morning before food.
Renal Impairment: CrCl (mL/min) below 30, contraindicated; 30-60, start treatment with individual components.
Hepatic Impairment: Severe, contraindicated; mild/moderate, caution.
Pregnancy, Lactation: See Notes below, individual components.
ADR: *Most common* (individual components), dizziness, headache, paraesthesia, somnolence, dysgeusia, visual impairment, diplopia, tinnitus, vertigo, palpitations, flushing, hypotension, cough, dyspnoea, GI disorders (abdominal pain, constipation, diarrhoea, dyspepsia, nausea, vomiting, change of bowel habit), pruritus, rash, rash maculo-papular, muscle spasms, ankle swelling, asthenia, oedema, fatigue.
Notes: See 2.1.1 ACEIs and Combinations.

> **Coverdine Tablets** *(Servier)* B. GMS.
> *Price,* (30) 5/1.25/5mg, €14.03. 5/1.25/10mg, €14.58. 10/2.5/5mg, €18.89. 10/2.5/10mg, €20.24.
> *Tablet,* perindopril arginine, indapamide, amlodipine 5/1.25/5(10), 10/2.5/5(10). White oblong f/c. Marked with logo. 5/1.25/5: Marked logo 2. 5/1.25/10: Marked logo 3. 10/2.5/5: Marked logo 4. 10/2.5/10: Marked logo 5. **Store:** No special conditions.

Perindopril (tosilate), Indapamide

ATC Code: C09BA04. **Sport:** Prohibited.
Driving: Caution (hypotension), see Notes below.
Indications: Essential hypertension not controlled with monotherapy.
Dose: Adult, Elderly: 1 tab (2.5mg/0.625mg) as single dose in morning before food; double dose after 1 month if BP not controlled.
Renal Impairment: CrCl (mL/min) below 30, contraindicated; 30-60, max. 2.5mg/0.625mg per day.
Hepatic Impairment: Severe, contraindicated.
Notes: See 2.1.1 ACEIs.

> **Perindopril Tosilate/Indapamide TEVA** *(TEVA)* B. GMS.
> *Price,* (30) 2.5/0.625mg, €6.39. 5/1.25mg, €7.14. 10/2.5mg, €4.88.
> *Tablet,* perindopril tosilate/indapamide 2.5/0.625mg, 5/1.25mg. White f/c. 2.5/0.625mg: Cap-shaped, scored (facilitates breaking). 5/1.25mg: Cap-shaped scored (divisible into equal halves). Marked P and I. 10/2.5mg: Round. *Lactose.* **Store:** Tightly closed to protect (moisture).

Perindopril (tert-butylamine)

ATC Code: C09AA04. **Sport:** Permitted.
Driving: Caution (hypotension), see Notes below.
Indications: Hypertension. Symptomatic CHF, adjunctive. Stable CAD, reduction of risk of cardiac events in patients with history of MI and/or revascularisation.
Dose: Adult: NOTE: Dosing is NOT the same for all perindopril salts.
Hypertension, 4mg once daily (morning). Strongly activated RAAS, diuretic co-admin, initially 2mg/day. After 1 month titrate to 8mg/day if needed.
CHF, initially 2mg in morning; titrate to 4mg once daily at 2-week interval.
Stable CAD, initially 4mg/day for 2 weeks, then 8mg/day if tolerated.
Elderly: *Hypertension,* initially 2mg; titrate at 1-month intervals to 4mg, then 8mg if needed. *CHF,* as for Adult.

Stable CAD, initially 2mg/day for 2 weeks, then 4mg/day if tolerated.
Renal Impairment: CrCl (mL/min) 30-60, initially 2mg/day; 15-30, 2mg every other day; below 15 (on haemodialysis), 2mg on dialysis day.
ADR: See Notes below.
Notes: See Perindopril (arginine, tosilate) above. See 2.1.1 ACEIs.
Interchangeability: Same strengths of all brands of perindopril tert-butylamine tabs listed below are deemed interchangeable.
Reference Price: (30) 2mg, €3.00. 4mg, €5.18. 8mg, €8.46.

> **Pendrex 2mg, 4mg, 8mg** *(Rowex)* B. GMS.
> *Price,* (30) see reference price above.
> *Tablet,* perindopril tert-butylamine. White round. Marked with strength. 4mg: Scored (divisible into equal halves).
> **Percarnil 4mg, 8mg** *(Accord)* B. GMS.
> *Price,* (30) see reference price above.
> *Tablet,* perindopril tert-butylamine. White. Marked PP; strength on reverse. 4mg: Oblong scored (divisible into equal halves). 8mg: Round. *Lactose.*
> **Perindopril Krka 4mg, 8mg** *(Krka)* B. GMS.
> *Price,* (30) see reference price above.
> *Tablet,* perindopril tert-butylamine. White (almost). 2mg: Round. 4mg: Oval scored (divisible into equal halves). 8mg: Round scored (facilitates breaking). *Lactose.*
> **Prindace 4mg, 8mg** *(Clonmel)* B. GMS.
> *Price,* (30) see reference price above.
> *Tablet,* perindopril tert-butylamine. White. 4mg: Rod-shaped scored. 8mg: Round. *Lactose.*

Perindopril (tert-butylamine), Indapamide

ATC Code: C09BA04. **Sport:** Prohibited.
Driving: Caution (hypotension), see Notes below.
Indications: Essential hypertension not controlled with monotherapy.
Dose: Adult, Elderly: 1 tab (4mg/1.25mg) daily as single dose in morning, before food. *Elderly,* as for Renal below.
Renal Impairment: CrCl (mL/min) 30 or below, contraindicated; 30-60 initiate with free combination.
Hepatic Impairment: Severe, contraindicated.
Notes: See 2.1.1 ACEIs.
Interchangeability: Same strengths of all brands of perindopril tert-butylamine/indapamide tabs listed below are deemed interchangeable.

> **Pendrex Plus** *(Rowex)* B. GMS.
> *Price,* (30) 4/1.25mg, €8.50.
> *Tablet,* perindopril tert-butylamine/indapamide 4/1.25mg. White oblong. Marked PI. *Lactose.*

Quinapril

ATC Code: C09AA06. **Sport:** Permitted.
Driving: Caution (hypotension), see Notes below.
Indications: Hypertension. CHF, adjunctive.
Dose: Adult, Elderly: *Hypertension,* initially 10mg/day; maintenance 20-40mg/day in 1 or 2 doses; max. 80mg/day. Diuretic co-admin, initially 5mg once daily.
CHF, initially, 5mg/day. Titrate to effective dose, up to 40mg/day in 1 or 2 doses; maintenance 10-20mg/day.
Child: Age 6-12 years, not recommended.
Renal Impairment: Hypertension, CrCl (mL/min) below 60, initially 5mg/day.
Hepatic Impairment: Caution.
Interactions: Effect of Quinapril on Other Drugs: Tetracyclines: *Reduced absorption (due to magnesium in quinapril formulation).* Drugs interacting with magnesium: *Avoid.*
ADR: *Most frequent,* headache, dizziness, cough, fatigue, rhinitis, nausea and/or vomiting, myalgia.
Notes: See 2.1.1 ACEIs.

> **Accupro 5mg, 10mg, 20mg, 40mg** *(Pfizer)* B. GMS.
> *Price,* (28) 5mg, €4.42. 10mg, €7.13. 20mg, €7.80. 40mg, €9.60.
> *Tablet,* quinapril HCl. Reddish-brown f/c scored (facilitates breaking). Marked with strength. 5mg: Oval. 10mg: Triangular. 20mg: Round. 40mg: Oval. *Lactose.*

Coversyl Arginine Plus *(Servier)* B. GMS.
Price, (30) 2.5/0.625mg, 5/1.25mg, see reference price above. 10/2.5mg, €11.98.

Stable CAD, initially 2mg/day for 2 weeks, then 4mg/day if tolerated.

Quinapril, Hydrochlorothiazide

ATC Code: C09BA06. **Sport:** Prohibited.
Driving: Caution (hypotension), see Notes below.
Indications: Essential hypertension not controlled with monotherapy.
Dose: **Adult,**   **Elderly:**   Initially   quinapril 10mg/hydrochlorothiazide 12.5mg/day; if required titrate to 20/12.5mg; maintenance, 10/12.5mg-20/12.5mg per day. Elderly, initiate with lowest dose.
Renal Impairment: CrCl (mL/min) below 40, contraindicated.
Notes: See 2.1.1 ACEIs.
  Accuretic (Pfizer) B. GMS.
  Price, (28) €7.08.
  Tablet, 20/12.5mg quinapril HCl/hydrochlorothiazide. Pink triangular f/c scored (facilitates breaking). Lactose.

Ramipril

ATC Code: C09AA04. **Sport:** Permitted.
Driving: Caution (hypotension), see Notes below.
Indications: Hypertension. CHF, adjunctive. Renal disease, renal complications of diabetes mellitus, glomerular diabetic nephropathy. Secondary prevention, post MI (clinically stable, with or without LVD). Reduction in (morbidity, mortality) in patients with atherothrombotic cardiovascular disease e.g. MI, stroke, diabetes with one cardiovascular risk factor.
Dose: Adult: Hypertension, initially 2.5mg/day; if needed titrate at 1-2 week intervals; max. 10mg/day; maintenance 2.5-10mg/day. Diuretic co-admin, initially 1.25mg/day.
CHF, initially 1.25mg/day; titrate at 1-2 week intervals; dose 2.5mg/day or more in 1 or 2 divided doses; max. 10mg/day.
Nephropathy, initially 1.25mg/day; double at 2-3 week intervals; max. 5mg/day. Diuretic co-admin, discontinue/reduce diuretic dose before initiating.
Prevention, MI, stroke or cardiovascular death, progression of microalbuminuria to overt nephropathy, initially 2.5mg/day; double after 1 week and then after 3 weeks; maintenance 10mg/day.
Post acute-MI, initiate during days 3-10 following AMI. Initially 5mg/day; titrate to 10mg/day after 2 days. If initial 5mg/day not tolerated, decrease to 2.5mg/day for 2 days before increasing. Maintenance 5-10mg/day in 2 divided doses. Admin, once daily unless otherwise specified; with or without food, with plenty of water; do not chew or crush tabs.
Elderly: Initially 1.25mg.
Child: No dosing recommendation.
Renal Impairment: CrCl (mL/min) above 30, initially 1.25mg/day; max. 5mg/day; below 10, initially 1.25mg/day (or every second day). Maintenance max. 2.5mg/day.
Hepatic Impairment: Max. 2.5mg/day.
ADR: Summary, persistent dry cough, reactions due to hypotension; serious, angioedema, hyperkalaemia, renal or hepatic impairment, pancreatitis, severe skin reactions, neutropenia, agranulocytosis.
Notes: See 2.1.1 ACEIs.
Interchangeability: Same strengths of all brands of ramipril caps/tabs listed below are deemed interchangeable.
Reference Price: (28) 1.25mg, €2.10; 2.5mg, €1.96; 5mg, €2.80; 10mg, €3.92. (30) 1.25mg, €2.25. 2.5mg, €2.10. 5mg, €3.00. 10mg, €4.20.
  Tritace 1.25mg, 2.5mg, 5mg, 10mg (SANOFI) B. GMS.
  Price, (28) 1.25mg, €2.10. 2.5mg, €2.80. 5mg, €3.64. 10mg, €4.90.
  Tablet, ramipril. Oblong scored both sides. 1.25mg, 10mg: White. 2.5mg: Yellow. 5mg: Red. Store: No special conditions.
  Ramic 2.5mg, 5mg, 10mg (Pinewood) B. GMS.
  Price, (28) see reference price above.
  Capsule, ramipril. Hard. Marked R/strength. 2.5mg: Light-grey/light-green. 5mg: Light-grey/green. 10mg: Light-grey/dark green.

Ramilo 1.25mg, 2.5mg, 5mg, 10mg (Rowex) B. GMS.
Price, (30) see reference price above.
Tablet, ramipril. White oblong biplanar scored (1.25mg, facilitates breaking; other strengths, divisible into equal halves; 10mg, divisible into equal doses). Marked R and strength.
Ramipril (Accord) Capsules (Accord) B. GMS.
Price, (28) see reference price above.
Capsule, ramipril 1.25mg, 2.5mg, 5mg, 10mg. Marked R/strength. Contains white powder. 1.25mg: Yellow/white. 2.5mg: Orange/white. 5mg: Scarlet/white. 10mg: Blue/white.
Ramipril Actavis 2.5mg, 5mg, 10mg (Accord) B. GMS.
Price, (28) see reference price above.
Capsule, ramipril. Contains white powder. Marked R/strength. 2.5mg, 5mg: Light-grey/green. 10mg: Light-grey/dark-green.
Ramipril Krka 1.25mg, 2.5mg, 5mg, 10mg (Krka) B. GMS.
Price, (30) see reference price above.
Tablet, ramipril. Oblong flat. 1.25mg, 10mg: White (whitish). 2.5mg: Yellow. 5mg: Pink. Lactose.
Ramipril TEVA 1.25mg, 2.5mg, 5mg, 10mg (TEVA) B. GMS.
Price, (28) see reference price above.
Tablet, ramipril. Round scored (divisible into equal halves). Marked with strength and RL. 1.25mg: White (off-white) scored (facilitates breaking). 2.5mg: Yellow. 5mg: Pink. 10mg: White (off-white).
Ramitace 2.5mg, 5mg, 10mg (Clonmel) B. GMS.
Price, (28) see reference price above.
Tablet, ramipril. Cap-shaped flat scored (divisible into equal halves). 2.5mg: Yellow. Marked R2. 5mg: Pink. Marked R3. 10mg: White. Marked R4. Lactose.

Ramipril, Felodipine

ATC Code: C09BB05. **Sport:** Permitted.
Driving: Caution (hypotension), see Notes below.
Indications: Essential hypertension not controlled with monotherapy.
Dose: Adult, Elderly: 1 tab (2.5mg/2.5mg)/day; max. 2 tabs (2.5mg/2.5mg) or 1 tab (5mg/5mg)/day. Admin, once daily; swallow tabs whole with liquid, do not crush or chew; without food or after light meal (not carbohydrate or fat rich).
Renal Impairment: CrCl (mL/min) below 20 or on dialysis, contraindicated.
Hepatic Impairment: Severe, contraindicated.
Notes: See 2.1.1 ACEIs.
Interchangeability: All brands of felodipine/ramipril Prolonged/R tabs are deemed interchangeable (includes parallel imports).
  Triapin 2.5/2.5mg, 5/5mg (SANOFI) A. GMS.
  Price, (28) 2.5/2.5mg, €17.78. 5/5mg, €13.22.
  Prolonged/R tablet, ramipril/felodipine. 2.5mg: Apricot. Marked H/OD. 5mg: Reddish/brown. Marked H/OE. Round. Marked with strength. Lactose.

Ramipril, Piretanide

ATC Code: C09BA05. **Sport:** Prohibited.
Driving: Caution (hypotension), see Notes below.
Indications: Essential hypertension not controlled with monotherapy.
Dose: Adult: 1 tab (5mg/6mg)/day. Inadequate BP control, titrate with individual components.
Elderly: Initially, half tab/day; max. 1 tab/day.
Renal Impairment: CrCl (mL/min) 30-60, titrate with individual components; maintenance, half tab/day; max. 1 tab/day.
SP: Ototoxicity, see Notes below (piretanide).
Notes: See 2.1.1 ACEIs, 2.9.2 Loop Diuretics (piretanide).
  Trialix Tablets (SANOFI) B. GMS.
  Price, (28) €14.69.
  Tablet, ramipril/piretanide 5mg/6mg. Oblong yellowish-white scored (facilitates breaking).

Trandolapril

ATC Code: C09AA10. **Sport:** Permitted.
Driving: Caution (hypotension), see Notes below.
Indications: Hypertension. Secondary prevention, post MI (clinically stable, with or without LVD). Cardiovascular prevention, reduction in morbidity and mortality patients with manifest atherothrombotic cardiovascular disease including MI/stroke, diabetes with one cardiovascular risk factor.
Dose: Adult, Elderly: Hypertension, initially 1mg/day; if needed titrate to max. 4mg/day.

2.1.2 Angiotensin II Antagonists (AIIAs, ARBs) and Combinations

LVD post-MI, initiate as early as day 3. Initially 0.5mg/day; titrate to max. 4mg/day. Diuretic co-admin, initially 0.5mg/day. Single dose once daily, with or without food.
Renal Impairment: CrCl (mL/min) below 30, initially 0.5mg/day. Dialysis, monitor BP; adjust dose if needed.
Hepatic Impairment: Initially 0.5mg/day.
ADR: *Common*, headache, dizziness, hypotension (patients with LV dysfunction following MI), cough, asthenia.
Notes: See 2.1.1 ACEIs.

Odrik 0.5mg, 1mg, 2mg *(BGP)* B. GMS.
Price, (28) 0.5mg, €3.95. 1mg, €4.85. 2mg, €4.30.
Capsule, trandolapril. Opaque hard. 0.5mg: Orange red/yellow. 1mg: Red/orange. 2mg: Red/red. *Lactose*. **Store:** Below 25 deg C; original pack.

Zofenopril

ATC Code: C09AA15. **Sport:** Permitted.
Driving: Caution (hypotension), see Notes below.
Indications: Hypertension. Secondary prevention, post MI (clinically stable, with or without LVD).
Dose: Adult: *Hypertension*, initially 15mg/day. Maintenance 30mg/day; max. 60mg/day in 1 or 2 divided doses. Diuretic co-admin, initially 7.5mg/day. Diuretics discontinued, initially 15mg/day.
Acute MI, initiate within 24 hours; evaluate after 6 weeks. Days 1 and 2, 7.5mg 12-hourly; days 3 and 4, 15mg 12-hourly; day 5 onwards, 30mg 12-hourly. Low systolic BP (120mmHg) at initiation or during first 3 days following MI, do not increase dose. Hypotension (100mmHg), continue at previously tolerated dose. *Admin*, unless specified, once daily with or without food.
Elderly: *Hypertension*, normal CrCl (mL/min), no adjustment; below 45, half Adult dose. *Post-MI*, over 75 years, caution.
Renal Impairment: CrCl (mL/min) below 45, half Adult dose. Dialysis, one-quarter adult dose. Dialysis post-MI, not recommended.
Hepatic Impairment: Mild/moderate, initially half Adult dose. Severe (with hypertension), not recommended. Post-MI, not recommended.
ADR: *Common*, dizziness, headache, cough, nausea, vomiting, fatigue.
Notes: See 2.1.1 ACEIs.

Zofenil 7.5mg, 30mg *(A.Menarini)* B. GMS.
Price, 7.5mg (12) €2.36. 30mg (28) €8.81.
Tablet, zofenopril. White. 7.5mg: Round. 30mg: Oblong scored (divisible into equal halves). *Lactose*.

2.1.2 - Angiotensin II Antagonists (AIIAs, ARBs) and Combinations

In This Chapter: *Azilsartan; candesartan, eprosartan, irbesartan, losartan, olmesartan, telmisartan, valsartan (and hydrochlorothiazide); valsartan, olmesartan, telmisartan (and amlodipine); valsartan (and sacubitril).*

Class Effects
Driving: See Notes below (ACEIs).
Pharmacology: Angiotensin II receptor antagonists (AIIAs) are also called angiotensin receptor blockers (ARBs). If BP not is not controlled on monotherapy consider using fixed combinations; initial dose titration with individual components is recommended. Fixed combinations are not for use as initial therapy.
CI: Children under 18 years, not recommended unless otherwise specified. Hypersensitivity to any member of class. Refractory hypokalaemia and/or hypercalcaemia. Symptomatic hyperuricaemia/gout. Cholestasis and biliary obstructive disorders, severe hepatic impairment. See Pregnancy, Lactation below.
Interactions: Effect of Other Drugs on AIIAs: *Co-admin contraindicated:* Aliskiren (in patients with diabetes mellitus or renal impairment GFR below 60mL/min/1.73m2). *Co-admin, limit (defined cases; close monitoring of renal function, potassium levels, BP):* AIIAs, ARBs, aliskiren (dual RAAS blockade). *Co-admin not recommended (hyperkalaemia):* Potassium-sparing diuretics, potassium supplements, table salt substitutes

containing potassium, ciclosporin and other immunosuppressants, indomethacin, heparin, epoetin, ketorolac, NSAIDs, trimethoprim (monitor renal function), co-trimoxazole (trimethoprim/sulfamethoxazole). *Enhanced hypotensive effect:* ALCOHOL, alprostadil, general anaesthetics, antidepressants, anxiolytics, antipsychotics (chlorpromazine, phenothiazines), other antihypertensives (guanethidine, methyldopa, vasodilators, ACEIs, AIIAs, adrenergic neurone blockers, alpha-blockers, beta-blockers, calcium channel blockers, diuretics, dopaminergics (levodopa), muscle relaxants (baclofen), nitrates. *Reduced hypotensive effect:* NSAIDs (including COX-2 inhibitors, acetylsalicylic acid above 3g/day, non-selective NSAIDs), oestrogens, carbenoxolone. *Increased renal impairment risk (caution especially elderly):* NSAIDs (ensure adequate hydration, monitor renal function). *Modest bioavailability reduction:* Antacids (aluminium, magnesium hydroxide). *Increased systemic exposure, caution:* Inhibitors of hepatic uptake transporter OATP1B1/OATP1B3 (rifampicin, ciclosporin) or hepatic efflux transporter MRP2 (ritonavir).
Combinations: *Thiazide absorption reduced:* Colestyramine, colestipol (allow dosing interval, 4 hours before or 4-6 hours after these drugs). *Symptomatic hyponatraemia (hyponatraemic effect of hydrochlorothiazide intensified):* Antidepressants, antipsychotics, antiepileptics.
Effect of AIIAs on Other Drugs: Lithium: *Co-admin not recommended (decreased excretion); reversible increases in lithium conc and toxicity (risk increased with diuretics); lithium renal clearance reduced by thiazides (toxicity risk increased with thiazide combination); if combination necessary, carefully monitor serum levels.* Antidiabetics: *Increased hypoglycaemic effect.* Pressor amines (adrenaline, noradrenaline): *Possible decreased response; clinical significance unknown.*
SP: Increased angioedema risk with dual RAAS blockage. If angioedema occurs with other drugs including ACEIs, discontinue; do not re-admin. Combination use especially in HF, see Notes below (ACEIs). Increased risk of severe hypotension and renal insufficiency in patients with bilateral renal artery stenosis or stenosis of the artery to a single functioning kidney when treated with medicinals affecting the renin-angiotensin-aldosterone system (RAAS).
Thiazides, sulfonamide-derived. Hypersensitivity to hydrochlorothiazide may occur with or without history of allergy or bronchial asthma. Exacerbation or activation of SLE, electrolyte imbalance, photosensitivity. Caution, impaired hepatic function or progressive liver disease as minor changes in fluid/electrolyte balance may precipitate hepatic coma. Associated with idiosyncratic acute transient myopia and acute angle-closure glaucoma. May decrease urinary calcium excretion.
Pregnancy, Lactation: *Pregnancy,* first trimester, not recommended; second and third trimesters, contraindicated. Not for initiation during pregnancy; if pregnancy planned, use alternative with established pregnancy safety profile. Pregnancy diagnosed, discontinue immediately, commence alternative. Monitor post-menarche patients for possibility of pregnancy. *Lactation,* not recommended (use alternatives with established safety profile; especially while nursing newborn or preterm infant). *Combinations,* see Notes below.
ADR: Hydrochlorothiazide, see Notes below.
Notes: See 2.1.1 ACEIs. See 2.9.5 Thiazides (hydrochlorothiazide) and 2.2.1 Calcium Channel Blockers (amlodipine).

Azilsartan

ATC Code: C09CA09. **Sport:** Permitted.
Driving: Caution (hypotension), see Notes below.
Indications: Essential hypertension.
Dose: Adult: 40mg once daily; max. 80mg if needed. Volume-depleted, initially 20mg. *Admin*, with or without food.
Elderly: 75 years and over, initially 20mg.
Renal Impairment: Severe, ESRD, caution. Not removed by dialysis.

Angiotensin II Antagonists (AIIAs, ARBs) and Combinations   2.1.2

Hepatic Impairment: Mild/moderate, as for Elderly above. Severe, not recommended.

ADR: Common, dizziness, diarrhoea, increased blood CPK.

Notes: See 2.1.2 AIIAs.

Edarbi 20mg, 40mg, 80mg *(Takeda)* B. GMS.
Price, (28) 20mg, €12.14. 40mg, €15.70. 80mg, €19.93.
Tablet, azilsartan medoxomil potassium. White round. Marked ASL and strength.

Candesartan

ATC Code: C09CA06. **Sport:** Permitted.
Driving: Caution (hypotension), see Notes below.

Indications: Primary hypertension (adults, children, adolescents age 6-18 years). Treatment (adults), heart failure (HF) and impaired left ventricular systolic function (LVEF 40% or less) when ACEIs are not tolerated or as add-on to ACEIs in patients with symptomatic HF despite optimal therapy, when mineralocorticoid receptor antagonists are not tolerated.

Dose: Adult, Elderly: *Hypertension,* initial and maintenance, 8mg once daily (with or without food); increase to 16mg/day; max. 32mg/day. Intravascular volume depletion or at risk for hypotension, initially 4mg/day. Antihypertensive effect less pronounced in black patients; up-titrate or use concomitant therapy.

HF, initially 4mg once daily; titrate by doubling dose at minimum 2-week intervals to highest tolerated dose; max. 32mg/day.

Child: *Hypertension,* age 6-18 years, initially 4mg once daily; if not controlled increase to 8mg/day (under 50kg) OR to 8mg then 16mg (over 50kg); doses above 32mg, no data. Volume depletion, initiate under close medical supervision at lower dose than above. Black patients, see Adult above. Age 1-6 years, limited data; under 1 year, contraindicated.

Renal Impairment: Initially, 4mg/day including haemodialysis patients; titrate according to response. CrCl (mL/min) below 15 (adults) or below 30 (children), no/limited data.

Hepatic Impairment: Mild/moderate, initially 2mg/day. Severe and/or cholestasis, contraindicated.

Interactions: Effect of Other Drugs on Candesartan: *Triple combination not recommended*: ACEI, mineralocorticoid receptor antagonist, candesartan (use only with specialist supervision).

ADR: *Most common,* indication hypertension (adults) dizziness, vertigo, headache, respiratory infection; (children) headache, dizziness, upper RTI, cough; indication HF (adults), hyperkalaemia, hypotension, renal impairment.

Notes: See 2.1.2 AIIAs.

Interchangeability: Same strengths of all brands of candesartan tabs listed below are deemed interchangeable.

Reference Price: (28) 4mg, €3.63. 8mg, €3.63. 16mg, €4.54.

Atacand 4mg, 8mg, 16mg *(AstraZeneca)* B. GMS.
Price, (28), 4mg, €7.79; 8mg, €9.89; 16mg, €13.36.
Tablet, candesartan cilexetil. Round scored (divisible into equal doses). 4mg: White. Marked A/CF; 004 on reverse. 8mg: Light pink. Marked A/CG; 008 on reverse. 16mg: Pink. Marked A/CH; 016 on reverse. *Lactose.*

Blopress 2mg, 4mg, 8mg, 16mg, 32mg *(Takeda)* B. GMS.
Price, (7) 2mg, €1.57; 4mg, €0.91. (28) 2mg, 6.27; 32mg, €13.28. 8mg, 16mg, see reference price above.
Tablet, candesartan cilexetil. Round. 2mg: White. 4mg: White scored both sides. 8mg: Light-pink scored. 16mg: Light-pink scored. Marked 16. 32mg: Light pink scored. Marked 32. *Lactose.*

Candesartan Actavis 4mg, 8mg, 16mg *(Accord)* B. GMS.
Price, (28), see reference price above.
Tablet, candesartan cilexetil. White scored (divisible into equal doses). Marked C and strength. *Lactose.*

Candesartan Krka 4mg, 8mg, 16mg *(Krka)* B. GMS.
Price, (28), see reference price above.
Tablet, candesartan cilexetil. Round scored (facilitates breaking). 4mg: White. 8mg: Pinkish-white. 16mg: Slightly-pink. *Lactose.*

Candesartan Mylan 4mg, 8mg, 16mg *(Gerard)* B. GMS.
Price, (28), see reference price above.
Tablet, candesartan cilexetil. White (off-white) round scored. Marked M. 4mg: Marked C1. 8mg*: Marked C5. 16mg*: Marked C6. *Lactose.* *(divisible into equal doses).

Candesartan TEVA 4mg, 8mg, 16mg *(TEVA)* B. GMS.
Price, (28), see reference price above.
Tablet, candesartan cilexetil. Cap-shaped scored (divisible into equal doses). 4mg: White (off-white). 8mg: Pink. 4mg, 8mg: Marked C and strength both sides. 16mg: Pink. Marked 16; C and C on reverse. *Lactose.*

Candist 4mg, 8mg, 16mg *(Clonmel)* B. GMS.
Price, (28), see reference price above.
Tablet, candesartan cilexetil. White scored (8mg, 16mg divisible into equal halves). Marked C and strength. *Lactose.*

Catasart 4mg, 8mg, 16mg *(Rowex)* B. GMS.
Price, (28), see reference price above.
Tablet, candesartan cilexetil. Round scored (divisible into equal halves). Marked with strength. 4mg: White. 8mg, 16mg: Pink mottled. *Lactose.*

Candesartan, Hydrochlorothiazide

ATC Code: C09DA06. **Sport:** Prohibited.
Driving: Caution (hypotension), see Notes below.

Indications: Primary hypertension not controlled with monotherapy.

Dose: Adult, Elderly: 1 tab/day. Hypotension risk (volume depletion), consider candesartan 4mg initially. Once daily in morning, with or without food.

Renal Impairment: CrCl (mL/min) 30 and above, titrate with 4mg candesartan cilexetil before combination.

Hepatic Impairment: Mild/moderate, as for Renal above.

Notes: See 2.1.2 AIIAs. See Candesartan above.

Interchangeability: Same strengths of all brands of candesartan/hydrochlorothiazide tabs listed below are deemed interchangeable.

Reference Price: 16/12.5mg (28) €4.84.

Atacand Plus *(AstraZeneca)* B. GMS.
Price, 16/12.5mg (28) €13.36.
Tablet, candesartan cilexetil/hydrochlorothiazide 16/12.5mg. Peach oval scored both sides. Marked A/CS. *Lactose.* **Store:** No special conditions.

Blopress Plus *(Takeda)* B. GMS.
Price, (28) 8/12.5mg, €10.38. 32/12.5mg, €14.36. 32/25mg, €15.54. 16/12.5mg, see reference price above.
Tablet, candesartan cilexetil/hydrochlorothiazide 8(16, 32)/12.5mg, 32/25mg. 8(16)/12.5: Oval scored (divisible into equal halves). Marked strength/C both sides. 8/12.5: White (off-white). 16/12.5: Light-pink flat. 32/12.5(25): Oval flat scored (facilitates breaking). 32/12.5: Light-yellow. Marked 32/C1. 32/25: Light-pink. Marked 32/C2. *Lactose.* **Store:** No special conditions.

Candesartan/Hydrochlorothiazide Actavis *(Accord)* B. GMS.
Price, (28), see reference price above.
Tablet, candesartan cilexetil/hydrochlorothiazide. 16/12.5mg. White scored (divisible into equal halves). Marked CH16. *Lactose.*

Candesartan/Hydrochlorothiazide Krka *(Krka)* B. GMS.
Price, (28), see reference price above.
Tablet, candesartan cilexetil/hydrochlorothiazide 16/12.5mg. Pale-pink oval scored (facilitates breaking). *Lactose.*

Candesartan/Hydrochlorothiazide TEVA *(TEVA)* B. GMS.
Price, (28), see reference price above.
Tablet, candesartan cilexetil/hydrochlorothiazide 16/12.5mg. Light-pink cap-shaped scored (facilitates breaking). Marked C 16 either side of score. *Lactose.*

Candist Plus *(Clonmel)* B. GMS.
Price, (28), see reference price above.
Tablet, candesartan cilexetil/hydrochlorothiazide 16/12.5mg. White scored (facilitates breaking). Marked CH16. *Lactose.*

Catasart Plus *(Rowex)* B. GMS.
Price, (28), see reference price above.
Tablet, candesartan cilexetil/hydrochlorothiazide 16/12.5mg. Apricot mottled oval scored (facilitates breaking). *Lactose.*

Eprosartan

ATC Code: C09CA02. **Sport:** Permitted.
Driving: Caution (hypotension), see Notes below.

Indications: Treatment, essential hypertension.

Dose: Adult, Elderly: 600mg once daily.

Renal Impairment: CrCl (mL/min) below 60, max. 600mg/day; below 30 or on dialysis, caution.

Hepatic Impairment: Mild/moderate, caution. Severe, not recommended.

27

2.1.2 Angiotensin II Antagonists (AIIAs, ARBs) and Combinations

ADR: *Very common,* headache; *common,* dizziness, rhinitis, allergic skin reactions, GI complaints, asthenia.

Notes: See 2.1.2 AIIAs.

Teveten 400mg, 600mg *(BGP)* B. GMS.
Price, 400mg (56) €23.36. 600mg (28) €17.50.
Tablet, eprosartan mesilate. f/c. 400mg: Oval light-pink. Marked 5044. 600mg: Capsule-shaped white. Marked 5046.

Eprosartan, Hydrochlorothiazide

ATC Code: C09DA02. **Sport:** Prohibited.
Driving: Caution (hypotension), see Notes below.
Indications: Essential hypertension not controlled with monotherapy.
Dose: Adult, Elderly: 1 tab/day in morning with or without food.
Hepatic Impairment: Not recommended.
Interactions: Effect of Other Drugs on Eprosartan, Hydrochlorothiazide Combination: *Antihypertensive effect potentiated*: Amifostine.
Notes: See 2.1.2 AIIAs. See Eprosartan above.

Teveten Plus *(BGP)* B. GMS.
Price, (28) €18.15.
Tablet, eprosartan, hydrochlorothiazide 600/12.5mg.
Butterscotch cap-shaped f/c. Marked 5147.

Irbesartan

ATC Code: C09CA04. **Sport:** Permitted.
Driving: Caution (hypotension), see Notes below.
Indications: Treatment, essential hypertension. Renal disease in hypertensives with type 2 diabetes mellitus.
Dose: Adult: *Hypertension,* initial and maintenance 150mg/day. If required titrate to 300mg/day or switch to combination.
Renal disease, initially 150mg/day; maintenance 300mg/day. *Admin,* once daily with or without food.
Elderly: Over 75 years, initially 75mg/day.
Renal Impairment: Haemodialysis, initially 75mg/day.
Hepatic Impairment: Severe, no data.
ADR: *Very common,* hyperkalaemia (usually in diabetics). *Common,* dizziness, orthostatic (dizziness, hypotension), nausea, vomiting, musculoskeletal pain, fatigue, increased plasma creatine kinase.
Notes: See 2.1.2 AIIAs.

Aprovel 75mg, 150mg, 300mg *(SANOFI)* B. GMS.
Price, (28) 75mg, €8.90. 150mg, €9.89. 300mg, €13.35.
Tablet, irbesartan. White (off-white) oval. Marked with heart. 75mg: Marked 2871. 150mg: Marked 2872. 300mg: Marked 2873. *Lactose.*
Ifirmasta 75mg, 150mg, 300mg *(Krka)* B. GMS.
Price, (28) 75mg, €7.13. 150mg, €7.92. 300mg, €10.68.
Tablet, irbesartan HCl. White oval f/c. *Castor oil.*
Irbesan 75mg, 150mg, 300mg *(Rowex)* B. GMS.
Price, (28) 75mg, €7.13. 150mg, €7.92. 300mg, €10.68.
Tablet, irbesartan. White oval f/c scored (facilitates breaking). Marked with strength. *Lactose.*
Irbesartan Accord 75mg, 150mg, 300mg *(Accord)* B. GMS.
Price, (28) 75mg, €7.13. 150mg, €7.92. 300mg, €10.68.
Tablet, irbesartan. White (off-white) oval f/c. Marked I and strength. *Lactose.*
Irbesartan Clonmel Tablets *(Clonmel)* B. GMS.
Price, (28) 75mg, €7.13. 150mg, €7.92. 300mg, €10.68.
Tablet, irbesartan 75mg, 150mg, 300mg. White oval f/c. *Lactose.*
Irprestan 75mg, 150mg, 300mg *(Accord)* B. GMS.
Price, (28) 75mg, €7.13. 150mg, €7.92. 300mg, €10.68.
Tablet, irbesartan. White elliptical f/c. Marked T and strength.

Irbesartan, Hydrochlorothiazide

ATC Code: C09DA04. **Sport:** Prohibited.
Driving: Caution (hypotension), see Notes below.
Indications: Essential hypertension not controlled with monotherapy.
Dose: Adult, Elderly: Usually 150/12.5mg/day. Use 300/12.5mg if insufficiently controlled by irbesartan 300mg or 150/12.5mg combination; if still uncontrolled, max. 300/25mg/day may be used.
Notes: See 2.1.2 AIIAs. See Irbesartan above.

CoAprovel *(SANOFI)* B. GMS.
Price, (28) 150/12.5mg, €9.90. 300/12.5mg, €13.36. 300/25mg, €21.42.
Tablet, irbesartan/hydrochlorothiazide 150(300)/12.5mg, 300/25mg. Oval. Marked with heart. 150/12.5: Marked 2775. 300/12.5: Marked 2776. Both peach. 300/25: Pink. Marked 2788. *Lactose.*
Ifirmacombi *(Krka)* B. GMS.
Price, (28) 150/12.5mg, €6.23. 300/12.5mg, €8.65. 300/25mg, €8.56.
Tablet, irbesartan/hydrochlorothiazide 150(300)/12.5mg, 300/25mg. f/c. 150/12.5: Pale-pink oval. 300/12.5: White cap-shaped. 300/25: Pale-pink cap-shaped.
Irprezide *(TEVA)* B. GMS.
Price, (28) 150/12.5mg, €6.23. 300/12.5mg, €8.65. 300/25mg, €8.56.
Tablet, irbesartan/hydrochlorothiazide 150(300)/12.5mg, 300/25mg. Oval pink f/c. Marked H; I on reverse.

Losartan

ATC Code: C09CA01. **Sport:** Permitted.
Driving: Caution (hypotension), see Notes below.
Indications: Treatment, essential hypertension. CHF and impaired left ventricular systolic function (LVEF 40% or less) when ACEIs not suitable or not tolerated. Renal disease in hypertensives with type 2 diabetes mellitus with proteinuria above 0.5g/day as part of antihypertensive treatment. Reduction in risk of stroke in hypertensives with ECG documented LVH.
Dose: Adult: *Hypertension,* initially 50mg/day; max. 100mg/day (morning) including type II diabetics with proteinuria (0.5g/day and above), may be admin with other antihypertensives, insulin and/or oral hypoglycaemics.
Heart failure, initially 12.5mg/day; titrate at weekly intervals (12.5mg/day, 25mg/day, 50mg/day, 100mg/day) to max. 150mg once daily if tolerated.
Stroke, reduction of risk (hypertensives with LVH), initially 50mg/day; if required titrate to 100mg/day or add low dose hydrochlorothiazide. Intravascular volume depletion, initially 25mg/day. *Admin,* once daily with or without food.
Elderly: Over 75 years, initially 25mg.
Child: *Hypertension,* age 6-18 years, limited data; if can swallow tabs, weight 20-50kg, 0.7mg/kg up to 25mg once daily; exceptionally 50mg/day; over 50kg, 50mg once daily; exceptionally 100mg/day.
Renal Impairment: *Child,* GFR (mL/min/1.73m2) below 30, not recommended. Recent transplantation, no data.
Hepatic Impairment: *Adult,* use lowest dose; severe, contraindicated; *child,* not recommended.
ADR: *Common,* anaemia, dizziness, vertigo, orthostatic hypotension, renal (impairment, failure), asthenia, fatigue, hyperkalaemia, increased (blood urea, serum creatinine, serum potassium), hypoglycaemia.
Notes: See 2.1.2 AIIAs.
Interchangeability: Same strengths of all brands of losartan film-coated (f/c) tabs listed below are deemed interchangeable.
Reference Price: (28) 50mg, €2.80. 100mg, €3.92.

Cozaar Tablets, Oral Susp 2.5mg/mL *(MSD)* B. GMS.
Price, (28) 12.5mg, €7.78. 50mg, €5.04. 100mg, €8.40. Oral susp (200mL) €43.20.
Tablet, losartan potassium 12.5mg, 50mg, 100mg. f/c. 100mg: White teardrop-shaped. Marked 960. 50mg: White oval scored (not intended for breaking). Marked 952. 12.5mg: Blue oval. Marked 11. *Lactose.* **Store:** Original container to protect (light, moisture).
Oral susp, as above 2.5mg/mL. White (off-white) powder; cloudy colourless solvent. *Benzoate, sorbitol, lactose.* **Store:** Below 25 degrees C (kit); refrigerate prepared susp.
Cosartal 50mg, 100mg *(Accord)* B. GMS.
Price, (28) see reference price above.
Tablet, losartan potassium. White round f/c scored (divisible into equal halves). 50mg: Marked 3L. 100mg: Marked 4L. *Mannitol.*
Cozatan 50mg, 100mg *(Clonmel)* B. GMS.
Price, (28) see reference price above.
Tablet, losartan potassium. White f/c cross-scored both sides (divisible into equal halves). 50mg: Round. 100mg: Oblong. *Lactose.*
Losartan (Accord) 25mg *(Accord)* B. GMS.
Price, (28) €3.26.
Tablet, losartan potassium. White (off-white) round f/c scored (facilitates breaking). Marked with strength. *Lactose.*

Angiotensin II Antagonists (AIIAs, ARBs) and Combinations   2.1.2

Losartan Krka 50mg, 100mg *(Krka)* B. GMS.
Price, (28) see reference price above.
Tablet, losartan potassium. White. 50mg: Round f/c scored (divisible into equal halves). 100mg: Oval. *Lactose*.
Losartan Pinewood Tablets *(Pinewood)* B. GMS.
Price, (28) 12.5mg, €3.11. 50mg, 100mg, see reference price above.
Tablet, losartan potassium. F/c round. 12.5mg: Blue. 50mg, 100mg: White. *Lactose*. **Store:** No special conditions.
Losartan TEVA 50mg, 100mg *(TEVA)* B. GMS.
Price, (28) see reference price above.
Tablet, losartan potassium. White oval slightly arched f/c scored (divisible into equal doses). Marked with strength. *Lactose*.
Lotanos 50mg, 100mg *(Rowex)* B. GMS.
Price, (28) see reference price above.
Tablet, losartan potassium. White f/c. 50mg: Oval notched each side. Marked 3. 100mg: Oblong with 3 notches. Marked 5.

Losartan, Hydrochlorothiazide

ATC Code: C09DA01. **Sport:** Prohibited.
Driving: Caution (hypotension), see Notes below.
Indications: Essential hypertension not controlled with monotherapy.
Dose: Adult, Elderly: Initially 1 tab (50/12.5)/day in morning. If required, titrate to 1 tab (100/12.5), then max. 1 tab (100/25)/day. Volume depletion, do not initiate with combination. *Admin*, with water, with or without food.
Notes: See 2.1.2 AIIAs. See Losartan above.
Interchangeability: Same strengths of all brands of losartan/hydrochlorothiazide film-coated (f/c) tabs listed below are deemed interchangeable.
Reference Price: (28) 50/12.5mg, €3.08. 100/12.5mg, 100/25mg, €4.20.

Cozaar Comp *(MSD)* B. GMS.
Price, (28) see reference price above.
Tablet, losartan potassium, hydrochlorothiazide 50(100)/12.5mg, 100/25mg. Oval f/c. 50/12.5: Yellow. Marked 717. 100/12.5: White. Marked 745. 100/25: White. Marked 747. *Lactose; potassium 8.48mg/(100/12.5), 4.24mg/(50/12.5) tab*.
Cosartal Plus *(Accord)* B. GMS.
Price, (28) see reference price above.
Tablet, losartan potassium/hydrochlorothiazide 50/12.5mg, 100/12.5mg, 100/25mg. 50/12.5: White round scored (divisible into equal halves). Marked LH1. 100/25: As for 50/12.5mg. Marked LH2. 100/12.5mg: Yellow round. Marked LH3.
Cozatan Comp *(Clonmel)* B. GMS.
Price, (28) see reference price above.
Tablet, losartan potassium/hydrochlorothiazide 50/12.5mg, 100/25mg. White f/c. 50/12.5: Round. 100/25: Oblong scored (divisible in equal halves). *Lactose*.
Losartan/Hydrochlorothiazide Bluefish *(Bluefish)* B. GMS.
Price, (28) see reference price above.
Tablet, losartan potassium/hydrochlorothiazide 50/12.5mg, 100/25mg. Yellow scored (facilitates breaking). 50/12.5: Oblong. 100/25: Round. *Lactose*.
Losartan/Hydrochlorothiazide Krka *(Krka)* B. GMS.
Price, (28) see reference price above.
Tablet, losartan potassium/hydrochlorothiazide 50(100)/12.5mg, 100/25mg. Oval f/c. 50/12.5: Yellow scored (facilitates breaking). 100/12.5: White. 100/25: Yellow. *Lactose*.
Losartan/Hydrochlorothiazide TEVA *(TEVA)* B. GMS.
Price, (28) see reference price above.
Tablet, losartan potassium/hydrochlorothiazide 50/12.5mg, 100/25mg. Yellow oval f/c, scored (divisible into equal doses). 50/12.5: Marked 5 and 0. 100/25: Marked 1 and 00. *Lactose*.
Losartan/Hydrochlorothiazide (Rowex) *(Rowex)* B. GMS.
Price, (28) see reference price above.
Tablet, losartan potassium/hydrochlorothiazide 50/12.5mg, 100/25mg. Round light-yellow f/c. *Lactose*.

Olmesartan

ATC Code: C09CA08. **Sport:** Permitted.
Driving: Caution (hypotension), see Notes below.
Indications: Treatment, essential hypertension (adults) *(all brands)*. Hypertension (children/adolescents age 6 to under 18 years) *(Benetor)*.
Dose: Adult: Initially 10mg/day; if needed titrate to 20mg/day; max. 40mg/day or use combination. *Admin*, once daily; with or without food with sufficient water, same time of day; do not crush.
Elderly: If max. 40mg/day is required, monitor BP.
Child: *Benetor*, age 6 to under 18 years, initially 10mg/day; may be increased to 20mg/day if BP not controlled. If

further BP reduction needed, increase to max. 40mg/day (35 kg and over); max. 20mg/day (under 35kg). age 1-5 years, no dose recommendation. *Admin*, once daily.
Other brands (except Benetor), under 18 years, no dose recommendation; under 1 year, not for use (safety concerns).
Renal Impairment: CrCl (mL/min) 20-60, 20mg/day; below 20, not recommended.
Hepatic Impairment: Moderate, initially 10mg/day; max. 20mg/day. Severe, not recommended.
CI: Biliary obstruction.
Interactions: Effect of Other Drugs on Olmesartan: *Reduced bioavailability*: Aluminium, magnesium (hydroxide). *Reduced systemic exposure*: Colesevelam (admin olmesartan 4 hours prior to colesevelam).
SP: Very rare cases of chronic diarrhoea with substantial weight loss reported; it patient develops symptoms, immediately discontinue; do not restart.
ADR: Summary, *most common*, headache, influenza-like symptoms, dizziness.
Notes: See 2.1.2 AIIAs.

Omesar 10mg, 20mg, 40mg *(A.Menarini)* B. GMS.
Price, (28) 10mg, €7.96. 20mg, €9.56. 40mg, €12.04.
Tablet, olmesartan medoxomil. White f/c. 10mg: Marked C13. 20mg: Marked C14 (both round). 40mg: Oval. Marked C15. *Lactose*. **Store:** No special conditions.
Benetor 10mg, 20mg, 40mg *(Daiichi Sankyo)* B. GMS.
Price, (28) 10mg, €7.96. 20mg, €9.56. 40mg, €12.04.
Tablet, olmesartan medoxomil. White f/c. 10mg: Marked C13. 20mg: Marked C14 (both round). 40mg: Oval. Marked C15. *Lactose*. **Store:** No special conditions.
Olmesartan (Accord) 10mg, 20mg, 40mg *(Accord)* B. GMS.
Price, (28) 10mg, €5.04. 20mg, €6.52. 40mg, €7.96.
Tablet, olmesartan medoxomil. White (off-white), f/c. 10mg: Round. Marked IO2. 20mg: Round. Marked IO3. 40mg: Oval. Marked IO4. *Lactose*. **Store:** No special conditions.
Olmesartan (Gerard) 10mg, 20mg, 40mg *(Gerard)* B. GMS.
Price, (28) 10mg, €5.04. 20mg, €6.52. 40mg, €7.96.
Tablet, olmesartan medoxomil. White f/c. Marked M. 10mg: Round. Marked O1. 20mg: Round. Marked O2. 40mg: Oval. Marked O4. **Store:** Below 25 deg C; original pack to protect (moisture).
Olmesartan Clonmel 10mg, 20mg, 40mg *(Clonmel)* B. GMS.
Price, (28) 10mg, €5.57. 20mg, €6.98. 40mg, €8.49.
Tablet, olmesartan medoxomil. White f/c. 10mg, 20mg: Round. 40mg: Oval. *Lactose*. **Store:** No special conditions.
Olmesartan Krka 10mg, 20mg, 40mg *(Krka)* B. GMS.
Price, (28) 10mg, €5.04. 20mg, €6.52. 40mg, €7.96.
Tablet, olmesartan medoxomil. White f/c round (except 40mg). 10mg: Marked S1. 20mg: Marked S2. 40mg: Oval. Marked S3. *Lactose*. **Store:** No special conditions.
Olmesartan Rowex 10mg, 20mg, 40mg *(Rowex)* B. GMS.
Price, (28) 10mg, €5.57. 20mg, €6.98. 40mg, €8.48.
Tablet, olmesartan medoxomil. White round (except 40mg). Marked with strength. 40mg: Oval. *Lactose*. **Store:** Below 30 deg C; original pack; protect (moisture).
Olmesartan TEVA 10mg, 20mg, 40mg *(TEVA)* B. GMS.
Price, (28) 10mg, €5.04. 20mg, €6.52. 40mg, €7.96.
Tablet, olmesartan medoxomil. White f/c round (except 40mg). Marked O and strength on reverse. 40mg: Oval. *Lactose*. **Store:** No special conditions.

Olmesartan, Amlodipine

ATC Code: C09DB02. **Sport:** Permitted.
Driving: Caution (hypotension), see Notes below.
Indications: Essential hypertension not controlled with monotherapy.
Dose: Adult: 1 tab/day. *Admin*, at same time, with or without food with liquid; do not chew.
Elderly: If max. 40mg olmesartan needed, monitor BP.
Renal Impairment: CrCl (mL/min) 20-60, max. 20mg olmesartan once daily; below 20, not recommended. Moderate, monitor potassium and creatinine.
Hepatic Impairment: Mild/moderate, caution. Initially 10mg olmesartan once daily; max. 20mg/day. Severe, contraindicated.
SP: ESRD, recent kidney transplant, no data.
ADR: Summary, *most common*, peripheral oedema, headache, dizziness.
Notes: See 2.1.2 AIIAs. See Olmesartan above.
Interchangeability: Same strengths of all brands of

2.1.2   Angiotensin II Antagonists (AIIAs, ARBs) and Combinations

olmesartan/amlodipine film-coated (f/c) tabs are deemed interchangeable (includes parallel imports).

Konverge Tablets *(A.Menarini)* B. GMS.
Price, (28) 20/5mg, €19.72. 40/5mg, €23.14. 40/10mg, €24.53.
Tablet, olmesartan medoxomil/amlodipine besilate 20/5mg, 40/5(10)mg. Round. 20/5: White. Marked C73. 40/5: Cream. Marked C75. 40/5: Brownish-red. Marked C77. **Store:** No special conditions.

Olmesartan, Amlodipine, Hydrochlorothiazide

ATC Code: C09DX03. **Sport:** Prohibited.
Driving: Caution (hypotension), see Notes below.
Indications: Essential hypertension not controlled with monotherapy.
Dose: Adult: 1 tab daily; max. 40/10/25mg per day. Titrate with individual components before initiation. *Admin*, swallow whole with water, same time of day, with or without food.
Elderly: Over 75 years, extreme caution, monitor BP.
Renal Impairment: CrCl (mL/min) 30-60, max. 20/5/12.5mg per day. Severe, contraindicated.
Hepatic Impairment: Mild, caution. Moderate, max. 20/5/12.mg once daily. Severe, cholestasis or biliary obstruction, contraindicated.
Notes: See Olmesartan, Amlodipine above. See 2.1.2 AIIAs.

Konverge Plus *(A.Menarini)* B. GMS.
Price, (28) 20/5/12.5mg, €20.91. 40/5/12.5mg, €25.25. 40/5/25mg, €25.22. 40/10/12.5(25)mg, €26.41.
Tablet, olmesartan medoxomil, amlodipine besilate, hydrochlorothiazide 20(40)/5/12.5mg, 40/10/12.5mg, 40/5(10)/25mg. f/c. ROUND: 20/5/12.5: Light-orange. Marked C51. 40/5/12.5: Light-yellow. Marked C53. 40/10/12.5: Greyish-red. Marked C55. OVAL: 40/5/25: Light-yellow. Marked C54. 40/10/25: Greyish-red. Marked C57. **Store:** No special conditions.

Olmesartan, Hydrochlorothiazide

ATC Code: C09DA08. **Sport:** Prohibited.
Driving: Caution (hypotension), see Notes below.
Indications: Essential hypertension not controlled with monotherapy.
Dose: Adult, Elderly: 1 tab (20/12.5)/ day or if not controlled 1 tab (20/25)/day (not controlled on olmesartan* 20mg/day) OR 1 tab (40mg/12.5mg)/day or if not controlled 1 tab (40mg/25mg)/day (not controlled on olmesartan* 40mg/day). *Admin*, swallow tabs whole with fluid, do not chew, take at same time each day. *(monotherapy).
Renal Impairment: CrCl (mL/min) 30-60, monitor; max. 20mg olmesartan once daily; below 30, contraindicated. 40mg dosage forms contraindicated.
Hepatic Impairment: Mild, use 40mg formulation with caution. Moderate, caution, initially 10mg olmesartan once daily; max. 20mg/day. Severe, 40mg contraindicated.
ADR: *Most common*, headache, dizziness, fatigue.
Notes: See 2.1.2 AIIAs. See Olmesartan above.

Omesar Plus *(A.Menarini)* B. GMS.
Price, (28) 20/12.5mg, €9.62. 20/25mg, €9.62. 40/12.5mg, €10.90. 40/25mg, €11.93.
Tablet, olmesartan medoxomil, hydrochlorothiazide 20/12.5(25)mg, 40/12.5(25)mg. Round f/c. 20/12.5: Reddish-yellow. Marked C22. 20/25: Pinkish. Marked C24; Oval f/c. 40/12.5: Reddish-yellow. Marked C23. 40/25: Pinkish. Marked C25. *Lactose*. **Store:** No special conditions.

Benetor Plus *(Daiichi Sankyo)* B. GMS.
Price, (28) 20/12.5mg, €9.62.
Tablet, olmesartan medoxomil, hydrochlorothiazide 20/12.5(25)mg. Round f/c. 20/12.5: Reddish-yellow. Marked C22. 20/25: Pinkish. Marked C24. *Lactose*. **Store:** No special conditions.

Olmesartan/Hydrochlorothiazide Clonmel *(Clonmel)* B. GMS.
Price, (28) 20/12.5mg, €7.05. 20/25mg, €7.28. 40/12.5mg, €8.49. 40/25mg, €8.74.
Tablet, olmesartan medoxomil, hydrochlorothiazide 20/12.5(25)mg, 40/12.5(25)mg. 20(40)/12.5mg: Beige round. 20(40)/25: Salmon oval scored (not intended for breaking). *Lactose*.

Olmesartan/Hydrochlorothiazide Krka *(Krka)* B. GMS.
Price, (28) 20/12.5mg, €6.57. 20/25mg, €6.85. 40/12.5mg, €7.96. 40/25mg, €8.06.
Tablet, olmesartan medoxomil, hydrochlorothiazide 20/12.5(25)mg, 40/12.5(25)mg. White (almost) f/c. 20/12.5mg: Round. Marked C1. 20/25mg: Oval. Marked C2. 40/12.5mg: Round. Marked C3. 40/25mg: Oval scored (facilitates breaking). *Lactose*. **Store:** Original pack to protect (moisture).

Olmesartan/Hydrochlorothiazide Rowex *(Rowex)* B. GMS.
Price, (28) 20/12.5mg, €7.05. 20/25mg, €7.28. 40/12.5mg, €8.49. 40/25mg, €8.74.
Tablet, olmesartan medoxomil, hydrochlorothiazide 20/12.5(25)mg, 40/12.5(25)mg. Yellow f/c oval (except 20/12.5mg). Marked L. 20/12.5mg: Round. Marked 346. 20/25mg: Marked 400. 40/12.5mg: Marked 347. 40/25mg: Marked 348. *Lactose*. **Store:** No special conditions.

Telmisartan

ATC Code: C09CA07. **Sport:** Permitted.
Driving: Caution (hypotension), see Notes below.
Indications: Treatment, essential hypertension. Reduction of cardiovascular morbidity in manifest atherothrombotic cardiovascular disease or diabetes with target organ damage.
Dose: Adult, Elderly: *Hypertension*, maintenance, 40mg/day; if required titrate to max. 80mg/day or switch to combination.
Cardiovascular prevention, 80mg/day. *Admin*, once daily.
Renal Impairment: CrCl (mL/min) below 30, not recommended.
Hepatic Impairment: Mild/moderate, max. 40mg/day. Severe, not recommended.
ADR: Increased incidence of sepsis (50 years and older). *Common*, none reported.
Notes: See 2.1.2 AIIAs.
Interchangeability: Same strengths of all brands of telmisartan f/c tablets listed below are deemed interchangeable.
Reference Price: (28) 20mg, €4.48. 40mg, €3.64. 80mg, €4.48.

Micardis Tablets *(Boehringer)* B. GMS.
Price, (28) 20mg, 40mg, see reference price above. 80mg, €7.00.
Tablet, telmisartan 20mg, 40mg, 80mg. 20mg: Round. Marked 50H. 40mg: Oblong. Marked 51H. 80mg: Oblong. Marked 52H. White. Marked with logo. *Sorbitol*. **Store:** Original pack; protect (moisture).

Telmisartan Actavis Tablets *(Accord)* B. GMS.
Price, (28) see reference price above.
Tablet, telmisartan 20mg, 40mg, 80mg. White. Marked T. 20mg: Round flat. 40mg: Oval scored (divisible in equal halves). 80mg: Oval. Marked T1.

Telmisartan Clonmel Tablets *(Clonmel)* B. GMS.
Price, (28) see reference price above.
Tablet, telmisartan 20mg, 40mg, 80mg. Yellow f/c. Marked strength; T on reverse. 20mg: Round. 40mg, 80mg: Cap-shaped. *Lactose*.

Telmisartan Mylan Tablets *(Gerard)* B. GMS.
Price, (28) see reference price above.
Tablet, telmisartan 20mg, 40mg, 80mg. White (off-white). Marked TN over strength; M on reverse. 20mg: Round. 40mg, 80mg: Oblong. **Store:** Original pack.

Telmisartan Rowex Tablets *(Rowex)* B. GMS.
Price, (28) see reference price above.
Tablet, telmisartan 20mg, 40mg, 80mg. White scored (divisible in equal halves). Marked with strength. 20mg: Round. 40mg, 80mg: Oblong. *Lactose*.

Telmisartan TEVA Tablets *(TEVA)* B. GMS.
Price, (28) see reference price above.
Tablet, telmisartan 20mg, 40mg, 80mg. White (off-white) oval. Marked 93. 20mg: Marked 7458. 40mg: Marked 7459. 80mg: Marked 7460. *Sorbitol*.

Tolura Tablets *(Krka)* B. GMS.
Price, (28) see reference price above.
Tablet, telmisartan 20mg, 40mg, 80mg. White (almost). 20mg: Round. 40mg: Oval. 80mg: Cap-shaped. *Lactose*, *sorbitol*.

Telmisartan, Amlodipine

ATC Code: C09DB04. **Sport:** Permitted.
Driving: Caution (hypotension), see Notes below.
Indications: Add-on therapy, essential hypertension not controlled with monotherapy. Replacement therapy, patients already receiving individual components.

Dose: Adult, Elderly: 1 tab/day; max. 1 tab (80mg/10mg) per day. *Admin*, with liquid, with or without food.

Renal Impairment: Severe or on dialysis, limited data. Caution (amlodipine, telmisartan are not dialysable).

Hepatic Impairment: Mild/moderate, caution max. 40mg telmisartan per day. Severe, contraindicated.

SP: Recent kidney transplant, no data.

ADR: Summary, *most common*, dizziness, peripheral oedema; *serious*, syncope (rare).

Notes: See 2.1.2 AIIAs. See Telmisartan above.

Twynsta (Boehringer) B. GMS.
Price, (28) 40/5mg, €16.56. 80/5mg, €18.83. 80/10mg, €19.06.
Tablet, telmisartan, amlodipine besilate 40/5mg, 80/5(10)mg. Blue and white oval 2-layer. Marked with logo on white layer. 40/5: Marked A1. 80/5: Marked A3. 80/10: Marked A4. *Sorbitol*.

Telmisartan, Hydrochlorothiazide

ATC Code: C09DA07. **Sport:** Prohibited.
Driving: Can influence; dizziness, drowsiness. Caution (hypotension), see Notes below.

Indications: Essential hypertension not controlled with monotherapy.

Dose: Adult, Elderly: 1 tab (40/12.5) per day; if not controlled 1 tab (80/12.5) per day. If needed 1 tab (80/25) per day. *Admin*, once daily with liquid, with or without food.

Renal Impairment: Mild/moderate, monitor serum (potassium, creatinine, uric acid). Recent kidney transplant, no data. CrCl (mL/min) below 30, contraindicated.

Hepatic Impairment: Mild/moderate, max. 40mg/12.5mg/day.

ADR: Summary, *most common*, dizziness; *serious*, angioedema.

Notes: See 2.1.2 AIIAs. See Telmisartan above.

Interchangeability: Same strengths of all brands of telmisartan/hydrochlorothiazide f/c tabs listed below are deemed interchangeable.

Reference Price: (28) 40/12.5mg, €5.60; 80/12.5mg, 80/25mg, €5.88.

MicardisPlus *(Boehringer)* B. GMS.
Price, (28) 40/12.5, see reference price above. 80/12.5(25)mg, €8.68.
Tablet, telmisartan, hydrochlorothiazide 40/12.5mg, 80/12.5(25)mg. 40/12.5: Marked H4. 80/12.5: Marked H8. Both red/white oval 2-layered. Marked with logo. 80/25: Yellow/white oval. Marked H9. *Lactose, sorbitol*. *Store*: Original pack to protect (light, moisture).

Actelsar HCT Tablets *(Accord)* B. GMS.
Price, (28) see reference price above.
Tablet, telmisartan, hydrochlorothiazide 40/12.5mg, 80/12.5(25)mg. White (almost). Oval. Marked TH. 80/12.5mg: Cap-shaped. Marked TH 12.5 both sides. 80/25mg: Oval. Marked TH; 25 on reverse.

Telmisartan/Hydrochlorothiazide Clonmel *(Clonmel)* B. GMS.
Price, (28) see reference price above.
Tablet, telmisartan, hydrochlorothiazide 40/12.5mg, 80/12.5(25)mg. White (almost) oval. Marked TH. 80/12.5mg: Marked 12.5. 80/25mg: Marked 25. *Lactose*.

Telmisartan/Hydrochlorothiazide Rowex *(Rowex)* B. GMS.
Price, (28) see reference price above.
Tablet, telmisartan, hydrochlorothiazide 40/12.5mg, 80/12.5(25)mg. Oval. Marked with telmisartan strength; hydrochlorothiazide strength on reverse. 40/12.5mg: Red. 80/12.5mg: White (off-white). 80/25mg: Yellow.

Telmisartan/Hydrochlorothiazide TEVA *(TEVA)* B. GMS.
Price, (28) see reference price above.
Tablet, telmisartan, hydrochlorothiazide 80/12.5(25)mg. Cap-shaped bilayered. 80/12.5mg: Red/white* scored (facilitates breaking). 80/25mg: Yellow/white* scored (divisible into equal doses). *(off-white). *Lactose*.

Tolucombi Tablets *(Krka)* B. GMS.
Price, (28) see reference price above.
Tablet, telmisartan, hydrochlorothiazide 40/12.5mg, 80/12.5(25)mg. Oval, two-layered. 40/12.5mg, 80/12.5mg: White (almost white, pinkish white) and pink marbled. 80/25mg: White (yellowish white) and yellow marbled. *Lactose, sorbitol*.

Valsartan

ATC Code: C09CA03. **Sport:** Permitted.
Driving: Caution (hypotension), see Notes below.

Indications: Treatment, essential hypertension; symptomatic HF or asymptomatic LV systolic dysfunction after recent MI (12 hours to 10 days); symptomatic HF (ACEIs or beta-blockers not tolerated) or add-on to ACEIs (mineralocorticoid receptor antagonists cannot be used).

Dose: Adult, Elderly: *Hypertension*, maintenance, 80mg/day; if required titrate to 160mg/day; max. 320mg/day; consider adding diuretic (hydrochlorothiazide) or fixed-combination. *Admin*, once daily.
Recent MI, initiate as early as 12 hours post-MI; initially 20mg twice daily; titrate to 40mg, 80mg and 160mg twice daily over next few weeks; max. target 160mg twice daily.
Heart failure, 40mg twice daily; titrate to 80mg then 160mg twice daily at minimum 2-week intervals to highest tolerated dose; max. 320mg/day in divided doses. With or without food, with fluid.

Child: Strength 40mg, *hypertension*, age 6-18 years, initially, weight 18-35kg, 40mg/day; max. 80mg/day; weight 35-80kg, 80mg/day; max. 160mg; weight 80-160kg, max. 320mg/day. Children unable to swallow tabs, use oral soln up to 80mg valsartan (27mL). *Congestive heart failure*, under 18 years, not recommended.
NOTE: Systemic exposure and peak plasma conc of valsartan is higher with soln compared to tabs. Not recommended to switch between tabs and oral solution unless clinically required.

Renal Impairment: *Adult*, CrCl (mL/min) above 10, no adjustment. *Child*, CrCl (mL/min) below 30 or on dialysis, not recommended.

Hepatic Impairment: *Adult/child*, mild/moderate, without cholestasis max. 80mg/day. Severe, biliary cirrhosis, cholestasis, contraindicated.

SP: Adverse events (hypotension, hyperkalaemia, decreased renal function) increased when used in combination with ACEIs. Triple combination (ACEI, valsartan and beta-blocker or potassium-sparing diuretic), not recommended (increased adverse events). Children, monitor renal function/serum potassium.

ADR: Hyperkalaemia (more frequent observed in children, adolescents aged 6-18 years with underlying chronic kidney disease). Post MI or HF, *common*, dizziness, dizziness, hypotension, orthostatic hypotension, renal failure/impairment.

Notes: See Class Effects 2.1.2 AIIAs.

Interchangeability: Same strengths of all brands of valsartan film-coated (f/c) tabs listed below are deemed interchangeable.

Reference price: (28) 40mg, €4.20. 80mg, €3.36. 160mg, €4.20. 320mg, €8.40.

Diovan Tablets, Oral Soln *(Novartis)* B. GMS.
Price, tabs (28), 40mg, €8.48; 80mg, €9.61; 160mg, €12.44; 320mg, €15.79. Oral soln (160mL) €8.29.
Tablet, valsartan 40mg, 80mg, 160mg, 320mg. Scored (facilitates breaking) except 40mg (divisible into equal doses). Marked NVR. 40mg: Yellow. Marked DO. 80mg: Pale-red round. Marked D/V. 160mg: Grey-orange ovaloid. Marked DX/DX. 320mg: Dark-grey-violet ovaloid. Marked DC/DC
Oral soln, as above 3mg/mL. Clear colourless (pale-yellow) soln. *Sucrose, parabens, poloxamer*.

Valsartan Actavis Tablets *(Accord)* B. GMS.
Price, (28) see reference price above.
Tablet, valsartan 40mg, 80mg, 160mg. Scored (divisible into equal halves.) f/c. Marked V either side of score. 40mg: Yellow oval. 80mg: Round pink. 160mg: Yellow oval. *Lactose, lecithin*.

Valsartan Krka Tablets *(Krka)* B. GMS.
Price, (28) see reference price above.
Tablet, valsartan 40mg, 80mg, 160mg. f/c. Scored (divisible into equal halves). 40mg: Round yellow-brown. 80mg: Round pink. 160mg: Oval yellow-brown. *Lactose*.

Valsartan Mylan Tablets *(Gerard)* B. GMS.
Price, (28) see reference price above.
Tablet, valsartan 40mg, 80mg, 160mg, 320mg. f/c. Marked VN; M on reverse. 40mg: Yellow oval scored*. Marked 1. 80mg: Pale-red round scored*. Marked 2. 160mg: Beige oval scored*. Marked 3. 320mg: Dark-grey oval. Marked 4. *(divisible into equal doses).
Store: No special conditions.

2.1.2 Angiotensin II Antagonists (AIIAs, ARBs) and Combinations

Valsartan TEVA Tablets *(TEVA)* B. GMS.
Price, (28) see reference price above.
Tablet, valsartan 40mg, 80mg, 160mg. Oval f/c scored (divisible into equal halves). Marked V and strength either side of score. 40mg, 160mg: Yellow. 80mg: Pink.
Valtan Tablets *(Clonmel)* B. GMS.
Price, (28) see reference price above.
Tablet, valsartan 40mg, 80mg, 160mg. Scored (divisible into equal halves) f/c. 40mg: Yellow round. 80mg: Pink round. 160mg: Yellow oblong. *Lactose.*
Vatan Tablets *(Rowex)* B. GMS.
Price, (28) see reference price above.
Tablet, valsartan 40mg, 80mg, 160mg. Scored (facilitates breaking; except 40mg which is divisible into equal halves) f/c. Marked NVR. 40mg: Yellow ovaloid. Marked D and O*. 80mg: Pale-red round. Marked D and V*. 160mg: Grey-orange ovaloid. Marked DX*. (*either side of score).

Valsartan, Amlodipine

ATC Code: C09DB01. **Sport:** Permitted.
Driving: Caution (hypotension), see Notes below.
Indications: Essential hypertension not controlled with monotherapy.
Dose: Adult: 1 tab/day with water, with or without food.
Elderly: Caution. Use lowest amlodipine dose available.
Renal Impairment: Mild/moderate, monitor potassium, creatinine. Severe, no data.
Hepatic Impairment: Mild/moderate (without cholestasis), max. 80mg valsartan/day; amlodipine, use lowest available dose. Severe, biliary cirrhosis or cholestasis, contraindicated.
SP: Recent kidney transplant, no data.
ADR: Summary, *most frequent/significant or severe,* nasopharyngitis, influenza, hypersensitivity, headache, syncope, orthostatic hypotension, oedema (including pitting, facial, peripheral), flushing, asthenia, hot flush.
Notes: See 2.1.2 AIIAs.
Interchangeability: Same strengths of all brands of valsartan/amlodipine tabs listed below are deemed interchangeable (includes parallel imports).
Exforge Tablets *(Novartis)* B. GMS.
Price, (28) 5/80mg, €19.16. 5/160mg, €21.70. 10/160mg, €22.72.
Tablet, amlodipine, valsartan 5/80(160)mg, 10/160mg. f/c. Marked NVR. 5/80: Round dark-yellow. Marked NV. 5/160: Dark-yellow oval. Marked ECE. 10/160: Light-yellow oval. Marked UIC.
Store: Below 30 deg C; original pack; protect (moisture).

Valsartan, Amlodipine, Hydrochlorothiazide

ATC Code: C09DX01. **Sport:** Prohibited.
Driving: Caution (hypotension), see Notes below.
Indications: Essential hypertension not controlled with monotherapy.
Dose: Adult: 1 tab daily; max. 320mg valsartan/10mg amlodipine/25mg hydrochlorothiazide.
Elderly: Mild/moderate, monitor potassium, creatinine. Severe, no data.
Renal Impairment: GFR (mL/min/1.73m2) below 30 or anuria, contraindicated (due to hydrochlorothiazide component).
Hepatic Impairment: Severe, contraindicated due to valsartan component. Mild/moderate without cholestasis, max 80mg valsartan/day, therefore *Exforge HCT* is not suitable. Use lowest amlodipine dose.
Notes: See 2.1.2 AIIAs. See Valsartan, Amlodipine above.
Exforge HCT Tablets *(Novartis)* B. GMS.
Price, (28) 5/160/12.5mg, €24.21. 5/160/25mg, €24.00. 10/160/12.5mg, €26.52.
Tablet, amlodipine besilate, valsartan, hydrochlorothiazide 5/160/12.5(25)mg, 10/160/12.5mg. Ovaloid f/c. Marked NVR. 5/160/12.5: White. Marked VCL. 5/160/25: Yellow. Marked VEL. 10/160/12.5: Pale-yellow. Marked VDL.

Valsartan, Hydrochlorothiazide

ATC Code: C09DA03. **Sport:** Prohibited.
Driving: Caution (hypotension), see Notes below.
Indications: Essential hypertension not controlled with monotherapy.
Dose: Adult, Elderly: 1 tab (80/12.5) per day; if not controlled 1 tab (160/12.5) per day. If still not controlled,

1 tab (160/25) per day, then 1 tab (320/12.5) per day to max. 1 tab (320/25) per day. Once daily in morning, with or without food with fluid.
Renal Impairment: Severe (GFR below 30mL/min) and anuria, contraindicated (due to hydrochlorothiazide component).
Hepatic Impairment: Mild/moderate without cholestasis, max. valsartan 80mg; no hydrochlorothiazide dose adjustment needed. Severe or with biliary cirrhosis and cholestasis, contraindicated.
CI: Refractory hypo- (kalaemia, natraemia), hyper- (calcaemia, uricaemia).
Notes: See Class Effects 2.1.2 AIIAs. See Valsartan above.
Interchangeability: Same strengths of all brands of valsartan/hydrochlorothiazide film-coated (f/c) tabs listed below are deemed interchangeable.
Reference price: (28) 80/12.5mg, €3.92. 160/12.5mg, 160/25mg, €4.48. 320/12.5mg, 320/25mg, €14.84.
Co-Diovan *(Novartis)* B. GMS.
Price, (28) 80/12.5mg, €9.61; 160/12.5mg, €12.88; 160/25mg, €13.13; 320/12.5mg, €46.46; 320/25mg, €47.89.
Tablet, valsartan, hydrochlorothiazide 80/12.5mg, 160/12.5(25)mg, 320/12.5(25)mg. Ovaloid f/c. 80/12.5: Light-orange. Marked HGH. 160/12.5: Dark-red. Marked HHH. Marked CG on reverse. 160/25: Brown. Marked HXH. 320/12.5: Pink. Marked HIL. 320/25: Yellow. Marked CTI. Marked NVR on reverse.
Co-Vatan Tablets *(Rowex)* B. GMS.
Price, (28) see reference price above.
Tablet, valsartan, hydrochlorothiazide 80/12.5mg, 160/12.5(25)mg. Ovaloid f/c. 80/12.5: Light-orange. Marked HGH; CG on reverse. 160/12.5: Dark-red. Marked HHH; CG on reverse. 160/25: Brown-orange. Marked HXH and NVR on reverse.
Valsartan/Hydrochlorothiazide (Actavis) *(Accord)* B. GMS.
Price, (28) see reference price above.
Tablet, valsartan, hydrochlorothiazide 80/12.5mg, 160/12.5(25)mg. Oval f/c. Marked V; H on reverse. 80/12.5mg: Pink. 160/12.5mg: Red. 160/25mg: Orange. *Lactose, lecithin.*
Valsartan/Hydrochlorothiazide Krka *(Krka)* B. GMS.
Price, (28) see reference price above.
Tablet, valsartan, hydrochlorothiazide 80(160)/12.5mg, 160/25mg. Oval f/c. 80/12.5: Pink. 160/12.5: Red-brown. 160/25: Light-brown. *Lactose.*
Valsartan Hydrochlorothiazide TEVA *(TEVA)* B. GMS.
Price, (28) see reference price above.
Tablet, valsartan, hydrochlorothiazide 80/12.5mg, 160/12.5(25)mg. Round f/c. 80/12.5: Pink. Marked 93; 7428 on reverse. *Sunset Yellow.* 160/12.5: Red. Marked VH. 160/25: Brown. Marked 93; 7430 on reverse.
Valtan Comp *(Clonmel)* B. GMS.
Price, (28) see reference price above.
Tablet, valsartan, hydrochlorothiazide 80/12.5mg. Pink oblong f/c. *Lactose.*

Valsartan, Sacubitril

ATC Code: C09DX04. **Sport:** Pending.
Driving: Minor influence; dizziness, fatigue.
Indications: Treatment (adults), symptomatic chronic heart failure with reduced ejection fraction.
Dose: Adult: 1 tab (49/51mg) twice daily; double dose at 2-4 weeks to target of 1 tab (97/103) twice daily if tolerated. Tolerability issues, decrease or discontinue. Patients not previously taking ACEI or ARB or other low dose medicinals, initiate with 24/26mg twice daily; titrate slowly. Serum potassium above 5.4mmoL/L or SBP below 100mmHg, do not initiate; SBP above 100mmHg to 110mmHg, initiate with 24/26mg. *Admin,* with or without food; swallow with glass of water.
Elderly: As for Renal below.
Child: Under 18 years, safety/efficacy not established.
Renal Impairment: Mild/moderate, more risk of hypotension. eGFR (mL/min/1.73m2) 30-60 and under 30*, initiate with 24/26mg twice daily. *(use with caution). ESRD, not recommended.
Hepatic Impairment: Moderate or with AST/ALT above 2xULN, caution; initiate with 24/26mg twice daily. Severe, biliary cirrhosis or cholestasis, not recommended.
CI: Angioedema with previous ACE or ARB therapy, hereditary or idiopathic angioedema.
Interactions: Effect of Other Drugs on Valsartan, Sacubitril: *Co-admin contraindicated:* ACEIs or AIIA (ARB) (do not initiate for at least 36 hours after discontinuing

ACE) (angioedema); aliskiren in patients with diabetes mellitus or with renal impairment (eGFR below 60mL/min/1.73m2) (increased adverse events). *Co-admin caution*: Rifampicin, ciclosporin, tenofovir, cidofovir, ritonavir.

Effect of Valsartan, Sacubitril on Other Drugs: Statins, PDE-5 inhibitors, potassium-sparing diuretics (triamterene, amiloride), mineralocorticoid antagonists (spironolactone, eplerenone), potassium supplements, salt substitutes, heparin: *Caution*. Lithium: *Co-admin not recommended*.

SP: *Monitor* blood pressure when initiating or titrating (symptomatic hypotension reported, especially in patients 65 years and older); serum potassium (especially with risk factors including renal impairment, diabetes mellitus, hypoaldosteronism, high potassium diet, on mineralocorticoid antagonists). Correct sodium and/or volume depletion before initiation.

Use may be associated with, decreased renal function increased by dehydration or NSAID co-admin; hyperkalaemia. Angioedema reported, discontinue immediately, do not re-administer. Black patients have increased susceptibility to angioedema. *Caution*, renal artery stenosis (monitor renal function); NYHA class IV (limited data).

Pregnancy, Lactation: Second and third trimester, contraindicated. See Notes below. Lactation, stop breastfeeding or stop drug.

ADR: Summary, *most common*, hypotension, hyperkalaemia, renal impairment. See SP above.

Notes: See Class Effects 2.1.2 AIIAs. See Valsartan above.

▼ **Entresto Tablets** *(Novartis)* B.
Price, not published by company (GMS-pending).
Tablet, sacubitril/valsartan 24/26mg, 49/51mg, 97/103mg as sacubitril valsartan sodium salt complex. Ovaloid f/c unscored. Marked NVR. 24/26mg: Violet white. Marked LZ. 49/51mg: Pale-yellow. Marked L1. 97/103mg: Light-pink. Marked L11. **Store:** Original pack; protect (moisture).

2.1.3 - Renin Inhibitors and Combinations

In This Chapter: *Aliskiren (and hydrochlorothiazide).*

Class Effects
Driving: See Notes below (ACEIs).
CI: Hypersensitivity to any member of the class.
SP: Angioedema. Symptomatic hypotension. Conditions pre-disposing to renal dysfunction including hypovolaemia due to blood loss, severe prolonged diarrhoea or prolonged vomiting, heart, liver or kidney disease. Acute renal failure reversible on discontinuation reported. Renal artery stenosis, caution. Dual RAAS blockade not recommended.
Pregnancy, Lactation: See, Notes below (ACEIs, hydrochlorothiazide).
Notes: See 2.1.1 ACEIs. See 2.9.5 Thiazides (hydrochlorothiazide).

Aliskiren
ATC Code: C09XA02. **Sport:** Permitted.
Driving: Caution (hypotension), see Notes below. Minor influence (dizziness, weariness)
Indications: Essential hypertension.
Dose: Adult: 150/12.5(25)mg daily or 300/12.5(25)mg daily if not controlled on monotherapy. *Admin*, swallow whole with water; once daily always with or always without food; preferably same time of day. Avoid admin with fruit juice and/or drinks containing plant extracts (including herbal tea).
Elderly: Initially 150mg; no additional BP reduction with 300mg in majority of elderly.
Child: Birth to under 2 years, contraindicated; age 2-6 years, safety concerns (potential aliskiren overexposure); age 6-17 years, safety and efficacy not established; no dose recommendation.
Renal Impairment: GFR (mL/min/1.73m2) below 30 or anuria, contraindicated. See Interactions below.
Hepatic Impairment: Severe, contraindicated.
CI: History of angioedema with aliskiren, refractory hypo-

(kalaemia, natraemia), hypercalcaemia, symptomatic hyperuricaemia.

Interactions: Effect of Other Drugs on Aliskiren: *Co-admin contraindicated*: ACEIs or AIIAs in patients with diabetes or renal impairment (GFR below 60mL/min/1.73m2); potent P-gp inhibitors (ciclosporin, itraconazole), other P-gp inhibitors (quinidine). *Co-admin not recommended*: Grapefruit and other fruit juices, herbal teas with plant extracts (aliskiren uptake inhibited); dual blockade with ARB, ACEI (hypertension, syncope, stroke, hyperkalaemia, changed renal function). *Co-admin caution*: Hypokalaemia (other kaliuretics, corticosteroids, laxatives, ACTH, amphotericin, carbenoxolone, penicillin G, salicylic acid derivatives); hyperkalaemia with potassium (supplements, -sparing diuretics, -containing salt substitutes), drugs increasing serum potassium (heparin), moderate P-gp inhibitors (ketoconazole, verapamil, clarithromycin, telithromycin, erythromycin, amiodarone). *Bioavailability decreased*: Irbesartan, P-gp inducers (St John's Wort, rifampicin). *Absorption reduced*: High fat meals. *Increased exposure*: CYP3AV inhibitors (also inhibit P-gp). *Anti-hypertensive effect reduced*: NSAIDs (caution, renal function especially elderly).

Effect of Aliskiren on Other Drugs: Digoxin: *Bioavailability slightly decreased*. Furosemide, torasemide: *Decreased exposure; monitor* (volume overload especially with CHF).

SP: Hyperkalaemia risk. CHF (NYHA III-IV), HF patients treated with furosemide, caution. Severe persistent diarrhoea, discontinue. Correct sodium and/or volume depletion before initiation. Signs of hypersensitivity or angioedema (breathing, swallowing difficulties, swelling of face, extremities, eyes, lips and/or tongue), discontinue. Dual RAAS blockade not recommended, see Interactions above. Uni- or bilateral renal artery stenosis or stenosis to solitary kidney, recent kidney transplant, no data.

Pregnancy, Lactation: Pregnancy, first trimester or women planning to become pregnant, not for use; second and third trimesters, contraindicated. Counsel women of childbearing potential about potential risk during pregnancy. Lactation, not recommended.

ADR: Summary, *most common*, diarrhoea; *common*, dizziness, arthralgia, hyperkalaemia; *serious*, anaphylactic reaction, angioedema.

Notes: See 2.1.3 Renin Inhibitors.

Rasilez 150mg, 300mg *(Novartis)* B. GMS.
Price, (28) 150mg, €21.52. 300mg, €26.57.
Tablet, aliskiren 150mg: Light-pink round. Marked NVR and IL. 300mg: Light-red ovaloid. Marked NVR and IU. **Store:** Below 30 deg C; original pack to protect (light).

Aliskiren, Hydrochlorothiazide
ATC Code: C09XA52. **Sport:** Prohibited.
Driving: Caution (hypotension), see Notes below.
Indications: Essential hypertension not controlled on monotherapy.
Dose: Adult, Elderly: 1 tab (150mg/12.5mg) per day; uncontrolled after 2-4 weeks, titrate to max. 300mg/25mg daily. *Admin*, see Notes below (aliskiren).
Child: See Notes below (aliskiren).
Renal Impairment: GFR (mL/min/1.73m2) below 30, contraindicated.
Hepatic Impairment: Mild/moderate, caution. Severe, contraindicated.
CI: Hypersensitivity to sulfonamide derivatives.
ADR: Summary, *most common*, diarrhoea.
Notes: See Aliskiren above. See 2.11.5 Thiazides.

Rasilez HCT *(Novartis)* B. GMS.
Price, (28) 150/12.5mg, €19.11. 150/25mg, €20.93. 300/12.5mg, €22.74. 300/25mg, €22.88.
Tablet, aliskiren, hydrochlorothiazide 150/12.5(25)mg, 300/12.5(25)mg. Ovaloid f/c. Marked NVR. 150/12.5: White. Marked LCI. 150/25: Pale-yellow. Marked CLL. 300/12.5: Violet. Marked CVI. 300/50: Light-yellow. Marked CVV. *Lactose*.

2.1.4 - Alpha-Blockers

In This Chapter: *Doxazosin, prazosin, terazosin.*

2.1.4   Alpha-Blockers

Class Effects

Driving: Caution (first dose hypotension).

Indications: Alfuzosin, indoramin and tamsulosin are indicated only for the management of benign prostatic hyperplasia (BPH), see Notes below.

CI: Children under 12 years, not recommended. Hypersensitivity to quinazolines (doxazosin, prazosin, terazosin). GI or oesophageal constriction, decreased diameter of lumen of GI tract with Prolonged/R formulations. History of orthostatic hypotension.

Interactions: Effect of Other Drugs on Alpha-Blockers: *Co-admin not recommended*: MAOIs, other alpha-1 blockers, general anaesthesia, highly protein bound drugs (digoxin, phenytoin, warfarin, indomethacin), sildenafil (allow 4-hour dosing interval). *Co-admin caution (hypotension)*: PDE-5 inhibitors (sildenafil, vardenafil, tadafil); to minimise postural hypotension risk, stabilise on alpha-blocker before initiating PDE-5 Inhibitors. *Enhanced hypotensive effect*: Other antihypertensives (ACEIs, AIIAs, adrenergic neurone blockers, beta-blockers, calcium channel blockers, diuretics, vasodilators). *Reduced antihypertensive effect*: Oestrogens, carbenoxolone, NSAIDS.

SP: First-dose hypotension; postural hypotension (dizziness, weakness, syncope). Hepatic impairment (caution); mild/moderate renal impairment, generally no dose adjustment. Caution (with all vasodilatory agents), acute cardiac conditions including pulmonary oedema due to aortic or mitral stenosis, heart failure (high output), right-sided HF (pulmonary embolism or pericardial effusion), left ventricular HF (low filling pressure). Half-life prolonged in CHF. LV failure with fall in cardiac output/systemic BP. History of micturition syncope, generally not recommended. Intraoperative Floppy Iris Syndrome (IFIS) observed during cataract surgery. Prolonged erections and priapism reported; seek medical advice. *Elderly*, use lowest effective dose; titrate with caution.

Pregnancy, Lactation: Pregnancy, if benefit outweighs risk (crosses placenta). Lactation, contraindicated unless otherwise stated.

ADR: *Commonly*, infection (respiratory, urinary tract), urinary incontinence, dizziness, postural (dizziness, hypotension), vertigo, headache, somnolence, rhinitis, bronchitis, dyspnoea, cough, diarrhoea, nausea, vomiting, gastritis, constipation, flatulence, fatigue, malaise, oedema, asthenia, dry mouth, palpitations, tachycardia, hypotension, pruritus, back pain, myalgia.

Notes: See 8.4.1 BPH (alfuzosin, indoramin, tamsulosin).

Doxazosin

ATC Code: C02CA04. **Sport**: Permitted.

Driving: Drowsiness.

Indications: Hypertension. BPH (not brands *Doxacar, Doxatan, Kamiren*).

Dose: Adult, Elderly: STANDARD/R, *hypertension*, initially, 1mg/day (1-2 weeks); titrate to 2mg/day (next 1-2 weeks). If needed, titrate at 1-2 week intervals to 4mg, 8mg, 16mg/day; maintenance 2-4mg/day; max. 16mg/day. *Admin*, once daily.

PROLONGED/R, *hypertension*, initially 4mg/day; titrate to max. 8mg/day if needed. Usually controlled with 4mg/day; may take up to 4 weeks to reach optimal effect. *Admin*, swallow whole with sufficient liquid; with or without food; do not crush, divide or chew.

BPH, usually Standard/R 2-4mg/day (initially 1mg/day to minimise postural hypotension risk; increase to 2mg, 4mg) OR Prolonged/R 4mg/day; max. 8mg/day. *Admin*, once daily.

Child: Safety/efficacy not established.

Renal Impairment: Not dialysable.

Hepatic Impairment: Caution. Severe, not recommended.

CI: BPH indication, hypotension (including orthostatic), concomitant urinary outflow obstruction, chronic UTI, bladder stones. Monotherapy, either overflow bladder or anuria with/without progressive renal insufficiency.

Interactions: Effect of Other Drugs on Doxazosin: Co-

admin caution: CYP3A4 inhibitors (clarithromycin, indinavir, itraconazole, ketoconazole, nefazodone, nelfinavir, ritonavir, saquinavir, telithromycin, voriconazole.

Effect of Doxazosin on Other Drugs: Dopamine, ephedrine, epinephrine (adrenaline), metaraminol, methoxamine, phenylephrine: *Blood pressure, vascular reactions may be reduced*. Protein-bound drugs (digoxin, phenytoin, warfarin, indomethacin): *Theoretical potential for interaction*.

SP: Exclude prostate carcinoma before initiating treatment of BPH symptoms. Diabetic autonomic neuropathy, caution. May influence plasma renin activity and vanillylmandelic acid urinary excretion. Highly protein bound (theoretical potential interaction with other protein bound drugs). Remaining shell of some Prolonged/R formulations may appear in stools (pass through GI tract).

ADR: See Notes below.

Notes: See 2.1.4 Alpha-Blockers.

Interchangeability: Same strengths of all brands of doxazosin Standard/R tabs and Prolonged/R tabs listed below are deemed interchangeable.

Reference Price: (28) 4mg SR (Prolonged/R) €3.68.

Cardura 1mg, 2mg, XL 4mg, 8mg *(Pfizer)* B. GMS.
Price, tabs (28) 1mg, €5.32. 2mg, €7.10. XL (28) 4mg, €7.94. 8mg, €14.14.
Standard/R tablet, doxazosin mesilate. Marked CN/strength; Pfizer logo on reverse. 1mg: Round. 2mg: Oblong. *Lactose*. **Store**: Below 30 deg C.
Prolonged/R tablet (XL), as above. White round with hole. Marked CXL/strength. **Store**: As above; original pack to protect (moisture).

Carsem XL 4mg *(TEVA)* B. GMS.
Price, (28), see reference price above.
Prolonged/R tablet, doxazosin mesilate. White round. Marked DL.

Doxacar Prolonged/R 4mg *(Gerard)* B. GMS.
Price, (28), see reference price above.
Prolonged/R tablet, doxazosin mesilate. White round. Marked DL.

Doxane XL 4mg *(Rowex)* B. GMS.
Price, (28), see reference price above.
Prolonged/R tablet, doxazosin mesilate. White round. Marked DL.

Doxatan 1mg, 2mg, 4mg, XL 4mg *(Clonmel)* B. GMS.
Price, tabs (28) 1mg €5.22. 2mg, €6.96. 4mg, €13.79. XL (28) 4mg, see reference price above.
Standard/R tablet, doxazosin mesilate. White scored. Marked D/strength. 1mg: Round. 2mg, 4mg: Oblong.
Prolonged/R tablet (XL), as above. White round. Marked DL.

Kamiren 4mg *(Krka)* B. GMS.
Price, (28), see reference price above.
Prolonged/R tablet, doxazosin mesilate. White round f/c.

Raporsin Prolonged/R 4mg, 8mg *(Accord)* B. GMS.
Price, 8mg (28) €7.07. 4mg, see reference price above.
Prolonged/R tablet, doxazosin mesilate. White round. Marked DH.

Prazosin

ATC Code: C02CA01. **Sport**: Permitted.

Driving: Caution.

Indications: Hypertension. BPH, CHF (adjunctive), Raynaud's Syndrome.

Dose: Adult, Elderly: *Hypertension*, initially 0.5mg (2-3 times daily) for 3-7 days (admin first dose in evening); then titrate to 1mg (2-3 times daily); maintenance 15mg/day; max. 20mg/day.

CHF, initially 0.5mg (2, 3 or 4 times daily); titrate to 4mg/day; maintenance 4mg-20mg/day.

Raynaud's, initially 0.5mg twice daily for 3-7 days; maintenance 1-2mg twice daily.

Renal Impairment: Initially 0.5mg/day.

Hepatic Impairment: As for Renal above.

Interactions: Effect of Prazosin on Other Drugs: Screening tests for phaeochromocytoma urinary vanillylmandelic acid (VMA), methoxyhydroxyphenyl glycol (MHPG) metabolites of noradrenaline: *False positive results risk*.

Pregnancy, Lactation: Lactation, caution.

Notes: See 2.1.4 Alpha-Blockers.

Hypovase 0.05mg, 1mg *(Pfizer)* B. GMS.
Price, (60) 0.5mg, €3.39. 1mg, €3.49.
Tablet, prazosin HCl. White marked Pfizer. 0.5mg: Unscored. 1mg: Scored both sides (divisible into equal halves). Marked M6.

Terazosin

ATC Code: G04CA03. **Sport:** Permitted.
Driving: Initial excessive hypotension, drowsiness.
Indications: Hypertension, BPH, symptomatic treatment.
Dose: Adult, Elderly: *Hypertension,* initially 1mg/day in evening; titrate to 2mg/day after 7-14 days; maintenance 5-10mg/day; max. 20mg/day.
BPH, initially 1mg/day in evening; if needed double dose at 1-week intervals; maintenance, max. 5-10mg.
CI: Quinazoline hypersensitivity.
ADR: *Common*, palpitation, tachycardia, vertigo, blurred vision/amblyopia, nausea, diarrhoea, asthenia, oedema including peripheral, chest pain, somnolence, dizziness, syncope, paraesthesia, headache, nasal congestion, rhinitis, dyspnoea, rash, pruritus, orthostatic hypotension *(both brands)*; erectile dysfunction *(Hytrin)*; nervousness, sinusitis, epistaxis, constipation, vomiting, back pain, urinary incontinence, impotence, light-headedness, extremity pain *(Terazosin Accord)*.
Notes: See 2.1.4 Alpha-Blockers.

Hytrin Starter, 2mg, 5mg, 10mg *(Concordia)* B. GMS.
Price, (28) 2mg, €16.58. 5mg, €22.39. 10mg, €31.49. Starter pack (7x1mg + 7x2mg), €9.13.
Tablet, terazosin hydrochloride dihydrate. Round flat. Marked with logo and triangular facets. 1mg: White. 2mg: Yellow. 5mg: Tan. 10mg: Blue. *Lactose*.

Terazosin 2mg, 5mg *(Accord)* B. GMS.
Price, (28) 2mg, €15.65. 5mg, €21.14.
Tablet, terazosin monohydrochloride dihydrate. Round flat. 2mg: Yellow scored (divisible into equal halves). 5mg: Light-pink scored (facilitates breaking). *Lactose*.

2.1.5 - Centrally Acting Antihypertensives

In This Chapter: *Clonidine.*

Class Effects
Clonidine is also used for migraine prophylaxis, menopausal flushing and part of the treatment regimen for opioid withdrawal.
CI: Hypersensitivity to any member of the class.

Clonidine (hypertension)

ATC Code: C02AC01. **Sport:** Permitted.
Driving: Dizziness, sedation, accommodation disorder.
Indications: Hypertension *(oral)*; hypertensive crisis *(IV)*.
Dose: Adult, Elderly: ORAL, initially 0.05-0.1mg 3-times daily; titrate gradually if required; usual range 0.3-1.2mg (divided doses).
PARENTERAL, acute hypertensive crisis 150-300mcg (1-2 amps) by slow IV injection over 10-15 minutes; repeat to max. 750mg (5 amps) in 24 hours.
Child: Under 18 years, not recommended.
Renal Impairment: Adjust dose according to degree of impairment or antihypertensive response.
CI: Severe bradyarrhythmia (sick sinus syndrome, second or third degree AV block). Phaeochromocytoma.
Interactions: Effect of Other Drugs on Clonidine: *Enhanced hypotensive effect*: Other antihypertensives (diuretics, vasodilators, beta-blockers, calcium channel blockers, ACEIs, AIIAs, alpha-blockers), other hypotensives (ALCOHOL, aldesleukin, alprostadil, general anaesthetics, anxiolytics and hypnotics, diazoxide, levodopa, MAOIs, minoxidil, thymoxamine, nitrates, nitroprusside, phenothiazines). *Effect antagonised*: TCADs, neuroleptics (with alpha-blocking properties), NSAIDs. *Bradycardia, rhythm disturbances*: Beta-blockers, digitalis glycosides. *Peripheral vascular disorders potentiated*: Beta-blockers. *Serious adverse reactions (including death)*: When used **off-label** with methylphenidate in children with ADHD (combination is not recommended).
SP: Sudden withdrawal, possible rebound hypertension; reduce dose gradually. Depression, Raynaud's disease, other peripheral vascular occlusive disease. Cerebrovascular or coronary insufficiency, mild/moderate bradyarrhythmia (low sinus rhythm with polyneuropathy and/or constipation). HF, renal insufficiency, monitor.

Agitation, restlessness, palpitations, nervousness, tremor, headache, abdominal symptoms. Decreased lacrimation (caution, contact lenses). *Off-label*, see Interactions above.
Pregnancy, Lactation: Pregnancy, if benefit outweighs risk. Lactation, not recommended.
ADR: *Very common*, dizziness, sedation, orthostatic hypotension, dry mouth. *Common*, depression, sleep disorder, headache, constipation, nausea, salivary gland pain, vomiting, erectile dysfunction, fatigue.
Notes: See 2.1.5 Centrally Acting Antihypertensives.

Catapres 100mcg *(Boehringer)* B. GMS.
Price, (100) €8.52.
Tablet, clonidine HCl. White round flat. Marked with logo; O1C/O1C on reverse. *Lactose*.
Catapres Parenteral *(Boehringer)* A. GMS.
Price, (5) €1.83.
Injection, clonidine 0.15mg/mL. Clear colourless soln.

2.1.6 - Adrenergic Neurone Blockers

In This Chapter: *Guanethidine.*

Class Effects
This class, including guanethidine are no longer used as they cause profound orthostatic hypotension. They prevent normal physiological release of noradrenaline from postganglionic sympathetic neurons, causing noradrenaline depletion in peripheral sympathetic nerve terminals. They do not control supine BP and may cause postural hypotension. There are no brands licensed in Ireland.

2.1.7 - Beta-Blockers and Combinations

In This Chapter: *Atenolol (and chlorthalidone, nifedipine), bisoprolol (and perindopril arginine), carvedilol, celiprolol, esmolol, labetalol, metoprolol, nebivolol (and hydrochlorothiazide), propranolol, sotalol, timolol (and bendroflumethiazide).*

Class Effects
Sport: According to the WADA Prohibited List 2017, beta-blockers (beta-2 agonists) are PROHIBITED in the following sports: *In-competition* only (*and *out-of competition* where indicated): Archery (WA)*, automobile (FIA), billiards (all disciplines) (WCBS), darts (WDF), golf (IGF), shooting (ISSF, IPC)*, skiing/snowboarding (FIS) (ski jumping, freestyle aerials/halfpipe and snowboard halfpipe/big air), underwater sports (CMAS) in constant-weight apnoea with/without fins, dynamic apnoea with/without fins, free immersion apnoea, Jump Blue apnoea, spearfishing, static apnoea, target shooting and variable weight apnoea. *Exceptions*: Inhaled salbutamol (max. 1600mcg over 24 hours; max. 800mcg every 12 hours), inhaled formoterol (max. 54mcg over 24 hours), inhaled salmeterol (max. 200mcg over 24 hours) (higher doses or other beta-2 agonists, the TUE Policy applies).
Pharmacology: Cardioselective beta-blockers (atenolol, betaxolol, bisoprolol, carteolol, celiprolol, esmolol, metoprolol, nebivolol). Non-cardioselective beta-blockers (carvedilol, labetalol, levobunolol, propranolol, sotalol, timolol).
Indications: Levobunolol and timolol are indicated in treatment of glaucoma and raised IOP. See Notes below. When beta-blockers are used in emergency or life-threatening situations always consult the manufacturers Full Prescribing Information.
CI: Children, not recommended unless otherwise specified. Hypersensitivity to any member of the class. Sick sinus syndrome, 2nd/3rd degree heart block unless pacemaker present, severe or symptomatic bradycardia (below 50 bpm), decompensated heart failure (HF), cardiogenic shock, acute obstructive airway disease (see SP below), asthma, SA block, metabolic acidosis, peripheral arterial occlusive disease, peripheral circulatory disorders (Raynaud's, intermittent claudication), congenital or acquired long QT syndromes, Torsades de Pointes, symptomatic hypotension (systolic below 100mmHg)

35

2.1.7 Beta-Blockers and Combinations

except due to arrhythmia. Untreated phaeochromocytoma, metabolic acidosis.

Interactions: Effect of Other Drugs on Beta-Blockers: *Hypotensive effect enhanced*: Other antihypertensives (ACEIs, AIIAs, adrenergic neurone blockers, alpha-blockers, calcium-channel blockers, diuretics, hydralazine, methyldopa, other beta-blockers including topical), ALCOHOL, aldesleukin, alprostadil, general anaesthetics, anxiolytics and hypnotics, baclofen, diazoxide, levodopa, MAOIs, minoxidil, moxonidine, nitrates, nitroprusside, phenothiazines, tizanidine, cimetidine. *Co-admin caution*: Baclofen, amifostine. *Co-admin not recommended*: Centrally acting antihypertensives (clonidine, methyldopa, moxonidine, rilmenidine). *Hypotensive effect antagonised*: Carbenoxolone, corticosteroids (not topical or inhaled), NSAIDs (not topical), oestrogens. *Severe hypotension and HF risk*: Dihydropyridines, verapamil and diltiazem (neither beta-blocker nor calcium channel blocker should be admin IV within 48 hours of discontinuing the other). *Severe hypertension*: Adrenaline, dobutamine, noradrenaline. *First-dose hypotension*: Prazosin. *Severe postural hypotension*: Moxisylyte. *Withdrawal hypertension*: Clonidine (rebound; if co-admin, discontinue several days after beta-blocker withdrawal). *Bradycardia risk*: Amiodarone, mefloquine, tizanidine, cardiac glycosides, fingolimod. *Arrhythmias*: Pilocarpine. *Increased AV conduction time, block (conduction disorders)*: Amiodarone, cardiac glycosides, diltiazem, Class I antiarrhythmics (disopyramide). *Myocardial depression*: Amiodarone, other antiarrhythmics, flecainide. *Increased peripheral vasoconstriction*: Ergotamine, methysergide.

Effect of Beta-Blockers on Other Drugs: Antidiabetics: *Hypoglycaemia signs masked*. Tropisetron; sultopride (co-admin contraindicated): *Caution, ventricular arrhythmia risk*. Myocardial depressants (chloroform, lidocaine, procainamide, halogenated anaesthetics), beta-adrenoreceptor stimulants (isoprenaline), alpha-adrenoreceptor stimulants (noradrenaline, adrenaline): reverses effects; increase the vasoconstrictor activities), quinidine: *Co-admin caution*. Class I antiarrhythmics (disopyramide), amiodarone: *May potentiate atrial conduction time and induce negative inotropic effect*. Oral hypoglycaemic agents, insulin: *Effects enhanced*. Sympathomimetics, xanthine bronchodilators: *Effect antagonised*. Verapamil, diltiazem (should not be admin IV within 48 hours of discontinuing the other), amiodarone: *Effects enhanced, cardiac failure risk*. Peripheral muscle relaxants (succinylcholine, tubocurarine): *Effect enhanced*. Iodated contrast products: *Compensatory cardiovascular reactions (hypotension, shock) may be impeded*.

Chlorthalidone Combinations: Lithium: *Reduced renal clearance*.

SP: CHF, caution sudden withdrawal; ischaemic heart disease, decrease gradually to prevent angina pectoris (exacerbation; increased number and/or duration of attacks). Worsening cardiac failure, fluid retention with dose increase; stop until clinically stable. Portal hypertension, increased encephalopathy risk. Caution, recent MI, asthma (history). May mask signs of thyrotoxicosis, diabetes tachycardia, tremor of hypoglycaemia; blood glucose control may worsen. Ocular changes (dry eyes), skin rashes. Severe reactions to a variety of allergens (especially with history of anaphylaxis to such allergens); may be unresponsive to usual adrenaline doses. Hypersensitivity reactions (angioedema, urticaria). Psoriasis aggravated. Stabilise dosing of other cardiovascular therapies (diuretics, digoxin, ACEIs, ARBs) for 2 weeks before initiating. Cardioselective beta-blockers have less effect on lung function; avoid with obstructive airways diseases unless necessary (caution); start at lowest possible dose; monitor for new symptoms (dyspnoea, exercise intolerance, cough).

Anaesthesia (warn anaesthetist); do not use agents causing cardiac depression (halothane, cyclopropane, trichloroethylene, ether, chloroform).

Pregnancy, Lactation: *Pregnancy*, generally not recommended; use only if benefit outweighs risk (reduced placental perfusion associated with growth retardation, intrauterine foetal death, immature and premature deliveries; may cause bradycardia, respiratory distress,

36

hypoglycaemia in foetus, newborn and breastfed infant). Monitor neonate for first 3 days of life. Neonatal cardiac decompensation, admin glucagon, hospitalise (ICU), admin isoprenaline. *Lactation*, generally not recommended; risk (hypoglycaemia, bradycardia) in newborns/infants cannot be excluded. *Diuretic combinations*, not recommended (pregnancy, lactation).

ADR: *Commonly*, bradycardia (may be very common), worsening HF, dizziness, headache, paraesthesia, hypotension, numbness or coldness of extremities, asthenia, fatigue, GI disturbances (nausea, vomiting, diarrhoea, constipation).

Notes: See 7.1 Glaucoma (levobunolol, timolol).

Atenolol

ATC Code: C07AB03. **Sport:** Prohibited (specific sports).
Driving: Dizziness, fatigue.

Indications: Hypertension, angina pectoris, arrhythmias, MI (early intervention, post MI).

Dose: Adult: *Hypertension*, initially 50mg/day; maintenance 100mg/day (single dose).
Angina pectoris, 100mg/day (1 or 2 divided doses).
Dysrhythmias, use oral atenolol, maintenance 50-100mg/day (single dose).
Acute MI, within 12 hours, 5-10mg by slow IV injection (1mg/mL), then after 15 minutes, 50mg orally. After 12 hours, 50mg, then 100mg once daily (6 days); long-term prophylaxis, 100mg/day. *Admin*, swallow tabs whole, with water, before meals.

Elderly: Consider dose reduction.

Renal Impairment: CrCl (mL/min) 15-35 (serum creatinine below 3-6mg/dL), 50mg/day; below 15 (serum creatinine above 6mg/dL), 25mg/day or 50mg/alternate days. Haemodialysis, 50mg after each dialysis.

SP: First-degree AV block, uncontrolled diabetes, phaeochromocytoma, psoriasis, severe hypersensitivity.

Notes: See 2.1.7 Beta-Blockers.

Tenormin 25mg, 50mg, 100mg *(AstraZeneca)* B. GMS.
Price, (28) 25mg, €1.71. 50mg, €2.19. 100mg, €2.79.
Tablet, atenolol. White round f/c. Marked with strength. 50mg, 100mg: Scored. *Store*: Below 25 deg C; original pack.

Atecor 25mg, 50mg, 100mg *(Rowex)* B. GMS.
Price, (30) 25mg, €1.79. 50mg, €2.30. 100mg, €2.93.
Tablet, atenolol. White round f/c scored (facilitates breaking). Marked with strength. *Lactose*.

Ateni 50mg, 100mg *(Gerard)* B. GMS.
Price, (28) 50mg, €2.15. 100mg, €2.73.
Tablet, atenolol. White f/c. Marked G; AT/strength on reverse.

Atenomel 25mg, 50mg, 100mg *(Clonmel)* B. GMS.
Price, (30) 25mg, €1.79. 50mg, €2.30. 100mg, €2.93.
Tablet, atenolol. White. 25mg: Marked C23. 50mg/100mg: Scored. 50mg: Marked C24. 100mg: Marked C25.

Trantalol 25mg, 50mg, 100mg *(Pinewood)* B. GMS.
Price, (30) 25mg, €1.79. 50mg, €2.30. 100mg, €2.93.
Tablet, atenolol. White. 25mg: Round flat scored. 50mg/100mg: Both f/c. 50mg: Marked 1U1. 100mg: Marked 2U1.

Atenolol, Chlorthalidone

ATC Code: C07CB03. **Sport:** Prohibited.
Driving: Dizziness, fatigue.

Indications: Hypertension not controlled with individual components alone.

Dose: Adult, Elderly: 1 tab (50/12.5) daily; inadequate response, increase to 1 tab (100/25) daily. *Elderly*, use lower strength.

Renal Impairment: Severe, contraindicated *(Tenoret, Tenoretic, Atenetic)*, caution *(Atecor-CT)*. Reduced efficacy in presence of renal insufficiency due to chlorthalidone.

CI: Severe (bradycardia, peripheral arterial circulatory disturbances, renal failure), hypotension, cardiogenic shock, metabolic acidosis, second or third degree AV block, sick sinus syndrome, untreated phaeochromocytoma, uncontrolled or digitalis/diuretic refractory heart failure, IV verapamil in previous 48 hours, hypokalaemia, precoma (hepatic, renal or Addison's disease), digitalis intoxication.

Interactions: Effect of Other Drugs on Atenolol, Chlorthalidone: *Increased antihypertensive effect (consider dose adjustment)*: Baclofen.

Pregnancy, Lactation: Contraindicated.

ADR: *Common*, bradycardia, cold extremities, GI disturbances (nausea related to chlorthalidone), fatigue; hyperuricaemia, hypo (natraemia, kalaemia), impaired glucose tolerance (related to chlorthalidone).

Notes: See Atenolol above. See 2.1.7 Beta-Blockers.

Tenoret, Tenoretic *(AstraZeneca)* B. GMS.
Price, (28) 50/12.5mg, €2.99. 100/25mg, €4.23.
Tablet, atenolol/chlorthalidone 50/12.5mg, 100/25mg. White f/c. 50/12.5: Marked Tenoret 50. 100/25: Scored. Marked Tenoretic.

Atecor CT *(Rowex)* B. GMS.
Price, (30) 50/12.5mg, €3.13. 100/25mg, €4.44.
Tablet, atenolol /chlorthalidone 50/12.5mg, 100/25mg. White round f/c scored (divisible into equal doses). *Lactose.*

Atenetic *(Gerard)* B. GMS.
Price, (28) 50/12.5mg, €2.93. 100/25mg, €4.15.
Tablet, atenolol/chlorthalidone 50/12.5mg, 100/25mg. White f/c. Marked G. 50/12.5: Marked AC62. 100/25: Marked AC125.

Atenolol, Nifedipine

ATC Code: C07FB03. **Sport:** Prohibited (specific sports).
Driving: Dizziness, fatigue.
Indications: Management, hypertension, angina pectoris.

Dose: Adult: *Hypertension*, 1 cap daily; titrate to 1 cap 12-hourly if needed.

Angina pectoris, 1 cap 12-hourly. *Admin*, do not take with grapefruit juice; swallow caps with water.

Elderly: *Hypertension*, max. 1 cap daily. *Angina*, max. 1 cap twice daily.

Renal Impairment: Max. 1 cap daily. CrCl (mL/min) 15, serum creatinine above 600 micromoL/L, contraindicated.

Hepatic Impairment: Severe, contraindicated.

CI: Bradycardia, cardiogenic shock, hypotension, metabolic acidosis, severe peripheral arterial disturbances, second or third degree heart block, untreated phaeochromocytoma, uncontrolled heart failure, severe aortic stenosis

Interactions: Effect of Other Drugs on Atenolol, Nifedipine Combination: *Co-admin contraindicated (exaggerated negative inotropic effects; severe hypotension, bradycardia, cardiac failure):* Calcium channel blockers with negative inotropic effects (verapamil, diltiazem). *Increased hypotension/cardiac failure risk:* Additional dihydropyridines (nifedipine).
SP: Ischaemic pain. Class I antiarrhythmics (disopyramide) and amiodarone may have potentiating effect on atrial-conduction time; negative inotropic effects induced.

Pregnancy, Lactation: Contraindicated.

ADR: *Common*, headache, bradycardia, cold extremities, vasodilation, GI disturbances, constipation.

Notes: See 2.1.7 Beta-Blockers. See Atenolol above. See 2.2.1 Calcium Channel Blockers (nifedipine).

NIF-TEN 50/20 *(AstraZeneca)* B. GMS.
Price, (28) €8.93.
Capsule, atenolol/nifedipine 50/20mg. Reddish-brown. *Lactose.*

Bisoprolol

ATC Code: C07AB07. **Sport:** Prohibited (specific sports).
Driving: Caution, initiation, dose change, alcohol co-admin.
Indications: Hypertension, angina pectoris. Stable CHF, adjunctive.

Dose: Adult: *Hypertension*, 10mg/day; range, 5-20mg/day.
Angina pectoris, 10mg/day; max. 20mg/day.
Stable CHF, without acute failure (adjunctive; if tolerated at each phase), initially 1.25mg/day (observe patient over 4 hours), then 2.5mg/day, then 3.75mg/day (at 1-week intervals); then 5mg/day, then 7.5mg/day (4-week intervals); then 10mg/day (maintenance/max.). *Discontinuation*, decrease dose divided into halves at weekly intervals. *Admin*, once daily (morning), with or without food; swallow whole with liquid; do not chew.

Elderly: Use lowest dose; uptitrate with caution.

Renal Impairment: CrCl (mL/min), below 20, max. 10mg/day. Dialysis, limited data. HF, caution.

Hepatic Impairment: Final stages, max. 10mg/day. HF, caution.

CI: Acute HF, HF decompensation (requiring IV inotropic therapy).

SP: Stable CHF, titrate slowly. Caution, insulin dependent diabetes mellitus (type I), restrictive cardiomyopathy, congenital heart disease, haemodynamically significant organic valvular disease, MI (within 3 months).
ADR: See Notes below.
Notes: See 2.1.7 Beta-Blockers.
Interchangeability: Same strengths of all brands of bisoprolol film-coated (f/c) tabs listed below are deemed interchangeable.
Reference Price: (28) 1.25mg, €2.40. 2.5mg, €1.68. 3.75mg, €3.36. 5mg, €1.96. 7.5mg, €4.20. 10mg, €2.52.

Cardicor Tablets *(Merck Serono)* B. GMS.
Price, (28) all strengths, see reference price above.
Tablet, bisoprolol hemifumarate 1.25mg, 2.5mg, 3.75mg, 5mg, 7.5mg, 10mg. Scored (divisible into 2 equal doses) f/c heart-shaped (except 1.25mg). 1.25mg: White round. 2.5mg: White. 3.75mg: Off-white. 5mg: White (yellowish). 7.5mg: Pale-yellow. 10mg: Light orange.

Bioscor 5mg, 10mg *(Niche)* B. GMS.
Price, (28) 5mg, 10mg, see reference price above.
Tablet, bisoprolol fumarate. Scored round. Marked BI/strength. 5mg: Pale-yellow. 10mg: Beige. *Lactose.*

Bisop Tablets *(Rowex)* B. GMS.
Price, (28) all strengths, see reference price above.
Tablet, bisoprolol fumarate 1.25mg, 2.5mg, 3.75mg, 5mg, 7.5mg, 10mg. Round f/c. Marked BIS/strength. 2.5mg: White, scored (divisible into equal halves). 3.75mg: Yellow-white scored f/c*. 5mg: Yellow cross-scored**. 7.5mg: Yellow scored*. 10mg: Apricot cross-scored**. *Lactose.* *(divisible into equal thirds), **(divisible into equal quarters).

Bisopine 5mg, 10mg *(Pinewood)* B. GMS.
Price, (28) 5mg, 10mg, see reference price above.
Tablet, bisoprolol fumarate. Mottled scored. Marked BI/strength. 5mg: Pale-yellow. 10mg: Beige. *Lactose.*

Bisoprolol (Actavis) Tablets *(Accord)* B. GMS.
Price, (28) 5mg, 10mg, see reference price above.
Tablet, bisoprolol fumarate 5mg, 10mg. Round mottled scored (divisible into equal halves). Marked BI/strength. 5mg: Pale yellow. 10mg: Beige. *Lactose.*

Bisoprolol (Niche) 2.5mg *(Niche)* B. GMS.
Price, (28) 2.5mg, see reference price above.
Tablet, bisoprolol fumarate. Scored (divisible into equal halves). Marked BI/strength. 2.5mg: White oblong u/c. *Lactose.*

Bisoprolol Krka Tablets *(Krka)* B. GMS.
Price, (28) 2.5mg, 5mg, 10mg, see reference price above.
Tablet, bisoprolol fumarate 2.5mg, 5mg, 10mg. Scored (divisible into equal doses) f/c. 2.5mg: Oval, white (almost). 5mg: Oval pale brownish-yellow. 10mg: Round pale brownish-yellow.

Bisoprolol Mylan Tablets *(Gerard)* B. GMS.
Price, (28) all strengths, see reference price above.
Tablet, bisoprolol fumarate 1.25mg, 2.5mg, 3.75mg, 5mg, 7.5mg, 10mg. Oval f/c scored or side-notched. Marked BL & (number); M on reverse. 1.25mg: White. Marked 1. 2.5mg: White. Marked 2*. 3.75mg: Cream. Marked 3. 5mg: Pale-yellow. Marked 4. 7.5mg: Pale-yellow. Marked 5. Pale-orange. Marked 6. *Lactose, tartrazine (5mg, 7.5mg), Sunset Yellow (10mg).* *(divisible into equal halves). **Store:** Original pack to protect (moisture); use within 30 days of opening bottles. Below 25 deg C (1.25mg, 2.5mg), 30 deg C (3.75mg, 7.5mg, 10mg).

Emcor 5mg, 10mg *(Merck Serono)* B. GMS.
Price, (28) 5mg, 10mg, see reference price above.
Tablet, bisoprolol fumarate. Heart-shaped f/c scored. 5mg: Yellowish-white. 10mg: Pale orange-light orange.

Bisoprolol, Perindopril Arginine

ATC Code: C09BX02. **Sport:** Prohibited (specific sports).
Driving: Caution, initiation, dose change, alcohol co-admin.
Indications: Treatment, hypertension and/or stable CAD (history of MI and/or revascularisation), stabilised on individual components (4 weeks). Not suitable for initial therapy.

Dose: Adult, Elderly: 1 tab (5/5mg, 5/10mg, 10/5mg, 10/10mg) per day. If stabilised on 2.5/2.5mg individual components, admin half 5/5mg tab per day. Changing dose, use individual components. *Elderly*, as for Renal. *Admin*, as single dose once daily; morning before food.

Renal Impairment: Use 5/5mg, CrCl (mL/min) 60 and above, 1 tab/day; under 60, half tab/day; below 30, use individual components.

Hepatic Impairment: No adjustment.

ADR: Summary, *most common*, (both components), headache, dizziness, abdominal pain, diarrhoea, constipation; (bisoprolol), worsening HF, hypotension, cold

2.1.7 Beta-Blockers and Combinations

extremities, asthenia, fatigue; (perindopril), vertigo, paraesthesia, visual disturbance, tinnitus, hypotension, cough, dyspnoea, nausea, vomiting, dysgeusia, dyspepsia, rash, pruritus, muscle cramp, asthenia.

Notes: For full prescribing information see individual components i.e. see Bisoprolol above and 2.1.1 Angiotensin Converting Enzyme Inhibitors (ACEIs) (perindopril arginine).

Cosimprel Tablets *(Servier)* B. GMS.
Price, (30) 5/5mg, 10/5mg, €7.70; 5/10mg, 10/10mg, €10.97.
Tablet, bisoprolol 5(10)mg, perindopril arginine 5(10)mg. Pink-beige bilayer f/c. Marked with logo; strength on reverse. 5/5mg, 5/10mg: Oblong scored (divisible into equal doses). 10/5mg: Round. 10/10mg: Oblong. **Store:** No special conditions.

Carvedilol

ATC Code: C07AG02. **Sport:** Prohibited (specific sports).
Driving: Dizziness; caution with ALCOHOL.
Indications: Hypertension, adjunctive in CHF.

Dose: Adult: *Hypertension*, initially 12.5mg/day for 2 days, then 25mg/day; max. 50mg/day (single or divided doses). *Angina pectoris*, initially 12.5mg twice daily for 2 days, then 25mg twice daily; max. 50mg twice daily.

CHF, initially 3.125mg twice daily (2 weeks); if tolerated, increase at 2 weekly intervals to 6.25mg twice daily, then 12.5mg twice daily, and then max. 25mg twice daily (patients below 85kg) OR 50mg twice daily (above 85kg). *Admin*, take tabs with fluid.

Elderly: *Hypertension*, initially 12.5mg/day; titrate to 50mg/day (single or divided doses) if needed. *Angina pectoris*, max. 50mg/day (single or divided doses). *CHF*, as for Adult above.

Renal Impairment: Monitor.

Hepatic Impairment: Clinically manifest dysfunction, contraindicated.

CI: Unstable/decompensated HF requiring IV inotropic support.

Interactions: Effect of Other Drugs on Carvedilol: *Co-admin not recommended (BP lowering, heart rate lowering potentiated)*: Clonidine. *Plasma levels decreased*: Rifampicin. *Monitor beta-blockade activity*: Amiodarone. *Hypotension, bradycardia risk*: Catecholamine depleting agents (reserpine, MAOIs). *Increased AV conduction disturbances*: Non-dihydropyridine calcium channel blockers, other antiarrhythmics. *Conduction disturbance risk*: Diltiazem.

Effect of Carvedilol on Other Drugs: Digoxin (increased monitoring, additive prolongation of AV conduction time), ciclosporin (average of 10-20% dose reaction required): *Plasma levels increased with co-admin*. Insulin, oral hypoglycaemics: *Effect enhanced, monitor blood glucose*.

SP: Reduced lacrimation, counsel contact lens users. Caution, Prinzmetal's variant angina. Severe cutaneous reactions reported; discontinue.

ADR: *Very common*, dizziness, headache, cardiac failure, hypotension, asthenia. *Common*, anaemia, bradycardia, hypervolaemia, fluid overload, oedema, visual impairment, decreased lacrimation, eye irritation, nausea, diarrhoea, vomiting, dyspepsia, pain (abdominal, extremity), oedema, pneumonia, bronchitis, upper RTI, UTI, weight increase, hypercholesterolaemia, impaired blood glucose control, syncope, presyncope, depression, impaired renal function/failure, dyspnoea, pulmonary oedema.

Notes: See 2.1.7 Beta-Blockers.

Eucardic Tablets *(Roche)* B. GMS.
Price, (28) 3.125mg, €3.96. 6.25mg, €3.72. 12.5mg, €5.16. 25mg, €6.18.
Tablet, carvedilol 3.125mg, 6.25mg, 12.5mg, 25mg. Round scored (divisible into equal halves). Marked BM. 3.125mg: Pink. Marked K1. 6.25mg: Pale-yellow. Marked F1. 12.5mg: Pale-peach. Marked H3. 25mg: Pale-beige. Marked D5. *Lactose, sucrose*. **Store:** Original pack to protect (moisture, light).

Carvedilol Krka Tablets *(Krka)* B. GMS.
Price, (28) 3.125mg, €3.88. 6.25mg, €4.61. 12.5mg, €5.05. 25mg, €6.05.
Tablet, carvedilol 3.125mg, 6.25mg, 12.5mg, 25mg. White. 3.125mg. 25mg*: Round. 6.25mg*: Oval. Marked S2. 12.5mg*: Oval. Marked S3. 25mg: Round scored*. *Lactose, sucrose*. *(scored, divisible into equal halves).

38

Celiprolol

ATC Code: C07AB07. **Sport:** Prohibited (specific sports).
Driving: Dizziness, fatigue; tremor, impaired vision, headache.
Indications: Hypertension, angina pectoris.

Dose: Adult, Elderly: Initially, 200mg/day; titrate to 400mg/day if required. *Elderly*, caution, decreased renal or hepatic function. Oral, once daily in morning 1-2 hours after food with water.

Renal Impairment: CrCl (mL/min) 15-40, monitor heart rate, reconsider with bradycardia (below 50-55 bpm); below 15, not recommended. Severe, consider dose reduction.

Hepatic Impairment: Limited data.

SP: If use in combination, monitor BP.

Pregnancy, Lactation: Pregnancy, if benefit outweighs risk; if admin within 48 hours of delivery of an obstetric patient, hypotension and bradycardia may be seen in infant. Lactation, not recommended.

Notes: See 2.1.7 Beta-Blockers.

Selectol 200mg, 400mg *(SANOFI)* B. GMS.
Price, (28) 200mg, €10.06. 400mg, €16.32.
Tablet, celiprolol HCl. White heart-shaped f/c. Marked with strength. 200mg: Scored. Marked with heart logo. 400mg: Marked Selectol. *Mannitol*.

Esmolol

ATC Code: C07AB09. **Sport:** Prohibited (specific sports).
Driving: Not relevant.
Indications: Short-term treatment of supraventricular tachycardia (except pre-excitation syndromes) and for rapid control of ventricular rate in atrial (fibrillation or flutter) (peri-, post-operative); tachycardia and hypertension (peri-operative).

Dose: Adult, Elderly: *Supraventricular tachycardia*, maintenance range 50-200mcg/kg/min; 25-300mcg/kg/min been used. Initially, loading dose 500mcg/kg/min (1 minute) then maintenance infusion 50mcg/kg/min (4 minutes); response, maintain 50mcg/kg/min; inadequate response, repeat loading as above, increase maintenance to 100mcg/kg/min (4 minutes). Inadequate response, continue repeating loading and increasing maintenance to 150mcg/kg/min, then 200mcg/kg/min.
Perioperative tachycardia and hypertension, intraoperative, 80mg bolus injection over 15-30 seconds, then 150mcg/kg/min infusion titrating to 300mcg/kg/min as needed; *upon awakening from anaesthesia*, 500mcg/kg/min by IV infusion (4 minutes) then 300mcg/kg/min by infusion; *post-operative* when time for titration available, loading of 500mcg/kg/min over 1 minute before each titration step to produce rapid onset (titrate by 50, 100, 150, 200, 250 and 300mcg/kg/min over 4 minutes).

Renal Impairment: Caution

Interactions: Effect of Other Drugs on Esmolol: *Plasma levels increased*: Morphine.

Notes: See 2.1.7 Beta-Blockers.

Brevibloc Premixed Parenteral 10mg/mL *(Baxter)* A.
Price, 10mL (5), €40.08.
Injection (100mg) or infusion (2500mg), esmolol HCl. Clear colourless (light-yellow) soln. *Sodium 28mg/vial (injection) or 700mg/bag (infusion)*. **Store:** Below 25 deg C; do not refrigerate or freeze.

Labetalol

ATC Code: C07AG01. **Sport:** Prohibited (specific sports).
Driving: Dizziness, fatigue.
Indications: Hypertension including hypertension of pregnancy, post-MI with angina pectoris; parenteral for severe hypertension, when rapid BP control is essential and in controlled hypotensive anaesthesia.

Dose: Adult: ORAL, *hypertension*, initially 100mg twice daily; titrate at 2-week intervals by 100mg if required. Maintenance 200mg twice daily; max. 800mg/day (2 divided doses). *Severe refractory hypertension*, max. 2400mg/day (3 or 4 divided doses). *Hypertension of pregnancy*, initially 100mg twice daily; increase at weekly intervals by 100mg twice daily; second/third trimester, titrate to dose range 100-400mg 3-times daily; max.

1200mg/day; do not exceed 2400mg/day. Oral following parenteral, initially 100mg orally. *Angina with hypertension*, dose required to control hypertension. *Admin*, with food.

PARENTERAL, IV route in hospital setting. *Bolus injection*, for rapid BP reduction, 50mg (IV over 1 minute); repeat 50mg at 5 minute intervals if required; max. 200mg. *Infusion*, dilute to 1mg/mL. *Hypertension (pregnancy)*, start infusion at rate 20mg/hour; double every 30 minutes if required; max. 160mg/hour. *Hypertensive episodes following acute MI*, start infusion at 15mg/hour; titrate gradually to max. 120mg/hour if needed. *Hypertension (other causes)*, start infusion at 2mg/min to achieve BP control, then stop infusion; range 50-200mg. Once BP is controlled, switch to oral.

Hypotensive anaesthesia, initially 10-20mg IV; after 5 minutes increase by 5-10mg if needed. Higher initial dose of 25-30mg in patients where halothane is contraindicated.

Elderly: Oral, initially 50mg twice daily. Parenteral, as for Adult above.

Interactions: Effect of Other Drugs on Labetalol: *Plasma levels increased*: Cimetidine, hydralazine, ALCOHOL.

SP: Severe hepatocellular injury (rare, monitor liver function). *Parenteral*, postural hypotension if patients are allowed to assume upright position within 3 hours of IV admin.

ADR: Most side effects are transient; include psychiatric, CNS disorders e.g. tremor (treatment of hypertension of pregnancy), impaired vision, dry eyes, cardiac and vascular disorders, bronchospasm (patients with asthma), GI and hepato-biliary disorders. See Notes below.

Notes: See 2.1.7 Beta-Blockers.

Trandate 100mg, 200mg *(RPH)* B. GMS.
Price, 100mg (56) €6.12; (250) €26.08. 200mg (56) €9.89; (250) €41.32.
Tablet, labetalol HCl. Orange round f/c. Marked Trandate/strength. *Lactose, parabens, Sunset Yellow.*
Trandate Parenteral *(RPH)* A. GMS.
Price, (5) €17.71
Injection, labetalol HCl 5mg/mL. Clear aqueous soln.

Metoprolol

ATC Code: C07AB02. **Sport:** Prohibited (specific sports).
Driving: Dizziness, fatigue.
Indications: *Oral*, treatment of hypertension, angina pectoris, adjunctive in thyrotoxicosis. Migraine prophylaxis. *Oral, parenteral*, arrhythmias especially supraventricular tachyarrhythmias. Reduction in mortality with definite or suspected acute MI.

Dose: Adult: ORAL, *hypertension*, initially 100mg (morning); if needed increase to 200mg/day (single or divided doses); max. 400mg/day.

Angina pectoris, 50-100mg 2 or 3-times daily. *Arrhythmias*, 50mg 2-3 times daily; can be increased to 300mg/day (divided doses); acute arrhythmias following IV admin, initiate oral 4-6 hours later at 50mg 3-times daily.

Thyrotoxicosis, 50mg 4-times daily.

Post MI, early intervention, commence oral 15 minutes after last IV with 50mg 6-hourly for 48 hours. Prophylaxis after MI, 100mg twice daily.

Migraine prophylaxis, 100-200mg/day (divided doses).

PARENTERAL, *tachyarrhythmia*, initially up to 5mg IV at rate 1-2mg/min; repeat at 5 minute intervals if needed; max. 10-15mg. Caution, systolic BP below 100mmHg. *MI, early intervention*, admin within 12 hours of onset of chest pain. Initially 5mg IV every 2 minutes; max. 15mg. Commence oral therapy 15 minutes after injection; 50mg orally 6-hourly for 48 hours.

Anaesthesia, 2-4mg slowly IV at induction, then 2mg as required; max. 10mg.

Elderly: Caution, excessive fall in BP or bradycardia may have more pronounced effects.

Hepatic Impairment: Severe, dose reduction may be required.

CI: Grade II or II AV block, acute/unstable decompensated HF, significant bradycardia (below 50 bpm), cardiogenic shock, sick-sinus syndrome, severe peripheral arterial diseases, systolic hypotension, severe bronchial asthma or COPD, untreated phaeochromocytoma, metabolic acidosis,

higher grade sinoatrial block. Suspected acute MI complicated by bradycardia, first-degree heart block or systolic BP below 100mmHg.

Interactions: Effect of Other Drugs on Metoprolol: *Co-admin contraindicated*: Anti-arrhythmics of the verapamil type. *Plasma levels increased*: Cimetidine. *Plasma levels decreased*: Rifampicin.

Effect of Metoprolol on Other Drugs: Lidocaine: Elimination impaired (parenteral).

SP: *Caution*, obstructive respiratory disorders, Prinzmetal's angina. Parenteral only for use in hospital setting with ECG and BP monitoring facilities.

ADR: Very common, (oral) pronounced BP drop and orthostatic hypotension (rarely with syncope), fatigue; (parenteral) bradycardia, postural disorders, cold extremities, palpitations.

Notes: See 2.1.7 Beta-Blockers.

Betaloc Parenteral *(AstraZeneca)* A.
Price, 5mL (5) 1mg/mL, €2.58.
Injection, metoprolol tartrate 1mg/mL. Clear colourless soln. *Sodium 3.6mg/mL; 17.8mg/5mL amp.* **Store:** Below 25 deg C; outer carton.
Metocor 50mg, 100mg *(Rowex)* B. GMS.
Price, (100) 50mg, €5.41. 100mg, €10.38.
Tablet, metoprolol tartrate. White round scored (divisible in equal halves). *Lactose.*

Nebivolol

ATC Code: C07AB12. **Sport:** Prohibited (specific sports).
Driving: Dizziness, fatigue.
Indications: Hypertension; congestive heart failure in the elderly (70 years and over), adjunctive to standard therapy.

Dose: Adult: *Hypertension*, 5mg/day. *Heart failure*, stable chronic, initially 1.25mg, then 2.5mg, then 5mg, then max. 10mg. *Admin*, once daily with fluid; with or without food; same time daily.

Elderly: Over 65 years, 2.5mg/day; titrate to 5mg/day if needed. Over 75 years, caution.

Renal Impairment: Initially 2.5mg daily; titrate to 5mg if required. Severe, not recommended.

Hepatic Impairment: Contraindicated.

Notes: See 2.1.7 Beta-Blockers.

Interchangeability: Same strengths of all nebivolol tabs listed below are deemed interchangeable.

NEBILET 5mg *(A.Menarini)* B. GMS.
Price, (28) €6.49.
Tablet, nebivolol HCl. White round cross-scored (divisible into equal quarters). *Lactose.* **Store:** No special conditions.
Nebimel 5mg *(Clonmel)* B. GMS.
Price, (28) €3.64.
Tablet, nebivolol HCl. White round cross-scored (divisible into equal quarters). *Lactose.* **Store:** Below 30 deg C.
Nebivolol TEVA 5mg *(TEVA)* B. GMS.
Price, (28) €3.64.
Tablet, nebivolol HCl. White (off-white) round quarter-scored (divisible into equal quarters). *Lactose.* **Store:** No special conditions.
Nebol 5mg *(Rowex)* B. GMS.
Price, (28) €3.64.
Tablet, nebivolol HCl. White (almost) round scored twice (divisible into equal doses). *Lactose.* **Store:** No special conditions.
Nelet 5mg *(Gerard)* B. GMS.
Price, (28) €3.64.
Tablet, nebivolol HCl. White rectangular quadrisected (divisible into equal doses). Marked N, L and 5. *Lactose.* **Store:** No special conditions.

Nebivolol, Hydrochlorothiazide

ATC Code: C07BB12. **Sport:** Prohibited.
Driving: Dizziness, fatigue.
Indications: Essential hypertension controlled on individual components.

Dose: Adult, Elderly: 1 tab (5mg/12.5mg or 5mg/25mg) per day. *Admin*, at same time of day; can be taken with food. *Elderly*, over 75 years, caution (limited data).

Notes: See 2.1.7 Beta-Blockers. See Nebivolol above. See 2.9 Diuretics (thiazides).

Nebilet Plus *(A.Menarini)* B. GMS.
Price, (28) 5/12.5mg, €7.31. 5/25mg, €7.37.
Tablet, nebivolol/hydrochlorothiazide 5mg/12.5(25)mg. Round

f/c. Marked with strength. 5/12.5: Almost pink. Scored (facilitates breaking). 5/25: Almost violet. *Lactose.* **Store:** No special conditions.

Propranolol

ATC Code: C07AA05. **Sport:** Prohibited (specific sports).
Driving: Dizziness, fatigue.

Indications: Treatment, essential and renal hypertension, angina pectoris, cardiac arrhythmia, essential tremor, anxiety and anxiety tachycardia, phaeochromocytoma, adjunctive in thyrotoxicosis; prophylaxis, post-MI (acute), migraine, upper GI bleeding (portal hypertension and oesophageal varices). IV indicated for emergency treatment, cardiac dysrhythmia, thyrotoxic crisis.

Dose: Adult, Elderly: ORAL, *hypertension,* initially 80mg twice daily; titrate at weekly intervals if required; range 160-320mg/day.

Angina, range 80-320mg/day, *anxiety, migraine, essential tremor,* range 80-160mg/day; *arrhythmias, anxiety, tachycardia, thyrotoxicosis,* range 30-160mg/day.

Post MI, commence treatment days 5-21 post MI. Initially, 40mg 4-times daily for 2-3 days; maintenance 160mg/day.

Portal hypertension, oesophageal varices, initially 40mg twice daily, range 80-320mg/day; titrate to 80mg twice daily depending on heart rate response; max. 160mg twice daily.

Phaeochromocytoma, propranolol only to be used in presence of effective alpha-blockade. Pre-operative, 60mg daily for 3 days. Non-operable malignant, 30mg daily. Divided doses.

PARENTERAL, initially 1mg (1mL) over 1 minute. Repeat at 2 minute intervals if required; max. 10mg (conscious patient) or 5mg (under anaesthesia).

Child: ORAL, *arrhythmias,* 0.25-0.5mg/kg 3 or 4 times daily; max. 1mg/kg 4-times daily; max. 160mg/day.

Migraine, under 12 years, 20mg 2-3 times daily; over 12 years, as for Adult above.

PARENTERAL, *arrhythmias,* 0.025-0.05mg/kg by slow injection. Repeat 3-4 times as required.

Renal Impairment: Increase dose interval.

Hepatic Impairment: Caution.

Interactions: Effect of Other Drugs on Propranolol: *Plasma levels increased:* Cimetidine, hydralazine. *Plasma levels decreased:* ALCOHOL. *Plasma levels increased or decreased:* Quinidine, propafenone, rifampicin, theophylline, warfarin, thioridazine, dihydropyridines.

Effect of Propranolol on Other Drugs: Lidocaine (IV): *Plasma levels increased.* Rizatriptan: *Increased exposure with co-admin; use rizatriptan 5mg dose.*

SP: Decompensated cirrhosis, caution.

ADR: *Common,* fatigue and/or lassitude, bradycardia, cold extremities, Raynaud's phenomenon, sleep disturbances, nightmares.

Notes: See 2.1.7 Beta-Blockers.

Inderal 10mg *(AstraZeneca)* B. GMS.
Price, 10mg (100) €1.30.
Standard/R tablet, propranolol HCl. Pink round f/c. Marked Inderal 10. *Lactose.* **Store:** Below 30 deg C.
Beta-Prograne 160mg, Half 80mg *(Tillomed)* B. GMS.
Price, (28) 160mg, €5.04. Half 80mg, €4.81.
Prolonged/R capsule, propranolol HCl. Contains microgranules. 160mg: White. 80mg: White/transparent. *Sucrose.* **Store:** Below 25 deg C; original pack.

Sotalol

ATC Code: C07AA07. **Sport:** Prohibited (specific sports).
Driving: Dizziness, fatigue.

Indications: Treatment, life-threatening ventricular arrhythmias (tachyarrhythmias, symptomatic non-sustained); prophylaxis, paroxysmal atrial tachycardia, atrial fibrillation, A-V nodal re-entrant tachycardia (using accessory pathways, supraventricular tachycardia post cardiac surgery). Maintenance, normal sinus rhythm following conversion of atrial (fibrillation or flutter).

Dose: Adult, Elderly: Initially 80mg in 1 or 2 divided doses; titrate gradually at 2-3 day intervals; maintenance 160-320mg/day in 2 divided doses, at 12-hour intervals. *Life-*

threatening refractory ventricular arrhythmias, 480-640mg/day only if benefit outweighs risk.

Renal Impairment: CrCl (mL/min) 30-60, half Adult dose; 10-30, quarter Adult dose; below 10, avoid.

Interactions: Effect of Other Drugs on Sotalol: *Additive Class II effects, co-admin not recommended:* Class Ia antiarrhythmics (disopyramide, quinidine, procainamide, flecainide), amiodarone, bepridil. *QT-interval prolongation risk, Torsades de Pointes:* Phenothiazines, TCADs, terfenadine, astemizole, erythromycin (IV), halofantrine, pentamidine, quinolone antibiotics. *Hypokalaemia:* Amphotericin B (IV), corticosteroids (systemic), some laxatives. *Hypotension/shock:* Floctafenine.

Effect of Sotalol on Other Drugs: Salbutamol, terbutaline, isoprenaline: *Increased dose may be required.*

SP: Re-treatment QTc interval above 450 msec, generally do not initiate. Prolonged QT interval, titrate cautiously.

ADR: *Summary, usually transient,* dyspnoea, fatigue, dizziness, headache, fever, excessive bradycardia and/or hypotension; *most significant,* those due to proarrhythmia, including Torsades de Pointes.

Notes: See 2.1.7 Beta-Blockers. See also 2.5 Antiarrhythmics.

Sotacor 80mg *(BMS)* B. GMS.
Price, (28) €1.73.
Tablet, sotalol HCl. Round white scored (divisible into equal halves). Marked with strength. *Lactose.* **Store:** Below 25 deg C; original pack to protect (light).
Sotoger 80mg, 160mg *(Gerard)* B. GMS.
Price, (28) 80mg, €1.68. 160mg, €3.34.
Tablet, sotalol HCl. White flat scored. Marked SL/strength. **Store:** Original pack to protect (light).

Timolol, Bendroflumethiazide

ATC Code: C07BA06. **Sport:** Prohibited.
Driving: Dizziness, fatigue.

Indications: Mild to moderate hypertension.

Dose: Adult: Range 1-4 tabs daily as single dose (morning) or 2 divided doses (morning, evening).

Elderly: Initially 1 tab daily; titrate according to response.

Renal Impairment: Consider dose adjustment.

Hepatic Impairment: As for Renal above.

Pregnancy, Lactation: Pregnancy, contraindicated. Lactation, not recommended.

Notes: See 2.1.7 Beta-Blockers. See 2.9 Diuretics (bendroflumethiazide).

Prestim 10/2.5mg *(Meda)* B. GMS.
Price, (30) €5.28. (100) €17.64.
Tablet, timolol maleate/bendroflumethiazide. White flat oval scored. Marked V PRE. **Store:** Below 25 deg C.

2.2.1 - Calcium Channel Blockers

In This Chapter: *Amlodipine, felodipine, lercanidipine (and enalapril combination), nifedipine, nimodipine (dihydropyridines); diltiazem, verapamil.*

Class Effects

Driving: Caution at start of treatment or in combination with ALCOHOL. Dizziness, headache, fatigue, nausea, ability to react.

Pharmacology: Dihydropyridines differ in therapeutic effect from verapamil and diltiazem. They are used to treat hypertension and angina pectoris as well as Raynaud's Phenomenon and aneurysmal subarachnoid haemorrhage.

CI: Children under 18 years, not recommended. Hypersensitivity to any member of the class. Hepatic impairment. Cardiogenic shock, bradycardia (below 50 bpm), second or third degree heart block, sick sinus syndrome, decompensated cardiac failure, aortic stenosis, during or within 1-month post-MI. Significant cardiac valvular obstruction, dynamic cardiac outflow obstruction, unstable angina pectoris (felodipine). Severe renal failure (ACEI, AIIA combinations), see Notes below.

Interactions: Effect of Other Drugs on Calcium Channel Blockers: *Co-admin not recommended (potentially dangerous):* Dantrolene IV. *Enhanced hypotensive effect:* Other antihypertensives (ACEIs, adrenergic neurone blockers, AIIAs, diuretics, hydralazine), beta-blockers (AV block, bradycardia risk; caution), alpha-blockers (strict BP monitoring), other hypotensives (ALCOHOL, general anaesthetics, antipsychotics, TCADs, clonidine, diazoxide, levodopa, MAOIs, methyldopa, minoxidil, thymoxamine, nitrate derivatives, nitroprusside, aldesleukin, antipsychotics). *Additive effect:* Other hypotensives, drugs causing bradycardia, other antiarrhythmics (only with close clinical and ECG monitoring), drugs with moderate protein binding.

Dihydropyridines: *Plasma levels increased (especially elderly); hypotension risk:* Grapefruit juice (co-admin not recommended), cimetidine, ranitidine, other CYP3A4 inhibitors (protease inhibitors, azole antifungals, macrolides e.g. erythromycin or clarithromycin, verapamil or diltiazem). *Plasma levels decreased (caution):* Phenobarbital, carbamazepine, other CYP3A4 inducers (phenytoin, fosphenytoin, primidone, rifampicin, St John's Wort), amiodarone, quinidine.

Effect of Calcium Channel Blockers on Other Drugs: Clopidogrel: *Effectiveness may be reduced (clinical significance unknown).*

Dihydropyridines: Digoxin, ciclosporin: *Increased plasma levels, monitor.*

SP: Diabetes (latent or manifest), adjustment in control may be needed; monitor carefully. *General anaesthesia,* inform anaesthetist (depression of cardiac contractility, conductivity and automaticity; vascular dilatation associated with enflurane, halothane, isoflurane may be potentiated by calcium channel blockers). *Caution,* increased plasma levels in elderly, renal/hepatic insufficiency; severe hepatic dysfunction, reduced LV function, first-degree heart block, bradycardia. Porphyria, acute, not recommended. Myasthenia gravis, exacerbation of muscle weakness. May be associated with mood changes including depression. Inhibitory effect on intestinal motility. See CI above.

Pregnancy, Lactation: Pregnancy, if benefit outweighs risk unless otherwise stated. Lactation, not recommended. Calcium antagonists may inhibit contractions of uterus during labour; risk of foetal hypoxia may occur if mother is hypotensive and uterine perfusion is reduced due to redistribution of blood-flow though peripheral vasodilation. AIIA combinations, see Notes below.

Notes: For combinations, see 2.1.7 Beta-Blockers, 2.1.1 ACEIs and 2.1.2 AIIAs (ARBs).

Amlodipine

ATC Code: C08CA01. **Sport:** Permitted.
Driving: Minor or moderate influence; dizziness, headache, fatigue, nausea (especially at initiation).
Indications: Hypertension. Chronic stable angina pectoris. Vasospastic (Prinzmetal's) angina.
Dose: Adult, Elderly: *Hypertension, angina pectoris,* initially 5mg/day; titrate to max. 10mg/day if needed. Co-admin (simvastatin), max. simvastatin 20mg/day. *Elderly,* caution with dose increase. *Admin,* once daily with liquid; with or without food.
Child: Age 6-17 years, initially 2.5mg once daily; if needed after 4 weeks increase to max. 5mg once daily. Under 6 years, no data.
Renal Impairment: No adjustment. Not dialysable.
Hepatic Impairment: Initiate at lower end of dose range. Severe, titrate slowly with caution.
CI: Severe hypotension, shock (including cardiogenic), LV outflow obstruction (high grade aortic stenosis), haemodynamically unstable HF following acute MI (first 28 days).
Interactions: Effect of Amlodipine on Other Drugs: Co-admin caution: CYP3A4 inducers (rifampicin, St John's Wort). See Notes below.
Effect of Amlodipine on Other Drugs: Simvastatin: *Increased exposure; see Dose above.* Ciclosporin: *Monitor levels (renal transplant patients on amlodipine); consider*

ciclosporin dose reduction. Tacrolimus: *Increased blood levels; consider tacrolimus dose reduction.*
SP: HF, increased pulmonary oedema incidence, possible increased future cardiovascular event risk, mortality. Patients susceptible to malignant hyperthermia and in hyperthermia management, avoid.
Pregnancy, Lactation: Pregnancy, use only if no safer alternative. Lactation, stop breastfeeding or stop drug; passes into breast milk.
ADR: Summary, *most common,* somnolence, dizziness, headache (at initiation), palpitations, flushing, abdominal pain, nausea, ankle swelling, oedema, fatigue.
Notes: See 2.2.1 Calcium Channel Blockers.
Interchangeability: Same strengths of all brands of amlodipine caps/tabs listed below are deemed interchangeable.
Reference Price: (28) 5mg, €2.16. 10mg, €3.24.

Istin 5mg, 10mg *(Pfizer)* B. GMS.
Price, (28) 5mg, €5.97. 10mg, €8.92.
Tablet, amlodipine besilate. White (off-white) emerald-shaped. Marked with Pfizer logo; AML-strength on reverse. 5mg: Scored (facilitates breaking). **Store:** Below 25 deg C.
Amlode 5mg, 10mg *(Rowex)* B. GMS.
Price, (28), see reference price above.
Tablet, amlodipine. White (almost) oblong scored (divisible into equal halves). Marked with strength. **Store:** Below 30 deg C; original pack to protect (light).
Amlodipine Bluefish 5mg, 10mg *(Bluefish)* B. GMS.
Price, (28), see reference price above.
Tablet, amlodipine besilate. White (almost) flat. Marked C. 5mg: Cylinder-shaped. Marked 58. 10mg: Round. Marked 59. **Store:** No special conditions.
Amlodipine Clonmel 5mg, 10mg *(Clonmel)* B. GMS.
Price, (28), see reference price above.
Tablet, amlodipine besilate. White round. 10mg: Scored (divisible into equal halves). **Store:** Original pack to protect (light).
Amlodipine Krka 5mg, 10mg *(Krka)* B. GMS.
Price, (28), see reference price above.
Tablet, amlodipine besilate. White round. 5mg: Sored (divisible into equal halves). **Store:** Original pack to protect (light).
Amlodipine Mylan 5mg, 10mg *(Gerard)* B. GMS.
Price, (28), see reference price above.
Tablet, amlodipine besilate. White round scored (divisible into equal halves). Marked with strength. **Store:** Original pack to protect (light).
Amlodipine Pfizer 5mg, 10mg *(Pfizer)* B. GMS.
Price, (28), see reference price above.
Tablet, amlodipine besilate. White (off-white) emerald-shaped. Marked AML and strength; Pfizer logo on reverse. 5mg: Scored (divisible into equal halves). **Store:** Below 25 deg C.
Amlodipine TEVA 5mg, 10mg *(TEVA)* B. GMS.
Price, (28), see reference price above.
Tablet, amlodipine besilate. White round scored (divisible into equal doses). Marked A and strength. **Store:** Below 25 deg C; original pack to protect (light).
Istolde 5mg, 10mg *(Accord)* B. GMS.
Price, (28), see reference price above.
Tablet, amlodipine besilate. White round flat u/c scored (divisible into equal halves). Marked AB/strength. **Store:** Below 25 deg C.

Diltiazem

ATC Code: C08DB01. **Sport:** Permitted.
Driving: Dizziness, malaise.
Indications: Treatment, mild to moderate hypertension; prophylaxis and treatment, angina pectoris including Prinzmetal's angina.
Dose: Adult: Hypertension, angina pectoris:
Adizem, SR, initially 60mg 3-times daily; titrate to 360mg/day if needed*. XL,* initially 240mg daily; titrate gradually to 300mg or 360mg/day if needed*.
Diltam Prolonged/R, initially 90mg twice daily.
Dilzem, SR, 90mg twice daily; titrate to 180mg twice daily if needed. *XL,* initially 180mg daily; titrate to 360mg/day if needed.
Admin, swallow Prolonged/R formulations whole with water; do not suck, crush or chew; with or without food. Tab membrane may pass through gut unchanged. Should not be taken at same time as an alcoholic beverage. *In unstable angina up to 480mg/day may be beneficial.
Elderly: Hypertension, angina pectoris:
Adizem, SR, 90mg twice daily*. XL,* 120mg daily*.

2.2.1   Calcium Channel Blockers

Diltam, as for Adult above.

Dilzem, SR, initially 60mg twice daily. *XL*, initially 120mg once daily*; do not increase if heart rate falls below 50 bpm. *Admin*, see Adult above. *(titrate slowly).

Child: Not recommended.

Renal Impairment: As for Elderly above. XL, initially 60mg twice daily.

Hepatic Impairment: AS for Renal above.

CI: Severe bradycardia (below 40 bpm), left ventricular failure with pulmonary congestion.

Interactions: Effect of Other Drugs on Diltiazem: *Co-admin contraindicated:* Dantrolene infusion, ivabradine. *Caution:* Warfarin, lithium, rifampicin. *Co-admin avoid:* Grapefruit juice. *Additive vasodilatory effect (may also increase rate of release of Modified/R preparations):* ALCOHOL. *Co-admin, consider dose adjustment:* H2-antagonists (initiation, discontinuation). *Diltiazem plasma levels decreased:* Phenytoin.

Effect of Diltiazem on Other Drugs: Digoxin, carbamazepine, ciclosporin, cilostazol, ivabradine, tacrolimus, theophylline, quinidine, moricizine, cisapride (ventricular arrhythmia risk), imipramine, nortriptyline, buspirone, statins CYP3A4 metabolic interaction (lovastatin, atorvastatin, simvastatin; raised creatine kinase, myopathy, rhabdomyolysis risk*), midazolam, triazolam, phenytoin: *Increased plasma levels.* TCADs: *Increased bioavailability.* Midazolam IV, alfentanil: *Slowed elimination.* Amiodarone: *AV conduction defects.* Halothane, isoflurane, enflurane: *Enhanced cardiac depression.* Lithium: *Increased neurotoxicity.* Methylprednisolone: *Consider dose adjustment.* *CYP3A4 not involved in fluvastatin, pravastatin, rosuvastatin metabolism.

SP: Mood changes (depression).

Pregnancy, Lactation: Pregnancy, contraindicated. Women of childbearing potential to ensure adequate contraception. Lactation, avoid; is excreted in breast milk.

ADR: *Very common,* peripheral oedema; *common,* headache, dizziness, AV block, palpitations, flushing, constipation, dyspepsia, gastric pain, nausea, erythema, pruritus, malaise, fatigue.

Notes: See 2.2.1 Calcium Channel Blockers.

Adizem SR, XL (Mundipharma) B. GMS.
Price, SR (56) 90mg, €10.72. 120mg, €11.92. 180mg, €17.85. XL (28) 120mg, €9.07. 180mg, €12.57. 240mg, €13.95. 300mg, €11.07.
Prolonged/R capsule, diltiazem HCl (SR) 90mg, 120mg, 180mg. Opaque hard gelatin; contains off-white spherical microgranules. Marked with strength. 90mg: White. 120mg: White/brown. 180mg: White/light brown. *Sucrose. Store:* Below 25 deg C.
Prolonged/R capsule, as above (XL) 120mg, 180mg, 240mg, 300mg. Hard gelatin. Marked DCR and strength. 120mg: Pale-pink/navy blue. 180mg: Dark-pink/royal blue. 240mg: Dark-red/blue. 300mg: Maroon/pale-blue. *Store:* As above.
Diltam 90mg (Rowex) B. GMS.
Price, (60) €13.01.
Prolonged/R tablet, diltiazem HCl. White round scored.
Dilzem SR, XL (TEVA) B. GMS.
Price, (56) 60mg, €6.72. 90mg, €12.57. 120mg, €14.35. XL (28) 120mg, €8.66. 180mg, €12.86. 240mg, €12.28.
Prolonged/R capsule, diltiazem HCl (SR) 60mg, 90mg, 120mg. Buff-coloured. Hard gelatin contains spherical white (off-white) beads. *Sucrose.*
Prolonged/R capsule, as above (XL) 120mg, 180mg, 240mg. White. Marked 'e'/strength. Hard gelatin contains spherical white (off-white) beads. *Sucrose.*

Felodipine

ATC Code: CO8CA02. **Sport:** Permitted.
Driving: Dizziness, fatigue.

Indications: Management, hypertension.

Dose: Adult, Elderly: Initially 5mg once daily increasing to 10mg/day or decreasing to 2.5mg/day depending on response; maintenance 5-10mg; max. 20mg. *Elderly,* initiate with lowest available dose. Oral once daily in morning, with or without food; swallow whole with water, do not crush or chew. Do not admin with grapefruit juice.

Hepatic Impairment: Elevated plasma levels; may respond to lower doses.

Interactions: Effect of Other Drugs on Felodipine: *Plasma levels decreased:* Efavirenz, nevirapine, St John's Wort (see Notes below).

Effect of Felodipine on Other Drugs: Tacrolimus: *Increased plasma levels.*

SP: Caution, severe LV dysfunction, propensity for tachycardia. Mild gingival enlargement in presence of gingivitis/periodontitis.

ADR: *Very common,* peripheral oedema. *Common,* headache, flush.

Notes: See 2.2.1 Calcium Channel Blockers.

Plendil 2.5mg, 5mg, 10mg (AstraZeneca) B. GMS.
Price, (28) 2.5mg, €6.80. 5mg, €6.32. 10mg, €9.60.
Prolonged/R tablet, felodipine. Round f/c. Marked with strength. 2.5mg: Yellow. Marked A/FL. 5mg: Pink. Marked A/FM. 10mg: Red-brown.   Marked   A/FE.   *Lactose, macrogolglycerol hydroxystearate.*

Lercanidipine

ATC Code: CO8CA13. **Sport:** Permitted.
Driving: Dizziness, asthenia, fatigue, somnolence.

Indications: Essential hypertension.

Dose: Adult, Elderly: Initially 10mg/day; titrate gradually to 20mg/day if required. *Elderly,* caution when initiating. Not to be taken with grapefruit juice. Oral once daily before food.

Renal Impairment: Caution when increasing to 20mg. CrCl (mL/min) below 10, not recommended.

Hepatic Impairment: As for Renal above. Severe, not recommended.

Interactions: Effect of Other Drugs on Lercanidipine: *Co-admin contraindicated (increased plasma levels):* Ketoconazole, itraconazole, ritonavir, erythromycin, troleandomycin, ciclosporin (mutually increased plasma levels), grapefruit juice (metabolism inhibited, enhanced hypotensive effect). *Co-admin caution:* Terfenadine, astemizole, class III antiarrhythmics (amiodarone, quinidine). *Increased absorption:* Midazolam. *Plasma levels decreased:* Metoprolol.

Effect of Lercanidipine on Other Drugs: Ciclosporin, digoxin (monitor), simvastatin: *Increased plasma levels.*

ADR: *Most common,* headache, dizziness, peripheral oedema, tachycardia, palpitations, flushing.

Notes: See 2.2.1 Calcium Channel Blockers.

Interchangeability: Same strengths of all brands of lercanidipine film-coated (f/c) tabs listed below are deemed interchangeable.

Reference Price: (28) 10mg, €3.18. 20mg, €4.76.

Zanidip 10mg, 20mg (Recordati) B. GMS.
Price, (28), 10mg, €5.91; 20mg, €9.64.
F/c tablet, lercanidipine HCl. Scored (facilitates breaking). 10mg: Yellow. 20mg: Pink round. *Lactose.*
Lecalpin 10mg, 20mg (Accord) B. GMS.
F/c tablet, lercanidipine HCl. Round scored (facilitates breaking). *Price,* see reference price above. Marked L. 10mg: Yellow. 20mg: Pink. *Lactose.*
Lercanidipine Clonmel 10mg, 20mg (Clonmel) B. GMS.
Price, see reference price above.
F/c tablet, lercanidipine hydrochloride hemihydrate. Round. 10mg: Yellow scored (facilitates breaking). 20mg: Pink scored (divisible into equal halves). *Lactose.*
Lercanidipine Mylan 10mg, 20mg (Gerard) B. GMS.
Price, see reference price above.
F/c tablet, lercanidipine HCl. Round scored (facilitates breaking). Marked LR. 10mg: Yellowish-brown. Marked 1. 20mg: Pink. Marked 2. *Lactose.*
Lercanidipine TEVA 10mg, 20mg (TEVA) B. GMS.
Price, see reference price above.
F/c tablet, lercanidipine HCl. Round scored (facilitates breaking). 10mg: Yellow. 20mg: Pink.

Lercanidipine, Enalapril

ATC Code: CO9BB02. **Sport:** Permitted.
Driving: Dizziness, asthenia, fatigue, somnolence.

Indications: Essential hypertension.

Dose: Adult, Elderly: If not controlled lercanidipine 10mg, titrate to 20mg or switch to fixed combination 10/10 (10mg enalapril, 10mg lercanidipine). If higher enalapril dose is needed use fixed combination 20/10 (20mg enalapril, 10mg lercanidipine). *Elderly,* as for Renal below. One tab in morning, 15 minutes before meals. Not to be taken with grapefruit.

Child: No relevant use.

Renal Impairment: Mild/moderate, caution. CrCl (mL/min) below 30 or haemodialysis, contraindicated.

Hepatic Impairment: As for Renal above. Severe, not recommended.

ADR: *Common*, dizziness, vertigo, cough.

Notes: See Lercanidipine above. See 2.1.1 ACEIs (enalapril).

Lercaril Tablets *(Recordati)* B. GMS.
Price, (28) 10/10mg, €10.17. 20/10mg, €11.83.
Tablet, lercanidipine HCl, enalapril maleate 10(20)/10mg. Round f/c. 10/10: White. 20/10: Yellow. *Lactose*.

Enalapril/Lercanidipine Krka Tablets *(Krka)* B. GMS.
Price, (28) 10/10mg, €5.29. 20/10mg, €5.72.
Tablet, enalapril maleate, lercanidipine HCl 10(20)/10mg. Round f/c. 10/10mg: White. 20/10mg: Yellow. *Lactose*.

Nifedipine

ATC Code: C08CA05. **Sport:** Permitted.
Driving: Caution, medication change or ALCOHOL combination.
Indications: Essential hypertension, treatment and prophylaxis of chronic stable and vasospastic (Prinzmetal's) angina pectoris, Raynaud's phenomenon.

Dose: Adult: STANDARD/R, *hypertension, chronic stable angina, Raynaud's Syndrome*, initially 5mg 3-times daily; if needed, increase after 2-3 days to 10mg 3-times daily; max. 20mg 3-times daily minimum of 2 hours between doses. *Admin*, oral with water.

PROLONGED/R, *Adalat LA, hypertension, angina pectoris*, guideline 20mg/day; max. 90mg/day. *Admin*, tab membrane may pass through GI tract unchanged; swallow tabs whole with water; do not crush or chew; once daily in morning.

Adalat, Nifed Retard, hypertension, angina pectoris, 10mg twice daily; titrate to 20mg twice daily if needed; max. 60mg/day. *Admin*, swallow whole with liquid; do not break or chew; do not take with grapefruit juice.

Elderly: Use lower maintenance doses.

Child: Under 18 years, no data.

Hepatic Impairment: Careful monitoring; consider dose reduction. Severe, caution. *Prolonged/R*, contraindicated.

CI: Cardiogenic shock, clinically significant aortic stenosis, unstable angina pectoris, MI (during or within 4 weeks), acute angina, malignant hypertension (safety not established), MI secondary prevention. *Prolonged/R*, GI/oesophageal obstruction, decreased lumen diameter of GI tract.

Interactions: Effect of Other Drugs on Nifedipine: *Co-admin contraindicated*: Rifampicin. *Co-admin caution*: IV magnesium sulfate in pregnant women. *Plasma levels increased*: Diltiazem, cisapride, nefazodone, quinupristin/dalfopristin, CYP3A4 inhibitors (erythromycin, azole antifungals, fluoxetine, indinavir, nelfinavir, ritonavir, amprenavir, saquinavir, valproic acid, nefazodone), ginkgo biloba. *Co-admin, monitor*: Quinidine.

Effect of Nifedipine on Other Drugs: Quinidine: *Plasma levels decreased*. Tacrolimus: *Plasma levels increased*.

SP: Caution, poor cardiac reserve; HF deterioration. Caution, very low BP, manifest HF, severe aortic stenosis. Ischaemic pain, discontinue. Diabetes mellitus. Dialysis with malignant hypertension and hypovolaemia, marked BP decrease. Obstructive symptoms without history of GI disorders with Prolonged/R formulations. *Immediate/R*, exaggerated BP fall, reflex tachycardia (complications, myocardial, cerebrovascular ischaemia), angina pectoris (start of treatment). *Standard/R*, in essential hypertension or chronic stable angina, Immediate/R nifedipine may result in dose-dependent increased cardiovascular complications (MI) and mortality risk.

Pregnancy, Lactation: Pregnancy, only severe hypertension unresponsive to standard therapy; lactation (Standard/R formulations), delay breastfeeding or milk expression for 3-4 hours after admin *(Adalat)*. Pregnancy, lactation, contraindicated *(Nifed)*. Not for use in women intending to fall pregnant *(both brands)*.

ADR: *Common*, headache, oedema (including peripheral), vasodilation, constipation, feeling unwell.

Notes: See 2.2.1 Calcium Channel Blockers.

Adalat 5mg, 10mg, LA, Retard *(Bayer)* B. GMS.
Price, (90) 5mg, €3.27. 10mg, €4.16. LA (28) 20mg, €5.68. 30mg, €5.98. 60mg, €9.28. Retard (56) 10mg, €8.10. 20mg, €6.90.
Standard/R capsule, nifedipine. Orange soft gelatin ovoid contains yellow viscous fluid. *Sunset Yellow*.
Prolonged/R tablet, as above (LA) 20mg, 30mg, 60mg, (Retard) 10mg, 20mg. Round f/c. *LA*: Pink. Marked Adalat/strength. *Sodium 8.3mg/20mg. Retard*: Grey-pink. Marked with Bayer cross. 10mg: Marked A10. 20mg: Marked 1U. *Lactose*.

Nifed 10mg, Retard 10mg, 20mg *(Rowex)* B. GMS.
Price, 10mg (100) €4.53. Retard 10mg (60) €8.49. 20mg (100) €19.11.
Standard/R capsule, nifedipine. Soft dark brown oblong.
Modified/R tablet (Retard), as above. Round slightly f/c. 10mg: Pink. *Mannitol*. 20mg: Pink (light-red). *Lactose*.

Nimodipine

ATC Code: C08CA06. **Sport:** Permitted.
Driving: Dizziness.
Indications: Prophylaxis, treatment of aneurysmal subarachnoid haemorrhage.

Dose: Adult, Elderly: ORAL/IV, *prophylaxis*, admin soln for infusion for 5-14 days then oral 60mg 4-hourly; total 360mg/day for 7 days OR initiate with oral 60mg 4-hourly. Commence within 4 days of onset of subarachnoid haemorrhage; continue for 21 days. *Treatment*, if cerebral ischaemia occurs, continue tabs to complete 21 days or substitute with infusion soln.

PARENTERAL, *treatment*, IV infusion 1mg/hour via central catheter for first 2 hours; then 2mg/hour for minimum 5 days, max. 14 days. Under 70kg and/or unstable BP, initially 0.5mg/hour.

Child: Under 18 years, safety/efficacy not established.

Hepatic Impairment: Severe or liver cirrhosis, increased bioavailability; effects and side-effects may be more pronounced; consider dose reduction.

CI: Unstable angina.

Interactions: Effect of Other Drugs on Nimodipine: *Co-admin contraindicated (efficacy significantly reduced)*: Rifampicin, phenobarbital, phenytoin, carbamazepine. *Co-admin not recommended*: Grapefruit juice. *Plasma levels increased*: Fluoxetine, nefazodone, erythromycin, ritonavir, ketoconazole, quinupristin/dalfopristin, cimetidine, valproic acid. *Monitor BP*: Erythromycin, ketoconazole, itraconazole, fluconazole, indinavir, ritonavir, saquinavir.

Effect of Nimodipine on Other Drugs: Zidovudine: *Plasma levels increased*.

SP: Cerebral oedema, severely raised intracranial pressure. Hypotension, caution. Unstable angina or within four weeks of acute MI, consider potential risk (reduced coronary artery perfusion and myocardial ischaemia) versus benefit (improvement of brain perfusion).

Pregnancy, Lactation: If benefit outweighs risk.

ADR: *Uncommon*, thrombocytopenia, allergic reaction, rash, headache, tachycardia, hypotension, vasodilation, nausea.

Notes: See 2.2.1 Calcium Channel Blockers.

Nimotop 30mg *(Bayer)* B. GMS.
Price, (100) €30.39.
Tablet, nimodipine. Yellow f/c. Marked with Bayer cross; SK on reverse. *Ethanol*.

Nimotop Parenteral *(Bayer)* A. HOS.
Price, 50mL (5) 0.2mg/mL, €63.96 (PTW).
Infusion, nimodipine 0.2mg/mL (0.02%). Clear yellow sterile conc for soln. *Ethanol, sodium 2.3mg/50mL vial*.

Verapamil

ATC Code: C08DA01. **Sport:** Permitted.
Driving: May affect reaction (initiation, dose change); blood alcohol (may increase levels, slow elimination), ALCOHOL effects exaggerated.
Indications: *Oral*, prophylaxis and/or treatment, angina pectoris (including Prinzmetal's); supraventricular tachycardia e.g. paroxysmal supraventricular tachycardia, atrial fibrillation/flutter with rapid ventricular response (except in WPW or LGL syndrome); mild/moderate essential

2.2.2　Potassium Channel Openers

hypertension. *Parenteral*, tachycardia (as for oral, including children); severe angina (not responsive to oral), severe hypertension, hypertensive crisis.

Dose: Adult, Elderly: Dose range for all indications, 240-360mg per day; max. 480mg (long-term); may be higher for short period. Do not discontinue abruptly.

ORAL, STANDARD/R, *angina* (including Prinzmetal's), 120mg 3 or 4-times daily; angina of effort, 80mg 3-times daily may be adequate. Dose below 120mg 3-times daily unlikely to be effective.

Supraventricular tachycardia and *essential hypertension*, 40-120mg 3-4 times daily depending on severity. Hypertension, max. 480mg/day (long-term). *Admin*, take with or shortly after meals with liquid; do not suck or chew or admin with grapefruit juice.

PROLONGED/R (SR), *hypertension*, 240mg in morning; increase after 1 week to 240mg 12-hourly, if needed; *elderly*, 120mg in morning; increase by 120mg at 1 week intervals if needed.

*Angina pectoris*s, 120-240mg twice daily. *Admin*, as for Standard/R.

PARENTERAL, initially 5mg by slow IV over 2 minutes (elderly, 3 minutes) with patient under constant observation; if needed, admin further 5mg after 5-10 minutes. Maintenance IV drip infusion, 5-10mg/hour; total 100mg/day. *Hypertensive crisis*, initially 0.05-0.1mg/kg/hour; titrate at 30-60 minute intervals until twice the dose or more is reached; max. 1.5mg/kg/day.

Child: PARENTERAL, newborn, 0.75-1mg; infants, 0.75-2mg; children, age 1-5 years, 2-3mg; age 6-14 years, 2.5-5mg. Injection should be given only until onset of action. Oral not recommended.

Renal Impairment: Caution, monitor. Not removed by haemodialysis.

Hepatic Impairment: Initiate with low dose (caution).. Severe, contraindicated; IV beta-blockers not for co-admin with Prolonged/R verapamil except in ICU.

CI: Cardiogenic shock, sick-sinus syndrome, second or third degree AV block (except with functioning pacemaker), with reduced ejection fraction (below 35%) and/or pulmonary wedge pressure above 20mmHg. Atrial fibrillation/flutter in presence of an accessory bypass tract (Wolff-Parkinson-White, Lown-Ganong-Levine syndromes) *(all oral formulations)*. Marked hypotension, LV failure, use within 7 days of acute MI *(Prolonged/R)*. Severe hypotension, ventricular tachycardia *(parenteral)*.

Interactions: Effect of Other Drugs on Verapamil: *Co-admin contraindicated*: Beta-adrenergic blockers (mutual potentiation of cardiovascular effects), ivabradine. *Co-admin caution*: Highly protein bound drugs. *Plasma levels increased (possible)*: Erythromycin, clarithromycin, telithromycin, HIV antivirals (ritonavir). *Plasma levels decreased*: Rifampicin, phenytoin. *Increased clearance*: Phenobarbital, sulfinpyrazone. *Increased exposure*: Atorvastatin, cimetidine, grapefruit juice. *Decreased exposure*: St John's Wort.

Effect of Verapamil on Other Drugs: Alpha-Blockers (prazosin, terazosin): *Additive hypotensive effect*. Quinidine, theophylline: *Decreased clearance*. Colchicine: *Co-admin, not recommended; increased exposure*; single report of paralysis (tetraparesis)*. Carbamazepine: *Increased exposure; carbamazepine side effects (diplopia, headache, ataxia, dizziness)*. Glyburide, buspirone, midazolam, metoprolol, propranolol, almotriptan, doxorubicin: *Increased exposure*. Statins** (atorvastatin, lovastatin, simvastatin), ciclosporin, everolimus, sirolimus, possibly tacrolimus; dabigatran (caution bleeding): *Plasma levels increased*. ALCOHOL: *Elevated plasma levels*. Lithium: *Possible reduced serum levels; possible increased sensitivity and enhanced neurotoxicity*. Digoxin: *Decreased clearance; increased exposure**. Neuromuscular blockers (anaesthesia): *Effect may be potentiated*. Aspirin: *Increased bleeding tendency*. *(reduce dose). **Fluvastatin, pravastatin, rosuvastatin, not CYP3A4 metabolised (interaction with verapamil less likely).

SP: *Caution*, acute MI complicated by bradycardia, marked hypotension, left ventricular dysfunction; SA nodal disease (older patients); neuromuscular transmission disorders (myasthenia gravis, Lambert-Eaton syndrome, advanced

Duchenne muscular dystrophy). *Extreme caution*, first degree AV block, bradycardia below 50 beats/min, hypotension below 90mmHg systolic, ventricular tachycardia (QRS complex above 0.12 sec). Treat acute cardiovascular side effects as for overdose (ICU measures). Verapamil affects AV and SA nodes, prolongs AV conduction time (see CI above). Fully digitalise HF patients before initiation.

Pregnancy, Lactation: Pregnancy, contraindicated unless considered essential. Lactation, only if essential to welfare of mother; potential for serious adverse reactions in nursing infants.

ADR: *Most common*, headache, dizziness, GI disorders (nausea, constipation, abdominal pain), bradycardia, tachycardia, palpitations, hypotension, flushing, peripheral oedema, fatigue.

Notes: See 2.2.1 Calcium Channel Blockers.

Isoptin 40mg, 80mg, 120mg, SR 240mg *(BGP)* B. GMS.
Price, (100) tabs 40mg, €2.29. 80mg, €3.66. 120mg, €5.84. SR (28) 240mg, €5.22.
Tablet, verapamil HCl. Round white f/c. 40mg: Marked 40; triangle on reverse. 80mg, 120mg: Scored (facilitates breaking). Marked Isoptin, strength; Knoll on reverse. **Store:** No special conditions.
Prolonged/R tablet, as above (SR). Oblong f/c light-green scored (divisible into equal halves). Marked with logo. *Sodium 32mg*.
Store: Below 25 deg C.

Isoptin Parenteral 2.5mg/mL *(BGP)* A. GMS.
Price, (5) €6.96.
Injection or infusion, verapamil HCl. Clear colourless sterile aqueous soln. *Sodium 17mg/amp*. **Store:** Below 30 deg C; outer carton to protect (light).

Veramil 40mg, 80mg, 120mg *(Orion)* B. GMS.
Price, (100) 40mg, €5.58. 80mg, €7.48. 120mg, €10.62.
Tablet, verapamil HCl. White f/c. Marked VL/strength. *Lactose, sucrose*.

Verap Prolonged/R 120mg, 240mg *(Rowex)* B. GMS.
Price, (30) 120mg, €5.71. 240mg, €5.12.
Prolonged/R tablet, verapamil HCl. F/c scored (not for breaking). 120mg: Beige round. 240mg: Green oblong. *Lactose*.

2.2.2 - Potassium Channel Openers

In This Chapter: *Nicorandil.*

Class Effects

Potassium-channel openers (potassium-channel activators) provide arterial vasodilation (reduces afterload). The nitrate component promotes venous relaxation (reduces preload).

CI: Hypersensitivity to any member of the class.

Nicorandil

ATC Code: C01DX16. **Sport:** Permitted.
Driving: BP-lowering effects, dizziness, feeling of weakness; increased with ALCOHOL, other antihypertensives.

Indications: Symptomatic treatment of stable angina pectoris, inadequately controlled or have contraindication or intolerance to first-line therapy (e.g. beta-blockers and/or calcium antagonists).

Dose: Adult, Elderly: Initially 10mg twice daily in morning and evening. Range 10-20mg twice daily; if needed titrate to max. 40mg twice daily. Patients prone to headache, initially 5mg twice daily. Tabs to be swallowed whole with liquid; with or without food.

Child: Not recommended. Safety/efficacy not established.

CI: Children, generally not recommended. Shock (including cardiogenic shock), severe hypotension, LV dysfunction with low filling pressure or cardiac decompensation, acute pulmonary oedema, hypovolaemia.

Interactions: Effect of Other Drugs on Nicorandil: *Co-admin contraindicated (can lead to serious BP drop)*: PDE-5 inhibitors (sildenafil, tadalafil, vardenafil), soluble guanylate cyclase stimulators (riociguat). *Co-admin caution*: Corticosteroids, acetylsalicylic acid, NSAIDS (increased GI ulceration risk); medicinals increasing potassium (hyperkalaemia, especially with moderate/severe renal impairment); dapoxetine (orthostatic tolerance). *Hypotensive effect enhanced*: ALCOHOL, TCADs, hydralazine, MAOIs, minoxidil, nitroprusside, other antihypertensives, other medicinals lowering BP.

SP: Avoid using in patients with depleted blood volume, low systolic BP (below 100mmHg), acute pulmonary oedema, acute MI with acute LVF and low filling pressure. Caution, heart failure (NYHA III or IV), G-6-PD deficiency). May cause serious skin, mucosal and eye ulceration; GI ulceration may develop into perforation, fistula or abscess formation; caution with diverticular disease. Stop nicorandil if ulceration develops on any part of the body.

Pregnancy, Lactation: Pregnancy, if considered essential. Lactation, not recommended; excreted in breast milk.

ADR: *Very common*, headache. *Common*, dizziness, nausea, vomiting, flushing, feeling of weakness, increased heart rate, rectal bleeding.

Notes: See 2.2.2 Potassium Channel Openers.

Ikorel 10mg, 20mg *(SANOFI)* B. GMS.
Price, (60) 10mg, €11.04. 20mg, €18.82.
Tablet, nicorandil. Round off-white faceted edges scored (divisible into equal halves). Marked IK/strength. *Mannitol.*

2.2.3 - Nitrates

In This Chapter: *Glyceryl trinitrate (parenteral, oromucosal, transdermal), isosorbide mononitrate, isosorbide dinitrate.*

Class Effects
Nitrates are both peripheral and coronary vasodilators used in treating angina pectoris, heart failure (HF), post-MI and during surgery for blood pressure (BP) control.

Driving: Caution (dizziness, syncope, fatigue, hypotension, decreased attention). Advise patient not to take ALCOHOL or use any psychoactive substances; caution at initiation, dose increase or when changing the product.

CI: Children, not recommended. Hypersensitivity to any member of the class. Acute MI with low filling pressure, acute circulatory failure (shock, vascular collapse), cardiogenic shock, severe (hypotension, anaemia, mitral stenosis, hypovolaemia), hypertrophic obstructive cardiomyopathy, constrictive pericarditis, cardiac tamponade, low cardiac filling pressure, increased intracranial pressure (cerebral haemorrhage, head trauma), closed angle glaucoma, extreme bradycardia, G-6-PD deficiency, toxic pulmonary oedema.

Interactions: Effect of Other Drugs on Nitrates: *Effect reduced (sublingual nitrates, due to decreased absorption):* TCADs, antimuscarinics, disopyramide. *Enhanced hypotensive effect:* Apomorphine, PDE-5 inhibitors used for ED or PAH (sildenafil, tadalafil, vardenafil; contraindicated in some cases), other antihypertensives (ACEIs, adrenergic neurone blockers, alpha-blockers, AIIAs, beta-blockers, including topical, calcium-channel blockers, including dihydropyridines, diuretics, methyldopa), ALCOHOL, aldesleukin, alprostadil, general anaesthetics, TCADs, baclofen, clonidine, diazoxide, hydralazine, levodopa, MAOIs, minoxidil, thymoxamine, nitroprusside, phenothiazines, tizanidine. *Hypotensive effect antagonised:* Carbenoxolone (not topical), NSAIDs, oestrogens.

SP: Tolerance to nitrates may occur; use lowest possible dose. Caution, hypothyroidism, severe liver or renal disease, hypothermia, malnutrition, orthostatic syndrome. Pericardial tamponade, low filling pressures (acute MI, LVF), dysregulation of orthostatic BP, increased intracranial pressure, severe cerebrovascular insufficiency, glaucoma, volume depletion (diuretic therapy). Avoid alcohol. Postural hypotension, syncope. Nitrates should not be stopped suddenly; both dosage and frequency should be tapered gradually. *Elderly,* caution hypotension/syncope.

Parenteral, arterial hypoxaemia due to severe anaemia including G6PD deficiency induced forms, caution nitroglycerin biotransformation reduced.

Pregnancy, Lactation: If benefit outweighs risk. There is data that nitrates are excreted in breast milk and may cause methaemoglobinaemia in infants.

ADR: *Commonly,* headache, nausea, hypotension (including orthostatic), facial flushing, tachycardia, diaphoresis, apprehension, restlessness, muscle twitching, retrosternal discomfort, palpitations, dizziness,

drowsiness, vertigo, abdominal pain, weakness, rash, asthenia. Paradoxical bradycardia.

Glyceryl Trinitrate (parenteral)
ATC Code: C01DA02. **Sport:** Permitted.
Driving: Dizziness, weakness, cardiac symptoms.

Indications: Rapid hypertension control during cardiac surgery; production and maintenance of controlled hypotension during surgery; myocardial ischaemia control during/after cardiovascular surgery. Unresponsive CHF secondary to acute MI. Unstable angina refractory to beta blockers, sublingual nitrates.

Dose: Adult, Elderly: *Surgery,* control of hypertension or to produce hypotension during surgery, initially 25mcg/min; increase at 5-minute intervals by 25mcg/min until desired BP drop achieved; range 10-200mcg/min; up to 400mcg/min has been used. *Peri-operative myocardial ischaemia,* initially 15-20mcg/min; increase by 10-15mcg/min if required.
Unresponsive CHF, initially 20-25mcg/min; decrease to 10mcg/min, or increase by 20-25mcg/min at 15-30 minute intervals if required; range 10-100mcg/min.
Unstable angina, initially 10mcg/min; increase by 10mcg/min at 30 minute intervals if required. *Admin* by slow IV infusion; dilute prior to infusion. Not for bolus injection.

Renal Impairment: Severe, additional dose adjustments may be needed.

Hepatic Impairment: As for Renal above.

Interactions: Effect of Other Drugs on Glyceryl Trinitrate (parenteral): *Co-admin contraindicated:* Phosphodiesterase inhibitors type 5 (PDE-5) (sildenafil, vardenafil, tadalafil), soluble guanylate cyclase stimulator (riociguat).

SP: Incompatible with polyvinyl chloride (PVC) or polyurethane (PU); induce loss of active substance. Do not mix with any other drug. Contains propylene glycol; caution acidosis; do not use for more than 3 successive days.

ADR: *Incidence unknown,* anxiety, restlessness, headache, dizziness, syncope, bradycardia (paradoxical), tachycardia, palpitations, hypotension, flushing, nausea, retching, abdominal pain, diaphoresis, muscle twitching, retrosternal discomfort.

Notes: See 2.2.3 Nitrates.

Glyceryl Trinitrate Parenteral *(Hospira)* A.
Price, (10) 10mg/10mL, €128.94. (1) 50mg/50mL, €30.22.
Infusion, glyceryl trinitrate 1mg/mL. Clear colourless odourless isotonic sterile soln.

Glyceryl Trinitrate (oromucosal)
ATC Code: C01DA02. **Sport:** Permitted.
Driving: See Notes below.

Indications: Treatment, acute angina pectoris. Prevention, inducible angina (physical effort, emotional stress, exposure to cold) *(both brands).* Emergency treatment of pulmonary oedema secondary to acute left ventricular failure until IV therapy can be instituted *(Nitrolingual).*

Dose: Adult, Elderly: *Both brands,* angina, at attack onset 1-2 metered doses (400-800mcg) to be sprayed under the tongue; if symptoms do not resolve repeat at 5 minute intervals, max. 3 doses at any one time. Prophylaxis, inducible angina, 1-2 metered doses (400-800mcg) immediately prior (2-3 minutes) to event.
Nitrolingual, left ventricular failure, 2 metered doses as quickly as possible. Admin, spray under the tongue; at rest in sitting position. *Elderly,* caution hypotension, syncope.

Renal Impairment: Severe, caution.

Hepatic Impairment: As for Renal above.

Interactions: Effect of Nitrates, Oromucosal on Other Drugs: Dihydroergotamine: *Increased bioavailability.* Heparin: *Reduced antithrombotic effect.* Organic nitrates (pre-treatment): *Higher dose of glyceryl trinitrate may be needed.*

SP: Careful monitoring (mitral stenosis, pericardial tamponade, orthostatic dysfunction), cerebrovascular disease, lung disease or cor pulmonale, MI. Caution, ambulant patients with angina and moderate to severe valvular aortic stenosis. Buccal, dental caries (prolonged use, poor dental hygiene).

Notes: See 2.2.3 Nitrates.

Glytrin Sublingual Spray *(Ayrton Saunders)* B. GMS.
Price, 200-dose (1) €4.20.
Sublingual spray, glyceryl trinitrate 400mcg/metered dose. Colourless soln.

Nitrolingual Pumpspray *(Merck Serono)* B. GMS.
Price, 200-dose (1) €5.48.
Oromucosal spray, glyceryl trinitrate 400mcg/dose. Clear colourless (slightly yellow) soln. 9.6mg ethanol/metered dose.

Glyceryl Trinitrate (transdermal)

ATC Code: C01DA02. **Sport:** Permitted.
Driving: See Notes below.
Indications: Prophylaxis, angina pectoris.
Dose: Adult, Elderly: Initially 1x 5mg or 1x 10mg patch daily; if needed increase to 2x 5mg patches or 2x 10mg patches daily.

Interactions: Effect of Other Drugs on Glyceryl Trinitrate (transdermal): *Reduced therapeutic response:* Acetylsalicylic acid, other NSAIDs. *BP lowering effect potentiated:* Acetyl salicylic acid, amifostine.

Effect of Glyceryl Trinitrate (transdermal) on Other Drugs: Dihydroergotamine: *Increased plasma levels.*

Notes: See 2.2.3 Nitrates.

Transiderm-Nitro Transdermal *(Novartis)* B. GMS.
Price, (28) 5mg, €4.72. 10mg, €6.39. (30) 15mg, €13.11.
Transdermal patch, glyceryl trinitrate 5mg, 10mg, 15mg. Flat foil-like sealed at edges. Off-white protective liner; greyish-orange backing film on reverse. 5mg: Marked CG DOD. 10mg: Marked CG DPD. 15mg: Marked CG EJE. *Lactose.*

Isosorbide

ATC Code: C01DA08. **Sport:** Permitted.
Driving: See Notes below.
Indications: *Oral,* management, angina pectoris, adjunctive, post acute-MI, chronic CHF. *Parenteral (IV),* unresponsive LV failure secondary to acute MI and various other aetiologies, severe or unstable angina pectoris. Intra-coronary, PTCA (facilitates prolongation of balloon inflation; to prevent or relieve coronary spasm).
Dose: Adult, Elderly: ORAL, STANDARD/R, initially 20mg/day; titrate to 30mg/day if needed; max. 120mg/day either twice daily (8-hour interval) or 3-times daily (6-hour interval) to allow nitrate-free period.
PROLONGED/R, 1 or 2 caps in morning; max. 120mg/day. Swallow whole with water; do not chew or crush; morning as single dose.
PARENTERAL (IV), slow infusion 2-12mg/hour; up to 20mg/hour may be required. Diluted soln should never be injected directly as bolus except for intra-coronary use.
INTRA-CORONARY, 1mg as bolus injection prior to balloon inflation; max. 5mg within 30-minute period.
CI: Closed angle glaucoma.
Interactions: Effect of Other Drugs on Isosorbide: *Co-admin contraindicated:* PDE-5 inhibitors (sildenafil, tadalafil, vardenafil). *Co-admin caution:* Sapropterin.
Effect of Isosorbide on Other Drugs: Dihydroergotamine: *Effect enhanced.*
SP: Not indicated for acute angina attacks where glyceryl trinitrate should be used. Monitor BP, pulse. Matrix of some Prolonged/R tabs may pass intact through GI tract. Parenteral, do not use if crystals are observed in the solution.
ADR: *Very common,* headache. *Common,* dizziness, tachycardia, hypotension, nausea.
Notes: See 2.2.3 Nitrates.

Elantan 10mg, 20mg, 40mg, LA *(Merus)* B. GMS.
Price, (56) 10mg, €4.78. 20mg, €6.09. 40mg, €9.94. LA (28) 25mg, €3.73. 50mg, €5.34.
Standard/R, isosorbide mononitrate. White flat upper side. Marked E/strength. 10mg: Rounded underside. 20mg: Scored. 40mg: Facet scored (facilitates breaking) with arc-shaped underside. *Lactose.*
Prolonged/R capsule (LA), as above 25mg, 50mg. Hard gelatin opaque. 25mg: Brown/white. 50mg: Brown/flesh-coloured containing white/beige odourless pellets. *Lactose, sucrose.*

Imdur 60mg *(AstraZeneca)* B. GMS.
Price, (28) €5.58.
Prolonged/R tablet, isosorbide mononitrate. Yellow oval f/c scored. Marked A/ID.

Isoket Parenteral *(Merus)* A.
Price, 0.5mg/mL, 50mL (1) €15.69. 1mg/mL 10mL (10) €59.11. 50mL (1) €29.33.
Injection or infusion, isosorbide dinitrate 0.5mg/mL soln and 1mg/mL conc for soln. Clear colourless soln. *Sodium 3.54mg/mL.*

Isomel SR 60mg *(Clonmel)* B. GMS.
Price, (28) €5.46.
Modified/R tablet, isosorbide mononitrate. Yellow oval f/c scored. Marked IM60.

Isomonit Retard 60mg *(Rowex)* B. GMS.
Price, (30) €5.85.
Prolonged/R tablet, isosorbide mononitrate. White round biplanar scored. *Lactose.*

Sormon Prolonged/R 60mg *(Gerard)* B. GMS.
Price, (28) €5.46.
Prolonged/R tablet, isosorbide mononitrate. Pale-yellow elliptical f/c scored (divisible into equal doses). Marked IM 60. *Lactose.*

2.2.4 - Pulmonary Arterial Hypertension (PAH), Idiopathic Pulmonary Fibrosis (IPF)

In This Chapter: Alprostadil, ambrisentan, bosentan, iloprost, macitentan, minoxidil, nintedanib, riociguat, sildenafil, tadalafil.

Class Effects

Discussed are vasodilators; may be direct-acting (antihypertensives), used in ischaemic heart disease (miscellaneous) or in cerebral and peripheral vascular disorders. Minoxidil is used in hair loss/regrowth. Alprostadil, sildenafil and tadalafil are used to treat erectile dysfunction (ED) and sildenafil to treat pulmonary arterial hypertension (PAH). Epoprostenol is a potent platelet aggregation inhibitor. Iloprost, a vasodilator, is indicated to treat PAH. Ambrisentan, macitentan are endothelin receptor antagonists (ERAs). Riociguat influences vascular tone, proliferation, fibrosis, inflammation.
CI: Hypersensitivity to any member of the class.
SP: With ERAs and severe PAH, switch to therapy indicated for severe condition (e.g. epoprostenol). Monitor, liver aminotransferases prior to initiation, then monthly for treatment duration; for dose-related Hb decrease.
Pregnancy, Lactation: Pregnancy, contraindicated; monthly pregnancy tests recommended. Women of childbearing potential to ensure adequate contraception. Pulmonary hypertension severely deteriorates with pregnancy (ambrisentan, bosentan, macitentan, riociguat).
Notes: See 10.8 Miscellaneous Dermatologicals (minoxidil). See 8.4.2 Erectile Dysfunction (alprostadil, sildenafil, tadalafil). See 2.6.8 Other Antiplatelets (epoprostenol).

Ambrisentan

ATC Code: C02KX02. **Sport:** Permitted.
Driving: Minor or moderate influence; hypotension, dizziness, asthenia, fatigue.
Indications: Treatment, PAH (WHO Class II, III) monotherapy or combination.
Dose: Adult, Elderly: *Monotherapy,* 5mg once daily; additional efficacy observed with 10mg (Class III symptoms); with connective tissue disease may require 10mg. *Combination* (tadalafil), titrate to 10mg/day; (ciclosporin A), max. 5mg once daily. *Admin,* swallow tabs whole with/without food; do not split, crush or chew.
Child: Under 18 years, not recommended.
Renal Impairment: CrCl (mL/min) below 30, initiate cautiously especially 10mg.
Hepatic Impairment: Severe (with or without cirrhosis) or AST and/or ALT above 3xULN, contraindicated.
CI: Idiopathic pulmonary fibrosis with or without secondary pulmonary hypertension.
Interactions: Effect of Other Drugs on Ambrisentan: *Co-admin caution:* Ciclosporin A, other PAH treatments (prostanoids, phosphodiesterase type V inhibitors). *Monitor closely:* Rifampicin initiation.

SP: Peripheral oedema (over 65 years) at 10mg dose. Pulmonary oedema (patients with veno-occlusive disease)

Pregnancy, Lactation: Lactation, contraindicated.

ADR: Summary, *most common*, peripheral oedema, fluid retention, headache (higher dose associated with a higher incidence); peripheral oedema (more severe age 65 years and over).

Notes: See 2.2.4 PAH, IPF.

Volibris 5mg, 10mg *(GSK)* A. HT.
Price, (30) 5mg, €2548.69. 10mg, €2571.52.
Tablet, ambrisentan. f/c. Marked GS. 5mg: Pale-pink square. Marked K2C. 10mg: Deep-pink oval. Marked KE3. *Lactose, lecithin, Allura red*. **Store:** No special conditions.

Bosentan

ATC Code: C02KX01. **Sport:** Permitted.
Driving: Hypotension, dizziness, blurred vision, syncope.
Indications: Treatment, PAH (WHO Class III). To reduce number of new digital ulcers (systemic sclerosis, ongoing digital ulcer disease).

Dose: Adult, Elderly: *PAH*, initially 62.5mg twice daily (4 weeks), then 125mg twice daily; max. 250mg twice daily (caution liver toxicity). *Admin*, morning and evening. Discontinue gradually halving dose for 3-7 days. *Systemic sclerosis*, as for PAH above, maintenance 125mg twice daily; max. 6 months.

Child: *PAH*, age 1 year and older, 2mg/kg morning and evening (starting and maintenance dose); neonates with persistent pulmonary hypertension of newborn, no dose recommendation. *Systemic sclerosis*, under 18 years, no data.

Hepatic Impairment: Moderate/severe, contraindicated.
CI: AST and/or ALT above 3xULN.
Interactions: Effect of Other Drugs on Bosentan: *Co-admin contraindicated**: Ciclosporin. *Co-admin not recommended**: Azole antifungals, tacrolimus, sirolimus, nevirapine. *Co-admin caution*: Sildenafil. *Plasma levels decreased*: Glibenclamide, rifampicin. *Increased (hepatotoxicity risk, haematological adverse events)**: Lopinavir + ritonavir, other boosted protease inhibitors. ***(plasma levels increased).

Effect of Bosentan on Other Drugs: Ciclosporin, glibenclamide, simvastatin: *Plasma levels reduced*. Coumarins (warfarin): *Monitor anticoagulant effect*. Oestrogen, progesterone (hormonal contraceptives): *Increased metabolism, possible contraceptive failure*.

SP: Initiate only if systemic systolic BP above 85mmHg. PAH (with HIV + antiretroviral treatment), cannot exclude increased long-term risk (hepatotoxicity, haematological adverse events). Pulmonary oedema, consider veno-occlusive disease. Fluid retention, monitor (weight gain).

Pregnancy, Lactation: Lactation, not recommended.

ADR: *Most frequent*, headache, oedema/fluid retention, elevated aminotransferases, anaemia, decreased Hb.

Notes: See 2.2.4 PAH, IPF.

Tracleer 62.5mg, 125mg *(Actelion)* A. HT.
Price, (56) 62.5mg, €2241.35. 125mg, €2348.88.
Tablet, bosentan monohydrate. Orange-white oval f/c. Marked with strength. 62.5mg: Round. 125mg: Oval. **Store:** Below 30 deg C (blisters).

Iloprost

ATC Code: B01AC11. **Sport:** Permitted.
Driving: Hypotension (dizziness) may seriously affect ability.
Indications: Treatment, adult primary pulmonary hypertension (NYHA Class III).

Dose: Adult, Elderly: Per inhalation, initially 2.5mcg delivered per mouthpiece of nebuliser, followed by 5mcg (second inhalation) 6-9 times daily; if poorly tolerated, reduce to 2.5mcg.

Child: Under 18 years, safety and efficacy not established.

Renal Impairment: CrCl (mL/min) 30 or less, as for Hepatic Impairment. Dialysis, cautious initial dose titration at 3-hourly intervals.

Hepatic Impairment: Initially, 2.5mcg at 3-4 hourly intervals; max. 6-times daily; if required titrate to 5mg at 3-4 hourly intervals.

CI: Effect on platelets might increase haemorrhage risk in active peptic ulcers, trauma, intracranial haemorrhage; severe coronary heart disease or unstable angina, MI within last 6 months, decompensated cardiac failure, severe arrhythmias, cerebrovascular events (TIA, stroke) within the last 3 months, pulmonary hypertension due to venous occlusive disease, congenital or acquired valvular defects with clinically relevant myocardial function disorders *not* related to pulmonary hypertension.

Interactions: Effect of Iloprost on Other Drugs: Vasodilators, other antihypertensives (ACEIs, AIIAs, adrenergic neurone blockers, alpha-blockers, beta-blockers, calcium channel blockers, diuretics, vasodilators): *Enhanced effect, hypotension risk*. Anticoagulants (heparin, coumarins), platelet aggregation inhibitors (acetylsalicylic acid, NSAIDs, ticlopidine, clopidogrel), glycoprotein IIb/IIIa antagonists (abciximab, eptifibatide, tirofiban): *Increased bleeding risk*.

SP: Unstable pulmonary hypertension with advanced right heart failure, systolic arterial hypotension below 85mmHg, not recommended. Syncope, acute pulmonary infections. Pulmonary bronchitis, severe asthma, COPD. Bronchospasm induction (especially with bronchial hyperactivity). Hypotension, pulmonary oedema; pulmonary vasodilators may worsen cardiovascular status in presence of pulmonary veno-occlusive disease. Avoid contact with skin/eyes or oral ingestion. Newborns, infants, pregnant women should not be subjected to *Ventavis* in room air.

Pregnancy, Lactation: Pregnancy, if benefit outweighs risk. Lactation, avoid.

ADR: *Very common*, bleeding events, headache, vasodilation, flushing, chest discomfort, cough, nausea, jaw pain/trismus, peripheral oedema.

Notes: See 2.2.4 PAH, IPF.

Ventavis Nebuliser Soln *(Bayer)* A. HT.
Price, 10mcg/mL (30) €500.76.
Nebuliser soln, iloprost trometamol 10mcg/mL. Clear colourless soln. *Ethanol 0.75mg/mL*.

Macitentan

ATC Code: C02KC04. **Sport:** Permitted.
Driving: Minor influence; headache, hypotension.
Indications: Long-term treatment (monotherapy or combination), PAH (WHO Class II, III).

Dose: Adult, Elderly: 10mg once daily. *Elderly*, over 75 years, caution. *Admin*, with or without food; swallow whole with water.

Child: Safety/efficacy not established.

Renal Impairment: Severe (with or without cirrhosis), contraindicated. Dialysis, not recommended.

Hepatic Impairment: Moderate, not recommended. Severe or AST/ALT above 3xULN, contraindicated.

Interactions: Effect of Other Drugs on Macitentan: *Co-admin avoid*: Strong CYP3A4 inducers (rifampicin, St John's Wort, carbamazepine, phenytoin). *Co-admin caution*: Strong CYP3A4 inhibitors (itraconazole, ketoconazole, voriconazole, clarithromycin, telithromycin, nefazodone, ritonavir, saquinavir).

SP: Monitor, LFTs prior to initiation; ALT, AST, signs of hepatic injury monthly; clinically relevant ALT/AST elevations or elevations with bilirubin above 2xULN or signs of liver injury (jaundice), discontinue. Severe anaemia, do not initiate; measure Hb prior to initiation then as needed. Monitor BP. Pulmonary oedema, consider pulmonary veno-occlusive disease.

Pregnancy, Lactation: Pregnancy, see Notes below; reliable contraception to be practised during and for 1 month after treatment. Lactation, contraindicated.

ADR: *Very common*, nasopharyngitis, bronchitis, headache, anaemia, oedema, fluid retention.

Notes: See 2.2.4 PAH, IPF.

▼ Opsumit 10mg *(Actelion)* A. HT.
Price, (30) €2811.37.
Tablet, macitentan. White (off-white) round f/c. Marked with strength. *Lactose, soya lecithin*. **Store:** Below 30 deg C.

2.2.4 Pulmonary Arterial Hypertension (PAH), Idiopathic Pulmonary Fibrosis (IPF)

Minoxidil (systemic)

ATC Code: C02DC01. **Sport:** Permitted.
Driving: Caution, especially at initiation (dizziness, fatigue, hypotension, decreased attention); alcohol co-admin.
Indications: Severe hypertension (symptomatic or with target organ damage), not controlled by combination (diuretic + sympathetic suppressant); not managed with (max. dose diuretic + two other antihypertensives). Not for use as sole agent.
Dose: *Adult: Hypertension*, initially 5mg/day (single or divided doses); if needed increase by 5-10mg at 3-day or more intervals to 20mg/day, then 40mg/day. If 50mg/day is reached, increase by 25mg/day to max. 100mg/day. Rapid BP reduction under hospital monitoring (continuous BP monitoring), increase by 5mg 6-hourly.
Elderly: Over 65 years, initially 2.5mg/day.
Child: 12 years and under (other treatment has failed), initially 0.2mg/kg (single or divided doses); if needed titrate at 3-day intervals by 0.1-0.2mg/kg/day; effective range 0.25-1mg/kg/day; max. 50mg/day.
Renal Impairment: Admin after or two hours before haemodialysis. Smaller doses may be required.
CI: Phaeochromocytoma.
Interactions: Effect of Minoxidil on Other Drugs: *Excessive BP reduction*: Guanethidine, bethanidine.
SP: Sodium and water retention. Not on dialysis, combine with diuretics e.g. hydrochlorothiazide, chlorthalidone, furosemide and/or restrict salt intake. Monitor bodyweight. Post MI, use minoxidil only after stable state established. Reflex tachycardia, angina pectoris may occur, use with beta-blocker. Hypertrichosis. ECG changes, thrombocytopenia, pericardial effusion, tamponade.
Pregnancy, Lactation: Pregnancy, women of childbearing potential not using contraception, not recommended. Lactation, stop breastfeeding or stop drug.
ADR: *Very common*, tachycardia, pericarditis, hypertrichosis, hair colour changes, abnormal ECG.
Notes: See 2.2.4 PAH, IPF.

▼ **Loniten 5mg** *(Pfizer)* B. GMS.
Price, (60) €16.25.
Tablet, minoxidil. White (light-tan) round scored (line has no function; do not break). Marked with strength; U either side of score on reverse. *Lactose*.

Nintedanib (pulmonary)

ATC Code: L01XE31. **Sport:** Permitted.
Driving: Minor influence; caution.
Indications: Treatment, Idiopathic Pulmonary Fibrosis (IPF).
Dose: Adult, Elderly: 150mg twice daily (12-hour intervals); 100mg twice daily only if 150mg twice daily is not tolerated; *Admin*, with food; swallow whole with water; do not crush or chew.
Child: Under 18 years, safety/efficacy not established.
Renal Impairment: Mild/moderate, no adjustment. CrCl (mL/min) under 30, not studied.
Hepatic Impairment: Mild, no adjustment; moderate/severe, not recommended.
CI: Peanut or soya hypersensitivity.
ADR: Summary, *most frequent*, diarrhoea, nausea, vomiting, abdominal pain, decreased (appetite, weight), increased liver enzymes.
Notes: See 13.1.6 Protein Kinase Inhibitors (nintedanib, oncology) for Interactions, SP and Pregnancy. See 2.2.4 PAH, IPF.

▼ **Ofev 100mg, 150mg** *(Boehringer)* A. HT.
Price, (60) 100mg, 150mg, €2733.17.
Soft capsule, nintedanib esilate. Opaque oblong soft gelatin. Marked with company symbol and strength. 100mg: Peach. 150mg: Brown. *Soya lecithin*. **Store:** Below 25 deg C; original pack to protect (moisture).

Riociguat

ATC Code: C02KX05. **Sport:** Pending.
Driving: Moderate influence (dizziness).
Indications: Adults with WHO Class II, III: Chronic thromboembolic pulmonary hypertension (CTEPH), inoperable or persistent or recurrent after surgical treatment; pulmonary arterial hypertension (PAH) (monotherapy or combination with ERA).
Dose: Adult: Initially 1mg 3-times daily (6-8 hours apart) for 2 weeks; increase by 0.5mg 3-times daily every 2 weeks to max. 2.5mg 3-times daily (if systolic BP is 95mmHg or above and no signs or symptoms of hypotension). If systolic BP drops below 95mmHg during titration, decrease by 0.5mg 3-times daily. Maintain on established individual dose unless hypotension occurs. *Admin*, with or without food; tabs may be crushed and mixed with water or soft food (e.g. apple sauce) and taken immediately; if prone to hypotension, not recommended to switch between fed or fasted intake. Treatment interruption for 3 days or more, restart at 1mg 3-times daily as above.
Smokers, advise to stop smoking due to risk of lower response; dose increase to max. 2.5mg 3-times daily may be needed if smoking or start smoking during treatment; dose decrease if smoking is stopped.
Elderly: Higher hypotension risk (caution during titration).
Child: Under 18 years, not recommended.
Renal Impairment: CrCl (mL/min) 30-50, as for Elderly; below 30, not recommended.
Hepatic Impairment: Moderate, as for Elderly above. Elevated aminotransferases (3xULN) or with elevated bilirubin (2xULN), not recommended. Severe, contraindicated.
CI: Systolic BP below 95mmHg at initiation.
Interactions: Effect of Other Drugs on Riociguat: *Co-admin contraindicated*: Nitrates, nitric oxide donors (amyl nitrite) in any form including recreational drugs (poppers), PDE-5 inhibitors (sildenafil, tadalafil, vardenafil). *Co-admin not recommended (increased riociguat exposure)*: Ketoconazole, itraconazole, ritonavir. *Co-admin caution (may increase exposure)*: Erlotinib, gefitinib, ciclosporin A. *Lower riociguat oral bioavailability*: Drugs increasing upper GI pH (dose antacids 2 hours before or 1 hour after riociguat). *Plasma levels decreased*: Bosentan, phenytoin, carbamazepine, phenobarbitone, St John's Wort). *Reduced exposure*: Cigarette smoking.
SP: Pulmonary veno-occlusive disease (PVOD), use of riociguat not recommended; signs of pulmonary oedema, possibly associated with PVOD, discontinue. Respiratory tract bleeding especially with anticoagulation therapy (monitor); *serious* and fatal in presence of risk factors (serious haemoptysis), assess risk/benefit of continued use. Hypotension risk, consider underlying conditions (on antihypertensives, resting hypotension, hypovolaemia, severe LV outflow obstruction, autonomic dysfunction).
Pregnancy, Lactation: Pregnancy, contraindicated; monthly pregnancy tests recommended. Women of childbearing potential to ensure adequate contraception. Lactation, stop breastfeeding during treatment.
ADR: Summary, *most common*, headache, dizziness, dyspepsia, peripheral oedema, nausea, diarrhoea, vomiting; *serious* haemoptysis, pulmonary haemorrhage (including fatal).
Notes: See 2.2.4 PAH, IPF.

▼ **Adempas Tablets** *(MSD)* A. HT.
Price, (42) 0.5mg, 1mg, 1.5mg, €1342.28; (84) 2mg, 2.5mg, €2683.51.
Tablet, Round. Marked with Bayer cross and strength; R on reverse. 0.5mg: White. 1mg: Pale-yellow. 1.5mg: Yellow-orange. 2mg: Pale-orange. 2.5mg: Red-orange. *Lactose*. **Store:** No special conditions.

Sildenafil (PAH)

ATC Code: G04BE03. **Sport:** Permitted.
Driving: Moderate influence (dizziness, altered vision).
Indications: Adult, pulmonary arterial hypertension (PAH) (WHO Class II, III); parenteral indicated if temporarily unable to take oral treatment. Age 1-17 years, primary PAH associated with congenital heart disease.
Dose: Adult, Elderly: 20mg orally with or without food OR 10mg IV as bolus injection 3-times daily. *Co-admin*, with CYP3A4 inhibitors (erythromycin, saquinavir), 20mg orally OR 10mg IV twice daily; with more potent CYP3A4 inhibitors (clarithromycin, telithromycin, nefazodone) 20mg orally or

10mg IV once daily. See Interactions below. Discontinuation, reduce gradually.

Child: ORAL, age 1-17 years, 20kg or under, 10mg 3-times daily; above 20kg, 20mg 3-times daily. PARENTERAL, under 18 years, not recommended.

Renal Impairment: CrCl (mL/min) below 30, no initial adjustment; reduce to 20mg orally or 10mg IV twice daily if not tolerated.

Hepatic Impairment: As for Renal above. Severe, contraindicated.

CI: Loss of vision in one eye due to non-arteritic anterior ischaemic optic neuropathy regardless of PDE-5 association. Recent history of stroke, MI; severe hypotension, BP below 90/50mmHg at initiation.

Interactions: Effect of Other Drugs on Sildenafil: *Co-admin contraindicated (hypotension)*: Nitric oxide donors (amyl nitrite), nitrates in any form including nicorandil, most potent CYP3A4 inhibitors (ketoconazole, itraconazole, ritonavir). *Co-admin caution*: IV epoprostenol, other pulmonary hypertension treatments (ambrisentan, iloprost), other PDE-5 inhibitors. *Caution, inhibitors (reduce clearance), inducers (increase clearance)*: P450(CYP) isoform (major route) and 2C9 (minor route). *Reduced clearance and/or increased oral bioavailability with co-admin*: CYP3A4 substrates and CYP3A4 substrates + beta-blockers. *Monitor efficacy*: CYP3A4 inducers (carbamazepine, phenytoin, phenobarbital, St John's Wort, rifampicin). *Decreased exposure*: Bosentan.

SP: Not recommended for use in PAH (severe, Class IV; related to primary idiopathic PAH; associated with connective tissue disease or congenital heart disease, secondary to sickle cell anaemia), other forms of PAH; known hereditary degenerative retinal disorders (*retinitis pigmentosa*). *Caution*, underlying conditions adversely affected by vasodilation (hypotension, fluid depletion, severe LV outflow obstruction, autonomic dysfunction), pre-existing cardiovascular risk factors (serious cardiovascular events reported), patients clinically or haemodynamically unstable, anatomical deformation of penis in males or conditions predisposing to priapism. In event of any sudden visual defect, discontinue immediately. Bleeding disorder or active peptic ulceration, careful benefit-risk assessment. Signs of pulmonary oedema, consider possible veno-occlusive disease.

Pregnancy, Lactation: Pregnancy, if strictly necessary. Women of childbearing potential to ensure adequate contraception. Lactation, not recommended.

ADR: *Very common*, headache, flushing, diarrhoea, dyspepsia, limb pain. See SP above.

Notes: See 2.2.4 PAH, IPF.

Interchangeability: Same strengths of all brands of sildenafil f/c tabs (20mg) listed below are deemed interchangeable.

Revatio 20mg, Oral Susp 10mg/mL *(Pfizer)* A. HT.
Price, (90) €254.26. Susp 10mg/mL (112mL) €281.18.
Tablet, sildenafil citrate. White round f/c. Marked Pfizer; RVT 20 on reverse. *Lactose*. **Store:** Below 30 deg C; original pack to protect (moisture).
Oral susp, as above. White (off-white) powder. *Sorbitol*. **Store:** Below 30 deg. Susp: Or refrigerate; do not freeze. Powder: Original pack to protect (moisture).
Revatio Parenteral *(Pfizer)* A.
Price, not published by company.
Injection, sildenafil 0.8mg/mL (20mL). Clear colourless soln. **Store:** No special conditions.
Granpidam 20mg *(Accord)* A. HT.
Price, (90) €203.41.
Tablet, sildenafil citrate. White (off-white) round. Marked 20. *Lactose*. **Store:** No special conditions.
Mysildecard 20mg *(Gerard)* A. HT.
Price, (90) €203.41.
Tablet, sildenafil citrate. White round f/c. Marked M; SL over 20 on reverse. **Store:** No special conditions.
Silcarfil 20mg *(Rowex)* A. HT.
Price, (90) €203.41.
Tablet, sildenafil citrate. White round f/c. Marked 20. **Store:** No special conditions.
Sildenafil Clonmel 20mg *(Clonmel)* A. HT.
Price, (90) €203.41.
Tablet, sildenafil citrate. Round f/c white. *Lactose*. **Store:** Original pack to protect (moisture).

Sildenafil TEVA 20mg *(TEVA)* A. HT.
Price, (90) €203.41.
Tablet, sildenafil citrate. White (off-white) round. Marked 20. **Store:** No special conditions.

Tadalafil (hypertension)

ATC Code: G04BE08. **Sport:** Permitted.
Driving: Negligible effect; dizziness.

Indications: Pulmonary arterial hypertension (PAH) (WHO Class II, III) (idiopathic; related to collagen vascular disease).

Dose: Adult, Elderly: 40mg once daily with or without food.

Child: Safety/efficacy not established.

Renal Impairment: Mild/moderate, initially 20mg once daily; titrate to 40mg/day based on efficacy and tolerability. Severe, not recommended.

Hepatic Impairment: Mild/moderate, initially 20mg once daily with caution. Severe, not recommended.

CI: See Notes below.

Interactions: Effect of Other Drugs on Tadalafil: *Co-admin contraindicated (hypotension)*: Organic nitrates, guanylate cyclase stimulators (riociguat). *Co-admin not recommended*: Other PDE-5 inhibitors, other alpha-blockers. *Co-admin caution*: Prostacyclin (or analogues). *Increased exposure*: Ketoconazole, ritonavir. *Decreased exposure*: Bosentan, rifampicin.

Effect of Tadalafil on Other Drugs: Doxazosin: *Increase hypotensive effect; co-admin not recommended*.

SP: Not recommended for use (aortic and mitral valve disease, pericardial constriction, restrictive or congestive cardiomyopathy, significant LVD, life-threatening arrhythmias, symptomatic CAD, uncontrolled hypertension, pulmonary veno-occlusive disease). Visual defects reported, retinal disorders. Cases of sudden hearing loss reported. Priapism reported; caution, use with anatomical deformity of penis or conditions predisposing to priapism. See Notes below.

Pregnancy, Lactation: Pregnancy, avoid. Lactation, not recommended.

ADR: *Very common*, headache, flushing, nasopharyngitis, nausea, dyspepsia, abdominal pain/discomfort, myalgia, back pain, extremity pain.

Notes: See Sildenafil above. See 2.2.4 PAH, IPF.

Adcirca 20mg *(Lilly)* A. HT.
Price, (56) €559.44.
Tablet, tadalafil. Orange almond-shaped f/c. Marked 4467. *Lactose*. **Store:** Below 30 deg C; original pack to protect (moisture).

2.2.5 - Peripheral Vascular Disorders

In This Chapter: *Cinnarizine, inositol nicotinate, naftidrofuryl.*

Class Effects

Cinnarizine is also used in the prevention and control of motion sickness.

SP: Not recommended for use in children.

Notes: See 2.2.4 Pulmonary Arterial Hypertension (PAH), Idiopathic Pulmonary Fibrosis (IPF). See also 3.8 Nausea and Vomiting, Vertigo, Motion Sickness (cinnarizine).

Cinnarizine (PVD)

ATC Code: N07CA02. **Sport:** Permitted.
Driving: Drowsiness.

Indications: Peripheral vascular disease (PVD), vasospastic disorders.

Dose: Adult, Elderly: PVD, 50-75mg two to 3-times daily. Oral, after meals.

Renal Impairment: Caution.

Hepatic Impairment: As for Renal above.

Interactions: Effect of Other Drugs on Cinnarizine: *Mutual sedative effect enhanced*: ALCOHOL (avoid), CNS depressants, TCADs.

SP: Epigastric discomfort (diminished if taken after food). Hypotension or CAD, caution (vasodilator). Parkinson's, use only if benefit outweighs risk of disease aggravation. Antihistamine effect may prevent otherwise positive

49

2.2.6 Miscellaneous Cardiac Preparations

reactions to dermal reactivity indicators if used up to 4 days prior to skin testing. Avoid using in porphyria.

Pregnancy, Lactation: Pregnancy, not advisable. Lactation, not recommended.

ADR: Common, somnolence.

Notes: See 2.2.5 Peripheral Vascular Disorders.

Stugeron 25mg (McNeil) B. GMS.
Price, (50) €4.44.
Tablet, cinnarizine. White. Marked Janssen; S/25 on reverse. Lactose, sucrose.

Inositol Nicotinate

ATC Code: C04AC03. **Sport:** Permitted.
Driving: Unlikely to impair.
Indications: Peripheral vascular disease (PVD), vasospastic disorders.

Dose: Adult, Elderly: 3g/day; if required titrate to 4g/day.

CI: Recent MI, acute phase of CVA.

SP: Cerebrovascular insufficiency.

Pregnancy, Lactation: Not recommended.

ADR: Flushing, dizziness, headache, nausea, vomiting, syncope, paraesthesia, rash, postural hypotension.

Notes: See 2.2.5 Peripheral Vascular Disorders.

Hexopal 500mg (Clonmel) B. GMS.
Price, (100) €21.89.
Tablet, inositol nicotinate. Round white scored. Marked with logo.

Naftidrofuryl

ATC Code: C04AX21. **Sport:** Permitted.
Driving: Unlikely to impair.
Indications: Peripheral vascular disease (PVD) with symptoms (intermittent claudication, cold extremities). Cerebral vascular disease to increase cerebral blood flow.

Dose: Adult, Elderly: 100-200mg 3-times daily. Caps to be swallowed whole during meals with sufficient water (to avoid oesophagitis).

Child: Not indicated for use.

Renal Impairment: Caution.

Hepatic Impairment: As for Renal above.

CI: Hyperoxaluria, recurrent calcium-containing stones.

Interactions: Effect of Naftidrofuryl on Other Drugs: Other Antihypertensives (ACEIs, AIIAs, adrenergic neurone blockers, alpha-blockers, beta-blockers, calcium channel blockers, diuretics, vasodilators): Enhanced effect, dose adjustment may be needed.

SP: Sufficient fluids should be taken to maintain adequate diuresis and to avoid development of calcium oxalate kidney stones.

Pregnancy, Lactation: Pregnancy, use not advised. Lactation, should not be used.

ADR: Nausea, epigastric pain, skin rash, insomnia. Hepatitis, calcium oxalate kidney stones.

Notes: See 2.2.5 Peripheral Vascular Disorders.

Praxilene 100mg (Merck Serono) B. GMS.
Price, (100) €11.36.
Capsule, naftidrofuryl hydrogen oxalate. Pale-pink hard gelatin. Marked Praxilene Lipha.

2.2.6 - Miscellaneous Cardiac Preparations

In This Chapter: Ivabradine, ranolazine, trimetazidine.

Class Effects
CI: Hypersensitivity to any member of the class.
SP: Not recommended for use in children under 18 years.

Ivabradine

ATC Code: C01EB17. **Sport:** Permitted.
Driving: Transient luminous phenomena, mainly phosphenes; consider night driving.
Indications: Treatment, chronic stable angina pectoris in adults with normal sinus rhythm (beta-blockers contraindicated or not tolerated). Chronic HF (NYHA II-IV) with systolic dysfunction, in sinus rhythm.

Dose: Adult: Chronic stable angina, initially 5mg twice daily; increase after 3-4 weeks, to 7.5mg twice daily if needed;

decrease 2.5mg twice daily if heart rate decreases persistently below 50 bpm at rest OR symptoms of bradycardia occur; persistent bradycardia below 50 bpm, discontinue.

Stable heart failure, initially 5mg twice daily; after 2 weeks titrate as for angina above. Heart rate is 50-60 bpm maintain 5mg twice daily. Admin, during meals.

Elderly: Age 75 years and over, initially 2.5mg twice daily.

Child: Under 18 years, safety/efficacy not established.

Renal Impairment: CrCl (mL/min) below 15, caution.

Hepatic Impairment: Moderate, caution. Severe, contraindicated.

CI: Resting heart rate below 60 bpm before treatment, cardiogenic shock, acute MI, severe hypotension (BP below 90/50mmHg), sick sinus syndrome, SA block, pacemaker dependant, unstable angina, third degree AV block.

Interactions: Effect of Other Drugs on Ivabradine: Co-admin contraindicated: Cytochrome CYP3A4 inhibitors (azole antifungals including ketoconazole, itraconazole; macrolides including oral clarithromycin and erythromycin, josamycin, telithromycin; HIV protease inhibitors including nelfinavir and ritonavir; nefazodone). Co-admin not recommended: Cardiovascular QT-prolonging drugs (quinidine, disopyramide, bepridil, sotalol, ibutilide, amiodarone), non-cardiovascular QT-prolonging drugs (pimozide, ziprasidone, sertindole, mefloquine, halofantrine, pentamidine, cisapride, erythromycin IV), heart rate reducing calcium channel blockers including verapamil and diltiazem. Plasma levels increased: CYP3A4 inhibitors, grapefruit juice. Plasma levels decreased: CYP3A4 inducers (rifampicin, barbiturates, phenytoin, St John's Wort).

SP: Not effective in cardiac arrhythmias; atrial fibrillation, cardiac arrhythmias interfering with sinus node function, second degree AV-block, post-stroke, not recommended. Do no initiate if resting heart rate is below 60 bpm. Chronic heart failure there is higher atrial fibrillation risk. Mild to moderate hypotension, congenital QT syndrome or treatment with QT prolonging drugs. Deterioration of visual function, consider cessation; patients with retinitis pigmentosa, caution.

Pregnancy, Lactation: Pregnancy and lactation, contraindicated. Women of childbearing potential to ensure adequate contraception.

ADR: Summary, most common, luminous phenomena (phosphenes) and bradycardia (dose dependent).

Notes: See 2.2.6 Miscellaneous Cardiac Preparations.

▼ **Procoralan 5mg, 7.5mg** (Servier) B. GMS.
Price, (56) 5mg, €46.15. 7.5mg, €46.26.
Tablet, ivabradine HCl. Salmon-coloured f/c scored. Marked with strength and triangle logo. 5mg: Oblong. Divisible into equal halves. 7.5mg: Triangular. Lactose.

Ranolazine

ATC Code: C01EB18. **Sport:** Permitted.
Driving: Dizziness, blurred vision, diplopia, confusional state, abnormal co-ordination, hallucination.
Indications: Add-on, treatment of stable angina pectoris not controlled by or intolerant to first-line anti-anginals.

Dose: Adult: Initially 375mg twice daily; titrate to 500mg twice daily after 2-4 weeks; if needed increase to max. 750mg twice daily. If not tolerated decrease; if symptoms do not resolve, discontinue. Co-admin, with simvastatin, max. simvastatin 20mg/day. Admin, swallow tabs whole; do not crush, break or chew; with or without food.

Elderly: Titrate with caution.

Renal Impairment: CrCl (mL/min) 30-80, titrate carefully; 30 or below, contraindicated.

Hepatic Impairment: Mild, titrate carefully. Moderate/severe, contraindicated.

Interactions: Effect of Other Drugs on Ranolazine: Co-admin contraindicated: Potent CYP3A4 inhibitors (itraconazole, ketoconazole, voriconazole, posaconazole, HIV protease inhibitors, clarithromycin, telithromycin, nefazodone), antiarrhythmics Class Ia (quinidine), Class III (dofetilide, sotalol) other than amiodarone. Careful dose titration with co-admin: Moderate CYP3A4 inhibitors (diltiazem, fluconazole, erythromycin), P-gp inhibitors (verapamil, ciclosporin). *Expected lack of efficacy with co-admin*: CYP3A4 inducers (rifampicin, phenytoin, phenobarbital, carbamazepine, St John's Wort). *Theoretical risk (ventricular arrhythmia)*: Drugs prolonging QTc interval including certain antihistamines (terfenadine, astemizole, mizolastine), antiarrhythmics (quinidine, disopyramide, procainamide), erythromycin, TCADs (imipramine, doxepin, amitriptyline).

Effect of Ranolazine on Other Drugs: P-gp, CYP3A4 sensitive substrates (simvastatin, see dose; lovastatin, atorvastatin) and CYP3A4 substrates with narrow therapeutic range (ciclosporin, tacrolimus, sirolimus, everolimus): *May increase plasma concentrations, monitor.* CYP2D6 substrates (TCADs, antipsychotics): *Exposure may be increased.* CYP2B6 substrates (bupropion, efavirenz, cyclophosphamide): *Caution with co-admin.* Digoxin, statins, metformin: *Plasma levels increased* (monitor digoxin levels).

SP: Elderly, low body weight (60kg or below), increased adverse event incidence, moderate/severe CHF (NYHA Class III-IV), titrate with caution. QTc prolongation, caution.

Pregnancy, Lactation: Pregnancy, use only if clearly necessary. Lactation, not recommended.

ADR: *Common,* dizziness, headache, constipation, vomiting, nausea, asthenia.

Notes: See 2.2.6 Miscellaneous Cardiac Preparations.

Ranexa 375mg, 500mg, 750mg *(A.Menarini)* A. GMS.
Price, (60) 375mg, €55.61; 500mg, 750mg, €55.61.
Prolonged/R tablet, ranolazine. Oval. Marked with strength. 375mg: Pale-blue. 500mg: Light-orange. 750mg: Pale-green. *Lactose* (750mg). **Store:** No special conditions.

Trimetazidine

ATC Code: C01EB15. **Sport:** Prohibited.
Driving: Dizziness, drowsiness.

Indications: Add-on therapy (adults), symptomatic treatment of stable angina pectoris, inadequately controlled or intolerant to first-line antianginal therapies.

Dose: Adult, Elderly: 20mg 3-times daily during meals. *Elderly,* as for Renal below.

Renal Impairment: CrCl (mL/min) 30-60, 20mg twice daily (morning, evening during meals); below 30, contraindicated.

CI: Parkinson's disease, Parkinsonian symptoms, tremors, RLS, other movement disorders.

SP: Not for initial treatment, angina/MI; not for use in pre-hospital phase or during first days of hospitalisation. Can cause or worsen Parkinsonism symptoms (tremor, akinesia, hypertonia), especially in elderly; occurrence of movement disorders, withdraw. Falls related to gait instability or hypotension especially with antihypertensives. Caution, where increased exposure expected (renal impairment, elderly over 75 years).

Pregnancy, Lactation: Pregnancy, avoid. Lactation, not recommended.

ADR: *Common,* dizziness, headache, abdominal pain, diarrhoea, dyspepsia, nausea, vomiting, rash, pruritus, urticaria, asthenia.

Notes: See 2.2.6 Miscellaneous Cardiac Preparations.

Vastarel 20mg *(Servier)* B. GMS.
Price, (90) €9.00.
Tablet, trimetazidine dihydrochloride. Red f/c. *Ponceau 4R, Sunset Yellow, mannitol.*

2.3 - Lipid Regulating Drugs

Class Effects
The principal groups of lipid regulating drugs are statins, fibrates, anion exchange resins (bile-acid sequestrants), nicotinic acid, omega-3-acid ethyl esters and ezetimibe. All should be used adjunctive to cholesterol-lowering dietary measures.

CI: Hypersensitivity to any member of the class.

2.3.1 - Anion Exchange Resins

In This Chapter: *Colesevelam, colestyramine.*

Class Effects
Bile acid sequestrants combine with intestinal bile acids to form an insoluble complex excreted in faeces. Increased faecal loss of bile acids leads to increased oxidation of cholesterol to bile acids resulting in decreased LDL-cholesterol.

Notes: See 2.3 Lipid Regulating Drugs.

Colesevelam

ATC Code: C10AC04. **Sport:** Permitted.
Driving: Unlikely to impair.

Indications: Primary hypercholesterolaemia (combination with a statin to provide additive LDL-cholesterol reduction). Adults with familial hypercholesterolaemia (with ezetimibe, with or without a statin). Monotherapy, elevated total cholesterol and LDL-cholesterol (statin inappropriate or not tolerated).

Dose: Adult, Elderly: *Monotherapy,* 6 tabs/day; max. 7 tabs/day. *Combination,* with statin, with or without ezetimibe, 4-6 tabs/day; max. 6 tabs/daily. 1 or 2 divided doses with/without food.

Child: Not recommended.

CI: Bowel or biliary obstruction.

Interactions: Effect of Other Drugs on Colesevelam: *Decreased colesevelam exposure*: Olmesartan (admin minimum 4 hours apart).

Effect of Colesevelam on Other Drugs: Ciclosporin: *Bioavailability reduced.* Fat soluble vitamins (A, D, E, K), oral contraceptive, levothyroxine, glibenclamide, glimepiride, glipizide, ursodeoxycholic acid: *Delayed or reduced absorption; other drugs should be admin 1 hour before or 4-6 hours after colesevelam (monitor patients on warfarin or similar anticoagulants).* Phenytoin: *Levels reduced.* Metformin (extended release): *Exposure increased.*

SP: Prior to initiation diagnose and/or treat secondary hypercholesterolaemia (poorly controlled diabetes mellitus, hypothyroidism, nephrotic syndrome, dysproteinaemias, obstructive liver disease). Triglyceride levels above 3.4 mmoL/L, caution due to triglyceride increasing effect. Caution, dysphagia, swallowing disorders, severe GI motility disorders, inflammatory bowel disease, liver failure, major GI tract surgery. May induce or worsen constipation.

Pregnancy, Lactation: Pregnancy, lactation, caution.

ADR: Summary, *most frequent,* flatulence, constipation.

Notes: See 2.3.1 Anion Exchange Resins.

Cholestagel 625mg *(Genzyme)* B. GMS.
Price, (180) €130.71.
Tablet, colesevelam HCl. Off-white cap-shaped f/c. Marked C625. **Store:** Tightly closed to protect (moisture).

Colestyramine

ATC Code: C10AC01. **Sport:** Permitted.
Driving: None known.

Indications: Reduction of plasma cholesterol in hypercholesterolaemia, particularly Fredrickson's Type II (high plasma cholesterol, normal or slightly elevated triglycerides). Relief of pruritus associated with (partial biliary obstruction, primary biliary cirrhosis), diarrhoea associated with (ileal resection, Crohn's disease, vagotomy, diabetic vagal neuropathy). Management, radiation-induced diarrhoea.

Dose: Adult, Elderly: *Hypercholesterolaemia, diarrhoea,* usually 12-24g (3-6 sachets) in 1-4 divided doses; max. 36g/day (9 sachets). If diarrhoea is induced by bile acid malabsorption and no response within 3 days, initiate alternative.

Pruritus, usually 4-8g/day (1-2 sachets); doses above 24g/day may interfere with normal fat absorption.

Not to be taken in dry form; mix with water or thin soup or pulpy fruit.

Child: Calculation for age 6-12 years, Dose=(Weight in kg) multiplied by (Adult Dose) divided by 70. Infants, children under 6 years, no data. Admin, as for Adult above.

CI: Complete biliary obstruction

Interactions: Effect of Colestyramine on Other Drugs:

2.3.2 Ezetimibe

Digitalis, tetracycline, chlorothiazide, warfarin, thyroxin, fat soluble vitamins (A, D, E, K): *Delayed or reduced absorption; other drugs should be admin 1 hour before or 4-6 hours after colestyramine*. Drugs undergoing enterohepatic recirculation: *Altered pharmacokinetics*.

SP: Children with familial hypercholesterolaemia, reduced serum folate levels. Interferes with absorption of fat soluble vitamins; increased bleeding tendency associated with Vitamin K deficiency. Hyperchloraemic acidosis with prolonged use.

Pregnancy, Lactation: No data.

ADR: *Most common*, constipation. See SP above.

Notes: See 2.3.1 Anion Exchange Resins.

Questran Powder Sachet 4g *(BMS)* B. GMS.
Price, (50) €20.52.
Sachet, colestyramine. Fine homogeneous cream (buff) powder for oral susp. Reconstitution with 150mL fluid forms uniform susp. *Sucrose* 3.79g/sachet.

2.3.2 - Ezetimibe

In This Chapter: *Ezetimibe*.

Class Effects
Ezetimibe selectively inhibits intestinal absorption of cholesterol and related plant sterols.

CI: Active liver disease, unexplained persistent elevations in serum transaminases.

Interactions: Effect of Other Drugs on Ezetimibe: *Co-admin caution*: Fibrates. *Decreased absorption*: Antacids (not clinically significant), colestyramine. *Plasma levels increased*: Ciclosporin (especially with renal impairment).

SP: Myopathy, rhabdomyolysis reported, usually with statins. Elevated liver enzymes (statin combinations). Cholelithiasis suspected, discontinue (fibrate combinations). Pre-disposing factors for rhabdomyolysis (renal impairment, hypothyroidism, hereditary muscular disorders, previous liver disease or substantial quantities of alcohol consumed, elderly over 70 years, situations where increased plasma levels may occur); measure CPK levels before initiation and if elevated (above 5xULN), do not initiate.

Pregnancy, Lactation: Ezetimibe monotherapy, use in pregnancy, if benefit outweighs risk; lactation, not recommended. Statin co-admin or fixed combinations with statins, contraindicated; women of childbearing potential to ensure adequate contraception.

ADR: *Commonly*, abdominal pain, diarrhoea, flatulence, fatigue *Statin co-admin*, increased ALT/AST, headache. *Fibrate co-admin*, abdominal pain.

Notes: See 2.3 Lipid Regulating Drugs. Statin combinations, see 2.3.5 Statins.

Ezetimibe

ATC Code: C10AX09. **Sport:** Permitted.
Driving: Dizziness.

Indications: Primary hypercholesterolaemia (with statin or monotherapy), homozygous familial hypercholesterolaemia (HoFH), homozygous sitosterolaemia (phytosterolaemia), adjunctive. Prevention of cardiovascular events (reduction of risk in coronary heart disease, acute coronary syndrome), adjunctive with statin.

Dose: Adult, Elderly: 10mg daily; prevention, 10mg/day with statin with proven cardiovascular benefit. *Co-admin*, admin ezetimibe minimum 2 hours before of 4 hours after bile acid sequestrants; statin co-admin, see individual statins for appropriate dose. *Admin*, with or without food, any time of day.

Child: Age 6-17 years, safety and efficacy not established, no dose recommendation; under 6 years, no data. Use only under specialist review.

Hepatic Impairment: Moderate or severe, not recommended.

SP: Safety and efficacy when co-admin with simvastatin above 40mg/day, age 10-17 years, no data.

ADR: *Common*, *monotherapy*, abdominal pain, diarrhoea, flatulence, fatigue; additional with *statin co-admin*, increased ALT and/or AST, headache, myalgia.

Notes: See 2.3.2 Ezetimibe.
Ezetrol 10mg *(MSD)* B. GMS.
Price, (28) €35.54.
Tablet, ezetimibe. White (off-white) cap-shaped. Marked 414. *Lactose*.

2.3.3 - Fibrates

In This Chapter: *Fenofibrate, gemfibrozil*.

Class Effects
For information regarding statin co-admin, see Notes below (statins).

CI: Biliary cirrhosis, severe hepatic or renal impairment, gall bladder disease, photoallergy or phototoxic reaction to ketoprofen.

Interactions: Effect of Fibrates on Other Drugs: Oral Anti-Coagulants: *Increased bleeding risk*. Statins, other fibrates: *Muscle toxicity risk (co-admin not recommended)*.

SP: Monitor liver function (transaminases). Increased risk of pancreatitis, muscle disorders with predisposing factors for rhabdomyolysis (over 70 years, history of muscular disorders, renal impairment, hypoalbuminaemia, hypothyroidism, high alcohol intake). Statin co-admin not recommended unless benefit outweighs risk.

Pregnancy, Lactation: Pregnancy, use only after careful benefit/risk assessment. Lactation, not recommended.

Notes: See 2.3 Lipid Regulating Drugs. See 2.3.5 Statins.

Fenofibrate

ATC Code: C10AB05. **Sport:** Permitted.
Driving: No or negligible effect.

Indications: Severe hypertriglyceridaemia (with or without low HDL-cholesterol), mixed hyperlipidaemia when statin contraindicated or not tolerated; high cardiovascular risk in addition to statin when triglycerides and HDL-cholesterol not adequately controlled.

Dose: Adult: *Micro*, 200mg/day as 1x200mg cap or 3x67mg caps (the dose can be titrated to 267mg/day as 4x67mg caps) OR *Supra*, 145mg once daily. *Admin*, during a meal; swallow whole.

Elderly: No renal impairment, as for Adult.

Child: Under 18 years, *Micro*, not recommended; *Supra*, contraindicated.

Renal Impairment: *Micro*, CrCl (mL/min) 20-60, 1x 67mg caps; 10-20, no dose recommendation. Creatinine above 50% ULN, interrupt treatment. Measure creatinine during first 3 months after initiation, then periodically. Severe, contraindicated.

Hepatic Impairment: Not recommended.

CI: Chronic or acute pancreatitis (exception, if due to severe hypertriglyceridaemia). Known gallbladder disease. Known photoallergy, phototoxicity.

Interactions: Effect of Fenofibrate on Other Drugs: Ciclosporin: *Renal impairment risk*. Co-admin of CYP2C19, CYP2A6, especially CYP2C9 metabolised drugs with narrow therapeutic index: *Consider dose adjustment*. Oral Anti-Coagulants: *Co-admin not recommended; if needed, reduce dose to about one-third at start of treatment; gradually adjust according to INR*. Glitazones: *Reversible paradoxical HDL-cholesterol reduction with co-admin*.

SP: Treat secondary causes of hypercholesterolaemia before initiation. *Liver Function*, monitor transaminases every 3 months during first year, then periodically. ASAT/ALAT above 3xULN, discontinue. Symptoms of hepatitis, discontinue. Pancreatitis.

ADR: *Common*, abdominal pain, nausea, vomiting, diarrhoea, flatulence, increased transaminases. See SP above.

Notes: See 2.3.3 Fibrates.
Lipantil Micro, Supra *(BGP)* B. GMS.
Price, Micro 67mg (90) €13.75. 200mg (30) €9.24. Supra 145mg (30) €8.07.
Capsule (Micro), fenofibrate 67mg, 200mg. Micronised. Hard gelatin. 67mg: Yellow. 200mg: Ochre. *Lactose*.
Tablet (Supra), fenofibrate 145mg. Nanoparticles. White oblong f/c. Marked 145; logo on reverse. *Sucrose, lactose, soy lecithin*.

Gemfibrozil

ATC Code: C10AB04. **Sport:** Permitted.
Driving: Caution.
Indications: Mixed dyslipidaemia, primary hypercholesterolaemia, primary prevention in males with increased non-HDL cholesterol and at high risk for first cardiovascular event.
Dose: Adult, Elderly: Range, 900mg as single dose to 600mg twice daily. Oral, before breakfast and half hour before evening meal.
Child: Not recommended.
Renal Impairment: CrCl (ml/min) 30-80, initially 900mg/day; below 30, not recommended.
Hepatic Impairment: Contraindicated.
Interactions: Effect of Other Drugs on Gemfibrozil: Co-admin contraindicated: Simvastatin, dasabuvir, repaglinide. Reduced bioavailability: Bile acid sequestrants, admin 2 hours apart. Increased myopathy and rhabdomyolysis risk: Colchicine.
Effect of Gemfibrozil on Other Drugs: Repaglinide (contraindicated), rosiglitazone (co-admin caution), hypoglycaemic agents (oral, insulin): Increased plasma levels, hypoglycaemic reactions. Bexarotene: Co-admin not recommended. Coumarin type vitamin K antagonist anticoagulants (warfarin, acenocoumarol, phenprocoumon): Caution, careful prothrombin time (INR) monitoring; anticoagulant dose may need reduction.
SP: Gallstone formation, cholelithiasis. Monitor serum lipids, blood count.
ADR: Very common, dyspepsia. Common, vertigo, headache, diarrhoea, vomiting, nausea, abdominal pain, constipation, flatulence, eczema, rash, fatigue.
Notes: See 2.3.3 Fibrates.

Lopid 300mg, 600mg *(Pfizer)* B. GMS.
Price, 300mg (100) €27.70. 600mg (56) €15.84.
Capsule, gemfibrozil. Hard gelatin white/maroon contains white powder. Marked Lopid 300.
Tablet, as above. White f/c elliptical.

2.3.4 - Omega-3-Fatty Acids

In This Chapter: Eicosapentaenoic acid (EPA), Docosahexaenoic acid (DHA).

Class Effects
Omega-3-fatty acids include omega-3-acid ethyl esters and omega-3-marine triglycerides.
CI: Hypersensitivity to any member of the class.
Notes: See 2.3 Lipid Regulating Drugs.

EPA, DHA

ATC Code: C10AX06. **Sport:** Permitted.
Driving: No or negligible effect.
Indications: Hypertriglyceridaemia as monotherapy (type IV) or combination with statins (type IIb/III) when insufficient control of triglycerides. Adjunctive, secondary prevention post-MI.
Dose: Adult, Elderly: Hypertriglyceridaemia, initially 2 caps/day; if required titrate to 4 caps/day. Post-MI, 1 cap/day. Elderly, over 70 years, limited data. Oral, with food.
Child: No data.
Renal Impairment: Caution.
Hepatic Impairment: Monitor ALAT/ASAT levels, especially at high doses.
Interactions: Effect of Omega-3-Acid Ethyl Esters on Other Drugs: Oral anti-coagulants, drugs affecting coagulation (aspirin, cephalosporins): Increased bleeding risk. Fibrates: Co-admin, no data.
SP: High haemorrhage risk patients.
Pregnancy, Lactation: Pregnancy, if benefit outweighs risk. Lactation, generally not recommended.
ADR: Common, abdominal distention/pain, constipation, diarrhoea, dyspepsia, flatulence, eructation, GORD, nausea, vomiting.
Notes: See 2.3.4 Omega-3-Fatty Acids.

Omega-3-Fatty Acids

Omacor 1000mg *(BGP)* B.
Price, (28) €17.77.
Capsule, EPA 460mg, DHA 380mg. Soft oblong transparent gelatin contains pale-yellow oil. Soy lecithin.

2.3.5 - Statins, Statin Combinations

In This Chapter: Atorvastatin (and combinations), fluvastatin, pravastatin, rosuvastatin, simvastatin (and combinations).

Class Effects
Statins (HMG-CoA Reductase Inhibitors) lower plasma cholesterol and lipoprotein serum levels by inhibiting HMG-CoA reductase and cholesterol biosynthesis in the liver. Ezetimibe inhibits intestinal cholesterol absorption.
Indications: Statin monotherapy, adjunctive to standard cholesterol lowering diet when response to diet and non-pharmacological treatments (exercise, weight reduction) and/or other treatment inadequate. Ezetimibe/statin fixed combinations, primary heterozygous familial and non-familial hypercholesterolaemia or mixed hyperlipidaemia, not adequately controlled with statin alone, already treated with a statin and ezetimibe. Homozygous Familial Hypercholesterolaemia (HoFH), adjunct to diet and other treatments (LDL apheresis).
CI: Children under 18 years unless otherwise specified. Active liver disease, impaired liver function, unexplained persistent serum transaminase elevations above 3xULN; myopathy, cholestasis.
Interactions: Effect of Other Drugs on Statins: Co-admin not recommended (caution): Macrolides (erythromycin, clarithromycin, telithromycin), azole antifungals (itraconazole, ketoconazole), HIV protease inhibitors, nefazodone; systemic fusidic acid (or within 7 days of stopping fusidic acid; rhabdomyolysis including fatal, see SP below). Co-admin avoid (caution): Fibrates, niacin*. Increased myopathy risk, adjust dose: Ciclosporin, danazol, fibric acid derivatives, fibrates (fenofibrate, gemfibrozil), amiodarone, verapamil, niacin*, nicotinic acid, other statins, ezetimibe, grapefruit juice (avoid). Plasma levels decreased: Colestyramine, colestipol, (ensure 4-hour dosing interval), antacids (magnesium, aluminium salts). *Lipid-lowering dose of 1g/day or above.
Effect of Statins on Other Drugs: Digoxin, warfarin: Monitor INR.
SP: Elevated liver enzymes, monitor; if ALT and AST exceed 3xULN, discontinue. Caution, liver disease, excessive ALCOHOL intake or history of liver disease; fatal/non-fatal hepatic failure reported.
Before treatment, measure creatine kinase if there are pre-disposing factors for rhabdomyolysis e.g. renal impairment, hypothyroidism, history of hereditary muscular disorders, muscular toxicity with statin or fibrate, liver disease, Asian patients, fibrate co-admin, substantial alcohol intake/abuse, age over 65 years (if CPK above 5xULN do not initiate), female gender, major surgery, sepsis, hypotension, excessive muscle exercise, severe metabolic, endocrine or electrolyte disorders. Pre-disposing factors present, prescribe with caution.
While on treatment, myopathy (muscular pain, weakness, cramps), CPK above 5xULN, rhabdomyolysis, discontinue; higher incidence at 80mg dose. Tendinopathy sometimes complicated by tendon rupture with some statins.
Co-admin, fibrates, amiodarone, verapamil, fusidic acid, amlodipine, diltiazem, increased myopathy and/or rhabdomyolysis risk. Statin treatment should be discontinued during fusidic acid treatment; reports of rhabdomyolysis (including fatalities); re-introduce statin seven days after last fusidic acid dose. Statin/niacin combination not recommended in Chinese patients.
Interstitial lung disease, with long-term treatment; signs/symptoms (dyspnoea, non-productive cough, fatigue, weight loss, fever); if suspected, discontinue.
Diabetes, evidence suggests statins as a class raise blood glucose. Fasting glucose 5.6-6.9mmol/L, BMI above 30kg/m2, raised triglycerides, hypertension, monitor.
Immune-mediated necrotising myopathy (IMNM) reported rarely during or after statin treatment.

53

2.3.5   Statins, Statin Combinations

In exceptional circumstances where prolonged systemic fusidic acid is needed (severe infection), the need for statin and fusidic co-admin should be considered on a case by case basis and under close medical supervision.

Pregnancy, Lactation: Contraindicated, including women of child-bearing potential not using appropriate contraception. Cholesterol and other products of cholesterol biosynthesis are essential for foetal development; potential risk of HMG-CoA reductase inhibition outweighs advantage of treatment during pregnancy.

ADR: *Commonly*, nasopharyngitis, allergic reactions, hyperglycaemia, headache, dizziness, pharyngolaryngeal pain, epistaxis, constipation, flatulence, dyspepsia, nausea, diarrhoea, myalgia, arthralgia, extremity pain, muscle spasm, joint swelling, back pain, asthenia, diabetes mellitus (depending on presence of risk factors); abnormal LFTs, increased creatine kinase.

Notes: See 2.3 Lipid Regulating Drugs. See 2.3.2 Ezetimibe.

Atorvastatin

ATC Code: C10AA05. **Sport:** Permitted.
Driving: Unlikely to impair.

Indications: Primary hypercholesterolaemia, including heterozygous familial and homozygous familial hypercholesterolaemia (HoFH), mixed hyperlipidaemia (Fredrickson Types IIa, IIb). Prevention, cardiovascular disease (adults) at high risk for first cardiovascular event.

Dose: Adult, Elderly: *Primary hypercholesterolaemia, mixed hyperlipidaemia, cardiovascular disease prevention,* usually 10mg/day.

Heterozygous familial hypercholesterolaemia, initially 10mg/day; titrate at 4-week intervals to 40mg/day; max. 80mg/day or add a bile acid sequestrant combined with 40mg dose. *HoFH*, up to 80mg/day.

Dose adjustments for co-admin (tipranavir, telaprevir, ciclosporin; max. atorvastatin 10mg/day), (lopinavir/ritonavir, clarithromycin; use lower atorvastatin maintenance; above 20mg atorvastatin*), (saquinavir, darunavir, itraconazole, fosamprenavir/ritonavir; use lower maintenance; above 40mg atorvastatin*), diltiazem, erythromycin, rifampicin, gemfibrozil, fenofibrate; dose* initiation or change). *Clinical monitoring required.

Admin, once daily at any time of the day, with or without food; avoid co-admin with grapefruit juice.

Child: *Hypercholesterolaemia,* age 10 years and above, 10mg/day; increase to 80mg/day, adjusting at 4-week or more intervals *(Lipitor, Atorvastatin Pfizer)* OR titrate to 20mg/day (about 0.5mg/kg) *(all other brands).* Under 10 years, not recommended. *Admin,* as for Adult above.

Hepatic Impairment: Moderate/severe, drug exposure increased; caution with substantial alcohol consumption and/or liver disease.

Interactions: Effect of Other Drugs on Atorvastatin: *Co-admin not recommended:* Grapefruit juice. *Increased plasma levels (increased myopathy risk), avoid:* Potent CYP3A4 inhibitors or transport proteins (ciclosporin, telithromycin, clarithromycin, delavirdine, stiripentol, ketoconazole, voriconazole, itraconazole, posaconazole, ritonavir, lopinavir, atazanavir, indinavir, darunavir); moderate CYP3A4 inhibitors (erythromycin, diltiazem, verapamil, fluconazole). *Co-admin caution:* Colchicine. *Increased myopathy risk:* Gemfibrozil, other fibric acid derivatives, boceprevir, erythromycin, niacin, ezetimibe, telaprevir, tipranavir/ritonavir combination. *Variable plasma concentrations:* CYP3A4 inducers (efavirenz, rifampicin, St John's Wort). *Possible increased exposure risk:* Verapamil, amiodarone. See Dose above.

Effect of Atorvastatin on Other Drugs: Oral contraceptives (norethisterone, ethinyl oestradiol): *Increased plasma levels.* Warfarin, digoxin: *Monitor closely.*

SP: Perform LFTs prior to initiation, then periodically; see Notes below. Risk factors predisposing to renal failure secondary to rhabdomyolysis (severe acute infection, hypotension, major surgery, trauma, severe metabolic, endocrine and electrolyte disorders, uncontrolled seizures), discontinue. Prior haemorrhagic stroke/lacunar

infarct, risk/benefit of atorvastatin 80mg uncertain; carefully consider potential haemorrhagic stroke risk before initiating. Paediatrics, no clinical significant effect on growth and sexual maturation observed.

ADR: *Common,* nasopharyngitis, allergic reactions, hyperglycaemia, headache, pharyngolaryngeal pain, epistaxis, constipation, flatulence, dyspepsia, nausea, diarrhoea, myalgia, arthralgia, extremity pain, muscle spasm, joint swelling, back pain, abnormal LFTs, increased creatine kinase.

Notes: See 2.3.5 Statins.

Interchangeability: Same strengths of all brands of atorvastatin film-coated (f/c) tabs listed below are deemed interchangeable. Exception, *Lipitor Chewable.*

Reference Price: (28) 10mg, €2.52. 20mg, €3.36. 40mg, €4.76. 80mg, €7.84.

Lipitor Tablets, Chewable *(Pfizer)* B. GMS.
Price, (28) 10mg, €3.47; 20mg, €5.46; 40mg, €9.14; 80mg, €10.53. Chewable (30) 10mg, €17.82. 20mg, €33.70.
F/c tablet, atorvastatin calcium trihydrate 10mg, 20mg, 40mg, 80mg. White round. Marked ATV/strength. *Lactose.* **Store:** No special conditions.
Chewable tab, as above 10mg, 20mg. White (off-white) with pink (purple) specks, round. Marked strength and LCT. *Aspartame.* **Store:** No special conditions.

Atorvas 10mg, 20mg, 40mg, 80mg *(Rowex)* B. GMS.
Price, (28), see reference price above.
F/c tablet, atorvastatin calcium. Light-yellow dappled glossy. Marked HLA/strength. 10mg, 20mg, 40mg: Round. 80mg: Oval.

Atorvastatin (Dexcel) Tablets *(Dexcel)* B. GMS.
Price, (28), see reference price above.
F/c tablet, atorvastatin calcium hemihydrate 10mg, 20mg, 40mg. White. 10mg, 20mg: Round. 40mg: Cap-shaped.

Atorvastatin (Pinewood) Tablets *(Pinewood)* B. GMS.
Price, (28), see reference price above.
F/c tablet, atorvastatin calcium trihydrate 10mg, 20mg, 40mg, 80mg. White oval. Marked with strength.

Atorvastatin Actavis Tablets *(Accord)* B. GMS.
Price, (28), see reference price above. 80mg, €7.84; (100) 10mg, €9.00; 20mg, €12.00; 40mg, €17.00.
F/c tablet, atorvastatin calcium 10mg, 20mg, 40mg, 80mg. White oval. Marked A; strength on reverse.

Atorvastatin Clonmel Tablets *(Clonmel)* B. GMS.
Price, (28), see reference price above.
F/c tablet, atorvastatin calcium trihydrate 10mg, 20mg, 40mg, 80mg. White (off-white) round. *Lactose.*

Atorvastatin Krka Tablets *(Krka)* B. GMS.
Price, (28), see reference price above.
F/c tablet, atorvastatin calcium 10mg, 20mg, 40mg, 80mg. White. 10mg, 20mg, 40mg. Round. 80mg: Cap-shaped. *Lactose.*

Atorvastatin Mylan Tablets *(Gerard)* B. GMS.
Price, (28), see reference price above.
F/c tablet, atorvastatin calcium 10mg, 20mg, 40mg, 80mg. White oval scored (except 10mg) (facilitates breaking). Marked with strength. *Lactose.* **Store:** Original pack to protect (light, moisture).

Atorvastatin Pfizer Tablets *(Pfizer)* B. GMS.
Price, (30) see reference price above. 80mg, €8.40.
F/c tablet, atorvastatin calcium trihydrate 10mg, 20mg, 40mg, 80mg. White round. Marked ATV/strength. *Lactose.* **Store:** No special conditions.

Atorvastatin TEVA Tablets *(TEVA)* B. GMS.
Price, (28), see reference price above.
F/c tablet, atorvastatin calcium 10mg, 20mg, 40mg, 80mg. White (off-white) elliptic smooth f/c.

Torvacol 10mg, 20mg, 40mg, 80mg *(Clonmel)* B. GMS.
Price, (28), see reference price above.
F/c tablet, atorvastatin calcium. White (off-white) scored (facilitates breaking). 10mg: Round. 20mg, 40mg: Oval. 80mg: Oblong. *Lactose.*

Acetylsalicylic Acid, Atorvastatin, Ramipril

ATC Code: C10BX06. **Sport:** Permitted.
Driving: Ramipril component (symptoms of reduced BP).

Indications: Secondary prevention of cardiovascular accidents (adults already controlled on monocomponents at equiv. dose).

Dose: Adult: Cardiovascular prevention, target maintenance dose of ramipril 10mg/day. *Admin,* once daily as single dose preferably after food; swallow with liquid; do not chew, crush or open capsule; avoid grapefruit juice.

Elderly: Very old, frail, caution.

Child: Under 18 years, contraindicated. Reye's syndrome

54

risk in children under 16 years with fever, flu or chicken-pox.
Renal Impairment: CrCl (mL/min) 60 and above, max. ramipril 10mg/day; 30-60, max. ramipril 5mg/day; below 30 or on haemodialysis, contraindicated.
Hepatic Impairment: Caution; max. ramipril 2.5mg/day. Severe or active impairment or unexplained serum transaminases about 3xULN, contraindicated.
CI: See Notes below for individual components.
Interactions: Effect of Other Drugs on Acetylsalicylic Acid, Atorvastatin, Ramipril: *Co-admin contraindicated*: Methotrexate (at dose 15mg/week or above), aliskiren, tipranavir, ritonavir, ciclosporin. *Co-admin, monitor*: NSAIDS, corticosteroids, SSRIs, antiplatelets, anticoagulants, ibuprofen. See Notes below for individual components.
SP: Monitor CK levels and LFTs prior to initiation, then periodically; transaminases above 3x ULN, discontinue. *Careful supervision*, hypersensitivity, known allergies, GI ulceration or bleeding, reduced liver and/or renal function, at hypotension risk, deterioration of cardiovascular circulation, G6PD deficiency, elevated uric acid, patients consuming substantial quantities of alcohol or liver disease. *Monitor*, signs of liver injury, renal impairment, serum potassium (at risk patients). Temporarily discontinue prior to elective major surgery. See Notes below.
Pregnancy, Lactation: Contraindicated including women of childbearing potential not using reliable contraception.
ADR: Summary, *most common*, GI complaints (aspirin); persistent cough, hypotension (ramipril); myalgia (statins). See notes below.
Notes: For individual components see 2.6.7 Non-Steroidal Antiplatelets, Aspirin, 2.3.5 Statins (atorvastatin), 2.1.1 ACEIs (ramipril).

Trinomia Capsules *(A.Menarini)* B. GMS.
Price, (28) 100/20: 2.5, €9.04; 5mg, €10.66; 10mg, €14.01. *Capsules*, acetylsalicylic acid, atorvastatin calcium trihydrate, ramipril 100/20/2.5(5)10)mg. Marked AAR and strength; caps contain 2x50mg acetylsalicylic white f/c tabs marked AS, 2x10mg atorvastatin greenish-brownish f/c tabs marked AT and 1x ramipril tab either 2.5mg, 5mg or 10mg, pale-yellow f/c marked R2 (2.5mg), R5 (5mg) or R1 (10mg). 100/20/2.5: Light-grey. 100/20/5: Pink/light-grey. 100/20/10: Pale-pink. *Lactose, soya lecithin*. **Store:** No special conditions.

Ezetimibe, Atorvastatin

ATC Code: C10BA05. **Sport:** Permitted.
Driving: Dizziness reported.
Indications: Prevention of cardiovascular events (reduction of risk in coronary heart disease, acute coronary syndrome). Hypercholesterolaemia (primary or mixed hyperlipidaemia). Homozygous familial hypercholesterolaemia (HoFH).
Dose: Adult, Elderly: *Hypercholesterolaemia and/or coronary heart disease, HoFH*, range 10/10mg/day to max. 10/80mg/day (usually 10/10mg once daily for hypercholesterolaemia).
Co-admin with, amiodarone, amlodipine, verapamil, diltiazem, erythromycin, fluconazole (consider a lower max. dose*); tipranavir/ritonavir (max. 10/10mg/day); lopinavir/ritonavir, clarithromycin, boceprevir, elbasvir or grazoprevir (max. 10/20mg/day*); saquinavir/ritonavir, itraconazole, fosamprenavir (lower maintenance doses recommended; 10/40mg/day*); rifampicin (avoid or*). Dosing with bile acid sequestrants should occur either 2 or more hours before or 4 or more hours after bile acid sequestrant. *Admin*, as single oral dose at any time of the day, with or without food. *with clinical monitoring.
Child: Safety/efficacy not established.
Hepatic Impairment: Caution. Acute liver disease or unexplained persistent elevations in serum transaminases (above 3xULN), contraindicated.
Interactions: Effect of Other Drugs on Ezetimibe, Atorvastatin Combination: *Co-admin not recommended*: Fibrates, grapefruit juice; systemic fusidic acid (or within 7 days of stopping fusidic acid). *Avoid co-admin (increased atorvastatin plasma levels)*: Ciclosporin, telithromycin, clarithromycin, delavirdine, stiripentol, ketoconazole, voriconazole, itraconazole, posaconazole, HIV protease

Statins, Statin Combinations 2.3.5

inhibitors (ritonavir, lopinavir, atazanavir, indinavir, darunavir). See Dose above.
Effect of Ezetimibe, Atorvastatin Combination on Other Drugs: Ciclosporin; warfarin, other coumarins, fluindione; digoxin: *Monitor*.
SP: Prior haemorrhagic stroke or lacunar infarct, atorvastatin 80mg risk/benefit is uncertain; carefully consider potential haemorrhagic stroke risk before initiating.
ADR: *Common*, diarrhoea, myalgia.
Notes: See Atorvastatin above and 2.3.2 Ezetimibe.

ATOZET Tablets *(MSD)* B. GMS.
Price, all strengths (30) €41.19.
Tablets, ezetimibe/atorvastatin 10mg/(20mg, 40mg, 80mg). White (off-white) cap-shaped f/c. 10/10: Marked 333. 10/20: Marked 333. 10/40: Marked 337. 10/80: Marked 357. *Lactose*. **Store:** Original pack to protect (oxygen).

Fluvastatin

ATC Code: C10AA04. **Sport:** Permitted.
Driving: Unlikely to impair.
Indications: Primary hypercholesterolemia or mixed dyslipidaemia. Secondary prevention of major adverse cardiac events in adults with CHD after percutaneous coronary interventions.
Dose: Adult, Elderly: *Dyslipidaemia*, range 20-80mg/day; LDL-C reduction goal below 25%, 20mg/day; LDL-C reduction goal above 25%, 40mg/day. If needed, uptitrate to 80mg/day.
Secondary prevention, 80mg/day. Oral with or after food, swallowed whole with little water at bedtime.
Child: Age 9 years and older; heterozygous familial hypercholesterolaemia, initially 20mg/day; titrate at 6-week intervals to max. 80mg/day.
Renal Impairment: CrCl (mL/min) below 30, limited data; above 40mg/day, initiate with caution.
Hepatic Impairment: Contraindicated.
Interactions: Effect of Other Drugs on Fluvastatin: *Decreased plasma levels*: Rifampicin. *Possible myotoxicity*: Colchicine.
Effect of Fluvastatin on Other Drugs: Oral sulphonylureas (glibenclamide): *Increased plasma levels*.
Notes: See 2.3.5 Statins.

Lescol 20mg, 40mg, XL 80mg *(Novartis)* B. GMS.
Price, (28) 20mg, €5.28. 40mg, €6.22. 40mg, €11.66. XL (28) 80mg, €8.25.
Capsule, fluvastatin sodium. Opaque. Marked XU/strength. 20mg: Reddish-brown/yellow. 40mg: Reddish brown/orange-yellow. *Soya lecithin*. **Store:** No special conditions.
Prolonged/R tablet, as above. Yellow round f/c. Marked LE; NVR on reverse. **Store:** Below 30 deg C; original pack; protect (moisture).

Pravastatin

ATC Code: C10AA03. **Sport:** Permitted.
Driving: Dizziness, visual disturbances.
Indications: Primary hypercholesterolaemia or mixed dyslipidaemia. Primary prevention, moderate or severe hypercholesterolaemia and at high risk of first cardiovascular event. Secondary prevention, MI history or unstable angina pectoris and with or without increased cholesterol levels. Post-transplant, reduction of hyperlipidaemia on immunosuppressive therapy following solid organ transplant.
Dose: Adult, Elderly: *Hypercholesterolaemia*, range 10-40mg/day; max 40mg/day.
Primary prevention, initial and maintenance, 40mg/day.
Post-transplant, initially 20mg/day; if required titrate to 40mg/day. Oral, once daily, preferably in evening, with or without food.
Elderly: No adjustment unless predisposing risk factors.
Child: *Heterozygous familial hypercholesterolaemia*, age 8-13 years, range 10-20mg/day; age 14-18 years, 10-40mg/day. Under 8 years, no data.
Renal Impairment: Moderate/severe, initially 10mg/day.
Hepatic Impairment: Significant, as for Renal above.

2.3.5 Statins, Statin Combinations

SP: Hypercholesterolaemia due to elevated HDL-cholesterol, not suitable.

Notes: See 2.3.5 Statins.

Interchangeability: Same strengths of all brands of pravastatin film-coated (f/c) tabs listed below are deemed interchangeable.

Reference Price: (28) 10mg, €2.80. 20mg, €3.64. 40mg, €5.32. (30) 10mg, €3.00. 20mg, €3.90. 40mg, €5.70.

Lipostat 10mg, 20mg, 40mg *(BMS)* B. GMS.
Price, (28) 10mg, €2.80. 20mg, €4.76. 40mg, €6.16.
F/c tablet, pravastatin sodium. Yellow cap-shaped scored. Marked with strength. *Lactose*. **Store:** Below 25 deg C; original pack to protect (light, moisture).

Pravamel 10mg, 20mg, 40mg *(Clonmel)* B. GMS.
Price, (30) see reference price above.
F/c tablet, pravastatin. Cap-shaped. Marked with strength. 10mg: Pink/peach. 20mg, 40mg: Yellow. **Store:** Below 25 deg C; original pack.

Pravastatin (Accord) 10mg, 20mg, 40mg *(Accord)* B. GMS.
Price, (28), see reference price above.
F/c tablet, pravastatin sodium. Cap-shaped. Yellow rounded-rectangular. Marked PDT and strength. *Lactose*. **Store:** Below 25 deg C; original pack to protect (light, moisture).

Pravastatin (Actavis) 10mg, 20mg, 40mg *(Accord)* B. GMS.
Price, (28), see reference price above.
F/c tablet, pravastatin sodium. Cap-shaped. Marked with heart; PV and strength on reverse. 20mg: Scored (divisible into equal halves). *Lactose*. **Store:** Below 25 deg C; original pack.

Pravastatin (TEVA) 10mg, 20mg, 40mg *(TEVA)* B. GMS.
Price, (28), see reference price above.
F/c tablet, pravastatin sodium. Round. Marked 93. 10mg: Pink. Marked 771. 20mg: Light-yellow. Marked 7201. 40mg: Light-green. Marked 7202. *Lactose*. **Store:** Below 30 deg C; original pack to protect (moisture).

Pravastatin Mylan 10mg, 20mg, 40mg *(Gerard)* B. GMS.
Price, (28), see reference price above.
F/c tablet, pravastatin sodium. Mottled round flat. Marked with strength. 10mg: Light-pink. 20mg: Light-yellow*. 40mg: Light-pink*. *scored (divisible into equal halves). *Lactose*. **Store:** Original pack to protect (moisture).

Pravat 10mg, 20mg, 40mg *(Pinewood)* B. GMS.
Price, (28), see reference price above.
F/c tablet, pravastatin sodium. Round unscored. Marked APO; PRA over strength on reverse. 10mg: Light-pink. 20mg: Off-white/light-yellow. 40mg: Light-green. *Lactose*. **Store:** Below 25 deg C; original pack.

Pravitin 10mg, 20mg, 40mg *(Rowex)* B. GMS.
Price, (30) 10mg, €3.00. 20mg, €5.10. 40mg, €6.60.
F/c tablet, pravastatin sodium. Yellow oval scored (10mg, to facilitate breaking; 20mg, 40mg, divisible into equal doses). Marked P/strength. **Store:** Below 25 deg C; original pack to protect (light, moisture).

Rosuvastatin

ATC Code: C10AA07. **Sport:** Permitted.
Driving: Dizziness.

Indications: Primary hypercholesterolaemia (Type IIa including heterozygous familial) or mixed dyslipidaemia (Type IIb), homozygous familial hypercholesterolaemia (adjunctive to diet, other measures) (from age 6 years). Prevention, major cardiovascular events (high risk for first cardiovascular event).

Dose: Adult: *Hypercholesterolaemia*, treatment, initial and maintenance, 5-10mg/day; if needed increase at 4-week intervals to 20mg/day; consider 40mg/day only with severe hypercholesterolaemia and at high cardiovascular risk, especially familial hypercholesterolaemia (recommend specialist supervision at 40mg initiation).
Prevention of cardiovascular events, 20mg/day. Race, predisposing factors to myopathy, initially 5mg (40mg contraindicated). Increased systemic exposure (Asian subjects, specific types of genetic polymorphism) *Admin*, oral once daily, any time of day, with or without food.

Elderly: Over 65 years, initially 5mg.

Child: Under specialist supervision, age 6-17 years (Tanner Stage under II-V): *Heterozygous* familial hypercholesterolaemia, initially 5mg/day. Age 6-9 years, range 5mg to max. 10mg/day*. Age 10-17 years, range 5mg to max. 20mg/day*. *(no safety/efficacy data above these doses). *Homozygous* familial hypercholesterolaemia, age 6-17 years, initially 5-10mg/day; increase to 20mg/day based on response. The 40mg tablet is not suitable for

paediatric patients. Under 6 years, not recommended. *Admin*, as for Adult above.

Renal Impairment: CrCl (mL/min) below 60, initially 5mg/day (40mg contraindicated); below 30, contraindicated.

Hepatic Impairment: Score (Child-Pugh) 7 or below, no increased systemic exposure; 8-9, increased systemic exposure; above 9, no data. Active liver disease (unexplained, persistent serum transaminase elevations; above 3xULN), contraindicated.

Interactions: Effect of Other Drugs on Rosuvastatin: *Co-admin contraindicated*: Fibrates (rosuvastatin 40mg dose), ciclosporin. *Co-admin not recommended*: Protease inhibitors (increased rosuvastatin exposure; decrease dose). *Co-admin caution*: Ezetimibe. *Plasma levels increased* (seek alternative or consider risk/benefit): Ciclosporin, ritonavir + (atazanavir, lopinavir, and/or tipranavir), clopidogrel, simeprevir. *Plasma levels decreased*: Erythromycin, baicalin.

Effect of Rosuvastatin on Other Drugs: Oral contraceptives, HRT: *Possible increased plasma levels.*

SP: Proteinuria, renal function deterioration. Increased rosuvastatin exposure; consider dose reduction (specific types of genetic polymorphisms). In children, evaluation of linear growth (height), weight, BMI and secondary characteristics of sexual maturation by Tanner staging limited to 2 years; after 2 years, no effect detected.

ADR: See Notes below.

Notes: See 2.3.5 Statins.

Interchangeability: Same strengths of all brands of rosuvastatin f/c tabs listed below are deemed interchangeable.

Reference Price: (28) 5mg, €5.88. 10mg, €7.28. 20mg, €11.76. 40mg, €12.32.

Crestor 5mg, 10mg, 20mg, 40mg *(AstraZeneca)* B. GMS.
Price, (28) 5mg, €13.77; 10mg, €17.84; 20mg, €27.64; 40mg, €28.39.
Tablet (f/c), rosuvastatin calcium. Marked ZD4522/strength. 5mg: Yellow round. 10mg, 20mg: Round pink. 40mg: Oval pink. *Lactose*. **Store:** Below 30 deg C (bottles, blisters).

Rosuva 5mg, 10mg, 20mg, 40mg *(Rowex)* B. GMS.
Price, (28), see reference price above.
F/c tablet, rosuvastatin calcium. Round. Marked RSV/strength. 5mg: Light-brown. 10mg, 20mg, 40mg: Brown. *Lactose*.

Rosuvastatin Accord Tablets *(Accord)* B. GMS.
Price, (28), see reference price above. (98) 5mg, €20.56. (500) 5mg, €104.91; 10mg, €129.99; 20mg, €210.00.
F/c tablet, rosuvastatin calcium 5mg, 10mg, 20mg, 40mg. Round (except 40mg). Marked R; strength on reverse. 5mg: Yellow. 10mg, 20mg: Pink. 40mg: Oval pink. *Lactose; Allura Red, Sunset Yellow (not 5mg).*

Rosuvastatin Actavis Tablets *(Accord)* B. GMS.
Price, (28), see reference price above.
F/c tablet, rosuvastatin calcium 5mg, 10mg, 20mg, 40mg. Round yellowish. Marked with strength. 5mg: Marked 15. *Lactose*.

Rosuvastatin Clonmel Tablets *(Clonmel)* B. GMS.
Price, (28), see reference price above.
F/c tablet, rosuvastatin calcium 5mg, 10mg, 20mg, 40mg. Round (except 40mg) white. 40mg: oval. *Lactose*. **Store:** Original pack; protect (light).

Rosuvastatin Krka Tablets *(Krka)* B. GMS.
Price, (28), see reference price above.
F/c tablet, rosuvastatin calcium 5mg, 10mg, 20mg, 40mg. White. 5mg, 10mg: Round. Marked with strength. 20mg: Round. 40mg: Cap-shaped. *Lactose*.

Rosuvastatin TEVA Tablets *(TEVA)* B. GMS.
Price, (28), see reference price above.
F/c tablet, rosuvastatin calcium 5mg, 10mg, 20mg, 40mg. Round. Marked N; strength on reverse. *Lactose*. 5mg: Orange. *Sunset Yellow*. 10mg, 20mg, 40mg: Light-pink. *Carmoisine*.

Simvastatin

ATC Code: C10AA01. **Sport:** Permitted.
Driving: Unlikely to impair.

Indications: Hypercholesterolaemia, primary or mixed dyslipidaemia, homozygous familial (HoFH), adjunct to diet and other appropriate measures. Cardiovascular prevention, patients with manifest atherosclerotic CVD or diabetes mellitus, with normal or increased cholesterol levels.

Dose: Adult, Elderly: Range, 5-80mg/day; adjust dose at 4-week intervals; max. 80mg/day (recommend only in severe hypercholesterolaemia and high risk for cardiovascular complications; increased myopathy risk). *Cardiovascular prevention*, usually 20-40mg/day. Hypercholesterolaemia, usually 10-20mg/day; if large LDL reduction required, initially 20-40mg/day. HFH, 40mg/day as single dose (evening).

Co-admin, with fibrates (except gemfibrozil or fenofibrate), simvastatin max. 10mg/day; amiodarone, amlodipine, verapamil, diltiazem, elbasvir, grazoprevir, max. simvastatin 20mg/day; lomitapide, simvastatin max. 40mg/day (HoFH patients). *Admin*, bile acid sequestrants, dose 2 hours before or 4 hours after. Oral, usually as single dose in evening.

Child: HoFH, age 10-17 years, boys Tanner Stage II and above; girls 1-year post-menarche, usually 10mg/day (evening); range 10-40mg; max. 40mg/day. Pre-pubertal children, limited data.

Renal Impairment: CrCl (mL/min) below 30, above 10mg/day, caution.

Interactions: Effect of Other Drugs on Simvastatin: *Co-admin contraindicated*: Potent CYP3A4 inhibitors e.g. azole antifungals (itraconazole, ketoconazole, posaconazole, voriconazole), HIV protease inhibitors (nelfinavir), macrolides (erythromycin, clarithromycin, telithromycin), boceprevir, telaprevir, nefazodone, medicinals containing cobicistat; gemfibrozil, ciclosporin, danazol, lomitapide (see Dose above). *Co-admin avoid*: Grapefruit juice. *Increased myopathy, rhabdomyolysis risk*: Amiodarone, amlodipine, fibrates (except fenofibrate), verapamil, diltiazem; colchicine (with renal insufficiency); OATP1B1 inhibitors (ciclosporin). *Rhabdomyolysis risk, co-admin not recommended*: Fusidic acid or within 7 days of stopping fusidic acid (if fusidic acid is essential discontinue statin during fusidic acid course). *Careful benefit/risk analysis*: Niacin (dose 1g/day or above), acipimox.

SP: Asian patients, use lowest dose necessary; combination with niacin (dose 1g/day or above) not recommended. Reduced hepatic transport protein function (inhibition by interaction medicines e.g. ciclosporin or SLCO1B1 gene allele carriers) can increase simvastatin systemic exposure (increased myopathy and rhabdomyolysis risk).

ADR: *Common*, increased (ALT, AST, blood CPK).

Notes: See 2.3.5 Statins.

Interchangeability: Same strengths of all brands of simvastatin film-coated (f/c) tabs listed below are deemed interchangeable.

Reference Price: (28) 10mg, €1.96. 20mg, €2.52. 40mg, €3.08. (30) 10mg, €2.10. 20mg, €2.70. 40mg, €3.30.

Zocor 10mg, 20mg, 40mg *(MSD)* B. GMS.
Price, (28) 10mg, €2.52; 20mg, €3.47; 40mg, €5.04.
Tablet, simvastatin. Oval f/c. Marked MSD. 10mg: Peach. Marked 735. 20mg: Tan. Marked 740. 40mg: Brick-red. Marked 749. *Lactose*. **Store:** Below 25 deg C; blister in outer carton to protect (moisture).

Simtan 5mg, 10mg, 20mg, 40mg, 80mg *(Clonmel)* B. GMS.
Price, (28) 5mg, €12.72, see reference price above.
Tablet, simvastatin. Oblong scored. Marked SV/strength on reverse. 5mg: Yellow. 10mg, 20mg 40mg: White.

Simvastatin Actavis 10mg, 20mg, 40mg *(Accord)* B. GMS.
Price, (28), see reference price above.
Tablet, simvastatin. Oval f/c scored (divisible into equal halves). 10mg: Peach. 20mg: Tan. 40mg: Brick-red. *Lactose*.

Simvastatin Bluefish Tablets *(Bluefish)* B. GMS.
Price, (28), see reference price above.
Tablet, simvastatin 10mg, 20mg, 40mg. Round f/c. Light-pink. 10mg: Marked 01. 20mg: Marked 02. 40mg: Pink. Marked 03. *Lactose*.

Simvastatin (Gerard) Tablets *(Gerard)* B. GMS.
Price, (30), see reference price above.
Tablet, simvastatin 10mg, 20mg, 40mg. Oval f/c. Marked G; SM and strength on reverse. 10mg: Dark-peach (pink) scored (facilitates breaking). 20mg: Dark-tan scored (divisible into equal doses). 40mg: Pink. *Lactose*.

Simvastatin KrKa 10mg, 20mg, 40mg *(Krka)* B. GMS.
Price, (28), see reference price above.
Tablet, simvastatin. White scored (divisible into equal halves). 10mg, 20mg: Oval. Marked with strength. 40mg: Round. *Lactose*.

Simvastatin TEVA Tablets *(TEVA)* B. GMS.
Price, (28), see reference price above.
Tablet, simvastatin 10mg, 20mg, 40mg, 80mg. Oval f/c scored. 10mg: Light-pink. 20mg: Tan. 40mg: Pink. *Lactose*.

Sivatin 10mg, 20mg, 40mg *(Rowex)* B. GMS.
Price, (30), see reference price above.
Tablet, simvastatin. Oval scored (divisible into equal doses) f/c. Marked with strength. 10mg: Pale-pink. Marked SIM. 20mg: Orange. 40mg: Red-brown. *Lactose*.

Ezetimibe, Simvastatin

ATC Code: C10BA02. **Sport:** Permitted.
Driving: Caution.

Indications: Prevention of cardiovascular events (reduction of risk in coronary heart disease, acute coronary syndrome). Hypercholesterolaemia (primary or mixed hyperlipidaemia) where combination is appropriate. Homozygous familial hypercholesterolaemia (HoFH).

Dose: Adult, Elderly: *Hypercholesterolaemia*, range 10/10mg/day to max. 10/80mg/day. Homozygous familial hypercholesterolaemia, cardiovascular risk reduction, 10/40mg (10/80mg only if benefit outweighs risk).

Co-admin with, amiodarone, amlodipine, verapamil, diltiazem, elbasvir or grazoprevir, niacin (lipid-lowering doses 1g/day or more), max. INEGY 10/20mg/day; lomitapide, max. INEGY 10/40/mg/day. *Admin*, bile acid sequestrants, either 2 or more hours before or 4 or more hours after. Oral, single dose in evening, with or without food; do not split tab.

Child: Adolescents 10 years and older, pubertal status boys Tanner Stage II and above; girls at least 1-year post-menarche; age 10-17 years, initially 10/10mg; max. 10/40mg/day. Once daily in evening. Under age 10 years, not recommended.

Renal Impairment: GFR (mL/1.73m2), 60 or below, 10/20mg once daily in evening.

Hepatic Impairment: Moderate to severe, not recommended.

Interactions: Effect of Other Drugs on Simvastatin, Ezetimibe Combination: *Co-admin contraindicated*: Potent CYP3A4 Inhibitors increasing exposure 5 fold or more (itraconazole, ketoconazole, posaconazole, voriconazole, erythromycin, clarithromycin, telithromycin, HIV protease inhibitors e.g. nelfinavir, nefazodone, drugs containing cobicistat, gemfibrozil, ciclosporin, danazol). *Co-admin not recommended*: Other fibrates; fusidic acid or within 7 days of stopping (if fusidic acid is essential discontinue statin during fusidic acid course). *Co-admin avoid*: Grapefruit juice. See Adult Dose (bile acid sequestrants, ciclosporin, danazol, niacin, amiodarone, verapamil, niacin, diltiazem, amlodipine). *Myopathy, rhabdomyolysis*: Colchicine + simvastatin co-admin. *Careful benefit/risk analysis*: Niacin (dose 1g/day or above), acipimox. *Increased simvastatin plasma levels*: BCRP inhibitors (elbasvir, grazoprevir); see Dose.

Effect of Simvastatin, Ezetimibe Combination on Other Drugs: Fusidic acid: *Co-admin not recommended (rhabdomyolysis); discontinue statin; re-introduce 7 days after last fusidic acid dose.*

SP: 10/80mg dose for use only when benefit outweighs risk in (severe hypercholesterolaemia, high risk for cardiovascular complications).

ADR: *Common*, increased (ALT and/or AST), myalgia.

Notes: See Simvastatin above and 2.3.2 Ezetimibe.

Interchangeability: Same strengths of all brands of ezetimibe/simvastatin tabs are deemed interchangeable (includes parallel imports).

INEGY Tablets *(MSD)* B. GMS.
Price, (28) 10(20mg), €38.45; (40mg), €39.29; (80mg), €40.98.
Tablet, ezetimibe/simvastatin 10mg/(20mg, 40mg, 80mg). White (off-white) cap-shaped. 10/20: Marked 312. 10/40: Marked 313. 10/80: Marked 315. *Lactose*. **Store:** Below 30 deg C; original pack/bottles tightly closed to protect (moisture, light).

2.4 - Sympathomimetics

In This Chapter: *Adrenaline (epinephrine), dobutamine, dopexamine, midodrine, noradrenaline (norepinephrine).*

Class Effects
Sympathomimetics mimic sympathetic nervous system agonists i.e. stimulate adrenergic receptors. In cardiology

2.4   Sympathomimetics

they are used in the management of acute heart failure and shock (septic, cardiogenic).

CI: Hypersensitivity to any member of the class.

Interactions: Effect of Other Drugs on Sympathomimetics: *Hypertensive effect antagonised:* Antipsychotics. *Increased toxicity risk:* Myelosuppressive drugs.

Effect of Sympathomimetics (class) on Other Drugs: Doxapram, oxytocin: *Increased hypertension risk.* Ergotamine, methysergide: *Increased ergotism risk.* MAOIs, moclobemide: *Hypertensive crisis risk.*

SP: Parenteral catecholamines, monitor infusion rate, heart rate and rhythm, arterial BP; initiate with ECG monitoring.

Adrenaline (epinephrine) (anaphylaxis)

ATC Code: C01CA24. **Sport:** Prohibited (in-competition; not prohibited in local admin or co-admin with local anaesthetics). **Driving:** Not applicable.

Indications: Acute bronchial spasm (acute asthma attacks). Hypersensitivity reactions (drugs, other allergens) *(Concordia).* Anaphylactic shock, cardiopulmonary resuscitation *(both brands).*

Dose: Adult: 1:1000 (Concordia), usually 0.3-0.5mg; can repeat at 15-20 minute intervals (2 doses), then 4-hourly as needed; caution, elderly. Severe allergic reactions, 1mg as single dose. *Resuscitation,* 0.3mg SC may be given after IV or intracardiac admin of 1:10000 dilution.

1:10000 (Aguettant), *cardiopulmonary resuscitation,* 10mL (1mg) IV or intraosseous; repeat every 3-5 minutes until return of spontaneous circulation. Endotracheal admin, last resort (no other route accessible), 20-25mL (2-2.5mg). Following cardiac surgery, 50-100mcg. *Acute anaphylaxis,* 1:10000 not recommended for IM use; 1:1000 to be used. IV bolus 0.05mg (0.5mL).

Admin, SC, IM or IV after dilution. IM preferred for initial treatment of anaphylaxis. IV generally used in ICU or Emergency Dept setting. 1:1000 (1mg/mL), not suitable for IV use and must be diluted to 1:10000 before IV use. Adrenaline 1:1000 should not be diluted to 1:10000 for use in cardiac resuscitation ('ready to use' 1:10000 should be used).

Elderly: Caution.

Child: 1:1000 (Concordia), over 12 years, 0.5mg IM; 6-12 years, 0.3mg IM; 6 months to 6 years, 0.15mg IM and under 6 months 0.01mg/kg IM. If needed, repeat at 5-15 minute intervals according to BP, pulse and respiratory function.

1:10000 (Aguettant), *cardiac arrest* (above 5kg), 10mcg/kg IV or intraosseous (max. 1mg as single dose); repeat every 3-5 minutes until return of spontaneous circulation. Endotracheal admin, last resort (no other route accessible), 100mcg/kg (max. 2.5mg). *Acute anaphylaxis,* not for use in neonates or infants under 5kg. *Admin,* see Adult above.

CI: Use during labour, with local anaesthesia of peripheral structures (digits, ear lobe). Presence of ventricular fibrillation, cardiac dilatation, coronary insufficiency, organic brain disease, arteriosclerosis (except if benefit outweighs risk) *(1:1000 Concordia).*

Interactions: Effect of Other Drugs on Adrenaline: *Co-admin not recommended:* Additive effects, increased toxicity (oxytocin, other sympathomimetics); effect potentiated (TCADs including imipramine). *Vasoconstriction, hypertensive effects antagonised (useful in adrenaline overdose):* Alpha-blockers (phentolamine). *Hypokalaemia potentiated:* Corticosteroids, potassium-depleting diuretics, aminophylline, theophylline. See SP below.

Effect of Adrenaline on Other Drugs: Antihypertensives: *Effect antagonised.*

SP: *Caution,* elderly, hyperthyroidism, diabetes mellitus, phaeochromocytoma, narrow angle glaucoma, hypokalaemia, hypercalcaemia, severe renal impairment, prostatic adenoma leading to residual urine, cerebrovascular disease, organic brain damage, shock (other than anaphylactic), hypertension, severe angina pectoris, obstructive cardiomyopathy, arrhythmias. *Prolonged admin,* injection-site necrosis, metabolic

acidosis, renal necrosis, adrenaline-fastness or tachyphylaxis. *Anaesthesia with halothane,* extreme caution (ventricular fibrillation). Accidental intravascular injection may result in cerebral haemorrhage (sudden BP rise). *Severe hypertension* and reflex bradycardia may occur with non-cardioselective beta-blockers (propranolol); also antagonise cardiac and bronchodilator effects of adrenaline. Adrenaline not for use to counteract circulatory collapse or hypotension caused by phenothiazines. Adrenaline-induced hyperglycaemia may lead to loss of blood sugar control in diabetics.

Pregnancy, Lactation: Pregnancy, only if clearly necessary. Lactation, avoid.

ADR: *Potentially severe* from effect on BP, cardiac rhythm; anginal pain, ventricular fibrillation, myocardial (ischaemia, infarction); severe hypertension may lead to cerebral haemorrhage, pulmonary oedema. Stress cardiomyopathy, bowel necrosis, pallor, thrombocytosis.

Notes: See 2.4 Sympathomimetics, 5.7 Anti-Allergic Drugs, 7.1 Glaucoma.

Adrenaline Parenteral 1mg/10mL *(Aguettant)* A.
Price, not published by company.
Injection (PFS), adrenaline acid tartrate 0.1mg/mL (1:10000). Clear colourless soln. *Sodium 3.54mg/mL.*

Adrenaline (Epinephrine) Parenteral *(Concordia)* A. GMS.
Price, (10) €2.91.
Injection, adrenaline acid tartrate 1mg/mL (1:1000). Clear colourless soln. *Essentially sodium-free; metabisulphite.*

Dobutamine

ATC Code: C01CA07. **Sport:** Prohibited (in-competition). **Driving:** Not applicable.

Indications: Adult, inotropic support in treatment of low output cardiac failure (MI, open heart surgery, cardiomyopathies, septic/cardiogenic shock). Can be used for cardiac stress testing when exercise stress testing is not feasible. Neonates to age 18 years, inotropic support in low cardiac output hypoperfusion (decompensated HF, following cardiac surgery, cardiomyopathies, cardiogenic/septic shock).

Dose: Adult, Elderly: *Inotropic support,* initially 2.5mcg/kg/min increasing at 10-30 minute intervals until desired response (range 2.5-10mcg/kg/min); dose as low as 0.5mcg/kg/min may be sufficient to elicit response; rarely, 40mcg/kg/min required. Continuous IV infusion; discontinue by reducing gradually.

Cardiac stress testing, incremental increase in infusion rates from 5mcg/kg/min to 10, 20, 30 and max. 40mcg/kg/min with each dose infused for 3 minutes. *Elderly,* increase by 5mcg/kg/min every 8 minutes.

Child: All ages, initially 5mcg/kg/min adjusted according to clinical response to 2-20mcg/kg/min; 0.5-1mcg/kg/min may be sufficient to elicit response. In children minimum effective dose is higher than for adults and max. tolerated dose lower than for Adult above. *Admin,* as for Adult above.

CI: Hypovolaemia, phaeochromocytoma. Sodium metabisulphite hypersensitivity.

Interactions: Effect of Other Drugs on Dobutamine: *Inotropic effect reversed:* Beta-blockers. *Caution:* Anaesthesia (cyclopropane, halothane, other halogenated anaesthetics). *Effect enhanced:* Entacapone.

Effect of Dobutamine on Other Drugs: Beta-blockers: *Effect counteracted.*

SP: Undue heart rate or systolic BP increase or arrhythmia precipitated, reduce dose or discontinue. May precipitate/exacerbate ventricular ectopic activity; patients with atrial flutter or fibrillation may develop rapid ventricular response. Caution, acute MI. Mechanical obstruction (dobutamine does not improve haemodynamics). Stress cardiomyopathy reported. Causes BP decrease, caution in severe hypotension complicating cardiogenic shock. Hypovolaemia (correct with whole blood or plasma). If arterial BP remains low, consider peripheral vasoconstrictor (dopamine, noradrenaline). *Children,* monitor closely; see Dose above.

Pregnancy, Lactation: If benefit outweighs risk.

ADR: *Very common,* increased heart rate, palpitations, angina pectoris, chest pain, ectopic heart beats, arrhythmia, ventricular tachycardia, coronary artery spasm,

ECG ST-segment elevation. *Children*, elevated systolic blood pressure, systemic hypertension or hypotension, tachycardia, headache, elevated pulmonary wedge pressure (pulmonary congestion, oedema).

Notes: See 2.4 Sympathomimetics.

Dobutamine Parenteral (Concordia) A. HOS.
Price, (5) €41.01 (PTW).
Infusion, dobutamine HCl 250mg/20mL. Clear colourless (almost colourless) sterile conc for soln. *Sodium Metabisulphite.*

Dopexamine

ATC Code: C01CA14. **Sport:** Prohibited (in-competition).
Driving: Not applicable.

Indications: Vasodilation (peripheral, renal), mild positive inotropic therapy in the treatment of HF (associated with exacerbation of chronic HF, cardiac surgery).

Dose: Adult, Elderly: Initially 0.5mcg/kg/min; titrate to 1mcg/kg/min; increase by 0.5-1mcg/kg/min up to 6mcg/kg/min; minimum 15-minute intervals. IV infusion through a cannula or catheter in a central or large peripheral vein.

Child: Not recommended.

CI: Phaeochromocytoma, thrombocytopenia, LV outlet obstruction (hypertrophic obstructive cardiomyopathy, aortic stenosis), hypovolaemia.

Interactions: Effect of Dopexamine on Other Drugs: Adrenaline, noradrenaline: *Effect enhanced.*

SP: Correct hypovolaemia, restrict sodium and fluid load. Severe hypotension, reduced systemic vascular resistance, ischaemic heart disease (post acute-MI, angina pectoris), hypokalaemia, hyperglycaemia, tachycardia, reports of partial tolerance, thrombophlebitis.

Pregnancy, Lactation: Not recommended.

ADR: Tachycardia, premature ventricular contractions, atrial fibrillation, bradycardia, worsening HF (asystole, cardiac arrest), angina, MI, cardiac enzyme changes, ECG changes. Hypotension, hypertension. Nausea, vomiting, tremor, headache, diaphoresis, Rarely (cardiac surgery) renal failure, ARDS, pulmonary oedema.

Notes: See 2.4 Sympathomimetics.

Midodrine

ATC Code: C01CA17. **Sport:** Prohibited (in-competition).
Driving: Caution.

Indications: Treatment, severe orthostatic hypotension due to autonomic nervous system dysfunction (corrective factors ruled out).

Dose: Adult, Elderly: Initially 2.5mg 2-3 times daily; increase in small increments at weekly intervals; maintenance, max. 30mg/day (divided doses). Last dose to be taken at least 4 hours before bedtime to reduce supine hypertension risk. Blood pressure above 180/100mmHg (either position), discontinue. *Elderly,* initiate with lowest dose.

Child: Not recommended.

Renal Impairment: Severe or acute renal disease, contraindicated.

CI: Hypertension, severe organic heart disease or CHF, thyrotoxicosis, phaeochromocytoma, acute (nephritis, renal disease), prostate hypertrophy with residual urine volume increased, proliferative diabetic retinopathy, urinary retention, hyperthyroidism, narrow angle glaucoma, obliterative or spastic vessel disease (cerebrovascular occlusions and spasms), vasovagal hypotension.

Interactions: Effect of Other Drugs on Midodrine: *Hypertensive effect enhanced*: Methyldopa, TCADs, antihistamines, thyroid hormones, MAOIs. *Effect antagonised*: Beta-blockers, alpha-blockers (prazosin, phentolamine).

Effect of Midodrine on Other Drugs: Digitalis, other glycosides, psycho-pharmaceuticals: *Bradycardia risk.* Mineralocorticoids, glucocorticoids: *Increased glaucoma or raised IOP risk.* Atropine: *BP raising effect enhanced.* Perphenazine, amiodarone, metoclopramide: *Increased systemic exposure.*

SP: Supine hypertension.

Pregnancy, Lactation: Not recommended.

ADR: *Very common*, piloerection, dysuria. *Common*, paraesthesia, supine hypertension with doses above 30mg/day, nausea, dyspepsia, vomiting, stomatitis, chills, rash, pruritus, flushing, urinary retention.

Notes: See 2.4 Sympathomimetics.

Midon 2.5mg, 5mg (Takeda) B. GMS.
Price, (100) 2.5mg, €30.30. 5mg, €46.41.
Tablet, midodrine HCl. Marked RPC and strength. 2.5mg: White. Marked 003. 5mg: Orange. Marked 004. *Sunset Yellow.*

Noradrenaline (norepinephrine)

ATC Code: C01CA03. **Sport:** Prohibited (in-competition).
Driving: Not applicable.

Indications: Acute hypotensive states. To restore BP following cardiac arrest.

Dose: Adult, Elderly: *Acute hypotension* (IV infusion via central venous catheter), soln equiv. to noradrenaline base 40mcg/mL; rate 0.16-0.33mL/min, adjust according to response.

Cardiac arrest, rapid IV or intracardiac injection 0.5-0.75mL of soln equiv. to noradrenaline base 100mcg/mL.

Interactions: Effect of Other Drugs on Noradrenaline: *Effect enhanced*: Dopexamine.

Effect of Noradrenaline on Other Drugs: Adrenergic Neurone Blockers: *Hypotensive effect antagonised.* TCADs: *Increased hypertension/arrhythmia risk.* Beta-Blockers (including topical), clonidine: *Hypertension risk.* MAOIs, other sympathomimetics: *Exaggerated response.*

SP: Hypertension, hypoxia, hypercapnia, hypovolaemia,

Pregnancy, Lactation: May reduce placental perfusion throughout pregnancy. Late pregnancy, provokes uterine contractions which can result in foetal asphyxia.

ADR: Hypertension, headache, peripheral ischaemia, Severe tissue irritant.

Notes: See 2.4 Sympathomimetics. See Adrenaline above.

Levophed Parenteral (Hospira) A.
Price, 2mL (6) 1mg/mL, €6.93.
Injection, noradrenaline acid tartrate 1mg/mL. Amps.

2.5 - Antiarrhythmics

In This Chapter: *Class I (a.b.c), Class II, Class III and Class IV Antiarrhythmics.*

Class Effects

Antiarrhythmics are a diverse group; many such as beta-blockers, digoxin, lidocaine, magnesium and phenytoin have a wide range of other clinical applications. A widely used classification of antiarrhythmics is that proposed by Vaughan Williams and later modified by Harrison. This classification is based on effects of the drug on electrical behaviour of myocardial cells during activity i.e. *Class Ia, Ib, Ic*, membrane stabilising drugs. *Class II*, beta-blockers. *Class III*, amiodarone and sotalol (also Class II). *Class IV*, calcium-channel blockers (includes verapamil but not dihydropyridines). Antiarrhythmics may also be classified clinically i.e. those acting on supraventricular arrhythmias *(verapamil)*, those acting on both supraventricular and ventricular arrhythmias *(disopyramide)*, and those acting on ventricular arrhythmias *(lidocaine).*

CI: Hypersensitivity to any members of the class. Cardiogenic shock. Pre-existing heart block (if no pacemaker is present).

SP: Life threatening, haemodynamically significant arrhythmia (difficult to treat, affected patients at high risk); initiate treatment in hospital. No evidence that prolonged suppression of ventricular premature contractions with antiarrhythmics prevents sudden death. Antiarrhythmics not shown to enhance survival in patients with ventricular arrhythmia; should not be prescribed for treatment of asymptomatic ventricular premature contractions, haemodynamically non-significant.

Pregnancy, Lactation: If benefit outweighs risk.

ADR: Nausea, vomiting, constipation, diarrhoea, dry mouth, drowsiness, dizziness, blurred vision, tremor, convulsion, psychiatric disorders, confusional state,

2.5.1   Class Ia Antiarrhythmics

hypotension, sinus node dysfunction, atrial fibrillation, conduction defects, arrhythmia exacerbation, pre-existing HF, Torsade de pointes, rash, arthralgia, fever, thrombocytopenia, liver damage, jaundice.

Phenylephrine

ATC Code: C01CA06. **Sport:** Permitted.
Driving: Not relevant.

Indications: Treatment, hypotension during spinal, epidural or general anaesthesia.

Dose: Adult, Elderly: IV bolus, 50-100mcg; repeat until desired effect. 1 bolus max. 100mcg. Continuous infusion, 25-50mcg/min; range 25-100mcg/min assessed effect.

Child: No data.

Renal Impairment: Lower doses may be needed.

Hepatic Impairment: Cirrhosis, higher doses may be needed.

CI: Severe hypertension or peripheral vascular disease (risk of ischaemic gangrene or vascular thrombosis). Severe hyperthyroidism.

Interactions: Effect of Other Drugs on Phenylephrine: *Co-admin contraindicated*: MAOIs (or within 2 weeks) (paroxysmal hypertension, fatal hyperthermia). *Co-admin not advisable*: Ergot alkaloids (dopaminergic, vasoconstrictor), TCADs, SNRIs, MAOIs type A (selective), linezolid, guanethidine, cardiac glycosides, quinidine, sibutramine, halogenated volatile anaesthetics; oxytocics (hypertension).

SP: Caution, diabetes mellitus, arterial hypertension, uncontrolled hyperthyroidism, coronary heart disease, chronic heart conditions, non-severe peripheral vascular insufficiency, bradycardia, partial heart block, tachycardia, arrhythmias, angina pectoris, aneurysm, closed angle glaucoma. Can reduce cardiac output, caution (arteriosclerosis, elderly, impaired cerebral or coronary circulation). Serious HF or cardiogenic shock, deterioration in HF (increased afterload). Caution, extravasation (tissue necrosis).

Pregnancy, Lactation: Late pregnancy or labour, may cause foetal hypoxia and bradycardia; see Interactions above. Breastfeeding possible with single bolus admin during childbirth.

ADR: Summary, *most common*, bradycardia, hypertensive episodes, nausea, vomiting.

Notes: See 2.4 Sympathomimetics.

> **Phenylephrine Parenteral 50mcg/mL** *(Aguettant)* A.
> *Price,* not published by company.
> *Injection (PFS),* phenylephrine HCl. Clear colourless soln. *Sodium 3.68mg/mL.*

2.5.1 - Class Ia Antiarrhythmics

In This Chapter: *Disopyramide.*

Class Effects

Class I drugs directly interfere with depolarisation of cell membranes. They also have local anaesthetic properties. They prolong the PR, QRS and QT-intervals on the ECG i.e. lengthen action potential duration.

CI: Children, not recommended. Second or third degree heart block and sinus node disease (if no pacemaker present). Bundle branch block associated with first degree AV block, double block, pre-existing long QT interval. Severe uncompensated CHF unless secondary to cardiac arrhythmia. Cardiogenic shock.

Interactions: Effect of Other Drugs on Class I Antiarrhythmics: *Co-admin contraindicated*: Other drugs liable to provoke ventricular arrhythmias.

SP: Structural heart disease, proarrhythmia, cardiac decompensation, significant HF. Aggravation of existing or emergence of new arrhythmia or development of AV/bifasicular block during treatment. Hypotension, hypoglycaemia, discontinue. Ventricular tachycardia and/or fibrillation, Torsade de pointes. Atrial flutter/tachycardia, digitalis intoxication, potassium imbalance.

ADR: Cardiac, proarrhythmic effects, intra-cardiac conduction abnormalities. Bradycardia, sinus block, severe

HF, cardiogenic shock with resulting low cardiac output. Epigastralgia, nausea, vomiting, anorexia, diarrhoea, impotence, psychiatric disorders, rash, anaphylactic-type urticaria, angioedema. Shock (parenteral). *Atropine-like effects* including dysuria, acute urinary retention, accommodation disorders, diplopia, dry mouth, constipation.

Notes: See 2.5 Antiarrhythmics.

Disopyramide

ATC Code: C01BA03. **Sport:** Permitted.
Driving: Caution; impaired ability to concentrate and react.

Indications: Treatment, various atrial and ventricular arrhythmias as monotherapy or in combination.

Dose: Adult: ORAL, STANDARD/R, initially 400-600mg/day; titrate to 800mg/day if required; 6-hourly in divided doses.

PROLONGED/R, 1 tab twice daily; do not crush or chew tabs.

PARENTERAL, IV, initially 2mg/kg bolus over minimum 5 minutes; max. 150mg. If conversion occurs transfer to oral 200mg immediately, then 200mg 8-hourly for 24 hours. Maintenance, 400-600mg/day. Total in 1 hour, 4mg/kg IV; max. 300mg; in 24 hours, max. 800mg. Initial bolus should be maintained by IV infusion, 20-30mg/hour (0.4mg/kg/hour); max. 800mg/day.

Elderly: As for Renal, Hepatic impairment.

Renal Impairment: *Standard/R*, CrCl (mL/min) 20-60, 100mg 8-hourly or 150mg 12-hourly; 8-20, 100mg 12-hourly; below 8mL/min, 150mg 24-hourly. *Modified/R*, CrCl (mL/min) below 40, not recommended.

Hepatic Impairment: Consider dose reduction.

CI: Sustained/R formulations (children; renal, hepatic impairment).

Interactions: Effect of Other Drugs on Disopyramide: *Co-admin not recommended*: Other antiarrhythmics (exceptions, beta-blockers for angina pectoris, digoxin with beta-blocker and/or verapamil for the control of atrial fibrillation). *Increased Torsades de Pointes and/or arrhythmia risk*: TCADs, IV (erythromycin, vincamine, sultopride) astemizole, cisapride, pentamidine, pimozide, sparfloxacin, terfenadine. *Plasma levels increased*: CYP3A4 inhibitors (macrolides, azole antifungals), CYP3A4 substrates (HIV protease inhibitors e.g. ritonavir, indinavir, saquinavir; theophylline, ciclosporin A, warfarin). *Plasma levels decreased*: CYP3A4 inducers (rifampicin, certain anticonvulsants). *Hypokalaemia and/or proarrhythmic risk*: Diuretics, amphotericin B, tetracosactrin, gluco- and mineralo-corticoids, stimulant laxatives.

Effect of Disopyramide on Other Drugs: Atropine, other anticholinergics, phenothiazines: *Potentiation of atropine-like effects.*

SP: Structural heart disease, aggravation of existing arrhythmia, emergence of new arrhythmia, AV or bifascicular block, urgent review. Hypotension, discontinue; resume at lower dose (monitor). Digitalis intoxication, caution. Monitor potassium, blood sugar levels. Atropine-like effects (ocular hypertension, narrow-angle glaucoma, acute urinary retention, paralytic ileus*, prostatic enlargement, myasthenia gravis, cognitive disorders*); avoid in glaucoma patients; history of glaucoma, measure IOP before initiating. *(elderly).

Pregnancy, Lactation: Pregnancy, if benefit outweighs risk; reported to stimulate contractions of pregnant uterus; passes into foetal circulation. Lactation, stop breastfeeding or drug; secreted in breast milk.

ADR: Rapid infusion may cause profuse sweating. Atropine-like effects.

Notes: See 2.5.1 Antiarrhythmics Class Ia.

> **Rythmodan Retard 250mg** *(SANOFI)* B. GMS.
> *Price,* (60) €19.00.
> *Prolonged/R tablet,* disopyramide phosphate. Whitish round f/c scored. Marked 013 and E; symbol on reverse. *Sucrose, glucose.*
> **Store:** Below 25 deg C.

2.5.2 - Class Ib Antiarrhythmics

In This Chapter: *Lidocaine.*

Class Effects

Phenytoin is also used in the control of cardiac arrhythmias and lidocaine for local anaesthesia.

Pharmacology: Class Ib drugs have limited effect on the rate of change of the depolarisation phase, shorten the repolarisation phase, shorten the QT-interval and elevate the fibrillation threshold.

CI: Children, with some exceptions. Hypersensitivity to local amide anaesthetics. Limited cardiac output (LVEF below 35%), first three months following MI.

SP: Sinus node dysfunction, conduction defects, bradycardia, hypotension, cardiac failure.

Pregnancy, Lactation: If benefit outweighs risk.

Notes: See 2.5.1 Class Ia Antiarrhythmics. See 3.1.4 Hydantoins (phenytoin). See 14.2 Local Anaesthesia (lidocaine).

Lidocaine (arrhythmias)

ATC Code: C01BB01. **Sport:** Permitted.
Driving: Not applicable.

Indications: Ventricular arrhythmias post MI and cardiac surgery. Local anaesthesia by infiltration, IV regional anaesthesia and nerve blocks.

Dose: Adult: *Arrhythmias*, initially 50-100mg IV at rate 25-50mg/min; after 5 minutes, admin second dose if needed; max. 200-300mg during a 1-hour period. Maintenance, IV infusion at rate 1-4mg/min (20-50mcg/kg/min). Switch to oral.
Local anaesthesia, max. 3mg/kg or 200mg whichever is lower. Continuous epidural, caudal or paracervical anaesthesia, max. dose should not be repeated at intervals under 90 minutes. IV regional anaesthesia (Bier's block), tourniquet should not be released until at least 20 minutes after admin.

Elderly: Consider adjustment.

Child: Loading dose 0.8-1mg/kg; if needed repeat up to 3-5mg/kg. Maintenance, IV infusion rate 10-50mcg/kg/min.

CI: Bradycardia, Stokes-Adams syndrome, porphyria. Severe degrees of sinoatrial, atrioventricular block or cardiac decompensation not dependent of tachyarrhythmias.

Interactions: Effect of Other Drugs on Lidocaine: *Renal/hepatic clearance reduced*: Propranolol, cimetidine. *Additive Cardiac Depressant Effects*: Other antiarrhythmics.

Effect of Lidocaine on Other Drugs: Suxamethonium: *Action prolonged*. Epidural admin lidocaine in combination with clonidine, adrenaline or clonidine plus adrenaline significantly reduces the Cmax of lidocaine.

SP: More frequent/serious arrhythmias. Toxicity due to accumulation. Intra-articular lidocaine may cause chondrotoxicity.

Notes: See 2.5.2 Antiarrhythmics Class Ib.

Lidocaine 1%, 2% Minijet *(IMS)* A.
Price, not published by company.
Injection, lidocaine HCl 10mg/mL. Clear colourless sterile soln.

2.5.3 - Class Ic Antiarrhythmics

In This Chapter: *Flecainide, propafenone.*

Class Effects

Class Ic drugs markedly prolong the PR and QRS intervals.

Indications: Ventricular tachyarrhythmias; AV nodal reciprocating tachycardia (unresponsive to beta-blockers or calcium channel blockers; absence of LVD); Wolff-Parkinson-White Syndrome *(flecainide, propafenone)*. Atrial fibrillation and atrial flutter (treatment need established; absence of LVD) *(flecainide)*.

CI: Children, not recommended. Hypersensitivity to any member of class. Left ventricular dysfunction or heart failure (regardless of arrhythmia type), history of MI (ventricular ectopics or tachycardia), atrial fibrillation, significant valvular heart disease, asymptomatic or symptomatic arrhythmias. Sinus node dysfunction, atrial conduction defects, second degree AV block, bundle

Class Ic Antiarrhythmics   2.5.3

branch or distal block (unless pacing rescue available). Electrolyte imbalance, known Brugada syndrome.

SP: Electrolyte disturbances, hepatic impairment, permanent pacemakers/temporary pacing electrodes, existing heart disease, history of MI, arterio-sclerotic heart disease, CHF. Atrial fibrillation following cardiac surgery.

Pregnancy, Lactation: If benefit outweighs risk.

ADR: AV block, MI, bradycardia, chest pain, fatigue, oedema, visual disturbances, dyscrasias, dyspnoea.

Notes: See Antiarrhythmics 2.5.1 Class Ia, 2.5.2 Class Ib.

Flecainide

ATC Code: C01BC04. **Sport:** Permitted.
Driving: Dizziness, visual disturbances.

Indications: Symptomatic ventricular tachycardia (life-threatening or disabling); premature ventricular contraction (resistant to other therapy); AV nodal reciprocating tachycardia (unresponsive to beta-blockers, calcium channel blockers); Wolfe-Parkinson-White Syndrome; paroxysmal atrial fibrillation and atrial flutter. *Parenteral* indicated when rapid control of above indications is needed.

Dose: Adult: ORAL, *supraventricular arrhythmias*, initially 50mg twice daily; increase to max. 300mg/day if needed. *Ventricular arrhythmias*, initially 100mg twice daily; titrate by 50mg/day every 4 days; max. 400mg/day. Reduce after 3-5 days to lowest dose to control arrhythmia.
PARENTERAL, initial bolus of 2mg/kg. Sustained ventricular tachycardia, CHF history, initially 2mg/kg over 30 minutes; follow with IV infusion, 1.5mg/kg/hour (hour 1) then 0.1-0.25mg/kg/hour (hour 2 onwards); max. duration 24 hours; max. in first 24 hours, 600mg.

Elderly: Rate of elimination may be reduced; consider when adjusting dose.

Renal Impairment: CrCl (mL/min) 35 or less, initially/max. 100mg/day or 50mg twice daily.

Hepatic Impairment: Significant, if benefit outweighs risk. Severe, not recommended.

CI: Amide hypersensitivity. See Notes below.

Interactions: Effect of Other Drugs on Flecainide: *Co-admin not recommended*: Sodium channel blockers. *Increased plasma levels*: Amiodarone (reduce flecainide dose by 50%), CYP2D6 inhibitors (antidepressants, neuroleptics, propranolol, ritonavir, some antihistamines, cimetidine, fluoxetine, quinine, terbinafine), cimetidine. *Additive negative inotropic effects*: Beta-blockers, other cardiac depressants. *Decreased plasma levels*: CYP2D6 inducers (phenytoin, phenobarbital, carbamazepine). *Increased arrhythmia risk*: TCADs, reboxetine (caution), clozapine. *Increased ventricular arrhythmia risk*: Anti-histamines (mizolastine, terfenadine), HIV protease inhibitors (ritonavir, lopinavir, indinavir; avoid co-admin). *Increased cardiac toxicity due to hypokalaemia*: Diuretics, corticosteroids, laxatives.

Effect of Flecainide on Other Drugs: Cardiac glycosides (digoxin), bupropion (reduce dose): *Plasma levels increased*.

SP: Recommended that IV treatment initiated in hospital; oral treatment under direct hospital or specialist supervision with (AV nodal reciprocating tachycardia, arrhythmias associated with WPW Syndrome, similar conditions with accessory pathways; paroxysmal atrial fibrillation in patients with disabling symptoms); all other indications, initiate in hospital. Continuous ECG monitoring recommended in all patients receiving bolus injection as flecainide prolongs QT-interval and widens the QRS complex. Brugada syndrome, consider discontinuation. Correct (electrolyte disturbances, severe bradycardia, pronounced hypotension) before initiation. Increases endocardial pacing thresholds; more marked on acute pacing threshold than on the chronic. Caution, permanent pacemakers or temporary pacing electrodes. Flecainide has a narrow therapeutic index and requires caution and close monitoring when switching to a different formulation. Dairy products may reduce absorption in children and infants.

Pregnancy, Lactation: If benefit outweighs risk.

ADR: *Very common*, dizziness, visual impairment (diplopia,

61

2.5.4 Class II Antiarrhythmics

blurred vision). *Common*, proarrhythmia, dyspnoea, asthenia, fatigue, pyrexia, oedema.

Notes: See 2.5.3 Antiarrhythmics Class Ic.

Tambocor 50mg, 100mg *(Meda)* B. GMS.
Price, (60) 50mg, €10.99. 100mg, €12.09.
Tablet, flecainide acetate. White. Marked 3M and TR/strength. 50mg: Round. 100mg: Scored (divisible into equal halves).

Tambocor Parenteral *(Meda)* A.
Price, 15mL (5) 10mg/mL, €29.20.
Injection or infusion, flecainide acetate 10mg/mL. Clear colourless soln. *Sodium 37.7mg/15mL amp.*

Flecainide 50mg, 100mg *(Gerard)* B. GMS.
Price, (60) 50mg, €10.78. 100mg, €11.85.
Tablet, flecainide acetate. White uncoated. Marked FC over strength; G on reverse. 100mg: Scored (facilitates breaking).

Propafenone

ATC Code: C01BC03. **Sport:** Permitted.
Driving: Caution; blurred vision, fatigue, postural hypotension.
Indications: Symptomatic supraventricular tachyarrhythmias requiring treatment (AV junctional tachycardia, supraventricular tachycardia with Wolff-Parkinson-White syndrome, paroxysmal atrial fibrillation). Severe symptomatic ventricular tachyarrhythmia, if considered life-threatening.

Dose: Adult: Initial and maintenance, weight 70kg or more, 450-600mg/day; titrate up to 900mg/day if needed. Under 70kg, significant QRS-complex widening or second or third degree AV block, consider dose reduction (5-12mg/kg/day), see Elderly below. *Admin*, in divided doses 2 or 3 times daily; swallow tabs whole, with liquid, after food.

Elderly: Initiate gradually (small incremental doses); no increase until after 5-8 days of therapy.

Child: Not recommended.

Renal Impairment: Titrate under ECG and plasma level monitoring.

Hepatic Impairment: As for Renal above.

CI: Known Brugada syndrome, MI within last 3 months, uncontrolled CHF with LVEF below 35%, cardiogenic shock unless caused by arrhythmia, severe symptomatic bradycardia, sinus node dysfunction, atrial conduction defects, second degree or more AV block or bundle branch block or distal block in absence of pacemaker, severe hypotension, electrolyte imbalance (potassium metabolism disorder), severe obstructive pulmonary disease, myasthenia gravis.

Interactions: Effect of Other Drugs on Propafenone: *Co-admin contraindicated*: Ritonavir. *Increased plasma levels*: Ketoconazole, cimetidine, quinidine, erythromycin, grapefruit juice, SSRIs (fluoxetine, paroxetine). *Decreased plasma levels*: Phenobarbital, rifampicin. *Effect potentiated*: Local anaesthetics, drugs inhibiting heart rate and/or contractility (beta-blockers, TCADs). *Proarrhythmic potential*: Amiodarone.

Effect of Propafenone on Other Drugs: Propranolol, metoprolol, desipramine, ciclosporin, digoxin, theophylline, drugs metabolised by CYP2D6 (venlafaxine): *Increased plasma levels*. Oral anticoagulants, coumarins: *Enhanced anticoagulant effect*. Digitalis: *Caution, toxicity*.

SP: Altered pacing/sensing threshold of artificial pacemakers, caution. Caution, asthmatics.

ADR: *Very common*, dizziness, cardiac conduction disorders, palpitations.

Notes: See 2.5.3 Antiarrhythmics Class Ic.

Arythmol 150mg, 300mg *(BGP)* B. GMS.
Price, 150mg (90) €8.77. 300mg (60) €12.53.
Tablet, propafenone HCl. White (off-white) f/c. Marked with strength.

Propafenone (Accord) 150mg, 300mg *(Accord)* B. GMS.
Price, 150mg (90) €4.37. 300mg (60) €6.26.
Tablet, propafenone HCl. White (off-white) round f/c. 300mg: Scored (divisible into equal halves).

2.5.4 - Class II Antiarrhythmics

In This Chapter: *Sotalol*.

62

Class Effects
Class II drugs are characterised by their beta-blocking activity (except of sotalol; predominantly Class III activity). They are used to treat arrhythmias.

Notes: See 2.1.7 Beta-Blockers.

2.5.5 - Class III Antiarrhythmics

In This Chapter: *Amiodarone*.

Class Effects
Class III drugs prolong the repolarisation phase of the action potential.

CI: Hypersensitivity to any member of class.

Notes: See Antiarrhythmics 2.5.1 Class Ia, 2.5.2 Class Ib and 2.5.3 Class Ic.

Amiodarone

ATC Code: C01BD01. **Sport:** Permitted.
Driving: Oral, unlikely to impair. Parenteral, not applicable.
Indications: *Oral, parenteral*, severe rhythm disorders (not responding to other therapy), atrial flutter and fibrillation, tachyarrhythmias of paroxysmal nature (supraventricular, nodal and ventricular tachycardias, ventricular fibrillation) when other drugs cannot be used. Tachyarrhythmias associated with Wolff-Parkinson-White Syndrome. *Oral*, prevention of ventricular arrhythmias in high-risk patients post-MI, with clinical signs of CHF and/or LVEF less than 40% receiving appropriate CHF treatment including ACEIs. Use minimum effective dose; initiate under hospital/specialist supervision. *Parenteral* for use when rapid response is required.

Dose: Adult: ORAL, initial stabilisation, 200mg 3-times daily for 1 week; reduce to 200mg twice daily for 1 week then maintenance of 200mg/day or less if appropriate.
PARENTERAL, prior to DC cardio-conversion, IV infusion, 5mg/kg over 20-120 minutes; repeat up to 1200mg (15mg/kg) per 24 hours. Extreme emergency, use slow IV injection, 150-300mg over minimum 3 minutes; do not repeat for at least 15 minutes. *Cardiopulmonary resuscitation*, shock resistant ventricular fibrillation, 300mg (or 5mg/kg) diluted in 20mL 5% dextrose and rapidly injected; additional 150mg (2.5mg/kg) IV may be considered if fibrillation persists. Adequate response, initiate oral concomitantly as loading dose 200mg 3-times daily.

Elderly: Use lowest dose, monitor thyroid function. May be more susceptible to bradycardia and conduction defects.

Child: Safety/efficacy not established. Under age 3 years, contraindicated (contains benzyl alcohol).

CI: Thyroid dysfunction. Iodine or amiodarone hypersensitivity. Sinus bradycardia, SA heart block, severe conduction disturbances, sinus node disease (unless pacemaker present). *Bolus injection*, severe respiratory failure, circulatory collapse, severe arterial hypotension; hypotension, HF, cardiomyopathy. See Child above.

Interactions: Effect of Other Drugs on Amiodarone: *Co-admin contraindicated* (Torsades de Pointes risk): Drugs prolonging QT-interval including Class Ia antiarrhythmics (quinidine, procainamide, disopyramide, bepridil), Class III antiarrhythmics (sotalol, bretylium), erythromycin (IV), co-trimoxazole, pentamidine (parenteral), vincamine, some neuroleptics, cisapride, some anti-psychotics (chlorpromazine, thioridazine, fluphenazine, pimozide, haloperidol, amisulpride, sertindole), lithium, TCADs (doxepin, maprotiline, amitriptyline), antihistamines (terfenadine, astemizole, mizolastine), anti-malarials (quinine, mefloquine, chloroquine, halofantrine). *Co-admin not recommended*: Potentiation of negative chronotropic properties, conduction slowing effects (beta-blockers, calcium channel blockers including diltiazem, verapamil), hypokalaemia risk (stimulant laxatives), severe (life-threatening) bradycardia, heart block (sofosbuvir alone or with daclatasvir, simeprevir or ledipasvir). *Co-admin avoid* (Torsades de Pointes risk): Fluoroquinolones. *Caution* (hypokalaemia and/or hypomagnesaemia risk): Diuretics, systemic corticosteroids, tetracosactide, amphotericin (IV).

Plasma levels increased: Grapefruit juice (avoid co-admin), other CYP3A4 inhibitors.

Effect of Amiodarone on Other Drugs: P-gp substrates (digitalis, dabigatran): *Consider dose adjustment, monitor*. CYP3A4/CYP2D6 substrates (ciclosporin, phenytoin, flecainide, lidocaine, tacrolimus, sildenafil, midazolam, triazolam, dihydroergotamine, ergotamine), fentanyl, statins metabolised by CYP3A4 (simvastatin, atorvastatin, lovastatin; increased risk of muscular toxicity): *Plasma levels increased*. Oral anticoagulants, coumarins, warfarin: *Plasma levels increased, enhanced anticoagulant effect*. General anaesthesia, high dose oxygen therapy: *Bradycardia unresponsive to atropine, hypotension, conduction disturbances, decreased cardiac output*.

SP: Amiodarone has low pro-arrhythmic effect. New arrhythmias, worsening of treated arrhythmias (sometimes fatal) reported. Bradycardia, conduction disturbances at high dose, especially elderly or during digitalis therapy (withdraw); severe bradycardia, consider pacemaker due to long amiodarone long half-life; caution with co-medication (see Interactions above). ECG changes (QT-prolongations, possible U-waves, deformed T-waves). Pulmonary toxicity (interstitial pneumonitis); suspected diagnosis, perform chest X-ray. Hepatic toxicity, monitor LFTs (transaminases); 3xULN, reduce dose or discontinue. Advise patients to moderate alcohol intake. Perform thyroid function tests prior to initiation; hyperthyroidism may occur. Peripheral sensory neuropathy and/or myopathy. Blurred/decreased vision, caution, optic neuropathy. Hypotension, decompensated cardiomyopathy, severe HF. Life threatening or even fatal cutaneous reactions, discontinue.

IV *injection* generally not advised due to haemodynamic effects associated with rapid injection; circulatory collapse may be precipitated by too rapid admin or overdose; use only in emergency. IV *infusion* preferable.

Pregnancy, Lactation: Pregnancy, contraindicated (except in exceptional circumstances), due to effect on foetal thyroid gland. Lactation, contraindicated.

ADR: *Very common*, corneal microdeposits, increased serum transaminases, photosensitivity; *common*, bradycardia, hyper-, hypothyroidism, constipation, extrapyramidal tremor, pulmonary toxicity, pigmentation of light exposed skin, eczema. Parenteral, *common*, bradycardia, eczema, injection-site reactions, decrease in blood pressure (hypotension or collapse with overdose or too rapid injection).

Notes: See 2.5.5 Antiarrhythmics Class III.

Cordarone X 100mg, 200mg *(SANOFI)* B. GMS.
Price, (28) 100mg, €5.19. 200mg, €7.06.
Tablet, amiodarone HCl. Round white scored (facilitates breaking). Marked with strength. *Lactose, iodine 37.5mg/100mg*. **Store:** Below 25 deg C.

Cordarone IV Parenteral *(SANOFI)* A.
Price, 30mL (10) 150mg/3mL, €20.81.
Injection, amiodarone HCl 50mg/mL. Clear pale-yellow conc for soln for IV injection/infusion. *Benzyl alcohol 60mg/amp*.

2.5.6 - Class IV Antiarrhythmics

Class Effects

Class IV drugs block the slow inward calcium current (calcium channel blockers) but not all calcium channel blockers have the same specific properties. Verapamil is typical of this class. Indicated for treatment of angina pectoris, arrhythmias, hypertension.

Notes: See 2.2.1 Calcium Channel Blockers.

2.5.7 - Class V Antiarrhythmics

Class Effects

Class V drugs reduce the slope of the slow diastolic depolarisation in pacemaker cells of SA node.

2.5.8 - Other Antiarrhythmics

In This Chapter: Adenosine, dronedarone, vernakalant.

Class IV Antiarrhythmics   2.5.6

Class Effects

Adenosine, slows conduction through the AV node; stimulation of A2 receptors results in peripheral vasodilation. It does not fit the Vaughan Williams classification. *Dronedarone* prevents atrial fibrillation or restores normal sinus rhythm. *Vernakalant* acts preferentially in the atria to prolong atrial refractoriness and to rate-dependently slow impulse conduction.

CI: Hypersensitivity to any member of the class. Second or third degree AV block, sick sinus syndrome except if pacemaker present.

SP: For use by qualified medical personnel in environment with monitoring and cardio-respiratory resuscitation equipment available.

Notes: See Antiarrhythmics 2.5.1 Class Ia, 2.5.2 Class Ib, 2.5.3 Class Ic.

Adenosine

ATC Code: C01BD01. **Sport:** Permitted.

Driving: Dizziness, fatigue, hypotension, decreased attention; ALCOHOL or psychoactive substance co-admin not recommended.

Indications: Rapid conversion to normal sinus rhythm of paroxysmal supraventricular tachycardias (adults, children), including those associated with accessory by-pass tracts (Wolff-Parkinson-White Syndrome). *Diagnostic aid*, broad or narrow complex supraventricular tachycardias. Sensitisation of intra-cavitary electrophysiological investigations.

Dose: Adult, Elderly: Initially, 3mg; if elimination of supraventricular tachycardia is not achieved within 1-2 minutes of dose 1, follow 6mg (dose 2), then 12mg (dose 3) by rapid IV bolus over 2 seconds. Additional or higher doses, not recommended. Directly into vein or proximal IV line.

Child: First bolus of 0.1mg/kg (max. 6mg) then increments of 0.1mg/kg as needed to achieve termination of supraventricular tachycardia (max. 12mg). *Admin*, see Adult above.

CI: Sick sinus syndrome, second or third degree AV block except with functioning pacemaker, chronic obstructive lung disease with bronchospasm, long QT syndrome, severe hypotension, decompensated HF.

Interactions: Effect of Other Drugs on Adenosine: *Co-admin contraindicated (action potentiated)*: Dipyridamole (if adenosine bolus essential, discontinue dipyridamole 24 hours before admin, or reduce adenosine dose significantly). *Competitive adenosine antagonists*: Aminophylline, theophylline, other xanthines (avoid 24 hours prior to adenosine admin); food/drink containing xanthines (tea, coffee, chocolate, cola) (avoid 12 hours prior to adenosine admin). *Possible interaction*: Drugs tending to impair cardiac conduction.

SP: Continuous ECG monitoring necessary during admin. Caution, left main coronary stenosis, uncorrected hypovolaemia, stenotic valvular heart disease, left to right shunt, pericarditis, pericardial effusion, autonomic dysfunction or stenotic carotid artery disease with cerebrovascular insufficiency. Recent MI, HF, minor conduction defects (first degree AV block, bundle branch block), transient aggravation during infusion. Atrial fibrillation/flutter, increased conduction down anomalous pathway, caution. Severe bradycardia, Torsades de pointes. Recent heart transplant (under 1 year), increased adenosine sensitivity. Bronchospasm.
Precautions, angina, severe bradycardia, severe hypotension, respiratory failure or asystole/cardiac arrest, discontinue immediately. Convulsion/seizure history, monitor.

Children, atrial arrhythmias may be triggered and might lead to ventricular acceleration in children with Wolff-Parkinson-White syndrome.

Pregnancy, Lactation: Pregnancy, if benefit outweighs risk. Lactation, not recommended.

ADR: *Very common*, flushing, bradycardia, sinus pause, atrial extrasystoles, AV block, ventricular excitability disorders, dyspnoea, chest pressure/pain, feeling of thoracic constriction/oppression. *Common*, headache,

2.6   Anticoagulants, Antiplatelets, Antithrombotics

dizziness, light-headedness, apprehension, nausea, burning sensation.

Notes: See 2.5.8 Other Antiarrhythmics.

Adenocor Parenteral *(SANOFI)* A.
Price, 2mL (6) 3mg/mL, €31.07.
Injection, adenosine 3mg/mL. Clear colourless soln. *Sodium 18mg (0.3mmoL)/2mL Vial.* **Store:** Below 25 deg C; do not refrigerate.

Dronedarone

ATC Code: C01BD07. **Sport:** Permitted.
Driving: None known.
Indications: Maintenance of sinus rhythm after successful cardioversion in clinically stable patients with paroxysmal or persistent atrial fibrillation, after alternatives considered.

Dose: Adult, Elderly: 400mg twice daily (1 tab morning and evening with food); do not admin with grapefruit juice. Can be initiated in outpatient setting. See SP below. *Elderly,* age 75 years and older, caution with co-morbidities. Swallow whole with water; cannot be divided into equal doses.

Child: Under 18 years, no data.

Renal Impairment: CrCl (mL/min) below 30, contraindicated.

Hepatic Impairment: Severe, contraindicated.

CI: Second or third degree AV block, complete bundle branch block, distal block, sinus node dysfunction, atrial conduction defects, sick sinus syndrome (except with functioning pacemaker). Bradycardia (below 50 bpm). AF duration 6 months or more and attempts to restore sinus rhythm no longer considered. Unstable haemodynamic conditions. HF or LV systolic dysfunction. Liver and lung toxicity related to previous amiodarone use. QTc Bazett interval above 500 milliseconds.

Interactions: Effect of Other Drugs on Dronedarone: *Co-admin contraindicated*: Potent CYP3A4 inhibitors (ketoconazole, itraconazole, voriconazole, posaconazole, telithromycin, clarithromycin, nefazodone, ritonavir), medicinals inducing Torsades de pointes (phenothiazines, cisapride, bepridil, TCADs, terfenadine, certain oral macrolides (erythromycin), Class I and III antiarrhythmics, dabigatran. *Co-admin Avoid*: Grapefruit juice. *Co-admin not recommended*: Potent CYP3A4 inducers (rifampicin, phenobarbital, carbamazepine, phenytoin, St John's Wort), dabigatran. *Co-admin caution*: Beta-blockers, calcium antagonists (ECG monitoring), statins (consider lower dosage; monitor for muscular toxicity signs), MAOIs (decrease clearance of active metabolite).

Effect of Dronedarone on Other Drugs: Digoxin: *Increased plasma levels; recommend digoxin dose halved (may precipitate symptoms associated with digoxin toxicity).* Sirolimus, tacrolimus: *Possible increased plasma levels; dose adjustment.* Anticoagulants: *Monitor INR.*

SP: Not for use in patients with left ventricular systolic dysfunction or with current or previous episodes of heart failure. Regularly assess cardiac, hepatic, pulmonary function. If AF reoccurs, consider discontinuation. Stop Class I or III antiarrhythmics (flecainide, propafenone, quinidine, disopyramide, dofetilide, sotalol, amiodarone) before initiation. Stable Class III or LVEF below 35%, not recommended; may induce moderate QTc Bazett prolongation. Correct potassium or magnesium deficiency before initiation and during therapy.

Hepatocellular injury, including life-threatening, reported. Perform LFTs before initiation, repeated monthly for 6 months, then at months 9, 12, then periodically. Measure plasma creatinine 7 days after initiation; if increased creatininaemia observed, use this value for new reference baseline.

Pregnancy, Lactation: Pregnancy, not recommended. Women of childbearing potential, ensure adequate contraception. Lactation, stop breastfeeding or stop drug.

ADR: Summary, *common reasons for discontinuation,* GI disorders; *most frequent,* diarrhoea, nausea, vomiting, fatigue, asthenia.

Notes: See 2.5.8 Other Antiarrhythmics.

MULTAQ 400mg *(SANOFI)* B. GMS.
Price, (60) €78.51.
Tablet, dronedarone HCl. White oblong f/c. Marked double wave; 4142 on reverse. *Lactose.*

Vernakalant

ATC Code: C01BG11. **Sport:** Permitted.
Driving: Dizziness within 2 hours of admin.
Indications: Rapid conversion of recent onset atrial fibrillation to sinus rhythm (adults), non-surgery patients (atrial fibrillation 7 days or less), post cardiac surgery (atrial fibrillation 3 days or less).

Dose: Adult, Elderly: Initially 3mg/kg IV*; if conversion to sinus rhythm does not occur after 15 minutes after initial dose, admin second 2mg/kg IV*. Cumulative doses above 5mg/kg should not be admin within 24 hours. Patients 113kg and above, do not exceed 339mg. *(IV infusion over 10 minutes using infusion pump; not for IV push or bolus). Monitor during infusion for sudden decrease in BP or heart rate.

Child: Under 18 years, no relevant use.

CI: Severe aortic stenosis, systolic BP below 100mg Hg, HF (NYHA III, IV), prolonged QT at baseline, severe bradycardia, sinus node dysfunction, IV rhythm control antiarrhythmics (Class I and III) within 4 hours prior to admin, acute coronary syndrome including MI within last 30 days.

Interactions: Effect of Other Drugs on Vernakalant: *Co-admin caution (increased atrial flutter risk)*: Oral antiarrhythmics (Class I, III). See Contraindications.

SP: Before initiation ensure adequate hydration, haemodynamic optimisation, anticoagulation, potassium levels corrected. During infusion, bradycardia and/or hypotension or ECG changes, discontinue, do not admin second infusion; CHF higher hypotension, ventricular arrhythmia risk, caution; NYHA III, IV, contraindicated. LVEF 35% or below, not recommended. Atrial flutter secondary to treatment, consider infusion continuation. Valvular heart disease, higher ventricular arrhythmia incidence.

Pregnancy, Lactation: Pregnancy, avoid use. Lactation, caution.

ADR: *Very common,* dysgeusia, sneezing. *Common,* paraesthesia, dizziness, headache, hypoaesthesia, bradycardia, atrial flutter, hypotension, cough, nasal discomfort, nausea, vomiting, oral paraesthesia, pruritus, hyperhidrosis, infusion site pain, feeling hot.

Notes: See 2.5.8 Other Antiarrhythmics.

Brinavess Parenteral *(Cardiome)* A. HOS.
Price, (1) 25mL, €398.04.
Infusion, vernakalant HCl 500mg (452.5mg free base) in 25mL vial (20mg/mL). Clear colourless (pale-yellow) soln. pH 5.5. *Sodium 80mg/vial.*

2.6 - Anticoagulants, Antiplatelets, Antithrombotics

Class Effects

Anticoagulants may be classed as direct (parenteral) e.g. heparin, low molecular weight heparins (LMWH), heparinoids (danaparoid), synthetic activated Factor X (Xa) inhibitors, hirudins and epoprostenol. Or indirect (oral) e.g. coumarins, warfarin.

If anticoagulant dose is missed or when switching from one anticoagulant to another, always consult the manufacturers Full Prescribing Information.

CI: Hypersensitivity to any members of the class. Acute bacterial endocarditis, active major bleeding disorders, thrombocytopenia (in patients with positive in-vitro aggregation test in the presence of enoxaparin), jaundice, active gastric or duodenal ulceration, hiatal ulceration, CVA (unless due to systemic emboli), threatened abortion, retinopathy, conditions with high uncontrolled haemorrhage risk (recent haemorrhagic stroke, subdural haematoma).

SP: Assess need for continuous prevention of thrombotic cardio- and cerebrovascular events based on available clinical guidance and national regulatory requirements.

Heparin-induced thrombocytopenia (history; with or without thrombosis), monitor platelets.

64

Increased haemorrhagic risk factors, impaired haemostasis, bleeding disorders (congenital, acquired), active ulcerative GI disease (or history of), recent (GI ulceration, ischaemic stroke), intra- (cranial or cerebral) haemorrhage, uncontrolled severe arterial hypertension, severe (liver, renal) impairment, diabetic retinopathy, recent (cerebral, spinal, ophthalmological) surgery or trauma, mechanical prosthetic heart valves, including pregnant women (no data), elderly, low body weight (women below 45kg, men below 57kg, monitor).

Neuraxial anaesthesia (spinal/epidural anaesthesia) or spinal/epidural puncture, risk of epidural or spinal haematoma (may result in long-term or permanent paralysis); risk increased by post-operative use of indwelling epidural catheters, co-admin of medicinals affecting haemostasis, traumatic or repeated epidural or spinal puncture. Monitor for signs/symptoms of neurological impairment (numbness or weakness of legs, bowel or bladder dysfunction).

Heparin, IV and SC route, monitor clotting time; IM, not recommended (haematoma). Heparin may cause suppression of adrenal aldosterone secretion (hyperkalaemia; especially in diabetes mellitus, chronic renal failure, pre-existing metabolic acidosis, raised plasma potassium, potassium-sparing drugs).

Pregnancy, Lactation: Pregnancy, only if clearly needed. Lactation, generally not recommended.

ADR: Haemorrhage, epistaxis, neuraxial haematoma (spinal/epidural anaesthesia), thrombocytopenia, local injection-site reactions, allergic reactions, increased platelet counts/liver enzyme levels. Heparin may cause febrile reactions, osteoporosis (prolonged use), late vasospastic reactions, hypoaldosteronism (increased plasma potassium), immune-mediated thrombocytopenia or thrombosis, priapism, hyperkalaemia.

2.6.1 - Heparin, Heparin Flush Solutions, Heparinoids

In This Chapter: *Danaparoid, enoxaparin, heparin, tinzaparin.*

Class Effects
Heparin flush solns are used to maintain patency of IV lines.

CI: Children, no data (heparin sodium); not recommended (enoxaparin, enoxaparin, tinzaparin).

Interactions: Effect of Other Drugs on Heparin/LMWH: *Co-admin avoid (enhanced anticoagulant effect):* Drugs affecting haemostasis (aspirin, NSAIDs, dextran solns, Vitamin K antagonists, ticlopidine, clopidogrel, glucocorticoids, thrombolytics, anticoagulants, anti-platelets). Danaparoid does not appear to interact unfavourably with oral anticoagulants, anti-platelets, thrombolytics.

SP: Premature infants, *use formulations without benzyl alcohol*. Renal, hepatic impairment, caution. NOTE: LMWH are not interchangeable (differ in manufacturing process, molecular weights, specific anti-Xa activities, units, dosage). Danaparoid anti-Xa units have a different relationship to clinical efficacy than those of heparin and LMWH. Compliance with dosage regimen and usage instructions for each product is required.

Pregnancy, Lactation: Heparin used during pregnancy has not been shown to affect the foetus. Increased risk of maternal bleeding; is excreted in breast milk. LMWH, pregnancy, if benefit outweighs risk; lactation, avoid. Danaparoid, caution; pregnancy and lactation, use only if no acceptable alternative.

ADR: LMWH: Haemorrhage (including major).

Notes: See 2.6 Anticoagulants, Antiplatelets, Antithrombotics.

Danaparoid
ATC Code: B01AB09. **Sport:** Pending.
Driving: Not known to affect.
Indications: Prevention and treatment, thrombo-embolic disorders where urgent parenteral anticoagulation is required due to development or history of heparin-induced

thrombocytopenia (HIT); prevention of deep vein thrombosis (DVT) in orthopaedic, major abdominal or thoracic surgery.

Dose: Adult, Elderly: *HIT, without thromboembolism*, dose depends on thrombotic risk; past HIT (more than 3 months before present admission), as for patients without HIT; acute HIT (less than 3 months) with circulating heparin-induced antiplatelet antibody, higher daily doses necessary, 2250-3750 anti-XA units SC in 3 divided doses (8-hourly) for 7-10 days.

Continuous renal replacement therapy, 2250 anti-XA units (under 55kg, 1500 anti-Xa units; above 90kg, 3750 anti-Xa units) IV as bolus, plus IV infusion of 400 anti-Xa units/hour for 4 hours, then 300 anti-Xa units/hour for 4 hours, then maintenance 150-200 anti-Xa units/hour for 5-7 days then convert to SC 750 anti-Xa units 2-3 times daily or oral anticoagulants. Intermittent renal haemodialysis*.

Vascular operation, invasive procedure by IV bolus, 90kg or under, 2250 anti-Xa units before procedure; above 90kg, 3750 anti-Xa units then no less than 6 hours post-operatively, 150-200 anti-Xa units by IV infusion for 5-7 days then convert to SC as above. *Cardiopulmonary procedures*, use for post-operative prophylaxis*.

Flush doses, dilute 1 amp in 50mL saline and use 5-10mL to flush intravascular lines/access ports.

Conversion to oral anticoagulants possible during SC and IV dosing schedules; advisable to start such therapy when only with adequate antithrombotic control with danaparoid.

Child: Experience limited to 36 children, age 2 weeks to 17 years.

Renal Impairment: Moderate, caution; severe, not recommended.

Hepatic Impairment: As for Renal above.

CI: Uncontrolled hypertension, patients receiving heparin for treatment rather than prophylaxis, local/regional anaesthesia in elective surgical procedure, CNS damage (brain, spinal cord, ophthalmic surgery). See Notes below.

SP: Cannot be neutralised by protamine or any other usual antagonists to limit bleeding. Not for IM admin.

ADR: *Common*, thrombocytopenia including heparin-induced, rash, post-procedural haemorrhage.

Notes: See 2.6.1 Heparin. *See Full Prescribing Information.

Organan Parenteral (Aspen) A.
Price, not published by company.
Injection or infusion, danaparoid sodium 1250 anti-factor Xa units/mL (0.6mL amp). Clear colourless (pale-yellow) aqueous soln. *Sulphite*.

Enoxaparin
ATC Code: B01AB05. **Sport:** Permitted.
Driving: Unlikely to impair.
Indications: Venous thromboembolic disorders (DVT, pulmonary embolism). Unstable angina, non-Q-wave MI. Orthopaedic, general surgery prophylaxis. Medical patients (acutely ill, bedridden); cardiac insufficiency, respiratory failure, severe infections. Haemodialysis. Acute STEMI (medical management, subsequent PCI).

Dose: Adult: PROPHYLAXIS, *surgery*, moderate risk, 20mg (2000 IU)/day*by SC injection (initial dose approx. 2 hours pre-operatively); higher risk (orthopaedic surgery), 40mg (4000 IU)/day* (initial dose 12 hours pre-operatively), average 7-10 days, hip replacement, 3 weeks; *medical patients*, 40mg/day* (6 to max. 14 days). *Admin*, once daily.

Haemodialysis, 1mg/kg (100 IU/kg) into arterial line at beginning of dialysis; admin another 0.5-1mg/kg (50-100 IU/kg) if fibrin rings found. Patients at high haemorrhage risk, 0.5mg/kg (50 IU/kg) for double vascular access or 0.75mg/kg (75 IU/kg) for single vascular access.

TREATMENT, *DVT, pulmonary embolism*, 1.5mg/kg (150 IU/kg) daily OR 1mg/kg (100 IU/kg) twice daily (5 days).

Unstable angina, non-Q-wave MI, 1mg/kg (100 IU/kg) 12-hourly with oral aspirin (100-325mg once daily) (2-8 days).

STEMI, single IV bolus 30mg plus 1mg/kg SC followed by 1mg/kg SC 12-hourly; max. 100mg for first two doses,

2.6.2 Synthetic Activated Factor X (Xa) Inhibitors

followed by 1mg/kg for remaining doses. *Admin*, SC (IV only when indicated).

Elderly: 80 years and older, monitor. STEMI, do not use bolus; initiate with 0.75mg/kg SC 12-hourly; max. 75mg for first two doses, then 0.75mg/kg for remaining doses.

Renal Impairment: CrCl (mL/min) below 30, reduce dose.

Hepatic Impairment: Caution.

SP: PCI, adhere to recommended intervals between admin.

ADR: *Most common*, haemorrhage (including major); some fatal; may occur with risk factors (organic lesions liable to bleed, invasive procedures, medications affecting haemostasis). In surgical patients, haemorrhage complications were considered major, if the haemorrhage caused a significant clinical event, if accompanied by Hb decrease of 2 g/dL (or above) or transfusion of 2 or more units of blood products. Always considered major (retroperitoneal, intracranial haemorrhage).

Notes: See 2.6.1 Heparin.

Clexane, Forte Parenteral *(SANOFI)* A. GMS.
Price, syringe 100mg/mL (10) 20mg, €21.01; 40mg, €37.68; 60mg, €52.27; 80mg, €64.64; 100mg, €80.61. Forte 150mg/mL (10) 120mg, €88.26. 150mg, €106.71.
Injection, enoxaparin sodium 100mg/mL, Forte 150mg/mL. Sterile colourless (pale-yellow) soln (PFS). **Store:** Below 25 deg C; do not refrigerate or freeze.

Heparin Sodium

ATC Code: C01BD01. **Sport:** Permitted.
Driving: Unlikely to impair.

Indications: Treatment and prophylaxis, thromboembolic disorders. Prevention of coagulation during transfusion or dialysis. Lipaemic effect may be used in prevention or treatment of fat embolism.

Dose: Adult, Elderly: PROPHYLAXIS, 5000 IU 2-6 hours pre-operative, then 5000 IU 8-hourly SC. *Pregnancy* prophylaxis, maintain plasma heparin levels between 0.1-0.4 units/mL (anti-Xa assay); whole blood clotting time, 15-20 minutes. Early Pregnancy, 5000 IU 8-hourly; third trimester, up to 10000 IU 2-3 times daily. Reduce dose during labour; post-partum, standard prophylactic dose. TREATMENT, 5000-10000 IU 4-hourly (bolus injection or continuous infusion). 5000 IU every 8-12 hours also used. IV or SC.

Notes: See 2.6.1 Heparin.

Monoparin Parenteral *(Fannin)* A.
Price, 0.2mL (10) 5000 IU/mL, €14.35.
Injection, heparin sodium 5000 IU/mL amp. *Preservative-free.*
Multiparin Parenteral *(Fannin)* A.
Price, 5mL (10) 1000 IU/mL, €26.72. 5000 IU/mL, €34.39
Injection, heparin sodium 1000 IU, 5000 IU multidose vials. *Benzyl alcohol.*

Heparin Sodium (flush soln)

ATC Code: B01AB01. **Sport:** Permitted.
Driving: Unlikely to impair.

Indications: 10 IU/mL, used as heparin flush to keep IV lines patent. 100 IU/mL, for IV admin into indwelling cannulae.

Dose: Adult, Elderly: *10 IU/mL,* 10-50 IU every 4-8 hours into catheter/cannula. *100 IU/mL,* fill cannula space once or twice daily using 2mL.

CI: Not for systemic use. Heparin hypersensitivity, haemorrhagic disease, current/history of heparin-induced thrombocytopenia.

Interactions: Effect of Other Drugs on Heparin Flush Solutions: Admixture with other drugs: *Inactivation of either active ingredient.*

SP: Should have no systemic anticoagulant effect as the IV line should be flushed through with saline.

Notes: See 2.6.5 Heparin Flush Solutions.

Hepsal Flush Solution *(Fannin)* A.
Price, 5mL (10) 10 IU/mL, €9.22.
Flush solution, heparin sodium 10 IU/mL.

Tinzaparin

ATC Code: B01AB10. **Sport:** Permitted.
Driving: No or negligible influence.
Indications: Prophylaxis, venous thromboembolism (VTE),

patients undergoing surgery (orthopaedic, general, oncological); non-surgical patients immobilised due to acute medical illness e.g. acute (heart failure, respiratory failure), severe infection, active cancer, rheumatic disease exacerbation. Prevention, clotting in extracorporeal circuits (haemodialysis, haemofiltration).

Dose: Adult: PROPHYLAXIS, surgery (moderate risk), 3500 anti-Xa IU 2 hours before surgery then once daily*; (high risk e.g. orthopaedic, cancer surgery), 4500 anti-Xa IU 12 hours before surgery then once daily*. Non-surgical (immobilised) patients, 3500 anti-Xa IU (moderate risk) or 4500 anti-Xa IU (high risk) once daily*. Very low or very high body weight, consider 50 anti-Xa IU per kg body weight once daily; admin 2 hours before surgery in surgical patients*. NOTE: Caution, neuraxial anaesthesia or lumbar puncture. See Full Prescribing Information.
Haemodialysis/filtration, (duration 4 hours or less), bolus 2000-2500 anti-Xa IU at start of dialysis; (duration more than 4 hours), 2500 anti-Xa IU at start of dialysis/filtration, then 750 anti-Xa IU per hour (continuous infusion). If needed adjust bolus gradually by 500 anti-Xa IU until satisfactory response; usual dose 2000-4500 anti-Xa IU. Concomitant transfusion (blood, conc red corpuscles), admin extra bolus of 500-1000 anti-Xa IU. Plasma anti-Xa level should be about 0.5 anti-Xa IU/mL one hour after admin.

Admin, SC injection. *(for as long as patient is considered a VTE risk).

Elderly: Caution, renal impairment.

Child: Under 18 years, no dose recommendation.

Renal Impairment: CrCl (mL/min) below 30, caution; below 20, weigh risk/benefit.

Hepatic Impairment: As for Renal above.

CI: Immune-mediated heparin-induced thrombocytopenia, patients receiving neuraxial anaesthesia.

Interactions: Effect of Other Drugs on Tinzaparin: *Effect potentially enhanced (avoid; monitor):* Platelet inhibitors (acetylsalicylic acid, NSAIDs), thrombolytics, Vitamin K antagonists, activated protein C, small molecule anti-Xa and IIa inhibitors.

SP: With epidural/spinal anaesthesia or spinal puncture, prophylactic heparin or LMWH rarely associated with epidural/spinal haematoma resulting in prolonged or permanent paralysis. *Platelets*, measure before initiation, then periodically (immune-mediated heparin-induced thrombocytopenia risk). *Hyperkalaemia*, risk factors (diabetes mellitus, chronic renal failure, pre-existing metabolic acidosis, hyperkalaemia pre-treatment, drugs elevating potassium, long-term use). LMWH should not be used interchangeably; exercise caution.

Pregnancy, Lactation: Pregnancy, can be used if clinically needed. Lactation, stop breastfeeding or stop drug.

ADR: *Most frequent*, haemorrhage events, anaemia secondary to haemorrhage, injection-site reactions.

Notes: See Class Effects 2.6.1 Heparin.

Innohep Parenteral *(LEO)* A. GMS.
Price, syringes (10) (x1000) 8 IU, €65.72; 10 IU, €77.16; 12 IU, €98.74; 14 IU, €104.11; 16 IU, €131.40; 18 IU, €129.94. Vials (10) (x1000) 10 IU (10) €132.40; 20 IU (1) €31.16. Injection (10) 2500 IU, €20.74. 3500 IU, €27.69. 4500 IU, €37.32.
Injection, tinzaparin sodium. Colourless (straw-coloured) aqueous soln. *Essentially sodium-free.* 10000 IU/mL vial. *Benzyl alcohol.* **Store:** Below 25 deg C.

2.6.2 - Synthetic Activated Factor X (Xa) Inhibitors

In This Chapter: *Apixaban, edoxaban, fondaparinux, rivaroxaban.*

Class Effects

These drugs are used in the prevention and management of venous thrombotic events or venous thromboembolism (VTE) e.g. deep vein thrombosis (DVT) and pulmonary embolism (PE).

CI: Children under 18 years, not recommended unless otherwise specified. Hypersensitivity to any member of the class. Active clinically significant bleeding or lesion or condition at significant risk of major bleeding (GI ulceration, malignant neoplasms, recent brain, spinal, ophthalmic injury or surgery, intracranial haemorrhage, oesophageal varices, arteriovenous malformations, vascular aneurysms, intraspinal or intracerebral vascular abnormalities).

Interactions: Effect of Other Drugs on Factor X (Xa) Inhibitors: *Co-admin caution, plasma levels increased (bleeding risk):* Strong CYP3A4 and P-gp inhibitors including azole antifungals (ketoconazole, itraconazole, voriconazole, posaconazole), protease inhibitors (ritonavir). *Co-admin caution, plasma levels decreased:* Strong CYP3A4 inducers (rifampicin, phenytoin, carbamazepine, phenobarbital, St John's Wort). *Co-admin caution (increased bleeding risk):* Drugs affecting haemostasis (NSAIDs, acetylsalicylic acid, platelet aggregation inhibitors, other antithrombotics).

SP: Hip fracture surgery, not recommended. *Haemorrhagic risk factors,* see Notes below.

Notes: See 2.6 Anticoagulants, Antiplatelets, Antithrombotics.

Apixaban

ATC Code: B01AF02. **Sport:** Permitted.
Driving: No or negligible influence.

Indications: *Prevention,* venous thromboembolism (VTE), in elective hip or knee replacement surgery; stroke and systemic embolism, adults with non-valvular atrial fibrillation (NVAF) with one or more risk factors. *Treatment* (and prevention of recurrence) of deep vein thrombosis (DVT) and pulmonary embolism (PE).

Dose: Adult, Elderly: *Prevention,* VTE in elective surgery (hip, knee), 2.5mg twice daily; initial dose 12-24 hours after surgery; duration, hip replacement (32-38 days), knee replacement (10-14 days). Stroke prevention, 5mg twice daily; reduce to 2.5mg twice daily with at least 2 risk factors (80 years and over, 60kg and under, serum creatinine 1.5mg/dL or more). Continue long-term.
Treatment, acute DVT and PE, 10mg twice daily (7 days), then 5mg twice daily; prevention, recurrent DVT and PE, 2.5mg twice daily initiated after completion of 6 months of treatment. Patients can stay on apixaban while being cardio-converted.

Switch from parenteral anticoagulants to *Eliquis* and vice versa can be done at next scheduled dose; do not take simultaneously. Switch from Vitamin K antagonists (VKA) to *Eliquis,* discontinue warfarin or other VKA therapy and start *Eliquis* when INR is below 2.

Admin, with water, with or without food. Tabs may be crushed and suspended in water, 5% dextrose in water (D5W), apple juice or mixed with apple puree (admin orally immediately) OR crushed and suspended in 60mL water or D5W (admin through nasogastric tube immediately). Crushed tabs are stable in water, D5W, apple juice and apple puree for up to 4 hours.

Renal Impairment: Moderate, no adjustment. Severe (CrCl 15-29 Ml/min), VTE, DVT, PE prevention, caution. Prevention of stroke and systemic embolism, 2.5mg twice daily. See Dose above (with risk factors). CrCl below 15mL/min, not recommended.

Hepatic Impairment: Mild/moderate or ALT/AST above 2xULN or total bilirubin 1.5xULN or above, caution. Severe, not recommended.

Interactions: Effect of Other Drugs on Apixaban: *Co-admin contraindicated:* Other anticoagulants including unfractionated heparin, LMWH (enoxaparin, dalteparin), heparin derivatives (fondaparinux), oral anticoagulants (warfarin, rivaroxaban, dabigatran). *Reduced exposure:* Activated charcoal.

SP: Use in acute ischaemic stroke, limited data. Prosthetic heart valves, with or without atrial fibrillation, not recommended. Use in DVT and PE in patients with active cancer, no data.

Pregnancy, Lactation: Pregnancy, not recommended. Lactation, stop drug or stop breastfeeding.

ADR: Summary, *common,* haemorrhage, contusion, epistaxis, haematoma.

Notes: See Class Effects 2.6.2 Synthetic Activated Factor X (Xa) Inhibitors.

Eliquis 2.5mg, 5mg *(BMS/Pfizer)* B. GMS.
Price, 2.5mg (20) €24.59; (60) €67.46. 5mg (28) €31.68; (56) €63.91.
Tablet, apixaban. (f/c). 2.5mg: Yellow round. Marked 893 and 2 and 1/2. 5mg: Pink oval. Marked 894 and 5. *Lactose.* **Store:** No special requirements.

Edoxaban

ATC Code: B01AF03. **Sport:** Permitted.
Driving: No or negligible effect.

Indications: Adults, *prevention,* stroke and systemic embolism, patients with nonvalvular atrial fibrillation (NVAF) with one or more risk factors (CHF, hypertension, age 75 years and older, diabetes mellitus, prior stroke or TIA); *treatment,* deep vein thrombosis (DVT) and pulmonary embolism (PE) and prevention of recurrence.

Dose: Adult: *Prevention* of stroke and systemic embolism, 60mg once daily (should be continued long-term).
Treatment (DVT, PE) and prevention of recurrence, 60mg once daily **following** initial parenteral anticoagulant for minimum 5 days; edoxaban not to be admin simultaneously. NVAF and VTE patients with one or more clinical factors*, 30mg once daily. *(moderate to severe renal impairment with CrCl 15-50mL/min; low body weight 60kg and under; P-gp inhibitor co-admin including ciclosporin, dronedarone, erythromycin, ketoconazole). *Admin,* with or without food.

Elderly: Co-admin with acetylsalicylic acid, caution.

Renal Impairment: CrCl (mL/min) above 50, no adjustment; 15-50, 30mg once daily; under 15 (ESRD) or on dialysis, not recommended.

Hepatic Impairment: Severe, not recommended. Mild/moderate, ALT/AST above 2x ULN, total bilirubin 1.5x ULN or above, 60mg once daily (caution);

CI: Hepatic disease associated with coagulopathy and clinically relevant bleeding risk.

Interactions: Effect of Other Drugs on Edoxaban: *Co-admin contraindicated:* P-gp inhibitors, see Dose above (other P-gp inhibitors, no data), other anticoagulants including unfractionated heparin, LMWH (enoxaparin, dalteparin), heparin derivatives (fondaparinux), oral anticoagulants (warfarin, rivaroxaban, apixaban, dabigatran). *Plasma levels decreased:* P-gp inducers (rifampicin, phenytoin, carbamazepine, phenobarbital, St John's Wort).

SP: *Monitor,* LFTs, creatinine clearance (prior to initiation); change in renal function suspected (hypovolaemia, dehydration, other medicine co-admin), monitor. *Lixiana 15mg* is not indicated as monotherapy (decreased efficacy). Should be stopped at least 24 hours before surgery. *Use not recommended,* with mechanical heart valves, as alternative to unfractionated heparin with PE and haemodynamically unstable. Safety and efficacy with active cancer not established. Edoxaban prolongs standard clotting tests e.g. prothrombin time (PT), INR, activated partial thromboplastin time (aPTT) by FXa inhibition

Pregnancy, Lactation: Pregnancy, contraindicated. Women of childbearing potential should avoid becoming pregnant during treatment.

ADR: Summary, *most common,* bleeding (cutaneous soft tissue haemorrhage, epistaxis, vaginal haemorrhage); can occur at any site and may be severe or even fatal.

Notes: See Class Effects 2.6.2 Synthetic Activated Factor X (Xa) Inhibitors.

▼ **Lixiana Tablets** *(Daiichi Sankyo)* B. GMS.
Price, (10) 15mg, €21.53. (28), 30mg, 60mg, €60.44.
Tablet, edoxaban tosilate. Round f/c. Marked DSC L and strength. 15mg: Orange. 30mg: Pink. 60mg: Yellow.

Fondaparinux

ATC Code: B01AX05. **Sport:** Permitted.
Driving: No data.

Indications: *Prevention, (1.5mg/0.3mL strength)* venous thromboembolic events (VTE) (adults) undergoing major orthopaedic surgery of lower limbs (hip fracture, major knee surgery, hip replacement), abdominal surgery at high risk of VTE complications (abdominal cancer surgery), medical patients at high VTE risk (immobilised due to acute illness e.g. cardiac insufficiency, acute respiratory disorders, acute infectious or inflammatory disease).

Treatment, (adults) *(1.5mg/0.3mL strength)* acute symptomatic spontaneous superficial-vein thrombosis of lower limbs without concomitant deep-vein thrombosis (DVT); *(2.5mg/0.5mL strength)* unstable angina or non-STEMI (urgent invasive management not indicated), STEMI (managed with thrombolytics or initially are to receive no other form of reperfusion therapy); *(5mg/0.4mL, 7.5mg/0.6mL, 10mg/0.8mL strengths)* acute DVT, acute pulmonary embolism (PE) except (haemodynamically unstable patients; or requiring thrombolysis or pulmonary embolectomy).

Dose: Adult, Elderly: *Prevention, surgery,* 2.5mg/day post-operative; initial dose 6 hours following surgical closure (5-9 days after surgery; hip fracture, up to additional 24 days); *medical,* 2.5mg/day (6-14 days).

Treatment, superficial-vein thrombosis, 2.5mg/day (minimum 30 days; max. 45 days); *unstable angina/non-STEMI,* 2.5mg/day SC; initiate soonest after diagnosis (max. 8 days or until hospital discharge if earlier); *STEMI,* 2.5mg/day; first dose IV* and then SC, as for non-STEMI; *acute DVT, PE,* 7.5mg/day (body weight 50-100kg); under 50kg, 5mg/day; over 100kg, 10mg/day; duration at least 5 days.

Special populations, 75 years and older and/or under 50kg and/or with renal impairment (CrCl 20-50mL/min), strict adherence to timing of first injection i.e. not earlier than 6 hours following surgical closure; superficial-vein thrombosis, under 50kg, not recommended.

Admin, once daily by deep SC injection (patient lying down); not for IM use. *IV admin (STEMI first dose) through existing IV line directly or using small volume (25 or 50mL) 0.9% saline minibag (infuse over 1-2 minutes).

Child: Under 17 years, not recommended.

Renal Impairment: *VTE prevention, superficial vein thrombosis,* CrCl (mL/min) below 20, contraindicated; 20-30 reduce to 1.5mg once daily; above 50, no adjustment. *Non-STEMI, STEMI,* CrCl (mL/min) below 20, contraindicated; above 20, no adjustment. *DVT, PE,* weight over 100kg and moderate impairment, after initial 10mg daily dose, consider reduction to 7.5mg; severe (CrCl below 30mL/min), not recommended.

Hepatic Impairment: VTE prevention, treatment DVT, PE, severe impairment, caution. Superficial vein thrombosis, not recommended.

CI: Acute bacterial endocarditis. See Notes below.

Interactions: Effect of Other Drugs on Fondaparinux: *Increased bleeding risk:* Other agents enhancing haemorrhage not for co-admin (desirudin, fibrinolytics, GP IIb/IIIa receptor antagonists, heparin, heparinoids); heparin or LMWH as follow-up therapy (admin first injection one day after fondaparinux).

SP: Heparin Induced thrombocytopenia type II (no data). Follow-up Vitamin K antagonist, continue fondaparinux until target INR reached. See Interactions above.

Pregnancy, Lactation: Pregnancy, if benefit outweighs risk. Lactation, not recommended; oral absorption by child unlikely.

ADR: Summary, *most common serious events,* bleeding complications at various sites, anaemia.

Notes: See Class Effects 2.6.2 Synthetic Activated Factor X (Xa) Inhibitors.

Arixtra Fondaparinux Parenteral *(Aspen)* A.
Price, not published by company.
Injection, fondaparinux sodium. Clear colourless soln (PFS). *Essentially sodium-free.* **Store:** Below 25 deg C; do not freeze.

Rivaroxaban

ATC Code: B01AF01. **Sport:** Permitted.
Driving: Minor influence (syncope, dizziness).

Indications: Prevention, venous thromboembolism (VTE) (elective hip or knee replacement surgery) (10mg). Prevention, stroke and systemic embolism (non-valvular atrial fibrillation with risk factors); treatment and prevention of recurrence, deep vein thrombosis (DVT) and pulmonary embolism (PE) (15mg, 20mg).

Dose: Adult, Elderly: 10mg strength: *VTE (elective surgery),* 10mg once daily, initial dose 6-10 hours after surgery; major hip surgery (5 weeks), knee (2 weeks). *Elderly,* may be at increased haemorrhagic risk.

15mg, 20mg strengths: *Prevention* (stroke, systemic embolism), 20mg once daily (max.); admin long-term. *Treatment, prevention of recurrence* (DVT, PE), 15mg twice daily (day 1-21) (max. 30mg/day), then max. 20mg once daily (day 22 onwards); individualise duration. *Admin,* with or without food; unable to swallow tabs, crush, mix with water or apple puree; may be given via gastric tube after correct tube placement.

Child: Under 18 years, not recommended.

Renal Impairment: CrCl (mL/min) 15-29, plasma levels significantly increased, caution increased bleeding risk; below 15, not recommended. CrCl 30-49 and receiving drugs increasing rivaroxaban plasma levels, caution.

CrCl(mL/min) 15-49: *Stroke prevention,* 15mg once daily. Treatment and prevention of DVT/PE, 15mg twice daily (3 weeks) then 20mg once daily.

Hepatic Impairment: Cirrhosis with moderate impairment, not with coagulopathy, caution.

CI: Hepatic disease associated with coagulopathy and clinically relevant bleeding risk.

Interactions: Effect of Other Drugs on Rivaroxaban: *Co-admin contraindicated:* Unfractionated heparin, LMWH (enoxaparin, dalteparin), heparin derivatives (fondaparinux), oral anticoagulants (warfarin, dabigatran, apixaban). *Co-admin caution:* Drugs affecting haemostasis (NSAIDs, acetylsalicylic acid, platelet aggregation inhibitors, other antithrombotics). See Renal above.

SP: At risk for ulcerative GI disease, consider prophylactic treatment. Routine monitoring of exposure is not required but levels measured with a calibrated quantitative anti-fact Xa assay may be useful (overdose, emergency surgery). *Xarelto* can be initiated or continued in patients requiring cardioversion. For all patients, confirmation should be sought prior to cardioversion that the patient has taken the medication as prescribed. To reduce potential bleeding risk associated with co-admin of rivaroxaban and neuraxial (epidural/spinal) anaesthesia or spinal puncture, placement or removal of epidural catheter or lumbar puncture is best performed when anticoagulant effect estimated to be low; minimum of 18 hours should elapse after last rivaroxaban admin before removal of epidural catheter; following catheter removal at least 6 hours should elapse before admin of next dose; traumatic puncture, delay rivaroxaban for 24 hours.

Pregnancy, Lactation: Pregnancy and lactation, contraindicated. Women of childbearing potential to avoid becoming pregnant during treatment.

ADR: Summary, *most common,* bleeding (epistaxis, GI haemorrhage); *common,* anaemia.

Notes: See 2.6.2 Synthetic Activated Factor X (Xa) Inhibitors.

▼ **Xarelto 10mg, 15mg, 20mg** *(Bayer)* A. GMS.
Price, 10mg (30) €68.51. 15mg (28) €64.11. 15mg (42) €96.16. 20mg (28) €64.11.
Tablet, rivaroxaban. 10mg: Light-red. 15mg: Red. 20mg: Brown-red. Round. Marked with BAYER-cross; strength and a triangle on reverse. *Lactose.* **Store:** No special conditions.

2.6.3 - Direct Thrombin Inhibitors, Reversal Agents

In This Chapter: *Hirudins (bivalirudin), dabigatran, idarucizumab.*

Class Effects

Hirudin, is a direct inhibitor of thrombin. Dabigatran is a potent competitive reversible direct thrombin inhibitor. Idarucizumab is a specific reversal agent for dabigatran.

CI: *Children,* no data. Hypersensitivity to any member of the class. Recent puncture of large vessels, blood vessel or organ anomaly, recent CVA, stroke or intracerebral surgery, bacterial endocarditis, advanced renal impairment, haemorrhagic diathesis, recent (major surgery, intracranial, GI, intraocular or pulmonary bleeding, active peptic ulcer), overt signs of bleeding, 65 years and older.

Pregnancy, Lactation: Not recommended.

Notes: See 2.6 Anticoagulants, Antiplatelets, Antithrombotics.

Bivalirudin

ATC Code: B01AE06. **Sport:** Permitted.
Driving: Not applicable.

Indications: Anticoagulant, patients undergoing percutaneous coronary intervention (PCI), including primary PCI with STEMI. Treatment, unstable angina/non-STEMI planned for urgent or early intervention.

Dose: Adult: *PCI, including STEMI undergoing primary PCI*, IV bolus 0.75mg/kg, 1.75mg/kg/hour IV infusion (duration of procedure and up to 4 hours post-PCI); then reduce dose to 0.25mg/kg/hour for an additional 4-12 hours as needed. *Angina, non-STEMI*, IV bolus 0.1mg/kg, then 0.25mg/kg/hour IV infusion; if medically managed, continue 0.25mg/kg/hour infusion for up to 72 hours. If proceeding to PCI, admin additional bolus 0.5mg/kg before procedure, then increase to 1.75mg/kg/hour infusion (procedure duration); following PCI, reduce to 0.25mg/kg/hour for 4-12 hours. If proceeding to coronary artery bypass graft (CABG) surgery off pump, continue IV infusion until time of surgery, then 0.5mg/kg bolus just prior to surgery, then 1.75mg/kg/hour infusion for surgery duration. If proceeding to CABG on pump, continue bivalirudin 1 hour prior to surgery, then discontinue and use unfractionated heparin. *Admin*, IV. Reconstitute initially to 50mg/mL bivalirudin; then further dilute in a total volume of 50mL to give 5mg/mL soln. Admin with aspirin and clopidogrel.

Elderly: Caution (age-related decreased renal function).

Child: Under 18 years, no indications.

Renal Impairment: GFR (mL/min) below 30 and dialysis-dependant, contraindicated. Mild/moderate (acute coronary syndrome), 0.1mg/kg bolus and 0.25mg/kg/hour infusion should not be adjusted. Moderate (GFR 30-59) undergoing PCI (treated with bivalirudin for ACS or not), admin lower infusion rate 1.4mg/kg/hour.

Interactions: Effect of Other Drugs on Bivalirudin: *Increased haemorrhage risk, monitor:* Coumarins, platelet aggregation inhibitors, other anticoagulants or antiplatelets (platelet inhibitors).

Effect of Bivalirudin on Other Drugs: Warfarin: *Monitor INR.*

SP: Not for IM use. Can be initiated 30 minutes after IV unfractionated heparin or 8 hours after SC LMW heparin; can be used with GPIIb/IIIa inhibitors. Prolonged PCI infusions not associated with increased bleeding rate. Acute stent thrombosis observed; mostly non-fatal; risk increased in first 4 hours after end of procedure (patients discontinuing bivalirudin after PCI or receiving reduced dose of 0.25mg/kg/hour). Admin errors may lead to fatal thrombosis.

ADR: Summary, *most frequent serious, fatal,* major haemorrhage (access site and non-access site, including intracranial), hypersensitivity (anaphylactic shock).

Notes: See 2.6.3 Direct Thrombin Inhibitors, Reversal Agents.

Angiox Parenteral 250mg (Medicines Co) A.
Price, not published by company.
Injection or infusion, bivalirudin. White (off-white) lyophilised powder for conc for soln.

Dabigatran

ATC Code: B01AE07. **Sport:** Permitted.
Driving: Not applicable.

Indications: *75mg, 110mg,* primary prevention, venous thromboembolic events (VTE) following elective total hip or knee replacement surgery. *110mg, 150mg,* prevention, stroke and systemic embolism with non-valvular atrial fibrillation with 1 or more risk factors (previous stroke or TIA; age 75 years or above, NYHA Class II or more; diabetes mellitus; hypertension). Treatment and prevention (recurrent), deep vein thrombosis (DVT) and pulmonary embolism (PE).

Dose: Adult: *VTE prevention, knee replacement,* initially 110mg within 1-4 hours after surgery then 220mg once daily (10 days); *hip,* as for knee (28-35 days). Co-admin with amiodarone, quinidine, verapamil, initially 75mg then 150mg once daily (2x 75mg); duration as above. Swallow whole with water (do not open cap); with or without food. *Stroke, systemic embolism,* 300mg/day; continue long-term.
Treatment and prevention (recurrent) DVT and PE, 150mg twice daily following treatment with parenteral anticoagulant for minimum 5 days; individualise duration according to risk factors.
Switching from other anticoagulants, discontinue the parenteral anticoagulant and start dabigatran 0-2 hours prior to time of next dose of alternate therapy would be due or at time of discontinuation of continuous treatment.
Elderly: *VTE prevention,* over 75 years, initially 75mg, then 150mg once daily. *Stroke, systemic embolism, DVT/PE treatment and prevention,* age 75-80 years and over, Adult dose can be used or consider 110mg twice daily based on individual assessment; 80 years and above, 110mg twice daily due to increased bleeding risk.
Child: Under 18 years, not recommended.
Renal Impairment: CrCl (mL/min) below 30, contraindicated; 30-50, for hip/knee replacement, initially 75mg, then 150mg once daily; co-admin with verapamil, reduce to 75mg/day. *Stroke prevention, DVT/PE,* 300mg/day; high bleeding risk, consider 110mg twice daily; co-admin with verapamil, reduce dose to 110mg twice daily. Renal function monitoring, impairment or age 75 years and above, evaluate function yearly or when function is expected to deteriorate.

Hepatic Impairment: If liver impairment or disease expected to impact on survival, contraindicated. Liver enzymes above 2xULN, not recommended.

CI: Conditions considered significant risk of major bleeding. Prosthetic heart valves requiring anticoagulant treatment.

Interactions: Effect of Other Drugs on Dabigatran: *Co-admin contraindicated:* Systemic ketoconazole, ciclosporin, itraconazole, dronedarone; anticoagulants including unfractionated heparin (UFH), heparin derivatives (fondaparinux, desirudin), LMWH (enoxaparin, dalteparin); oral anticoagulants (warfarin, rivaroxaban, apixaban) except under specific circumstance of switching anticoagulant therapy. *Co-admin not recommended:* Protease inhibitors and combinations, tacrolimus. *Co-admin caution (reduced plasma levels):* P-glycoprotein inducers (rifampicin, St John's Wort, carbamazepine, phenytoin). *Co-admin caution (plasma levels increased, consider dose reduction):* Strong P-gp inhibitors (amiodarone, posaconazole, verapamil, quinidine, clarithromycin, ticagrelor). *Increased bleeding risk:* Thrombolytic agents, GPIIb/IIIa receptor antagonists, ticlopidine, prasugrel, dextran, sulfinpyrazone, rivaroxaban, vitamin K antagonists (UFH can be admin at doses necessary to maintain a patent central venous or arterial catheter), aspirin, clopidogrel, NSAIDs (notably with elimination half-life above 12 hours), SSRIs, SNRIs. *Stagger co-admin (2-hour interval):* Ticagrelor.

SP: Caution, conditions with increased bleeding risk or drugs affecting haemostasis by inhibiting platelet aggregation. Bleeding can occur at any site during therapy. Life-threatening or uncontrolled bleeding, when rapid reversal of anticoagulation effect of dabigatran is needed, the specific reversal agent (idarucizumab) is available.
Increased dabigatran levels associated with (decreased renal function, age 75 years and older, body weight under 50kg, co-medication, diseases or procedures with haemorrhagic risk). Patients undergoing surgery or invasive procedures at increased bleeding risk; consider temporary discontinuation. Spinal anaesthesia, epidural, lumbar puncture, observe for neurological signs and symptoms of spinal or epidural haematoma. Post-op, restart after surgery as soon as adequate haemostasis established. Hip fracture surgery, not recommended. MI risk.

Pregnancy, Lactation: Pregnancy, only if clearly necessary. Lactation, stop breastfeeding.

ADR: *Common,* anaemia, decreased Hb, epistaxis,

2.6.4   Heparin Antagonists

haemorrhage, abdominal pain, diarrhoea, dyspepsia, nausea, abnormal LFTs.

Notes: See 2.6.3 Direct Thrombin Inhibitors, Reversal Agents.

Pradaxa Capsules *(Boehringer)* A. GMS.
Price, (10) 75mg, €11.85; 110mg, €11.75; 150mg, €11.56. (60) 75mg, €66.39; 110mg, €68.23; 150mg, €68.66.
Hard capsule, dabigatran etexilate (as mesilate) 75mg, 110mg, 150mg. Opaque; contain yellowish pellets. Marked with company symbol, R and strength. 75mg: White. 110mg: Light-blue. 150mg: Light-blue/white. **Store:** Original pack to protect (moisture).

Idarucizumab

ATC Code: Pending. **Sport:** Permitted.
Driving: Not relevant.

Indications: Specific reversal agent for dabigatran when rapid anticoagulant reversal is needed (emergency surgery, urgent procedures, life-threatening or uncontrolled bleeding). Does not reverse effects of other anticoagulants.

Dose: Adult, Elderly: 5g (2 x 2.5g/50mL); a second 5g may be considered if there is recurrence of clinically relevant bleeding*, if potential re-bleeding would be life-threatening*, second emergency surgery or urgent procedure is needed*. Dabigatran etexilate can be re-initiated 24 hours after idarucizumab if patient is clinically stable and adequate haemostasis achieved. *(and have prolonged clotting times). *Admin,* IV as two consecutive infusions over 5-10 minutes each or as bolus injection.

Child: Under 18 years, safety/efficacy not established.

Renal Impairment: No adjustment.

Hepatic Impairment: No adjustment.

SP: For hospital use only. Anaphylaxis or other serious allergic reaction, discontinue. Reversing dabigatran exposes patient to thrombotic risk of underlying disease; resume therapy as soon as medically appropriate to reduce risk. Transient proteinuria (physiological reaction to renal protein overflow) after bolus/short-term admin.

Pregnancy, Lactation: Pregnancy, may be used if benefit outweighs risk. Lactation, not known whether excreted into human milk.

ADR: No adverse reactions identified.

Notes: See 2.6.3 Direct Thrombin Inhibitors, Reversal Agents.

▼ **Praxbind Parenteral** *(Boehringer)* A. HOS.
Price, 2 x 50mL, €2565.39 (PTW).
Injection or infusion, idarucizumab 2.5g/50mL. Produced by rDNA technology. Clear (slightly opalescent) colourless (slightly yellow) soln. *Sorbitol; sodium 25mg/vial.*

2.6.4 - Heparin Antagonists

In This Chapter: *Protamine sulfate.*

Class Effects
Protamines are low molecular weight proteins. Administered alone protamine sulfate has an anticoagulant effect. Administered with strongly acid heparin, strongly basic protamine combines to form a stable salt, resulting in loss of anticoagulant activity of both drugs.

Indications: Treatment, overdosage or haemorrhage during heparin or LMWH therapy. To counteract anticoagulant effect of heparin or LMWH before emergency surgery. To reverse anticoagulant effects of heparin in cardiopulmonary bypass procedures.

CI: Hypersensitivity to any member of the class.

SP: Admin can cause anaphylactic reactions; facilities for resuscitation and treatment of shock should be available. If given too rapidly, may cause severe hypotension. Risk factors for hypersensitivity (fish allergy; previous protamine insulin, protamine sulphate/chloride; infertility in men; medical history of vasectomy). Excessive dosage or given in absence of heparin/LMWH may prolong coagulation time. Thrombocytopenia may be aggravated. Rebound anticoagulant effect of heparin/LMWH with haemorrhage reported despite initial neutralisation; rebound bleeding responds to further protamine sulphate doses. Prolonged procedures requiring repeated protamine sulphate doses,

monitor clotting parameters (activated clotting time, platelet count).

Pregnancy, Lactation: Pregnancy, not recommended unless clinical condition strongly requires use. Lactation, discontinue.

ADR: *Most serious,* hypotension, pulmonary hypertension, anaphylactic reactions.

Protamine Sulfate

ATC Code: V03AB14. **Sport:** Permitted.
Driving: No or negligible influence.

Dose: Adult, Elderly: Slow IV injection over 10 minutes or constant slow IV infusion. Max. bolus dose 7000 anti-heparin IU/50mg protamine sulfate. *Heparin neutralisation,* 1mL (10mg protamine sulfate) will neutralise approx. 1400 IU heparin. *LMWH neutralisation,* 1mL protamine sulfate (10mg) per 1000 anti Xa IU LMWH. *Cardiopulmonary bypass,* generally 0.1mL-0.2mL (1-2mg) protamine sulfate IV for each 100 units heparin given. *Elderly,* no data.

Child: Under 18 years, safety/efficacy not established.

Renal Impairment: No data.

Hepatic Impairment: No data.

Notes: See 2.6.4 Heparin Antagonists.

Protamine Sulphate LEO Parenteral *(LEO)* A. HOS.
Price, 5mL (5) 1400 anti-heparin IU/mL, €44.29 (PTW).
Injection or infusion, protamine sulfate anti-heparin 1400 IU/mL (10mg/mL). Clear colourless soln.

2.6.5 - Oral Anticoagulants

In This Chapter: *Warfarin.*

Class Effects
Indirect anticoagulants depress hepatic vitamin K-dependent synthesis of coagulation factors II (prothrombin), VII, IX and X and anticoagulant protein C and cofactor protein S. Warfarin, a coumarin, is an indirect anticoagulant; it does not have any effect on established thrombus. The onset of action is slow.

Indications: Treatment and prophylaxis, venous thrombosis, pulmonary embolism. Prophylaxis, systemic embolisation (rheumatic heart disease, atrial fibrillation).

CI: Children, not recommended. Hypersensitivity to any member of the class. Use within 3 days of surgery. Any condition where haemorrhage risk greater than clinical benefit of anticoagulation. Pregnancy.

Interactions: Effect of Other Drugs on Warfarin: *Effect enhanced (monitor):* Protein bound drugs (diuretics, oral anti-diabetics, anti-inflammatories, amiodarone), drugs increasing affinity for hepatic receptor sites (D-thyroxine), liver enzyme inhibitors (ALCOHOL), anabolic steroids, cimetidine, aspirin, other NSAIDs, clofibrate, simvastatin, sulphinpyrazone, chloral hydrate, aminoglycosides, chloramphenicol, macrolides (erythromycin, clarithromycin, azithromycin), quinolones (ciprofloxacin, nalidixic acid), miconazole, HIV protease inhibitors (indinavir, ritonavir), 5-fluorouracil, SSRIs (fluvoxamine, fluoxetine), disulfiram, paracetamol, decreased Vitamin K intake. *Plasma levels decreased (increase dose):* Barbiturates, phenytoin, oestrogens, oral contraceptives. *Effect reduced:* Colestyramine, carbamazepine, glutethimide, phenazone, griseofulvin, rifampicin, St John's Wort *(Hypericum perforatum*; contraindicated). *Increased bleeding risk:* Cranberry juice.

SP: Severe hypertension, warfarin resistance.

Pregnancy, Lactation: Contraindicated especially first trimester (risk of warfarin embryopathy or 'foetal warfarin syndrome') and third trimester (fatal bleeding, still birth).

Notes: See 2.6 Anticoagulants, Antiplatelets, Antithrombotics.

Warfarin

ATC Code: B01AA03. **Sport:** Permitted.
Driving: No influence.

Dose: Adult: Initially, 5-10mg/day for 2 days then according to prothrombin time; maintenance range 3-9mg/day.

Elderly, initiate at lower dose. *Admin*, oral at same time each day.
Renal Impairment: Caution.
Hepatic Impairment: As for Renal above.
SP: Monitor INR if changing brands. Calciphylaxi reported.
ADR: Fever, hypersensitivity, cerebral (haemorrhage, subdural haematoma), haemorrhage, haemothorax, epistaxis.
Notes: See 2.6.5 Oral Anticoagulants.

> **Warfant 1mg, 3mg, 5mg** *(Concordia)* B. GMS.
> *Price*, (100) 1mg, €3.34. 3mg, €5.43. 5mg, €7.68.
> *Tablet*, warfarin sodium clathrate. Scored (facilitates breaking). Marked with logo and W/strength. 1mg: Brown. 3mg: Blue. 5mg: Pink. *Lactose*.

> **Warfarin TEVA 1mg, 3mg, 5mg** *(TEVA)* B. GMS.
> *Price*, (100) 1mg, €3.11. 3mg, €5.08. 5mg, €7.18.
> *Tablet*, warfarin sodium clathrate. Flat cap-shaped scored (facilitates breaking). Marked Warfarin and Taro; strength on reverse. 1mg: Brown. 3mg: Blue. 5mg: Pink. *Lactose*.

2.6.6 - Antiplatelets Excluding Heparin

In This Chapter: *Abciximab, ticagrelor.*

Class Effects
These drugs reduce platelet aggregation. Generally used to prevent further thromboembolic events post-MI, ischaemic stroke, TIA, unstable angina; also primary prevention of thromboembolic events in patients at risk. Generally, for hospital use only under specialist care.
CI: Children under 18 years, not recommended. Hypersensitivity to any members of the class. Active/recent (within 30 days) internal GI or GU bleeding, haemorrhagic stroke, stroke within 2 years, intracranial disease (neoplasm, arteriovenous malformation, aneurysm), recent within 2 months, intracranial or intraspinal surgery or trauma, major surgery, known bleeding diathesis, severe uncontrolled or malignant hypertension, pre-existing thrombocytopenia.
Interactions: Effect of Other Drugs on Thrombolytics: *Increased bleeding risk*: Iloprost, other thrombolytics, anticoagulants, antiplatelets.
SP: Increased bleeding risk with trauma, surgery, treatment with aspirin, heparin, glycoprotein IIb/IIIa inhibitors, NSAIDs including COX-2 inhibitors. Children, under 18 years, not recommended (generally no data available). *Caution* all potential bleeding sites (arterial/venous puncture sites, catheter insertion sites, cutdown sites, needle puncture sites, central/peripheral nervous system, retroperitoneal sites). Thrombocytopenia.
Pregnancy, Lactation: If benefit outweighs risk. Lactation, not recommended, insufficient data.
ADR: Increased bleeding risk.
Notes: See 2.6 Anticoagulants, Antiplatelets, Antithrombotics.

Abciximab
ATC Code: B01AC13. **Sport:** Permitted.
Driving: Not applicable.
Indications: Adjunctive to heparin and acetylsalicylic acid (adults), prevention, ischaemic complications associated with percutaneous coronary intervention (PCI); short-term reduction in MI risk in unstable angina not responding to full conventional therapy or scheduled for PCI.
Dose: Adult: IV, initially 0.25mg/kg bolus, immediately followed by 0.125mcg/kg/min continuous infusion; max. 10mcg/min. *Unstable angina*, commence bolus followed by infusion 24 hours prior to intervention; conclude 12 hours after. *Prevention of ischaemic cardiac complications*, bolus 10-60 minutes prior to intervention; follow with infusion for 12 hours. Aspirin dose, not less than 300mg/day.
Elderly: Over 65 years, if benefit outweighs risk. Over 80 years, not recommended.
Renal Impairment: Severe, only if benefit outweighs risk. Haemodialysis, contraindicated.
Hepatic Impairment: Severe, not recommended.

CI: Hypersensitivity to murine monoclonal antibodies or papain. Vasculitis, hypertensive retinopathy.
Interactions: Effect of Other Drugs on Abciximab: *Increased bleeding incidence/risk*: Heparin, other thrombolytics.
SP: Use weight adjusted heparin regimen. Pulmonary (alveolar) haemorrhage, discontinue; spontaneous GI bleeding, pretreat with H2-antagonist/liquid antacids, antiemetics; for rapid haemostasis, admin platelets. Allergic reactions including anaphylaxis, thrombocytopenia.
Pregnancy, Lactation: Pregnancy, if clearly necessary. Lactation, stop breastfeeding.
ADR: Summary, *most frequent*, bleeding, back pain, hypotension, nausea, chest pain, vomiting, headache, bradycardia, fever (pyrexia), puncture-site pain, thrombocytopenia. Cardiac tamponade, pulmonary (mostly alveolar) haemorrhage, adult respiratory distress syndrome rarely reported.
Notes: See 2.6.6 Antiplatelets Excluding Heparin.

> **ReoPro Parenteral** *(Janssen-Cilag)* A. HOS.
> *Price*, 5mL (1) €292.11 (PTW).
> *Injection or infusion*, abciximab 2mg/mL. Colourless clear liquid.
> **Store:** Refrigerate; do not freeze; do not shake.

Ticagrelor
ATC Code: B01AC24. **Sport:** Permitted.
Driving: No or negligible influence; dizziness reported.
Indications: Adjunctive, prevention of atherothrombotic events in Acute Coronary Syndromes (ACS) or history of MI and high risk of developing an atherothrombotic event.
Dose: Adult, Elderly: Initially 180mg as single loading dose, then 90mg twice daily with aspirin (unless contraindicated). *Admin*, with or without food. Swallowing difficulty, crush tabs to fine powder, mix with half glass of water; drink immediately; rinse glass with further half glass of water and drink. Can be admin via nasogastric tube.
Renal Impairment: Dialysis, not recommended.
Hepatic Impairment: Moderate to severe, contraindicated.
Interactions: Effect of Other Drugs on Ticagrelor: *Co-admin contraindicated (increased exposure)*: Strong CYP3A4 inhibitors (ketoconazole, clarithromycin, nefazodone, ritonavir, atazanavir). *Co-admin not recommended*: Simvastatin, lovastatin (doses above 40mg/day); cisapride, ergot alkaloids. *Co-admin caution*: Medicinals altering haemostasis, P-gp inhibitors (verapamil, quinidine, ciclosporin); SSRIs (paroxetine, sertraline, citalopram) (increased bleeding risk). *Decreased exposure*: CYP3A inducers (phenytoin, carbamazepine, phenobarbital).
Effect of Ticagrelor on Other Drugs: Digoxin, ciclosporin: *Monitor*.
SP: Known bleeding risk, use if benefit outweighs risk. Inform surgeon/dentist before surgery. Caution, if at risk for bradycardia, hyperuricaemia, gouty arthritis. Dyspnoea (caution, asthma or COPD). Monitor renal function after 1 month, then routinely (especially elderly over 75 years). Co-admin with high-dose aspirin not recommended. Platelet transfusion did not reverse antiplatelet effect of ticagrelor; desmopressin unlikely to be effective in managing clinical bleeding events.
Pregnancy, Lactation: Pregnancy, not recommended. Women of childbearing potential, ensure adequate contraception. Lactation, stop breastfeeding or stop drug.
ADR: Summary, *most common*, bleeding, dyspnoea.
Notes: See 2.6.6 Antiplatelets Excluding Heparin.

> **Brilique 90mg** *(AstraZeneca)* B. GMS.
> *Price*, (56) €65.02.
> *Tablets*, ticagrelor. Round yellow f/c. Marked 90 and T.

2.6.7 - Non-Steroidal Antiplatelets, Aspirin

In This Chapter: *Aspirin.*

Class Effects
Aspirin is an antithrombotic (inhibits platelet activation); may inhibit thrombus formation in the arterial circulation.
Indications: Acetylsalicylic acid (aspirin), an

2.6.8   Other Antiplatelets

antithrombotic, is also used for short-term pain relief, pyrexia and inflammation reduction at analgesic doses. See Notes below.

CI: Children under 16 years, unless specifically indicated (Reye's syndrome risk which can be fatal). Hypersensitivity to aspirin or NSAIDs (hypersensitivity reactions with previous admin). Haemorrhage diathesis, coagulation disorders, cerebral haemorrhage, active peptic ulceration/haemorrhage, liver cirrhosis, severe cardiac insufficiency (HF), severe renal disorder.

SP: Caution, symptoms of asthma, rhinitis, urticaria with previous aspirin or NSAID admin.

Notes: See 4.2.1 Non-Opioid Analgesics (acetylsalicylic acid). See 2.6 Anticoagulants, Antiplatelets, Antithrombotics.

Acetylsalicylic Acid (aspirin) (antiplatelet)

ATC Code: B01AC06. **Sport:** Permitted.
Driving: None known.

Indications: *Caprin, Nu-Seals, Aspirin (Clonmel)*, secondary prevention (unstable angina or ischaemic stroke and MI history).

Nuprin, Aspirin (Clonmel), secondary prevention (MI, TIA, CVA). Prevention, cardiovascular morbidity, graft occlusion after CABG. Except in acute phase, unstable angina pectoris, coronary angioplasty.

Nuasa, Aspirin (Clonmel), stable and unstable angina pectoris to reduce MI risk. Secondary prophylaxis post MI. Thrombosis prophylaxis post vascular surgery. Secondary prevention (TIA, stroke) if intracerebral haemorrhage excluded.

Dose: Adult: *Nu-Seals, Caprin*, 75mg/day. For rapid absorption 150mg can be chewed *(Nu-Seals)* OR 225mg/day for first two days of treatment *(Caprin)*, then 75mg daily.

Nuprin, Aspirin (Clonmel), 75-160mg once daily. Secondary prevention (TIA, CVA), 75-325mg once daily.

Nuasa, 75-150mg per day. Thrombosis prophylaxis post vascular surgery, 100-300mg/day. Swallow whole with water; do not crush or chew unless specified.

Elderly: Caution, higher risk for adverse events. Use lowest effective dose for shortest duration.

Child: See Notes below.

Renal Impairment: Severe, avoid.

Hepatic Impairment: As for Renal above.

CI: See Notes below.

Interactions: Effect of Other Drugs on Acetylsalicylic Acid: Co-admin contraindicated: Methotrexate (doses above 15mg/week). *Co-admin not recommended:* Warfarin, heparin, other NSAIDs, antacids (cause premature drug release with enteric coat). *Nephrotoxicity risk increased:* Diuretics. *Reduced metabolism and elimination:* Probenecid. *Increased absorption rate (no special precautions):* Metoclopramide. *Increased GI bleeding risk:* Corticosteroids, warfarin, SSRIs, clopidogrel, dipyridamole, ALCOHOL, nicorandil. *Increased hepatotoxicity:* Gold.

Effect of Acetylsalicylic Acid on Other Drugs: Antihypertensives, diuretics: *Reduced effect.* Cardiac glycosides: *Increased cardiac failure risk, reduced GFR, increased plasma levels.* Lithium, methotrexate: *Decreased excretion.* Ciclosporin: *Increased nephrotoxicity risk.* Aminoglycosides: *Reduced renal function, decreased elimination, increased plasma levels.* Oral hypoglycaemic agents: *Metabolism inhibited, prolonged half-life, increased hypoglycaemia risk.* Phenytoin, valproate: *Effect enhanced, no special precautions.* Spironolactone: *Natriuretic effect decreased.* Probenecid, sulphinpyrazone, other uricosurics: *Uricosuric effect inhibited.* Warfarin, heparin: *Co-admin not recommended, anticoagulant effect enhanced.* Uricosurics: *Effect inhibited.* Thiopental anaesthesia: *Effects potentiated.*

SP: Impaired cardiac function, dehydration, peptic ulceration, inflammatory bowel disease, coagulation abnormalities. May induce GI haemorrhage. Elderly particularly susceptible to NSAID adverse effects. May precipitate bronchospasm or induce asthma attacks. Hypertension. Stroke treatment, exclude cerebral

haemorrhage before aspirin admin. Prolonged/R, unsuitable for short-term pain relief. *Ibuprofen* co-admin may inhibit effect of low dose aspirin on platelet aggregation; no firm data (regular ibuprofen use); no likely clinical effect (occasional use).

Pregnancy, Lactation: If benefit outweighs risk; with medical advice. Third trimester, avoid analgesic doses; use in last 2 weeks, increased foetal/neonatal haemorrhage risk. Regular or high doses may result in constriction or premature closing of foetal ductus arteriosus. Lactation, not recommended; is excreted in breast milk.

ADR: *Common,* increased bleeding tendency, dyspepsia, peptic ulcer perforation or GI bleeding; nausea, vomiting, diarrhoea, flatulence, constipation, abdominal pain, melaena, haematemesis, ulcerative stomatitis, colitis and Crohn's disease exacerbation.

Notes: See 2.6.7 Non-Steroidal Antiplatelets, Aspirin.

Nu-Seals 75mg *(Alliance)* B. GMS.
Price, (28) €1.94. (56) €3.90. (100) €6.93.
Tablet, acetylsalicylic acid. Smooth white g/r. Marked with strength.
Aspirin (Clonmel) 75mg *(Clonmel)* B. GMS.
Price, (28) €1.03.
Tablet, acetylsalicylic acid. Oval white g/r, f/c.
Aspirin Krka 75mg *(Krka)* B. GMS.
Price, (28) €1.03.
Tablet, acetylsalicylic acid. Pink round g/r f/c. *Lactose.* **Store:** Below 25 deg C. Original pack to protect (light).
Caprin 75mg *(Pinewood)* B. GMS.
Price, (100) €3.66.
Tablet, acetylsalicylic acid. e/c. *Lactose.*
Nuasa 75mg *(Uniphar)* B. GMS.
Price, (30) €1.10.
Tablet, acetylsalicylic acid. White g/r round coated. *Lactose.*
Nuprin 75mg *(Accord)* B. GMS.
Price, (28) €1.03. (56) €2.05. (100) €3.66.
Tablet, acetylsalicylic acid. Oval white f/c, g/r.

2.6.8 - Other Antiplatelets

In This Chapter: *Clopidogrel (acetylsalicylic acid combination), epoprostenol, prasugrel.*

Class Effects

Clopidogrel and *prasugrel* inhibit platelet aggregation. *Epoprostenol* is a potent inhibitor of platelet aggregation and is also a potent vasodilator.

CI: Children under 18 years, not recommended. Hypersensitivity to any member of class. Severe pathological bleeding. *Acetylsalicylic acid (aspirin),* hypersensitivity to NSAIDs, syndrome of asthma, rhinitis, nasal polyps; third trimester of pregnancy.

Interactions: Effect of Other Drugs Acetylsalicylic Acid (Aspirin): *Platelet aggregation reduced:* Metamizole.

Effect of Acetylsalicylic Acid (Aspirin) on Other Drugs: Uricosurics (benzbromarone, probenecid, sulfinpyrazone): *Caution, effect inhibited (competitive uric acid elimination).* Methotrexate: *Caution dose above 20mg/week; inhibited renal clearance; possible bone marrow toxicity.* ACEIs, acetazolamide, anticonvulsants (phenytoin, valproic acid), beta-blockers, diuretics, oral hypoglycaemics: *Interactions reported (anti-inflammatory acetylsalicylic acid doses).* Tenofovir: *Increased renal failure.*

SP: *Acetylsalicylic acid,* caution, asthma/allergic disorders, increased risk of hypersensitivity reactions; gout (low dose acetylsalicylic acid may increase urate conc); children under 18 years, (Reye's syndrome). *Ibuprofen* may inhibit effect of low dose aspirin on platelet aggregation; no firm data for regular ibuprofen use; occasional use, no likely clinically relevant effect. *Cross-reactivity among thienopyridines reported (clopidogrel, ticlopidine, prasugrel).*

Pregnancy, Lactation: First and second trimester, caution, use only if considered essential. Third trimester, avoid completely (acetylsalicylic acid combinations contraindicated). Lactation, generally not recommended.

Acetylsalicylic acid combinations, from sixth month of pregnancy, all prostaglandin synthesis inhibitors may expose foetus to cardiopulmonary toxicity with premature ductus arteriosus closure and pulmonary hypertension;

renal dysfunction, may progress to failure with oligo-hydroamniosis or expose mother and neonate at end of pregnancy to possible prolongation of bleeding time even at low doses, inhibition of uterine contractions/delayed or prolonged labour.

Notes: See 2.6 Anticoagulants, Antiplatelets, Antithrombotics. See also 4.2.1 Non-Opioid Analgesics (acetylsalicylic acid).

Clopidogrel

ATC Code: B01AC04. **Sport:** Permitted.
Driving: None known.

Indications: *Secondary prevention,* atherothrombotic events after MI (from few days until less than 35 days), ischaemic stroke (from 7 days until less than 6 months) or established peripheral arterial disease. Acute coronary syndrome (with acetylsalicylic acid): Non-ST segment elevation acute coronary syndrome (unstable angina or non-Q-wave MI), ST segment elevation acute MI (medically treated patients eligible for thrombolytic therapy). *Prevention,* atherothrombotic and thromboembolic events (including stroke) in atrial fibrillation (with acetylsalicylic acid).

Dose: Adult: *Non-STEMI acute coronary syndrome,* initially clopidogrel 300mg single loading dose (with acetylsalicylic acid); maintenance, 75mg/day (with acetylsalicylic acid 75-325mg/day; recommended max. 100mg/day).
STEMI (acute), loading dose as above, then 75mg/day (with acetylsalicylic acid, with or without thrombolytics). Initiate combined therapy as early as possible; continue for 4 weeks.
Atrial fibrillation, 75mg once daily (with acetylsalicylic acid 75-100mg/day). Admin as single daily dose, with or without food.

Elderly: *STEMI (acute)* over 75 years, initiate without loading dose.

Child: Under 18 years, no data.

Renal Impairment: Caution.

Hepatic Impairment: Moderate, caution. Severe, contraindicated.

CI: Active bleeding (peptic ulcer, intracranial haemorrhage).

Interactions: Effect of Other Drugs on Clopidogrel: *Increased bleeding risk:* Warfarin (co-admin not recommended); glycoprotein IIb/IIIa, acetylsalicylic acid, heparin, other thrombolytics, NSAIDs including COX-2 inhibitors (co-admin, caution), SSRIs (caution). *Plasma levels of active clopidogrel metabolite decreased (clinical relevance unknown; co-admin not recommended):* CYP2C19 inhibitors (omeprazole, esomeprazole, fluvoxamine, fluoxetine, moclobemide, voriconazole, fluconazole, ticlopidine, carbamazepine, efavirenz).

Effect of Clopidogrel on Other Drugs: Phenytoin, tolbutamide, CYP2C9 substrates: *Potential risk, increased plasma levels.*

SP: Increased bleeding risk from trauma, surgery, occult/GI, intraocular bleeding, haematological disturbances. Discontinue 7 days prior to elective surgery. Advise patients to report unusual bleeding (site, duration). Acquired haemophilia reported following clopidogrel use; if confirmed, discontinue. Allergic cross-reactivity reported among thienopyridines (ticlopidine, prasugrel).

Pregnancy, Lactation: Pregnancy, preferable not to be used. Breastfeeding should not continue during treatment.

ADR: *Common,* haematoma, epistaxis, GI haemorrhage GI, diarrhoea, abdominal pain, dyspepsia, bruising, puncture site bleeding.

Notes: See 2.6.8 Other Antiplatelets.

Interchangeability: Same strengths of all brands of clopidogrel f/c tablets listed below are deemed interchangeable.

Reference Price: 75mg (28) €5.04.

Plavix 75mg, 300mg *(SANOFI)* B. GMS.
Price, 75mg (28) €7.56. HOS: 300mg, €155.40 (PTW).
Tablet, clopidogrel hydrogen sulfate. Pink f/c. 75mg: Round. Marked 75; 1171 on reverse. 300mg: Marked 300; 1332 on reverse. *Lactose, castor oil.* **Store:** Below 30 deg C.

Clodel 75mg *(Rowex)* B. GMS.
Price, see reference price above.
Tablet, clopidogrel HCl. Pink round f/c. *Castor oil.* **Store:** Below 25 deg C; original pack to protect (moisture, light).
Clopidogrel (Accord) 75mg *(Accord)* B. GMS.
Price, see reference price above.
Tablet, clopidogrel hydrogen sulphate. Pink round f/c. *Castor oil.* **Store:** No special conditions.
Clopidogrel Actavis 75mg *(Accord)* B. GMS.
Price, (28), see reference price above. (100) €18.00.
Tablet, clopidogrel besilate. Pink round f/c. Marked II. *Lactose, lecithin containing soya oil.* **Store:** No special conditions.
Clopidogrel Krka 75mg *(Krka)* B. GMS.
Price, see reference price above.
Tablet, clopidogrel HCl. Pink round f/c. *Castor oil.* **Store:** Original pack to protect (moisture, light).
Clopidogrel Mylan 75mg *(Gerard)* B. GMS.
Price, see reference price above.
Tablet, clopidogrel HCl. Pink round f/c. *Castor oil.* **Store:** Original pack to protect (moisture, light).
Clopidogrel TAD 75mg *(Clonmel)* B. GMS.
Price, see reference price above.
Tablet, clopidogrel HCl. Pink round f/c. *Castor oil.* **Store:** Original pack to protect (moisture, light).
Clopidogrel TEVA 75mg *(TEVA)* B. GMS.
Price, see reference price above.
Tablet, clopidogrel HCl. Pink round f/c. *Castor oil.* **Store:** No special conditions.

Clopidogrel, Acetylsalicylic Acid (aspirin)

ATC Code: B01AC30. **Sport:** Permitted.
Driving: None known.

Indications: *Secondary prevention,* atherothrombotic events (adults already taking clopidogrel + acetylsalicylic acid). Fixed dose combination, continuation therapy in non-STEMI acute coronary syndrome, ST segment elevation acute MI.

Dose: Adult, Elderly: Admin 75mg/75mg as single daily dose with or without food. Initiate with separate components, see Notes below (clopidogrel). *Admin,* oral, with/without food.

Child: Under 18 years, not recommended.

Renal Impairment: Mild/moderate, caution. Severe (CrCl below 30mL/min), contraindicated.

Hepatic Impairment: Mild/moderate, may have bleeding diatheses, caution; severe, contraindicated.

CI: See Notes below (clopidogrel).

SP: See Notes below.

Pregnancy, Lactation: See Notes below.

ADR: Summary, *most common,* bleeding (mostly during first month of treatment).

Notes: See Clopidogrel above. See 2.6.8 Other Antiplatelets (acetylsalicylic acid).

DuoPlavin Tablets *(SANOFI)* B. GMS.
Price, (28) €13.19.
Tablet, clopidogrel hydrogen sulfate 75mg, acetylsalicylic acid 75mg. Yellow oval f/c. Marked C75 on; A75 on reverse. *Lactose, castor oil.* **Store:** Below 25 deg C.

Epoprostenol

ATC Code: B01AC08. **Sport:** Permitted.
Driving: Pulmonary hypertension may affect.

Indications: Treatment, pulmonary arterial hypertension (PAH) (idiopathic or heritable, associated with connective tissue disease; patients with WHO Class III-IV to improve exercise capacity) *(both strengths).* Haemodialysis in emergency situations (risk of exacerbating bleeding with heparin, or heparin contraindicated).

Dose: Adult: *PAH, acute dose-ranging* (peripheral or central venous line), initially 2 nanograms/kg/min. If required titrate at intervals of 15 minutes or more, by 2 nanograms/kg/min to max. tolerated infusion rate (MTIR). *Long-term* (central venous catheter), initially 4 nanograms/kg/min less than MTIR established in acute dose ranging. If MTIR is 5 nanograms/kg/min or less, start long-term infusion at 1 nanogram/kg/min.
Renal dialysis (continuous infusion only), prior to dialysis, 4 nanograms/kg/min IV for 15 minutes. During dialysis, 4 nanograms/kg/min into arterial inlet of dialyser. Stop infusion at end of dialysis. NOTE: Not for bolus injection.

Elderly: Over 65 years, limited data.

2.6.9 Antithrombotics, Enzymes and Proteins

Child: Under 18 years, safety/efficacy not established.
CI: CHF arising from severe LVD. Pulmonary oedema development during dose-ranging.
Interactions: Effect of Other Drugs on Epoprostenol: *Vasodilation enhanced:* Other vasodilators. *Increased bleeding risk:* NSaIDs.
Effect of Epoprostenol on Other Drugs: Heparin, other anticoagulants: *Action potentiated, monitor.* Digoxin: *Transient increased plasma levels after epoprostenol initiation (may be clinically significant if digoxin-toxicity prone).*
SP: Final infusion soln has high pH, avoid extravasation. Potent inhibitor of platelet aggregation, consider increased risk for haemorrhagic complications. Hypotension, change in heart rate, elevated serum glucose. Avoid, abrupt infusion withdrawal or interruption. *Renal dialysis,* hypotension, avoid use of acetate buffer. Patients with spontaneous or drug-induced haemorrhagic diatheses, caution haemorrhagic risk. *Pulmonary hypertension,* acute treatment, hospital only.
Pregnancy, Lactation: Can be used in women who choose to continue their pregnancy, despite the known risk of PAH during pregnancy. Lactation, discontinue breastfeeding.
ADR: *Very common,* headache, facial flushing, nausea, vomiting, diarrhoea, pain (jaw, unspecified).
Notes: See 2.6.8 Other Antiplatelets. For other vasodilators, see 2.2.4 PAH, IPF.

> **Flolan Parenteral 0.5mg, 1.5mg** *(GSK)* A. HT.
> *Price,* (1) 0.5mg, €67.72. 1.5mg, €149.69.
> *Infusion,* epoprostenol sodium. White (off-white) freeze-dried powder. Clear colourless solution (pH 10.3-10.8) for soln. *Sodium* (0.5mg and 1.5mg) 55.9mg *(solvent pH 10.5);* 73mg *(solvent pH 12.5).* **Store:** Below 25 deg C (powder, solvent); do not freeze; original pack.

Prasugrel

ATC Code: B01AC22. **Sport:** Permitted.
Driving: No or negligible effect.

Indications: Prevention of atherothrombotic events in adults, patients undergoing primary or delayed PCI (with acetyl salicylic acid).
Dose: Adult: Age 18 years and older, initially, single 60mg loading-dose; then maintenance 10mg once daily with acetylsalicylic acid 75-325mg daily. In UA/N-STEMI where coronary angiography is performed within 48 hours after admission, admin loading-dose only at the time of PCI. Tabs should not be broken or crushed, with or without food.
Elderly: Age 75 years and older, use if benefit outweighs risk or under 60kg body weight, initiate as for Adult; maintenance 5mg/day.
Renal Impairment: Caution, increased bleeding risk.
Hepatic Impairment: Mild/moderate, as for Renal above. Severe, contraindicated.
CI: Active pathological bleeding, stroke/TIA.
Interactions: Effect of Other Drugs on Prasugrel: *Co-admin caution (potential bleeding risk):* Coumarin derivatives (warfarin), NSAIDs. *Increased bleeding risk:* Oral anticoagulants, clopidogrel, fibrinolytics.
SP: Age 75 years and older or under 60kg, propensity to bleed especially if co-admin with medicinals that may increase risk; advise patients or report unusual bleeding. Urgent CABG, weigh benefit/risk. Elective surgery, see Notes below (clopidogrel). Hypersensitivity, angioedema.
Pregnancy, Lactation: Pregnancy, if benefit outweighs risk. Lactation, not recommended.
ADR: *Common,* anaemia, haematoma, epistaxis, haemorrhage, rash, ecchymosis, haematuria, puncture site haemorrhage/haematoma, contusion.
Notes: See Clopidogrel above. See 2.6.8 Other Antiplatelets.

> **Efient 5mg, 10mg** *(Daiichi Sankyo)* B. GMS.
> *Price,* (28) 5mg, €48.09. 10mg, €49.26.
> *Tablet,* prasugrel HCl. Double-arrow-shaped f/c. Marked with strength. 5mg: Yellow. Marked 4760. 10mg: Beige. Marked 4759. *Lactose.*

2.6.9 - Antithrombotics, Enzymes and Proteins

In This Chapter: *Alteplase, tenecteplase.*

Class Effects

Fibrinolytics, also called thrombolytics, are used in the treatment of thrombo-embolic disorders including MI, peripheral arterial thrombo-embolism and venous thrombo-embolism (DVT, pulmonary embolism). Alteplase and tenecteplase are recombinant tissue plasminogen activators (r-tPAs).

CI: Significant bleeding disorder, known haemorrhagic diathesis, haemorrhage (intracranial, subarachnoid, CVA), stroke, TIA. Major surgery, biopsy of parenchymal organ, significant trauma (acute MI, cranium, head), CNS damage (neoplasm, aneurysm, intracranial or spinal surgery), traumatic external heart massage, obstetrical delivery, recent puncture of a non-compressible blood-vessel (subclavian or jugular vein puncture), oral anticoagulants treatment, hypertension (severe, uncontrolled), acute (pancreatitis, pericarditis, bacterial endocarditis), ulcerative GI disease, arterial aneurysm, arterial/venous malformations, severe liver disease (hepatic failure, cirrhosis, active hepatitis, oesophageal varices), prolonged cardiopulmonary resuscitation, neoplasms with increased bleeding risk.

Interactions: Effect of Other Drugs on Fibrinolytics: *Increased haemorrhage risk:* Coumarins, oral anticoagulants, platelet aggregation inhibitors, unfractionated heparin or LMWH, other anticoagulants or drugs affecting platelet formation or function (acetylsalicylic acid, ticlopidine, clopidogrel, abciximab, allopurinol, anabolic steroids, androgens, dipyridamole, thyroid hormones, volatile oils, quinidine, clofibric acid derivatives, phenylbutazone, indomethacin, aryl acetic acid, aryl propionic acid derivatives, tetracyclines, valproic acid, thiouracil, sulfonamides), vitamin K antagonists, dextrans (co-admin), GPIIb/IIIa antagonists. *Admixture not recommended:* Any other soln (including heparin).
SP: See CI above. Hypersensitivity reactions possible with intravenous protein products which may be acute and life-threatening; ensure presence of life-support facilities. Wit protein products, record the name of batch number of product to maintain link between patient and batch.
Pregnancy, Lactation: Pregnancy, if benefit outweighs risk. Lactation, not known if excreted in breast milk.
ADR: Bleeding, superficial (punctures, damaged blood vessels, haematoma) or internal bleeding (GI or GU, retro-peritoneum, CNS, parenchymatous organs). Intracranial haemorrhage, ecchymosis, thrombotic embolisation, epistaxis, nausea, vomiting, gingival bleeding, hypotension, increased temperature, fever, chills, cholesterol crystal embolisation. Allergic-anaphylactic reactions, rash, flushing, dyspnoea. Cardiac failure, recurrent ischaemia, angina, cardiac arrest, cardiogenic shock, reinfarction, valve disorders, pulmonary embolism. Class related CNS events.

Alteplase

ATC Code: B01AD02. **Sport:** Permitted.
Driving: Caution.

Indications: Thrombolytic treatment in acute (MI, massive pulmonary embolism with haemodynamic instability, ischaemic stroke) *(Actilyse).* Thrombolytic treatment of occluded central venous access devices (including dialysis) *(Actilyse Cathflo).*
Dose: Adult: *Actilyse, acute-MI, 90-minute accelerated regimen* started within 6 hours after symptom onset, 15mg by IV bolus, then 50mg infused over 30 minutes; followed by 35mg over 60 minutes; max 100mg. Body weight under 65kg, 15mg by IV bolus, then 0.75mg/kg infusion over 30 minutes, max. 50mg; followed by 0.5mg/kg over 60 minutes, max. 35mg. *3-hour regimen* started 6-12 hours after symptom onset, 10mg by IV bolus, then 50mg infused over 60 minutes; followed by 10mg over 30 minutes until max. 100mg over 3 hours. Body weight under 65kg, max. 1.5mg/kg.
Actilyse, pulmonary embolism, total 100mg in 2 hours.

74

Initially 10mg by IV bolus over 1-2 minutes, followed by 90mg by IV infusion over 2 hours. Body weight under 65kg, max. 1.5mg/kg.

Actilyse, acute ischaemic stroke, initiate within 4.5 hours of symptom onset (negative benefit risk ratio beyond 4.5 hours). Recommended 0.9mg/kg by IV infusion over 60 minutes with 10% total dose admin as initial IV bolus. max. 90mg. Adjunctive with heparin and aspirin.

Actilyse Cathflo, up to 2mg (reconstituted to 1mg/mL) instilled into the occluded central venous device up to 2-times for any one occlusion to restore function which have become dysfunctional due to thrombotic occlusion. Body weight under 30kg, instil volume corresponding to 110% of internal lumen volume of device; max. total 2mg. If central venous access function not restored at 120 minutes after first dose, a second dose of equal amount may be instilled.

Elderly: *Actilyse, acute stroke,* over 80 years, not recommended.

Child: *Actilyse, acute stroke,* under 18 years, not recommended; *Cathflo,* as for Adult above.

CI: Gentamicin hypersensitivity. See also Notes below.

Interactions: Effect of Other Drugs on Alteplase: *Anaphylactoid risk enhanced:* ACEIs. See Notes below. *Co-admin not recommended (Cathflo):* Heparin (does not improve rate of catheter function).

SP: NOTE: *Actilyse Cathflo 2mg* is not indicated for use in MI, acute PE or acute ischaemic stroke. Caution, use in patients at risk for bleeding events.

Anaphylactoid reactions, potentially dangerous haemorrhage (cerebral), discontinue. Recent biopsy, major vessel puncture, IM injection, cardiac massage for resuscitation, haemorrhagic retinopathy, conditions with increased risk of haemorrhage, weigh risk/benefit. Intracranial haemorrhage risk increase in elderly. Avoid using rigid catheters. Treatment with platelet aggregation inhibitors should not be initiated within the first 24 hours following thrombolysis with alteplase.

ADR: *Indication MI,* reperfusion arrhythmias; *indication stroke,* intracerebral/intracranial haemorrhage; *occluded catheters,* sepsis, catheter-related complications.

Notes: See 2.6.9 Antithrombotics, Enzymes and Proteins.

Actilyse Parenteral, Cathflo 2mg *(Boehringer)* A. HOS.
Price, (1) 10mg, €138.00; 20mg, €233.12; 50mg, 516.32; Cathflo 2mg, €220.28 (PTW).
Injection or infusion, alteplase. 10mg, 20mg, 50mg. Colourless (pale-yellow) lyophilised powder cake. Solvent for soln. *Latex (stopper),* gentamicin trace. **Store:** Before reconstitution, store below 25 deg C.
Cathflo 2mg injection or infusion, as above. Solvent not included. **Store:** Refrigerate.

Protein C

ATC Code: B01AD12. **Sport:** Permitted.
Driving: No influence.

Indications: Severe congenital protein C deficiency, purpura fulminans and coumarin induced skin necrosis; short-term prophylaxis when (surgery or invasive therapy is imminent; while initiating coumarin therapy or when coumarin therapy alone is insufficient or not feasible).

Dose: Adult, Elderly: Initially 60-80 IU/kg for determination of recovery and half-life advised. Individualise dose based on laboratory assessment. 100% Protein C activity should be achieved initially then maintained above 25% for duration of treatment. Individual responses differ widely and coagulation parameters should be checked regularly. *Admin,* by IV injection; max. rate 2mL/min.

Child: As for Adult above. *Admin,* by IV injection; max. rate 2mL/min; under 10kg bodyweight, max. 0.2mL/Kg/min.

Renal Impairment: Monitor closely.

Hepatic Impairment: Monitor closely.

CI: Mouse protein or heparin hypersensitivity (except for control of life-threatening thrombotic complications).

Interactions: Effect of Other Drugs on Protein C: *Transient hypercoagulable state before desired anticoagulant effect:* Vitamin K antagonist anticoagulants (warfarin).

SP: Consider hepatitis A and B vaccination for patients in regular or repeated receipt of human plasma-derived

Protein C products. May contain trace amounts of heparin; may induce allergic reaction with rapidly decreased thrombocytes or heparin induced thrombocytopenia (HIT); if HIT suspected, determine number of thrombocytes and stop therapy if needed. Bleeding episodes observed.

Pregnancy, Lactation: Weigh risk/benefit.

ADR: Advise patient of early signs of hypersensitivity.

Notes: See 2.6.9 Antithrombotics, Enzymes and Proteins.

CEPROTIN Parenteral *(Baxalta)* A.
Price, not published by company.
Injection, Protein 1000 IU*. From human plasma purified by mouse monoclonal antibodies. White (cream) powder or friable solid and solvent for soln. *One IU of Protein C equates to amidolytically measured activity of Protein C in 1mL normal plasma. *Sodium chloride 88mg, sodium citrate 44mg per vial.*
Store: Refrigerate; do not freeze.

Tenecteplase

ATC Code: B01AD11. **Sport:** Permitted.
Driving: Caution.

Indications: Suspected MI with persistent ST elevation or recent left Bundle Branch Block within 6 hours after the onset of acute MI symptoms.

Dose: Adult: Dose calculated according to body weight; max. 50mg (10000 IU) as single IV bolus over approx. 10 seconds. Adjunctive with heparin (unfractionated), enoxaparin, acetylsalicylic acid. Treatment to be initiated soonest after onset of symptoms.

Elderly: Over 75 years, caution.

Child: Under 18 years, not recommended.

CI: Dementia. See Notes below.

Interactions: Effect of Other Drugs on Tenecteplase: *Increased bleeding risk:* GPIIb/IIIa antagonists.

SP: Body weight under 60kg. Arrhythmias. Re-admin, not recommended.

ADR: Reperfusion arrhythmias.

Notes: See 2.6.9 Antithrombotics, Enzymes and Proteins.

Metalyse Parenteral *(Boehringer)* A. HOS.
Price, (1) 8000 IU (40mg) €703.04. 10000 IU (50mg) €990.81 (PTW).
Injection, tenecteplase. White (off-white) powder and solvent for soln. Clear colourless (slightly yellow) soln when reconstituted.
Notes: Incompatible with dextrose infusion soln. Potency expressed in units (U) using reference standard specific for tenecteplase and not comparable with units used for other thrombolytics.

2.7 - Anti-Fibrinolytics and Haemostatics

In This Chapter: *Eltrombopag, eptacog alfa (recombinant coagulation factor VIIa), Factor VIII Inhibitor Bypassing Activity, human fibrinogen, efmoroctocog alfa, octocog alfa (recombinant human coagulation factor VIII), nonacog alfa (recombinant coagulation factor IX), romiplostim, tranexamic acid.*

Class Effects

Antifibrinolytics are a diverse group of drugs used to prevent haemorrhage. Other indications include: *Desmopressin,* management of haemorrhage (mild to moderate haemophilia, Von Willebrand's disease type I and IIA undergoing surgery or following trauma); diagnosis and treatment of cranial diabetes insipidus; to establish renal concentration capacity. *Oxidised cellulose,* to control capillary bleeding. *Vitamin K,* to treat haemorrhage or threatened haemorrhage associated with low prothrombin or factor VII blood levels; antidote to anticoagulant coumarin type drugs. See Notes below.

CI: Hypersensitivity to any member of the class.

SP: Treatment under supervision of physician experienced in haemophilia treatment.

Intravenous protein products, including (eptacog, octocog, nonacog alfa, efmoroctocog alfa; Factor VIII), allergic-type hypersensitivity reactions possible; early hypersensitivity signs (difficult breathing, shortness of breath, swelling, hives, itching, chest tightness, bronchospasm, laryngospasm, wheezing, hypotension, blurred vision,

2.7   Anti-Fibrinolytics and Haemostatics

anaphylaxis). When admin, record name and batch number of product to maintain a link between patient and batch.
Thrombopoietin-receptor agonists (TPO-R agonists) (eltrombopag, romiplostim), theoretical concern is stimulation of progression of existing haematopoietic malignancies. *Factor VIII* (efmoroctocog alfa, octocog alfa, Factor VIII), formation of neutralising antibodies (inhibitors) to factor VIII is a known management complication (high inhibitor levels, Factor VIII may not be effective).
Notes: See 11.6.4 Posterior Pituitary Hormones (desmopressin). See 16.3.9 Vitamin K.

Eltrombopag

ATC Code: B02BX05. **Sport:** Pending.
Driving: Dizziness, lack of alertness.
Indications: Chronic immune thrombocytopenic purpura (ITP) in patients (1 year and above) refractory to other treatments (corticosteroids, immunoglobulins). Treatment (adults), thrombocytopenia associated with chronic hepatitis C (HCV) infection (optimal interferon-based therapy not possible); acquired severe aplastic anaemia (refractory to prior treatment or unsuitable for stem cell transplantation).
Dose: Adult: *Chronic ITP,* initially 50mg once daily; patients with East Asian ancestry, initiate at 25mg once daily; max. 75mg/day. Adjust dose* at minimum 2-week intervals based on platelet count.
HCV-associated thrombocytopenia, initially 25mg once daily; East Asian ancestry, mild hepatic impairment, no adjustment. Increase* at 2-week intervals, max. 100mg/day. *Admin,* oral minimum 2 hours before or 4 hours after antacids, dairy products or other calcium-containing foods, mineral supplements (iron, calcium, magnesium, aluminium, selenium, zinc).
Severe aplastic anaemia, initially 50mg once daily; patients with East Asian ancestry, initiate at 25mg once daily; haematological response requires dose titration up to 150mg and may take 16 weeks. Adjust dose* at minimum 2-week intervals based on platelet count.
NOTE: Powder for oral susp (if available) may lead to higher eltrombopag exposure than tablet formulation; if switching formulation, monitor platelet counts weekly for 2 weeks. *(standard dose adjustment is 25mg once daily, either increase or decrease).
Elderly: Age 65 years and older, possible greater sensitivity. Age 75 years and older, limited data (caution).
Child: Age 6-17 years, as for Adult above. Age 1-5 years, initially 25mg once daily. Under 1 year, not recommended; insufficient data. *Admin,* see Adult above.
Renal Impairment: Caution/close monitoring, serum creatinine and/or urinalysis.
Hepatic Impairment: Caution in presence of hepatic disease. ITP, Child-Pugh 5 or above, use only if benefit outweighs risk of portal venous thrombosis. If necessary, initiate at 25mg once daily; wait 3 weeks before increasing dose. HCV, initiate as above; wait 2 weeks before increasing dose.
Interactions: Effect of Other Drugs on Eltrombopag: *Co-admin caution:* Topotecan, lopinavir/ritonavir, methotrexate (decreased eltrombopag conc). *Eltrombopag exposure decreased:* Ciclosporin. *Dose minimum 4 hours apart:* Polyvalent cations, antacids, dairy products/high calcium foods, mineral supplements (see Dose above). *Co-admin, monitor platelets:* Other medicinals used for ITP (corticosteroids, danazol, and/or azathioprine, IV immunoglobulin, anti-D immunoglobulin). *Eltrombopag plasma levels:* Increased (fluvoxamine); decreased (rifampicin).
Effect of Eltrombopag on Other Drugs: Statins: *Consider dose reduction with co-admin; monitor statin side effects.*
SP: Increased adverse event risk (potentially fatal hepatic decompensation, thromboembolic events), in thrombocytopenic HCV patients with liver disease (advanced chronic or model for end stage). Measure serum ALT, AST, bilirubin prior to initiation, 2-weekly (during dose adjustment), monthly (with stable dosing). Discontinue if ALT increases to 3xULN (normal liver function) OR 3x baseline (or more) or 5xULN whichever is lower (with pre-

treatment elevated transaminases) AND are (progressive OR persistent for 4 weeks or more OR with increased direct bilirubin OR with clinical symptoms of liver injury or hepatic decompensation).
Caution, thromboembolism risk factors (inherited or acquired, advanced age, prolonged immobilisation, malignancies, contraceptives, HRT, surgery/trauma, obesity, smoking). May increase risk for development or progression of reticulin fibres within bone marrow; monitor morphology. Exclude myelodysplastic syndrome (MDS). Cataracts.
Pregnancy, Lactation: Pregnancy, not recommended. Women of childbearing potential to ensure adequate contraception. Lactation, stop breastfeeding or stop drug.
ADR: Summary, *most important serious,* hepatotoxicity, thrombotic and thromboembolic events; *most common,* headache, anaemia, decreased appetite, insomnia, cough, nausea, diarrhoea, alopecia, pruritus, myalgia, pyrexia, fatigue, flu-like illness, asthenia, chills, peripheral oedema.
Notes: See 2.7 Anti-Fibrinolytics and Haemostatics.

> **Revolade 25mg, 50mg** *(Novartis)* A. HT.
> *Price,* (28) 25mg, €1020.04. 50mg, €2043.58.
> *Tablet,* eltrombopag olamine. Round f/c. Marked GS/strength. 25mg: White. Marked NX3. 50mg: Brown. Marked UFU. **Store:** No special conditions.

Efmoroctocog Alfa

ATC Code: B02BD02. **Sport:** Permitted.
Driving: No influence.
Indications: Treatment and prophylaxis of bleeding in patients (all ages) with haemophilia A (congenital factor VIII deficiency).
Dose: Adult: Dose and duration of substitution therapy is based on severity of factor VIII deficiency, location and extent of bleeding and patient clinical condition.
'On-demand' treatment, calculated using the formula: Required units = body weight (kg) x desired factor VIII rise (%) (IU/dL) x 0.5 (IU/kg per IU/dL). *Haemorrhage,* early haemarthrosis, muscle or oral bleed, Factor VIII level required (%) (IU/dL), 20-40; repeat infusion every 12-24 hours, for minimum 1 day. More extensive haemarthrosis, muscle bleed, haematoma, 30-60; repeat every 12-24 hours for 3-4 days. Life-threatening haemorrhages, 60-100; repeat every 8-24 hours until resolved.
Surgery, minor, including tooth extraction, 30-60 every 24 hours for at least 1 day. Major, 80-100 (pre- and post-operative); repeat injection every 8-24 hours until adequate wound healing, then for at least another 7 days to maintain Factor VIII activity at 30-60% (IU/dL).
Prophylaxis (long-term), recommended 50 IU/kg every 3-5 days; adjust dose on patient response in range 25-65 IU/kg. *Admin,* IV over several minutes; max. 10mL/min.
Elderly: 65 years and older, limited experience.
Child: Under 12 years, more frequent or higher doses may be needed; 12 years and over, as for Adult above.
SP: Substitution therapy may increase cardiovascular risk in patients with existing cardiovascular risk factors. If central venous access is required, complications risk (local infection, bacteraemia, catheter site thrombosis).
Pregnancy, Lactation: Use only if clearly indicated.
ADR: Summary, hypersensitivity or allergic reactions (rarely); may progress to severe anaphylaxis (including shock).
Notes: See 2.7 Anti-Fibrinolytics and Haemostatics.

> ▼ **ELOCTA Parenteral** *(SOBI)* A.
> *Price,* not published by company.
> *Injection,* efmoroctocog alfa (human coagulation factor VIII) IU (250, 500, 1000, 1500, 2000, 3000). White (off-white) powder or cake; water for injection clear colourless soln. *Sodium* 14mg/vial. **Store:** Refrigerate; do not freeze.

Eptacog Alfa

ATC Code: B02BD08. **Sport:** Permitted.
Driving: Unlikely to impair.
Indications: Treatment and prophylaxis of bleeding in congenital haemophilia with inhibitors to coagulation factors VIII or IX above 5 Bethesda Units (BU) or where a high anamnestic response to factor VIII or factor IX admin

is expected. Acquired haemophilia. Factor VII deficiency. Glanzmann's thrombasthenia.

Dose: Adult, Elderly: *Haemophilia A or B,* initially 90mcg/kg body weight by IV bolus over 2-5 minutes every 2-3 hours. *Mild to moderate* bleeding episode, 2-3 injections of 90mcg/kg at 3-hour intervals to achieve haemostasis, if needed 1 additional dose (90mcg/kg) OR single injection of 270mcg/kg; max. 24 hours. *Serious* bleeding episode, initially 90mcg/kg 2-hour intervals. *Invasive procedures/surgery,* initially 90mcg/kg immediately before intervention; repeat after 2 hours and then at 2-3 hour intervals for 24-48 hours; major surgery, continue at 2-4 hour intervals for 6-7 days.

Acquired haemophilia, initially 90mcg/kg; if required further injection can be given, dose interval 2-3 hours.

Factor VII deficiency, surgery or invasive procedures, 15-30mcg/kg every 4-6 hours.

Glanzmann's thrombasthenia, surgery/invasive procedures, 90mcg/kg 2-hourly; range 80-120mcg/kg.

Child: *Haemophilia A or B,* as for Adult above; higher doses may be required as children have faster clearance.

CI: Hypersensitivity to mouse, hamster or bovine protein.

Interactions: Effect of Other Drugs on Eptacog alfa: *Co-admin not recommended:* Prothrombin complex conc; rFVIIa and rFXIII.

SP: Atherosclerotic disease, crush injury, septicaemia or DIC. Monitor prothrombin time and factor VII coagulant activity before and after admin; if factor VIIa activity fails to reach expected level or bleeding not contained after treatment, suspect antibody formation. Thrombosis reported in factor VII deficient patients.

Pregnancy, Lactation: Pregnancy, if benefit outweighs risk. Lactation, caution.

ADR: *Uncommon,* venous thromboembolic events, rash, pruritus, decreased therapeutic response, pyrexia.

Notes: See 2.7 Anti-Fibrinolytics and Haemostatics.

NovoSeven Parenteral *(Novo Nordisk)* A.
Price, not published by company.
Injection, eptacog alfa (activated) 50 KIU (1mg), 100 KIU (2mg), 250 KIU (5mg). Recombinant coagulation factor VIIa (rFVIIa) produced by rDNA technology. White lyophilised powder. Clear colourless solvent for soln. *Sucrose.*

FEIBA (Factor VIII inhibitor bypassing activity)

ATC Code: B02BD03. **Sport:** Permitted.
Driving: No or negligible effect.
Indications: Treatment, bleeding in haemophilia A patients*; and haemophilia B patients* (no other specific treatment available); bleeding in non-haemophiliacs with acquired Factor VIII inhibitors. Prophylaxis, haemophilia A patients* (had significant bleed or at high risk of significant bleeding). *(with inhibitors).

Dose: Adult, Elderly: General guideline, 50-100 U/kg; a single dose of 100 U/kg body weight and max. 200 U/kg/day not be exceeded unless bleeding justifies higher dose. *Admin,* slow IV infusion; max. infusion rate 2 U/kg/min.

Spontaneous bleeding, joint, muscle, soft tissue haemorrhage, 50-75 U/kg 12-hourly; severe (retroperitoneal haemorrhage), 100 U/kg 12-hourly. Mucous membrane haemorrhage, 50 U/kg 6-hourly; if bleeding does not stop, increase to 100 U/kg*. Other severe haemorrhage (CNS bleeding), 100 U/kg 12-hourly; may be admin 6-hourly until improvement*.

Surgery, initially 100 U/kg pre-operatively, then 50-100 U/kg after 6-12 hours; post-operative maintenance, 50-100 U/kg 6-12 hourly*. *(max. 200 U/kg/day).

Prophylaxis, haemophilia A patients with inhibitors with failed immune tolerance induction (ITI) or not considered, 70-100 U/kg every other day; increase to 100 U/kg/day or decrease. Prophylaxis with inhibitors during ITI, 50-100 U/kg twice daily (can admin with Factor VIII) until inhibitor titre is below 2 Bethesda units.

Child: As for Adult; under 6 years, limited experience.

CI: Disseminated Intravascular Coagulation (DIC), acute thrombosis or embolism including MI.

Interactions: Effect of Other Drugs on Factor VIII Inhibitor Bypassing Activity: *Co-admin not recommended:* Antifibrinolytics (allow 6-12 hour after *Feiba* admin).

SP: A sufficient number of functionally intact platelets (thrombocytes) are necessary for efficacy. Thrombotic and thromboembolic events (DIC, venous thrombosis, pulmonary embolism, MI, stroke) have occurred; risk increased with high doses; use with caution (history of coronary heart disease, liver disease, DIC, arterial or venous thrombosis, post-operative immobilisation, elderly, neonates). 100 U/kg, monitor carefully. Signs of thrombotic or thromboembolic events, significant changes (BP, pulse rate, respiratory distress, coughing or chest pain), discontinue immediately. Inhibitor haemophilia or with acquired inhibitors, may have increased bleeding tendency and thrombosis risk at the same time. Response to bypassing agents can vary. If inhibitor levels rise, do not reintroduce.

Pregnancy, Lactation: If benefit outweighs risk.

ADR: Allergic-type hypersensitivity reactions (urticaria, angioedema, GI manifestations, bronchospasm, BP drop); can be severe, systemic (anaphylaxis, circulatory shock).

Notes: See 2.7 Anti-Fibrinolytics and Haemostatics.

FEIBA Parenteral *(Baxalta)* A.
Price, not published by company.
Infusion, FEIBA (U) 25 U, 50 U per mL. Also Factors II, IX, X (non-activated), VII (activated). White (off-white, pale green) powder; solvent for soln. *Sodium approx. 80mg/500(1000) U; 200mg/2500 U.* **Store:** Below 25 deg C; do not freeze.

Human Fibrinogen

ATC Code: B02BB01. **Sport:** Permitted.
Driving: No or negligible effect.
Indications: Treatment, bleeding in patients with congenital hypo-, or afibrinogenemia with bleeding tendency.

Dose: Adult, Elderly: If fibrinogen level is not known, recommend initially 70mg/kg IV. Dose of fibrinogen = [Target level (g/L) - measured level (g/L) divided by [0.017 (g/L per mg/kg body weight)]. Target level (1g/L) for minor events (epistaxis, intramuscular bleed, menorrhagia) and maintain for 3 days; target level (1.5g/L) for major events (head trauma, intracranial haemorrhage) and maintain for 7 days. *Admin,* by IV infusion or injection; max. rate 5mL/min.

Child: Limited data, as for Adult above.

SP: Thrombosis risk (high or repeated dosing). *Caution,* weigh risk benefit in patients with (coronary heart disease, MI, liver disease, peri- or post-operative, neonates, risk of thromboembolic events, DIC). Allergic or anaphylactic-type reactions, discontinue immediately.

Pregnancy, Lactation: Based on experience in treating obstetric complications, no harmful effects on course of pregnancy of health of foetus or neonate are expected. Lactation, stop drug or stop breastfeeding.

ADR: *Rarely,* allergic reactions, increased body temp; *very rarely,* thromboembolic episodes.

Notes: See 2.7 Anti-Fibrinolytics and Haemostatics.

Riastap 1g Parenteral *(CSL Behring)* A.
Price, not published by company.
Injection or infusion, human fibrinogen. White powder for soln. *Sodium 164mg/vial.*

Octocog Alfa

ATC Code: B02BD02. **Sport:** Permitted.
Driving: No influence.
Indications: Treatment and prophylaxis, bleeding in haemophilia A (congenital factor VIII deficiency) (all ages).

Dose: Adult, Elderly: *Haemorrhage,* early haemarthrosis, muscle or oral bleed, dose expressed as Factor VIII level required (%) (IU/dL), 20-40; repeat infusion every 12-24 hours (minimum 1 day); more extensive haemarthrosis, muscle bleed, haematoma, 30-60; repeat every 12-24 hours (3-4 days); life-threatening haemorrhage (intracranial, throat, severe abdominal), 60-100; repeat every 8-24 hours until resolved.

Surgery, minor (tooth extraction), 30-60 every 24 hours (at least 1 day); major, 80-100 pre- and post-operative; repeat infusion every 8-24 hours until adequate wound healing,

2.7 Anti-Fibrinolytics and Haemostatics

then for at least another 7 days to maintain Factor VIII activity at 30-60% (IU/dL) (bolus infusion) OR *Kogenate*, raise Factor VIII activity pre-surgery with initial bolus, followed immediately with continuous infusion (in IU/kg/hour).

Scheduled prophylaxis, severe haemophilia A, 20-60 IU/kg body weight; intervals of 2-3 days. *Admin*, IV over several minutes; max. 2mL/min (*Kogenate*), 10mL/min (*Advate*) or continuous infusion (*Kogenate*).

Child: *Kogenate*, as for Adult above. *Advate*, under 6 years, as for Adult above; *haemorrhage*, early haemarthrosis, more extensive haemarthrosis, repeat every 8-24 hours; life-threatening haemorrhage, every 6-12 hours; *surgery*, minor, repeat every 12-24 hours; major, repeat every 6-24 hours. *Prophylaxis*, under 6 years, 20-50 IU Factor VIII per kg bodyweight, 3-4 times weekly.

CI: Mouse, hamster protein hypersensitivity.

SP: Hypersensitivity, discontinue use; seek medical advice (may contain traces of mouse or hamster protein). Catheter-related complications with central venous access. Cardiovascular events, monitor. Misapplication of *Advate* (intra-arterially or paravenously) may lead to mild, short-term injection-site reactions (bruising, erythema). *Kogenate* does not contain Von Willebrand's factor; not indicated for Von Willebrand's disease.

Pregnancy, Lactation: Only if clearly indicated; based on rare occurrence of haemophilia A in women, experience of use during pregnancy and lactation, is not available.

ADR: *Very common*, Factor VIII inhibitor formation (neutralising antibodies).

Notes: See 2.7 Anti-Fibrinolytics and Haemostatics.

Kogenate Bayer Parenteral *(Bayer)* A.
Price, not published by company.
Injection or infusion, octocog alfa (human coagulation factor VIII) 250 IU, 500 IU, 1000 IU. Dry white (slightly yellow) powder/cake. *Sucrose; sodium below 23mg/vial*. Solvent for soln. Potency (IU) determined using 1-stage clotting assay against FDA Mega standard calibrated against WHO International Units (IU) standard.
Store: Refrigerate; do not freeze; may be stored below 25 deg C for max. 12 months.

ADVATE Parenteral *(Baxalta)* A.
Price, not published by company.
Injection, octocog alfa (human coagulation factor VIII) (IU) (2mL) 250; (5mL) 500. 1000, 1500, 2000, 3000. White (off-white) powder. Clear colourless soln. *Sodium 10mg/vial (2mL, 5mL)*.
Store: Refrigerate; do not freeze.

Nonacog Alfa

ATC Code: B02BD09. **Sport:** Permitted.
Driving: No data.

Indications: Treatment and prophylaxis, bleeding in patients (all ages) with haemophilia B (congenital factor IX deficiency).

Dose: Adult: Formula: Number of Factor IX IU required = body weight (kg) X desired Factor IX increase (%) or (IU/dL) X reciprocal of observed recovery.

Haemorrhage, early haemarthrosis, muscle or oral bleed, Factor IX level required (%) (IU/dL), 20-40; repeat every 24 hours (minimum 1 day) until resolved or healing achieved. More extensive haemarthrosis, muscle bleed, haematoma, 30-60; repeat every 24 hours (3-4 days). Life-threatening bleeds, 60-100; repeat every 8-24 hours until resolved.

Surgery, minor including tooth extraction, 30-60; every 24 hours (minimum 1 day); major, 80-100 pre- and post-operative; repeat every 8-24 hours until adequate wound healing, then for another 7 days to maintain a factor IX activity of 30-60% (IU/dL).

Long-term prophylaxis, severe haemophilia B, previously treated patients, 40 IU/kg (range 13-78 IU/kg); intervals of 3-4 days (shorter dosage intervals or higher doses may be needed in some cases, especially younger patients). Slow IV infusion (4mL/min) after reconstitution; continuous infusion not recommended. Hypersensitivity, decrease infusion rate or stop.

Elderly: Over 65, individualise dose.

Child: Age under 6 years, 'on-demand' treatment and surgery, limited data. Mean dosage for prophylaxis as 63.7 (+/- 19.1) IU/kg at intervals of 3-7 days; younger patients,

shorter dosage intervals or higher doses may be needed. *Admin*, as for Adult above.

CI: Hypersensitivity to hamster proteins.

SP: Allergic-type hypersensitivity possible. Factor IX inhibitors, increased anaphylaxis risk. Major deletion mutations of factor IX gene, monitor for hypersensitivity. Thrombosis, DIC risk; thrombotic complications, liver disease, post-operative, neonates, risk of thrombotic phenomena or DIC. Agglutination of RBCs in tube or syringe.

Pregnancy, Lactation: Pregnancy, breastfeeding, use only if clearly indicated.

ADR: *Very common*, headache, cough, pyrexia; *common*, hypersensitivity, dizziness, dysgeusia, phlebitis, flushing, vomiting, nausea, rash, urticaria, chest discomfort, infusion-site reaction or pain.

Notes: See 2.7 Anti-Fibrinolytics and Haemostatics.

BeneFIX Parenteral *(Pfizer)* A.
Price, not published by company.
Infusion, nonacog alfa 250 IU, 500 IU, 1000 IU. White (almost) powder. *Sucrose*. Clear colourless solvent for soln.

Romiplostim

ATC Code: B02BX04. **Sport:** Pending.
Driving: Moderate influence: dizziness.

Indications: Treatment, adult chronic (idiopathic) thrombocytopenic purpura (ITP) in patients refractory to other treatments (corticosteroids, immunoglobulins).

Dose: Adult, Elderly: Age 18 years and over, initially, 1mcg/kg based on actual body weight, SC once weekly; base further dose adjustments in 1mcg increments, on platelet counts. *Elderly*, caution.

Renal Impairment: Caution.

Hepatic Impairment: Moderate/severe, use only if benefit outweighs risk; portal vein thrombosis.

CI: Hypersensitivity to *E. coli*-derived proteins.

SP: Exclude diagnosis of Myelodysplastic Syndromes. Reoccurrence of thrombocytopenia and bleeding after treatment discontinuation; restart ITP treatment according to current guidelines. Increased bone marrow reticulin; examine for cellular morphological abnormalities. Platelet counts above normal, risk for thrombotic or thromboembolic complications; caution known thromboembolism risk; portal vein thrombosis. Loss of response, investigate causative factors, immunogenicity, increased bone marrow reticulin. Monitor red and white blood cells; combination with other ITP treatment, monitor platelets. Concurrent anaemia and leucocytosis may occur. Evaluate patients periodically; decide continued therapy on an individual basis and in non-splenectomised patients include evaluation relative to splenectomy. NOTE: Medication errors reported (caution).

Pregnancy, Lactation: Pregnancy, women of childbearing potential not using contraception, not recommended. Lactation, stop drug or stop breastfeeding.

ADR: Summary, *most serious*, thrombocytopenia reoccurrence and bleeding after treatment cessation, increased bone marrow reticulin, thrombotic and/or thromboembolic complications, medication errors, progression of existing MDS to AML; *most common*, hypersensitivity reactions (rash, urticaria, angioedema), headache.

Notes: See 2.7 Anti-Fibrinolytics and Haemostatics.

Nplate Parenteral *(Amgen)* A. HOS.
Price, (1) €590.15 (PTW).
Injection, romiplostim 250mcg. Produced by rDNA technology. White powder for soln.

Tranexamic Acid

ATC Code: B02AA02. **Sport:** Permitted.
Driving: None known/no studies.

Indications: Prevention and treatment of haemorrhage due to general or local fibrinolysis (adults, children from 1 year). Specific indications, *(parenteral)*, menorrhagia, metrorrhagia, GI bleeding, haemorrhagic urinary disorders; surgery (prostate, urinary tract), ear, nose and throat (adenoidectomy, tonsillectomy, dental extractions), gynaecological, obstetric, thoracic, abdominal, other major surgical interventions (cardiovascular); haemorrhage due to fibrinolytic admin; *oral*, surgery (prostatectomy, bladder), menorrhagia, epistaxis, conisation of cervix, traumatic hyphaemia, hereditary angioedema, dental extractions (haemophiliacs), upper GI haemorrhage.

Dose: Adult, Elderly: ORAL, local fibrinolysis, 15-25mg/kg bodyweight 2-3 times daily. *Prostatectomy*, commence with parenteral, then oral 1g 3-4 times daily until macroscopic haematuria no longer present; *menorrhagia*, 1-1.5g 3-4 times daily or 3-4 days; *epistaxis*, 1g 3-times daily for 7 days where recurrent bleeding is anticipated; *conisation of cervix*, 1.5g 3-times daily; *traumatic hyphaemia*, 1-1.5g 3-times daily (based on 25mg/kg 3-times daily).

Angioedema (hereditary), 1-1.5g 2-3 times daily intermittently or continuously depending on whether patient has prodromal symptoms; *haemophilia* (dental extractions), 1-1.5g 8-hourly; *upper GI haemorrhage*, 1g by slow IV injection 6-hourly for 3 days; then 1-1.5g orally, 6-hourly for a further 3-4 days.

PARENTERAL, local fibrinolysis (standard treatment), 0.5-1g IV 2-3 times daily. General fibrinolysis (standard treatment), 1g IV every 6-8 hours (15mg/kg body weight). *Admin*, by slow IV injection (1mL/min). Not for IM admin.

Child: Limited data, region of 20mg/kg/dose.

Renal Impairment: Serum creatinine (micromoL/L), 120-249, 15mg/kg (oral) or 10mg/kg* (parenteral) twice daily (12-hourly); 250-500, 15mg/kg (oral) or 10mg/kg* (parenteral) 24-hourly; above 500, 5mg/kg* (parenteral) 24-hourly. Severe, contraindicated (accumulation risk). *(body weight).

Hepatic Impairment: No dose adjustment.

CI: Subarachnoid haemorrhage (oral), fibrinolytic conditions following consumption coagulopathy; venous or arterial thrombosis, convulsions (history of). Intrathecal and intraventricular injection, intracerebral application (risk of cerebral oedema and convulsions).

SP: *Caution*, haematuria from upper urinary tract, urethral obstruction risk; when intravascular coagulation is in progress; patients receiving oral contraceptives (increased thrombosis risk). With high thrombosis risk, only if (strong medical indication, strict medical supervision); investigate risk factors of thromboembolic disease. Irregular menstrual bleeding, use only when cause established.

Rapid IV injection (dizziness and/or hypotension). Visual disturbances (long-term parenteral treatment, conduct regular ophthalmic examinations). Cases of convulsion reported (high IV doses); history of convulsions, use not recommended.

Pregnancy, Lactation: Pregnancy, first trimester not recommended; throughout, use only if benefit outweighs risk. Lactation, not recommended.

ADR: *Rarely (oral)* , colour vision disturbances, retinal artery occlusion, thromboembolic events, allergic skin reactions. *Common (parenteral)*, diarrhoea, vomiting, nausea.

Notes: See 2.7 Anti-Fibrinolytics and Haemostatics.

Cyklokapron 500mg *(Meda)* B. GMS.
Price, (60) €16.23.
Tablet, tranexamic acid. White cap-shaped f/c scored. Marked CY.
Cyklokapron Parenteral *(Pfizer)* A. GMS.
Price, (10) 500mg, €16.92.
Injection or infusion, tranexamic acid 500mg (100mg/mL). Clear colourless aqueous soln. **Store:** Do not freeze.

2.8 - Positive Inotropes

Class Effects
Positive cardiac inotropes are used for the management of both acute and chronic HF as they increase the force of myocardial contraction e.g. cardiac glycosides, phosphodiesterase inhibitors. Sympathomimetics are also employed as inotropes.

2.8.1 - Cardiac Glycosides

In This Chapter: *Digoxin.*

Class Effects
Digoxin increases contractility of the myocardium by direct

activity. The effect is proportional to dose in the lower range and some effect may be achieved at low dose.

CI: Hypersensitivity to any member of the class.

Notes: See 2.8 Positive Inotropes.

Digoxin
ATC Code: C01AA05. **Sport:** Permitted.
Driving: Caution.

Indications: Chronic cardiac failure where the dominant problem is systolic dysfunction (therapeutic benefit greatest in patients with ventricular dilatation) or accompanied by atrial fibrillation. Supraventricular arrhythmias, particularly atrial flutter and fibrillation where a major benefit is reduction of ventricular rate.

Dose: Adult: ORAL, *rapid oral loading*, 0.75-1.5mg as single dose (less urgency, admin in 2 divided doses 6 hours apart); *slow oral loading*, 0.25-0.75mg daily for 1 week; maintenance usually 0.125-0.25mg/day but 0.0625mg may suffice.

PARENTERAL, *emergency parenteral loading*, 0.5-1mg in divided doses by IV infusion over 10-20 minutes; maintenance 0.125-0.75mg/day. Tailor dose according to age, lean body weight, renal function. Switch oral to IV, reduce dose by 33%.

Elderly: Avoid hypokalaemia, monitor serum levels. Consider dose reduction.

Child: ORAL, if cardiac glycosides have not been given in preceding 2 weeks, *loading dose* over 24 hours, preterm neonates (under 1.5kg), 25mcg/kg/24-hours; (1.5-2.5kg), 30mcg/kg/24-hours; term neonates to 2 years, 45mcg/kg/24-hours. Children 2-5 years, 35mcg/kg/24-hours; 5-10 years, 25mcg/kg/24-hours. *Maintenance*, preterm neonates, 20% of 24-hour loading dose (IV or oral) per day. Term neonates, children 10 years, 25% of 24-hour loading dose (IV or oral) per day.

PARENTERAL (IV), *loading dose* over 24 hours, preterm neonates, under 1.5kg, 20mcg/kg; 1.5kg-2.5kg, 30mcg/kg; term neonates to 2 years, 35mcg/kg. Children 2-5 years, 35mcg/kg; 5-10 years, 25mcg/kg. *Maintenance*, as for oral. If cardiac glycosides have been given in the 2 preceding weeks, optimum loading doses will be less.

Renal Impairment: Consider dose reduction.

CI: Known hypersensitivity to digoxin or other digitalis glycosides. Intermittent complete heart block or second degree AV block (especially with history of Stokes-Adams attacks). Arrhythmias due to cardiac glycoside intoxication; supraventricular associated with an accessory AV pathway (Wolff-Parkinson-White syndrome), ventricular tachycardia or fibrillation. Hypertrophic obstructive cardiomyopathy.

Interactions: Effect of Other Drugs on Digoxin: *Increased AV conduction time*: Beta-blockers. *Increased sensitivity* (hypokalaemia): Diuretics, lithium, corticosteroids, carbenoxolone, suxamethonium. *Arrhythmias*: Calcium (especially IV). *Plasma levels increased*: Amiodarone, flecainide, prazosin, propafenone, quinidine, spironolactone, macrolides (erythromycin, clarithromycin), tetracyclines, gentamicin, itraconazole, quinine, trimethoprim, alprazolam, indomethacin, propantheline, nefazodone, atorvastatin, ciclosporin, epoprostenol, carvedilol, verapamil, felodipine (possibly all dihydropyridines), tiapamil, ACEIs (increase or no change), P-glycoprotein inhibitors. *Plasma levels decreased*: St John's Wort, antacids, bulk laxatives, kaolin-pectin, acarbose, neomycin, penicillamine, rifampicin, some cytostatics, metoclopramide, sulfasalazine, salbutamol, adrenaline, colestyramine, phenytoin.

SP: Digoxin toxicity may precipitate arrhythmias. When incomplete AV block, anticipate rapid progression in the block; in complete heart block, idioventricular escape rhythm may be suppressed. SA disorder (sick sinus syndrome), digoxin may exacerbate sinus bradycardia or cause sinoatrial block.

Digoxin admin immediately following MI, not contraindicated. Avoid in HF associated with cardiac amyloidosis, myocarditis. Should not be used in constrictive pericarditis. Caution in presence of thyroid disease; adjust dose. Treat underlying thiamine deficiency in beri-beri.

2.8.2　Phosphodiesterase Inhibitors

At therapeutic doses, PR interval prolongation, ST segment depression, false ST-T changes on ECG. Monitor serum electrolytes, renal function (serum creatinine). Patients with severe respiratory distress (increased myocardial sensitivity to digitalis glycosides); hypokalaemia sensitises myocardium to cardiac glycosides; hypoxia, hypomagnesaemia, hypercalcaemia increases myocardial sensitivity to cardiac glycosides.

Parenteral, IM route painful, associated with muscle necrosis. Rapid IV can cause vasoconstriction (hypertension and/or reduced coronary flow).

Cardioversion, risk of provoking dangerous arrhythmias with direct current cardioversion increased in presence of digitalis toxicity.

Pregnancy, Lactation: If benefit outweighs risk. Dosage may be less predictable. Not contraindicated in pregnancy or breast feeding.

ADR: *Common*, CNS disturbances, dizziness, visual disturbances (blurred or yellow vision), arrhythmia, conduction disturbances, bi/trigeminy, PR-prolongation, sinus bradycardia, nausea, vomiting, diarrhoea, skin rash (urticarial, scarlatiniform).

Notes: See 2.8.1 Cardiac Glycosides.

> **Lanoxin 250mcg, PG 62.5mcg, Elixir** *(Aspen)* B. GMS.
> *Price*, (500) 250mcg, €9.04. PG 62.5mcg, €8.48. Elixir (60mL) €5.79.
> *Tablet*, digoxin. Round. 62.5mcg: Blue. Marked D06. 250mcg: White scored. Marked DO25. *Lactose*.
> *Oral soln*, as above 50mcg/mL. Clear bright yellow lime flavoured. *Parabens, sucrose, ethanol.*
>
> **Lanoxin Parenteral** *(Aspen)* A. GMS.
> *Price*, (5) €4.02.
> *Injection*, digoxin 500mcg/2mL. Clear colourless sterile aqueous soln. *Ethanol 0.104mL/mL, less than 23mg sodium.*

2.8.2 - Phosphodiesterase Inhibitors

In This Chapter: *Enoximone.*

Class Effects
Phosphodiesterase inhibitors are positive inotropes which also have vasodilating effects. They are generally used for the management of severe heart failure.

Pregnancy, Lactation: If benefit outweighs risk. Breast feeding, no data.

Notes: See 2.8 Positive Inotropes.

Enoximone

ATC Code: C01CE03. **Sport:** Permitted.
Driving: Caution.
Indications: Congestive heart failure.
Dose: Adult, Elderly: Initially 0.5mg/kg; rate max. 12.5mg/min. Repeat after 30 minutes if needed.
Child: Not recommended.
Renal Impairment: Reduce dose.
Hepatic Impairment: Monitor.
SP: Monitor platelets. BP, ECG, heart rate.
Pregnancy, Lactation: Not recommended.
Notes: See 2.8.2 Phosphodiesterase Inhibitors.

> **Perfan Parenteral** *(Myogen)* A.
> *Price*, 20mL (10) 5mg/mL, €179.90
> *Injection*, enoximone 5mg/mL. Clear yellow conc for soln. *Ethanol.*

2.9 - Diuretics

Class Effects
Diuretics promote the excretion of water and electrolytes by the kidneys. There are five main groups of diuretics, carbonic anhydrase inhibitors, loop, osmotic, potassium sparing and thiazide diuretics. They are used in the treatment of hypertension, HF, oedema and ascites.

CI: Children, not recommended unless otherwise specified. Hypersensitivity to any member of the class.

2.9.1 - Carbonic Anhydrase Inhibitors

In This Chapter: *Acetazolamide.*

Class Effects
Weak diuretics used mainly in treating raised IOP. Now seldom used in management of heart failure and certain oedematous conditions.

Indications: Congestive heart failure, drug induced oedema, premenstrual tension. Glaucoma.

Notes: See 7.1.2 Carbonic Anhydrase Inhibitors (acetazolamide).

2.9.2 - Loop Diuretics

In This Chapter: *Bumetanide, frusemide, piretanide and combinations.*

Class Effects
Loop diuretics produce intense diuresis of short duration.

CI: Children unless otherwise stated. Hypersensitivity to any member of the class, sulfonamides and/or thiazides (potential cross-sensitivity with loop diuretics). Electrolyte imbalance or depletion, severe hypo- (kalaemia, natraemia, volaemia) or dehydration, anuria, renal failure with anuria. Renal failure due to nephrotoxic or hepatotoxic agents, or associated with hepatic coma. Pre-comatose and comatose states associated with hepatic encephalopathy. Porphyria. *Combinations* (amiloride, potassium salts), hyperkalaemia, Addison's disease.

Interactions: Effect of Other Drugs on Loop Diuretics: *Effect decreased*: NSAIDs, phenytoin. *Effect attenuated*: Probenecid.

Effect of Loop Diuretics on Other Drugs: Acetazolamide, amphotericin, carbenoxolone (not topical), corticosteroids (not topical, inhalation), corticotrophin, thiazides, reboxetine, sympathomimetics, theophylline: *Hypokalaemia risk*. Aminoglycosides, cisplatin, other ototoxic drugs: *Otoxicity risk, co-admin not recommended*. Cephalosporins: *Nephrotoxicity risk*. Lithium: *Reduced excretion, increased plasma levels, toxicity risk*. Amiodarone, cardiac glycosides, disopyramide, flecainide, quinidine, sotalol: *Cardiac toxicity risk (due to hypokalaemia)*. Nephro-, cytotoxics: *Monitor closely*. Antidiabetics, lidocaine, mexiletine: *Effect antagonised*. Chloral hydrate: *Sensations of heat, sweating attacks, restlessness, nausea, increased BP, tachycardia with IV furosemide admin with 24 hours after chloral hydrate*. ACEI, AIIAs: *First-dose hypotension risk*.

SP: Orthostatic hypotension, acute hypotensive episodes; correct hypotension, hypovolaemia before initiation. *Monitor*, elderly (caution, electrolyte disturbances), serum (sodium, potassium, creatinine), hypovolaemia, dehydration, electrolyte and acid-base disturbances, blood profile, bone marrow depression, partial obstruction of urinary outflow (increased urine production may aggravate), hypotension, at risk for pronounced fall in BP, latent or manifest diabetes (furosemide may induce hyperglycaemia), hyperuricaemia and gout may be induced, hepatorenal syndrome, hypoproteinaemia, nephrolithiasis, acute porphyria, premature infants.

Pregnancy, Lactation: Contraindicated.

ADR: Headache, dizziness, vertigo, syncope, postural hypotension, paraesthesia, fatigue, asthenia, dry mouth, thirst, dysaesthesia, fever, nausea, gastric irritation, flatulence, vomiting, constipation, diarrhoea, ulcer, acute pancreatitis, dehydration, hypo- (natraemia, kalaemia, chloraemia, calcaemia, magnesaemia), hyper- (kalaemia, uricaemia, glycaemia), gout, diabetes mellitus, metabolic alkalosis, allergic reactions, rash, urticaria, bullous lesions, urticaria, photosensitivity, vasculitis, hypotension including orthostatic, thrombocytopenia, leucopenia, agranulocytosis, pancytopenia, aplastic anaemia, renal impairment or failure, hypotension, tachy-, bradycardia, AV block, hearing disturbances, ototoxicity, tinnitus, jaundice, liver damage, intrahepatic cholestasis, increased transaminases, anaphylactic, anaphylactoid reactions.

Notes: See 2.9 Diuretics, 2.9.4 Potassium-Sparing Diuretics and 16.3.4 Potassium.

Bumetanide

ATC Code: C03CA02. **Sport:** Prohibited.
Driving: Dizziness.
Indications: Oedema of congestive heart failure, hepatic cirrhosis, renal disease, nephrotic syndrome.
Dose: Adult: Initially 0.5-2mg/day; if needed increase according to response. Oral, single or divided doses.
Elderly: Slower elimination; titrate according to response.
Renal Impairment: Severe or progressive or elevated BUN or creatinine, caution.
Hepatic Impairment: Severe, caution.
Interactions: Effect of Bumetanide on Other Drugs: Digitalis glycosides, non-depolarising neuromuscular blockers: *Increased sensitivity (hypokalaemia)*. PPIs: *Hypomagnesaemia*. Other antihypertensives (including diuretics), other hypotensives (TCADs, MAOIs): *Effect potentiated*.
SP: Musculoskeletal pain especially with severe chronic renal failure, high doses.
ADR: *Common*, electrolyte imbalance, dizziness, orthostatic hypotension, vertigo, fatigue, lethargy, somnolence, asthenia, malaise, abdominal pain, nausea, muscle spasm, pain, myalgia, micturition disorder.
Notes: See 2.9.2 Loop Diuretics.

Burinex 1mg, 5mg *(LEO)* B. GMS.
Price, (28) 1mg, €2.13. 5mg, €9.75.
Tablet, bumetanide. White flat round u/c scored. 1mg: Marked 133; logo on reverse. 5mg: Marked 5mg. *Lactose.* **Store:** Below 30 deg C.

Frusemide

ATC Code: C03CA01. **Sport:** Prohibited.
Driving: Caution; reduced mental alertness may impair ability.
Indications: Oedema of CHF, hepatic cirrhosis, renal disease, nephrotic syndrome, hypertension.
Dose: Adult: ORAL, initially 40mg as single dose daily or alternate days. *Oedema, mild,* 20mg/day or 40mg on alternate days; *resistant,* 80mg/day; *severe,* titrate gradually to 600mg/day; max 1500mg/day.
PARENTERAL, initially, 20-50mg IM or slow IV injection (max. 4mg/min); increase by 20mg at 2-hour intervals; above 50mg, admin by slow IV infusion.
Elderly: Caution, eliminated more slowly; initiate with 20mg.
Child: ORAL, range 1-3mg/kg; max. 40mg/day. Premature infants, monitor; may precipitate nephrocalcinosis or nephrolithiasis. Infants (first weeks of life), increased risk of persistence of patent ductus arteriosus. Brand *Furosemide Bristol,* contraindicated for use in children.
PARENTERAL, range 0.5-1.5mg/kg/day; max. 20mg/day.
Renal Impairment: PARENTERAL (IV), serum creatinine above 5mg/dL, infusion rate max. 2.5mg/min. CrCl (mL/min), below 30, contraindicated.
Interactions: Effect of Other Drugs on Frusemide: *Co-admin caution:* Risperidone (consider risk/benefit); avoid dehydration (see SP). *Absorption decreased:* Sucralfate (allow 2-hour dosing interval). *Sodium retention:* Corticosteroids. *Hyponatraemia:* Carbamazepine, aminoglutethimide. *Hypotension, decreased renal function:* ACEIs. *Severe diuresis:* Metolazone. *Ototoxic drugs:* Increased ototoxicity risk.
Effect of Frusemide on Other Drugs: Cardiac glycosides, other hypotensives, drugs inducing QT-interval prolongation: *Furosemide-induced hypokalaemia (cardiac arrhythmias).* Cisplatin: *Increased nephrotoxicity, ototoxicity.* Salicylates: *Increased toxicity.* Sympathomimetics (adrenaline, noradrenaline): *Effect reduced.* Curare-type muscle relaxants, theophylline: *Effects increased.* Liquorice: *Hyperkalaemia risk.* Hypoglycaemics: *Consider dose adjustment.* Levothyroxine: *Increased free thyroid hormones, then overall decrease in total levels (monitor).*
SP: Symptomatic hypotension (dizziness, fainting, loss of consciousness), especially (elderly, concomitant medication, conditions causing hypotension). Ototoxicity (infusion rates above 4mg/min). Bone marrow depression.

Elderly, with dementia, higher incidence of mortality observed (furosemide + risperidone). May exacerbate or activate SLE.
ADR: Decreased glucose tolerance, impaired electrolytes, cholesterol serum levels (decreased HDL-cholesterol, increased LDL-cholesterol) and triglycerides. Hypovolaemia, dehydration (especially elderly). Obstruction of urinary outflow aggravated. Injection-site reactions.
Notes: See 2.9.2 Loop Diuretics.

Lasix Parenteral 20mg/2mL *(SANOFI)* A. GMS.
Price, (5) €1.61.
Injection or infusion, frusemide. Clear colourless aqueous soln. *Sodium 6.14mg/2mL.*
Furosemide 20mg, 40mg *(Clonmel)* B. GMS.
Price, (100) 20mg, €3.29. (500) 40mg, €10.53.
Tablet, furosemide. White (almost) round scored (facilitates breaking). *Lactose.*
Furosemide Bristol 40mg *(Gerard)* B. GMS.
Price, (28) €0.58. (100) €3.38.
Tablet, furosemide. Round white (off-white) scored (facilitates breaking). Marked F and strength; BL on reverse.
Furosemide Parenteral 20mg, 50mg *(Concordia)* A.
Price, (10) 20mg/2mL, €2.75. 50mg/5mL, €5.67 (PTW).
Injection or infusion, furosemide 10mg/mL. Clear colourless sterile soln. *Sodium 3.64mg/mL.*

Frusemide, Amiloride

ATC Code: C03EB01. **Sport:** Prohibited.
Driving: Caution.
Indications: Management of fluid retention where potassium conservation required.
Dose: Adult, Elderly: Initially 1 LS tab *(20mg frusemide, 2.5mg amiloride);* titrate to 2 tablets if required or switch to 1 tab *(40mg frusemide, 5mg amiloride);* titrate to 2 tabs* if required. *Usually taken in morning but in this case can be taken morning and noon. Elderly,* caution (serious side effects with electrolyte disturbances); consider dose reduction.
Renal Impairment: CrCl (mL/min) below 30, acute failure, anuria, contraindicated.
Interactions: Effect of Other Drugs on Frusemide, Amiloride Combination: *Co-admin not recommended:* Potassium supplements, spironolactone, triamterene. *Co-admin caution (consider risk/benefit):* Risperidone.
SP: See Notes below (Frusemide).
ADR: *Very common,* nausea. *Common,* hypokalaemia, gout attack, thrombosis, rash, urinary retention (acute retention in patients with partial obstruction of urinary outflow).
Notes: See 2.9.2 Loop Diuretics. See Frusemide above.

Frumil, Low Strength *(SANOFI)* B. GMS.
Price, (28) €2.00. (56) €3.91. Low Strength. (28) €4.19.
Tablet, frusemide/amiloride 40mg/5mg (20mg/2.5mg). Orange round. 40/5: Scored u/c. Marked Frumil. 20/2.5: Flat. Marked LS. *Lactose.*

Piretanide

ATC Code: C03CA03. **Sport:** Prohibited.
Driving: Reduced mental alertness may impair (individual cases); most likely at initiation, dose change, interaction with alcohol.
Indications: Oedema of CHF, hepatic cirrhosis, renal disease, nephrotic syndrome, hypertension. Oedema in children.
Dose: Adult: *Oedema,* initially 6mg daily; max. 30mg. *Hypertension (mild, moderate),* initially 6mg daily (2-4 weeks); titrate at 2-4 week intervals to max. 18mg/day if needed; maintenance, 6mg/day.
Elderly: Initially 3mg/day.
Hepatic Impairment: Severe liver disease, caution hepatic coma; co-admin potassium-sparing agents.
Interactions: Effect of Piretanide on Other Drugs: Other anti-hypertensives, cardiac glycosides, non-depolarising muscle relaxants, uricosurics: *Dose adjustment.* ACEIs: *Co-admin, monitor.* Salicylates, curare-type muscle relaxants: *Effect increased.* Pressor amines: *Effect decreased.*
SP: Monitor carefully with: Hypotension, diabetes mellitus (regular blood sugar tests), gout (regular uric acid level checks), obstructed urinary flow (prostatic hypertrophy, hydronephrosis, ureteric stenosis), cirrhosis of liver with

2.9.3　Osmotic Diuretics

renal impairment, hypoproteinaemia (nephrotic syndrome), advanced cerebral and/or coronary sclerosis. Prolonged treatment, regularly check (serum creatinine, urea, uric acid, glucose and electrolytes especially potassium, sodium, calcium, chloride and bicarbonate).

Pregnancy, Lactation: Not for use in first trimester; safety in later phases, insufficient data. Lactation, not for use; excreted in breast milk.

ADR: See Notes below.

Notes: See 2.9.2 Loop Diuretics.

Arelix 6mg *(SANOFI)* B. GMS.
Price, (20) €4.67.
Tablet, piretanide. Yellowish-white oblong scored (divisible into equal halves). Marked with logo; ARE on reverse. **Store:** Below 25 deg C; original pack; protect (light).

urinary output, fluid balance, central venous pressure, electrolyte balance. Evaluate cardiovascular status before admin (sudden expansion of extracellular fluid may lead to sudden CHF). May lower serum sodium (aggravate hyponatraemia); may obscure inadequate hydration, hypovolaemia.

Pregnancy, Lactation: Not for use unless clearly necessary.

ADR: Hypersensitivity reactions, fluid and electrolyte imbalance. See Full Prescribing Information.

Notes: See 2.9.3 Osmotic Diuretics.

Mannitol Parenteral *(Baxter)* A.
Price, (1) viaflex 10%, 500mL, €3.11. 20%, 500mL, €4.69.
Infusion, mannitol 100(200)g/L. Clear colourless soln free from particles. **Store:** Do not refrigerate or freeze.

2.9.3 - Osmotic Diuretics

In This Chapter: *Mannitol.*

Class Effects
Generally used in management of cerebral oedema and for urgent or short-term reduction of IOP.

CI: Hypersensitivity to any member of the class.

Mannitol

ATC Code: B05BC01. **Sport:** Prohibited.
Driving: Not applicable.

Indications: Osmotic diuretic: Diuresis in prevention and/or treatment of oliguric phase of acute renal failure (before irreversible failure established). Reduction: Intracranial pressure and cerebral oedema (blood-barrier intact); elevated IOP. Elimination of renally excreted toxic substances (poisoning).

Dose: Adult, Elderly: *Acute renal failure,* range, 50-200g (500-2000mL/day) by IV infusion over 24 hours; max. 50g on any 1 occasion; usually 50-100g/24-hour achieves adequate response. *Reduction of intracranial pressure, cerebral volume and IOP,* usually 1.5-2g/kg body weight infused over 30-60 minutes. Pre-operative, 1.5 hours before surgery. *Poisoning,* adjust dose to maintain urinary output of minimum 100mL/hour and positive fluid balance of 1-2 litres. Initial loading dose, approx. 25g. *Admin,* IV through admin set with a final in-line filter. Rate adjusted to maintain urine flow of 30-50mL/hour. Emergency situations, max. infusion rate as high as 200mg/kg infused over 5 minutes; after 5 minutes adjust to urine flow as above; max 200g/24 hours. May cause vein damage (check osmolarity); admin via large peripheral or preferably central vein.

Child: Test dose, 200mg/kg over 3-5 minutes. Treatment dose, range 0.5-1.5g/kg; repeat once or twice after 4-8 hours if needed. Cerebral, ocular oedema, admin this dose over 30-60 minutes. *Admin,* as for Adult above.

Renal Impairment: Adults and children, admin a test dose of 200mg/kg over 3-5 minutes; response is adequate if 30-50mL/hour of urine is excreted for 2-3 hours. Inadequate response, repeat test dose; inadequate response to second test dose, discontinue; assess for established renal failure.

CI: Pre-existing plasma hyperosmolarity, anuria, severe (dehydration, HF, pulmonary congestion or pulmonary oedema, active intracranial bleeding (except during craniotomy), disturbance of blood-brain barrier.

Interactions: Effect of Other Drugs on Mannitol: *Effect potentiated:* Other diuretics. *Cumulative nephrotoxicity:* Ciclosporin, aminoglycosides.

Effect of Mannitol on Other Drugs: Lithium, methotrexate, drugs renally reabsorbed: *Increased elimination.* Neuromuscular blockers, agents causing QT-prolongation, digoxin: *Altered effects due to electrolyte imbalance.* Neurotoxic agents (aminoglycosides): *May potentiate neurotoxicity.* Tubocurarine: *Enhanced effect.* Oral anticoagulants: *Reduced effect.*

SP: *Monitor:* For deterioration in renal, cardiac, pulmonary function, CNS toxicity (severe adverse events, discontinue),

2.9.4 - Potassium-Sparing Diuretics

In This Chapter: *Amiloride, spironolactone.*

Class Effects
Potassium-sparing diuretics generally have a weak diuretic effect; usually used in combination with loop or thiazide diuretics.

CI: Hypersensitivity to any member of the class. Hyperkalaemia, anuria, acute renal insufficiency, significant renal compromise, anuria, Addison's disease.

Interactions: Effect of Other Drugs on Potassium-Sparing Diuretics and Aldosterone Antagonists: *Co-admin contraindicated:* Eplerenone. *Effect decreased:* NSAIDs including COX-2 inhibitors.

Effect of Potassium-Sparing Diuretics and Aldosterone Antagonists on Other Drugs: ACEIs, AIIAs, ciclosporin, indomethacin, systemic NSAIDs, potassium salts, tacrolimus, trilostane, other potassium-sparing diuretics: *Hyperkalaemia risk.* Chlorpropamide (plus thiazide): *Hyponatraemia risk.* Lithium: *Reduced excretion, increased lithium plasma levels.*

SP: Monitor fluids, electrolytes. *Elderly,* potential obstruction of urinary tract, hyponatraemia, increased blood urea, hyperkalaemia (caution, arrhythmias), metabolic acidosis.

Pregnancy, Lactation: Pregnancy, if benefit outweighs risk. Lactation, not recommended. Thiazide combinations, see Notes below (thiazides).

ADR: Elevated plasma potassium, electrolyte disturbances, nausea, vomiting, abdominal pain, diarrhoea, constipation, drowsiness, lethargy, headache, mental confusion, ataxia, drug fever, skin rash.

Notes: See 2.9 Diuretics, see 2.9.5 Thiazides and 2.9.2 Loop Diuretics.

Amiloride

ATC Code: C03DB01. **Sport:** Prohibited.
Driving: Caution.

Indications: Oedema of cardiac, renal or hepatic origin, hypertension.

Interactions: Effect of Amiloride on Other Drugs: Carbenoxolone (not topical): *Ulcer-healing effect inhibited.*

Notes: See 2.9.4 Potassium-Sparing Diuretics.

Spironolactone

ATC Code: C03DA01. **Sport:** Prohibited.
Driving: Caution.

Indications: Oedema of CHF including severe HF (NYHA III-IV), hypertension, hepatic cirrhosis with ascites and oedema, malignant ascites, nephrotic syndrome, diagnosis and treatment of primary aldosteronism.

Dose: Adult: *CHF,* initially 100mg/day (single or divided dose); titrate gradually to 200mg/day if needed; maintenance, 75-200mg/day. Severe CHF (with standard therapy), initially 25mg/day (once daily); if tolerated increase to 50mg/day; if 25mg/day not tolerated, reduce to 25mg every other day.

Hepatic cirrhosis with ascites, oedema, urinary Na+/K+

82

ratio above 1, admin 100mg/day; ratio below 1, admin 200-400mg/day.

Malignant ascites, initially 100-200mg/day; increase to 400mg/day if severe.

Nephrotic syndrome, maintenance 100-200mg/day.

Diagnosis, treatment of primary aldosteronism, long test, 400mg/day (3-4 weeks). Short test, 400mg/day (4 days). After diagnosis, 100-400mg/day in preparation for surgery.

Essential hypertension, initially 50-100mg/day; increase at 2-week intervals to 200mg/day if need. *Admin*, once daily with food unless otherwise specified.

Elderly: Consider dose reduction.

Child: Initially, 1-3mg/kg/day (divided doses); limited data.

Renal Impairment: Severe, caution.

Hepatic Impairment: As for Renal above.

Interactions: Effect of Other Drugs on Spironolactone: *Co-admin contraindicated:* Eplerenone. *Co-admin avoid:* Carbenoxolone, lithium. *Effect antagonised, reduced:* Acetylsalicylic acid. *Hyperkalaemic metabolic acidosis:* Ammonium chloride, colestyramine. *Hyperkalaemia:* NSAIDs, trimethoprim/sulfamethoxazole, other potassium-sparing diuretics, potassium supplements.

Effect of Spironolactone on Other Drugs: Digoxin (half-life increased), cardiac glycosides, other antihypertensives, hypotensive agents: *Dose adjustment may be needed.* Noradrenaline: *Vascular responsiveness reduced.* Anaesthesia (regional, general): *Caution.* Antipyrine: *Metabolism enhanced.*

SP: Caution, elderly, urinary tract obstruction, electrolyte imbalance. Reversible hyperchloraemic metabolic acidosis with decompensated hepatic cirrhosis even with normal renal function. Hyperkalaemia (concomitant medication, renal failure). Caution, in severe HF hyperkalaemia may be fatal; monitor potassium and creatinine 1-week post initiation and/or dose increase, monthly (3 months), quarterly (1 year), then 6-monthly.

Pregnancy, Lactation: Pregnancy, if benefit outweighs risk. Lactation, avoid (metabolite canrenone is detected in breast milk).

ADR: Gynaecomastia, breast soreness, menstrual irregularities, impotence.

Notes: See 2.9.4 Potassium-Sparing Diuretics.

Aldactone 25mg, 50mg 100mg *(Pfizer)* A. GMS.
Price, 25mg (100) €7.61. 50mg (100) €20.11. 100mg (28) €8.15; (100) €28.23.
Tablet, round f/c; peppermint odour. Marked Searle. 25mg: Buff. Marked 39. 50mg: White. Marked 916. 100mg: Buff. Marked 134. **Store:** Below 30 deg C.

Spironolactone 25mg, 50mg 100mg *(Accord)* A. GMS.
Price, (100) 25mg, €4.33; 50mg, €8.05. 100mg (30) €3.50; (100) €11.30.
Tablet, spironolactone. White (pale-white) round f/c. 25mg: Marked AD. 50mg: Marked AE. 100mg: Marked AF. *Lactose*. **Store:** No special conditions.

2.9.5 - Thiazides

In This Chapter: *Bendroflumethiazide, hydrochlorothiazide (and combinations), indapamide.*

Class Effects

Thiazides inhibit sodium and chloride reabsorption (in kidney tubule) with corresponding increased potassium excretion.

Indications: Oedema of cardiac, renal or hepatic origin, hypertension.

CI: Children. Hypersensitivity to any member of class. Severe electrolyte imbalance (hypokalaemia, hyperchloraemia). Precoma associated with hepatic cirrhosis, Addison's disease, severe hepatic or renal impairment or anuria, Thiazides and bendroflumethiazide are sulphonamides, caution sulfonamide hypersensitivity.

Interactions: Effect of Other Drugs on Thiazides: *Co-admin, monitor:* Nephrotoxic drugs. *Absorption reduced:* Colestipol, colestyramine. *Additive effects:* Other anti-

hypertensives (guanethidine, methyldopa, beta-blockers, vasodilators, calcium channel blockers, ACEIs, ARBs, direct renin inhibitors), other hypotensives. *Effect reduced:* NSAIDs including COX-2 inhibitors. *Increased hyperuricaemia (gout complications):* Ciclosporin.

Effect of Thiazides on Other Drugs: Acetazolamide, amphotericin, carbenoxolone (not topical), corticosteroids (not topical, inhalation), loop diuretics, reboxetine, sympathomimetics, theophylline: *Hypokalaemia risk.* Amiodarone, cardiac glycosides, disopyramide, flecainide, quinidine: *Increased cardiac toxicity and/or hypokalaemia.* Antidiabetics (insulin, oral antidiabetics): *Hypoglycaemic effect antagonised, adjust dose.* Metformin: *Caution, lactic acidosis risk.* Beta-blockers, diazoxide: *Increased hyperglycaemia risk.* Calcium salts: *Hypercalcaemia risk.* Chlorpropamide + potassium-sparing diuretics, carbamazepine: *Hyponatraemia risk.* Lithium: *Reduced excretion, increased plasma levels.* Sotalol: *Ventricular arrhythmia risk.* ALCOHOL, barbiturates, narcotics: *Co-admin caution, orthostatic hypotension.* Tubocurarine: *Effect potentiated.* Amantadine: *Increased adverse event risk.* Cytotoxics (cyclophosphamide, methotrexate): *Reduced renal excretion (myelosuppressive effect potentiated).* Tetracyclines (probably not doxycycline): *Increased risk of tetracycline-induced urea increase.* Digitalis glycosides: *Hypokalaemia or hypomagnesaemia; digitalis-induced cardiac arrhythmias.* Pressor amines (noradrenaline): *Reduced response.*

SP: Monitor fluid, electrolytes. Avoid inadequate potassium supplementation or excessive fluid loss (monitor potassium). Caution (elderly, potential urinary tract obstruction, renal or hepatic impairment). Hyper- (uricaemia, glycaemia), gout.

Thiazides, only fully effective when renal function is normal or only minimally impaired. Photosensitivity. Idiosyncratic reaction with sulfonamides or derivatives (transient myopia and acute angle-closure glaucoma); hydrochlorothiazide is a sulfonamide can cause idiosyncratic reactions e.g. acute transient myopia, acute angle-closure glaucoma. Symptoms include (acute onset of decreased visual acuity, ocular pain); may occur within hours to weeks of initiation. Untreated acute angle-closure glaucoma can lead to permanent vision loss, discontinue immediately.

Pregnancy, Lactation: Pregnancy, if benefit outweighs risk. Thiazides cross placental barrier, may decrease placental perfusion, increase uterine inertia, and inhibit labour. Prolonged exposure during third trimester can reduce maternal plasma volume and uteroplacental blood flow; may cause foeto-placental ischaemia, growth retardation. Hypoglycaemia, thrombocytopenia in neonates. NOT for use for gestational oedema/hypertension or pre-eclampsia. Lactation, not recommended. Thiazides appear in human milk; may inhibit lactation. Can produce hypokalaemia, haemolysis, hypersensitivity (sulfonamide properties).

ADR: *Commonly* (hydrochlorothiazide), hyper- (glycaemia, uricaemia); hypo- (natraemia, kalaemia); light-headedness, vertigo, glycosuria, weakness, increased (cholesterol, triglycerides).

Notes: See 2.9 Diuretics.

Bendroflumethiazide, Potassium Salts

ATC Code: C03AB01. **Sport:** Prohibited.
Driving: No or negligible effect; dizziness.

Indications: Oedema of cardiac, renal or hepatic origin, hypertension.

Dose: Adult: *Centyl K*, hypertension, 1-2 tabs/day. Oedema, initially 1-4 tabs/day; maintenance 1-2 tabs/day. *Low Centyl K*, hypertension, 1 tab/day. Oral, once daily in morning with full glass of water or fluid.

CI: Established arthritis urica. GI ulceration or obstruction. See Notes below.

SP: Oesophageal, small bowel ulceration. Bendroflumethiazide is a sulphonamide, caution hypersensitivity. Long-term treatment, monitor potassium levels, fluid, electrolytes (especially elderly).

2.9.6   Aldosterone Antagonists

ADR: *Most frequent*, dizziness (including orthostatic hypotension, vertigo), headache, fatigue; hypokalaemia, electrolyte disturbances (with long-term treatment).

Notes: See 2.9.5 Thiazides.

Centyl K, Low Centyl K *(LEO)* B. GMS.
Price, (250) €33.59. Low (250) €18.24.
Modified/R tablet, bendroflumethiazide/potassium chloride. Oval f/c. 2.5mg/573mg: Green. 1.25mg/573mg: Light-yellow.

Hydrochlorothiazide, Amiloride

ATC Code: C03EA01. **Sport:** Prohibited.
Driving: Caution.

Indications: Oedema of cardiac, renal or hepatic origin, hypertension.

Dose: Adult: 1 tab once daily.

ADR: Usually associated with diuresis, thiazide therapy or underlying disease.

Notes: See 2.9.5 Thiazides, 2.9.4 Potassium-Sparing Diuretics (amiloride).

Moduret 25/2.5mg *(MSD)* B. GMS.
Price, (28) €1.11.
Tablet, hydrochlorothiazide/amiloride HCl. Off-white diamond-shaped scored. Marked 923. *Lactose*.

Indapamide

ATC Code: C03BA11. **Sport:** Prohibited.
Driving: Reactions related to decreased blood pressure.

Dose: Adult, Elderly: 1 tab/day. Oral, once daily in morning; swallow whole with water, do not chew. *Elderly*, use only if renal function normal or only minimally impaired.

Renal Impairment: CrCl (mL/min) below 30, contraindicated.

Hepatic Impairment: Severe, contraindicated.

CI: Sulfonamide hypersensitivity.

Interactions: Effect of Other Drugs on Indapamide: *Reduced effect*: NSAIDs including systemic COX-2 inhibitors, salicylic acid (high dose, 3g/day), corticosteroids, systemic tetracosactide. *Hypotension/acute renal failure*: ACEIs. *Increased effect*: Baclofen, imipramine-like antidepressants and neuroleptics (orthostatic hypotension risk).

Effect of Indapamide on Other Drugs: Class Ia antiarrhythmics (quinidine, hydroquinidine, disopyramide), Class III antiarrhythmics (amiodarone, sotalol, dofetilide, ibutilide), phenothiazines (chlorpromazine, cyamemazine, levomepromazine, thioridazine, trifluoperazine), benzamides (amisulpride, sulpiride, sultopride, tiapride), butyrophenones (droperidol, haloperidol), bepridil, cisapride, diphemanil, erythromycin (IV), halofantrine, mizolastine, pentamidine, sparfloxacin, moxifloxacin, vincamine IV: *Increased ventricular arrhythmia, Torsades de Pointes risk*. Amphotericin B (IV), gluco- and mineralocorticoids (not topical), tetracosactide, stimulant laxatives: *Hypokalaemia risk*. Digitalis: *Increased toxicity*. Potassium-sparing diuretics (amiloride, spironolactone, triamterene): *Hyper-, hypokalaemia risk*. Metformin: *Lactic acidosis risk*. Calcium (salts): *Hypercalcaemia risk*. Ciclosporin, tacrolimus: *Increased plasma creatinine*. Allopurinol: *Increased hypersensitivity risk*.

ADR: *Common*, maculopapular rash.

Notes: See 2.9.5 Thiazides.

Natrilix SR 1.5mg *(Servier)* B. GMS.
Price, (30) €2.85.
Prolonged/R tablet, indapamide. White round f/c. *Lactose*.

Icorvida SR 1.5mg *(Krka)* B. GMS.
Price, (30) €2.71.
Prolonged/R tablet, indapamide. White round f/c. *Lactose*.

2.9.6 - Aldosterone Antagonists

In This Chapter: *Eplerenone*.

Class Effects
Notes: See 2.9 Diuretics.

Eplerenone

ATC Code: C03DA04. **Sport:** Prohibited.
Driving: Dizziness.

Indications: Addition to standard therapy, to reduce risk of cardiovascular mortality and morbidity: Stable patients with LVD (LVEF 40% or less) and clinical evidence of HF after recent MI; NYHA Class II chronic heart failure and LVEF 30% or less.

Dose: Adult, Elderly: Post MI and NYHA class II HF, initially 25mg/day; titrate to 50mg/day within 4 weeks (take into account serum potassium levels). Commence within 3-14 days post acute-MI. Co-admin (amiodarone, diltiazem, verapamil), initially and max. 25mg/day. *Admin*, once daily. *Elderly*, monitor serum potassium.

Child: Safety/efficacy not established.

Renal Impairment: CrCl (mL/min) 30-60, initially 25mg every other day; below 50, caution; below 30 (eGFR below 30mL/min/1.73m2), contraindicated. Not dialysable. Adjust dose based on potassium level, monitor.

Hepatic Impairment: Monitor serum potassium. Severe, contraindicated.

CI: Hypersensitivity to any member of the class. Serum potassium above 5mmoL/L at initiation.

Interactions: Effect of Other Drugs on Eplerenone: *Co-admin contraindicated (hyperkalaemia risk)*: ACEIs, AIIAs (ARBs), potassium-sparing diuretics, potassium supplements, strong CYP3A4 inhibitors (ketoconazole, itraconazole, ritonavir, nelfinavir, clarithromycin, telithromycin, nefazodone). *Co-admin not recommended (plasma levels decreased)*: Strong CYP3A4 inducers (St John's Wort, rifampicin, carbamazepine, phenytoin, phenobarbital). *Hyperkalaemia, impaired renal function risk*: Ciclosporin, tacrolimus, NSAIDs, trimethoprim. *Increased hypotensive effect or postural hypotension risk*: Alpha-blockers (prazosin, alfuzosin), TCADs, neuroleptics, amifostine, baclofen. *Decreased hypotensive effect*: Glucocorticoids, tetracosactide. *Increased plasma levels (co-admin at max eplerenone dose 25mg*: Mild/moderate CYP3A4 inhibitors (erythromycin, saquinavir, amiodarone, diltiazem, verapamil, fluconazole).

Effect of Eplerenone on Other Drugs: Lithium: *Co-admin not recommended (if necessary monitor lithium plasma levels)*. Digoxin, warfarin: *Caution, when dosed near the upper limit of therapeutic range*.

SP: Hyperkalaemia risk in elderly, diabetics.

Pregnancy, Lactation: Pregnancy, caution. Lactation, stop breastfeeding or stop drug.

ADR: *Common*, hyper- (kalaemia, cholesterolaemia), insomnia, dizziness, syncope, headache, LVF, atrial fibrillation, hypotension, cough, diarrhoea, nausea, constipation, vomiting, rash, pruritus, muscle spasm, back pain, renal impairment, asthenia, increased blood (urea, creatinine).

Notes: See 2.9.6 Aldosterone Antagonists.

Inspra 25mg, 50mg *(Pfizer)* B. GMS.
Price, (28) both strengths, €30.24.
Tablet, eplerenone. Yellow f/c. Marked Pfizer; NSR over strength on reverse. *Lactose*. **Store:** No special precautions.

Eplerenone 25mg, 50mg *(Accord)* B. GMS.
Price, (30) both strengths, €24.19.
Tablet, eplerenone. Yellow f/c diamond-shaped. 25mg: Marked E1. 50mg: Marked E2. *Lactose*.

Eplerenone Actavis 25mg, 50mg *(Accord)* B. GMS.
Price, (30) both strengths, €24.19.
Tablet, eplerenone. Light-yellow round f/c. Marked E9RN and strength. *Lactose*.

Eplerenone Mylan 25mg *(Gerard)* B. GMS.
Price, (28) €24.19.
Tablet, eplerenone. Round f/c yellow. Marked M one side. 25mg: Marked EP1. *Lactose*.

Eplerenone Rowex 25mg, 50mg *(Rowex)* B. GMS.
Price, (28) both strengths, €24.19.
Tablet, eplerenone. Light-yellow round f/c. Marked E9RN and strength. *Lactose*.

Central Nervous System Drugs

3.1 - Antiepileptics

Class Effects

Driving: Use of antiepileptics may provide seizure control so that a patient may be eligible to hold a driving licence; warn of risk of transient drowsiness especially with polytherapy; with anticonvulsants, possibility of impaired reaction time. *General warning*, advise patient to take their medication as prescribed; NOT to (stop suddenly and to inform their doctor if they do so; drink alcohol; drive during first days of treatment or after dose change). *Decision to treat*, once made, the drug choice depends on efficacy for particular seizure type, co-morbidity, other medications and age.

Indications: For clobazam, diazepam and lorazepam information (also indicated for management of seizures), see Notes below.

CI: Hypersensitivity to any member of the class.

SP: Suicidal ideation and behaviour, reported with antiepileptics; monitor (signs); consider appropriate treatment; if signs emerge, advise patients (caregivers) to seek medical advice. See Notes below. Titrate dose according to individual response; withdraw gradually to prevent rebound seizures; adjunctive, withdraw or introduce gradually. Increased seizure frequency or onset of new types, severe life-threatening systemic hypersensitivity, drug rash with eosinophilia and systemic symptoms (DRESS) reported with antiepileptics. Anticonvulsant Hypersensitivity Syndrome (AHS) associated with anticonvulsants. *Phenytoin* and other anticonvulsants been shown to affect bone mineral

Antiepileptics   3.1

metabolism; increased risk of osteomalacia, bone fractures, osteoporosis, hypocalcaemia, hypophosphataemia with long-term treatment.

Pregnancy, Lactation: For all anti-epileptics, in offspring of women treated with epilepsy, prevalence of malformations is 2-3 times greater than rate of approx. 3% in general population (cleft palate, cardiovascular malformations, neural tube defects); increased malformations noted with polytherapy. Folic acid supplementation recommended; antiepileptic drugs reported to aggravate folic acid deficiency. Bleeding disorders in newborn; admin vitamin K as preventative in last few weeks of pregnancy and to newborn.

Unless otherwise stated, *pregnancy*, use only if clearly necessary (if benefit outweighs risk) and as monotherapy, if possible, for at least for first trimester; *lactation*, stop breastfeeding or stop drug. Women of childbearing potential to ensure adequate contraception.

Notes: See also 3.3 Antidepressants and Anxiolytics (suicidality).

3.1.1 - Barbiturates

In This Chapter: *Phenobarbital, primidone.*

Class Effects

Driving: See Notes below.

Interactions: Effect of Other Drugs on Barbiturates: *Increased CNS depression*: ALCOHOL, barbiturates, other CNS depressants. *Plasma levels decreased*: St John's Wort. *Plasma levels increased*: Valproic acid.

SP: Suicide, see Notes below. Prolonged admin (psychological dependence, addiction; severe withdrawal). *Caution*, infants, elderly, malnourished, marked renal or hepatic dysfunction, shock, respiratory depression, Addison's disease. Cumulative effect, chronic poisoning (headache, depression, slurred speech).

Pregnancy, Lactation: See Notes below.

ADR: Respiratory depression, sedation, unsteadiness, vertigo, incoordination, allergic skin reaction, folate deficiency (prolonged admin), megoblastic anaemia. Subtle mood changes, impaired cognition and memory, mental depression. Nystagmus, ataxia (high doses), altered LFTs. Paradoxical excitement, irritability, hyper-excitability in children, elderly.

Notes: See 3.1 Antiepileptics.

Phenobarbital

ATC Code: N03AA02. Sport: Permitted.
Driving: Drowsiness, incoordination.

Indications: Anticonvulsant (all forms of epilepsy except absence seizures).

Dose: Adult, Elderly: 60-180mg/day; plasma conc. 10-40mcg/mL usually required. *Admin*, at night.

Child: 5-8mg/kg/day.

Renal Impairment: Severe, not recommended.

Hepatic Impairment: As for Renal above.

CI: Porphyria. Severely impaired respiratory function.

Interactions: Effect of Other Drugs on Phenobarbital: *Effect antagonised*: Antipsychotics (haloperidol, chlorpromazine, thioridazine), antidepressants. *Increased toxicity*: Other anti-epileptics.

Effect of Phenobarbital on Other Drugs: Mianserin, TCADs (nortriptyline): *Metabolism accelerated*. Carbamazepine, clonazepam, lamotrigine, phenytoin (may also rise), valproate, ethosuximide: *Plasma levels lowered*. Anticoagulants (warfarin), antibiotics (doxycycline, metronidazole), beta-blockers (propranolol), verapamil, nifedipine, prednisolone, dexamethasone, cimetidine, methadone, pethidine, sex hormones (oral contraceptives), antivirals (indinavir, saquinavir), antiarrhythmics (disopyramide, quinidine), antifungals (griseofulvin, itraconazole), digoxin, folic acid (high doses), theophylline: *Metabolism altered*.

ADR: *Most frequent*, sedation.

Notes: See 3.1.1 Barbiturates. See 3.1 Antiepileptics (pregnancy, lactation).

3.1.2 Benzodiazepines

Phenobarbital 15mg, 30mg *(Clonmel)* A. GMS.
Price, (250) 15mg, €5.23. 30mg, €6.06.
Tablet, phenobarbital. Round. 15mg: Pale-yellow scored (divisible into equal halves). 30mg: White. 60mg: Pale-orange. *Lactose.*

Primidone

ATC Code: N03AA03. **Sport:** Permitted.
Driving: Possible impaired reaction time.
Indications: Grand mal and psychomotor (temporal lobe) epilepsy. Management, focal or Jacksonian seizures, myoclonic jerks and akinetic attacks.

Dose: Adult, Elderly: Initially 125mg late in evening; increase at 3-day intervals by 125mg to 500mg/day; then by 250mg (children under 9 years, 125mg) to max. 1500mg/day (children 1000mg/day). *Admin*, daily dose in divided doses (morning, evening).
Child: Initiation, see Adult above. Average daily maintenance, age up to 2 years, 250-500mg/day; 2-5 years, 500-750mg/day; 6-9 years, 750-1000mg/day; over 9 years, as for Adult above. *Admin*, see Adult above.
Renal Impairment: Caution. May need reduced dose.
Hepatic Impairment: As for Renal above.
CI: Phenobarbitone hypersensitivity. Porphyria.
Interactions: Effect of Other Drugs on Primidone: *Plasma levels mutually increased:* Chloramphenicol, felbamate, nelfinavir, metronidazole, sodium valproate. *Free phenobarbitone levels may be affected:* Theophylline. *Additive CNS depressant effect:* ALCOHOL, opiates, barbiturates.
Effect of Primidone on Other Drugs: Androgens, beta-antagonists, carbamazepine, ciclosporin, clozapine, chloramphenicol*, corticosteroids, glucocorticosteroids, cyclophosphamide, dicoumarins, digitoxin, doxycycline, ethosuximide, etoposide, felbamate*, granisetron, lamotrigine, losartan, methadone, metronidazole*, mianserin, montelukast, nelfinavir*, nimodipine, oral-contraceptives, oxcarbazepine, phenytoin, quinidine, rocuronium, sodium valproate*, tiagabine, theophylline*, topiramate, TCADs, vecuronium, warfarin, zonisamide; *Plasma levels lowered and/or shorter half-life.* Paracetamol: *Increased hepatotoxicity* *(mutual interaction).
SP: Impaired respiratory function, as for Renal above. Partially metabolised to phenobarbitone; prolonged admin, potential for tolerance, dependence, withdrawal if stopped abruptly. May affect Vitamin D metabolism (predispose to bone disease); supplement with long-term treatment. Megaloblastic anaemia on discontinuation. Suicidal ideation.
Pregnancy, Lactation: See Notes below.
ADR: *Common*, drowsiness, listlessness, ataxia, visual disturbance, nystagmus, nausea; *less common*, headache, dizziness, vomiting, allergic reactions (skin).
Notes: See 3.1.1 Barbiturates. See 3.1 Antiepileptics (pregnancy, lactation).

Mysoline 250mg *(Fannin)* B. GMS.
Price, (100) €17.28.
Tablet, primidone. Round white scored (divisible into equal halves). Marked on one face. **Store:** Below 25 deg C; in outer carton, tightly closed to protect (light, moisture).

3.1.2 - Benzodiazepines

In This Chapter: *Clonazepam, midazolam.*

Class Effects
Notes: See 3.1 Antiepileptics. For benzodiazepine class effects, see 3.3.5 Benzodiazepine Anxiolytics.

Clonazepam

ATC Code: N03AE01. **Sport:** Permitted.
Driving: Slowed reactions; aggravated by alcohol; impaired cognitive function.
Indications: All forms of epileptic disease and seizures, especially absence seizures (petit mal), tonic-clonic (grand mal), partial (focal), myoclonus.
Dose: Adult: Initially, max. 1mg/day (3 divided doses);

maintenance, 4-8mg (single dose in evening). Larger doses, up to max. 20mg/day can be given.
Elderly: Especially sensitive to central depressants and may experience confusion; initially max. 0.5mg/day in 3 or 4 divided doses.
Child: Initially, age 1-5 years, max. 250mcg/day; over 5 years, max. 500mcg/day maintenance, age 5-12 years, 3-6mg; 1-5 years, 1-3mg/day; under 1 year, 500mcg-1mg.
Renal Impairment: Caution.
Hepatic Impairment: Severe, not recommended.
CI: Insufficiency (acute pulmonary, severe respiratory), sleep apnoea syndrome, myasthenia gravis. Coma. Known drug or alcohol abuse.
Interactions: Effect of Other Drugs on Clonazepam: *Co-admin not recommended:* ALCOHOL (severe sedation, respiratory and/or cardiovascular depression). *Enhanced side-effects (sedation, apathy, toxicity):* Other anti-epileptics (hydantoins, phenobarbitone; sodium valproate, development of absence status epilepticus). *Reduced clearance (action potentiated):* Hepatic enzyme inhibitors (cimetidine). *Increased clearance (action reduced):* Hepatic enzyme inducers (phenytoin, phenobarbital, carbamazepine, valproate, rifampicin). *Mutual potentiation of effects (consider dose adjustment):* Other centrally acting drugs (anticonvulsants, anaesthetics, hypnotics, psychoactive drugs, some analgesics, muscle-relaxants).
Effect of Clonazepam on Other Drugs: Phenytoin, primidone: *Increased serum levels.*
SP: Caution, chronic pulmonary insufficiency, elderly, debilitation, spinal or cerebellar ataxia, acute alcohol intoxication, porphyria. Extreme caution, alcohol or drug abuse. Dependence with prolonged use. Loss or bereavement, psychological adjustment may be inhibited. *Infants, small children,* increased production of saliva and bronchial secretion. Pre-existing respiratory disease (COPD), co-admin with other centrally acting medications or anticonvulsants.
ADR: Allergic reactions, premature secondary sex characteristics (children), psychiatric disorders (e.g. impaired concentration, restlessness, confusional state, disorientation, depression); paradoxical reactions, weigh benefit/risk; CNS disorders (e.g. somnolence, slowed reaction, muscular hypotonia, dizziness, ataxia, co-ordination disturbance); diplopia (long-term treatment), nystagmus; cardiac failure including arrest, respiratory depression (especially IV admin); infants/young children with degree of mental impairment, increased saliva/bronchial secretion production; nausea, urticaria; pruritus, rash, transient hair loss, pigmentation changes, angioedema; muscle weakness, incontinence, ED; fatigue, tiredness, lassitude, increased fall risk, decreased platelet count.
Notes: See 3.1.2 Benzodiazepines.

Rivotril 0.5mg, 2mg *(Roche)* A. GMS.
Price, tabs (100) 0.5mg, €4.50. 2mg, €8.51.
Tablet, clonazepam. Round scored. Marked Roche/strength. 0.5mg: Pinkish-buff. 2mg: White. *Lactose.*

Midazolam (epilepsy)

ATC Code: N05CD08. **Sport:** Permitted.
Driving: Major influence; sedation, amnesia, impaired (attention, muscular function).
Indications: Prolonged, acute, convulsive seizures (age 3 months to 18 years); age 3-6 months, use in hospital.
Dose: Adult: Not for Adult use.
Child: Age 3-6 months (hospital) and 6-12 months, 2.5mg (yellow*); 1-5 years, 5mg (blue*); 5-10 years, 7.5mg (purple*); 10-18 years, 10mg (orange*). Oromucosal use; insert into space between gum and cheek. Not for IV use. Under 3 months, safety/efficacy not established. NOTE: Carers to admin only 1 single dose; if seizure has not stopped within 10 minutes after admin, seek emergency medical assistance; do not give second or repeat dose without prior medical advice. *Label colour.
Renal Impairment: Chronic failure, caution (elimination may be delayed; effects prolonged).
Hepatic Impairment: Mild/moderate, caution as for Renal above. Severe, contraindicated.

CI: Myasthenia gravis, severe respiratory insufficiency, sleep apnoea syndrome.

Interactions: Effect of Other Drugs on Midazolam: *Clearance reduced:* Fentanyl, cimetidine, ranitidine, omeprazole. *Enhanced sedation/respiratory depression:* Other antiepileptics, nabilone. *Increased midazolam levels:* Saquinavir, HIV protease inhibitors. *Metabolism accelerated:* Xanthines. See SP below.

Effect of Midazolam on Other Drugs: Levodopa: *Inhibition.* Baclofen: *Potentiation.* Interactions for oromucosal midazolam probably similar to IV, see Notes below.

SP: Caution, chronic (respiratory insufficiency), renal failure), impaired (hepatic, cardiac) function. Debilitated, consider lower doses. Alcohol or drug abuse, avoid. Anterograde amnesia.

Pregnancy, Lactation: High doses (last trimester, during labour), maternal or foetal adverse reactions reported (aspiration of fluids and stomach contents during labour in mother; irregularities in foetal heart rate, hypotonia, poor sucking, hypothermia, respiratory depression in new-born); use only if clearly necessary. Lactation, passes into breast milk; may not be necessary to stop breast feeding following a single dose.

ADR: *Common,* sedation, somnolence, depressed levels of consciousness, respiratory depression, nausea, vomiting.

Notes: See 3.1.2 Benzodiazepines. See also 14.1.3 Other Anaesthetic Adjuncts (midazolam IV).

Buccolam Oromucosal Soln *(Shire)* A. GMS.
Price, prefilled oral syringe (4) 2.5mg, €91.03. 5mg, €93.03. 7.5mg, €95.03. 10mg, €94.14.
Oromucosal soln, midazolam 2.5mg, 5mg, 7.5mg, 10mg. Clear colourless. **Store:** Do not refrigerate or freeze.

3.1.3 - GABAergic Drugs

In This Chapter: *Gabapentin, pregabalin, tiagabine, vigabatrin.*

Class Effects
Notes: See 3.1 Antiepileptics.

Gabapentin

ATC Code: N03AX12. **Sport:** Permitted.
Driving: Drowsiness, dizziness.
Indications: Epilepsy (adjunctive or monotherapy), treatment of partial seizures with or without secondary generalisation. Neuropathic pain (diabetic neuropathy, post-herpetic neuralgia).

Dose: Adult: *Epilepsy,* initially, titrate by 300mg once daily (day 1), 300mg twice daily (day 2), 300mg 3-times daily (day 3) and then increase by 300mg/day every 2-3 days; max. 3600mg/day (2-3 divided doses); up to 4800mg/day tolerated. Max. 12 hours between doses to prevent breakthrough seizures.
Neuropathic pain, titrate as for *Epilepsy* above or 900mg/day; max. 3600mg/day. *Admin,* oral with or without food, 3 divided doses daily; swallow whole with a glass of water.

Elderly: As for Renal below.

Child: *Epilepsy,* age 6-12 years, initially 10-15mg/kg/day (titrate) over 3 days; effective dose, 25-35mg/kg/day (3 divided doses); up to 50mg/kg/day tolerated. Over 12 years, as for Adult above. *Neuropathic pain,* not recommended.

Renal Impairment: CrCl (mL/min) over 80, 900-3600mg/day; 50-79, 600-1800mg/day; 30-49, 300-900mg/day; 15-29, 150-600mg/day; below 15, 150mg/day or 300mg/day every other day.

Interactions: Effect of Other Drugs on Gabapentin: *Bioavailability reduced:* Antacids (aluminium, magnesium); dose 2 hours after antacids. *CNS depression risk (increased gabapentin conc):* Morphine (consider dose reduction of either gabapentin or opioid).

SP: Suicidality, see Notes below. Acute pancreatitis (discontinue). Not effective against primary generalised seizures (absences); long-term therapy, if benefit outweighs risk; withdraw gradually over 1 week; cases of

abuse, dependence*. Dizziness, somnolence; could increase accidental injury (falls) in the elderly; loss of consciousness, confusion, mental impairment*. Concomitant opioid treatment, observe for signs of CNS depression (somnolence, sedation, respiratory depression). Severe, life-threatening, systemic hypersensitivity reactions (DRESS)*; signs of hypersensitivity, discontinue. Gabapentin can cause anaphylaxis (difficulty breathing, swelling of lips, throat and tongue, hypotension requiring emergency treatment); discontinue, seek medical care. False positive readings of total urine protein by dipstick tests. Haemodialysis patients (ESRD), myopathy with elevated creatine kinase levels. *(reported).

ADR: Adults, *very common,* viral infection, somnolence, dizziness, ataxia, fatigue, fever. *Children,* respiratory tract infections, otitis media, convulsions, bronchitis.

Notes: See 3.1 Antiepileptics.

Neurontin Capsules, Tablets *(Pfizer)* B. GMS.
Price, (100) 100mg, €13.42. 300mg, €31.14. 400mg, €36.03. 600mg, €56.46. 800mg, €68.62.
Capsule, gabapentin 100mg, 300mg, 400mg. Opaque hard containing white (off-white) powder. Marked Neurontin/strength and PD. 100mg: White. 300mg: Yellow. 400mg: Orange. *Lactose.* **Store:** Below 30 deg C.
Tablet, as above 600mg, 800mg. White elliptical f/c scored (divisible into equal halves). Marked NT. 600mg: Marked 16. 800mg: Marked 26. **Store:** Below 25 deg C.
Gabapentin (Accord) 600mg, 800mg *(Accord)* B. GMS.
Price, (100) 600mg, €45.17. 800mg, €54.90.
Tablet, gabapentin. White (off-white) oval/cap-shaped (f/c). 600mg: Marked G1. 800mg: Marked G2.
Gabapentin (Gerard) Capsules *(Gerard)* B. GMS.
Price, (100) 100mg, €10.75. 300mg, €24.90. 400mg, €28.81.
Capsule, gabapentin 100mg, 300mg, 400mg. 100mg: White. 300mg: Yellow. 400mg: Orange. *Lactose.* **Store:** Below 25 deg C.
Gabapentin TEVA 600mg, 800mg *(TEVA)* B. GMS.
Price, (100) 600mg, €45.17. 800mg, €54.90.
Tablet, gabapentin. White (off-white) oval f/c. Marked 93. 600mg: Marked 7173. 800mg: Marked 7174.
Gabin 100mg, 300mg, 400mg *(Rowex)* B. GMS.
Price, (100) 100mg, €10.75. 300mg, €24.90. 400mg, €28.81.
Capsule, gabapentin. Hard opaque filled with white powder. 200mg: White. 300mg: Yellow. 400mg: Orange.
Neurostil 100mg, 300mg, 400mg *(TEVA)* B. GMS.
Price, (100) 100mg, €10.75. 300mg, €24.90. 400mg, €28.81.
Capsule, gabapentin. Marked GAB/strength and logo. 100mg: White. 300mg: Yellow. 400mg: Orange.

Pregabalin

ATC Code: N03AX16. **Sport:** Permitted.
Driving: Dizziness, somnolence.
Indications: Epilepsy, in treatment of partial seizures with or without secondary generalisation; generalised anxiety disorder (GAD). Neuropathic pain (diabetic neuropathy, post-herpetic neuralgia) *(Lyrica, Pregabalin Sandoz).*

Dose: Adult: *Epilepsy, neuropathic pain,* initially 150mg/day; if needed titrate at 1-week intervals to 300mg/day; max. 600mg/day. GAD, initially 150mg/day; titrate to 300mg/day after 1 week, then to 450mg/day after another week; max. 600mg/day after an additional week. Oral in 2-3 divided doses, with or without food.

Elderly: Over 65 years, consider dose reduction.

Child: Under 17 years, not recommended.

Renal Impairment: CrCl (mL/min) over 60, initially 150mg, max. 600mg/day; 30-60, initially 75mg, max. 300mg (2 or 3 divided doses); below 30, initially 25-50mg, max. 150mg (1 or 2 divided doses); below 15, initially 25mg, max. 75mg once daily. Supplementary following haemodialysis, initially 25mg; max. 100mg (single dose).

Interactions: Effect of Pregabalin on Other Drugs: Oxycodone: *Additive impairment of cognitive and gross motor function.* CNS-influencing medicinals: *Effects potentiated.*

SP: Diabetics who gain weight may need hypoglycaemic dose adjusted. Hypersensitivity reactions e.g. angioedema, discontinue. Dizziness, somnolence increasing risk of accidental fall (elderly). Visual changes (vision loss, blurring, changed visual acuity). CHF reported (mostly elderly or cardiovascular compromised treated for neuropathic pain). Increased CNS adverse events when

3.1.3 GABAergic Drugs

used for central neuropathic pain due to spinal cord injury. Reduced lower GI function. Encephalopathy.

ADR: *Very common*, dizziness, somnolence, headache.

Notes: See 3.1 Antiepileptics.

Lyrica Capsules *(Pfizer)* A. GMS.
Price, (56) 25mg, €26.38; 75mg, 150mg, 300mg, €44.13. (84) 25mg, €39.57; 50mg, 100mg, 200mg, €66.18.
Capsule, pregabalin 25mg, 50mg, 75mg, 100mg, 150mg, 200mg, 300mg. Hard capsule. Marked Pfizer, PGN/strength. 25mg, 50mg, 150mg: White. 50mg: Marked with black band. 75mg, 300mg: White/orange. 100mg: Orange. 200mg: Light-orange. 300mg: White/light-orange. *Lactose.* Store: No special conditions.

Brieka Capsules *(Accord)* A. GMS.
Price, (56) 25mg, €10.55; 75mg, €19.99; 150mg, €27.55; 300mg, €35.28. (84) 25mg, €15.82; 50mg, €31.65; 100mg, €38.83; 200mg, €52.93.
Capsules, pregabalin 25mg, 50mg, 75mg, 100mg, 150mg, 200mg, 300mg. Hard. Marked PGB and strength. 25mg, 150mg: White. 50mg: White. Marked with black line. 75mg, 300mg: White/orange. 100mg: Orange. 200mg: Light-orange.

Pregabalin Accord Capsules *(Accord)* A. GMS.
Price, (56) 25mg, €10.55; 75mg, €19.99; 150mg, €27.55; 300mg, €35.29. (84) 50mg, €31.67; 100mg, €38.83; 200mg, €52.93.
Capsules, pregabalin 25mg, 50mg, 75mg, 100mg, 150mg, 200mg, 300mg. Hard opaque. Marked PG (cap) and strength (body). 25mg, 50mg, 150mg: White/white. 75mg: Red/white. 100mg: Red/red. 200mg: Orange/orange. 300mg: Red/white.

Pregabalin Clonmel Capsules *(Clonmel)* A. GMS.
Price, (56) 25mg, €10.55; 75mg, €19.99; 150mg, €27.55; 300mg, €35.28. (84) 50mg, €31.65; 100mg, €38.83; 200mg, €52.93.
Capsules, pregabalin 25mg, 50mg, 75mg, 100mg, 150mg, 200mg, 300mg. Hard. Marked PGB and strength. 25mg, 150mg: White. 50mg: White. Marked with black line. 75mg, 300mg: White/orange. 100mg: Orange. 200mg: Light-orange.

Pregabalin Krka Capsules *(Krka)* A. GMS.
Price, (56) 25mg, €10.55; 75mg, €19.99; 150mg, €27.55; 300mg, €35.29. (84) 50mg, €31.65; 100mg, €38.83; 200mg, €52.93.
Capsules, pregabalin 25mg, 50mg, 75mg, 100mg, 150mg, 200mg, 300mg. Hard capsule containing white (off-white powder). Marked P strength. 25mg: White. 50mg: White/bright yellow. 75mg: Brownish-yellow. 100mg: Reddish-brown. 150mg: White/yellowish-brown. 200mg: Brown. 300mg: White/dark-brown.

Pregabalin Mylan Capsules *(Gerard)* A. GMS.
Price, (56) 25mg, €10.55; 75mg, €19.99; 150mg, €27.55; 300mg, €34.04. (84) 50mg, €31.65; 100mg, €38.83; 200mg, €52.93.
Capsule, pregabalin. Hard opaque; filled with white (off-white) powder. Marked MYLAN and PB and strength. 25mg, 150mg, 300mg: Light peach/white. 50mg: Dark-peach/white. 75mg, 200mg: Light-peach. 100mg: Dark-peach. *Store:* Original pack to protect (moisture).

Pregabalin Sandoz Capsules *(Rowex)* A. GMS.
Price, (56) 25mg, €10.55; 75mg, €19.99; 150mg, €27.55; 300mg, €35.28. (84) 50mg, €31.65; 100mg, €38.83; 200mg, €52.93.
Capsule, pregabalin. Hard opaque; filled with white (nearly white) powder. 25mg: Yellow-brown. 50mg: Light-yellow. 75mg: Red/white. 100mg: Red. 150mg: White. 200mg: Pale-orange. 300mg: Red/pale yellow-brown.

Pregabalin TEVA Capsules *(TEVA)* A. GMS.
Price, (56) 25mg, €10.55; 75mg, €19.99; 150mg, €27.55; 300mg, €35.29. (84) 50mg, €31.65; 100mg, €38.83; 200mg, €52.93.
Capsules, pregabalin. Hard opaque; contains white (off-white) powder. Marked with strength. 25mg, 50mg, 150mg: Ivory. 75mg, 300mg: Pink/ivory. 100mg: Pink. 200mg: Flesh-coloured. *Store:* No special conditions.

Pregabalin Wockhardt Capsules *(Pinewood)* A. GMS.
Price, (56) 25mg, €10.55; 75mg, €19.99; 150mg, €27.55; 300mg, €35.28. (84) 50mg, €31.61; 100mg, €38.83; 200mg, €52.93.
Capsule, pregabalin. Hard; contain white (off-white) powder. Marked with strength. 25mg, 150mg: White. 50mg: White/pinkish-orange. 75mg, 300mg: Brownish-red/white. 100mg: Brownish-red. 200mg: Pinkish-orange. *Lactose.*

Vigabatrin

ATC Code: N03AG04. **Sport:** Permitted.
Driving: Drowsiness, visual field defects.
Indications: Epilepsy (adjunctive or monotherapy), treatment of partial seizures with or without secondary generalisation. Monotherapy in infantile spasms (West's syndrome).

Dose: Adult: Initially 1g/day; increase by 0.5g at 1-week intervals if needed; max. 3g/day. Oral, once or twice daily, before or after meals.

Elderly: As for Renal below.

Child: Initially 40mg/kg/day. Maintenance, weight 10-15kg, 0.5-1g/day; 15-30kg, 1-1.5g/day; 30-50kg, 1.5-3g/day; above 50kg, 2-3g/day. *Infants,* monotherapy for infantile spasms, initially 50mg/kg/day; titrate over 1 week if needed to up to 150mg/kg/day.

Renal Impairment: CrCl (mL/min) below 60, caution.

CI: Pre-existing clinically significant visual field defects, generally not recommended.

Interactions: Effect of Other Drugs on Vigabatrin: *Co-admin not recommended*: Other retinotoxic drugs.

Effect of Vigabatrin on Other Drugs: Phenytoin: *Gradual reduction in plasma levels.*

SP: Visual field defects (VFD), occur in about one third of patients; males at greater risk; mild to severe, onset usually after months to years of vigabatrin treatment. Perimetry seldom possible in children under 9 years, weigh benefit against risk. *Encephalopathic symptoms,* sedation, stupor, confusion in association with non-specific slow wave activity on EEG. Increased seizure frequency or onset of new types of seizures. Caution, history of psychosis, depression or behavioural problems. In treatment of infantile spasms, abnormal brain MRIs (high doses), movement disorders (dystonia, dyskinesia, hypertonia). Altered LFTs.

Pregnancy, Lactation: Pregnancy, use only if clearly necessary. Women of childbearing potential to ensure adequate contraception. Lactation, not recommended.

ADR: Summary, *about 50% of patients,* CNS (sedation, drowsiness, fatigue, impaired concentration; excitation or agitation in children); *some patients,* increased seizure frequency including status epilepticus. Visual field defects, see SP above.

Notes: See 3.1 Antiepileptics.

Sabril 500mg, Sachets 500mg *(SANOFI)* B. GMS.
Price, tabs (100) €55.56. Sachets (50) €30.88.
Tablet, vigabatrin. White (off-white) oval f/c scored (facilitates breaking). Marked Sabril.
Sachet, as above. White (off-white) granular powder for oral soln.

Tiagabine

ATC Code: N03AG06. **Sport:** Permitted.
Driving: Dizziness, other CNS-related symptoms.
Indications: Epilepsy (adjunctive or monotherapy), treatment of partial seizures with or without secondary generalisation.

Dose: Adult, Elderly: Age 12 years and over, initially 5-10mg; increase at 1-week intervals by 5-10mg/day; maintenance, *with enzyme inducers,* 30-50mg/day OR *without enzyme inducers,* 15-30mg/day. Admin, oral, initially (single or 2 divided doses), with meals; maintenance (2-3 divided doses). *Elderly,* caution.

Child: Under 12 years, not recommended.

Hepatic Impairment: Mild to moderate, reduce dose and/or increase dosing interval. Severe, contraindicated.

Interactions: Effect of Other Drugs on Tiagabine: *Enhanced metabolism:* CYP450 inducers (phenytoin, carbamazepine, phenobarbitone, primidone, rifampicin).

SP: Generalised epilepsy, use not recommended. Aggravation of absences. Recurrence of behavioural problems, increased seizure frequency and/or onset of new seizure types, new onset seizures, status epilepticus. Ecchymosis, perform FBC. Visual field defects.

ADR: Dizziness, tremor, visual field defects, somnolence, depressed mood, unspecific nervousness, concentration difficulties, diarrhoea, platelet, bleeding disorders (ecchymosis), tiredness.

Notes: See 3.1 Antiepileptics.

Gabitril 5mg, 10mg, 15mg *(TEVA)* B. GMS.
Price, (100) 5mg, €54.63. 10mg, €100.60. 15mg, €149.84.
Tablet, tiagabine hydrochloride monohydrate. White oval f/c scored. 5mg: Marked 251. 10mg: Marked 252. 15mg: Marked 253. *Lactose.*

3.1.4 - Hydantoins

In This Chapter: *Fosphenytoin, phenytoin.*

Class Effects

CI: Hypersensitivity to other hydantoins.

SP: *Pro-Epanutin* dose is always expressed as phenytoin sodium equivalent (PE = phenytoin sodium equivalent). When *Pro-Epanutin* is dosed as PE, no dose adjustment should be made when substituting *Pro-Epanutin* for phenytoin sodium or vice versa (oral or parenteral). *Pro-Epanutin* admin differs from parenteral phenytoin sodium. Admin *Pro-Epanutin* IV (max. 150mg PE/min); max. phenytoin IV infusion rate 50mg/min.

Suicide, see Notes below. Hypersensitivity Syndrome (HSS) or Drug Reaction with Eosinophilia and Systemic Symptoms (DRESS) reported with anticonvulsants including phenytoin; may be fatal or life-threatening.

Pregnancy, Lactation: Phenytoin (other antiepileptics) may produce congenital abnormalities in offspring of a small number of epileptic patients; not for use first-line during pregnancy, especially early (weigh risk benefit). Congenital abnormalities (cleft lip/palate, heart malformations); foetal hydantoin syndrome (prenatal growth deficiency, microcephaly, mental deficiency) in children born to mothers receiving phenytoin, barbiturates, alcohol, or trimethadione. See Notes below.

Notes: See 3.1 Antiepileptics.

Fosphenytoin

ATC Code: N03AB05. **Sport:** Permitted.
Driving: Dizziness, drowsiness.

Indications: Control of *status epilepticus* of the tonic-clonic (grand mal) type; prevention and treatment, seizures in connection with neurosurgery and/or head trauma. Substitute for oral phenytoin (oral admin not possible or contraindicated).

Dose: Adult: NOTE: Phenytoin sodium equivalents (PE): 1.5mg fosphenytoin equiv. to 1mg PE (phenytoin sodium equivalent). IV admin rate for fosphenytoin 50-100mg PE/min; max. 150mg PE/min even in emergency. Max. IV infusion rate for phenytoin 50mg/min. CAUTION: Dosing errors; note mg/mL strength, product name, preparation, infusion/admin errors, incorrect dose calculations; always express dose as mg PE.

Status epilepticus, following diazepam or lorazepam, 15mg PE/kg IV infusion as single loading dose, rate 100mg to max. 150mg PE/min. Maintenance, max. 5mg PE/kg/day by IV infusion or IM injection (single or 2 divided doses); infusion rate max. 100mg PE/min.

Treatment, seizure prophylaxis, 10-15mg PE/kg as single loading dose by IV infusion, rate max. 100mg PE/min. Maintenance, 4-5mg PE/kg/day by IV infusion OR IM injection (single or 2 divided doses).

Temporary substitution of oral phenytoin, same dose and frequency as for oral, admin IV or IM; infusion rate 50-100mg PE/min; max. 5 days.

Elderly: Consider 10-25% reduction in dose or rate.

Child: NOTE: Age 5 years and over, use same milligram (mg) PE/kg as for Adult; only by IV infusion. *Status epilepticus*, following diazepam or lorazepam, loading dose 15mg PE/kg single dose IV infusion, rate 2-3mg PE/kg/min; max rate 3mg PE/kg/min or 150mg PE/min (whichever is slower). Maintenance 4-5mg PE/kg/day by IV infusion or IM injection (single or 4 divided doses); rate 1-2mg PE/kg/min (max. 100mg PE/min).

Treatment or seizure prophylaxis, 10-15mg PE/kg as single loading dose IV infusion, rate 1-2mg PE/kg/min, max. 3mg PE/kg/min (max. 150mg PE/min). Maintenance as for status epilepticus above.

Temporary substitution of oral phenytoin, see Adult above. Recommended infusion rate 1-2mg PE/kg/min or max. 100mg PE/min.

Renal Impairment: Except for status epilepticus, consider 10-25% reduction in dose or rate.

Hepatic Impairment: As for Renal above.

CI: Sinus bradycardia, sino-atrial block, second or third degree A-V block, Adams-Stokes syndrome, acute intermittent porphyria.

Interactions: Effect of Fosphenytoin on Other Drugs: *Delavirdine: Co-admin contraindicated (possible loss of virological response).*

SP: Caution, hypotension and severe myocardial insufficiency; hypotension following IV admin (high dose and/or high infusion rate). Cardiac monitoring with IV loading doses (elderly, children, especially infants, gravely ill). Acute cerebrovascular events, increased hypotension risk (monitor). Oedema, discolouration and pain distal to injection site (purple glove syndrome); may be associated with extravasation; may develop several days after injection. Confusional states or irreversible cerebellar dysfunction and/or atrophy may occur (plasma phenytoin levels sustained above optimal range and/or long-term use); excessive levels, reduce dose; discontinue if symptoms persist.

ADR: *Most important*, cardiovascular collapse and/or CNS depression, hypotension; *most common*, nystagmus, dizziness, pruritus, paraesthesia, headache, somnolence, ataxia.

Notes: See Phenytoin below. See 3.1.4 Hydantoins.

> **Pro-Epanutin Parenteral** *(Pfizer)* A.
> *Price*, 75mg/mL (10x10mL), €439.08.
> *Injection*, fosphenytoin sodium 75mg/mL. Clear colourless (pale-yellow) sterile soln. Store: Refrigerate; store undiluted at room temperature (max. 24 hours).

Phenytoin

ATC Code: N03AB02. **Sport:** Permitted.
Driving: Caution; dizziness, drowsiness.

Indications: Control, tonic-clonic seizures (grand mal), partial seizures (focal including temporal lobe). Prophylaxis and treatment, seizures with neurosurgery and/or severe head injury. Trigeminal neuralgia, second-line to carbamazepine. Treatment, cardiac arrhythmias (life-threatening ventricular, secondary to digitalis intoxication); first line not effective.

Dose: Adult: ORAL, initially 3-4mg/kg/day; maintenance 200-500mg/day (single or divided doses).

PARENTERAL, *status epilepticus*, following diazepam, 10-15mg/kg loading, IV max. rate 50mg/min; maintenance 100mg orally or IV 6-8 hourly. *Admin*, slow IV injection through large vein.

Arrhythmias, initially 3.5-5mg/kg IV, rate as above. If needed, repeat once.

Neurosurgery, no previous phenytoin, 100-200mg IM 4-hourly, prophylactically and 48-72 hours post-operative. Maintenance 300mg. *Admin*, IM; max. 1 week.

Elderly: Over 65 years, caution. Phenytoin clearance is decreased slightly in elderly; lower or less frequent dosing may be required.

Child: ORAL, *infants, children*, initially, 5mg/kg/day (2 divided doses); max. 300mg/day; maintenance 4-8mg/kg. *Neonates*, absorption following oral admin unpredictable; metabolism may be depressed, monitor serum levels.

PARENTERAL IV, *neonates*, 15-20mg/kg loading IV produces serum conc 10-20mg/L; slow admin, rate 1-3mg/kg/min. *Children*, as for Adult (tend to metabolise phenytoin quicker than adults).

Renal Impairment: See SP below.

Hepatic Impairment: Reduced dose may be needed to prevent accumulation. Hepatotoxicity incidence may be higher in black patients. See SP below.

CI: Sinus bradycardia, SA block, second and third degree AV block, Adams-Stokes syndrome. Avoid intra-arterial admin (high pH).

Interactions: Effect of Other Drugs on Phenytoin: *Plasma levels increased:* CYP2C9 inhibition (fluconazole, ketoconazole, miconazole, itraconazole; glibenclamide), CYP2C19 inhibition (felbamate), CYP2C9/19 inhibition (azapropazone, fluvoxamine, nifedipine, sertraline, ticlopidine, tolbutamide), unknown mechanism (acute ALCOHOL intake, amiodarone, amphotericin B, chloramphenicol, high dose diltiazem, disulfiram, fluoxetine, cimetidine, halothane, isoniazid, methylphenidate, oestrogens, omeprazole,

3.1.5 Carboxamides

phenothiazines, phenylbutazone, salicylates, succinimides ethosuximide, sulfonamides, trazodone, viloxazine). *Plasma levels decreased:* Unknown mechanism (chronic ALCOHOL intake, diazoxide, folic acid, sucralfate, nelfinavir, theophylline, vigabatrin, St John's Wort), CYP2C9/19 induction (rifampicin). *Plasma levels increased and/or decreased:* Unknown mechanism (antineoplastic agents, carbamazepine, chlordiazepoxide, ciprofloxacin, diazepam, phenobarbital, valproic acid, sodium valproate, antacids). *Seizure threshold lowered:* Paroxetine, sertraline.

Effect of Phenytoin on Other Drugs: Delavirdine: *Co-admin contraindicated (loss of virological response).* Teniposide, ciclosporin, erythromycin, methadone, pancuronium, vecuronium, nicardipine, nifedipine, praziquantel, verapamil (CYP3A4 induction), chlorpropamide (CYP2C9/19 induction), theophylline (CYP1A2 induction), doxycycline, rifampicin, tetracycline, warfarin, azole antifungals, corticosteroids, digoxin, nimodipine, quinidine, furosemide, glibenclamide, oestrogens, oral contraceptives, lamotrigine, paroxetine, clozapine, Vitamin D: *Blood levels and/or effects altered.* Glibenclamide, tolbutamide: *Consider dose adjustment; phenytoin increases serum glucose levels.*

SP: Abrupt withdrawal may precipitate *status epilepticus.* Not effective for absence (petit mal) seizures; if tonic-clonic (grand mal) and absence seizures are present together, use combined treatment. Phenytoin may, precipitate or aggravate absence and myoclonic seizures, affect glucose metabolism, inhibit insulin release; not indicated for metabolic seizures. Suicide, see Notes below. Hypersensitivity Syndrome or DRESS (fever, rash, lymphadenopathy); life-threatening cutaneous reactions (Stevens-Johnson syndrome, toxic epidermal necrolysis), discontinue. Impaired liver function, reduce dose to prevent accumulation and toxicity. Haematopoietic complications (fatal). Above optimal serum levels may produce confusional states or irreversible cerebellar dysfunction and/or atrophy. Chronic treatment, Vitamin D deficiency risk. Porphyria exacerbation. Reduced serum folate levels. Hyperglycaemia.

Increased unbound phenytoin fraction with renal or hepatic disease, or hypoalbuminaemia. Caution interpretation of total phenytoin plasma conc. Unbound phenytoin conc may be elevated with hyperbilirubinaemia. Unbound phenytoin conc may be more useful in these patients.

Parenteral, IV admin max. 50mg/min (adult), 1-3mg/kg/min (neonates). Cardiovascular collapse and/or CNS depression. Atrial and ventricular conduction depression, ventricular fibrillation, respiratory arrest, tonic seizures (caution elderly, seriously ill). Hypotension. Injection site soft tissue irritation/inflammation. NOTE: 100mg phenytoin sodium is equiv. to 92mg of phenytoin on molecular weight basis; not necessarily biologically equivalent.

Pregnancy, Lactation: IV management of status epilepticus in pregnancy, weigh risk/benefit (potential adverse effects upon foetus especially hypoxia), make control imperative in shortest possible time. Phenytoin crosses placenta. Breastfeeding not recommended. See Notes below.

ADR: Anaphylactoid reaction, anaphylaxis, DRESS. CNS reactions (usually dose-related), GI (hepatic, vomiting, nausea, constipation), dermatological (sometimes with fever); rash through to severe cutaneous reactions, connective tissue disorders, haematopoietic complications (fatal), musculoskeletal (bone metabolism), secondary hyperparathyroidism. Injection site reactions; Purple Glove Syndrome.

Notes: See 3.1.4 Hydantoins.

Epanutin Capsules, Infatabs, Oral Susp *(Pfizer)* B. GMS.
Price, caps 25mg (28) €1.19; (500) €12.30. 50mg (28) €1.20; (500) €12.56. 100mg (84) €7.51; (500) €16.38. 300mg (28) €7.51; (100) €10.19. Infatabs 50mg (100) €6.88; (112) €13.10; (200) €23.39. Susp 30mg/5mL (500mL) €7.91.
Capsule, phenytoin sodium 25mg, 50mg, 100mg, 300mg. Gelatin opaque contains white powder. Marked EPANUTIN/strength. 25mg: White/purple. 50mg: White/flesh-coloured. 100mg: White/orange. 300mg: White/dark green. *Lactose.* **Store:** Below 25 deg C.

Chewable tablet (Infatab), phenytoin. Yellow triangular scored (facilitates breaking). Marked P-D007. *Sucrose, Sunset Yellow.* **Store:** Below 25 deg C.
Oral susp, as above 30mg/5mL. Viscous cherry red. *Sucrose, ethanol, Carmoisine, Sunset Yellow.* **Store:** Below 25 deg C.
Epanutin Ready Mixed Parenteral *(Pfizer)* A. GMS.
Price, (10) €52.15.
Injection or infusion, phenytoin sodium 50mg/mL. Clear colourless sterile soln. *Ethanol, sodium 24.6mg/5mL.* **Store:** Below 25 deg C.

3.1.5 - Carboxamides

In This Chapter: *Carbamazepine, eslicarbazepine, oxcarbazepine, rufinamide.*

Class Effects
CI: Hypersensitivity to any member of the class, carboxamide derivatives.
SP: HLA-A*3101 or HLA-B*1502 allele in individuals of descent various population groups (Han Chinese, Thai, European, Japanese) associated with risk of carbamazepine-induced cutaneous reactions e.g. Stevens-Johnson syndrome, TEN, drug rash with eosinophilia (DRESS) or less severe generalised exanthematous pustulosis (AGEP) and maculopapular rash (with oxcarbazepine or eslicarbazepine); screen for allele before initiating. **Suicide,** see Notes below.
Pregnancy, Lactation: See Notes below.
Notes: See 3.1 Antiepileptics.

Carbamazepine
ATC Code: N03AF01. **Sport:** Permitted.
Driving: Caution; impaired ability to react; dizziness, drowsiness, ataxia, diplopia, impaired accommodation, blurred vision.
Indications: Epilepsy, generalised tonic-clonic, partial seizures. Paroxysmal pain of trigeminal neuralgia, deafferentation pain. Alcohol withdrawal symptoms. Treatment, mania and prophylaxis, manic depressive illness unresponsive to lithium.
Dose: Adult: *Epilepsy,* 100-200mg once or twice daily; titrate slowly to 800-1200mg/day if required; up to 1600-2000mg/day may be needed.
Trigeminal neuralgia, deafferentation pain, usually 200mg 3-4 times daily; may be increased gradually until satisfactory clinical response (up to 1600mg daily in some instances); max. recommended dose 1200mg/day.
Alcohol withdrawal, 600-800mg/day; 1200-1600mg/day may be required with delirium tremens.
Treatment (mania), prophylaxis (manic-depressive illness), initially 100-200mg/day; titrate slowly to max. 1600mg/day (800-1600mg); usual range 400-600mg/day. Divided doses.
Admin Standard/R tabs in 2-4 divided doses during, after or between meals, with fluid. Prolonged/R in 2 divided doses, do not chew.
Elderly: Caution. Trigeminal neuralgia, initially 100mg twice daily.
Child: *Epilepsy,* 10-20mg/kg/day in several divided doses. Age 1 year and under, usually 100-200mg/day; 1-5 years, 200-400mg/day; 5-10 years, 400-600mg/day; 10-15 years, 600-1000mg/day. Children 5 years and under, use liquid. Prolonged/R tabs not recommended.
Renal Impairment: Caution.
Hepatic Impairment: Caution.
CI: AV conduction abnormalities, bone marrow depression, hepatic porphyrias.
Interactions: Effect of Other Drugs on Carbamazepine: *Co-admin contraindicated:* MAOIs (or within 2 weeks), St John's Wort. *Plasma levels increased:* Analgesics/anti-inflammatories (dextropropoxyphene, ibuprofen), danazol, erythromycin, clarithromycin, desipramine, fluoxetine, fluvoxamine, nefazodone, paroxetine, trazodone, viloxazine, stiripentol, vigabatrin, itraconazole, ketoconazole, fluconazole, voriconazole, loratadine, terfenadine, olanzapine, isoniazid, protease inhibitors, ritonavir, acetazolamide, diltiazem, verapamil; possibly cimetidine, omeprazole; oxybutynin, dantrolene, ticlopidine, grapefruit juice; nicotinamide in adults, only

high doses; ciprofloxacin. *Carbamazepine metabolite levels increased*: Loxapine, quetiapine, primidone, progabide, valproic acid, valnocamide, valpromide. *Plasma levels decreased*: Methsuzimide, oxcarbazepine, phenobarbitone, phensuximide, phenytoin, fosphenytoin, primidone; possibly clonazepam; cisplatin, doxorubicin, rifampicin, theophylline, aminophylline, St John's Wort, albendazole, cyclophosphamide, lapatinib, temsirolimus, aripiprazole, paliperidone, tadalafil, tacrolimus, sirolimus. *Effect antagonised*: Mefloquine. *Bioavailability altered*: Isotretinoin.

Effect of Carbamazepine on Other Drugs: Analgesics/anti-inflammatories (buprenorphine, methadone, paracetamol, phenazone, tramadol), antibiotics (doxycycline, rifabutin), oral anticoagulants (warfarin, phenprocoumon, dicoumarol, acenocoumarol), antidepressants (bupropion, citalopram, mianserin, nefazodone, sertraline, trazodone, TCADs including imipramine, amitriptyline, nortriptyline, clomipramine), antiemetics (aprepitant), antiepileptics (clobazam, clonazepam, ethosuximide, felbamate, lamotrigine, oxcarbazepine, primidone, tiagabine, topiramate, valproic acid, zonisamide), azole antifungals (itraconazole, voriconazole), anthelmintics (praziquantel), antineoplastics (imatinib, cyclophosphamide, lapatinib, temsirolimus), antipsychotics (clozapine, haloperidol, bromperidol, olanzapine, quetiapine, risperidone, ziprasidone, aripiprazole, paliperidone), protease inhibitors (indinavir, ritonavir, saquinavir), anxiolytics (alprazolam, midazolam), asthma drugs (theophylline), hormonal contraceptives (possible contraceptive failure), cardiovascular (digoxin, dihydropyridine calcium channel blockers including felodipine, isradipine), statins (simvastatin, atorvastatin, lovastatin, cerivastatin), corticosteroids (prednisolone, dexamethasone), drugs used in ED (tadalafil), immunosuppressants (ciclosporin, everolimus), thyroid (levothyroxine), other (gestrinone, tibolone, toremifene): *Plasma levels decreased*. Phenytoin: *Plasma levels increased and/or decreased*. Paracetamol, acetaminophen: *Bioavailability decreased*. Isoniazid: *Increased hepatotoxicity*. Lithium, metoclopramide, haloperidol, thioridazine: *Increased neurological ADRs*. Some diuretics (hydrochlorothiazide, frusemide): *Hyponatraemia*. Non-depolarising muscle relaxants (pancuronium): *Effect antagonised*. Alcohol: *CNS side effects exacerbated*.

SP: HLA-B*1502 allele, see Notes below. Agranulocytosis, aplastic anaemia, decreased platelet or WBC counts, obtain base-line full blood counts and then periodically; leucopenia (severe, progressive, with symptoms), discontinue. *Counsel patient* to consult medical advice if haematological, dermatological, hepatic reactions (fever, sore throat, rash, mouth ulcers, easy bruising, petechial or purpuric haemorrhage), occur. Rash (macular or maculopapular exanthemata); severe skin reactions (Stevens-Johnson syndrome, toxic epidermal necrolysis or Lyell's syndrome), discontinue; do not restart. Hypersensitivity (multi-organ, systemic); cross-hypersensitivity (oxcarbazepine, phenytoin). Seizures, mixed (absences, typical or atypical), monitor plasma levels; seizure exacerbation, discontinue. Perform LFTs before initiation then periodically (especially with liver disease, elderly). Baseline and periodic urinalysis and BUN recommended. Hyponatraemia, hypothyroidism, glaucoma; latent psychosis activation, agitation, confusion (elderly). Reduced efficacy of combined oral contraceptive. Monitor plasma levels (increased seizure frequency, pregnancy, children, adolescents, suspected absorption disorders, for verification of compliance, suspected toxicity).

ADR: Summary, *very common, common* (especially is initial dose too high, or elderly), CNS (dizziness, headache, ataxia, drowsiness, fatigue, diplopia), GI (nausea, vomiting), allergic skin reactions. See SP above.

Notes: See 3.1.5 Carboxamides.

Tegretol Tablets, SR, Oral Susp *(Novartis)* B. GMS.D*.
Price, tabs (100) 100mg*, €4.49. 200mg*, €7.29. 400mg* (50) €6.02; (56) €8.26. SR Prolonged/R tabs (50) 200mg*, €4.42. 400mg*, €7.10. Oral Susp 100mg/5mL (300mL) €5.07.
Tablet, carbamazepine 100mg, 200mg, 400mg. White. 100mg:

Round scored. Marked Geigy; B/W on reverse. 200mg: Round scored. Marked GG; G/K on reverse. 400mg: Rod-shaped. Marked CG/CG; LR/LR on reverse. **Store:** Below 25 deg C; original pack; protect (moisture).
Prolonged/R tablet (SR), as above 200mg, 400mg. Oval slightly f/c, g/r scored both sides (divisible into equal halves). 200mg: Beige-orange. Marked H/C; C/G on reverse. 400mg: Brownish-orange. Marked ENE/ENE; G/CG on reverse. *Castor oil*. **Store:** Below 30 deg C as above.
Oral susp, as above 100mg/5mL. White susp; aromatic odour; caramel flavour. *Parabens, sorbitol*. **Store:** Below 30 deg C; bottle in outer carton; protect (light).

Eslicarbazepine

ATC Code: N03AF04. **Sport:** Permitted.
Driving: Dizziness, somnolence, visual disorders.
Indications: Monotherapy, partial-onset seizures* (adults, newly diagnosed epilepsy). Adjunctive, partial-onset seizures* (over 6 years and above). *(with or without secondary generalisation).
Dose: Adult: Monotherapy or adjunctive, initially 400mg/day; increase to 800mg/day after 1-2 weeks; based on response increase to 1200mg/day. Monotherapy, some patients may benefit from 1600mg/day. *Admin*, once daily with or without food.
Elderly: No adjustment or as for Renal below. Monotherapy 1600mg/day regimen not recommended.
Child: Above 6 years, 10mg/kg/day once daily; increase weekly or bi-weekly by 10mg/kg/day up to 30mg/kg/day based on response; max. 1200mg once daily. Body weight 60kg and above, as for Adult above. Under 6 years, safety/efficacy not established. *Admin*, see Adult above.
Renal Impairment: CrCl (mL/min) above 60, no adjustment; 30-60, initially 200mg (or 5mg/kg*) once daily OR 400mg (10mg/kg*) every other day for 2 weeks then 400mg once daily; below 30, not recommended. *(children above age 6 years).
Hepatic Impairment: Mild/moderate, no adjustment. Severe, not recommended.
Interactions: Effect of Other Drugs on Eslicarbazepine: *Co-admin not recommended*: Oxcarbazepine (over-exposure to active metabolites), carbamazepine (increased adverse reaction risk). *Increased/decreased exposure*: Phenytoin (may require increased eslicarbazepine dose/decreased phenytoin dose), lamotrigine (no dose adjustment), topiramate (no dose adjustment). **Effect of Eslicarbazepine on Other Drugs:** Hormonal contraceptives: *Decreased efficacy (use additional non-hormonal methods)*. Substrates of CYP3A4 (simvastatin) and CYP2C19 (phenytoin), rosuvastatin: *Metabolism induced, may need dose increase (monitor cholesterol)*. Warfarin: *Monitor INR*. MAOIs: *Interaction theoretically possible*.
SP: Somnolence, dizziness, accidental injury risk. Hypersensitivity signs and/or rash, discontinue. Hyponatraemia with increasing dose, pre-existing renal disease, medicinals causing hyponatraemia; monitor serum sodium before/during treatment. PR prolongation caution, low thyroxine levels, cardiac conduction abnormalities, medicinals causing PR prolongation.
Pregnancy, Lactation: See Notes below.
ADR: Summary, *most common*, dizziness, somnolence, headache, nausea.
Notes: See 3.1.5 Carboxamides.
Zebinix 800mg *(Eisai)* B. GMS.
Price, (30) €138.42.
Tablet, eslicarbazepine acetate. White oblong scored (divisible into equal halves). Marked ESL/strength. **Store:** No special conditions.

Oxcarbazepine

ATC Code: N03AF02. **Sport:** Permitted.
Driving: Dizziness, somnolence, ataxia, diplopia, visual disturbances, blurred vision, hyponatraemia, depressed levels of consciousness.
Indications: Partial seizures with or without secondary generalised tonic-clonic seizures.
Dose: Adult, Elderly: Monotherapy and adjunctive, initially 600mg/day (8-10mg/kg/day); increase by max. 600mg/day at 1-week intervals if needed; range 600-

91

3.1.6   Miscellaneous Antiepileptics

2400mg/day; 1200mg/day usually effective, 2400mg/day in refractory cases; above 2400mg/day, no data. *Elderly*, as for Renal; monitor sodium levels. *Admin*, oral in 2 divided doses with or without food; oral susp and tabs may be interchanged at equal doses.

Child: Monotherapy and adjunctive, over 6 years, initially, 8-10mg/kg/day in 2 divided doses. In adjunctive trials, maintenance 30-46mg/kg/day achieved over 2 weeks increasing by max. 10mg/kg/day at weekly intervals; median maintenance 30mg/kg/day. Under 6 years, not recommended.

Renal Impairment: CrCl (mL/min) below 30, initiate at 300mg/day.

Hepatic Impairment: Severe, no data.

Interactions: Effect of Other Drugs on Oxcarbazepine: *Plasma levels decreased:* Carbamazepine, phenobarbitone, phenytoin, valproic acid. *Co-admin not recommended:* MAOIs. *Monitor sodium levels:* Diuretics, desmopressin, NSAIDs (indomethacin). *Increased sedative effect, caution:* ALCOHOL. *Increased adverse events risk:* Lamotrigine.

Effect of Oxcarbazepine on Other Drugs: Drugs metabolised by CYP2C19 (phenobarbitone, phenytoin): *Plasma levels increased, reduce dose.* Dihydropyridines, oral contraceptives (ethinyloestradiol, levonorgestrel), antiepileptics (carbamazepine): *Plasma levels reduced, efficacy reduced.* Lithium: *Enhanced neurotoxicity.*

SP: Hypersensitivity Class I immediate reactions (rash, pruritus, urticaria, angioedema, anaphylaxis); carbamazepine cross hypersensitivity, severe skin reactions (Stevens-Johnson syndrome, toxic epidermal necrolysis, erythema multiform). HLA-B*1502 allele individuals (Han Chinese, Thai, other Asians) and HLA-A*3101 allele individuals (European, Japanese) associated with risk of severe cutaneous reactions; Multi-organ hypersensitivity without history of carbamazepine hypersensitivity. Monitor serum sodium (hyponatraemia); fluid retention (in cardiac insufficiency, secondary HF). Cardiac conduction disturbances, hepatitis, agranulocytosis, aplastic anaemia, pancytopenia. Long-term use, bone metabolism affected. Seizure aggravation especially in children. Hypothyroidism. Plasma level monitoring of oxcarbazepine or active metabolite routinely not warranted unless clearance suspected.

Pregnancy, Lactation: See Notes below.

ADR: Summary, *most common*, somnolence, headache, dizziness, diplopia, nausea, vomiting, fatigue. See SP above.

Notes: See 3.1.5 Carboxamides.

Trileptal Tablets, Oral Soln *(Novartis)* B. GMS.
Price, tabs (50) 150mg, €9.02. 300mg, €14.627. 600mg, €27.60. Susp 60mg/mL (250mL) €30.64.
Tablets, oxcarbazepine 150mg, 300mg, 600mg. Ovaloid f/c scored (facilitates breaking). 150mg: Pale grey-green. Marked T/D; C/G on reverse. 300mg: Yellow. Marked TE/TE; CG/CG on reverse. 600mg: Light-pink. Marked TF/TF; CG/CG on reverse.
Oral susp, as above 60mg/mL. Off-white (slightly reddish-brown). *Parabens, sorbitol.*

Rufinamide

ATC Code: N03AF03. **Sport:** Permitted.
Driving: Dizziness, somnolence, blurred vision.
Indications: Seizures associated with Lennox-Gastaut syndrome.

Dose: Adult, Elderly: Initially 400mg/day; increase by 400mg every 2 days to max. 1800mg/day (30-50kg) OR 2400mg/day (50-70kg) OR 3200mg/day (70.1kg and over). Withdraw gradually reducing dose by 25% every 2 days. Consider dose reduction (patients under 30kg) who are initiated on valproate. *Admin*, oral with food; two equally divided doses morning, evening.

Child: Over 4 years AND under 30kg NOT receiving valproate, initially 200mg/day; titrate by 200mg/day increments every 2 days; max. 1000mg/day. Under 30kg ALSO receiving valproate, which decreases rufinamide clearance, initially 200mg/day; after minimum 2 days, titrate by 200mg/day to max. 600mg/day. Over 4 years OR over 30kg, as for Adult above.

Hepatic Impairment: Mild/moderate, caution; severe, not recommended.

Interactions: Effect of Other Drugs on Rufinamide: *Co-admin (increased plasma levels):* Valproate.

Effect of Rufinamide on Other Drugs: Oral contraceptives: *Use additional safe and effective contraceptive method; plasma levels decreased.* Drugs metabolised by cytochrome P450 enzymes, drugs with narrow therapeutic window (warfarin, digoxin): *Monitor, dose adjustments may be needed*

SP: Withdraw gradually. New seizures, increased status epilepticus frequency, assess risk/benefit. Advise patients/carers (dizziness, somnolence, ataxia, gait disturbances; accidental falls). Serious hypersensitivity (fever, rash with other organ system involvement; lymphadenopathy, abnormal LFTs, haematuria), monitor or discontinue (DRESS, Stevens-Johnson syndrome). Congenital short QT Syndrome, caution; further shortening QTc duration risk.

Pregnancy, Lactation: See Notes below.

ADR: *Very common*, somnolence, headache, dizziness, nausea, vomiting, fatigue. See SP above.

Notes: See 3.1.5 Carboxamides.

Inovelon 100mg, 200mg, 400mg, Oral Susp *(Eisai)* A. GMS.
Price, tabs (10) 100mg, €5.42. (60) 200mg, €63.70; 400mg, €105.78. Susp 40mg/mL (460mL) €107.79.
Tablet, rufinamide. Pink ovaloid f/c scored both sides (divisible into equal halves). 100mg: Marked E261. 200mg: Marked E262. 400mg: Marked E263. *Lactose.*
Oral susp, as above 40mg/mL. White slightly viscous. *Parabens, sorbitol.*

3.1.6 - Miscellaneous Antiepileptics

In This Chapter: *Brivaracetam, ethosuximide, lacosamide, lamotrigine, levetiracetam, perampanel, retigabine, topiramate, valproate, zonisamide.*

Class Effects
Notes: See 3.1 Antiepileptics.

Brivaracetam

ATC Code: N03AX23. **Sport:** Permitted.
Driving: Minor or moderate influence; somnolence, dizziness, other CNS symptoms.
Indications: Adjunctive, partial-onset seizures with or without secondary generalisation (from age 16 years).
Dose: Adult: ORAL, initially 50mg/day or 100mg/day based on required seizure reduction versus potential side effects. Range 50-200mg/day. Discontinuation, gradually by 50mg/day weekly; after 1 week at 50mg/day, reduce to 20mg/day for final week. *Admin*, daily dose in equally divided doses (morning, evening), with or without food. Tabs, swallow whole with liquid. Oral soln, can be diluted in water or juice just before admin; a nasogastric tube or gastrostomy tube may be used.
PARENTERAL, as for oral admin above; use longer than 4 days, no experience. *Admin*, IV bolus without dilution OR diluted and admin as 15-minute IV infusion. Do not mix with other medicinals.

Elderly: No dose adjustment; 65 years and older, limited experience.

Child: Age 16 years and over, as for Adult above. Under 16 years, safety/efficacy not established.

Renal Impairment: No adjustment. ESRD on dialysis, not recommended (no data).

Hepatic Impairment: Increased exposure. Consider initially 50mg/day; max. 150mg/day (in two divided doses) for all stages of impairment.

CI: Pyrrolidone derivative hypersensitivity.

Interactions: Effect of Other Drugs on Brivaracetam: *Co-admin not recommended:* ALCOHOL. *No benefit observed:* Levetiracetam. *Possible increased plasma levels:* Strong CYP2C19 inhibitors (fluconazole, fluvoxamine). *Plasma levels decreased :* Rifampicin (consider brivaracetam dose adjustment), anti-epileptics (carbamazepine, phenobarbital, phenytoin) (no dose adjustment), St John's Wort (caution).

Effect of Brivaracetam on Other Drugs: CYP2C19 substrates (lansoprazole, omeprazole, diazepam), CYP2B6 substrates (efavirenz). OAT3 transporters: *Plasma levels may be increased.*

SP: Suicidal ideation, see Notes below. Type I hypersensitivity reported.

Pregnancy, Lactation: Pregnancy, use only if clearly necessary. Women of childbearing potential to ensure adequate contraception. Lactation, stop breastfeeding or stop drug.

ADR: Summary, *most frequent,* somnolence, dizziness; somnolence and fatigue (with increasing dose); *most frequent for discontinuation,* dizziness, convulsion.

Notes: See 3.1 Antiepileptics.

▼ **Briviact Tablets, Oral Soln, Parenteral** *(UCB)* A. GMS.
Price, tabs (14) 10mg, €42.26; (56), 25mg, 50mg, 75mg, 100mg, €158.00. Oral soln 300mL, €178.60. Parenteral 5mL (10), €352.32.
Tablet, brivaracetam 10mg, 25mg, 50mg, 75mg, 100mg. Oval (except 10mg). Marked u and strength. 10mg: Round white (off-white). 25mg: Grey. 50mg: Yellow. 75mg: Purple. 100mg: Green-grey. *Lactose* **Store:** No special conditions.
Oral soln, as above 10mg/mL. Slightly viscous, clear colourless (yellowish). *Sodium 1.16mg/mL; sorbitol, parabens.* **Store:** As above.
Injection or infusion, as above 10mg/mL. Clear colourless soln. *Sodium 3.8mg/mL.* **Store:** As above.

Ethosuximide

ATC Code: N03AD01. **Sport:** Permitted.
Driving: May impair mental and/or physical abilities.

Indications: Absence seizures when they co-exist with grand mal and other forms of epilepsy.

Dose: Adult, Elderly: Initially 500mg/day; if required increase by 250mg every 5-7 days. Control usually achieved with 1000-1500mg/day; occasionally 2000mg may be needed.

Child: Over 6 years, as for Adult above. Infants, children 0-6 years, initially 250mg/day; optimum 20mg/kg/day; max. 1000mg. Effective plasma levels range 40-100mcg/mL. Once daily; larger doses can be divided morning, evening.

Renal Impairment: Caution.

Hepatic Impairment: As for Renal above.

CI: Succinimide hypersensitivity.

Interactions: Effect of Other Drugs on Ethosuximide: *Plasma levels increased or decreased:* Valproic acid.
Effect of Ethosuximide on Other Drugs: Phenytoin: *Serum levels increased.*

SP: Blood dyscrasias may be fatal. Autoimmune disorders (SLE). Advise to contact physician if signs of infection develop (sore throat, fever).

ADR: *Common,* decreased appetite, headache, ataxia, dizziness, somnolence, abdominal pain/discomfort, GI disorder, nausea, vomiting, erythematous rash, urticaria.

Notes: See 3.1 Antiepileptics.

Zarontin Syrup 250mg/5mL *(Essential Pharma)* B. GMS.
Price, (200mL) €54.00.
Oral syrup, ethosuximide. Clear slightly yellowish/pinkish dye-free raspberry-flavour. *Sucrose, glucose.* **Store:** Below 25 deg C.

Lacosamide

ATC Code: N03AX18. **Sport:** Permitted.
Driving: Dizziness, blurred vision.

Indications: Adjunctive, partial-onset seizures with/without secondary generalisation in epileptics. Parenteral, alternative when oral temporarily not feasible.

Dose: Adult: ORAL, initially 50mg twice daily; titrate to 100mg twice daily after 1 week. Maintenance, increase by 50mg twice daily every week to max. 200mg twice daily. With or without food. Discontinuation, taper by 200mg/week.

PARENTERAL, direct dose conversion from oral. Infuse over 15-60 minutes twice daily.

Elderly: As for Renal below.

Child: Under 16 years, safety/efficacy not established.

Renal Impairment: CrCl (mL/min) above 30, no adjustment; consider 200mg loading dose; titrate further with caution; 30 and below and ESRD, max. maintenance

250mg/day (initially 100mg/day, then 50mg twice daily for one week). Haemodialysis, supplement of 50% of daily dose at end of dialysis.

Hepatic Impairment: Mild/moderate, max. 300mg/day. Consider 200mg loading dose; titrate further with caution. Severe, pharmacokinetics not evaluated; use only if benefit outweighs risk.

CI: Second or third degree AV block.

Interactions: Effect of Other Drugs on Lacosamide: *Caution:* Drugs associated with PR prolongation (carbamazepine, lamotrigine, pregabalin), Class I antiarrhythmics, strong enzyme inducers (rifampicin, St John's Wort; may reduce systemic exposure). *Formation of odesmethyl metabolite catalysed:* CYP2C9, CYP2C19, CYP3A4 (in vitro data). *Possible increased systemic exposure:* Strong CYP2C9 inhibitors (fluconazole), CYP3A4 (itraconazole, ketoconazole, ritonavir, clarithromycin).

SP: Accidental injury or falls due to dizziness. PR interval prolongation, caution with conduction problems or severe cardiac disease (MI, HF), especially elderly. Advise patients of symptoms of second-degree or higher AV block (slow or irregular pulse, feeling lightheaded, fainting), atrial fibrillation and flutter (palpitations, rapid or irregular pulse, shortness of breath); counsel to seek medical advice. Multi-organ hypersensitivity reactions (DRESS), discontinue.

ADR: *Very common,* dizziness, headache, diplopia, nausea. Incidence of CNS effects e.g. dizziness may be higher after a loading dose.

Notes: See 3.1 Antiepileptics.

Vimpat Tablets, Syrup 10mg/mL *(UCB)* B. GMS.
Price, tabs 50mg (14) €11.42. 100mg (14) €22.42. (56) €87.81. 150mg (14) €32.77; (56) €130.84. 200mg (56) €167.86. Syrup (200mL) 10mg/mL, €33.81.
Tablet, lacosamide 50mg, 100mg, 150mg, 200mg. Oval f/c. Marked SP; strength on reverse. 50mg: Pinkish. 100mg: Dark-yellow. 150mg: Salmon. 200mg: Blue. **Store:** No special conditions.
Syrup, as above. Clear slightly yellow (yellow-brown). *Parabens, sorbitol, aspartame, sodium 1.96mg/mL.* **Store:** Do not refrigerate.

Vimpat Parenteral 10mg/mL *(UCB)* A.
Price, not published by company.
Infusion, lacosamide. Clear colourless soln. *Sodium 2.99mg/mL.* **Store:** Below 25 deg C.

Lamotrigine

ATC Code: N03AX09. **Sport:** Permitted.
Driving: Dizziness, diplopia.

Indications: Monotherapy or adjunctive, partial and generalised seizures (tonic-clonic, associated with Lennox-Gastaut Syndrome (age 2 years and over). Monotherapy, typical absence seizures (age 2-12 years). Prevention, depressive mood episodes in Bipolar I disorder (age 18 years and over) where predominantly depressive episodes experienced.

Dose: Adult, Elderly: *Epilepsy, monotherapy,* initially 25mg/day (2 weeks), then 50mg/day (2 weeks), once daily; increase by max. 50-100mg every 1-2 weeks if needed; maintenance 100-200mg/day once daily or 2 divided doses; may need 500mg/day.

Adjunctive, **WITH** valproate, initially 25mg/day on alternate days (2 weeks), then 25mg once daily (2 weeks); increase by max. 25-50mg every 1-2 weeks if needed; maintenance usually 100-200mg/day once daily or 2 divided doses.

WITHOUT valproate, WITH lamotrigine glucuronidation inducers*, initially 50mg once daily (2 weeks), then 100mg/day in 2 divided doses (2 weeks); increase by max. 100mg every 1-2 weeks if needed; maintenance 200-400mg/day in 2 divided doses; may need 700mg/day. **WITHOUT** valproate, WITHOUT lamotrigine glucuronidation inducers*, initially 25mg/day (2 weeks), then 50mg/day (2 weeks), once daily; increase by max. 50-100mg every 1-2 weeks if needed; maintenance 100-200mg/day once daily or 2 divided doses.

Bipolar disorder (monotherapy OR adjunctive), **WITHOUT** valproate and WITHOUT lamotrigine glucuronidation inducers*, initially 25mg once daily (2 weeks), then 50mg once daily or 2 divided doses (2 weeks), then 100mg once daily or 2 divided doses, to max. 200mg/day (usual target dose); range 100-400mg.

93

3.1.6 Miscellaneous Antiepileptics

Adjunctive, **WITH** valproate, initially 25mg on alternate days (2 weeks), then 25mg once daily (2 weeks); then once daily or in 2 divided doses, 50-100mg/day; max. 200mg/day. **WITHOUT** valproate and **WITHOUT** lamotrigine glucuronidation inducers*, initially 50mg/day once daily (2 weeks); then in 2 divided doses, 100mg/day (2 weeks), then weekly, 200-300mg/day, 400mg/day if needed. Gradual withdrawal not required. Withdrawal of concomitant medicinals, and dosing recommendations for women taking hormonal contraceptives, see manufacturers Full Prescribing Information.

*Lamotrigine glucuronidation inducers (phenytoin, carbamazepine, phenobarbitone, primidone, rifampicin, lopinavir + ritonavir).

Child: *Epilepsy,* age 2-12 years, *monotherapy,* initially 0.3mg/kg/day (2 weeks), then 0.6mg/kg/day; titrate by max. 0.6mg/kg/day every 1-2 weeks if needed; maintenance, usually 1-15mg/kg/day; max. 200mg/day. Once daily or 2 divided doses.

Adjunctive, **WITH** valproate, initially 0.15mg/kg/day once daily (2 weeks), then 0.3mg/kg/day once daily (2 weeks). Titrate by max. of 0.3mg/kg increments every 1-2 weeks if needed; maintenance, usually 1-5mg/kg/day once daily or 2 divided doses; max. 200mg/day. **WITHOUT** valproate, **WITH** lamotrigine glucuronidation inducers*, initially 0.6mg/kg/day in 2 divided doses (2 weeks), then 1.2mg/kg/day in 2 divided doses (2 weeks). Titrate by max. 1.2mg/kg increments every 1-2 weeks if needed. Maintenance, usually 5-15mg/kg/day once daily or 2 divided doses; max. 400mg/day. **WITHOUT** valproate, WITHOUT lamotrigine glucuronidation inducers*, initially 0.3mg/kg/day (2 weeks), then 0.6mg/kg/day; titrate by max. 0.6mg/kg every 1-2 weeks; maintenance, 1-10mg/kg/day; max. 200mg/day once daily or in 2 divided doses. Under 2 years, not recommended. Withdraw gradually. Swallow tabs whole, do not chew or crush. *Lamotrigine glucuronidation inducers, see Adult above.

Bipolar Disorder, under 18 years, use not recommended (no significant efficacy; increased suicidality); over 18 years, as for Adult above.

Renal Impairment: Caution, glucuronide metabolite accumulation.

Hepatic Impairment: Reduce initial escalation and maintenance doses by 50% in mild/moderate, and by 75% in severe.

Interactions: Effect of Other Drugs on Lamotrigine: *Plasma levels decreased (initiation), increased (following withdrawal) plasma levels:* Oral contraceptives. *Enhanced rash risk; reduced metabolism, increased half-life (glucuronidation inhibited*):* Valproate. *Glucuronidation induced*:* Phenytoin, carbamazepine, phenobarbitone, primidone, rifampicin, atazanavir/ritonavir, lopinavir/ritonavir, ethinyloestradiol + levonorgestrel combination. *Glucuronidation not* induced:* Oxcarbazepine, felbamate, gabapentin, levetiracetam, pregabalin, zonisamide, lithium, bupropion, olanzapine, aripiprazole. *Co-admin with medical advice:* Other lamotrigine-containing medicinals. *Consider dose increase or decrease:* Atazanavir/ritonavir, lopinavir/ritonavir (added to lamotrigine maintenance, not taking glucuronidation inducers OR discontinued). *(significantly).

Effect of Lamotrigine on Other Drugs: Carbamazepine (reduce dose): *Dizziness, ataxia, diplopia, blurred vision, nausea.* Hormonal contraceptives: *Decreased efficacy.* Metformin, gabapentin, varenicline: *Plasma levels increased.*

SP: Skin reactions, rash e.g. Stevens-Johnson Syndrome, toxic epidermal necrolysis, DRESS (potentially fatal) reported; risk higher in children. Rash associated with high initial lamotrigine dose (excess of dose escalation) and/or valproate co-admin; may be part of hypersensitivity syndrome (fever, lymphadenopathy, facial oedema, blood/liver abnormalities; rarely, DIC, multiple organ failure; if develops, discontinue immediately; do not restart. Assess need for escalation to maintenance dose when restarting therapy. *Clinical worsening and suicide risk,* suicidal ideation/behaviour reported; monitor, advise

94

patients and caregivers to seek medical advice; bipolar disorder, monitor (initiation, dose change). Not indicated for acute treatment of manic or depressive episode.

Pregnancy, Lactation: Pregnancy, data does not suggest substantial increase in major congenital malformations risk; too limited to exclude oral cleft risk. If considered necessary, use lowest possible dose. Lactation, passes into breast milk; use if benefit outweighs risk.

ADR: *Very common,* headache, skin rash.

Notes: See 3.1 Antiepileptics.

Lamictal Tabs, Chewable/Dispersible *(GSK)* B. GMS.
Price, tabs (56) 25mg, €13.62. 50mg, €21.37. 100mg, €36.87. 200mg, €66.36. Chew/Disp 2mg (30) €6.09. 5mg (28) €4.60. (56) 25mg, €13.62. 50mg, €20.52. 100mg, €36.87. 200mg, €66.92.
Tablet, lamotrigine 25mg, 50mg, 100mg, 200mg. Pale yellowish-brown elliptical. Marked strength, GS. 25mg: Marked EC7. 50mg: Marked EE1. 100mg: Marked EE5. 200mg: Marked EE7. *Lactose.* *Chewable dispersible tablet,* as above 2mg, 5mg, 25mg, 50mg, 100mg, 200mg. White (off-white) slightly mottled elliptical (not 2mg, 5mg); blackcurrant odour. Marked with strength and GS (not 2mg). 2mg: Round. Marked LTG; 2 super-ellipses on reverse. 5mg: Elongated. Marked CL2. 25mg: Marked CL5. 50mg: Marked CX7. 100mg: Marked CL7. 200mg: Marked EC5.

Lamoro 25mg, 50mg, 100mg, 200mg *(Pinewood)* B. GMS.
Price, (60) 25mg, €11.67. 50mg, €18.32. 100mg, €31.60. 200mg, €56.87.
Dispersible tablet, lamotrigine. White (off-white) round plain both sides. *Mannitol, aspartame.*

Larig 25mg, 50mg, 100mg, 200mg *(Rowex)* B. GMS.
Price, (56) 25mg, €10.90. 50mg, €17.10. 100mg, €29.49. 200mg, €53.08.
Dispersible tablet, lamotrigine. White (off-white) modified-square. Marked L/strength. *Sorbitol.*

Levetiracetam

ATC Code: N03AX14. **Sport:** Permitted.
Driving: Minor or moderate influence (somnolence, other CNS symptoms).

Indications: Monotherapy, partial onset seizures with or without secondary generalisation, in newly diagnosed epilepsy. Adjunctive, partial onset seizures with or without secondary generalisation; myoclonic seizures in Juvenile Myoclonic Epilepsy; primary generalised tonic-clonic seizures in Idiopathic Generalised Epilepsy.

Dose: Adult: ADD-ON THERAPY (age 12 and over, weighing 50kg or more), initially 500mg twice daily (can be started on day 1 of treatment); titrate in 500mg twice daily increments every 2-4 weeks; max. 1500mg twice daily. Swallow tabs with sufficient quantity of liquid, with or without food, in 2 equally divided doses. Oral soln may be diluted in a glass of water or baby's bottle. Soln for IV infusion to be diluted in minimum 100mL of compatible diluent; admin over 15 minutes. Convert oral to IV or IV to oral directly without titration.

MONOTHERAPY (age 16 years and over), initially 250mg twice daily; titrate to 500mg twice daily after 2 weeks; if needed increase in 250mg twice daily increments every 2 weeks; max. 1500mg twice daily.

Discontinue gradually; adults and adolescents, 50kg and over, decrease by 500mg twice daily every 2-4 weeks; under 50kg and older than 6 months, decrease by max. 10mg/kg twice daily every 2 weeks; infants under 6 months, decrease by 7mg/kg twice daily every 2 weeks.

Elderly: Over 65 years, as for Renal below.

Child: ADD-ON THERAPY, infants (1 month to under 6 months), using oral soln (100mg/mL and 1mL oral syringe), initially 7mg/kg twice daily; if needed titrate by 7mg/kg twice daily every 2 weeks; max. 21mg/kg twice daily. Infants (6-23 months), children (4-11 years), adolescents (12-17 years) (under 50kg), 10-30mg/kg twice daily; (50kg and over), as for Adult above. Admin, see Adult above.

MONOTHERAPY, under 16 years, not recommended; 16 years and over, as for Adult above.

Renal Impairment: Adults and adolescents (50kg and over), CrCl (mL/min) above 80, 500-1500mg twice daily; 50-79, 500-1000mg twice daily; 30-49, 250-750mg twice daily; below 30, 250-500mg twice daily. ESRD, 250-500mg twice daily; undergoing dialysis*, 500-1000mg once daily. *(750mg loading dose recommended on day 1 of treatment; supplemental dose of 250-500mg following

dialysis). For dosing in infants, children, adolescents (under 50kg), see manufacturers Full Prescribing Information.
Hepatic Impairment: Severe, reduce daily maintenance by 50% if CrCl (mL/min) below 60.
CI: Hypersensitivity to pyrrolidone derivatives.
Interactions: Effect of Other Drugs on Levetiracetam: *Renal clearance or primary metabolite inhibited:* Probenecid. *Decreased efficacy:* Macrogol (leave 1-hour dosing interval before or after levetiracetam).
Effect of Levetiracetam on Other Drugs: Methotrexate: *Decreased clearance (monitor levels).*
SP: Suicide, see Notes below. Tablet formulation not for use in infants, children under 6 years. Acute kidney injury. Decreased blood cell counts, usually at initiation; monitor with (weakness, pyrexia, recurrent infection, coagulation disorder).
Pregnancy, Lactation: Physiological changes during pregnancy may decrease levetiracetam concentration, especially in third trimester.
ADR: Summary, *most frequent,* nasopharyngitis, somnolence, headache, fatigue, dizziness (safety profile similar across age groups).
Notes: See 3.1 Antiepileptics.

Keppra 250mg, 500mg, 1000mg, Oral Soln *(UCB)* B. GMS.
Price, tabs (60) 250mg, €21.30. 500mg, €37.36. 1000mg, €72.87. Oral soln 100mg/mL (300mL) €52.03; Syringe 150mL, (1mL syringe) €42.02; (3mL syringe) €43.22.
Tablet, levetiracetam. Oblong f/c scored. Marked UCB/strength. 250mg: Blue. 500mg: Yellow. 1000mg: White.
Oral soln, as above 100mg/mL. Clear liquid. *Parabens, maltitol.*
Store: In original bottle; protect from light.
Keppra Parenteral *(UCB)* A. HOS.
Price, (10) 100mg/mL, €124.83 (PTW).
Infusion, levetiracetam 100mg/mL. Clear colourless sterile conc for soln. *Sodium 57mg (2.5mmoL) per max. single dose.*
Levetiracetam Accord Tablets *(Accord)* B. GMS.
Price, (60) 250mg, €17.04. 500mg, €29.88. 1000mg, €58.29.
Tablet, levetiracetam 250mg, 500mg, 1000mg. Oval f/c scored (divisible into equal halves). 250mg: White. Marked L64. 500mg: Yellow. Marked L65. 1000mg: White. Marked L67.
Levetiracetam Bluefish Tablets *(Bluefish)* B. GMS.
Price, (60) 250mg, €17.04. 500mg, €29.88. 1000mg, €58.29.
Tablet, levetiracetam. Oval f/c scored (divisible into equal halves). 250mg: White (off-white). Marked L64. 500mg: Yellow. Marked L65. White (off-white). Marked L67.
Levetiracetam Clonmel Tablets *(Clonmel)* B. GMS.
Price, (60) 250mg, €17.04. 500mg, €29.88. 1000mg, €58.29.
Tablet, levetiracetam 250mg, 500mg, 1000mg. Oblong f/c with breaking notch (divisible into equal halves). 250mg: Blue. 500mg: Yellow. 1000mg: White.

Perampanel

ATC Code: N03AX22 **Sport:** Permitted.
Driving: Moderate influence; dizziness, somnolence.
Indications: Adjunctive, partial-onset seizures with/without secondary generalisation; primary generalised tonic-clonic seizures, patients with idiopathic generalised epilepsy.
Dose: Adult: Initially 2mg/day; increase by 2mg (weekly or every 2 weeks) to maintenance 4-8mg/day (partial onset seizures) OR 8mg/day (primary generalised tonic-clonic seizures). Depending on response and/or tolerability, increase to 12mg/day. *Admin,* as single oral dose at bedtime; with or without food; swallow whole with water; do not crush or chew; cannot be split. Discontinue gradually to avoid rebound seizures.
Elderly: Caution if polymedicated.
Child: Age 12 years and over, as for Adult above; under 12 years, no data.
Renal Impairment: Moderate, severe, on haemodialysis, not recommended.
Hepatic Impairment: Mild/moderate, initiate at 2mg; increase at minimum 2-week intervals; max. 8mg/day. Severe, not recommended.
Interactions: Effect of Other Drugs on Perampanel: *Plasma levels decreased:* CYP450 inducers (carbamazepine, phenytoin, oxcarbazepine, rifampicin, St John's Wort), felbamate. *Plasma levels increased:* CYP450 inhibitors (ketoconazole).
Effect of Perampanel on Other Drugs: Progestative-

containing hormonal contraceptives: *Effectiveness reduced at perampanel 12mg/day.* Midazolam: *Exposure decreased.*
SP: Increased falls (elderly). Aggressive, hostile behaviour (may be increased by CNS depressant co-admin); significant changes in mood or behaviour, reduce dose or discontinue. Potential for substance abuse.
Pregnancy, Lactation: Pregnancy, not recommended. Women of childbearing potential to ensure adequate contraception. Lactation, stop breastfeeding or stop drug.
ADR: *Very common* dizziness, somnolence.
Notes: See 3.1 Antiepileptics.

Fycompa Tablets *(Eisai)* B. GMS.
Price, (7) 2mg, €26.99. (28) 4mg, €116.63; 6mg, €120.75; 8mg, €125.80; 10mg, €130.35; 12mg, €131.30.
Tablet, perampanel 2mg, 4mg, 6mg, 8mg, 10mg, 12mg. Round f/c. Marked with strength. 2mg: Orange. Marked E275. 4mg: Red. Marked E277. 6mg: Pink. Marked E294. 8mg: Purple. Marked E295. 10mg: Green. Marked E296. 12mg: Blue. Marked E297. *Lactose.* **Store:** No special conditions.

Retigabine

ATC Code: N03AX21 **Sport:** Permitted.
Driving: Dizziness, somnolence, diplopia, blurred vision.
Indications: Adjunctive, drug-resistant partial onset seizures with/without secondary generalisation (adults) where other drug therapy not adequate or not tolerated.
Dose: Adult: Initially 300mg/day; increase by max. 150mg/week to maintenance 600-1200mg/day. *Admin,* 3 divided doses with or without food; swallow tabs whole, do not crush or chew.
Elderly: Over 65 years, initially 150mg/day; titrate by max. 150mg every week; max. 900mg/day.
Child: Under 18 years, no data.
Renal Impairment: CrCl (mL/min) below 50, reduce initial and maintenance dose by 50%; initially 150mg/day titrating by max. 50mg every week to max. 600mg/day. ESRD on dialysis, admin 3 daily doses as usual on dialysis day with single supplemental dose immediately after dialysis; breakthrough seizures towards end of dialysis, consider additional supplemental dose at start of subsequent dialysis session.
Hepatic Impairment: Moderate/severe, initially 150mg; during titration, increase by 50mg every week to max. 600mg/day.
Interactions: Effect of Other Drugs on Retigabine: *Reduced systemic exposure:* Phenytoin, carbamazepine. *Possible visual effects (blurred vision):* ALCOHOL.
Effect of Retigabine on Other Drugs: Digoxin: *Plasma levels may be increased.* Anaesthetics (thiopental sodium): *Increased duration.*
SP: Ocular tissue (including retina) pigment changes (discolouration); reversibility of retinal pigmentation after discontinuation reported; sometimes pigment changes of skin, lips, nails. Macular abnormality with features of vitelliform maculopathy identified. Vision abnormalities (field constriction, loss of central sensitivity, reduced visual acuity) reported. Perform comprehensive ophthalmic examination at baseline, then every 6 months.
Urinary retention, dysuria, hesitation, caution. QT-interval prolongation with other drugs prolonging QT-interval, CHF, ventricular hypertrophy, hypokalaemia, hypomagnesaemia, over 65 years; recommend ECG before initiation. May interfere with laboratory tests for serum/urine bilirubin.
ADR: *Most frequent (leading to discontinuation),* dizziness, somnolence, fatigue, confusional state. For pigment changes, see SP above.
Notes: See 3.1 Antiepileptics.

Trobalt Tablets *(GSK)* B. GMS.
Price, 50mg (21) €5.23; (84) €20.88. 100mg (21) €10.23; (84) €40.91. (84) 200mg, €80.35. 300mg, €119.73. 400mg, €149.21. Initiation Pack: 50mg x 21 + 100mg x 42, €25.36.
Tablet, retigabine 50mg, 100mg, 200mg, 300mg, 400mg. Round (50mg, 100mg), oblong (200mg, 300mg, 400mg) f/c. Marked RTG and strength. 50mg, 400mg: Purple. 100mg, 300mg: Green. 200mg: Yellow.

3.1.6 Miscellaneous Antiepileptics

Topiramate

ATC Code: N03AX11. **Sport:** Permitted.

Driving: Drowsiness, dizziness, visual disturbances, blurred vision.

Indications: Partial onset seizures with or without secondary generalised and primary generalised tonic-clonic seizures, monotherapy; adjunctive, for seizures associated with Lennox-Gastaut Syndrome. Migraine prophylaxis, intolerant or unresponsive to other treatment.

Dose: Adult, Elderly: *Epilepsy, monotherapy*, initially 25mg at night (1 week); increase by 25-50mg/day at 1-2 week intervals to 100-200mg/day; max 500mg/day; refractory forms, may require up to 1000mg/day. *Adjunctive*, as above; minimum effective, 200mg/day; range 200-400mg/day. *Admin*, in 2 divided doses.

Migraine, initially 25mg nightly (1 week); increase by 25mg/day at 1-week intervals to recommended 100mg/day in 2 divided doses; 50mg/day has been beneficial; up to 200mg/day has been used. *Admin*, swallow tabs whole with or without food or sprinkle the contents of a capsule on a small amount (1 teaspoon) of soft food and swallow immediately.

Child: *Epilepsy, monotherapy*, 6 years and over, initially 0.5-1mg/kg nightly for 1 week; titrate at 1-2 week intervals by 0.5-1mg/kg/day; initial target dose 100mg/day (about 2mg/kg/day in children 6-16 years). *Adjunctive*, 2 years and above, initially 25mg nightly or less, based on range 1-3mg/kg/day for 1 week; titrate at 1-2 week intervals by 1-3mg/kg/day to achieve response; up to 30mg/kg/day been well tolerated. Children over 16 years, as for Adult above. Admin in 2 divided doses.

Renal Impairment: CrCl (mL/min) 70 or less, caution; admin half usual starting and maintenance dose. Haemodialysis, admin on dialysis days, supplemental dose (half daily dose), in divided doses, at beginning and end of dialysis.

Hepatic Impairment: Moderate/severe, caution.

Interactions: Effect of Other Drugs on Topiramate: *Co-admin not recommended*: CNS depressants, ALCOHOL. *Decreased plasma levels*: Phenytoin, carbamazepine, St John's Wort. *Adjust dose*: Hydrochlorothiazide. *Nephrolithiasis risk*: Nephrolithiasis predisposing agents. *Co-admin (hyperammonaemia, hypothermia)*: Valproic acid.

Effect of Topiramate on Other Drugs: Phenytoin, carbamazepine, valproic acid, phenobarbital, primidone: *Occasional changes in plasma levels*. Digoxin, metformin, pioglitazone, glyburide, lithium: *Monitor*. Oral contraceptives: *Decreased efficacy, breakthrough bleeding*.

SP: Ensure adequate hydration to reduce nephrolithiasis risk, heat-related adverse events. Nephrolithiasis predisposition, hypercalciuria history; increased renal stone formation risk, renal colic/pain, flank pain.

Acute myopia with secondary angle-closure glaucoma (decreased visual acuity and/or ocular pain, bilateral myopia, anterior chamber shallowing, hyperaemia, increased IOP with or without mydriasis, supraciliary effusion, anterior displacement of lens and iris). Visual field defects reported independent of elevated IOP. Weight loss or inadequate gain (consider dietary supplement). Altered laboratory tests.

Reported with topiramate treatment: Hyperchloraemic, non-anion gap, metabolic acidosis (decreased serum bicarbonate without respiratory alkalosis); acidosis predisposing factors (renal disease, severe respiratory disorders, status epilepticus, diarrhoea, surgery, ketogenic diet) may be additive to bicarbonate lowering effect. Hyperammonaemia with/without encephalopathy (dose-related); more frequent with valproic acid co-admin.

Pregnancy, Lactation: Contraindicated if not using a highly effective contraception method.

ADR: *Very common*, nasopharyngitis, depression, paraesthesia, somnolence, dizziness, nausea, diarrhoea, fatigue, weight increase/decrease.

Notes: See 3.1. Antiepileptics. See 4.1.3 Migraine Prophylaxis for other drugs used.

Topamax Tablets, Sprinkle Cap *(Janssen-Cilag)* B. GMS.
Price, tabs (60) 25mg, €13.59. 50mg, €22.82. 100mg, €42.41. 200mg, €78.92. Sprinkle (60) 15mg, €13.18. 25mg, €15.16.
Tablet, topiramate 25mg, 50mg, 100mg, 200mg. Round f/c. Marked TOP; strength on reverse. 25mg: White. 50mg: Light-yellow. 100mg: Yellow. 200mg: Salmon. *Lactose*. **Store:** Below 25 deg C; original pack to protect (moisture).
Sprinkle capsule, as above 15mg, 25mg. Hard gelatin; contains small white (off-white) spheres. White/clear. Marked TOP/strength. *Sucrose*. **Store:** As above.

Valproate Sodium

ATC Code: N03AG01. **Sport:** Permitted.

Driving: Drowsiness (especially in combination).

Indications: Epilepsy (generalized, partial, other), manic episode in bipolar disorder (lithium contraindicated, not tolerated). Parenteral (IV), short-term (oral not possible).

Dose: Adult: ORAL, *epilepsy, monotherapy*, initially 600mg/day (10-15mg/kg); titrate by 200mg at 3-day intervals to range 1000-2000mg/day (20-30mg/kg); max. 2500mg/day. Above 50mg/kg*. Adjunctive, with liver enzyme inducers (phenytoin, phenobarbitone, carbamazepine), increase by 5-10mg/kg/day.

Bipolar disorder, initially 750mg/day (20mg/kg/day); maintenance, 1000-2000mg/day. Above 45mg/kg/day*. *Admin*, 2 divided doses; coated tabs, swallow whole; Prolonged/R, admin once or twice daily; swallow tabs whole; tabs/granules, do not crush or chew; uncoated tabs may be crushed.

PARENTERAL, already treated, continue current dose OR 400-800mg (up to 10mg/kg) by continuous or repeated infusion; max. 2500mg/day. *Admin*, direct, slow (over 3-5 minutes) IV injection or infusion using separate IV line. Replace with oral as soon as possible.

NOTE: If adequate control achieved, Epilim Chrono formulations are interchangeable with other Epilim conventional or Prolonged/R formulations on equivalent daily dose basis. *Female* children, adolescents, women of childbearing potential, for specialist initiation (other treatments ineffective, not tolerated; consider risk/benefit). Preferably monotherapy, at lowest effective dose, possibly Prolonged/R formulation to avoid high peak plasma conc; daily dose divided into at least 2 doses. *(monitor carefully)*. See Pregnancy below.

Elderly: Adjust according to clinical response.

Child: ORAL, epilepsy, *over 20kg*, initially 400mg/day (irrespective of weight). Titrate until control is achieved, dose usually 20-30mg/kg/day; max. 35mg/kg/day; *under 20kg*, initially 20mg/kg/day; increase only if plasma valproic acid levels can be monitored; over 40mg/kg/day, monitor; under 3 years, monotherapy recommended. Manic episodes in bipolar disorder, under 18 years, no data.
PARENTERAL IV, range 20-30mg/kg/day. If monitoring available increase to 40mg/kg/day. Over 40mg/kg/day, monitor. Admin, see Adult above.

Renal Impairment: Consider dose adjustment.

Hepatic Impairment: Caution. Severe, contraindicated.

CI: Active liver disease, porphyria; mitochondrial disorders (Alpers-Huttenlocher Syndrome), children under age 2 years suspected of having mitochondrial disorders; urea cycle disorders.

Interactions: Effect of Other Drugs on Valproate: *Plasma levels increased (free valproic acid)*: Highly protein bound agents (salicylates, acetylsalicylic acid). *Decreased plasma levels*: Phenytoin, phenobarbital, carbamazepine, carbepenem antibiotics, (imipenem, meropenem, panipenem; co-admin not recommended), rifampicin. *Increased plasma levels*: Felbamate (decreased clearance), cimetidine, erythromycin. *Increased metabolism, convulsing effect*: Mefloquine, chloroquine. *Decreased absorption*: Colestyramine. *Encephalopathy and/or hyperammonaemia (with co-admin)*: Topiramate (monitor carefully).

Effect of Valproate on Other Drugs: Neuroleptics (antipsychotics), MAOIs, antidepressants, benzodiazepines: *Effect potentiated*. Phenobarbital, primidone: *Increased plasma levels, increased sedation*. Phenytoin: *Plasma levels decreased, phenytoin free-form increased (possible overdose symptoms); clinical* monitoring recommended. Carbamazepine, zidovudine: Toxic effects potentiated. Lamotrigine: Metabolism reduced, half-life increased; toxicity risk. Warfarin, other coumarins (Vitamin K dependent anticoagulants): Anticoagulant effect increased. Felbamate: Mean clearance decreased.

SP: Females, see Dose above, see also Pregnancy below. Severe hepatic failure reported (infants and young children most at risk); signs are non-specific, sudden onset (asthenia, malaise, anorexia, lethargy, oedema, drowsiness, repeated vomiting, abdominal pain), epilepsy, recurrence of seizures, withdraw immediately. Pancreatitis, severe (young at risk). Blood tests (prior to initiation, before surgery, with spontaneous bruising).

SLE, use if benefit outweighs risk. Hyperammonaemia, metabolic investigations before initiation. Weight gain. Extrapyramidal disorders which may not be reversible (including Parkinsonism). ALCOHOL intake not recommended. Long-term use, decreased bone mineral density reported.

Pregnancy, Lactation: Pregnancy, not for use in women of childbearing potential or pregnant women unless alternatives are ineffective or not tolerated because of its high teratogenic potential (developmental disorder risk in infants exposed in utero); weigh risk/benefit. Inform female patient (risk with use during pregnancy, need for effective contraception, regular treatment review, to seek medical advice if planning or becomes pregnant). If used during pregnancy, use lowest effective dose divided through the day or Prolonged/R formulations; initiate prenatal monitoring, folate supplements (may decrease risk of neural tube defects). Children exposed in utero at high risk of serious developmental disorders and/or congenital malformations. If taking valproate, recommended that women are enrolled in the Irish Epilepsy & Pregnancy Register, Freephone 1800 320 820. Lactation, breastfeeding can be envisaged.

ADR: Very common, nausea, tremor.

Notes: See 3.1 Antiepileptics.

▼ **Epilim Tablets (Enteric Coated, Crushable, Chrono), Chronosphere Granules, Oral Soln** (SANOFI) B. GMS.
Price, tabs (100) 200mg, €7.10. 500mg, €14.09. Crushable (100) 100mg, €4.98. Chrono (100) 200mg, €8.91. 300mg, €13.01. 500mg, €20.30. Chronosphere Granules (30) 100mg, €3.07; 250mg, €4.33; 500mg, €7.65.
Tablet, sodium valproate (Enteric) 200mg, 500mg, (Crushable) 100mg. Crushable: White (off-white) round flat scored (facilitates breaking). Enteric Coated g/r: Lilac. **Store:** Below 30 deg C (Enteric Coated), 25 deg C (Crushable); original pack; leave tabs in foil until just before admin.
Prolonged/R granules and tablet, sodium valproate, valproic acid (Chronosphere Granules) 100mg, 250mg, 500mg; (Chrono) tablet 200mg, 300mg, 500mg. Granules: Off-white (slightly yellow), waxy; in sachet. Tablet (Chrono): Violet oblong f/c. **Store:** Below 25 deg C (granules); below 30 deg C and then as above (Chrono). Oral soln or syrup, as above 200mg/5mL. Clear red cherry flavour. Parabens, sorbitol, Ponceau 4R; sucrose (syrup).
▼ **Epilim Parenteral** (SANOFI) A. HOS.
Price, (1) 400mg, €7.74 (PTW).
Injection or infusion, sodium valproate 400mg/vial. Sterile off-white freeze dried powder and solvent for soln (95mg/mL). **Store:** Below 25 deg C.

Zonisamide

ATC Code: N03AX15. **Sport:** Permitted.
Driving: Drowsiness, concentration difficulty.
Indications: Treatment of partial seizures, with or without secondary generalisation as monotherapy (adults, newly diagnosed epilepsy) or adjunctive (age 6 years and older).

Dose: Adult, Elderly: MONOTHERAPY, initially 100mg once daily (week 1 + 2), then 200mg/day (week 3 + 4), then 300mg/day (week 5 + 6); maintenance 300mg/day; if higher dose needed, increase at 2-week intervals, in 100mg increments; max. 500mg/day.
ADJUNCTIVE, with CYP3A4 inducers, initially 50mg/day in 2 divided doses (week 1), then 100mg/day in 2 divided doses (week 2), then increase at weekly intervals, in 100mg increments (week 3-5); maintenance usually 300-500mg/day (once daily or 2 divided doses). Without CYP3A4 inducers OR with renal or hepatic impairment, initially 50mg/day in 2 divided doses (week 1+2), then

100mg/day in 2 divided doses (week 3+4), then increase at weekly intervals, in 100mg increments (week 5-10); maintenance usually 300-500mg/day (once daily or 2 divided doses). Elderly, caution. Admin, with/without food.
Child: Age 6 years and above, adjunctive with CYP3A4 inducers, 1mg/kg/day (week 1) then increase at weekly intervals by 1mg/kg; maintenance, (weight 20-55kg), 6-8mg/kg/day, (weight above 55kg), 300-500mg/day. Without CYP3A4 inducers, 1mg/kg/day (weeks 1 + 2), then increase at 2-weekly intervals by 1mg/kg; maintenance, (weight 20-55kg), 6-8mg/kg/day, (weight above 55kg), 300-500mg/day. Admin once daily.

Renal Impairment: Caution. Acute renal failure, significant impairment, sustained increase in serum creatinine, discontinue. See Dose above.
Hepatic Impairment: Severe, not recommended. Mild/moderate, caution. See Dose above.
CI: Hypersensitivity to sulfonamides.
Interactions: Effect of Other Drugs on Zonisamide: Increased urolithiasis risk: Drugs causing urolithiasis. Dose adjustment: Phenytoin, carbamazepine, phenobarbitone, rifampicin (potent enzyme inducers). Increased body temp: Carbonic anhydrase inhibitors (topiramate), anticholinergics.

Effect of Zonisamide on Other Drugs: Carbonic anhydrase inhibitors (topiramate): Insufficient data to exclude interactions.
SP: Serious rash, including Stevens-Johnson syndrome (SJS); additional caution with other antiepileptics as they may also induce skin rash. SJS and Drug-Induced Hypersensitivity Syndrome (DIHS) more common, 65 years and over. Immune-based reactions to sulfonamides (rash, allergic reaction, major haematological disturbances; zonisamide contains sulfonamide group). Urolithiasis, increased (fluid intake, urine output) may reduce risk; pancreatitis, muscle pain/weakness (monitor for muscle damage markers). Decreased sweating, elevated body temperature, mainly paediatrics (keep child cool, avoid heavy exercise, hydrate; especially in hot weather). Hyperchloraemic, non-anion gap, metabolic acidosis; risk appears more frequent and severe in younger patients. See Interactions above.
ADR: Very common, anorexia, agitation, irritability, confusional state, depression, ataxia, dizziness, memory impairment, somnolence, diplopia, decreased bicarbonate.
Notes: See 3.1 Antiepileptics.
Zonegran 25mg, 50mg, 100mg (Eisai) A. GMS.
Price, (14) 25mg, €9.94. (56) 50mg, €52.68; 100mg, €70.39.
Capsule, zonisamide. Hard opaque. Marked Zonegran/strength. 25mg: White/white. 50mg: White/grey. 100mg: White/red; Sunset Yellow E110, Allura Red E129.

3.2 - Antipsychotics and Antimanics

Class Effects
Driving: Inform patient of effects of this medication on reaction time and may cause side effects that may impair driving (dizziness, drowsiness, sleepiness, blurred/double vision, reduced alertness); advise not to drive until effect of medication is known; not to drink alcohol or use other psychoactive substances when taking this medicine.
Interactions: Effect of Other Drugs on Antipsychotics: Increased QT-prolongation: Drugs increasing QT-interval, Class Ia antiarrhythmics (quinidine, hydroquinidine, disopyramide), Class III antiarrhythmics (amiodarone, sotalol, dofetilide, ibutilide), certain neuroleptics including phenothiazines (chlorpromazine, cyamemazine, thioridazine), benzamides (amisulpride, sulpiride, tiapride), butyrophenones (droperidol, haloperidol), other neuroleptics (pimozide); other agents: bepridil, cisapride, diphemanil, mizolastine, vincamine IV, macrolides (erythromycin), antihistamines (terfenadine, astemizole), quinolones (gatifloxacin, moxifloxacin, sparfloxacin), halofantrine, pentamidine.
SP: Suicide, occurrence of suicidal behaviour is inherent in psychotic illness, either early after initiation or with therapy switch; close supervision, see Notes below (antidepressants). With antipsychotic treatment,

3.2.1 Phenothiazines

improvement in clinical condition may take several days to some weeks; monitor. Increased cerebrovascular adverse events seen in dementia population with some atypical antipsychotics (cannot exclude for other antipsychotics or patient populations). *Neuroleptic Malignant Syndrome (NMS)* (hyperthermia, muscle rigidity, autonomic instability, altered consciousness, elevated CPK) is associated with neuroleptics; hyperthermia, discontinue all antipsychotics. *Hormonal,* hyperprolactinaemia may be associated with galactorrhoea, gynaecomastia, oligomenorrhoea, amenorrhoea. Impaired sexual function, erection, ejaculation; increased libido. Leucopenia, neutropenia, agranulocytosis reported with antipsychotics (monitor). *Elderly with dementia,* treated with antipsychotics (typical, atypical) at increased risk of death, incidence of cerebrovascular adverse events, venous thromboembolism (VTE) including pulmonary embolism and DVT; hypotension or sedation risk. Consider dose reduction with renal insufficiency. Cases of sudden death reported with antipsychotics.

Withdrawal, acute withdrawal symptoms including nausea, vomiting, sweating, insomnia with abrupt cessation; recurrence of psychotic symptoms, emergence of involuntary movement disorders (akathisia, dystonia, dyskinesia). Always withdraw gradually.

Pregnancy, Lactation: Newborns of mothers treated with neuroleptics/antipsychotics in late pregnancy (third trimester) or during labour may show signs of intoxication (lethargy, tremor, hyper-excitability; have a low Apgar score); extrapyramidal and/or withdrawal symptoms; monitor. Agitation, hypertonia, hypotonis, somnolence, respiratory distress, feeding disorder reported; bradycardia, tachycardia, meconium ileus, delayed meconium passage, abdominal bloating.

Notes: See 3.3 Antidepressants and Anxiolytics.

3.2.1 - Phenothiazines

In This Chapter: *Chlorpromazine, fluphenazine, levomepromazine, prochlorperazine, trifluoperazine.*

Class Effects

Typical antipsychotics include phenothiazines. Phenothiazines have pronounced sedative, antimuscarinic and extrapyramidal effects; are also use in the management of allergic states and as anti-emetics, see Notes below (sedating antihistamines).

CI: Hypersensitivity to any member of the class. Children, not recommended unless otherwise specified.

Interactions: Effect of Other Drugs on Phenothiazines: *Decreased GI absorption:* Antacids (admin 2 hours apart). *Increased CNS depression (increased sedation):* ALCOHOL, hypnotics, sedatives, analgesics, narcotics. *Enhanced anticholinergic effects:* Anti-Parkinsonian drugs, other anticholinergics. *Avoid:* Drugs prolonging QT-interval.

Effect of Phenothiazines on Other Drugs: Beta-blockers (plasma levels mutually increased), thiazides, ACEIs, other antihypertensives: *Enhanced hypotensive effect.* Guanethidine, clonidine: *Antihypertensive action blocked.* Adrenaline, other sympathomimetics, anti-Parkinsonian effect of L-Dopa, anticonvulsants: *Effect antagonised.* TCADs: *Metabolism impaired (mutually increased plasma levels).* Antidiabetic agents: *Altered control.* Oral anticoagulants: *Effect diminished.* Quinidine, other antiarrhythmics: *Enhanced cardiac-depressant effects.* Corticosteroids, digoxin, neuromuscular blockers: *Enhanced absorption.* Lithium: *Increased extrapyramidal side effects, neurotoxicity.*

SP: *Suicide,* NMS, VTE, Elderly with Dementia, see Notes below (antipsychotics). *Extrapyramidal,* symptoms may occur; tardive dyskinesia (greater risk in elderly, especially female); likely to be severe in children. *Caution,* existing liver disease, jaundice. Cardiac arrhythmias, subarachnoid haemorrhage, mitral insufficiency, risk factors for (stroke, cardiovascular disease), history of QT-prolongation (drugs prolonging QT-interval, monitor ECG), hypotension. Metabolic abnormalities e.g. including hypo- (kalaemia, calcaemia, magnesaemia), starvation, modification of insulin and glucose response (monitor). Alcohol abuse,

hyperthyroidism, thyrotoxicosis, myasthenia gravis, prostatic hypertrophy, phaeochromocytoma, blood dyscrasias, VTE. Extremes of temperature (phenothiazines interfere with thermoregulation). CNS, depression, epilepsy, conditions predisposing to convulsions (alcohol withdrawal, brain damage, organic brain syndrome), caution, may lower seizure threshold. Parkinson's' disease. Severe respiratory disease.

Prolonged use, monitor eye changes, haemapoeisis, liver function, myocardial conduction defects.

Pregnancy, Lactation: Pregnancy, if considered essential by physician. Use lowest possible dose for the shortest duration. Lactation, not recommended. Effect on neonates, see Notes below (antipsychotics).

ADR: Most commonly, CNS related. Drowsiness, seizures; extrapyramidal symptoms, Parkinsonian signs and/or symptoms (hypersalivation, tremor, gait/speech abnormalities, dysphagia); tardive dyskinesia (rhythmical involuntary movements of tongue, face, mouth, jaw); depression, sedation, agitation, drowsiness, insomnia, headache, confusion, vertigo, grand mal seizures, exacerbation of psychotic symptoms, paradoxical effects of excitement. GI (constipation, nausea, vomiting, dry mouth, anorexia, dyspepsia, paralytic ileus, appetite/weight changes). Hyperprolactinaemia, may cause galactorrhoea, gynaecomastia, oligo- or amenorrhoea. Cardiac (coronary insufficiency, hypotension including postural, tachycardia, syncope; myocardial conduction defects, QT-prolongation, ventricular arrhythmia, cardiac arrest, Torsades de pointes). Blood dyscrasias, leucopenia. Pruritus, photosensitivity. Long-term use, monitor eye changes, retinal artery occlusion. ED, altered sexual function, loss of libido, priapism. Liver (jaundice, elevated liver enzymes). Hypoglycaemia and/or diabetes. Syndrome of inappropriate ADH secretion; peripheral oedema, erythema, swelling, tender lumps; altered body temperature regulation, renal failure (caution), sudden death. Anticholinergic effects (blurred vision, urinary retention, decreased sweating).

Notes: See 3.2 Antipsychotics, Antimanics. See 5.7.1 Sedating Antihistamines.

Chlorpromazine

ATC Code: N05AA01. **Sport:** Permitted.
Driving: Not recommended.

Indications: Management, anxiety and tension, agitation, depression, behavioural disturbances and subnormality, schizophrenia, other psychoses (mania and hypomania, psychopathy). Terminal illness, nausea and vomiting, senile irritability, intractable hiccup, eclampsia and pre-eclampsia. Pre- and post-anaesthetic, pre-medication, adjunctive to anaesthesia, and induction of hypothermia. Control of central effects of certain drugs (LSD).

Dose: Adult: *Psychiatric,* ORAL, initially 25mg 3-times daily or 75mg at bedtime; titrate daily by 25mg increments if required; usual range 75-300mg/day; up to 1g/day may be required. PARENTERAL (if available), acute symptom relief, 25-50mg by deep IM injection every 6-8 hours. *Hiccups,* ORAL, 25-50mg 3-4 times daily. PARENTERAL, 25-50mg by slow infusion. *Induction of hypothermia* to prevent shivering, IM; 25-50mg every 6-8 hours. *Nausea and vomiting* of terminal illness, ORAL and IM, 10-25mg every 4-6 hours.

Elderly: Psychiatric, nausea and vomiting of terminal illness, ORAL, one third to one half Adult dose; uptitrate gradually. PARENTERAL (IM), use lowest Adult dose.

Child: *Psychiatric,* ORAL, age 1-5 years, 0.5mg/kg every 4-6 hours; max. 40mg/day; 6-12 years, one third to one half adult dose; max. 75mg/day. PARENTERAL (IM), age 1-12 years, 0.5mg/kg 6-8 hours; max. 40mg/day. *Induction of hypothermia,* IM, age 1-12 years, initially 0.5-1mg/kg; maintenance 0.5mg/kg every 4-6 hours. *Nausea and vomiting of terminal illness,* ORAL and IM, age 1-12 years, 0.5mg/kg every 4-6 hours; max. 40mg/day (1-5 years), 75mg/day (6-12 years). Under 1 year, not recommended unless life-saving.

CI: Risk of angle-closure glaucoma, urinary retention. Coma due to direct CNS depressants (alcohol, barbiturates, opiates). Concomitant haemotoxic drugs. Parkinson's except under exceptional circumstances.

Interactions: Effect of Chlorpromazine on Other Drugs: Drugs prolonging QT-interval (antidepressants, other antipsychotics): *Increased arrhythmia risk.* CNS depressants (ALCOHOL, anaesthetics), antihypertensives, anticholinergics: *Effects accentuated.* Desferrixoamine: *Co-admin caution (transient metabolic encephalopathy/loss of consciousness observed with co-admin of prochlorpromazine).*

Pregnancy, Lactation: Labour, withhold until labour established and cervix dilated 3-4cm.

Notes: See 3.2.1 Phenothiazines.

Clonactil 25mg, 50mg, 100mg *(Clonmel)* B. GMS.
Price, (250) 25mg, €11.55. 50mg, €19.42. 100mg, €34.68.
Tablet, chlorpromazine HCl. White f/c. Marked name/strength.
Chlorpromazine Elixir *(Pinewood)* B. GMS.
Price, (1L) €3.00
Oral soln, chlorpromazine 25mg/5mL. Amber-brown; spearmint odour/flavour.

Fluphenazine

ATC Code: N05AB02. **Sport:** Permitted.
Driving: Not recommended.

Indications: Long-term management, chronic schizophrenia, disturbed elderly, severe anxiety tension states, personality disorders. Not indicated for nonpsychotic disorders for short-term therapy.

Dose: Adult: Initially 12.5mg, then 25mg every 2-4 weeks; range 12.5mg to max. 100mg. If doses above 50mg are needed, increase succeeding doses cautiously by 12.5mg Deep IM.

Elderly: Initially 6.25mg.

Renal Impairment: Failure, not recommended.

Hepatic Impairment: Caution. As for Renal above.

CI: Cerebral atherosclerosis, phaeochromocytoma, severe cardiac insufficiency, concomitant hypnotics, existing blood dyscrasias, subcortical brain damage. Cross sensitivity may occur with other phenothiazines.

Interactions: Effect of Other Drugs on Fluphenazine: *Co-admin contraindicated:* CNS depressants. *Effects increased/prolonged:* CYP450 2D6 substrates or inhibitors including anti-arrhythmics, SSRIs, TCADs, antipsychotics, beta-blockers, protease inhibitors, opiates, cimetidine, ecstasy (MDMA).

Effect of Fluphenazine on Other Drugs: Metrizamide: *Discontinue fluphenazine decanoate 48 hours prior to or for 24 hours after melopgraphy; metrizamide-induced seizures.*

SP: Not shown to be effective in management of behavioural complications in mentally retarded patients. Severely agitated patients may be treated initially with a rapid-action phenothiazine (gluphenazine); when acute symptoms subside, 25mg of *Modecate* may be admin. Respiratory disease, narrow angle glaucoma, elderly, myasthenia gravis, prostatic hypertrophy. *Caution*, with liver disease, cardiac arrhythmias, mitral insufficiency

ADR: *Most frequent,* extrapyramidal symptoms.

Notes: See 3.2.1 Phenothiazines.

Modecate Parenteral *(BMS)* A. GMS.
Price, (1) €30.24.
Injection, fluphenazine decanoate 25mg/mL, (conc) 100mg/mL. Clear yellow oily conc soln. *Benzyl alcohol 15mg/mL, sesame oil.*
Notes: Patient to carry treatment card indicating dose.

Levomepromazine

ATC Code: N05AA02. **Sport:** Permitted.
Driving: Not recommended.

Indications: Treatment, schizophrenia, other major psychoses (mania, hypomania). Adjunctive, severe terminal pain with accompanying anxiety, restlessness or distress.

Dose: Adult, Elderly: Usually 12.5-25mg IM or IV (after dilution with equal volume normal saline); severe agitation, up to 50mg every 6-8 hours. Continuous SC infusion, 25-200mg/day over 24-hour period via syringe driver.

CI: Coma (particularly associated with CNS depressants).

Risk of (closed angle glaucoma, urinary retention related to urethroprostatic disorders), agranulocytosis.

Interactions: Effect of Other Drugs on Levopromazine: *Co-admin contraindicated:* Haemotoxic drugs, dopaminergic agonists (amantadine, apomorphine, bromocriptine, cabergoline, entacapone, lisuride, pergolide, piribedil, pramipexole, quinagolide, ropinirole): except in Parkinson's Disease (but co-admin inadvisable). See Notes below.

Effect of Levopromazine on Other Drugs: Drugs metabolised by CYP450 2D6: *Increased plasma levels.*

Pregnancy, Lactation: Pregnancy, women of childbearing potential not using contraception, not recommended. Lactation, contraindicated.

ADR: *Starting at low doses,* postural hypotension, anticholinergic effects, sedation or drowsiness, indifference, anxiety, mood changes. *At higher doses,* early onset dyskinesia, extrapyramidal syndrome, tardive dyskinesia, hyperprolactinaemia, altered (temperature regulation, glucose tolerance), weight gain.

Notes: See 3.2.1 Phenothiazines.

Nozinan Parenteral *(SANOFI)* A. GMS.
Price, (10) €9.31.
Injection or infusion, levomepromazine HCl 25mg/mL. Clear bright pale-yellow soln. *Sulphite.* **Store:** Below 25 deg C; amp in outer carton.

Prochlorperazine

ATC Code: N05AB04. **Sport:** Permitted.
Driving: Drowsiness.

Indications: Acute vertigo (Meniere's syndrome), nausea and vomiting, migraine, anxiety states, phobias, schizophrenia, acute mania, similar psychotic reactions.

Dose: Adult: ORAL, *Meniere's Syndrome, nausea and vomiting,* 10-40mg/day. *Schizophrenia, other psychoses,* 75-100mg/day. Divided doses.
PARENTERAL (IM), *migraine, nausea and vomiting,* 12.5mg then oral after 6 hours if needed. *Schizophrenia, psychotic disorders,* 25-75mg. *Admin,* divided doses.

Elderly: Caution, use lowest dose.

Child: Contraindicated (dystonic reactions after cumulative 0.5mg/kg dose).

Renal Impairment: Avoid.

Hepatic Impairment: Contraindicated.

Interactions: Effect of Prochlorperazine on Other Drugs: *Co-admin (transient metabolic encephalopathy; loss of consciousness):* Deforoxamine.

SP: Agranulocytosis; unexplained fever, caution NMS.

Notes: See 3.2.1 Phenothiazines. For other drugs used, see 4.1 Migraine.

Stemetil 5mg, 25mg *(SANOFI)* B. GMS.
Price, 5mg (250) €11.98. 25mg (56) €6.97.
Tablet, prochlorperazine maleate. Off-white (pale-cream) smooth almost matt. Marked Stemetil/strength. *Lactose.*
Stemetil Parenteral 12.5mg/mL *(SANOFI)* A. GMS.
Price, (10) 12.5mg/mL, 1mL, €4.35. 2mL, €5.49.
Injection, prochlorperazine mesilate. Clear bright almost colourless (very pale-yellow). *Sulphite.*

Trifluoperazine

ATC Code: N05AB06. **Sport:** Permitted.
Driving: Drowsiness, dizziness, visual disturbances.

Indications: Low dose, management of anxiety states (short-term, adjunctive), symptomatic treatment of nausea and vomiting; high dose, treatment of symptoms and relapse prevention in schizophrenia and other psychoses especially of paranoid type but not depressive psychoses.

Dose: Adult, Elderly: *Low dose,* 2-4mg/day; may be increased to 6mg/day. *High dose,* initially 5mg twice daily; may be increased to 15mg/day after 1 week; further 5mg increases may be made at 3-day intervals; max. 30mg/day. After satisfactory control, reduce gradually to effective maintenance. *Elderly* and frail, reduce starting dose by at least half.

Child: Age 6-12 years, low dose, 1-4mg/day. High dose requirements, 5mg/day; increase with caution at minimum 3-day intervals. Divided doses.

99

3.2.2   Other Typical Antipsychotics

Hepatic Impairment: Liver dysfunction, jaundice, liver disease, not recommended.

CI: Coma (especially due to other CNS depressants), existing blood dyscrasias, uncontrolled cardiac decompression, liver damage. See Interactions below.

Interactions: Effect of Other Drugs on Trifluoperazine: *Co-admin contraindicated*: Cytotoxics, other haemotoxic drugs. *Co-admin avoid*: Neuroleptics.

SP: Tardive dyskinesia, NMS, discontinue. Eye changes (pigmentary retinopathy), haemapoeisis, liver function, myocardial conduction defects. Bone marrow suppression, jaundice with previous phenothiazines, use if benefit outweighs risk. Angina pectoris, narrow angle glaucoma, myasthenia gravis, prostatic hypertrophy, risk factors for stroke, caution. Hyperpigmentation.

ADR: Extrapyramidal symptoms more common at higher doses; likely to be severe in children.

Notes: See 3.2.1 Phenothiazines.

> Stelazine 1mg, 5mg, Syrup *(Concordia)* B. GMS.
> Price, (112) 1mg, €2.97. 5mg, €4.23. Syrup (200mL) €2.08.
> Tablet, trifluoperazine HCl. Blue f/c. 1mg: Marked FW231. 5mg: Marked FW241. Sucrose.
> Oral syrup, as above 1mg/5mL. Clear yellow; peach aroma. Sorbitol, Sunset Yellow.

3.2.2 - Other Typical Antipsychotics

In This Chapter: *Flupenthixol, haloperidol, zuclopenthixol.*

Class Effects

CI: Children unless otherwise specified.

SP: Suicide, NMS, Elderly with dementia, VTE, see Notes below (antipsychotics). Extrapyramidal effects, tardive dyskinesia, see Notes below (phenothiazines).

Pregnancy, Lactation: Pregnancy, only if considered essential (risk/benefit). Lactation, if essential (risk/benefit); passes into breast milk. See Notes below (antipsychotics).

Notes: See 3.2.1 Phenothiazines. See 3.2. Antipsychotics, Antimanics.

Flupenthixol Decanoate

ATC Code: N05AF01. **Sport:** Permitted.
Driving: Impairment in general attention and concentration.
Indications: Schizophrenia and allied paranoid psychoses.

Dose: Adult: *Injection (20mg/mL),* usually 20-40mg every 2-4 weeks. *Conc injection (100mg/mL),* usual dose is between 50mg every 4 weeks and 300mg every 2 weeks; increase to 400mg weekly if required before reducing to maintenance levels. Deep IM injection in upper outer buttock or lateral thigh.

Elderly: Lower end of dosage range.

CI: Comatose states, depressed levels of consciousness (alcohol intoxication, barbiturates, opiates), circulatory collapse, senile confusional states.

Interactions: Effect of Other Drugs on Flupenthixol: *Increased QT-prolongation risk*: Diuretics (hypokalaemia). *Increased extrapyramidal disorder risk*: Metoclopramide, piperazine.

Effect of Flupenthixol on Other Drugs: Levodopa, adrenergic drugs: *Effect reduced.* ALCOHOL, barbiturates, other CNS depressants: *Sedative effects enhanced.* General anaesthetics: *Effects potentiated.*

ADR: *Very common*, somnolence, akathisia, hyperkinesia, hypokinesia, dry mouth.

Notes: See 3.2.2 Other Typical Antipsychotics.

> Depixol Parenteral *(Lundbeck)* A. GMS.
> Price, (10) 20mg/mL, €12.26. 100mg/mL, €50.49.
> Depot injection, cis (z)-flupenthixol decanoate 20mg/mL (1mL). Conc 100mg/mL (1mL). Clear colourless (slightly yellow) practically particle-free. **Store:** Protect from light.

Haloperidol

ATC Code: N05AD01. **Sport:** Permitted.
Driving: Drowsiness, impaired alertness; may be potentiated by ALCOHOL.
Indications: Long-term management, behavioural disorders, schizophrenia, hypomania and mania, allied

conditions *(parenteral).* Management of schizophrenia, hypomania, mania, agitation, psychotic illness, paranoid psychosis, childhood behaviour disorders especially mentally retarded, and severe motor tics and Gilles de la Tourette Syndrome, intractable hiccup, control of severe nausea and vomiting (excluding hyperemesis gravidarum) *(oral).*

Dose: Adult: ORAL, usual initial dose 1.5-20mg/day depending on patient and severity of disorder; usual maintenance 3-10mg/day. *Gilles de la Tourette Syndrome,* initially 2mg/day increasing to 6-50mg/day then decrease to maintenance around 4mg/day. *Admin,* oral.

DEPOT PARENTERAL, initially 50mg every 4 weeks increasing if needed by 50mg increments up to 200mg every 4 weeks; titrate by 50mg increments to 200mg every 4 weeks; if 2-weekly admin is preferred, halve dose. *Admin,* by deep (gluteal region) IM injection (NOT for IV admin); provides 1 month of therapy.

Elderly: ORAL, may be more sensitive to haloperidol; use lower max. and maintenance doses. Half adult starting dose may be sufficient.

DEPOT PARENTERAL, initiate with low doses, 12.5mg-25mg every 4 weeks; increase according to patient response.

Child: ORAL, initially 0.025-0.05mg/kg/day; max. 10mg; maintenance 0.05mg/kg body weight. Risk of extrapyramidal symptoms. DEPOT PARENTERAL, no relevant use.

Renal Impairment: Caution.

Hepatic Impairment: Caution.

CI: Comatose states, Parkinson's disease, cardiac disorders (recent acute MI, uncompensated heart failure, arrhythmias treated with Class IA and II antiarrhythmics), QTc prolongation, history of ventricular arrhythmia or Torsades de pointes, uncorrected hypokalaemia *oral, parenteral*; CNS depression (alcohol, depressant drugs); butyrophenone or sesame oil hypersensitivity, bradycardia, second or third degree heart block *(parenteral).*

Interactions: Effect of Other Drugs on Haloperidol: *Co-admin contraindicated*: QT-prolonging drugs including antiarrhythmics (Class IA, III), sparfloxacin, moxifloxacin, erythromycin IV, amitriptyline, maprotiline, phenothiazines, pimozide, sertindole, terfenadine, cisapride, bretylium, quinine, mefloquine. *Co-admin not recommended*: Drugs causing electrolyte imbalance (diuretics causing hypokalaemia). *Encephalopathy-like syndrome*: Lithium (monitor levels, keep below 1mmoL/L). *Enhanced sedation, mental disturbances*: Methyldopa. *Reduced plasma levels*: Enzyme inducers CYP3A4 and CYP2D6 (itraconazole, venlafaxine, alprazolam, fluvoxamine, sertraline, chlorpromazine, promethazine, carbamazepine, phenobarbital, rifampicin, quinidine, buspirone, fluoxetine).

Effect of Haloperidol on Other Drugs: CNS depressants (ALCOHOL, hypnotics, sedatives, strong analgesics): *Effect potentiated.* Levodopa: *Antiparkinson effect impaired; CNS effects enhanced.* Adrenaline, other sympathomimetics; phenindione: *Effect antagonised.* Adrenergic neurone blockers (guanethidine): *Hypotensive effect reversed.* TCADs: *Metabolism inhibited, increased plasma levels.* Anticonvulsants: *Increase dose.* Indomethacin: *Severe drowsiness.*

SP: NOT indicated in dementia patients. Sudden death reported with antipsychotics; increased risk in elderly with dementia-related psychosis.

Caution, CYP2D6 slow metabolisers during use with CYP450 inhibitors; avoid co-admin with other antipsychotics; thyrotoxic patients, those with arteriosclerosis with lesions of basal ganglia, more prone to extrapyramidal symptoms; severe cardiac disorders (possible transient hypotension). Cardiac risk factors (assess risk/benefit); conduct baseline ECG (prior to and during therapy).

Pregnancy, Lactation: Pregnancy, only if considered essential. Lactation, if essential (if benefit outweighs risk); passes into breast milk. See Notes below (antipsychotics).

ADR: Oral, *common*, extrapyramidal symptoms, tardive dyskinesia (rhythmical involuntary movements).

Parenteral, *most common*, extrapyramidal disorder, insomnia, agitation, hyperkinesia, headache.

Notes: See 3.2.2 Other Typical Antipsychotics.

Haldol Decanoate Parenteral *(Janssen-Cilag)* A. GMS.
Price, (5) 50mg/mL, €24.29. 100mg/mL, €37.03. HOS: 50mg/mL, €22.49 (PTW).
Depot IM injection, haloperidol decanoate 50mg (100mg)/1mL. Slightly (amber, viscous) oily soln. Benzyl alcohol, sesame oil.

Serenace Tablets *(TEVA)* A. GMS.
Price, tabs (30) 1.5mg, €1.29. 5mg, €2.39. 10mg, €4.82. 20mg, €14.01.
Tablet, as above 1.5mg, 5mg, 10mg, 20mg. Round. Marked Norton, strength, Serenace. 1.5mg: White. 5mg: Bright pink. 10mg: Pale pink. 20mg: Dark pink.

Zuclopenthixol

ATC Code: N05AF05. **Sport:** Permitted.
Driving: Impairment in general attention, concentration. Not recommended (parenteral).

Indications: Schizophrenia particularly with agitation or aggression. Initial treatment, acute psychoses including mania and exacerbation of chronic psychoses.

Dose: ORAL, usually 20-30mg/day; if needed, titrate to max. 150mg/day.
PARENTERAL (deep IM injection), *injection* (200mg/mL), range 200-400mg every 2-4 weeks; *conc* (500mg/mL), range 250-500mg every 1-4 weeks. max. 600mg/week. Previous treatment with depot neuroleptics, initially 100mg. *Maintenance,* switch to oral 2-3 days after last injection or to depot admin at same time as last injection.

Elderly: Consider dose reduction; max. 100mg per injection.

Interactions: Effect of Other Drugs on Zuclopenthixol: *Decreased clearance:* CYP2D6 inhibitors.

SP: Extrapyramidal reactions, anti-Parkinson agents should not be routinely prescribed. Severe atherosclerosis, myocardial insufficiency, patients who are excitable or overactive, convulsive disorders, severe respiratory disease, Parkinson's disease (admin may induce exacerbation), advanced hepatic disease, history of narrow-angle glaucoma (caution). Long-acting depot antipsychotics, caution use in combination with other myelosuppressive agents.

ADR: Usually dose-dependent. *Very common,* somnolence, akathisia, hyper/hypokinesia, dry mouth.

Notes: See Flupenthixol Decanoate above. See 3.2.2 Other Typical Antipsychotics.

Clopixol *(Lundbeck)* A. GMS.
Price, (100) 10mg, €5.73.
Tablet, zuclopenthixol dihydrochloride. Round f/c. 10mg: Light-red-brown. Lactose, castor oil.

Clopixol Parenteral *(Lundbeck)* A. GMS.
Price, injection 200mg/mL (10) €23.04. 500mg/mL (5) €27.68.
Depot injection, zuclopenthixol decanoate, triglycerides 200mg/mL; (Conc) 500mg/mL. Clear yellowish sterile oily soln.
Store: Protect from light.

3.2.3 - Atypical Antipsychotics

In This Chapter: *Amisulpride, aripiprazole, asenapine, clozapine, olanzapine (including pamoate), paliperidone, quetiapine, risperidone, sulpiride, ziprasidone.*

Class Effects

Atypical antipsychotics have a reduced tendency to cause extrapyramidal side effects seen with older antipsychotics.

CI: Hypersensitivity to any member of the class. Not recommended in children under 18 years unless otherwise stated.

Interactions: Effect of Other Drugs on Atypical Psychotics: *Co-admin caution:* CNS depressants (narcotics, anaesthetics, analgesics, sedative antihistamines, barbiturates, benzodiazepines, other anxiolytics, clonidine), ALCOHOL. *Caution, QT-prolongation, Torsades de Pointes risk:* Drugs causing pronounced bradycardia (beta-blockers, some calcium channel blockers including diltiazem and verapamil, clonidine, guanfacine, digitalis), drugs inducing electrolyte imbalance especially hypokalaemia (hypokalaemic diuretics, stimulant laxatives, intravenous amphotericin B,

Atypical Antipsychotics 3.2.3

glucocorticoids, tetracosactides), decreased intracardiac conduction, prolonged QT-interval (quinidine, disopyramide, procainamide, propafenone, amiodarone, sotalol; amitriptyline, maprotiline, quinine, mefloquine), drugs enhancing Torsades de Pointes risk. *Hypotension risk:* Antihypertensives.

SP: Suicide, NMS, VTE, Elderly with dementia, see Notes below (antipsychotics). *When switching antipsychotics always consult the manufacturers Full Prescribing Information. Caution,* epilepsy, history of seizures (seizure threshold may be lowered), increased risk of cerebrovascular events. QT-prolongation, risk of serious ventricular arrhythmias (Torsade de pointes), enhanced by pre-existing bradycardia (below 55 bpm), electrolyte imbalances (hypo- kalaemia, magnesaemia, calcaemia), congenital or acquired long QT-interval. History of MI, ischemic heart disease, HF, conduction abnormalities, cerebrovascular disease, conditions predisposing to hypotension (dehydration, hypovolaemia) or hypertension (accelerated or malignant). If signs/symptoms of tardive dyskinesia appear, reduce dose or discontinue. Antidopaminergics used in Parkinson's patients may worsen disease. *Metabolic parameters,* assess at initiation and manage changes; altered glucose tolerance; signs/symptoms of hyperglycaemia (polydipsia, polyuria, polyphagia, weakness); diabetics, monitor for worsening glucose control. Monitor lipids for increased (triglycerides, cholesterol). Weight gain. Increased appetite.

Pregnancy, Lactation: Pregnancy, only if clearly necessary; monitor neonates. Lactation, contraindicated unless otherwise stated. See Notes below (antipsychotics).

Notes: See 3.2.1 Phenothiazines. See 3.2 Antipsychotics and Antimanics.

Amisulpride

ATC Code: N05AL05. **Sport:** Permitted.
Driving: Somnolence, blurred vision.

Indications: Schizophrenia.

Dose: Adult: Acute psychotic episodes, 400-800mg/day; above 800mg/day, no greater efficacy, higher rates of extrapyramidal symptoms; predominantly negative symptoms, 50-300mg/day. Once daily; above 300mg, admin in 2 divided doses.

Elderly: Caution, hypotension, sedation risk.

Child: Up to puberty, under 15 years, contraindicated.

Renal Impairment: CrCl (mL/min) 30-60, half dose; 10-30, one third of dose; below 10, contraindicated.

CI: Concomitant prolactin-dependent tumours (pituitary gland prolactinomas, breast cancer), phaeochromocytoma. See Interactions below.

Interactions: Effect of Other Drugs on Amisulpride: *Co-admin contraindicated (Torsades de Pointes risk):* Class Ia antiarrhythmics (quinidine, disopyramide, procainamide), Class III antiarrhythmics (amiodarone, sotalol), bepridil, cisapride, sultopride, thioridazine, methadone, erythromycin (IV), vincamine (IV), halofantrine, pentamidine, sparfloxacin. *Co-admin not recommended:* ALCOHOL (enhanced central effects). *Co-admin avoid:* Neuroleptics. *Reciprocal antagonism:* Levodopa. *Caution:* Pimozide, haloperidol, imipramine, lithium.

Effect of Amisulpride on Other Drugs: Dopamine agonists (levodopa): *Effect antagonised.*

SP: Amisulpride induces QT-interval prolongation which is known to potentiate risk of serious ventricular arrhythmias (Torsades de Pointes). Caution, with known cardiovascular disease or family history of QT-prolongation, significant bradycardia, congenital QT-interval prolongation, electrolyte imbalance (hypokalaemia, hypomagnesaemia). See also Interactions above.
Anticholinergic activity, caution (prostatic enlargement, narrow-angle glaucoma, impaired peristalsis, constipation, intestinal obstruction, faecal impaction, paralytic ileus). May increase prolactin levels, caution (breast cancer); benign pituitary tumour observed.

ADR: *Very common,* dose-related extrapyramidal symptoms (tremor, rigidity, hypokinesia, hypersalivation, akathisia, dyskinesia).

3.2.3   Atypical Antipsychotics

Notes: See 3.2.3 Atypical Antipsychotics. See Sulpiride below.

Solian Tablets *(SANOFI)* B. GMS.
Price, (60) 50mg, €10.84. 100mg, €21.66. 200mg, €39.60. 400mg, €86.67.
Tablets, amisulpride 50mg, 100mg, 200mg, 400mg. White (off-white) round flat-faced scored* (facilitates breaking). Marked AMI/strength. *Lactose*. *(except 50mg). **Store:** No special conditions.

Amisulpride Mylan Tablets *(Gerard)* B. GMS.
Price, (60) 50mg, €8.67. 100mg, €21.66. 200mg, €31.68. 400mg, €86.65.
Tablet, amisulpride. White (off-white) f/c scored (divisible into equal doses): 50mg, 200mg: Round. 400mg: Cap-shaped. *Lactose*. **Store:** No special conditions.

Aripiprazole

ATC Code: N05AX12. **Sport:** Permitted.
Driving: Caution, until effect known.

Indications: Schizophrenia *(all brands)*. Moderate to severe manic episodes in Bipolar I Disorder; prevention, new manic episodes *(Abilify, Aripiprazole Sandoz, Lemilvo)*. Rapid control of agitation and disturbed behaviours in schizophrenia or manic episodes in Bipolar I Disorder *(IM parenteral)*. Maintenance treatment of schizophrenia in adults stabilised with oral aripiprazole *(Maintena)*.

Dose: Adult: ORAL, *schizophrenia* (all brands), initially, 10mg or 15mg/day (10 or 15mL oral soln); maintenance, 15mg/day; range, 15-30mg/day (10-30mL oral soln); max. 30mg/day; *manic episodes* (*Abilify, Aripiprazole Sandoz*), initially 15mg/day; max. 30mg/day; prevention of recurrence of manic episodes (bipolar I disorder), continue at same dose. *Admin*, once daily with or without food; swallowing difficulties, use soln or orodispersible.
PARENTERAL IM, initially 9.75mg (1.3mL) as single IM injection; range 5.25-15mg; lower dose, 5.25mg (0.7mL) may be given*. If needed, admin a second injection 2 hours after first*; max. 3 injections in any 24-hours. Max. 30mg/day (including all formulations). *Admin*, IM, deltoid or deep gluteus maximus; avoid adipose regions; NOT for IV or SC admin.
PARENTERAL Prolonged/R *(Maintena)*, 400mg as a once monthly single injection (no sooner than 26 days after previous injection). After first injection, maintain 10-20mg oral for 14 consecutive days to maintain therapeutic levels. With CYP2D6 poor metabolisers, initially 300mg; with strong CYP3A4 inhibitors, reduce to 200mg. Adverse reactions, consider reducing to 300mg. *Admin*, only by a healthcare professional; IM route; not for IV or SC admin. *(based on clinical status).

Elderly: Consider dose reduction *(oral, IM)*. Over 65 years, safety/efficacy not established *(Prolonged/R parenteral)*.

Child: *Schizophrenia*, age 15 years and older, initially 2mg/day (2 days), increase to 5mg/day (another 2 days); recommended 10mg/day; range 10-30mg/day; max. 30mg/day. *Manic episodes (Bipolar I disorder)* (brands *Abilify, Aripiprazole Sandoz*), age 13 years and older, using oral soln, initially 2mg/day (2 days); then 5mg/day (2 days), then 10mg/day. No dose recommendation, autistic disorder (under 18 years), tics associated with Tourette's (age 6-18 years). *Admin*, once daily with/without food. Parenteral, no experience under 18 years *(parenteral IM)* or under 17 years *(Prolonged/R parenteral)*.

Hepatic Impairment: Severe, cautious dosing; oral formulations preferred (30mg/day).

Interactions: Effect of Other Drugs on Aripiprazole: Co-admin caution: Medicinals causing QT-prolongation or electrolyte imbalance. *Sedation*: ALCOHOL (increased), parenteral antipsychotics and parenteral benzodiazepine (excessive). *Reduced absorption*: Famotidine. *Increased plasma levels*: Quinidine, fluoxetine, paroxetine, ketoconazole, itraconazole, HIV protease inhibitors. *Plasma levels decreased*: Carbamazepine, rifampicin, rifabutin, phenytoin, phenobarbital, primidone, efavirenz, nevirapine and St John's Wort. *Serotonin syndrome risk*: Other serotonergics (SSRIs, SNRIs).

Effect of Other Drugs on Aripiprazole: Certain antihypertensives: *Enhanced effect (due to alpha-1 adrenergic receptor antagonism)*.

SP: Not indicated for dementia-related psychosis.

Pathological gambling, serotonin syndrome, reported. Akathisia, Parkinsonism observed (paediatric trials); also increased somnolence and fatigue incidence. Weight gain. *Parenteral*, orthostatic hypotension.

Pregnancy, Lactation: Lactation, not recommended.

ADR: Summary, *most common*, (oral) akathisia, nausea; (parenteral IM) nausea, dizziness, somnolence; (parenteral Prolonged/R) increased weight, akathisia, insomnia, injection-site pain.

Notes: See 3.2.3 Atypical Antipsychotics.

Interchangeability: Same strengths of all brands of aripiprazole tabs/orodispersible tabs and oral soln listed below are deemed interchangeable.

Abilify Tablets, OroDisp, Oral Soln *(Otsuka)* A. GMS.
Price, (28) tabs 5mg, €93.58. 10mg, 15mg, €97.08. 30mg, €194.16. OroDisp 10mg, €97.47. 15mg, €99.68. Soln 1mg/mL (150mL) €109.03.
Tablet, aripiprazole 5mg, 10mg, 15mg. Marked A- and strength. 5mg: Rectangular blue. Marked 007. 10mg: Rectangular pink. Marked 008. 15mg: Round yellow. Marked 009. 30mg: Round pink. Marked 011. *Lactose*.
OroDisp, as above 10mg, 15mg. Round. Marked A and strength. 10mg: Pink. Marked 640. 15mg: Yellow. Marked 641. *Aspartame*.
Oral soln, as above 1mg/mL. Clear colourless (light yellow). *Fructose, sucrose, parabens*.

Abilify Maintena Parenteral *(Lundbeck)* A. GMS.
Price, (1) 400mg, €292.02. PFS, €314.12.
Prolonged/R suspension for injection, aripiprazole 200mg/mL. White (off-white) powder; clear solvent soln.

Abilify IM Parenteral *(Lundbeck)* A.
Price, not published by company.
IM (only) injection, aripiprazole 7.5mg/mL. Clear colourless aqueous soln.

Aripiprazole Oral Soln *(Pinewood)* A. GMS.
Price, 150mL, €54.24.
Oral soln, aripiprazole 1mg/mL. Clear colourless (light-yellow). *Fructose, sucrose, parabens*.

Aripiprazole Accord Tablets *(Accord)* A. GMS.
Price, (28) 5mg, €21.00. 10mg, 15mg, €23.80. 30mg, €40.60.
Tablet, aripiprazole 5mg, 10mg, 15mg, 30mg. u/c. Marked A and strength. 5mg: Blue rectangular. 10mg: Pink rectangular. 15mg: Yellow round. 30mg: Pink round. *Lactose*.

Aripiprazole Clonmel Tablets *(Clonmel)* A. GMS.
Price, (28) 5mg, €21.00. 10mg, 15mg, €23.80. 30mg, €40.60.
Tablet, aripiprazole 5mg, 10mg, 15mg, 30mg. Round flat with scattered specks. 5mg: Pale-blue. 10mg: Pale-pink. 15mg: Pale-yellow. *Lactose*.

Aripiprazole Focus Tablets *(Krka)* A. GMS.
Price, (28) 5mg, €21.00. 10mg, 15mg, €23.80. 30mg, €40.60.
Tablet, aripiprazole 5mg, 10mg, 15mg, 30mg. Marked A and strength (not 5mg). 5mg: Blue round. 10mg: Light-pink rectangular. 15mg: Light-yellow (brownish-yellow) round. 30mg: Light-pink round. *Lactose*.

Aripiprazole Sandoz Tablets *(Rowex)* A. GMS.
Price, (28) 5mg, €21.00. 10mg, 15mg, €23.80. 30mg, €40.60.
Tablets, aripiprazole. Round mottled. Marked SZ. 5mg: Blue. Marked 444. 10mg: Pink. Marked 446. 15mg: Yellow. Marked 447. 30mg: Pink. Marked 449. *Lactose*.

Aripiprazole TEVA Tablets *(TEVA)* A. GMS.
Price, (28) 5mg, €21.00. 10mg, 15mg, €23.80. 30mg, €40.60.
Tablets, aripiprazole. Round (except 10mg, oblong), scored (except 5mg) (divisible into equal doses). Marked with strength. 5mg, 15mg: Light-yellow. 10mg, 30mg: Pink (light-pink). *Lactose*.

Lemilvo Tablets *(Accord)* A. GMS.
Price, (28) 5mg, €21.00. 10mg, 15mg, €23.80. 30mg, €40.60.
Tablet, aripiprazole. White. Marked ZL; strength on reverse. 5mg, 15mg, 30mg: Round. 10mg: Cap-shaped. *Lactose*.

Asenapine

ATC Code: N05AH05. **Sport:** Permitted.
Driving: Somnolence, sedation.

Indications: Moderate to severe manic episodes in bipolar I disorder (adults).

Dose: Adult: Monotherapy, initially 10mg twice daily morning and evening; decrease to 5mg twice daily according to response. Combination, initially 5mg twice daily; can be increased to 10mg twice daily depending on response. Place under tongue and allow to dissolve completely; do not chew, swallow or crush tab. Avoid eating or drinking for 10 minutes after admin.

Elderly: Caution. Over 65 years, limited data.

Child: Limited data; no dose recommendation.

Renal Impairment: CrCl (mL/min) below 15, no data.

Hepatic Impairment: Moderate, caution. Severe, not recommended.

Interactions: Effect of Other Drugs on Asenapine: Co-admin caution: Fluvoxamine, medicinals that are both substrates and inhibitors of CYP2D6.

Effect of Asenapine on Other Drugs: Antihypertensives: *Effect enhanced.* Levodopa, dopamine agonists: *Effect antagonised.*

SP: Not indicated for dementia-related psychosis; elderly with dementia-related psychosis treated with antipsychotics are at increased risk of death. Orthostatic hypotension. Tardive dyskinesia. Known cardiovascular disease or QT-prolongation, caution. Dysphagia. Parkinson's, weight benefit/risk.

ADR: Summary, *most frequent,* anxiety, somnolence.

Notes: See 3.2.3 Atypical Antipsychotics.

Sycrest Sublingual 5mg, 10mg *(Lundbeck)* A. GMS.
Price, (60) both strengths, €113.08.
Sublingual tablet, asenapine maleate. White (off-white) round. Marked with strength.

Clozapine

ATC Code: N05AH02. **Sport:** Permitted.
Driving: Sedation, lowered seizure threshold.

Indications: Treatment-resistant schizophrenia; patients with severe, untreatable neurological adverse reactions to other antipsychotics. Psychotic disorders of Parkinson's disease.

Dose: Adult: *Schizophrenia,* initially 12.5mg once or twice daily (day 1), then 25mg once or twice daily (day 2); if needed/tolerated, increase within 2-3 weeks by 25-50mg to 300mg/day; can be further increased by 50-100mg at half-weekly or weekly intervals. Range 200-450mg/day in divided doses; max. 900mg/day. Maintenance, 200mg or less, once daily (evening). Discontinuation, withdraw over 1-2 weeks. Re-starting therapy, more than 2 days since last dose, initiate with 12.5mg once or twice daily (day 1) then titrate as above.
Psychotic disorders in Parkinson's Disease, initially 12.5mg (evening); increase by 12.5mg (max. 2 per week); max. 50mg only in exceptional cases, 100mg/day (never exceed). Discontinuation, reduce by 12.5mg at a time, over 1-2 weeks. Titrate cautiously. Use divided dosing to minimise (hypertension, seizure, sedation) risk. Generally, not for use in combination (other antipsychotics).

Elderly: Age 60 years and older, initially 12.5mg once daily (day 1); increase by max. 25mg/day.

Child: Under 16 years, not recommended.

Renal Impairment: Severe, contraindicated.

Hepatic Impairment: Active or progressive liver disease, hepatic failure, contraindicated. Stable pre-existing disorders, regular LFTs.

CI: Patients unable to undergo regular blood tests, toxic and/or idiosyncratic granulocytopenia and/or agranulocytosis (except from previous chemotherapy), concurrent treatment with substances causing agranulocytosis, impaired bone marrow function, uncontrolled epilepsy, alcoholic/other toxic psychoses, drug intoxication, comatose conditions, circulatory collapse and/or CNS depression, severe cardiac disorders (myocarditis), paralytic ileus. See Renal/Hepatic Impairment above.

Interactions: Effect of Other Drugs on Clozapine: *Bone marrow suppression, increased risk and/or severity, contraindicated:* Bone marrow suppressants (carbamazepine, chloramphenicol, sulfonamides including co-trimoxazole, phenylbutazone, penicillamine, cytotoxics; antipsychotics, long-acting depot injection; increased myelosuppression); ALCOHOL (increased sedation). *Increased circulatory collapse risk:* Benzodiazepines. *Enhanced central effects:* MAOIs, CNS depressants (narcotics, benzodiazepines, antihistamines). *Increased NMS risk:* Lithium. *Constipation risk:* Drugs causing constipation/with anticholinergic properties (some antipsychotics, antidepressants, Parkinson's treatments). *Increased plasma levels:* CYP1A2 inhibitors (caffeine, fluvoxamine, paroxetine), CYP2D6 inhibitors (fluoxetine, sertraline), CYP3A4 inhibitors (azole antifungals,

cimetidine, erythromycin, HIV protease inhibitors), sudden smoking cessation. *Decreased plasma levels:* CYP450 inducers (carbamazepine, co-admin not recommended; phenytoin, rifampicin). *Consider clozapine dose adjustment:* Hormonal contraceptives (initiation and/or discontinuation), ciprofloxacin, perazine.

Effect of Clozapine on Other Drugs: Highly protein bound drugs (warfarin, digoxin): *Increased plasma levels.* Anticholinergics, antihypertensives: *Action potentiated.* Noradrenaline: *Effect reduced.* Adrenaline: *Effect reversed.* Valproic acid: *Seizures (including onset in non-epileptics).*

SP: Can cause agranulocytosis. Limit use to: Schizophrenia (non-responsive or intolerant to other antipsychotics), psychosis in Parkinson's disease (other treatments have failed); patients with normal leucocytes (WBC count 3500/mm3, ANC 2000/mm3 or more) and where regular WBC counts and absolute neutrophil counts (ANC) can be performed weekly (first 18 weeks), then every 4 weeks. Advise patients to report signs of infection (flu-like symptoms, fever, sore throat); may indicate neutropenia. Eosinophilia, thrombocytopenia, discontinue. Increased myocarditis risk, cardiomyopathy (rarely fatal; risk greatest in first 2 months); if suspected discontinue; do not re-expose to clozapine. MI (fatal) reported. Orthostatic hypotension, with/without syncope, collapse, cardiac and/or respiratory arrest, pericarditis or pericardial effusion, persistent tachycardia at rest, palpitations, arrhythmias, chest pain, other signs/symptoms of HF, symptoms mimicking MI, flu-like symptoms. Caution, QT-prolongation, cerebrovascular events. Epilepsy, monitor (dose-related convulsions). Anticholinergic effects, temperature (dysregulation, elevations), thromboembolism (avoid immobilisation). Metabolic changes, hyperglycaemia, dyslipidaemia.

Pregnancy, Lactation: Women of childbearing age to ensure adequate contraception.

ADR: Summary, *most serious,* agranulocytosis, seizure, cardiovascular effects, fever; *most common,* drowsiness/sedation, dizziness, tachycardia, constipation, hypersalivation.

Notes: See 3.2.3 Atypical Antipsychotics.

Clozaril 25mg, 100mg *(BGP)* A.
Price, (84) 25mg, €57.03. 100mg, €228.12.
Tablet, clozapine. Yellow round flat angle-scored (divisible into equal halves). Marked SANDOZ. 25mg: Marked L/O. 100mg: Marked Z/A. *Lactose.* NOTE: Supply restricted in Ireland to hospital and retail pharmacies registered with the Clozaril Patient Monitoring Service (CPMS); Clozaril is not sold to, or distributed through wholesalers. Prescribers and pharmacists should adhere to brand prescribing and dispensing; patients to be registered only with the monitoring service for that brand. *Ireland Official Recommendations:* UK/IRL CPMS provides centralised leucocyte and neutrophil count monitoring, mandatory for all patients in the UK and Ireland treated with clozapine; use is restricted to patients registered with CPMS. Monitor white cell count with differential count weekly (first 18 weeks), 2-weekly intervals (weeks 18-52), then at 4-week intervals (if stable neutrophil counts after 1 year). Monitor for 4 weeks after discontinuation. NOTE: *CPMS,* Tel +353 1 662 1141.

Denzapine Tablets, Oral Susp *(Clonmel)* A.
Price, (84) 25mg, €40.00. 100mg, €160.00. (50) 50mg, €47.62. 200mg, €90.48. Oral Susp 50mg/mL (100mL) €95.24.
Tablet, clozapine 25mg, 50mg, 100mg, 200mg. 25mg, 50mg, 100mg: Yellow round flat. Marked with strength. 25mg: Scored (divisible into equal halves). 50mg, 100mg: Scored*. 200mg: Large oval yellow scored*. Marked 200. *Lactose.* *(facilitates breaking)
Oral susp, as above 50mg/mL. Free-flowing yellow. *Sorbitol, parabens.* NOTE: *Denzapine Monitoring Service* call 0845 009 2440 (UK) or 1800 936 081 (Ireland).

Olanzapine

ATC Code: N05AH03. **Sport:** Permitted.
Driving: Somnolence, dizziness. Prolonged/R parenteral, advise not to drive for remainder of day after injection.

Indications: Oral, schizophrenia, moderate/severe manic episode, prevention of recurrence in patients with bipolar disorder. Parenteral (Depot), maintenance treatment of schizophrenia sufficiently stabilised with oral olanzapine during acute treatment.

Dose: Adult: ORAL, *schizophrenia,* initially 10mg/day.

3.2.3 Atypical Antipsychotics

Manic episodes, initially 15mg as single dose monotherapy or 10mg/day adjunctive. *Prevention of recurrence* bipolar disorder, initially 10/day; range 5-20mg/day; titrate at 24-hour intervals. Smokers, see Interactions below. Admin with or without food; dissolve orodispersible in saliva in mouth or disperse in glass of water.

PROLONGED/R PARENTERAL (DEPOT), switch from *oral (10mg/day)*, initially 210mg/2-weeks OR 405mg/4-weeks; maintenance 150mg/2-weeks OR 300mg/4-weeks; *oral (15mg/day)*, initially 300mg/2-weeks; maintenance 210mg/2-weeks OR 405mg/4-weeks; *oral (20mg/day)*, initial and maintenance 300mg/2-weeks. Deep IM gluteal injection; after each admin observe for minimum 3 hours for signs/symptoms of overdose.

Elderly: ORAL, over 65 years, initially 5mg/day when clinical factors warrant.

PROLONGED/R PARENTERAL, over 65 years, not recommended unless well-tolerated oral regimen established; consider lower starting dose (150mg/4-weeks); over 75 years, initiation not recommended.

Renal Impairment: Oral, initially 5mg/day. Prolonged/R Parenteral, as for Elderly (over 65 years) above.

Hepatic Impairment: Oral, mild/moderate, cirrhosis, initially 5mg/day; uptitrate with caution. Prolonged/R Parenteral, moderate as for Renal above.

CI: Narrow angle glaucoma.

Interactions: Effect of Other Drugs on Olanzapine: *Co-admin not recommended*: Parenteral benzodiazepines and IM olanzapine; potential for excessive sedation, cardiorespiratory depression; rare cases, death (admin 1 hour apart). *Caution*: CNS depressants, ALCOHOL, drugs with haemodynamics similar to IM olanzapine (other antipsychotics oral/parenteral, benzodiazepines). *Reduced plasma levels (metabolism induced)*: CYP1A2 inducers (carbamazepine, cigarette smoking). *Plasma levels increased*: CYP1A2 inhibitors (fluvoxamine, ciprofloxacin). *Decreased bioavailability*: Activated charcoal (admin 2 hours apart). *Safety/efficacy not evaluated (IM)*: ALCOHOL or drug intoxication.

Effect of Olanzapine on Other Drugs: Direct and indirect dopamine agonists: *Effect antagonised.*

SP: Not indicated for dementia-related psychosis and/or behavioural disturbances. Altered lipids, monitor (baseline, 12 weeks, then every 5 years). Low incidence of anticholinergic effects (caution prostatic hypertrophy, paralytic ileus). *Risk factors* for increased mortality (over 65 years, dysphagia, sedation, malnutrition, dehydration, pulmonary conditions including pneumonia, with/without aspiration, benzodiazepine co-admin). Cerebrovascular adverse events; elevated hepatic aminotransferases, ALT/AST, hepatic impairment, hepatitis, (monitor liver enzymes; signs of liver damage, discontinue). Low leucocyte and/or neutrophil counts, drugs causing neutropenia, history of drug-induced bone marrow depression radiation and/or chemotherapy, hypereosinophilic conditions, myeloproliferative disease. VTE, avoid immobilisation. Hyperglycaemia (monitor, baseline, 4, 8 and 12 weeks, then quarterly).

Parenteral Prolonged/R (Depot), not for use in acutely agitated or severely psychotic state. Potential overdose risk, observe for 3 hours post admin; if parenteral benzodiazepines are essential for post-injection adverse reaction management, monitor (excessive sedation, cardiorespiratory depression). See Interactions above. Sudden cardiac death reported.

ADR: *Very common*, weight gain, somnolence, orthostatic hypotension, elevated plasma prolactin levels.

Notes: See 3.2.3 Atypical Antipsychotics.

Interchangeability: Same strengths of all brands of olanzapine tablets, coated tablets, film-coated (f/c) tablets, orodispersible tablets listed below are deemed interchangeable.

Reference Price: (28 tabs/orodispersible tabs) 2.5mg, €5.60; 5mg, €9.00; 7.5mg, €13.50; 10mg, €18.00; 15mg, €27.00; 20mg, €36.00. (56 tabs) 7.5mg, €27.00.

Zyprexa Tablets, Velotab *(Lilly)* A. GMS.
Price, (28) tabs 2.5mg, €22.52; 5mg, €31.75; 10mg, €63.51; 15mg, €99.89. (56) 7.5mg, €95.27. Velotab 5mg, €38.10; 10mg, €76.22; 15mg, €119.46; 20mg, €122.84.
Tablet, olanzapine 2.5mg, 5mg, 7.5mg, 10mg, 15mg. Marked LILLY. Round white coated (15mg, 20mg, elliptical). 2.5mg: Marked 4112. 5mg: Marked 4115. 7.5mg: Marked 4116. 10mg: Marked 4117. 15mg: Blue. Marked 4415. 20mg: Pink. Marked 4420. *Lactose*. **Store:** Original pack; protect (light, moisture).
OroDisp tablet (Velotab), as above 5mg, 10mg, 15mg, 20mg. Yellow round freeze-dried. *Aspartame, mannitol, parabens.* **Store:** See above.

Zypadhera Parenteral *(Lilly)* A. HOS.
Price, (1) 210mg, €175.67; 300mg, €244.96; 405mg, €323.09 (PTW).
Prolonged/R injection, olanzapine pamoate. Yellow solid powder; clear colourless (slightly yellow) solvent for soln. **Store:** Do not refrigerate or freeze.

Olanzapine Accord Tablets *(Accord)* A. GMS.
Price, (28) 2.5mg, €5.04. 5mg, €8.12. 7.5mg, €12.33. 10mg, €13.17. 15mg, €21.00.
Tablet, olanzapine 2.5mg, 5mg, 7.5mg, 10mg, 15mg. Round f/c white (off-white) except 15mg, 20mg. 5mg: Marked 01. 7.5mg: Marked 02. 10mg: Marked 03. 15mg: Light-blue. *Lactose*.

Olanzapine Actavis Tablets, OroDisp *(Accord)* A. GMS.
Price, tabs, OroDisp (28) 2.5mg, €5.04. 5mg, €8.12. 7.5mg, €12.33. 10mg, €13.17. 15mg, €21.00. Tabs (56) 7.5mg, €24.65.
Tablet, olanzapine 2.5mg, 5mg, 7.5mg, 10mg, 15mg, 20mg. f/c. 2.5mg: Marked 0. 5mg: Marked 01. 7.5mg: Marked 02. 10mg: Marked 03 (all round white). 15mg: Blue. 20mg: Pink (both oval. Marked 0). *Lactose, lecithin soya*.
OroDisp tablet, as above 5mg, 10mg, 15mg, 20mg. Round yellow. 5mg: Marked 0. 10mg: Marked 01. 15mg: Marked 02. 20mg: Marked 03. *Aspartame*.

Olanzapine Clonmel Tablets *(Clonmel)* A. GMS.
Price, (28) 2.5mg, €5.04. 5mg, €8.12. 7.5mg, €12.33. 10mg, €13.17. 15mg, €21.00. 20mg, €26.32. (56) 7.5mg, €24.65.
Tablet, olanzapine 2.5mg, 5mg, 7.5mg, 10mg, 15mg, 20mg. White f/c. Round: 2.5mg: Marked 0. 5mg: Marked 01. 7.5mg: Marked 02. 10mg: Marked 03. Oval. Marked 0: 15mg: Light-blue. 20mg: Light-pink. *Lactose, soya lecithin*.

Olanzapine Glenmark Tablets, OroDisp *(Rowex)* A. GMS.
Price, tabs, OroDisp (28) 2.5mg, €5.04. 5mg, €8.12. 10mg, €13.17. 15mg, €21.00. 20mg, €26.32. Tabs (56) 7.5mg, €24.65.
Tablet, olanzapine 2.5mg, 5mg, 7.5mg, 10mg, 15mg. Yellow round flat. 2.5mg: Marked I. 5mg: Marked 2. 7.5mg: Marked 3. 10mg: Marked OL; 4 on reverse. 15mg: Marked OL; 5 on reverse. *Aspartame*.
OroDisp tablet, as above 5mg, 10mg, 15mg, 20mg. Yellow round flat. Marked OL (not 5mg). 5mg: Marked 2. 10mg: Marked 4. 15mg: Marked 5. 20mg: Marked 6. *Aspartame*.

Olanzapine Mylan Tablets *(Gerard)* A. GMS.
Price, (28) 2.5mg, €5.04. 5mg, €8.12. 10mg, €13.17. 15mg, €21.00. (56) 7.5mg, €24.65.
Tablet, olanzapine 2.5mg, 5mg, 7.5mg, 10mg, 15mg. White f/c. Marked OZ over strength; G on reverse. 2.5mg-10mg: Round. 15mg: Elliptical. *Lactose, soya lecithin*. **Store:** Below 25 deg C.

Olanzapine TEVA Tablets, OroDisp *(TEVA)* A. GMS.
Price, tabs, OroDisp(28) 2.5mg, €5.04. 5mg, €8.12. 10mg, €13.17. 15mg, €21.00. 20mg, €26.32. Tabs (56) 7.5mg, €24.65.
Tablet, olanzapine 2.5mg, 5mg, 7.5mg, 10mg, 15mg, 20mg. f/c. Marked OL and strength. 2.5-10mg: White round. 15mg: Light-blue. 20mg Pink (both oval). *Lactose*.
OroDisp tablet, as above 5mg, 10mg, 15mg, 20mg. Round, yellow. *Lactose, sucrose, aspartame*.

Rolyprexa Tablets, DisTab *(Rowex)* A. GMS.
Price, tabs, OroDisp(28) 2.5mg, €5.04. 5mg, €8.12. 10mg, €13.17. 15mg, €21.00. 20mg, €26.32. Tabs (56) 7.5mg, €24.65.
Tablet, olanzapine 2.5mg, 5mg, 7.5mg, 10mg, 15mg, 20mg. 2.5mg, 7.5mg: White round f/c. 5mg, 10mg: White round f/c notched*. 15mg: Light-blue oval notched*. 20mg: Pink oval notched* *Lactose*. (division into equal halves).
OroDisp tablet (DisTab), as above10mg, 15mg, 20mg. Yellow round. *Lactose*.

Zalasta Tablets, OroDisp *(Krka)* A. GMS.
Price, tabs, OroDisp(28) 2.5mg, €5.04. 5mg, €8.12. 10mg, €13.17. 15mg, €21.00. 20mg, €26.32. Tabs (56) 7.5mg, €24.65.
Tablet, olanzapine 2.5mg, 5mg, 7.5mg, 10mg, 15mg. Round slightly-yellow with possible individual spots. Marked with strength (except 2.5mg). *Lactose*.
OroDisp tablet, as above 5mg, 10mg, 20mg. Round yellow marbled with possible individual spots. *Aspartame*.

Paliperidone

ATC Code: N05AX13. **Sport:** Permitted.
Driving: Potential nervous system and visual effects.
Indications: Schizophrenia (age 15 years and older), schizoaffective disorder (adults) *(oral)*. Maintenance, schizophrenia (adults) stabilised with paliperidone or risperidone *(Xeplion)* or stable on 1-monthly paliperidone injectable *(Trevicta)*.

Dose: Adult: ORAL, *schizophrenia*, 6mg/day; increase by 3mg/day (intervals usually of more than 5 days); range 3-12mg/day; *schizoaffective disorder*, 6mg once daily; range 6-12mg; titrate at 3mg/day at intervals usually of more than 4 days. *Admin*, once daily (morning), swallow whole with liquid; do not chew, break or crush; always in fasting state OR always with breakfast. Tablet shell and insoluble core eliminated in stool.
PARENTERAL, *Xeplion* (1-monthly), initially 150mg (day 1) and 100mg 1-week later (day 8) IM deltoid. Admin third dose 1 month after second initiation dose. Maintenance 75mg; range 25-150mg. Overweight/obese may require dose in upper range. After the second dose, admin maintenance doses either deltoid or gluteal. NOT for SC or IV admin. *Trevicta* (3-monthly), initiate in place of next scheduled 1-monthly paliperidone (+/- 7days); use 3.5-fold higher dose than 1-monthly e.g. 50mg (1-monthly), use 175mg (3-monthly); 75mg (1-monthly), use 263mg (3-monthly); 100mg (1-monthly), use 350mg (3-monthly); 150mg (1-monthly) use 525mg (3-monthly). *Admin*, IM every 3 months (+/- 2 weeks).

Elderly: As for Renal below. Caution, dementia with stroke risk factors. *Trevicta*, over 35 years, not data.

Child: ORAL, *schizophrenia* (age 15 years and older), 3mg once daily (morning); max. 6mg (weight under 51kg) OR 12mg (weight 51kg and over). Increase by 3mg/day at intervals of 5 days or more. Schizophrenia (age 12-14 years), schizoaffective disorder (age 12-17) years, safety and efficacy not established; under 12 years, no relevant use. PARENTERAL, under 18 years, no data.

Renal Impairment: CrCl (mL/min) 50-79, oral initially 3mg/day; increase to 6mg/day based on response OR parenteral 100mg (day 1) and 75mg one week later using 1-month paliperidone. Maintenance 50mg, range 25-100mg; 10-49, oral only, initially 1.5mg every day; increase to 3mg/day based on response; below 10, not recommended.

Hepatic Impairment: Severe, caution.

CI: Risperidone hypersensitivity.

Interactions: Effect of Other Drugs on Paliperidone: *Co-admin not recommended*: Risperidone (additive paliperidone exposure). *Co-admin caution*: Drugs prolonging QT-interval e.g. Class I antiarrhythmics (quinidine, disopyramide), Class III antiarrhythmics (amiodarone, sotalol), antihistamines, antipsychotics, antimalarials (mefloquine), other centrally acting drugs (anxiolytics, most antipsychotics, hypnotics, opiates, ALCOHOL), drugs lowering seizure threshold (phenothiazines, butyrophenones, TCADs, SSRIs, tramadol, mefloquine, clozapine). *Altered absorption*: Drugs affecting GI transit time. *Additive orthostatic hypotension risk*: Other antipsychotics, TCADs. *Re-evaluate dose*: Carbamazepine (initiation, discontinuation), rifampicin, St John's Wort. *Paliperidone Parenteral (caution)*: Risperidone or oral paliperidone co-admin for extended time.

Effect of Paliperidone on Other Drugs: Levodopa, other dopamine agonists: *Effect antagonised*.

SP: GI obstruction (caution, dysphagia), conditions reducing GI transit time, cerebrovascular adverse events. Parkinson's Disease or Dementia with Lewy Bodies, increased NMS risk (weigh risk/benefit). Priapism (advise to seek urgent attention if not resolved in 3-4 hours), altered body temperature regulation. Anti-emetic effect may mask sign/symptoms of overdose. Hypersensitivity reactions *(parenteral)*. *Paediatrics*, monitor closely (sedative effects, extrapyramidal symptoms, other movement disorders); evaluate endocrine status regularly. *Parenteral*, not for use when immediate symptom control needed; caution, inadvertent injection into blood vessel. See Notes below (risperidone).

Atypical Antipsychotics 3.2.3

ADR: Paliperidone is active metabolite of risperidone. Postural orthostatic tachycardia syndrome noted with paliperidone. See Notes below (risperidone).

Notes: See 3.2.3 Atypical Antipsychotics. See Risperidone below.

INVEGA 3mg, 6mg, 9mg *(Janssen-Cilag)* A. GMS.
Price, (28) 3mg, €101.28. 6mg, €108.30. 9mg, €129.38.
Prolonged/R tablet, paliperidone. Trilayer cap-shaped. Marked PAL/strength. 3mg: White Lactose. 6mg: Beige. 9mg: Pink.

Trevicta Prolonged/R Parenteral *(Janssen-Cilag)* A. GMS.
Price, (1) 175mg, €668.54. 263mg, €913.84. 350mg, €1154.61. 525mg, €1656.58.
Prolonged/R injection (3-monthly), paliperidone palmitate 175mg, 263mg, 350mg, 525mg. White (off-white) susp. pH neutral.

Xeplion Prolonged/R Parenteral *(Janssen-Cilag)* A. GMS.
Price, (1) 50mg, €217.46. 75mg, €296.06. 100mg, €374.88. 150mg, €536.82.
Prolonged/R injection, paliperidone palmitate 50mg, 75mg, 100mg, 150mg. White (off-white). pH neutral. PFS.

Quetiapine

ATC Code: N05AH04. **Sport:** Permitted.
Driving: Do not drive until individual susceptibility known.
Indications: Schizophrenia, bipolar disorder (manic episodes, major depressive episode, prevention of recurrence of manic or depressed episodes) *(all formulations)*. Adjunctive, major depressive episodes in Major Depressive Disorder (MDD) with sub-optimal response to antidepressant monotherapy *(Prolonged/R)*.

Dose: Adult: NOTE: Different dosing schedules exist for each indication.
STANDARD/R, *schizophrenia*, 50mg (day 1), 100mg (day 2), 200mg (day 3), 300mg (day 4); then titrate to usual effective dose, 300-450mg/day; range 150-750mg/day.
Bipolar disorder, manic episodes, 100mg (day 1), 200mg (day 2), 300mg (day 3) and 400mg (day 4); titrate up to 800mg/day by day 6, increments max. 200mg/day; range 200-800mg/day; usual effective dose 400-800mg/day. Admin daily dose in 2 divided doses, with or without food; *major depressive episodes*, 50mg (day 1), 100mg (day 2), 200mg (day 3), 300mg (day 4); recommended dose 300mg/day; may be titrated up to 600mg. Once daily at bedtime to reduce daytime sedation. *Recurrence prevention*, continue with dose providing response; range 300-800mg/day; use lowest dose.
PROLONGED/R, *schizophrenia*, 300mg (day 1), 600mg (day 2); recommended 600mg/day; may be increased to 800mg/day; effective range, 400-800mg. Admin once daily 1 hour before food.
Bipolar disorder, manic episodes, as for schizophrenia; *major depressive episodes*, 50mg/day (day 1), 100mg (day 2), 200mg (day 3), 300mg (day 4); recommended 300mg/day. Admin at bedtime. *Recurrence prevention*, continue same dose as for acute treatment; range 300-800mg/day at bedtime. Use lowest effective dose.
Major Depressive Disorder (MDD), add-on, 50mg (day 1 and 2), 150mg (day 3 and 4). Use lowest effective dose; antidepressant effect seen at 150-300mg/day. Admin prior to bedtime. Prolonged/R formulations should be swallowed whole and not crushed or chewed.

Elderly: Prolonged/R (XR, XL), *Major Depressive Disorder*, 50mg/day (days 1-3); titrate to 100mg/day (day 4), 150mg/day (day 8). Use lowest effective dose; if increase to 300mg/day required this should not be prior to day 22.

Child: Under 18, not recommended.

Hepatic Impairment: Standard/R, initially 25mg/day; titrate daily with 25-50mg/day increments if required. Prolonged/R, initially 50mg/day; titrate by 50mg/day increments to effective dose.

Interactions: Effect of Other Drugs on Quetiapine: *Co-admin not recommended (plasma levels increased)*: CYP3A4 inhibitors (HIV-protease inhibitors, azole antifungals, erythromycin, clarithromycin, nefazodone). *Co-admin caution*: Other centrally acting drugs, ALCOHOL, drugs causing (QT-prolongation, electrolyte imbalance). *Plasma levels decreased (use only if benefit outweighs risk)*: CYP3A4 inducers (carbamazepine, phenytoin) (any change in inducer should be gradual; if required replace

3.2.3 Atypical Antipsychotics

with non-inducer e.g. valproate). *Increased pyramidal events*: Lithium.

SP: Children, adolescents (age 10-17 years), higher adverse event frequency (increased appetite, serum prolactin elevation, vomiting, rhinitis, syncope) or different implications (extrapyramidal symptoms, irritability) identified in adults (increased BP); thyroid function changes observed. Tardive dyskinesia, may worsen/arise after discontinuation. Sedation. *Caution*, sleep apnoea syndrome (overweight or obese, male, history of or receiving other CNS depressants), cardiovascular, cerebrovascular, conditions predisposing to hypotension (quetiapine may induce hypotension), history of seizures, co-admin of medications with anti-cholinergic effect, caution (urinary retention, prostatic hypertrophy, intestinal obstruction), history or alcohol or drug abuse (misuse reported). *Reported*, cardiomyopathy, myocarditis, dysphagia (aspiration pneumonia risk), constipation. *Consider*, slower titration (especially elderly, younger patients); severe neutropenia, agranulocytosis (presence of infection or fever especially without predisposing factors). False positive enzyme immunoassays (methadone, TCADs). Pancreatitis. Metabolic parameters, see Notes below.

ADR: Summary, *most common*, somnolence, dizziness, headache, dry mouth, withdrawal symptoms, elevated (serum triglycerides, total cholesterol predominantly LDL-cholesterol), decreased (HDL-cholesterol, Hb), weight gain, extrapyramidal symptoms. See SP above.

Notes: See 3.2.3 Atypical Antipsychotics.

Interchangeability: Same strengths of all brands of quetiapine film-coated (f/c) Standard/R tabs and Prolonged/R tabs listed below are deemed interchangeable.

Reference Price: Standard/R (60) 25mg, €5.40. 100mg, €11.40. 200mg, €17.40. 300mg, €25.20. Prolonged/R (60) 50mg, €16.20. 150mg, €24.60. 200mg, €31.80. 300mg, €49.80. 400mg, €60.60.

Seroquel Tablets, XR Tablets *(AstraZeneca)* A. GMS.
Price, (60) 25mg, €23.32; 100mg, €58.28; 200mg, €66.43; 300mg, €108.51. Prolonged/R (XR) (60) 50mg, €25.92. 150mg, €98.86. 200mg, €51.65. 300mg, €67.32. 400mg, €90.21.
Standard/R f/c tablet, quetiapine fumarate 25mg, 100mg, 200mg, 300mg. Round (except 300mg). Marked SEROQUEL and strength. 25mg: Peach. 100mg: Yellow. 200mg: White. 300mg: White cap-shaped. *Lactose*.
Prolonged/R tablet (XR), as above 50mg, 150mg, 200mg, 300mg, 400mg. Marked R/strength. 50mg: Peach. 150mg: White. 200mg: Yellow. 300mg: Pale-yellow. 400mg: White. *Lactose*.

Geroquel 25mg, 100mg, 200mg *(Gerard)* A. GMS.
Price, (60) see reference price above.
Standard/R f/c tablet, quetiapine fumarate 25mg, 100mg, 200mg, 300mg. Round. Marked Q over strength (25mg marked only Q). 25mg: Peach. 100mg: Yellow. 200mg: White. *Lactose*.

Notiabolfen XL 200mg, 300mg, 400mg *(Accord)* A. GMS.
Price, (60) see reference price above.
Prolonged/R tablet (XL), quetiapine hemifumarate. Round. 200mg: Yellow. Marked I2. 300mg: Light-yellow. Marked Q300. 400mg: White. Marked I4. *Lactose, sodium*.

Quentiax SR Tablets *(Krka)* A. GMS.
Price, tabs see reference price above. 300mg, €67.32.
Prolonged/R f/c tablet (SR), quetiapine hemifumarate 50mg, 150mg, 200mg, 300mg. 50mg: White cap-shaped. Marked 50. 150mg: Pink (orange) round. 200mg: Yellow (brown) oval. 300mg: Pale brownish-yellow. *Lactose, sodium*.

Quetex, XR Tablets *(Rowex)* A. GMS.
Price, (60) see reference price above.
Standard/R f/c tablet, quetiapine fumarate 25mg, 50mg 100mg, 200mg, 300mg. Round (except 300mg). Marked with strength. 25mg: Salmon-pink. 100mg: Yellow scored*. 200mg: White scored*. 300mg: White oval scored*. *Lactose*. *(divisible into equal quarters)*.
Prolonged/R tablet (XR), quetiapine fumarate 50mg, 150mg, 200mg, 300mg, 400mg. Round f/c. 50mg: Peach-coloured. Marked Q50. 200mg: Yellow. Marked I2. 300mg: Light-yellow. Marked Q300. 400mg: White. Marked I4. *Lactose, sodium 3.5mg/200mg tab, 5.3mg/300mg tab, 7.1mg/400mg tab*.

Quetiapine (Accord) Tablets *(Accord)* A. GMS.
Price, (60) see reference price above.
Standard/R f/c tablet, quetiapine fumarate 25mg, 100mg, 200mg, 300mg. Round (except 300mg). 25mg: Pink. 100mg: Yellow. 200mg: White (off-white). 300mg: Cap-shaped white (off-white). Marked 300. *Lactose*.

Quetiapine Actavis Tablets *(Accord)* A. GMS.
Price, (60) see reference price above.
Standard/R f/c tablet, quetiapine fumarate 25mg, 100mg, 200mg, 300mg. Round (25mg, 100mg). Marked Q. 25mg: Light-orange. 100mg: Yellow. 200mg, 300mg: White oval. 300mg: Marked 300. *Lactose*.

Quetiapine Krka Tablets *(Krka)* A. GMS.
Price, (60) see reference price above.
Standard/R f/c tablet, quetiapine hemifumarate 25mg, 100mg, 200mg, 300mg. Round (except 300mg). 25mg: Pale-red. 100mg: Yellow-brown. 200mg: White. 300mg: White cap-shaped. *Lactose*.

Seropia, XR Tablets *(Clonmel)* A. GMS.
Price, (60) see reference price above.
Standard/R f/c tablet, quetiapine fumarate 25mg, 100mg, 200mg, 300mg. Round (except 300mg) scored (except 25mg, 200mg) (divisible into equal halves). 25mg: Peach. 100mg: Yellow. 200mg: White. 300mg: White cap-shaped. *Lactose*.
Prolonged/R (XR) tablet, as above 50mg, 150mg, 200mg, 300mg, 400mg. White (off white). Marked with strength. 50mg: Round. 150mg, 200mg, 300mg: Oblong. 400mg: Oval. *Lactose*.

Tevaquel, XL Tablets *(TEVA)* A. GMS.
Price, (60) see reference price above. Standard/R 300mg, €64.80.
Standard/R f/c tablet, quetiapine fumarate 25mg, 100mg, 200mg, 300mg. Round (except 300mg). Marked with strength. 25mg, 100mg: Light-orange. 200mg: White (off-white). 300mg: Pale-yellow cap-shaped. *Lactose, Sunset Yellow (25mg, 100mg)*.
Prolonged/R tablet (XL), quetiapine fumarate 50mg, 200mg, 300mg, 400mg. Cap-shaped f/c. Marked Q and strength. 50mg: Brown. 200mg: Yellow. 300mg: Light-yellow. 400mg: White.

Risperidone

ATC Code: N05AX08. **Sport:** Permitted.
Driving: CNS, visual effects.

Indications: Schizophrenia; moderate to severe manic episodes in bipolar disorder. Short-term treatment (up to 6 weeks) persistent aggression (patients with moderate to severe Alzheimer's dementia), persistent aggression (conduct disorder). Schizophrenia, parenteral maintenance.

Dose: Adult: ORAL, *schizophrenia*, initially 2mg/day (day 1); increase to 4mg/day (day 2); maintenance, range 4-6mg/day; above 10mg/day no additional efficacy; over 16mg/day, not recommended. Admin in 1-2 divided doses.
Bipolar mania, initially 2mg/day; increase by 1mg/day at minimum 24-hour intervals; range 1-6mg once daily.
Behavioural disturbances, persistent aggression in Alzheimer's dementia, initially 0.25mg twice daily; titrate by 0.25mg twice daily increments every other day; optimum 0.5mg twice daily; 1mg twice daily has been beneficial. With or without food. OroDisp tabs not to be divided. Film-coated tabs to be taken with fluid.
PARENTERAL, 25mg every 2 weeks; max. 50mg every 2 weeks. Deep IM deltoid or gluteal injection (not for IV use). Conversion oral to IM, stabilised on 4mg oral, switch to 25mg IM; above 4mg oral, consider 37.5mg IM.
Elderly: ORAL, schizophrenia, bipolar mania, initially 0.5mg twice daily; titrate by 0.5mg twice daily increments to 1-2mg twice daily.
PARENTERAL (IM), initially 25mg every 2 weeks. Dementia, see Adult above.
Child: ORAL, age 5-18 years. *Conduct, other disruptive behaviour disorders*, 50kg or more, initially 0.5mg/day; titrate by 0.5mg/day increments every second day if needed; optimum 1mg/day; range 0.5-1.5mg/day. 50kg or less, initially 0.25mg/day; titrate by 0.25mg increments as above; optimum 0.5mg/day; range 0.25-0.75mg/day. Admin once daily.
Autism, age 5 years and over, adolescents, under 20kg, initially 0.25mg/day (days 1-3); titrate by 0.25mg (days 4-14); titrate at 2-week intervals to max. 1.5mg/day. 20kg or more, initially 0.5mg (days 1-3); titrate by 0.5mg (days 4-14); titrate at 2-week intervals to max. 2.5mg/day or 3.5mg/day (over 45kg). Under 5 years, not recommended.
Renal Impairment: As for Elderly above. Consider, half initial and maintenance doses; titrate slowly with caution.
Hepatic Impairment: As for Renal above.
Interactions: Effect of Other Drugs on Risperidone: *Co-admin caution*: Other centrally acting drugs. *Plasma levels decreased*: Carbamazepine, CYP3A4 and/or P-gp inducers. *Plasma levels increased*: Phenothiazines, TCADs, beta-

blockers, CYP2D6 inhibitors (fluoxetine, paroxetine, quinidine), haloperidol. *Increased bioavailability*: Cimetidine, ranitidine. *Higher elderly mortality*: Furosemide. See Notes below.

Effect of Risperidone on Other Drugs: Levodopa, other dopamine agonists: *Effect antagonised.*

SP: Cardiovascular disorders (titrate gradually). Parkinson's Disease, Lewy body dementia (use only if benefit outweighs risk). Change in timing of dose may improve impact on sedation. Antiemetic effect may mask overdose of certain medicines or conditions (intestinal obstruction, Reye's syndrome, brain tumour). Intraoperative Floppy Iris Syndrome observed during cataract surgery. Hyperprolactinaemia; evaluate prolactin plasma level if evidence of possible prolactin-related side-effects (gynaecomastia, menstrual disorders, anovulation, fertility disorder, decreased libido, erectile dysfunction, and galactorrhoea). *Children*, measure baseline weight before initiation; monitor regularly. *Parenteral*, avoid injection into blood vessel. If hypersensitivity reactions occur, discontinue.

ADR: *Most frequent*, insomnia, sedation, somnolence, parkinsonism, headache. *Children/adolescents*, similar to adults. *Parenteral*, serious injection-site reactions.

Notes: See 3.2.3 Atypical Antipsychotics.

Interchangeability: Same strengths of all brands of risperidone oral soln and tabs (f/c, orodispersible) listed below are deemed interchangeable.

Reference Price: (20) 0.5mg, €2.20; 1mg, €2.41. (60) 2mg, €11.34; 3mg, €16.46; 4mg, €22.94. (28) 6mg, €25.62. Oral soln 1mg/mL (100mL) €23.73.

Risperdal Quicklet, Oral Soln *(Janssen-Cilag)* A. GMS.
Price, tabs 1mg (60) €7.23, other strengths, oral soln, see reference price above. Quicklet (28) 1mg, €3.37. 2mg, €5.29. 3mg, €7.68. 4mg, €10.70.
F/c tablet, risperidone 0.5mg, 1mg, 2mg, 3mg, 4mg, 6mg. Oblong (except 6mg) scored (facilitates breaking). Marked RIS/strength; JANSSEN may be on reverse. 0.5mg: Brownish-red. 1mg: White. 2mg: Orange. 3mg: Yellow. 6mg: Round yellow. *Lactose, Sunset Yellow (2mg, 6mg).*
OroDisp tablet (Quicklet), as above 1mg, 2mg, 3mg, 4mg. 1mg, 2mg: Square light-coral. 3mg, 4mg: Round coral. Marked R/strength. *Aspartame.*
Oral soln, as above 1mg/mL. Clear colourless.

Risperdal Consta Parenteral *(Janssen-Cilag)* A. GMS.
Price, (1) 25mg €103.37. 37.5mg, €143.59. 50mg, €187.35.
Prolonged/R Injection, risperidone 25mg, 37.5mg, 50mg. IM injection. Powder: White (off-white) free-flowing. Diluent: Clear colourless aqueous soln. *Sodium 3mg/mL reconstituted soln.*

Perdamel Tablets *(Clonmel)* A. GMS.
Price, tabs 1mg (60) €7.23, see reference price above.
Tablet, 0.5mg, 1mg, 2mg, 3mg, 4mg. Oblong f/c scored (divisible into equal halves). Marked R; strength on reverse. 0.5mg: Brownish-red. 1mg: White. 2mg: Salmon. 3mg: Yellow. 4mg: Light-green. *Lactose, Sunset Yellow (3mg, 6mg).*

Risperidone (Accord) Tablets *(Accord)* A. GMS.
Price, tabs 1mg (60) €7.23, see reference price above.
Tablet, risperidone 0.5mg, 1mg, 2mg, 3mg, 4mg. Cap-shaped (except 0.5mg, 3mg). 0.5mg: Round brick-red. 1mg: White (off-white). 2mg: Light-orange. 3mg: Light-yellow oval scored (facilitates breaking). 4mg: Green. *Lactose, Sunset Yellow (2mg).*

Rispeva Tablets *(TEVA)* A. GMS.
Price, tabs 1mg (60) €7.23, see reference price above.
Tablet, risperidone 0.5mg, 1mg, 2mg, 3mg, 4mg. Round f/c scored (all divisible into equal doses). Marked RIS and strength. 0.5mg: Brownish-red. 1mg: White. 2mg: Tan. 3mg: Yellow. 4mg: Green. *Lactose.*

Rispone Tablets, Oral Soln *(Rowex)* A. GMS.
Price, tabs 1mg (60) €7.23, see reference price above.
Tablet, risperidone 0.5mg, 1mg, 2mg, 3mg, 4mg, 6mg. f/c. 0.5mg: Red oval breaking-notched*. 1mg: White. 2mg: Pink. 3mg: Yellow. 4mg: Dark-pink. Oblong scored*. 6mg: Yellow oval breaking-notched (divisible (6mg) into equal halves). *(divisible into equal halves). *Lactose.*
Oral soln, as above 1mg/mL. Clear colourless.

Sulpiride

ATC Code: N05AL01. **Sport:** Permitted.
Driving: May cause sedation; ability can be impaired.
Indications: Schizophrenia.
Dose: Adult, Elderly: Predominantly positive symptoms, initially 400mg twice daily; max. 1200mg twice daily. Predominantly negative symptoms, as well as depression,

initially 400mg twice daily; reduction to 200mg twice daily normally increases alerting effect. Mixed positive and negative symptoms, usually 400-600mg twice daily. *Elderly*, as for Renal below.

Renal Impairment: Initiate at lowest dose; titrate slowly.

CI: Phaeochromocytoma, acute porphyria, concomitant prolactin-dependent tumours (pituitary gland prolactinomas, breast cancer).

Interactions: Effect of Other Drugs on Sulpiride: *Co-admin contraindicated, reciprocal antagonism*: Levodopa or antiparkinsonian drugs (including ropinirole). *Enhanced sedative effect, co-admin not recommended*: ALCOHOL. *Torsades de Pointes risk, QT-interval prolonged*: Drugs causing bradycardia (beta-blockers, diltiazem, verapamil, clonidine, digitalis), drugs inducing hypokalaemia (hypokalaemic diuretics, stimulant laxatives, IV amphotericin B, glucocorticoids, tetracosactides), Class Ia antiarrhythmics (quinidine, disopyramide), Class III antiarrhythmics (amiodarone, sotalol), pimozide, haloperidol, imipramine antidepressants, cisapride, thioridazine, IV erythromycin, pentamidine. *Postural hypotension risk*: Other antihypertensives. *Caution*: CNS depressants (narcotics, analgesics, sedative H1-antihistamines, barbiturates, benzodiazepines and other anxiolytics, clonidine), lithium. *Absorption decreased*: Antacids, sucralfate (admin 2 hours apart).

Effect of Sulpiride on Other Drugs: Metoclopramide: *Response modified.*

SP: Increased motor agitation at high doses; hypomania, convulsions, extrapyramidal reactions. Sulpiride may increase prolactin levels, caution with history/family history of breast cancer (monitor).

ADR: *Common*, hyperprolactinaemia, insomnia, sedation or drowsiness, extrapyramidal disorder, Parkinsonism, tremor, akathisia, increased hepatic enzymes, breast pain, galactorrhoea, weight gain.

Notes: See 3.2.3 Atypical Antipsychotics.

Dolmatil 200mg, 400mg *(SANOFI)* B. GMS.
Price, (100) 200mg, €20.90. 400mg, €45.90.
Tablet, sulpiride. White scored. 200mg: Round. Marked D200. 400mg: Stick-shaped f/c scored (facilitates breaking). Marked SLP400. *Lactose.*

Ziprasidone

ATC Code: N05AE04. **Sport:** Permitted.
Driving: Somnolence. May influence.
Indications: Schizophrenia. Manic or mixed episodes of moderate severity in bipolar disorder.

Dose: Adult, Elderly: Schizophrenia, bipolar mania, acute, 40mg twice daily; titrate to max. 80mg twice daily (as early as day 3); max. 160mg/day. Maintenance, 20mg twice daily. *Admin*, with food. *Elderly*, over 65 years, consider lower starting dose.

Child: Bipolar mania, age 10-17 years, acute, single 20mg dose (day 1) with food; then as 2 divided daily doses, titrating over 1-2 weeks to target range 120 to max. 160mg/day (weight 45kg and above) OR 60mg/day to max. 80mg/day (weight under 45kg).

Hepatic Impairment: Consider lower doses; severe, caution.

CI: QT-interval prolongation, congenital long QT-syndrome, recent MI, uncompensated HF. Arrhythmias treated with Class Ia and III antiarrhythmics.

Interactions: Effect of Other Drugs on Ziprasidone: *Co-admin contraindicated*: Drugs prolonging QT-interval (Class Ia and III antiarrhythmics), arsenic trioxide, halofantrine, levomethadyl acetate, mesoridazine, thioridazine, pimozide, sparfloxacin, gatifloxacin, moxifloxacin, dolasetron mesilate, mefloquine, sertindole, cisapride. *Co-admin caution*: Other centrally acting drugs, ALCOHOL, serotonergics (SSRIs; serotonin syndrome). *Plasma levels increased*: Ketoconazole, other potent CYP3A4 inhibitors (unlikely to be of clinical importance). *Plasma levels decreased*: Carbamazepine.

SP: Drug reaction with eosinophilia and systemic symptoms (DRESS), Stevens-Johnson syndrome; severe cutaneous adverse reactions, discontinue.

ADR: *Most common* (in clinical trials), insomnia,

3.2.4 Antimanic Drugs

somnolence, headache, agitation (schizophrenia); sedation, headache, somnolence (bipolar mania). See SP above.

Notes: See 3.2.3 Atypical Antipsychotics.

Geodon 20mg, 40mg, 60mg, 80mg *(Pfizer)* A. GMS.
Price, (56) 20mg, €75.73. 40mg, €75.54. 60mg, €86.97. 80mg, €114.70.
Capsule, ziprasidone HCl. Marked Pfizer, ZDX/strength. 20mg, 80mg: Blue/white. 40mg: Blue. 60mg: White. *Lactose.* **Store:** Below 30 deg C.

3.2.4 - Antimanic Drugs

In This Chapter: *Lithium.*

Class Effects

CI: Hypersensitivity to any member of the class.

Lithium

ATC Code: N05AN01. **Sport:** Permitted.
Driving: Reaction-time affected; consider adverse reaction profile.
Indications: Treatment and prophylaxis, mania, bipolar affective disorders, recurrent depression. Treatment, aggressive or self-mutilating behaviour.

Dose: Adult: *Priadel,* initially 400-1200mg/day as single dose morning or bedtime or as 2 divided doses for 4-7 days; adjust dose to serum lithium range 0.5-1.5mmoL/L. Tabs should not be crushed or chewed.

NOTE: Bioavailability varies from product to product particularly retard or slow release preparations; change of product should be regarded as initiation of new treatment. Lithium has narrow therapeutic window; regular plasma lithium monitoring obligatory; do not initiate unless adequate monitoring facilities available.

Elderly: *Priadel,* under 50kg, initially 200-400mg; increase by 200-400mg every 3-5 days to achieve serum level range 0.8-1mmoL/L (range 800-1800mg/day). Prophylaxis, range 0.4-2.5mmoL/L (range 600-1200mg/day).

Child: Not recommended.

Renal Impairment: Mild/moderate, lithium excretion reduced; monitor. Severe, contraindicated.

CI: Hypothyroidism (untreated, untreatable), cardiac disease (with rhythm disorder), Brugada syndrome (family history of), low body sodium (dehydrated, low sodium diet, Addison's disease).

Interactions: Effect of Other Drugs on Lithium: *Plasma levels increased (reduced renal clearance), toxicity risk:* Drugs which may cause renal impairment (monitor lithium levels). *Co-admin avoid:* Drugs prolonging QT-interval including amisulpride, Class Ia antiarrhythmics (disopyramide, procainamide, quinidine), Class III antiarrhythmics (amiodarone, sotalol), arsenic trioxide, artemisinin derivatives, cisapride, erythromycin (IV), haloperidol, pimozide, sertindole, terfenadine, thioridazine, antipsychotics. *Co-admin caution:* Drugs lowering epileptic threshold (SSRIs, TCADs, antipsychotics, anaesthetics, theophylline); thiazides (paradoxical antidiuretic effect with possible water retention/lithium intoxication), other diuretics (including herbal), loop diuretics (furosemide, bumetanide, etacrynic acid; less likely to cause lithium retention) (caution), drugs affecting electrolyte balance (steroids, sodium bicarbonate salts), NSAIDs including COX II inhibitors, antibiotics (tetracyclines, metronidazole, co-trimoxazole), drugs affecting RAS (ACEIs, AIIAs). *Plasma levels decreased (increased renal clearance):* Osmotic diuretics, carbonic anhydrase inhibitors, xanthines (theophylline, caffeine), products containing high sodium content (sodium bicarbonate), calcium channel blockers. *Interactions perhaps not due to increased/decreased plasma levels (neurotoxic effects):* Antipsychotics (including atypical antipsychotics olanzapine, clozapine), carbamazepine, phenytoin, methyldopa, clonazepam, triptan derivatives/SSRIs (serotonin syndrome); calcium channel blockers, neuromuscular blockers (neurotoxic effects).

SP: Before initiation, evaluate renal function (primarily excreted by kidney), cardiac and thyroid function (patients should be euthyroid; monitor periodically. Use lowest effective dose; adjust according to serum lithium levels to provide adequate control and prevent toxicity; monitor more frequently (dose or formulation change, intercurrent disease or infection, change in fluid or sodium intake, drugs altering lithium renal clearance or changing electrolyte balance i.e. sodium and fluid intake). Caution, electrolyte imbalances in hot weather or work environment, infectious diseases including colds, influenza, gastro-enteritis, UTI. Low sodium diets, not recommended. Elderly particularly liable to lithium toxicity; caution, excretion may be reduced. Discontinue 24 hours before major surgery.

Signs of acute lithium toxicity (sedation, coarse tremor, vomiting, diarrhoea), discontinue immediately. Convulsion risk increased (epileptics, drugs lowering seizure threshold). Benign intracranial hypertension (persistent headache and/or visual disturbances). May unmask or aggravate Brugada syndrome.

NOTE: Clear instructions of symptoms of toxicity should be given to patients on long-term lithium therapy; polyuria or polydipsia, episodes of nausea, vomiting, diarrhoea, excessive sweating and/or other conditions leading to salt/water depletion, including severe dieting.

Pregnancy, Lactation: *Pregnancy,* avoid unless considered essential, especially first trimester; harmful to foetus (neonatal severe cardiovascular system abnormalities, hypothyroidism); if necessary, ensure lowest plasma levels. Increased lithium clearance in second and third trimesters, adjust dose. Women of childbearing potential should use adequate contraception. If pregnancy planned, strongly recommend discontinuing lithium. Monitor fluid balance during labour; titrate dose after delivery. *Lactation,* contraindicated; lithium passes extensively into breast milk.

ADR: Dose related; less common at plasma level below 1mmoL/L. Adverse reactions usually subside with temporary reduction or lithium discontinuation. Mild GI effects (nausea), general discomfort, vertigo initially; fine hand tremors, polyuria, mild thirst may persist.

Notes: See 3.2.4 Antimanic Drugs.

Priadel 200mg, 400mg *(SANOFI)* A. GMS.
Price, (100) 200mg, €2.80. 400mg, €4.71.
Prolonged/R tablet, lithium carbonate. White. 200mg: Cap-shaped scored. Marked P200. 400mg: Round scored (divisible into equal halves). Marked Priadel. *Mannitol*

3.3 - Antidepressants and Anxiolytics

Class Effects

A wide range of drug classes are used in the treatment of depressive states. Certain anxiolytics (benzodiazepines) may also be used. See Notes below (anxiolytics).

CI: Hypersensitivity to any member of the class.

SP: Antidepressants and Suicidality: Depression is associated with increased risk of suicidal thoughts, self-harm, and suicide or suicide-related events; risk persists until significant remission occurs, monitor closely. With all antidepressants, suicide risk may increase in early stages of recovery or with dose changes. History of suicide-related events or those exhibiting significant degree of suicidal ideation prior to treatment initiation at greater risk and need careful monitoring. Possibility of increased suicide risk in young adults including suicide attempts/thoughts and hostility (predominantly aggression, oppositional behaviour, anger) were more frequently observed in clinical trials with children and adolescents. Other psychiatric conditions treated with antidepressants can also be associated with increased suicide risk.

Notes: See 3.3.5 Benzodiazepine Anxiolytics.

3.3.1 - Tricyclic, Tetracyclic Antidepressants

In This Chapter: *Amitriptyline, clomipramine, dosulepin (dothiepin), lofepramine, trimipramine. Related antidepressants, trazodone.*

Class Effects

Driving: Inform patient of effects of this medication on reaction time and that it can cause side effects that may impair driving (dizziness, drowsiness, sleepiness,

108

blurred/double vision, reduced alertness). Advise patient not to drive until effect of medication is known; not to drink alcohol or use other psychoactive substances when taking this medicine.

CI: Children under 18 years unless otherwise specified. Recent MI, heart block, cardiac arrhythmias, severe (liver, renal) disease. Closed-angle glaucoma, existing urinary retention, prostatic hypertrophy, acute psychosis and/or mania.

Interactions: Effect of Other Drugs on Tricyclic, Tetracyclic and Related Antidepressants: *Co-admin, not recommended:* MAOIs (with or within 14 days of cessation). *Plasma levels increased:* Antipsychotics, cimetidine, oestrogens (increased toxicity), methylphenidate, quinidine, SSRIs, disulfiram, ritonavir, fluconazole. *Plasma levels decreased:* Carbamazepine, barbiturates, phenytoin, nicotine, rifampicin. *Reduced antidepressant effect:* Oestrogens. *Increased antimuscarinic side effect risk:* Other antimuscarinics, antihistamines (sedation), clozapine. *Increased CNS effects:* Sibutramine. *Severe cardiac arrhythmias:* Thioridazine. *Hyperpyrexia:* Anticholinergics, neuroleptics (especially during hot weather). *Increased ventricular arrhythmia risk/Torsades de Pointes, caution:* Non-antiarrhythmics prolonging QT-interval (macrolides, cisapride, malaria agents, terfenadine, neuroleptics).

Effect of Tricyclic, Tetracyclic and Related Antidepressants on Other Drugs: Guanethidine, bethanidine, debrisoquine, methyldopa, clonidine: *Effect reduced.* Sympathomimetics, including topical (adrenaline, ephedrine, isoprenaline, noradrenaline, phenylephrine, phenylpropanolamine: *Cardiovascular effects potentiated.* ALCOHOL, tramadol, opioid analgesics (sedation), CNS depressants (barbiturates, benzodiazepines): *Increased CNS side effects.* Anticholinergics (atropine, biperiden, levodopa, phenothiazines), antipsychotics with anticholinergic action: *Hyper-excitation, delirium, glaucoma.* Antiarrhythmics (quinidine type): *Co-admin not recommended.* Phenytoin: *Elevated serum levels.* Anaesthetics: *Increased arrhythmia/hypotension risk; inform anaesthetist.* Amphetamines, baclofen, thyroid hormones, coumarins: *Effect potentiated.* Anticonvulsants: *Potentiation or reduction of effect.* Antiarrhythmics (Class 1a), other antipsychotics, moxifloxacin and terfenadine (avoid co-admin): *Increased arrhythmia risk/potentiation.*

SP: Suicide, see Notes below (antidepressants). *Caution,* cardiovascular disease, QT-prolongation (medicinals prolonging QT-interval, congenital long QT-syndrome, bradycardia, uncorrected electrolyte imbalance), heart-block, arrhythmias, recovery period post MI. Diabetes, altered glycaemic control. Epilepsy, factors lowering seizure threshold (brain damage), porphyria, blood dyscrasias. Elective surgery, discontinue before; emergency, inform anaesthetist. Electroconvulsive therapy, caution. Antimuscarinic effects (urinary retention, prostatic hyperplasia, chronic constipation, narrow-angle glaucoma, phaeochromocytoma). Hyperthyroidism. Impaired liver function or severe hepatic adverse events (potentially fatal). Long-term, increased dental caries. Schizophrenia, psychotic symptoms aggravated. Bipolar disorder, mania. *Elderly,* caution, agitation, confusion, postural hypotension; pharmacogenic psychoses; more prone to adverse events. Increased bone fracture risk. Withdrawal symptoms, insomnia, irritability, excessive perspiration with abrupt withdrawal; withdraw gradually. Serotonin syndrome may occur when TCADs are used with other serotonergics (may be fatal) (neuromuscular excitation, autonomic changes, changed mental state).

Pregnancy, Lactation: Pregnancy, if benefit outweighs risk. Withdrawal symptoms, respiratory depression, agitation reported in neonates born to mothers taking tricyclic antidepressants during last trimester. Lactation, stop nursing or stop drug.

ADR: Arrhythmias, conduction defects, hypotension, postural hypotension, tachycardia, clinically irrelevant ECG changes, drowsiness, confusion, anxiety, dizziness, tremor, headache, paraesthesia, nausea, vomiting, abdominal disorder, diarrhoea, anorexia, hepatic dysfunction, elevated LFTs, allergic reactions, photosensitivity, pruritus, weight gain, disturbances of libido and potency, breast disorders, gynaecomastia, taste disturbance, tinnitus. Serious, bone marrow depression, agranulocytosis, cholestatic jaundice, hypomania, convulsions. Anticholinergic effects, dry mouth, accommodation disturbances, constipation, urinary retention. *Phenothiazine combination,* QT-prolongation, cardiac arrhythmias (ventricular fibrillation/tachycardia), sudden unexplained death, cardiac arrest and Torsades de pointes. See Notes below (phenothiazines).

Notes: See 3.3 Antidepressants and Anxiolytics. See 3.2.1 Phenothiazines.

Amitriptyline

ATC Code: N06AA09. **Sport:** Permitted.
Driving: Caution.

Indications: Depressive illness.

Dose: Adult: Initially 75mg/day in divided doses or single dose at night; titrate to 150mg/day if needed. *Hospitalised,* initially 100mg/day; titrate to 200mg/day, 300mg/day may be needed. Maintenance, 50-100mg at bedtime; use lowest effective dose.

Elderly: Initially 30-75mg/day in divided doses or at bedtime.

Notes: See 3.3.1 Tricyclic, Tetracyclic Antidepressants.

Amitriptyline 25mg *(Clonmel)* A. GMS.
Price, (500) €14.80.
Tablet, amitriptyline HCl. Round yellow s/c. *Lactose.*

Clomipramine

ATC Code: N06AA04. **Sport:** Permitted.
Driving: Blurred vision, somnolence, disturbed attention, confusion, disorientation, aggravated depression, delirium.

Indications: Endogenous depression e.g. manic depression, periodic and involutional depression, reactive and neurotic depression. Obsessional and phobic states. Adjunctive, cataplexy associated with narcolepsy.

Dose: Adult: *Depression,* initially 10mg/day; titrate gradually to 30-150mg/day; usual range 30-75mg, max. 250mg. *Obsessional or phobic states,* initially 25mg/day; titrate over 2 weeks to 100-150mg/day.

Cataplexy associated with narcolepsy, adjunctive, initially 10mg/day; titrate to 50mg/day.

Admin with or without food as single dose at bedtime or divided doses; do not break tabs. Interchange standard and prolonged release at equiv. dose.

Elderly: Age 65 years and older, initially 10mg/day; titrate cautiously to 30-75mg/day.

Child: Not recommended.

Renal Impairment: Severe, caution.

Hepatic Impairment: Caution. Severe, not recommended.

Interactions: Effect of Other Drugs on Clomipramine: *Increased plasma levels:* Alprazolam, disulfiram, cimetidine, grapefruit juice, cranberry juice. *Increased exposure (clomipramine and N-demethylated metabolite accumulation), consider dose adjustment:* Terbinafine, valproate. *Decreased plasma levels:* St John's Wort.

SP: NOTE: QTc prolongation and serotonergic toxicity, adhere to recommended dose; caution, dose increase, co-admin with serotonergic agents. Recent convulsions, low convulsion threshold, pre-existing agitation exacerbation. Adrenal medulla tumours. Panic disorders, paradoxical initial increase in anxiety. Avoid abrupt discontinuation.

ADR: May be difficult to distinguish certain undesirable events from symptoms of depression (fatigue, disturbed sleep, agitation, anxiety, constipation, dry mouth).

Notes: See 3.2.3 Atypical Antipsychotics.

Anafranil 10mg, 25mg, 50mg, SR 75mg *(Novartis)* A. GMS.
Price, (84) 10mg, €3.70; 25mg, €7.47. (56) 50mg, €9.24. SR 75mg (28) €7.16.
Capsule, clomipramine HCl. Hard gelatin opaque. Marked with Geigy logo. 10mg: Greyish-yellow/caramel. 25mg: Brownish-orange/caramel. 50mg: Light-grey/caramel. *Lactose.*
Prolonged/R tablet, as above. Pink cap-shaped f/c scored. Marked CG; GD on reverse. *Castor oil.*

3.3.2 Monamine Oxidase Inhibitors

Dosulepin (dothiepin)

ATC Code: N06AA16. **Sport:** Permitted.
Driving: Caution.
Indications: Depression, associated anxiety.
Dose: Adult: Usually 75-150mg/day in divided doses or as single dose at night. *Hospitalised*, usually 25-50mg 3-times daily or 75-150mg as single dose at night; up to 225mg/day.
Elderly: Initially, 50-75mg/day. Titrate with caution; half normal adult dose may be sufficient.
Child: Not recommended.
Notes: See 3.3.1 Tricyclic, Tetracyclic Antidepressants.

> **Prothiaden 25mg, 75mg** *(Teofarma)* A. GMS.
> *Price*, caps 25mg (100) €4.98; (500) €23.76. Tabs 75mg (28) €3.91; (100) €13.31.
> *Capsule*, dosulepin HCl. Hard red/brown gelatin containing white (off-white) powder. Marked P25. *Lactose*.
> *Tablet*, as above. SC red. Marked P75. *Sucrose, glucose.*

Lofepramine

ATC Code: N06AA07. **Sport:** Permitted.
Driving: Ability may be affected especially with ALCOHOL.
Indications: Depressive illness, including states associated with panic disorder.
Dose: Adult: Usually 70mg twice or 3-times daily; max. 70mg per dose. Depression, anxiety states associated with panic disorder, initially 70mg daily for first week.
Elderly: Consider lower dose.
Child: Not recommended.
CI: Mania, risk of paralytic ileus. Acute alcoholic, hypnotic, analgesic, psychotropic drug poisoning, acute deliria.
Interactions: Effect of Lofepramine on Other Drugs: Digitalis glycosides: *Higher arrhythmia risk.*
SP: Blood dyscrasias, porphyria, susceptibility to paralytic ileus.
ADR: Testicular pain, bone marrow depression (rare).
Notes: See 3.3.1 Tricyclic, Tetracyclic Antidepressants.

> **Gamanil 70mg** *(Creo Pharma)* A. GMS.
> *Price*, (56) €12.57.
> *Tablet*, lofepramine HCl. Round lacquered brown-violet f/c scored (facilitates breaking). *Lactose, Ponceau 4R.*

Trazodone

ATC Code: N06AX05. **Sport:** Permitted.
Driving: Drowsiness, sedation, dizziness, confusional states, blurred vision.
Indications: Depression including accompanied by anxiety.
Dose: Adult: Age 18 years and over, initially 75-150mg as single dose in evening or divided doses after food* during the day. Increase slowly to optimal control (as high as 600mg); doses above 300mg only to be admin if hospitalised. *to decrease side-effects.
Elderly: Initially 100mg/day in divided doses or as a single dose at night; may be increased according to tolerance/efficacy; avoid single doses above 100mg; 300mg/day rarely exceeded.
Renal Impairment: Severe, caution.
Hepatic Impairment: Caution, especially severe; monitor liver function periodically.
CI: Alcohol/hypnotics intoxication, acute MI.
Interactions: Effect of Other Drugs on Trazodone: *Undesirable effects more common*: St John's Wort.
SP: Severe hepatic disorders with potential fatal outcome, consider discontinuation.
ADR: Adverse events are of unknown frequency and cannot be estimated from available data.
Notes: See 3.3.1 Tricyclic, Tetracyclic Antidepressants.

> **Molipaxin 50mg, 100mg, 150mg** *(SANOFI)* B. GMS.
> *Price*, caps 50mg (84) €19.13. 100mg (56) €22.52. Tabs 150mg (28) €12.83.
> *Capsule*, trazodone HCl. Hard gelatin opaque contains white powder. Marked with logo. 50mg: Violet/green. Marked R365B. 100mg: Violet/fawn. Marked R365C. *Lactose*.
> *Tablet*, as above. Salmon-pink scored. Marked Molipaxin 150. *Lactose*.

Trimipramine

ATC Code: N06AA06. **Sport:** Permitted.
Driving: Not recommended.
Indications: Depressive illness, especially with sleep disturbance, anxiety, or agitation.
Dose: Adult: Usually 50-100mg/day as single dose 2 hours before bedtime; titrate to 150-300mg/day if needed; reduce after 4-6 weeks to maintenance 75-150mg.
Elderly: Initially half adult dose; increase gradually, caution, falls/confusion.
Child: Under 18 years, not recommended.
Renal Impairment: Lower dose recommended.
Hepatic Impairment: As for Renal above.
Interactions: Effect of Other Drugs on Trimipramine: *Co-admin contraindicated*: MAOI (or within 14 days), sultopride (increased ventricular arrhythmia risk), selegiline (increased serotonin syndrome risk). *Co-admin not advisable*: ALCOHOL (increased sedative effect); clonidine and guanfacine (antihypertensive effect inhibited); alpha and beta sympathomimetics including adrenaline, noradrenaline, dopamine for systemic action by parenteral route (paroxysmal hypertension, possible ventricular arrhythmia); sulpiride (QT-prolongation risk); haloperidol, pimozide, sertindole, ziprasidone (increased cardiac side effect risk). *Co-admin caution*: Drugs prolonging QT-interval (Class IA and III antiarrhymics, macrolides, fluoroquinolones, some antifungals, some antipsychotics), drugs inducing hypokalaemia (hypokalaemic diuretics, stimulant laxatives, glucocorticoids, tetracosactides), drugs causing bradycardia (beta-blockers, diltiazem, verapamil, clonidine, digitalis). *Mutually increased plasma levels/convulsion risk*: Citalopram, fluoxetine, fluvoxamine, paroxetine, sertraline. *Reduced absorption or increased elimination*: Zopiclone. *Serotonin syndrome risk*: Serotonergics (SSRIs, SNRIs, MAOIs, lithium, triptans, tramadol, linezolid, L-tryptophan, St John's Wort).
Effect of Trimipramine on Other Drugs: Antiepileptics, carbamazepine: *Risk of generalised convulsive episodes*. Valproic acid, valpromide: *Adjust dose, clinical supervision.* Baclofen: *Increased muscular hypotonia risk*. Guanethidine (ocular route): *Antihypertensive effect reduced*.
SP: Caution, in elderly or patients with cardiovascular disorders or renal insufficiency.
ADR: Mainly drowsiness or sedation (antihistamine effect) more pronounced at the start of treatment, anti-cholinergic effects, hypotension (particularly orthostatic), CNS irritability, GI upset (constipation), dryness of the mouth, accommodation difficulties, dysuria, micturition disorders, urinary retention, perspiration, impotence.
Notes: See 3.3.1 Tricyclic, Tetracyclic Antidepressants.

> **Surmontil 25mg, 50mg** *(SANOFI)* A. GMS.
> *Price*, 25mg (50) €4.79. 50mg (28) €6.21.
> *Tablet*, trimipramine maleate. White (pale-yellow) round f/c. Marked Surmontil; 25 on reverse. *Lactose*.
> *Capsule*, as above. Opaque green hard gelatin containing white (almost) powder (powder plug). Marked SU 50.

3.3.2 - Monamine Oxidase Inhibitors

In This Chapter: *Moclobemide, tranylcypromine.*

Class Effects

Pharmacology: The MAOIs, rasagiline and selegiline are MAO-B inhibitors used to treat Parkinson's Disease.
CI: Use in children. Liver damage, cardiovascular disease, cerebrovascular disease, phaeochromocytoma, blood dyscrasias.
Interactions: Effect of Other Drugs on MAOIs: *Co-admin contraindicated*: Other MAOI (allow 2-week interval after stopping MAOI). *Co-admin not recommended*: Selegiline, pethidine; TCADs and tetracyclics (contraindicated for some members of class), dextromethorphan, tapentadol, nefazodone, trazodone. *Co-admin avoid*: High ALCOHOL intake. *Metabolism prolonged (reduce dose)*: Cimetidine. *Serotonin Syndrome risk*: Drugs enhancing serotonin (clomipramine).

110

Effect of MAOIs on Other Drugs: Sympathomimetics (amphetamine, dopamine, levodopa, phenylephrine, ephedrine, pseudoephedrine): *Effect enhanced, hypertension risk.* Buspirone: *Hypertension risk.* Opiates: *Effect potentiated.* Antihypertensives: *Caution; interactions, including those with food can occur up to 14 days after MAOIs have been discontinued.*

SP: Suicide, see Notes below (antidepressants). NOTE: Avoid consumption of tyramine-rich food (cheese especially aged or matured, meat, protein rich foods, yeast extracts, smoked foods, pickled herrings, liver, Chianti wine, beer). Dietary restrictions need not be as strict with RIMAs. High levels of tyramine may cause severe hypertensive reactions. Depression with excitation/agitation. Serotonin syndrome (hyperthermia, confusion, hyperreflexia, myoclonus). Epilepsy, depressive episodes in bipolar disorders, manic episodes provoked. Thyrotoxicosis, phaeochromocytoma (hypertensive reactions). Hypersensitivity (rash, oedema). Hyponatraemia (usually elderly; possibly inappropriate ADH secretion); consider if drowsiness, confusion or convulsions develop. Elderly, more prone to adverse events.

Pregnancy, Lactation: Use only if benefit outweighs risk.

ADR: Sleep disturbances, agitation, anxiety, restlessness or irritability, headache, dizziness, paraesthesia, nausea, dry mouth, diarrhoea, constipation, vomiting, visual disturbances, oedema, rash, pruritus, urticaria, flushing, orthostatic hypotension, elevated liver enzymes. Serotonin Syndrome. See SP above.

Notes: See 3.3 Antidepressants and Anxiolytics. See also 3.5.3 Selective MAOIs (rasagiline, selegiline).

Moclobemide

ATC Code: N06AG02. **Sport:** Permitted.
Driving: Monitor individual reaction initially.
Indications: Depressive illness.
Dose: Adult, Elderly: Usually 300mg/day in 2 or 3 divided doses; max. 600mg/day; after 4 weeks reduce slowly to 150mg/day. *Admin,* after food.
Hepatic Impairment: Severe, reduce dose to half or one third.
CI: Acute confusional states.
Interactions: Effect of Other Drugs on Moclobemide: *Co-admin contraindicated:* Selegiline, bupropion, triptans, pethidine, tramadol, dextromethorphan, linezolid. *Co-admin not recommended:* Sibutramine, dextropropoxyphene. *Caution:* St John's Wort (may increase serotonin), drugs enhancing serotonin (venlafaxine, fluvoxamine, clomipramine, citalopram, escitalopram, paroxetine, sertraline, bupropion).
Effect of Moclobemide on Other Drugs: Opiates: *Opiate effect potentiated; consider dose adjustment.* Cimetidine: *Reduce moclobemide dose to half or one-third.* PPIs (omeprazole), fluoxetine, fluvoxamine, trimipramine, maprotiline: *Plasma levels increased.* Sympathomimetics: *Action may be intensified and prolonged.*
SP: Confusional states. Hyponatraemia (usually in elderly) rare. Depressive patients with excitation or agitation as predominant feature, not to be treated with moclobemide alone; only in combination with a sedative (benzodiazepine). Treatment may exacerbate schizophrenic symptoms in depressives with schizophrenic or schizoaffective psychoses. Use with caution in epileptics. Insomnia, nervousness at beginning of treatment; mania or hypomania, interrupt or initiate alternative. When switching from SSRIs to moclobemide, take into account half-life of SSRI.
Notes: See 3.3.2 MAOIs.

Manerix 150mg *(Meda)* A. GMS.
Price, (30) €12.07.
Tablet, moclobemide. Oblong pale-yellow f/c scored. Marked 150. *Lactose.*

Tranylcypromine

ATC Code: N06AF04. **Sport:** Permitted.
Driving: May affect ability.
Indications: Treatment of symptoms of depressive illness especially where phobic symptoms are present or where

---

other types of antidepressants have failed. Recommended for mild depressive states resulting from temporary situational difficulties.
Dose: Adult: Initially 10mg morning and afternoon; if response inadequate after first week, add 10mg at midday and continue for at least a week; 30mg/day should be exceeded with caution. Satisfactory response achieved, reduce to maintenance 10mg/day. With electroconvulsive therapy, 10mg twice daily during the series, then 10mg/day maintenance. *Admin,* with preferably a half a glass of water.
Elderly: Caution, use lowest dose.
SP: Cardiovascular disease, history of drug/alcohol dependence. Caution, in cardiovascular disease where physical activity should be regulated (anginal pain may be suppressed), epilepsy (may affect convulsive threshold). Discontinue minimum two weeks before elective surgery.
Pregnancy, Lactation: Pregnancy, if considered essential. Lactation, stop drug or stop breastfeeding.
ADR: *Most frequent,* insomnia.
Notes: See Class Effects 3.3.2 MAOIs.

Parnate 10mg *(Concordia)* A. GMS.
Price, (28) €15.97.
Tablet, tranylcypromine sulfate. Geranium-red s/c. Marked FW 251. *Carmoisine, Ponceau 4R, sucrose.*

3.3.3 - SSRIs, SNRIs

In This Chapter: *Citalopram, duloxetine, escitalopram, fluoxetine, fluvoxamine, paroxetine, reboxetine, sertraline, venlafaxine.*

Class Effects

Pharmacology: Selective Serotonin Reuptake Inhibitors (SSRIs) and Serotonin and Noradrenaline Reuptake Inhibitors (SNRIs) (duloxetine, venlafaxine) are less sedative than TCADs and have fewer cardiac adverse events. Reboxetine is a Selective Noradrenaline Reuptake Inhibitor.
Indications: Duloxetine *(Yentreve)* is also indicated for treatment of stress urinary incontinence.
CI: Not recommended in children and adolescents under 18 years, unless otherwise specified and then should be used with caution.
Interactions: Effect of Other Drugs on SSRIs/SNRIs: *Co-admin contraindicated:* MAOI irreversible (selegiline, iproniazid); stop SSRI at least 7 days before MAOI; stop MAOI at least 14 days before starting SSRI OR minimum 24 hours for reversible MAOIs (RIMAs); RIMAs (moclobemide, linezolid, methylthioninium chloride/methylene blue) caution serotonin syndrome; linezolid can be co-admin with paroxetine or fluvoxamine if facilities available (observation for serotonin syndrome, BP monitoring). *Co-admin contraindicated (unless serotonin syndrome, Neuroleptic Malignant Syndrome monitoring available):* Other serotonergic antidepressants, 5HT-agonists (sumatriptan, tramadol, tryptophan, oxitriptan, other triptans), opiates. *Co-admin not recommended (enhanced serotonergic effects):* Other SSRIs or SNRIs, clomipramine, amitriptyline, St John's Wort, venlafaxine, pethidine, lithium, linezolid. *Mutual high doses (caution):* Cimetidine. *QT-prolongation risk:* Drugs prolonging QT-interval (quinidine, amiodarone, sotalol, dofetilide, thioridazine, erythromycin, some antihistamines, moxifloxacin), drugs inducing hypo-(kalaemia, magnesaemia).
Effect of SSRIs/SNRIs on Other Drugs: Anticoagulants, drugs affecting platelets (NSAIDs, acetylsalicylic acid, ticlopidine), drugs increasing haemorrhage risk (atypical antipsychotics, phenothiazines, most TCADs, dipyridamole): *Increased bleeding risk.* Insulin, hypoglycaemics: *Consider dose adjustment.* Mivacurium, suxamethonium: *Neuromuscular blocking action may be prolonged.*
SP: Suicide, see Notes below (antidepressants). Mania/hypomania, patients entering manic phase, caution, discontinue. Paradoxical anxiety, aggression. Seizures, epilepsy (contraindicated for some members of class, see individual drugs); ECT, CHD, caution. Psychoses. Serotonin syndrome (agitation, tremor, hallucinations,

3.3.3   SSRIs, SNRIs

coma), autonomic instability (tachycardia, labile BP, hyperthermia), neuromuscular aberrations (hyperreflexia, incoordination) or GI symptoms (nausea, vomiting, diarrhoea); severe form can resemble Neuroleptic Malignant Syndrome (NMS); may be life-threatening (increased risk with co-admin or serotonergics, drugs impairing serotonin metabolism, antipsychotics, other dopamine antagonists). Hyponatraemia (SIADH), caution (elderly, cirrhosis, drugs causing hyponatraemia, altered fluid balance). Akathisia, psychomotor restlessness. Bleeding abnormalities, haemorrhage. Diabetes, altered glycaemic control; consider antidiabetic dose adjustment. Elderly, increased bone fracture risk. Always withdraw slowly; avoid abrupt discontinuation. Mydriasis, caution with raised IOP or risk of acute narrow-angle glaucoma.

Pregnancy, Lactation: *Pregnancy*, if benefit outweighs risk. After maternal use in later stages of pregnancy, risk of discontinuation symptoms in neonates e.g. respiratory distress, cyanosis, apnoea, seizures, temperature instability, feeding difficulty, vomiting, hypoglycaemia, hypertonia, hypotonia, hyperreflexia, tremor, jitteriness, irritability, lethargy, constant crying, somnolence, difficulty sleeping (either serotonergic effects or discontinuation symptoms); complications may begin immediately or within 24-hours after delivery; duration depends on half-life. Use in late pregnancy may increase risk of persistent pulmonary hypertension (PPHN) of newborn. *Lactation*, if benefit outweighs risk OR stop drug or stop breastfeeding; if considered necessary, use lowest dose. Pregnancy and lactation, contraindicated or not recommended for some members of class, see individual drugs below.

ADR: Weight or appetite increase/decrease, increased (blood cholesterol, CPK); palpitation, postural hypotension, tachycardia, hypertension including postural; tremor, headache, dizziness, paraesthesia, migraine; abnormal accommodation/vision, raised IOP; tinnitus; GI disorders e.g. nausea, dry mouth, constipation, diarrhoea, dyspepsia, vomiting, abdominal pain, flatulence, increased salivation; micturition disorder, polyuria; increased sweating, rash, pruritus; somnolence, insomnia, agitation, nervousness, sleep disorders, abnormal dreaming, amnesia, anxiety; decreased libido, sexual dysfunction, impotence; impaired concentration, anorexia, apathy, confusion; rhinitis, sinusitis, pharyngitis; skin reactions (e.g. purpura, ecchymosis), anaphylactoid reactions, vasculitis, serum sickness-like reaction, photosensitivity, erythema multiforme, Stevens-Johnson Syndrome; asthenia, taste perversion, fatigue, yawning, muscle spasm, SIADH, gynaecological disorder.

Notes: See 3.3 Antidepressants and Anxiolytics.

Citalopram

ATC Code: N06AB04. **Sport:** Permitted.
Driving: Unlikely to impair.

Indications: Depressive illness in initial phase and as maintenance against relapse or recurrence *(Cipramil, Citalopram Actavis and Niche)*. Major depressive episode *(Ciprager, Ciprotan, Citrol, Citalopram Bluefish, and Teva)*. Panic disorder with or without agoraphobia *(Cipramil, Ciprager, Citrol, Citalopram Niche)*.

Dose: Adult: *Depression*, TABLETS, initially 20mg/day; titrate to max. 40mg/day if required; DROPS, initially 16mg/day; titrate to max. 32mg/day.

Panic disorder, TABLETS, initially 10mg/day (1 week); increase by 10mg/day to 20mg/day, max. 40mg/day; DROPS, 8mg/day (1 week); titrate to 16mg/day; max. 32mg/day. Poor CYP2C19 metabolisers, adjust dose. Oral, once daily morning or evening with fluid; with or without food. Drops, mix with water or juice.

NOTE: Oral drops have approx. 25% higher bioavailability compared to tabs (10mg tab = 8mg or 4 drops).

Elderly: Age 65 years and over, half recommended adult dose; TABLETS, 10mg to max. 20mg/day or DROPS 8mg to max. 16mg/day.

Renal Impairment: CrCl (mL/min) below 30, caution.

Hepatic Impairment: Tabs, mild/moderate, initially 10mg/day for first two weeks; increase to max. 20mg/day if needed. Drops, max. 16mg/day. Severe, careful dose titration.

CI: Known QT-interval prolongation, congenital long QT-syndrome.

Interactions: Effect of Other Drugs on Citalopram: *Co-admin contraindicated*: Drugs prolonging QT-interval including antiarrhythmics (Class IA, II), antipsychotics (phenothiazine derivatives, pimozide, haloperidol), TCADs, antimicrobials (sparfloxacin, moxifloxacin, erythromycin IV, pentamidine, anti-malarials particularly halofantrine), antihistamines (astemizole, mizolastine), pimozide. *Co-admin caution*: CYP2C19 inhibitors (omeprazole, esomeprazole, fluvoxamine, lansoprazole, ticlopine), cimetidine.

Effect of Citalopram on Other Drugs: CYP2D6 substrates with narrow therapeutic index (flecainide, propafenone, metoprolol), antidepressants (desipramine, clomipramine, nortriptyline).

SP: Dose dependent QT-prolongation.

ADR: *Very common*, dry mouth, nausea, increased sweating.

Notes: See Class Effects 3.3.3 SSRIs, SNRIs.

Interchangeability: Same strengths of all brands of citalopram film-coated (f/c) tabs and oral drops 40mg/mL listed below are deemed interchangeable.

Reference Price: Tabs (28) 10mg, €10.96. 20mg, €2.80. 40mg, €5.60.

> **Cipramil 10mg, 20mg, Drops** *(Lundbeck)* A. GMS.
> *Price*, (28) 10mg, €4.62; 20mg, €7.24. Drops (15mL) €13.17.
> *Tablet*, citalopram hydrobromide. White f/c. 10mg: Round. Marked CL. 20mg: Oval scored (divisible into equal halves). Marked C and N either side of score. *Lactose.* **Store:** Below 25 deg C.
> *Oral drops*, citalopram HCl 40mg/mL (1mL=20 drops; 1 drop=2mg citalopram). Clear, nearly colourless (yellowish) soln with bitter taste. *Parabens, ethanol.* **Store:** Below 25 deg C; bottle in outer pack to protect (light).
>
> **Ciprager 10mg, 20mg 40mg** *(Gerard)* A. GMS.
> *Price*, (28) see reference price above.
> *Tablet*, citalopram hydrobromide. White f/c. 10mg: Round. Marked CL. 20mg: Oval scored*. Marked C and N either side of score. 40mg: Oval scored*. Marked CM and 40 either side of score. *Divisible into equal halves. *Lactose.* **Store:** No special conditions.
>
> **Ciprotan 10mg, 20mg** *(Clonmel)* A. GMS.
> *Price*, (28) see reference price above.
> *Tablet*, citalopram hydrobromide. White round f/c. *Mannitol.* **Store:** No special conditions.
>
> **Citalopram Actavis 10mg, 20mg** *(Accord)* A. GMS.
> *Price*, (28) see reference price above.
> *Tablet*, citalopram hydrobromide. Round white f/c. 20mg: Scored (divisible into equal halves). *Mannitol.* **Store:** Below 25 deg C.
>
> **Citalopram Bluefish 10mg, 20mg** *(Bluefish)* A. GMS.
> *Price*, (28) see reference price above.
> *Tablet*, citalopram hydrobromide. White f/c. 10mg: Round. 20mg: Oval scored (divisible into equal halves). *Lactose.* **Store:** No special conditions.
>
> **Citalopram TEVA 10mg, 20mg, 40mg** *(TEVA)* A. GMS.
> *Price*, (28) see reference price above.
> *Tablet*, citalopram hydrobromide. White f/c. 10mg: Round. 20mg, 40mg: Oval scored (divisible into equal halves). *Lactose.* **Store:** Below 25 deg C.
>
> **Citrol 10mg, 20mg, 30mg** *(Rowex)* A. GMS.
> *Price*, (28) 10mg, 20mg see reference price above. 30mg, €15.00.
> *Tablet*, citalopram hydrobromide. White f/c. 10mg: Round. 20mg, 30mg: Oblong scored (divisible into equal halves). Marked C/strength. *Lactose.* **Store:** No special conditions.

Duloxetine (CNS)

ATC Code: N06AX21. **Sport:** Permitted.
Driving: Sedation, dizziness.

Indications: Treatment, major depressive disorder (MDD), generalised anxiety disorder (GAD), diabetic peripheral neuropathic pain.

Dose: Adult: *Major depressive disorder*, initial and maintenance, 60mg/day.
Generalised anxiety disorder, initially 30mg/day; insufficient response, increase to 60mg.
Diabetic peripheral neuropathic pain, initially 60mg/day. Oral, once daily with or without food.

Elderly: MDD, GAD, caution at dose 120mg/day (limited data).

Child: MDD, under 18 years not recommended. GAD, age

7-17 years, safety/efficacy not established. Neuropathic pain, no data.

Renal Impairment: CrCl (mL/min) below 30, contraindicated.

Hepatic Impairment: Liver disease resulting in hepatic impairment, contraindicated.

CI: Uncontrolled hypertension, hypertensive crisis risk.

Interactions: Effect of Other Drugs on Duloxetine: *Plasma levels increased, co-admin contraindicated:* Potent CYP1A2 inhibitors (fluvoxamine, ciprofloxacin, enoxacin), irreversible non-selective MAOI. *Co-admin caution:* Drugs metabolised by CYP2D6 (risperidone, TCADs including nortriptyline, amitriptyline, imipramine) especially with narrow therapeutic window (flecainide, propafenone, metoprolol). *Plasma levels decreased:* Smoking. *Caution:* ALCOHOL, sedatives (benzodiazepines, morphinomimetics, antipsychotics, phenobarbital, sedative antihistamines). *Co-admin (adverse events more common):* St John's Wort.

Effect of Duloxetine on Other Drugs: Oral anticoagulants, antiplatelets: *Increased bleeding risk.* Warfarin: *Increased INR reported (no effect in steady state conditions, healthy volunteers).*

SP: Hypertension/other cardiac disease, monitor, hypertensive crisis risk. Conditions compromised by increased heart rate or increased BP, caution. Neuropathic pain, evaluate treatment response after 2 months; if inadequate initial response, additional response unlikely.

Pregnancy, Lactation: Lactation, not recommended.

ADR: Summary, *most common,* nausea, headache, dry mouth, somnolence, dizziness.

Notes: See Class Effects 3.3.3 SSRIs, SNRIs.

Interchangeability: Same strengths (30mg, 60mg) of all brands of duloxetine g/r capsules listed below are deemed interchangeable.

Reference Price: (28) 10mg, €2.24.

Cymbalta 30mg, 60mg *(Lilly)* A. GMS.
Price, (28) 30mg, €11.07. 60mg, €18.45.
Capsule, duloxetine HCl. Hard opaque g/r. Marked with strength. 30mg: White/blue. Marked 9543. 60mg: Green/blue. Marked 9542. *Sucrose.* **Store:** Below 30 deg C; original pack.

Aritavi 30mg, 60mg *(Accord)* A. GMS.
Price, (28) 30mg, €5.61; 60mg, €8.40.
Capsule, duloxetine HCl. Hard opaque g/r. Marked DLX and strength. 30mg: Grey/blue. 60mg: Grey/white. *Sucrose.* **Store:** Below 25 deg C.

Duloxetine Clonmel 30mg, 60mg *(Clonmel)* A. GMS.
Price, (28) 30mg, €5.61; 60mg, €8.40.
Capsule, duloxetine HCl. Hard g/r hard; contains off-white g/r pellets. 30mg: White/dark-blue. 60mg: Green/dark-blue. *Sucrose.*

Duloxetine Krka 30mg, 60mg *(Krka)* A. GMS.
Price, (28) 30mg, €5.61; 60mg, €8.40.
Capsule, duloxetine HCl. Hard g/r hard; contains white (almost) pellets. Marked with strength: 30mg: White/dark-blue. 60mg: Yellowish-green/dark-blue. *Sucrose.*

Duloxetine Mylan 30mg, 60mg *(Gerard)* A. GMS.
Price, (28) 30mg, €5.61; 60mg, €8.40.
Capsule, duloxetine HCl. Hard opaque g/r. Marked MYLAN over DL and strength. 30mg: Blue/white. 60mg: Blue/yellow. *Sucrose.*

Duloxetine TEVA 30mg, 60mg *(TEVA)* A. GMS.
Price, (28) 30mg, €5.61; 60mg, €8.40.
Capsule, duloxetine HCl. Hard opaque g/r; filled with white (yellow) coated pellets. Marked with strength. 30mg: Blue/white. 60mg: Blue/light-green. *Sucrose.*

Escitalopram

ATC Code: N06AB10. **Sport:** Permitted.
Driving: Unlikely to impair.

Indications: See Dose below.

Dose: Adult: *Major depressive episode, generalised anxiety disorder, OCD,* usually 10mg/day; if needed increase to max. 20mg/day.

Panic disorder (with or without agoraphobia), initially 5mg/day (1 week); then increase to 10mg/day; max. 20mg/day.

Social anxiety disorder, 10mg/day; after 2-4 weeks, decrease to 5mg/day or increase to max. 20mg/day.

Admin as single daily dose, with or without food.

Elderly: Over 65 years, initially 5mg once daily; max. 10mg/day.

Renal Impairment: CrCl (mL/min) below 30, caution.

Hepatic Impairment: Mild/moderate, initially 5mg/day (first 2 weeks); increase to 10mg/day if needed. Severe, caution.

CI: Known QT-interval prolongation, congenital long QT-syndrome.

Interactions: Effect of Other Drugs on Escitalopram: *Caution, seizure threshold lowered*: Antidepressants (TCADs, SSRIs), neuroleptics (phenothiazines, flupentixol, zuclopenthixol, haloperidol), mefloquine, bupropion, tramadol. *Plasma levels increased*: CYP2C19 inhibitors (omeprazole, esomeprazole, fluvoxamine, lansoprazole, ticlopidine), cimetidine.

Effect of Escitalopram on Other Drugs: CYP2D6 substrates with narrow therapeutic index (flecainide, propafenone, metoprolol), antidepressants (desipramine, clomipramine, nortriptyline), antipsychotics (risperidone, thioridazine, haloperidol): *Plasma levels increased, dose adjustment.* CYP2C19 substrates: *Caution.*

SP: Coronary heart disease. Discontinue over 1-2 weeks; abrupt withdrawal, discontinuation symptoms. Seizures for first time or increased frequency, discontinue. Dose-dependent QT-interval prolongation; caution, Torsade de Pointes risk (uncompensated HF, recent MI, bradyarrhythmia, predisposition to hypo- (kalaemia, magnesaemia), concomitant illness/medicines, female gender).

ADR: *Very common,* headache, nausea.

Notes: See Class Effects 3.3.3 SSRIs, SNRIs.

Interchangeability: Same strengths of all brands of escitalopram film-coated/orodispersible tabs listed below are deemed interchangeable.

Reference Price: (28) 5mg, €3.64. 10mg, €3.64. 15mg, €4.76. 20mg, €6.44.

Lexapro 5mg, 10mg, 15mg, 20mg *(Lundbeck)* A. GMS.
Price, (28) 5mg, €10.58. 10mg, €16.93. 15mg, €25.63. 20mg, €33.88.
Tablet, escitalopram oxalate. White f/c. 5mg: Round. Marked EK. 10mg, 15mg, 20mg: Oval scored (divisible into equal halves). Marked EL, EM, EN respectively.

Esciprex 5mg, 10mg, 15mg, 20mg *(Rowex)* A. GMS.
Price, (28) 5mg, 10mg, €3.64. 15mg, €4.76. 20mg, €6.44.
Tablet, escitalopram oxalate. 5mg, 10mg, 15mg, 20mg. White f/c. 5mg: Round. 10mg: Oval scored (divisible into equal halves). 15mg: Oval scored (twice) (divisible into 3 equal doses). 20mg: Round cross-scored (divisible into equal quarters and doses). *Lactose.*

Escitalopram Actavis Tablets *(Accord)* A. GMS.
Price, (28) see reference price above.
Tablet, escitalopram oxalate 5mg, 10mg, 15mg, 20mg. Oval (except 5mg) f/c white. Marked E. 5mg: Round. 10mg, 15mg, 20mg: Scored (divisible into equal doses).

Escitalopram (Accord) Tablets *(Accord)* A. GMS.
Price, (28) see reference price above.
Tablet, escitalopram oxalate 5mg, 10mg, 20mg. White (off-white) f/c. 5mg: Round. 10mg: Oval. Marked 1 and 0 either side of score*. 20mg: Oval, scored*. *(divisible into equal halves).

Escitalopram (Cipla) Tablets *(Cipla)* A. GMS.
Price, (28) see reference price above.
Tablet, escitalopram oxalate 5mg, 10mg, 20mg. White (off-white) round. Marked E and strength. 20mg: Scored (divisible into equal halves).

Escitalopram Krka Tablets *(Krka)* A. GMS.
Price, (28) see reference price above.
Tablet, escitalopram oxalate 5mg, 10mg, 15mg, 20mg. Oval (except 5mg, 15mg) white f/c. Marked with strength. 5mg, 15mg: Round. 10mg, 20mg: Scored (divisible into equal doses). *Lactose.*

Escitalopram (TEVA) Tablets *(TEVA)* A. GMS.
Price, (28) see reference price above.
Tablet, escitalopram oxalate 5mg, 10mg, 15mg, 20mg. White f/c. 5mg: Marked 93; 7414 on reverse. 10mg: Scored*. Marked 9 and 3; 7415 on reverse. 15mg: Scored (facilitates breaking). Marked S and C; 15 on reverse. 20mg: Scored*. Marked 9 and 3; 7463 on reverse. *(divisible into equal halves)

Escitalpro Tablets *(Gerard)* A. GMS.
Price, (28) see reference price above.
Tablet, escitalopram oxalate 5mg, 10mg, 15mg, 20mg. White oblong (except 5mg) f/c. Marked EC and strength; G on reverse. 5mg: Round. 10mg, 15mg, 20mg: Scored (divisible into equal doses). *Lactose.* **Store:** Below 25 deg C; original pack.

Etalopro Tablets *(Clonmel)* A. GMS.
Price, (28) see reference price above.
Tablet, escitalopram oxalate 5mg, 10mg, 15mg, 20mg. Oval (except 5mg) f/c. 5mg: Round. 10mg, 20mg: Scored (divisible into equal halves). 15mg: Scored (facilitates breaking).

113

3.3.3   SSRIs, SNRIs

Fluoxetine

ATC Code: N06AB03. Sport: Permitted.
Driving: Caution.

Indications: See Dose below.

Dose: Adult: *Major depressive episodes, OCD,* initially 20mg/day; titrate to max. 60mg/day if required. Doses above 80mg/day not evaluated.
Bulimia nervosa, 60mg/day. *Admin,* oral as single or divided dose, during or between meals. Caps and soln are bioequivalent.

Elderly: Generally 40mg/day; max. 60mg/day.

Child: *Moderate to severe major depressive episode* (unresponsive to psychotherapy), age 8-18 years, initiate under specialist supervision. Initially 10mg/day (2.5mL oral soln); after 1-2 weeks, increase to 20mg/day if needed. Therapeutic effect may be achieved with lower doses in lower-weight children.

Renal Impairment: Mild/moderate, 20mg every second day; GFR (mL/min) below 10, not recommended.

Hepatic Impairment: 20mg every second day.

Interactions: Effect of Other Drugs on Fluoxetine: *Co-admin contraindicated*: Metoprolol used in CHF. *Plasma level changes, toxicity risk*: Phenytoin.

Effect of Fluoxetine on Other Drugs: Diazepam: *Plasma levels increased.* Tamoxifen: *Reduced endoxifen conc (active metabolite of tamoxifen); avoid co-admin with any SSRI.* See Notes below (escitalopram).

SP: Acute cardiac disease. Age 8-18 years, monitor height, weight. QT interval prolongation reported; caution, congenital QT syndrome, history of QT prolongation, conditions predisposing to arrhythmias (hypokalaemia, hypomagnesaemia, bradycardia, acute MI, uncompensated HF, increased fluoxetine exposure due to hepatic impairment, medicinals prolonging QT interval).

Pregnancy, Lactation: Possible increased risk of cardiovascular defects when used in first trimester. See Notes below (SSRIs, SNRIs).

ADR: Summary, *most common,* headache, nausea, insomnia, fatigue, diarrhoea.

Notes: See Class Effects 3.3.3 SSRIs, SNRIs. See Escitalopram above.

Interchangeability: Same strengths of all brands of fluoxetine caps listed below are deemed interchangeable.

Reference Price: (30) 20mg, €3.60.

> Prozac 20mg, Oral Soln *(Lilly)* A. GMS.
> Price, (30), see reference price above. Liq (70mL) €4.86.
> Capsule, fluoxetine HCl. Hard gelatin. 20mg: Green/yellow. Marked Lilly 3105.
> Oral soln, as above 20mg/5mL. Clear colourless; mint odour. Ethanol, sucrose 3g/5mL.
> Fluzac 20mg *(Rowex)* A. GMS.
> Price, (30), see reference price above.
> Capsule, fluoxetine HCl. Opaque light-green hard gelatin.
> Gerozac 20mg, 60mg *(Gerard)* A. GMS.
> Price, (30) 20mg, see reference price above. 60mg, €10.80.
> Capsule, fluoxetine HCl. Opaque. Marked FL/strength. 20mg: Light-green/purple. Marked with alpha symbol. 60mg: Light-yellow. Marked G. *Lactose.*
> Prozamel 20mg *(Clonmel)* A. GMS.
> Price, (30), see reference price above.
> Capsule, fluoxetine HCl. Green.
> Prozit 20mg *(Pinewood)* A. GMS.
> Price, (30), see reference price above.
> Capsule, fluoxetine HCl. Olive green. Marked FLE20.

Fluvoxamine

ATC Code: N06AB08. Sport: Permitted.
Driving: Caution.

Indications: See Dose below.

Dose: Adult: *Major depressive episode,* initially 50-100mg as single dose in the evening; usual effective dose 100mg/day; max. 300mg/day. Above 150mg/day, admin in divided doses. *OCD,* initially 50mg/day; range 100-300mg/day; max. 300mg/day. *Admin,* swallow whole with water without chewing.

Child: *OCD,* over 8 years, initially 25mg/day; titrate every 4-7 days in 25mg increments to max. 200mg/day. Above

50mg/day, admin in divided doses with larger dose at bedtime.

Renal Impairment: Caution.

Hepatic Impairment: As for Renal above.

Interactions: Effect of Other Drugs on Fluvoxamine: *Co-admin contraindicated*: Tizanidine.

Effect of Fluvoxamine on Other Drugs: Terfenadine, astemizole, cisapride: *Plasma levels increased, increased QT-prolongation/Torsade de Pointes risk.* TCADs (clomipramine, imipramine, amitriptyline), neuroleptics (clozapine, olanzapine), propranolol: *Consider dose reduction.* CYP1A2 substrates with narrow therapeutic index (tacrine, theophylline, methadone, mexiletine), CYP2C substrates (phenytoin), CYP3A4 substrates (carbamazepine, ciclosporin): *Monitor, consider dose adjustment.* Warfarin: *Plasma levels and prothrombin times significantly increased.* Thioridazine: *Cardiac toxicity.* Caffeine (reduce intake), ropinirole, benzodiazepines (triazolam, midazolam, alprazolam, diazepam): *Caution.*

SP: Post acute-MI, caution.

ADR: *Common,* anorexia, agitation, nervousness, anxiety, insomnia, somnolence, tremor, headache, dizziness, palpitations, tachycardia, abdominal pain, constipation, diarrhoea, dry mouth, dyspepsia, nausea, vomiting, hyperhidrosis, sweating, asthenia, malaise.

Notes: See Class Effects 3.3.3 SSRIs, SNRIs.

> Faverin 50mg, 100mg *(BGP)* A. GMS.
> Price, 50mg (60) €17.30. 100mg (30) €13.80.
> Tablet, fluvoxamine maleate. White (off-white) f/c scored (divisible into equal halves). 50mg: Round. Marked 291. 100mg: Oval. Marked 313.

Paroxetine

ATC Code: N06AB05. Sport: Permitted.
Driving: Unlikely to impair.

Indications: See Dose below.

Dose: Adult: *Major depressive episode,* initially 20mg daily; if needed titrate in 10mg increments to max. 50mg/day.
OCD, initially 20mg/day; titrate as above to 40mg/day; max. 60mg/day.
Panic disorder (with or without agoraphobia), initially 10mg/day, then as for OCD.
Anxiety (social anxiety disorder/social phobia, generalised anxiety disorder, post-traumatic stress disorder), initially 20mg/day; titrate as above to max. 50mg/day. Admin once daily in the morning with food. Swallow tablet rather than chew.

Elderly: Max. 40mg/day.

Renal Impairment: CrCl (mL/min) below 30, use lowest dose.

Hepatic Impairment: Use lowest dose.

Interactions: Effect of Other Drugs on Paroxetine: *Reduced absorption (Seroxat Liquid)*: Drugs increasing gastric pH (PPIs, antacids, H2-antagonists). *Plasma levels reduced*: Fosamprenavir + ritonavir (short-term). *Co-admin with serotonergic drugs, Serotonin Syndrome risk*: L-tryptophan, triptans, tramadol, linezolid, methylthioninium chloride (methylene blue), SSRIs, lithium, pethidine, St John's Wort *(Hypericum perforatum).*

Effect of Paroxetine on Other Drugs: Procyclidine, TCADs (clomipramine, nortriptyline, desipramine), phenothiazines (perphenazine; thioridazine, co-admin not recommended), risperidone, certain Type 1c antiarrhythmics (propafenone, flecainide), metoprolol (co-admin not recommended), pimozide: *Plasma levels increased.* Endoxifen (one of tamoxifen most important metabolites): *Reduced concentrations (avoid paroxetine use during tamoxifen treatment).*

SP: Akathisia (psychomotor restlessness). History of mania, caution. Withdrawal symptoms on discontinuation.

ADR: *Very common,* nausea, sexual dysfunction.

Notes: See Class Effects 3.3.3 SSRIs, SNRIs.

Interchangeability: Same strengths of all brands of paroxetine film-coated (f/c) tabs listed below are deemed interchangeable.

Seroxat 10mg, 20mg, 30mg, Oral Susp *(GSK)* A. GMS.
Price, 10mg (28) €9.37. 20mg (30) €7.48. 30mg (30) €11.23. Susp €11.93.
Tablet, paroxetine hydrochloride hemihydrate. f/c. 10mg: Round white (pinkish) scored*. Marked FC1; GS on reverse. 20mg: White oval scored*. Marked SEROXAT 20. 30mg: Blue oval scored (facilitates breaking). Marked SEROXAT 30. *(divisible into equal halves).
Oral susp, as above 20mg/10mL. Bright orange viscous; orange odour. *Parabens, Sunset Yellow E110, sorbitol.*
Paroser 20mg *(Pinewood)* A. GMS.
Price, (30) €7.33.
Tablet, paroxetine HCl. White oval f/c scored (divisible into equal halves). Marked 20. *Lactose.*
Parox 10mg, 20mg, 30mg *(Rowex)* A. GMS.
Price, (30) 10mg, €7.04. 20mg, €7.33. 30mg, €11.01.
Tablet, paroxetine HCl. Round (except 30mg) f/c. Marked PX and strength. 10mg: White. 20mg: White scored (divisible into equal halves). 30mg: Oval blue scored (divisible into equal doses).

Reboxetine

ATC Code: N06AX18. **Sport:** Permitted.
Driving: Caution until effect known.
Indications: Depressive illness/major depression.
Dose: Adult, Elderly: Initially 8mg/day; after 3-4 weeks titrate to 10mg/day if required; max. 12mg/day in 2 divided doses. *Elderly,* not recommended.
Renal Impairment: Initially 4mg/day.
Hepatic Impairment: As for Renal above.
Interactions: Effect of Other Drugs on Reboxetine: *Plasma levels increased, co-admin not recommended:* Potent CYP3A4 inhibitors (ketoconazole, nefazodone, erythromycin, fluvoxamine). *Co-admin not evaluated:* TCADs, MAOIs, SSRIs, lithium. *Increased BP:* Ergot derivatives. *Hypokalaemia:* Diuretics (potassium losing).
SP: Serious concomitant systemic illnesses. Does not appear to potentiate effect of alcohol.
ADR: *Very common,* insomnia, dizziness, dry mouth, constipation, nausea, hyperhidrosis.
Notes: See Class Effects 3.3.3 SSRIs, SNRIs.

Edronax 4mg *(Pfizer)* A. GMS.
Price, (60) €25.30.
Tablet, reboxetine. White round scored (divisible into equal halves). Marked P and U; 7671 on reverse.

Sertraline

ATC Code: N06AB06. **Sport:** Permitted.
Driving: Caution.
Indications: See Dose below.
Dose: Adult, Elderly: *Major depressive episodes* (treatment, prevention of recurrence), *OCD,* initially 50mg/day; increase to 100mg/day if needed. *Panic disorder* (with or without agoraphobia), *post traumatic stress disorder, social anxiety disorder,* initially 25mg/day; titrate to 50mg/day after 1 week. All indications, increase by 50mg at 1-week intervals; max. 200mg/day. *Admin,* as single daily dose.
Child: Not for use under age 18 years except in OCD (age 6-17 years). Age 6-12 years, initially 25mg/day, increasing to 50mg/day after 1 week; age 13-17 years, initially 50mg/day, titrating by 50mg/day increments and 1 week intervals; max. 200mg/day. Monitor patients for appearance of suicidal symptoms.
Hepatic Impairment: Severe, contraindicated.
Interactions: Effect of Other Drugs on Sertraline: *Co-admin not recommended:* ALCOHOL; grapefruit juice (avoid). *Co-admin caution:* Fentanyl (general anaesthesia, chronic pain). *Plasma levels decreased:* Phenytoin. *Increased QTc prolongation and/or ventricular arrhythmia risk:* Other drugs prolonging QTc interval (some antipsychotics, antibiotics). **Effect of Sertraline on Other Drugs:** Pimozide: *Co-admin contraindicated (increased pimozide levels).* Phenytoin, lithium: *Monitor levels.*
SP: Switching from other antidepressants or anti-obsessional drugs, caution. False-positive urine immunoassay screening for benzodiazepines. QTC prolongation and Torsade de Pointes reported; majority in patients with risk factors (caution).

Pregnancy, Lactation: Contraindicated. Women of child-bearing potential to use adequate contraception.
ADR: *Most common,* nausea.
Notes: See Class Effects 3.3.3 SSRIs, SNRIs.
Interchangeability: Same strengths of all brands of sertraline film-coated (f/c) tabs listed below are deemed interchangeable.
Reference Price: (28) 50mg, €3.64; 100mg, €5.04; (30) 50mg, €3.90; 100mg, €5.40.

Lustral 50mg, 100mg *(Pfizer)* A. GMS.
Price, (28) 50mg, €13.64. 100mg, €20.46.
Tablet, sertraline HCl. White cap-shaped f/c. Marked Pfizer; ZLT/strength on reverse. 50mg: Scored (divisible into equal doses).
Depreger 50mg, 100mg *(Gerard)* A. GMS.
Price, (28), 50mg, €3.08; 100mg, €4.48.
Tablet, sertraline HCl. White (off-white) cap-shaped f/c scored (divisible into equal doses). Marked ST/strength; G on reverse.
Store: Original pack.
Seretral 50mg, 100mg *(TEVA)* A. GMS.
Price, (30) 50mg, €3.30; 100mg, €4.80.
Tablet, sertraline HCl. 50mg: Elliptical scored (divisible into equal halves). Marked 9 and 3. 50mg: Light-blue. Marked 7176. 100mg: Light-yellow. Marked 7177. **Store:** No special conditions.
Serimel 50mg, 100mg *(Clonmel)* A. GMS.
Price, (28), 50mg, €3.08; 100mg, €4.48.
Tablet, sertraline HCl. White cap-shaped f/c scored. Marked with strength. **Store:** No special conditions.
Serlan 50mg, 100mg *(Rowex)* A. GMS.
Price, (28), 50mg, €3.08; 100mg, €4.48.
Tablet, sertraline HCl. White cap-shaped f/c scored. Marked SE/strength. **Store:** No special conditions.
Sertraline Actavis 50mg, 100mg *(Accord)* A. GMS.
Price, (28), 50mg, €3.08; 100mg, €4.48.
Tablet, sertraline HCl. White scored f/c. 50mg: Oval. Marked L. 100mg: Round. Marked C. *Lactose.* **Store:** Below 25 deg C.
Sertraline Bluefish 50mg, 100mg *(Bluefish)* A. GMS.
Price, (28), 50mg, €3.08; 100mg, €4.48.
Tablet, sertraline HCl. White cap-shaped f/c. Marked A. 50mg: Scored (facilitates breaking). Marked 81. 100mg: Marked 82. **Store:** Original pack.
Sertraline Krka 50mg, 100mg *(Krka)* A. GMS.
Price, (28), 50mg, €3.08; 100mg, €4.48.
Tablet, sertraline HCl. White oval f/c scored (divisible into equal halves). 50mg: Oval. Marked S3. 100mg: Round. **Store:** No special conditions.

Venlafaxine

ATC Code: N06AX16. **Sport:** Permitted.
Driving: Unlikely to impair.
Indications: Major depressive episode, generalised anxiety disorder (GAD), panic disorder with or without agoraphobia, social anxiety disorder.
Dose: Adult: STANDARD/R, *major depressive episode,* initially 75mg/day in 2 or 3 divided doses; if required increase at 2-week intervals to max. 375mg/day.
PROLONGED/R, *major depressive episodes,* as for Standard/R, admin once daily.
Generalised anxiety disorder (GAD), social anxiety disorder, 75mg once daily; if needed increase at 2-week intervals to max. 225mg/day.
Panic disorder (with or without agoraphobia), initially 37.5mg/day for 7 days, then 75mg/day; no response, may benefit from max. 225mg/day increasing as for GAD. Admin with food; swallow whole with fluid; do not divide, crush or chew.
Elderly: Caution, use lowest effective dose.
Renal Impairment: GFR (mL/min) 30-80, consider dose reduction; below 30 and haemodialysis, reduce by 50%.
Hepatic Impairment: Mild/moderate, consider 50% dose reduction. Severe, use if benefit outweighs risk, consider dose reduction of more than 50%.
Interactions: Effect of Other Drugs on Venlafaxine: *Co-admin not recommended:* Weight loss agents (including phentermine). *Co-admin caution:* Metoprolol. *Increased exposure:* Ketoconazole. *Co-admin, adverse events more common:* Nefazodone, SSRIs, triptans.
Effect of Venlafaxine on Other Drugs: Indinavir: *Plasma levels decreased, clinical significance not known.* Desipramine: *Increased exposure.* Haloperidol: *Clearance*

3.3.4 Other Antidepressants

decreased; increased exposure. Warfarin: *Potentiated anticoagulant effect.*

SP: Recent MI, unstable heart disease, hypertension (screen, control pre-existing hypertension before initiation), history of drug abuse, underlying conditions exacerbated by increased heart rate (increased heart rate can occur at higher doses), increased serum cholesterol. QTc prolongation, Torsade de Pointed, ventricular tachycardia, cardiac arrhythmias (fatal) reported especially with overdose or patients with risk factors.

ADR: *Summary, very common,* nausea, dry mouth, headache, sweating (including night sweats). *Paediatric,* suicidal ideation, hostility, self-harm (in clinical trials).

Notes: See 3.3.3 SSRIs, SNRIs.

Interchangeability: Same strengths of all brands of venlafaxine Standard/R tablets and Prolonged/R capsules and/or tablets listed below are deemed interchangeable.

Reference Price: Standard/R (56) 37.5mg, €5.04; 75mg, €7.84. Prolonged/R (28) 37.5mg, €4.48; 75mg, €3.36; 150mg, €5.60.

Efexor XL 37.5mg, 75mg, 150mg *(Pfizer)* A. GMS.
Price, XL 37.5 (7), €2.10; (28) 75mg, €12.02; 150mg, €20.27. *Prolonged/R capsule,* venlafaxine HCl. Opaque. Marked W/strength. 37.5mg: Light-grey/peach. 75mg: Peach. 150mg: Dark-orange. **Store:** Below 30 deg C.
Ireven 75mg, 150mg *(TEVA)* A. GMS.
Prolonged/R capsule, venlafaxine HCl. Opaque hard; containing 2 (75mg) or 3 (150mg) white round f/c tabs. Marked VEN/strength. 75mg: Flesh/flesh. 150mg: Scarlet/scarlet.
Vedixal 37.5mg, 75mg, XL *(Rowex)* A. GMS.
Price (56) 37.5mg, €5.04; 75mg, €7.84. XL (28) see reference price above.
Standard/R tablet, venlafaxine HCl 37.5mg, 75mg. Oblong pale-red-brown (brownish). 37.5mg: Marked 3. 75mg: Scored (divisible into equal halves). Marked 7 on each half. *Lactose.*
Prolonged/R capsule (XL), as above 37.5mg, 150mg. 37.5mg: Light-grey. 150mg: Dark-orange. Contain white (off-white) pellets.
Venex XL 37.5mg, 75mg, 150mg *(Clonmel)* A. GMS.
Price, (28) see reference price above.
Prolonged/R capsule, venlafaxine HCl. Hard contains white (off-white) granules. *Sucrose.* 37.5mg: Orange/transparent. *Ponceau 4R red.* 75mg: Yellow/transparent; 150mg: Buff/transparent. *Sunset Yellow.*
Venlablue XL 75mg, 150mg *(Bluefish)* A. GMS.
Price, (28) see reference price above.
Prolonged/R capsule, venlafaxine HCl. Hard opaque; contains 6 (75mg) or 12 (150mg) white (off-white) round f/c mini 12.5mg tabs. Marked with radial bands. 75mg: Peach. 150mg: Dark orange *Allura red, Sunset Yellow.*
Venlafaxine TEVA 37.5mg, 75mg *(TEVA)* A. GMS.
Price, (56) 37.5mg, €5.04; 75mg, €7.84.
Standard/R tablet, venlafaxine HCl. Mottled peach round flat scored. Marked 9 and 3 either side of score. 37.5mg: Scored (facilitates breaking). Marked 7380. 75mg: Scored (divisible into equal halves). Marked 7382. *Lactose.*
Venlafex XL 37.5mg, 75mg, 150mg *(Krka)* A. GMS.
Price, (28) see reference price above.
Prolonged/R capsule, venlafaxine HCl. Hard gelatin opaque contains white (off-white) pellets. 37.5mg: White/brownish-rose. 75mg: Light-pink. 150mg: Brownish-orange. *Sucrose.*
Venlofex PR 75mg, 150mg *(Gerard)* A. GMS.
Price, (28) see reference price above.
Prolonged/R capsule, venlafaxine HCl. Opaque hard. Marked VEN/strength. 75mg: Flesh. 150mg: Scarlet. **Store:** No special conditions.
Vensir XL 75mg, 150mg *(Rowex)* A. GMS.
Price, (28) see reference price above.
Prolonged/R capsule, venlafaxine. Hard with thick and thin radial circular band on body and cap; filled with 6 (75mg) or 12 (150mg) white (off-white) round coated mini 12.5mg tabs. 75mg: Peach opaque/peach opaque. 150mg: Dark orange/dark orange.

3.3.4 - Other Antidepressants

In This Chapter: *Agomelatine, mirtazapine.*

Class Effects
Carbamazepine, flupentixol and lamotrigine are also used to treat depressive states.

CI: Hypersensitivity to any member of the class. Use in children under 18 years.

SP: Suicide, see Notes below (antidepressants).

116

Pregnancy, Lactation: See Notes below (SSRIs, SNRIs).

Notes: See 3.3 Antidepressants (SSRIs, SNRIs). See 3.2 Antipsychotics, Antimanics (carbamazepine, flupentixol). See 3.1 Antiepileptics (lamotrigine).

Agomelatine
ATC Code: N06AX22. **Sport:** Permitted.
Driving: Dizziness, somnolence common.
Indications: Major depressive episodes.
Dose: Adult: 25mg/day; titrate to 50mg/day after 2 weeks if needed; weight benefit/risk of dose increase to 50mg with LFT monitoring (elevated transaminase risk). Discontinuation, no dose tapering needed. Oral, with/without food once daily at bedtime.
Elderly: No dose adjustment; age 75 years and older, not recommended.
Child: Age 7 and older, no data.
Renal Impairment: Moderate/severe, caution.
Hepatic Impairment: Cirrhosis, active liver disease, contraindicated.
Interactions: Effect of Other Drugs on Agomelatine: *Co-admin contraindicated:* Potent CYP1A2 inhibitors (fluvoxamine, ciprofloxacin). *Co-admin caution (increased exposure):* Moderate CYP1A2 inhibitors (propranolol, grepafloxacin, enoxacin). *Co-admin not advisable:* ALCOHOL.
SP: Perform LFTs at initiation (above 3xULN, do not initiate), then at week 3, week 6 (end of acute phase), week 12, week 24 (end of maintenance phase), then when indicated clinically; increased serum transaminases, repeat LFTs within 48 hours (above 3xULN, discontinue). Jaundice, discontinue. Caution, obese or overweight or non-alcoholic fatty liver disease, or high ALCOHOL consumption or treated with medicinals associated with hepatic injury. Elderly with dementia, not recommended. Mania, hypomania, caution; discontinue if manic symptoms develop. Discontinuation symptoms may be experienced after SSRI/SNRI cessation. Agomelatine can be started immediately while tapering SSRI/SNRI dose.
ADR: *Common,* anxiety, headache, dizziness, somnolence, insomnia, migraine, nausea, diarrhoea, constipation, abdominal pain, vomiting, hyperhidrosis, back pain, fatigue, increased (ALAT and/or ASAT).
Notes: See 3.3.4 Other Antidepressants.
Valdoxan 25mg *(Servier)* B. GMS.
Price, (28) €38.88.
Tablet, agomelatine. Orange-yellow oblong f/c. Marked with logo. *Lactose.*

Mirtazapine
ATC Code: N06AX11. **Sport:** Permitted.
Driving: Impaired concentration, alertness.
Indications: Major depressive episodes.
Dose: Adult, Elderly: Initially 15-30mg/day; effective dose range 15-45mg/day. *Admin,* oral tabs once daily, preferably at night before going to bed; admin with fluid, swallow whole without chewing. Place orodispersible tabs on the tongue and swallow with or without water. *Elderly,* increase dose with caution.
Renal Impairment: CrCl (mL/min) below 40, clearance decreased.
Hepatic Impairment: Clearance decreased.
Interactions: Effect of Other Drugs on Mirtazapine: *Co-admin contraindicated:* MAOI (or within 2 weeks after discontinuation). *Co-admin caution (increased serotonin effects):* Serotonergic active substances (L-tryptophan, triptans, tramadol, linezolid, methylene blue, SSRIs, venlafaxine, lithium, St John's Wort). *Sedating properties increased:* Antipsychotics, antihistamine H1-antagonists, opioids, ALCOHOL. *Increased clearance (consider dose increase):* CYP3A4 inducers (carbamazepine, phenytoin). *Increased plasma levels (consider dose reduction):* Cimetidine, HIV protease inhibitors, azole antifungals, erythromycin, nefazodone. *Increased QT-prolongation risk:* Drugs prolonging QTc interval (some antipsychotics, antibiotics).
Effect of Mirtazapine on Other Drugs: Warfarin: *Increased INR (monitor).*

SP: Bone marrow depression. Jaundice, discontinue. Conditions needing supervision include epilepsy/organic brain disorder, hepatic/renal impairment, cardiac disease (conduction disturbances, angina pectoris, recent MI), low BP, diabetes mellitus. Take into account worsening psychotic symptoms depressive phase when treated may transform into manic phase, withdrawal symptoms, micturition disturbances, akathisia/psychomotor restlessness. QT-prolongation, Torsades de Pointes, ventricular tachycardia, sudden death reported, usually with overdose or presence of risk factors. Hyponatraemia, SIADH, serotonin syndrome.

ADR: *Very common*, increased appetite/weight, somnolence, sedation, headache, dry mouth. *Paediatrics*, *common*, weight gain, urticaria, hypertriglyceridaemia.

Notes: See 3.3.1 Tricyclic, Tetracyclic Antidepressants. See 3.3.3 SSRIs, SNRIs.

Interchangeability: Same strengths of all brands of mirtazapine film-coated (f/c) tabs/orodispersible tabs listed below are deemed interchangeable.

Reference Price: (30) 15mg, €3.60; 30mg, €5.40; 45mg, €9.00. (28) 30mg, €5.04.

Zispin 30mg, SolTab *(MSD)* A. GMS.
Price, (30) 30mg, €8.70. SolTab 15mg, €4.88. 30mg, €9.75. 45mg, €14.62.
Tablet, mirtazapine. Red/brown oval f/c scored (divisible into equal halves). Marked Organon; TZ-5 on both sides of score on reverse. *Lactose.* **Store:** Below 30 deg C; original pack; protect (light, moisture).
OroDisp tablet (SolTab), as above 15mg, 30mg, 45mg. Round white. 15mg: Marked TZ1. 30mg: Marked TZ2. 45mg: Marked TZ4. *Sucrose, aspartame, mannitol.* **Store:** Original pack; protect (light, moisture).

Mirap 15mg, 30mg, 45mg, DisTab *(Rowex)* A. GMS.
Price, (30) tabs, DisTab, 15mg, €3.60. 30mg, €4.80. 45mg, €7.80.
Tablet, mirtazapine. f/c. 15mg, 30mg: Oblong scored (divisible into equal doses). 15mg: Yellow. 30mg: Beige. 45mg: White round. *Lactose.*
OroDisp tablet (DisTab), as above 15mg, 30mg, 45mg. White (off-white) flat round. *Aspartame, sulphites.*

Mirtazapine Activis 15mg, 30mg, 45mg *(Accord)* A. GMS.
Price, (30) 15mg, €3.60. 30mg, €4.80. 45mg, €7.80.
Tablet, mirtazapine. Oval scored f/c. 15mg: Yellow. 30mg: Brownish. 45mg: White. Marked I. *Lactose.*

Mirtazapine Bluefish Tablets *(Bluefish)* A. GMS.
Price, (30) 15mg, €3.60. 30mg, €4.80. 45mg, €7.80.
OroDisp tablet, mirtazapine 15mg, 30mg, 45mg. White round. Marked A. 15mg: Marked 36. 30mg: Marked 37. 45mg: Marked 38. *Aspartame.*

Zismirt 30mg, Orotab 15mg, 30mg, 45mg *(Gerard)* A. GMS.
Price, tabs (28) 30mg, €4.48; OroTab (30) 15mg, 3.60. 30mg, €4.80; 45mg, €7.80.
Tablet, mirtazapine. Buff f/c (facilitates breaking). Marked MR and 30; G on reverse. *Lactose.* **Store:** Original pack.
OroDisp tablet, as above. White round. Marked A. 15mg: Marked 36. 30mg: Marked 37. 45mg: Marked 38. *Aspartame.* **Store:** No special conditions.

3.3.5 - Benzodiazepine Anxiolytics

In This Chapter: *Alprazolam, bromazepam, chlordiazepoxide, clobazam, diazepam, lorazepam, prazepam.*

Class Effects

A number of drug classes are indicated in the management of anxiety disorders, see Notes below.

Driving: Caution; sedation, amnesia, impaired concentration, impaired muscular function; if insufficient sleep duration occurs, the risk of impaired alertness may be increased. ALCOHOL may intensify impairment.

Indications: In anxiety disorders and/or insomnia, benzodiazepines are only indicated when the disorder is severe, disabling or subjecting the individual to extreme distress.

CI: Hypersensitivity to any member of the class. Children under 18 years, unless otherwise specified. Myasthenia gravis, severe respiratory insufficiency or depression, sleep apnoea syndrome, severe hepatic insufficiency (may precipitate encephalopathy) *(rectal, oral, parenteral).* Acute pulmonary insufficiency. Phobic or obsessional states,

chronic psychoses, primary treatment of psychotic disease; monotherapy to treat depression or anxiety associated with depression (may precipitate suicide) *(oral, parenteral).*

Interactions: Effect of Other Drugs on Benzodiazepines: Co-admin not recommended, enhanced sedative effect *(severe sedation, clinically relevant respiratory and/or cardio-vascular depression):* ALCOHOL. *Enhanced central depressive effects:* Antipsychotics, hypnotics, anxiolytics/sedatives, antidepressants, narcotic analgesics (also enhanced euphoria, increased psychological dependence), anti-epileptics, anaesthetics, sedative antihistamines, clozapine. *Plasma levels increased (action potentiated):* Hepatic enzyme inhibitors (cimetidine, omeprazole, ketoconazole, fluvoxamine, fluoxetine) (applies to lesser degree to those metabolised only by conjugation). *Plasma levels decreased:* Hepatic enzyme inducers (rifampicin). *Increased sedative effects (faster absorption following oral admin):* Cisapride.

Effect of Benzodiazepines on Other Drugs: Phenytoin: *Metabolic elimination changed.*

SP: Suicide, benzodiazepines should not be used alone to treat depression or anxiety associated with depression; suicide may be precipitated, see Notes below (antidepressants). Tolerance and/or dependence risk increases with dose, treatment duration, alcohol or drug abuse (history), personality disorders; avoid if dependent on CNS depressants including alcohol (except in acute withdrawal reactions); tolerance to alcohol, other CNS depressants may be decreased. Anterograde amnesia. Psychiatric and paradoxical reactions (caution, children and elderly); restlessness, agitation, irritability, aggressiveness, delusion, rages, nightmares, hallucinations, psychoses, inappropriate behaviour, somnambulism, other nightly unconscious behaviours e.g. eating, driving. *Special populations,* children, careful assessment; minimum duration. Elderly, debilitated, very ill, respiratory insufficiency, limited pulmonary reserve, possibility of apnoea and/or cardiac arrest. Chronic hepatic diseases, reduce dose. Increased risk for falls and fractures (hip) in elderly (myorelaxant effect). Loss or bereavement, psychological adjustment may be inhibited. Rebound insomnia and anxiety on withdrawal.

Withdrawal symptoms (headaches, muscle pain, extreme anxiety, tension, restlessness, confusion, irritability; severe cases, derealisation, depersonalisation, hyperacusis, numbness and tingling of extremities, hypersensitivity to light, noise and physical contact, hallucinations, epileptic seizures). Greater risk with abrupt discontinuation; always decreased gradually. Use for shortest duration possible. Long-term chronic use not recommended. Severe anaphylactic and/or anaphylactoid reactions; angioedema (tongue, glottis, larynx). May lead to potentially fatal respiratory depression.

Pregnancy, Lactation: First and third trimesters, not recommended; use only if benefit outweighs risk. High dose during second and third trimester (decreased foetal active movements, variability of cardiac rhythm). Use in late phase of pregnancy or during labour, effects on the neonate expected (hypothermia, hypotonia, foetal heart rate irregularities, poor sucking, moderate respiratory depression). Chronic use in late pregnancy, risk of withdrawal/floppy infant syndrome in the newborn infant. Lactation, not recommended.

ADR: Decreased appetite, sedation, somnolence, ataxia, dysarthria, slurred speech, headache, tremor, anterograde amnesia. Paradoxical reactions, more likely in children and elderly; confusion, emotional poverty, alertness decreased, depression, libido increased or decreased. Risk of fall/fractures in elderly, nausea, dry mouth, hypersalivation, constipation, diplopia, blurred vision, hypotension, circulatory depression, irregular heart rate, increased transaminases and ALP, incontinence, urinary retention, skin reaction, vertigo, cardiac arrest, jaundice. Chronic use, physical dependence; discontinuation may result in withdrawal or rebound phenomena. See SP above.

Notes: See 2.1.7 Beta-Blockers, 3.2 Antipsychotics, Antimanics, 3.3 Antidepressants and Anxiolytics and 3.1.3 GABAergic Drugs.

3.3.5 Benzodiazepine Anxiolytics

Alprazolam

ATC Code: N05BA12. **Sport:** Permitted.
Driving: Caution. See Notes below.
Indications: Anxiety.
Dose: Adult, Elderly: Initially 0.5-1mg in divided doses; increase by max. 1mg at 3-4 day intervals to optimum range 3-4mg/day. Discontinuation, reduce slowly by no more than 0.5mg every 3 days.
Elderly: Including debilitated patients, initially 0.25mg twice daily; titrate gradually.
Notes: See 3.3.5 Benzodiazepine Anxiolytics.
Interchangeability: Same strengths of all brands of alprazolam tablets listed below are deemed interchangeable.

Xanax 250mcg, 500mcg, 1mg *(Pfizer)* A. GMS.
Price, (100) 0.25mg, €2.28. 0.5mg, €4.38. 1mg, €9.16.
Tablet, alprazolam. Oval scored. Marked Upjohn. 0.25mg: White. Marked 29. 0.5mg: Pink. Marked 55. 1mg: Lavender. Marked 90. *Lactose.*
Alprazolam (Rowex) 0.25mg, 0.5mg, 1mg *(Rowex)* A. GMS.
Price, (100) 0.25mg, €2.22. 0.5mg, €4.30. 1mg, €8.97.
Tablet, alprazolam. Oblong scored (divisible into equal doses). Marked APZM and strength. 0.25mg: White. 0.5mg: Pink. 1mg: Light-blue. *Lactose.* **Store:** Below 25 deg C; blister in outer carton to protect (light).
Gerax 250mcg, 500mcg, 1mg *(Gerard)* A. GMS.
Price, (100) 0.25mg, €2.22. 0.5mg, €4.30. 1mg, €8.97.
Tablet, alprazolam. Oval scored (facilitates breaking). Marked AL/strength; G on reverse. 250mcg: White. 500mcg: Pale-pink. 1mg: Light-blue. *Lactose.*

Bromazepam

ATC Code: N05BA08. **Sport:** Permitted.
Driving: Caution. See Notes below.
Indications: Anxiety.
Dose: Adult: Usual range 3-18mg/day. *Hospitalised,* up to max. 60mg/day. Oral, in divided doses.
Elderly: Half adult dose.
Child: Under 12 years, safety/efficacy not established.
Renal Impairment: Caution.
Hepatic Impairment: Caution.
Notes: See 3.3.5 Benzodiazepine Anxiolytics.

Lexotan 1.5mg, 3mg *(Roche)* A. GMS.
Price, (30) 1.5mg, €2.19. 3mg, €2.62.
Tablet, bromazepam. Cylindrical biplanar scored (divisible into equal doses). Marked Roche/strength. 1.5mg: Off-white (slightly yellow). 3mg: Pale-red slightly speckled. *Lactose.*

Chlordiazepoxide

ATC Code: N05BA02. **Sport:** Permitted.
Driving: Caution. See Notes below.
Indications: Anxiety. Control of muscle spasm. Alcohol withdrawal.
Dose: Adult: *Anxiety states* including muscle spasm, usually 30mg/day; max. 100mg/day in divided doses.
Alcohol withdrawal, 25-100mg. If required repeat after 2-4 hours. Patients with organic brain damage or respiratory impairment, see Elderly below. Max. duration 4 week including tapering off.
Elderly: Half adult dose (max).
Renal Impairment: As for Elderly above.
Hepatic Impairment: As for Elderly above. Severe, contraindicated.
CI: Spinal or cerebral ataxia.
Interactions: Effect of Other Drugs on Chlordiazepoxide: *Increased respiratory depression:* Sodium oxybate.
ADR: *Common,* sedation, dizziness, somnolence, ataxia, fatigue, balance disorder.
Notes: See 3.3.5 Benzodiazepine Anxiolytics.

Librium 5mg, 10mg *(Meda)* A. GMS.
Price, (100) 5mg, €5.80. 10mg, €8.07.
Capsule, chlordiazepoxide HCl. Marked LIB/strength. 5mg: Green/yellow. 10mg: Green/black. *Lactose.*

Clobazam

ATC Code: N05BA09. **Sport:** Permitted.
Driving: Caution. See Notes below.
Indications: Anxiety. Epilepsy, adjunctive.
Dose: Adult: *Anxiety,* usually 20-30mg/day in divided doses or single dose at night; severe, up to 60mg/day. Debilitated patients, see Elderly below.
Epilepsy, initially 10-20mg daily; titrate with 10mg increments; max. 60mg/day. Swallow with liquid; do not break tab; do not chew.
Elderly: *Anxiety,* 10-20mg daily; titrate gradually.
Child: Age 6 years and over, initially 5mg/day; maintenance 0.3-1mg/kg/day; titrate gradually.
Renal Impairment: Titrate gradually; increased responsiveness and higher susceptibility to adverse events.
Hepatic Impairment: As for Renal above.
CI: History of alcohol or drug dependence. Children 6 months to 3 years, exceptional use only.
Interactions: Effect of Other Drugs on Clobazam: *Caution:* Lithium. *Effect enhanced:* Carbamazepine, phenytoin.
Effect of Clobazam on Other Drugs: Phenytoin, valproic acid: *Plasma levels altered, monitor.* Muscle relaxants, analgesics, nitrous oxide: *Effects enhanced.*
Notes: See 3.3.5 Benzodiazepine Anxiolytics.

Frisium 10mg *(SANOFI)* A. GMS.
Price, (100) €7.02.
Tablet, clobazam. White round scored. Marked Hoechst; B and GL on reverse. *Lactose.*

Diazepam

ATC Code: N05BA01. **Sport:** Permitted.
Driving: Caution. See Notes below.
Indications: Adjunctive, control of muscle spasm associated with cerebral spasticity. Epilepsy. Premedication before general anaesthesia or sedation in minor surgery. Anxiety. Insomnia. Severe anxiety or agitation (delirium tremens), convulsions of status epilepticus, or where rapid onset of action is required.
Dose: Adult: ORAL, adults (debilitated patients, see Elderly below), *anxiety,* usually 2-5mg 2-3 times daily; max. 30mg/day (divided doses); *insomnia,* 5-15mg before bedtime; *muscle spasm,* 2-15mg/day (2-4 divided doses); *cerebral spasticity,* 2-60mg/day (divided doses).
Alcohol withdrawal, 5-20mg repeated once within 2-4 hours if needed OR 10mg 3-4 times on day 1; then usually 5mg 3-4 times daily as needed.
Premedication, 5-20mg pre-operative.
PARENTERAL, admin by slow IV injection (1mL/min), IM injection or IV infusion (minimum 4mL/hour). *Severe anxiety or agitation,* 10mg repeated 4-hourly; acute *muscle spasm,* 0.1-0.3mg/kg IV every 1-4 hours or IV infusion 3-10mg/kg every 24 hours; *convulsions,* 10-20mg IV or IM; *status epilepticus,* initially 0.15-0.25mg/kg IV repeated in 30-60 minutes; if required follow with IV infusion 3mg/kg over 24 hours.
Premedication, 0.1-0.2mg/kg IV.
RECTAL, 10mg; no response after 5 minutes, repeat.
Elderly: Half adult dose (extended half-life).
Child: ORAL, usually 0.1-0.3mg/kg/day in 2-4 divided doses. Tension/irritability in *cerebral spasticity,* 2-40mg/day in divided doses. *Premedication,* 2-10mg pre-operative.
PARENTERAL, convulsions 0.2-0.3mg/kg IV or IM OR 1mg per year of life.
RECTAL, 1-3 years, 5mg; over 3 years, 10mg. Under 6 months, use with extreme caution; only if no alternative.
Hepatic Impairment: Reduce dose.
Notes: See 3.3.5 Benzodiazepine Anxiolytics.

Anxicalm 2mg, 5mg, 10mg *(Clonmel)* A. GMS.D.
Price, (90) 2mg, €2.10. 5mg, €2.24. 10mg, €4.11.
Tablet, diazepam. Scored. Marked D/strength. 2mg: White. 5mg: Yellow. 10mg: Blue.
Diazemuls Emulsion Parenteral *(Accord)* A. GMS.
Price, (10) €7.78.
Injection, diazepam 5mg/mL. Sterile white opaque oil-in-water emulsion. *Soya-bean oil.*

Diazepam Actavis 2mg, 10mg *(Accord)* A. GMS.D.
Price, (100) 2mg, €2.33. 10mg, €4.57.
Tablet, diazepam. White round flat. Marked D and strength. 10mg: Scored (divisible into equal halves). *Lactose.*
Stesolid Rectal Tubes *(Accord)* A. GMS.
Price, (5) 5mg, €5.82. 10mg, €7.29.
Rectal soln, diazepam 5mg (2mg/mL), 10mg (4mg/mL). Clear colourless (yellowish). *Benzoic acid, propylene glycol.*

Lorazepam

ATC Code: N05BA06. **Sport:** Permitted.
Driving: Caution. See Notes below.
Indications: *Oral,* short-term treatment, anxiety states associated with psychosomatic, organic and psychotic illness; insomnia associated with anxiety. Premedication before operative dentistry and general surgery. *Parenteral,* acute (anxiety states, excitement, mania), premedication (as for oral including minor invasive investigations), control of status epilepticus.
Dose: Adult: ORAL, *anxiety,* 1-4mg daily in divided doses; *insomnia,* 1-2mg before bedtime. *Premedication* (dentistry, general surgery), 2-3mg the night before surgery; then 2-4mg 1-2 hours before surgery.
PARENTERAL, *acute anxiety,* 0.025-0.03mg/kg (1.75-2.1mg for average 70kg man), repeat 6-hourly; *status epilepticus,* 4mg IV. *Premedication,* 0.05mg/kg (3.5mg for average 70kg man), 30-45 minutes before surgery IV OR 1-1.5 hours before surgery IM. May be admin IM or IV but IV route is preferred; avoid injection into small veins and intra-arterial injection; not for long-term chronic use.
Elderly: Including debilitated patients, half Adult dose may be sufficient.
Child: ORAL, age 5-13 years, *premedication,* 0.5-2.5mg at 0.05mg/kg to the nearest 0.5mg according to weight, not less than 1 hour before operation.
PARENTERAL, *status epilepticus,* 2mg IV; acute anxiety, under 12 years, not recommended.
Renal Impairment: Lower doses may be sufficient.
Hepatic Impairment: Mild/moderate, lower doses may be sufficient. Severe, contraindicated.
CI: *Parenteral,* vehicle constituent hypersensitivity (propylene glycol, polyethylene glycol, benzyl alcohol), severe pulmonary insufficiency, out-patient use unless accompanied, children under 3 years (benzyl alcohol). Myasthenia gravis, sleep apnoea syndrome *(both formulations).*
Interactions: Effect of Other Drugs on Lorazepam: *Excessive stupor, reduced respiratory rate, hypotension risk:* Loxapine. *Marked sedation, excessive salivation, ataxia risk:* Clozapine. *Increased plasma levels:* Sodium valproate. *More rapid onset, prolonged effect:* Probenecid. *Sedative effect reduced:* Theophylline, aminophylline.
ADR: *Very common,* sedation, drowsiness, fatigue.
Notes: See 3.3.5 Benzodiazepine Anxiolytics.

Ativan 1mg, Parenteral *(Pfizer)* A. GMS.
Price, (100) €3.27. Injection (10) €5.07.
Tablet, lorazepam. Round flat white scored (divisible into equal halves). Marked 1.0. *Lactose.*
Injection, as above 4mg/mL. Clear colourless soln. *Benzyl alcohol.*
Store: Refrigerate.

Prazepam

ATC Code: N05BA11. **Sport:** Permitted.
Driving: Caution. See Notes below.
Indications: Anxiety.
Dose: Adult: Initially 30mg/day as single or divided dose; range 10-60mg/day.
Elderly: Including debilitated patients, half adult dose.
Renal Impairment: Half adult dose.
Hepatic Impairment: Half adult dose; severe, contraindicated.
Interactions: Effect of Other Drugs on Prazepam: *Plasma levels increased (increased effect):* Oral contraceptives.
Notes: See 3.3.5 Benzodiazepine Anxiolytics.

Centrax 10mg *(Pfizer)* A. GMS.
Price, (60) €4.07.
Tablet, prazepam. White scored (divisible into equal halves). *Lactose.*

3.4 - Hypnotics

3.4.1 - Benzodiazepine Hypnotics

In This Chapter: *Flurazepam, lormetazepam, nitrazepam, temazepam, triazolam.*

Class Effects
Driving: May have major influence. Caution; sedation, amnesia, impaired (concentration, alertness), dizziness. ALCOHOL may intensify impairment.
Indications: Benzodiazepines are only indicated for insomnia when the disorder is severe, disabling or subjecting the individual to extreme distress. For short-term treatment.
CI: Hypersensitivity to any member of the class. Children under 18 years, unless otherwise specified. Myasthenia gravis, severe (respiratory, hepatic, acute pulmonary) insufficiency, sleep apnoea syndrome, phobic or obsessional states, chronic psychosis.
SP: Myorelaxant effect, caution (elderly); increased risk of falls (ataxia, muscle weakness, dizziness, somnolence or sleepiness, fatigue). Chronic respiratory or pulmonary insufficiency, use lower dose, respiratory depression risk. Psychiatric and paradoxical reactions, restlessness, agitation, irritability, aggressiveness, delusion, rages, nightmares, hallucinations, psychoses, inappropriate abnormal behaviour, other behaviour disorders (discontinue). More likely in elderly/children, organic brain syndrome. May induce anterograde amnesia, caution (elderly, debilitated). Not recommended for primary treatment of psychotic illness, sleep disorders associated with depression. May unmask depression; may precipitate suicide. Dependence with high doses and prolonged use especially with history of alcohol/drug abuse or marked personality disorder; monitor (avoid routine repeat prescriptions). Always use for shortest duration possible. Rebound insomnia and anxiety may occur on withdrawal; may be accompanied by (mood changes, anxiety or sleep disturbances, restlessness); always withdraw gradually. See Notes below.
Notes: See 3.3.5 Benzodiazepine Anxiolytics.

Flurazepam

ATC Code: N05CD01. **Sport:** Permitted.
Driving: Caution. See Notes below.
Indications: Insomnia.
Dose: Adult: 15-30mg just before going to bed; 15mg usually optimal. Chronic pulmonary insufficiency, consider dose reduction.
Elderly: Including debilitated patients, initially max. 15mg; reduce dose if organic brain changes present.
Child: Not recommended.
Renal Impairment: Reduce dose.
Hepatic Impairment: Reduce dose; severe, contraindicated.
CI: Myasthenia gravis, severe (respiratory, pulmonary, hepatic) insufficiency, sleep apnoea syndrome, phobic or obsessional states, chronic psychosis.
SP: Max. duration 4 weeks in insomnia, then re-evaluate.
ADR: *Common,* somnolence during day, emotional poverty, reduced alertness, confusional state, fatigue, headache, dizziness, muscle weakness, ataxia, diplopia.
Notes: See 3.4.1 Benzodiazepine Hypnotics.

Dalmane 15mg, 30mg *(Meda)* A. GMS.
Price, (30) 15mg, €3.76. 30mg, €8.68.
Capsule, flurazepam HCl. Marked ICN/strength. 15mg: Grey/yellow. 30mg: Black/grey. *Lactose.*
Dalmapm 15mg, 30mg *(Pinewood)* A. GMS.
Price, (30) 15mg, €2.32. 30mg, €4.07.
Capsule, flurazepam monohydrochloride. Hard gelatin. Marked FLU/strength. 15mg: Ivory/light yellow. 30mg: Grey/black.

Lormetazepam

ATC Code: N05CD06. **Sport:** Permitted.
Driving: Caution. See Notes below.
Indications: Insomnia.

3.4.2 Zolpidem, Zopiclone

Dose: Adult: Initially, 1mg as single dose; dose may be doubled. Admin with liquid before bedtime. Mild/moderate chronic respiratory insufficiency or hepatic insufficiency, consider dose reduction. Duration few days to 2 weeks, max. 4 weeks.

Elderly: Max. 0.5mg as single dose.

Child: Under 18 years, only with careful assessment.

Renal Impairment: Severe, caution.

Hepatic Impairment: Mild/moderate, consider dose reduction. Severe, caution.

CI: Acute ALCOHOL intoxication, hypnotics, analgesics, psychotropic drugs. See Notes below.

SP: Spinal and cerebellar ataxia, caution. Myorelaxant effect, caution danger of falls, especially elderly getting up at night.

Notes: See 3.4.1 Benzodiazepine Hypnotics.

Noctamid 1mg *(Bayer)* A. GMS.
Price, (30) €3.80.
Tablet, lormetazepam. Round white flat scored (divisible into equal halves). Marked CF in a regular hexagon. *Lactose.*

Nitrazepam

ATC Code: N05CD02. **Sport:** Permitted.
Driving: Caution. See Notes below.
Indications: Insomnia.

Dose: Adult: 5-10mg at bedtime. *Hospitalised,* a single dose of 20mg may be given. Pulmonary insufficiency, chronic renal/hepatic disease, dosage may need reduction. Organic brain changes, max. 5mg.

Elderly: Including debilitated patients, doses not to exceed half those normally recommended.

Renal Impairment: As for Elderly above.

Hepatic Impairment: As for Elderly above.

Notes: See 3.4.1 Benzodiazepine Hypnotics.

Mogadon 5mg *(Meda)* A. GMS.D.
Price, (30) €1.20.
Tablet, nitrazepam. Round white scored. Marked ICN. *Lactose.*

Temazepam

ATC Code: N05CD07. **Sport:** Permitted.
Driving: Caution. See Notes below.
Indications: Insomnia. Premedication.

Dose: Adult: *Insomnia,* 10-20mg at bedtime; exceptionally 30-40mg.
Premedication, 20-40mg admin 30-60 minutes before procedure.

Elderly: 10mg; exceptionally 20mg.

Interactions: Effect of Other Drugs on Temazepam: *Sedative effect enhanced:* Disulfiram.

Notes: See 3.4.1 Benzodiazepine Hypnotics.

Nortem 10mg, 20mg *(TEVA)* CD. GMS.D.
Price, (28) 10mg, €2.00. 20mg, €3.08.
Tablet, temazepam. White (off-white) flat scored. Marked with logo; TMZ/strength on reverse. *Mannitol, lactose.*

Triazolam

ATC Code: N05CD05. **Sport:** Permitted.
Driving: Caution. See Notes below.
Indications: Insomnia.

Dose: Adult: Previously untreated, initially 125mcg; usually max. 250mcg at bedtime just before going to bed.

Elderly: Including debilitated, initially 125mcg to decrease over-sedation, dizziness or impaired co-ordination.

Hepatic Impairment: Mild/moderate, caution. Severe, contraindicated.

CI: Sleep apnoea syndrome.

Interactions: Effect of Other Drugs on Triazolam: *Co-admin contraindicated:* Nefazodone, ketoconazole, itraconazole, efavirenz, HIV protease inhibitors. *Co-admin caution:* Isoniazid, fluvoxamine, sertraline, paroxetine, diltiazem, verapamil, other CNS depressants. *Co-admin not recommended:* ALCOHOL, other azole antifungals. *Activity enhanced (consider dose reduction):* Cimetidine, verapamil, diltiazem, erythromycin, other macrolides (clarithromycin, triacetyloleandomycin). *Enhanced clinical effects:* Oral contraceptives, imatinib, aprepitant. *Effect*

reduced: Rifampicin, carbamazepine. *Dose-reduction or discontinuation with co-admin:* Ritonavir. *Increased bioavailability:* Grapefruit juice.

SP: Generally, use for 7-10 days; longer than 2 weeks requires complete re-evaluation of patient.

ADR: *Common,* somnolence, dizziness, ataxia, headache.

Notes: See 3.4.1 Benzodiazepine Hypnotics.

Halcion 125mcg, 250mcg *(Pfizer)* A. GMS.
Price, (30) 0.125mg, €2.12. 0.25mg, €2.29.
Tablet, triazolam. Elliptical. 125mcg: Lavender. Marked Upjohn10. 250mcg: Powder-blue scored. Marked with logo and 17. *Lactose.*

3.4.2 - Zolpidem, Zopiclone

Class Effects

Treatment for insomnia is only indicated when the disorder is severe, disabling or subjecting the individual to extreme distress. Treatment duration should be as short as possible.

CI: Hypersensitivity to any member of the class. Children under 18 years. Acute and/or severe, respiratory insufficiency.

SP: Suicide, benzodiazepines or benzodiazepine-like drugs should not be used alone to treat depression or anxiety associated with depression (may precipitate suicide), see Notes below (antidepressants). These drugs should be taken immediately before going to bed or in bed. Treatment should be as short as possible and only if the condition is debilitating or causing severe distress.

Pregnancy, Lactation: Pregnancy, not recommended; late phase of pregnancy/labour use may affect neonate (hypothermia, hypotonia, moderate respiratory depression but severe reported). Chronic use in latter stages of pregnancy, infants may develop withdrawal symptoms; severe neonatal respiratory depression reported. Lactation, not recommended (passes into breast milk). See Notes below (benzodiazepine anxiolytics).

ADR: Evidence of dose-relationship for adverse events (CNS, GI). Occur more frequently in the elderly.

Notes: See 3.3 Antidepressants and Anxiolytics.

Zolpidem

ATC Code: N05CF02. **Sport:** Permitted.
Driving: Major influence; next-day psychomotor impairment, drowsiness.
Indications: Short-term treatment, insomnia (adults).

Dose: Adult: Max. 10mg taken immediately at bedtime as a single dose; do not repeat during same night.

Elderly: Including debilitated patients, 5mg admin as for Adult; max. 10mg.

Child: Under 18 years, insufficient data to support use.

Hepatic Impairment: As for Elderly above; severe, contraindicated (may contribute to encephalopathy).

CI: Acute and/or severe respiratory insufficiency.

Interactions: Effect of Other Drugs on Zolpidem: *Co-admin not recommended (increased zolpidem blood levels):* Fluvoxamine, ciprofloxacin, ALCOHOL. *CNS depression enhanced (increased drowsiness, next day psychomotor impairment, including driving):* Antipsychotics (neuroleptics), hypnotics, anxiolytics, sedatives, muscle relaxants, antidepressants, narcotic analgesics, antiepileptics, anaesthetics, sedative antihistamines. *Visual hallucinations:* Bupropion, desipramine, fluoxetine, sertraline, venlafaxine. *Sedative effects may be enhanced:* Ketoconazole. *Possible interactions:* CYP3A4 substrates or inducers.

SP: Next day psychomotor impairment, including driving ability, is increased if (admin less than 8 hours before activities requiring mental alertness; higher than recommended dose; co-admin with other CNS depressants, drugs increasing blood levels of zolpidem, alcohol or illicit drugs). Drowsiness and decreased level of consciousness or awareness may lead to falls and severe injuries. Somnambulism reported.

ADR: *Common,* somnolence, headache, dizziness, exacerbated insomnia, cognitive disorders such as memory

disorders, fatigue, diarrhoea, nausea, vomiting, abdominal pain, back pain, respiratory tract infection (upper, lower).
Notes: See 3.4.2 Zaleplon, Zolpidem, Zopiclone.

Stilnoct 5mg, 10mg *(SANOFI)* A. GMS.
Price, (28) 5mg, €1.52. 10mg, €3.05.
Tablet, zolpidem tartrate. White f/c. 5mg: Round. 10mg: Oblong scored. Marked SN10. *Lactose.*
Nytamel 5mg, 10mg *(Clonmel)* A. GMS.
Price, (28) 5mg, €1.49. 10mg, €2.98.
Tablet, zolpidem tartrate. White oval f/c. Marked ZIM/strength. 10mg: Scored.
Zoldem 10mg *(Gerard)* A. GMS.
Price, (28) €2.98.
Tablet, zolpidem tartrate. White (off-white) cap-shaped f/c scored (divisible into equal doses). Marked ZM10; G on reverse. *Lactose.*
Zolpidem Tartrate TEVA 5mg *(TEVA)* A. GMS.
Price, (28) €2.85.
Tablet, zolpidem tartrate. White oval f/c. Marked ZIM; strength on reverse. *Lactose.*
Zolnod 10mg *(Rowex)* A. GMS.
Price, (30) €3.20.
Tablet, zolpidem tartrate. White f/c scored oblong.

Zopiclone

ATC Code: N05CF01. **Sport:** Permitted.
Driving: Sedation, amnesia, impaired (concentration, muscular function); impaired alertness.
Indications: Short-term treatment, insomnia.
Dose: Adult: Recommended 7.5mg just before bedtime. Chronic respiratory insufficiency, as for Elderly below.
Elderly: Initiate with 3.75mg; if needed titrate to 7.5mg
Child: Under 18 years, safety/efficacy not established.
Renal Impairment: As for Elderly above.
Hepatic Impairment: As for Elderly above.
Interactions: Effect of Other Drugs on Zopiclone: *Co-admin not recommended:* Alcohol (enhanced sedative/CNS depressive effect). *Accelerated absorption, faster hypnotic effect:* Erythromycin. *Increased plasma levels:* Metoclopramide; CYP3A4 inhibitors (erythromycin, clarithromycin, ketoconazole, itraconazole, fluconazole, tacrolimus, ritonavir; consider dose reduction; caution, elderly). *Plasma levels decreased:* Atropine. *Plasma levels decreased, reduced effect:* Rifampicin, phenytoin, carbamazepine.
Effect of Zopiclone on Other Drugs: Muscle relaxants: *Effect enhanced.*
SP: Somnambulism and other behaviours (with amnesia for event), reported; increased risk with ALCOHOL co-admin.
ADR: *Common,* drowsiness during following day, reduced alertness, headache, dizziness, bitter taste.
Notes: See 3.4.2 Zaleplon, Zolpidem, Zopiclone.
Interchangeability: Same strengths of all brands of zopiclone f/c tablets listed below are deemed interchangeable.
Reference Price: (28) 3.75mg, €2.16; 7.5mg, €3.24.

Zimovane 7.5mg *(Meda)* A. GMS.
Price, (28) €3.97.
Tablet, zolpiclone. White elliptical f/c scored (divisible into equal halves). *Lactose.* **Store:** Below 30 deg C; original pack to protect (light).
Zileze 3.75mg, 7.5mg *(Chiesi)* A. GMS.
Price, (28) both strengths, €2.80.
Tablet, zopiclone. f/c. Marked ZOC/strength. 3.75mg: Orange. 7.5mg: White. *Lactose.* **Store:** Below 25 deg C; outer carton to protect (light).
Zimoclone 7.5mg *(Gerard)* A. GMS.
Price, (28) €2.80.
Tablet, zopiclone. White oval f/c scored (divisible into equal halves). Marked ZZ; 7.5 on reverse. **Store:** Below 25 deg C; original pack.
Zopitan 3.75mg, 7.5mg *(Clonmel)* A. GMS.
Price, (28) both strengths, €2.80.
Tablet, zopiclone. f/c. Marked ZOC/strength. 3.75mg: Orange. 7.5mg: White scored both sides. **Store:** Below 25 deg C; original pack to protect (moisture).
Zorclone 7.5mg *(TEVA)* A. GMS.
Price, (28) €2.80.
Tablet, zopiclone. White round f/c scored (divisible into equal doses). Marked ZOC 7.5. *Lactose.* **Store:** Below 25 deg C; original pack.

3.4.3 - Other Drugs Used In Sleep Disorders

In This Chapter: *Melatonin, sodium oxybate.*

Class Effects

CI: Hypersensitivity to any member of the class. Use in children unless otherwise specified.

Melatonin

ATC Code: N05CH01. **Sport:** Permitted.
Driving: Drowsiness.
Indications: Short-term treatment of primary insomnia, characterised by poor sleep quality (patients aged 55 years or over).
Dose: Adult, Elderly: 2mg once daily 1-2 hours before bedtime; may be continued for up to 13 weeks. *Admin,* swallow tabs whole, after food.
Child: Under 18 years, not recommended.
Renal Impairment: Caution.
Hepatic Impairment: Not recommended.
Interactions: Effect of Other Drugs on Melatonin: *Co-admin avoid (metabolism inhibited; plasma levels increased):* Fluvoxamine, 5- or 8-methoxypsorelen (5- and 8-MOP), cimetidine, oestrogens (contraceptives, HRT), quinolones. *Plasma levels decreased:* Cigarette smoking, CYP1A2 inducers (carbamazepine, rifampicin). *Effect on sleep reduced:* ALCOHOL.
Effect of Melatonin on Other Drugs: Benzodiazepines, non-benzodiazepines (zaleplon, zolpidem, zopiclone): *Enhanced sedative properties.* Imipramine: *Increased feeling of tranquillity, difficulty in performing tasks.* Thioridazine: *Increased feelings of 'muzzy-headedness'.*
SP: Autoimmune disease, not recommended.
Pregnancy, Lactation: Not recommended.
ADR: *Most common,* headache, nasopharyngitis, back pain, arthralgia.
Notes: See 3.4.3 Other Drugs Used In Sleep Disorders.

Circadin 2mg *(Flynn)* A.
Price, (21) €14.51.
Prolonged/R tablet, melatonin. White (off-white) round. *Lactose.*

Sodium Oxybate

ATC Code: N07XX04. **Sport:** Permitted.
Driving: Major influence. See SP below.
Indications: Narcolepsy with cataplexy.
Dose: Adult: Initially 4.5g/day in 2 equal doses of 2.25g; titrate to max. 9g/day in 2 equal doses; adjust up or down in 1.5g/day increments and at 2-week intervals. *Co-admin with valproate,* reduce sodium oxybate dose by 20% starting with 3.6g/night admin in 2 equal divided doses of 1.8g; monitor response and tolerability. Admin 2-3 hours after food, at bedtime; first dose getting into bed, second dose 2.5-4 hours later; if stopped for 14 days or more, restart from lowest dose. NOTE: Use only measuring syringe provided which is graduated in grams (g).
Elderly: Monitor closely.
Renal Impairment: Consider reduction of dietary sodium.
Hepatic Impairment: Halve dose.
CI: Major depression. Succinic semialdehyde dehydrogenase deficiency. Current opioid or barbiturate treatment.
Interactions: Effect of Other Drugs on Sodium Oxybate: *CNS-depression and/or respiratory depression:* Other CNS depressants, ALCOHOL, benzodiazepines (avoid). *Potential interaction, consider dose reduction:* Drugs stimulating or inhibiting GHB dehydrogenase (valproate, phenytoin, ethosuximide, topiramate). *Caution:* Antidepressants, TCADs.
SP: *Xyrem* has the potential to induce respiratory depression; BMI 40kg/m2 or more, higher sleep apnoea risk. Potential for abuse, evaluate history of drug abuse (specialist use). Not for use in porphyria or epilepsy. Confusion, psychosis, paranoia, hallucinations, agitation; caution, depressive illness and/or suicide attempt. Urinary or faecal incontinence. Rarely withdrawal symptoms. Heart

121

failure, hypertension, compromised renal function, reduce dietary sodium intake. Driving not recommended for 6 hours after admin.

Pregnancy, Lactation: Pregnancy, not recommended; first trimester, possible increased risk of spontaneous abortion; second and third trimester, no indication of malformative or foeto/neonatal toxicity. Lactation, not recommended; not known if excreted in breast milk.

ADR: Summary, *most common*, dizziness, nausea, headache; *most serious*, suicidal attempt, psychosis, respiratory depression, convulsion.

Notes: See 3.4.3 Other Drugs Used In Sleep Disorders.

> **Xyrem Oral Soln 500mg/mL** *(UCB)* CD. HT.
> Price, (180mL) €377.39.
> Oral soln, sodium oxybate. Clear (opalescent). *Sodium range 0.82g/(4.5g/day)* to *1.6g/(9g/day)* dose. **Store:** Use within 24 hours after dilution.

3.5 - Parkinson's Disease, Restless Legs Syndrome

Class Effects

Driving: Most of the drugs used in the treatment of these disorders have major influence on ability to drive or operate machinery; may cause dizziness, symptomatic orthostatic hypotension through to somnolence and/or sudden sleep onset episodes. Instruct patients to refrain from driving until symptoms/episodes have resolved.

CI: Hypersensitivity to any member of the class.

SP: *Impulse control disorders* e.g. pathological gambling, compulsive shopping, increased libido, hypersexuality; principally in Parkinson's patients treated with dopamine agonists and other dopaminergic drugs (generally reversible with dose reduction or discontinuation). Involuntary movements and mental disturbances; observe for depression with concomitant suicidal tendencies; past or current psychoses, caution. All dopamine agonists should be withdrawn gradually. Patients with Parkinson's disease have higher risk of melanoma development; consider periodic skin examinations.

3.5.1 - Dopaminergics Used In Parkinson's Disease

In This Chapter: *Ergot alkaloids and related dopamine agonists (apomorphine, bromocriptine, cabergoline, pramipexole, ropinirole, rotigotine), dopamine reuptake inhibitor (tetrabenazine).*

Class Effects

Driving: See Notes below.

CI: Children under 18 years. Hypersensitivity to ergot alkaloids.

Interactions: Effect of Other Drugs on Ergot Alkaloids and Related Drugs: *Co-admin not recommended (reduced efficacy)*: Dopamine antagonists including neuroleptics, phenothiazines, butyrophenones (haloperidol), thioxanthenes (flupentixol, zuclopenthixol), metoclopramide, sulpiride.

Effect of Ergot Alkaloids and Related Drugs on Other Drugs: Levodopa: *Efficacy enhanced.*

SP: Impulse control disorders, see Notes below. Fibrotic and serosal inflammatory disorders. Cardiac valvulopathy. Retroperitoneal fibrosis. Severe cardiovascular disease, Raynaud's syndrome, peptic ulcer, GI bleeding, serious, particularly psychotic mental disease, caution. Hypotension, postural hypotension, syncope. Somnolence, episodes of sudden sleep onset (particularly in Parkinson's). With sudden withdrawal, neuroleptic malignant syndrome (NMS) or withdrawal symptoms (taper treatment). Dopaminergic adverse reactions (hallucinations, dyskinesia, peripheral oedema) generally higher in combination with levodopa in Parkinson's patients. *Restless Legs Syndrome*, dopaminergics can result in augmentation; earlier onset of symptoms in evening, increased severity, spread to other body parts.

Pregnancy, Lactation: Pregnancy, if clearly indicated and if benefit outweighs risk. Lactation, not recommended

(inhibits lactation). Women of childbearing age not wishing to conceive, advise use of reliable contraceptive method.

ADR: Application site reactions (transdermal), see SP above.

Notes: See 3.6 Parkinson's Disease, RLS.

Apomorphine

ATC Code: N04BC07. **Sport:** Permitted.

Driving: Somnolence and/or sudden sleep episodes.

Indications: Disabling motor fluctuations ('on-off' phenomenon) in Parkinson's disease.

Dose: Adult: Initially 1mg; inadequate response after 30 minutes, admin 2mg; uptitrate by minimum 40-minute intervals to satisfactory response; once determined, single SC injection may be admin at first signs of 'on-off' phenomenon. Max. 100mg/day. Max. bolus 10mg. Establish patient on domperidone (20mg 3-times daily) for minimum 2 days before initiation. Admin SC by intermittent bolus injection.

Elderly: Caution during initiation.

Hepatic Impairment: Not recommended.

CI: Respiratory depression, dementia, psychotic illness. Intermittent apomorphine not suitable if 'on' response to levodopa marred by severe dyskinesia or dystonia.

Interactions: Effect of Other Drugs on Apomorphine: *Co-admin caution*: Drugs with narrow therapeutic window. *Effect antagonised*: Neuroleptics (clozapine).

Effect of Apomorphine on Other Drugs: Antihypertensives: *Effect potentiated*.

SP: Caution, renal, pulmonary, cardiovascular disease; patients prone to nausea and vomiting. Exacerbation of neuropsychiatric disturbances. Somnolence, sudden sleep onset episodes.

Pregnancy, Lactation: Not recommended.

ADR: Injection site (local induration, erythema, tenderness, ulceration, pruritus), nausea, vomiting, sedation, somnolence, neuropsychiatric (confusion, visual hallucinations). Postural hypotension, dyskinesias during 'on' periods, Coombs' positive haemolytic anaemia, breathing difficulties. Eosinophilia.

Notes: See 3.5.1 Dopaminergics Used In Parkinson's Disease.

> **APO-go Parenteral** *(Clonmel)* B.
> Price, (5) Pens 10mg/mL, €232.52. PFS 5mg/mL, €152.33.
> Injection, apomorphine. Clear colourless soln. *Metabisulphite*.

Bromocriptine

ATC Code: N04BC01. **Sport:** Permitted.

Driving: Hypotensive reactions, reduced alertness, somnolence, sudden sleep episodes.

Indications: *Treatment*, idiopathic Parkinson's disease, prolactin secreting adenomas (macroadenomas, microadenomas), hyperprolactinaemia (hypogonadism and/or galactorrhoea), female infertility. *Adjunctive* to surgery and/or radiotherapy to reduce circulating growth hormone levels in acromegaly. *Prevention or suppression* of post-partum lactation only when medically indicated (not for routine suppression of lactation or relief of post-partum pain and engorgement).

Dose: Adult, Elderly: Except for lactation prevention, to minimise side-effects, use gradual introduction schedule i.e. initially 1.25mg at bedtime, increasing after 2-3 days to 2.5mg at bedtime; then by 1.25-2.5mg at 2-3 day intervals until 2.5mg twice daily achieved. Always admin during a meal.

Lactation prevention, 2.5mg on first day of delivery, then 2.5mg twice daily for 14 days; lactation suppression, 2.5mg on first day increasing after 2-3 days to 2.5mg twice daily for 14 days (gradual introduction not necessary in these indications).

Hypogonadism, galactorrhoea syndrome, infertility, usually 7.5mg/day (divided doses); up to 30mg/day; infertility without elevated serum prolactin levels, usually 2.5mg twice daily.

Acromegaly, prolactinomas, titrate by 2.5mg daily at 2-3 day intervals (2.5mg 8-hourly, 2.5mg 6-hourly, 5mg 6-

hourly); final dose usually 20-60mg daily (acromegaly), 30mg (prolactinomas).

Parkinson's Disease, 1.25mg (week 1), 2.5mg (week 2) at bedtime; 2.5mg twice daily (week 3), 2.5mg 3-times daily (week 4) then increase by 2.5mg every 3-14 days; usually 10-40mg daily.

Child: Under 15 years, not recommended.

CI: Hypertension (uncontrolled; of pregnancy including eclampsia, pre-eclampsia, pregnancy-induced; post-partum and in puerperium); suppression of lactation or other non-life threatening indications, patients with (CAD, other severe cardiovascular conditions, symptoms/history of severe psychiatric disorders). Long-term treatment, evidence of cardiac valvulopathy.

Interactions: Effect of Other Drugs on Bromocriptine: *Plasma levels increased:* Erythromycin, josamycin, other macrolides, octreotide. *Reduced tolerability:* ALCOHOL.

SP: Conditions not associated with hyperprolactinaemia, use lowest dose to relieve symptoms and avoid impaired luteal function. GI bleeding, ulceration, withdraw. Hypotensive reactions (reduced alertness), somnolence, sudden sleep onset. Monitor for impulse control disorders. Use postpartum for lactation inhibition associated with (hypertension, MI, seizures, stroke, psychological disorders), sometimes preceded by severe headache and/or visual disturbances; monitor BP. If hypertension is severe, progressive, or unremitting headache (with or without visual disturbances) or evidence of CNS toxicity, discontinue. Prolactin-secreting adenomas, evaluate pituitary function; secondary adrenal insufficiency, use corticosteroid substitution. Macroprolactinoma, visual field impairment.

ADR: *Common*, headache, drowsiness, dizziness, nasal congestion, nausea, constipation, vomiting.

Notes: See 3.5.1 Dopaminergics Used In Parkinson's Disease.

Parlodel 2.5mg, 5mg *(Meda)* B. GMS.
Price, 2.5mg (30) €6.96. 5mg (100) €45.18.
Tablet, bromocriptine mesilate 2.5mg. Whitish round scored (divisible into equal halves). Marked 2.5 MG. *Lactose.* **Store:** Below 25 deg C; blister in outer carton.
Capsule, as above 5mg. Opaque light-blue/white. Marked 5mg. *Lactose.* **Store:** Below 25 deg C; original pack to protect (light, moisture).

Cabergoline

ATC Code: N04BC06, G02CB03. **Sport:** Permitted.
Driving: Somnolence and/or sudden sleep episodes, impaired alertness.

Indications: Parkinson's disease, hyperprolactinaemia in females (amenorrhoea, oligomenorrhoea, anovulation, galactorrhoea); prolactin-secreting pituitary adenomas, idiopathic hyperprolactinaemia, or empty sella syndrome; suppression of lactation.

Dose: Adult, Elderly: *Cabaser, Parkinson's disease*, initially 1mg/day; increase slowly by 0.5-1mg/day at weekly (initially) or bi-weekly intervals; recommended 2-3mg/day. Single daily dose with food.

Dostinex, hyperprolactinaemia, initially 0.5mg/week in 1 or 2 doses (Mon, Thurs); increase by 0.5mg/week and 1-month intervals to usual 1mg/week; range 0.25-2mg/week; max. 3mg/week. Up to 4.5mg/week has been used. Above 1mg/week, divided doses.

Inhibition, puerperal lactation, day 1 post-partum; range 1mg as single dose. Suppression, established lactation, 0.25mg 12-hourly for 2 days; total 1mg.

Child: Under 16 years, not recommended.

Renal Impairment: ESRD or haemodialysis, caution.

Hepatic Impairment: Severe, caution; max. 1mg/day. See CI below.

CI: Evidence of cardiac valvulopathy. Hepatic insufficiency, toxaemia of pregnancy, puerperal psychosis. Pulmonary, pericardial, retroperitoneal fibrotic disorders.

Interactions: Effect of Other Drugs on Cabergoline: *Co-admin contraindicated (Dostinex):* Antipsychotics. *Co-admin not recommended:* Other ergot alkaloids (long-term treatment) *(Cabaser).* Increased adverse effects:

Macrolides (erythromycin). *Symptomatic hypotension:* Co-admin (other antihypertensives).

SP: Caution, severe cardiovascular disease, Raynaud's syndrome, peptic ulcer, GI bleeding, serious psychotic disorders, postural hypotension; fibrotic and serosal inflammatory disorders (pleuritis, pleural effusion, pleural fibrosis, pulmonary fibrosis, pericarditis, pericardial effusion, cardiac valvulopathy, retroperitoneal fibrosis; prolonged usage). Abnormally increased ESR in association with pleural effusion/fibrosis.

Before initiating long-term treatment, cardiac evaluation including echocardiography, baseline ESR, lung function/chest X-ray, renal function prior to initiation; valvular regurgitation; fibrotic valvular disease detected, do not initiate. Sudden sleep onset, impulse control disorders, see Notes below.

Pregnancy, Lactation: Pregnancy, use only if clearly needed. Use adequate contraception during treatment. Due to long half-life, women intending to become pregnant should stop drug 1 month before intended conception. Lactation, not recommended.

ADR: *Very common*, valvulopathy (including regurgitation) and related disorders (pericarditis, pericardial effusion), nausea *(both brands)*; peripheral oedema *(Cabaser)*; headache, dizziness, vertigo, dyspepsia, gastritis, abdominal pain, asthenia, fatigue *(Dostinex).*

Notes: See 3.5.1 Dopaminergics Used In Parkinson's Disease.

Cabaser 1mg, 2mg *(Pfizer)* A. GMS.
Price, (20) 1mg, €34.22. 2mg, €47.13.
Tablet, cabergoline. White oval concave scored (divisible into equal halves). Marked 7. 1mg: Marked 01. 2mg: Marked 02. *Lactose.*

Dostinex 0.5mg *(Pfizer)* A. GMS.
Price, (8) €26.95.
Tablet, cabergoline. Cap-shaped flat white scored. Marked P and U; 700 on reverse. *Lactose.*

Pramipexole

ATC Code: N04BC05. **Sport:** Permitted.
Driving: Major influence (hallucinations, somnolence, sudden sleep episodes).

Indications: Treatment, Parkinson's Disease *(all brands)*. Restless Legs Syndrome (RLS) *(brand Mirapexin)*.

Dose: Adult, Elderly: Dose stated as BASE: *Parkinson's Disease*, STANDARD/R, initially, 0.264mg/day; increase every 5-7 days to 0.264mg/day (week 1), 0.54mg/day (week 2) and 1.05mg/day (week 3). If needed increase by 0.54mg at weekly intervals to max. 3.5mg/day. Maintenance, range 0.264mg to max. 3.3mg/day. Discontinuation, decrease by 0.54mg/day until 0.54mg/day is reached, then reduce by 0.264mg/day.

Dose stated as BASE: *Parkinson's Disease*, PROLONGED/R, initially 0.26mg/day; increase every 5-7 days to 0.26mg/day (week 1), 0.52mg/day (week 2), 1.05mg/day (week 3). If needed, increase by 0.52mg at weekly intervals; max. 3.15mg/day. NOTE: Doses above 1.05mg, increased somnolence incidence. Maintenance, range 0.26mg; max. 3.15mg/day. Discontinuation, decrease by 0.52mg/day until 0.52mg/day is reached; then reduce by 0.26mg/day. Switch, Standard/R to Prolonged/R overnight at same daily dose.

Dose stated as BASE: *Restless Legs Syndrome*, STANDARD/R, initially 0.088mg once daily 2-3 hours before bedtime; if needed, increase every 4-7 days to max. 0.54mg/day.

Admin, swallow tabs whole with water, with or without food. STANDARD/R, usually in 3 divided doses. PROLONGED/R, once daily; do not chew, divide or crush.

Child: No relevant use.

Renal Impairment: Dose stated as BASE: Standard/R, *Parkinson's*, CrCl (mL/min) 20-50, initially 0.088mg twice daily; max. 1.57mg/day; 20, initially 0.088mg/day as single dose; max. 1.1mg/day. Reduce dose by same percentage as CrCl declines. *RLS*, CrCl (mL/min) above 20, no adjustment.

Prolonged/R, CrCl (mL/min) 30-50, initially 0.26mg every other day; if needed, increase by 0.26mg at weekly intervals; max 1.57mg/day; below 30, not recommended.

Interactions: Effect of Other Drugs on Pramipexole: Co-

3.5.1 Dopaminergics Used In Parkinson's Disease

admin avoid: Other antipsychotics. Reduced clearance (consider dose reduction): Cimetidine, amantadine, mexiletine, zidovudine, cisplatin, quinine, procainamide. Additive effects: Other sedating medication, ALCOHOL.

Effect of Pramipexole on Other Drugs: Levodopa (co-admin): Reduce dose; maintain dose of other anti-Parkinsonian drugs while increasing Mirapexin dose.

SP: Hallucinations (mostly visual), dyskinesia, somnolence, episodes of sudden sleep onset (especially with Parkinson's), behavioural changes (binge eating), psychotic disorders (use only if benefit outweighs risk), vision abnormalities (monitor), severe cardiovascular disease (caution; monitor BP, hypotension risk). Restless Legs Syndrome (augmentation). Mania, delirium can occur (consider dose reduction or tapered discontinuation). Dopamine dysregulation Syndrome (DDS), an addictive disorder, resulting in excessive use in some patients treated with dopaminergics; warn patients and caregivers of potential DDS risk before initiation. Dopamine agonist withdrawal syndrome; always taper off dose.

Remnants in faeces may resemble intact Mirapexin Prolonged/R tabs; reassess patient response to therapy.

ADR: Most common (Parkinson's), nausea, dyskinesia (more frequent in combination with levodopa), hypotension, dizziness, somnolence, insomnia, constipation, hallucination, headache, fatigue; (RLS), nausea*, headache, dizziness, fatigue*. *(more common in women).

Notes: See 3.5.1 Dopaminergics Used In Parkinson's Disease.

Mirapexin Tablets, PR (Boehringer) B. GMS.
Price, 0.088mg (30) €3.95. 0.18mg (100) €26.29. 0.7mg (100) €105.40. PR (30) 0.26mg, €15.27. 0.52mg, €30.55. 1.05mg, €61.10. 2.1mg, €122.19. 3.15mg, €183.29.
Standard/R tablet (base), pramipexole dihydrochloride monohydrate 0.088mg, 0.18mg, 0.7mg. Flat white. Marked with code. **Strength:** 0.088mg: Round. 0.18mg: Oval scored*. 0.7mg: Round scored*. *both sides (divisible into equal halves). **Store:** Below 30 deg C; original pack; protect (light).
Prolonged/R (base), as above 0.26mg, 0.52mg, 1.05mg, 2.1mg, 3.15mg. White (off-white). Marked with logo. 0.26mg: Round. Marked P1. 0.52mg: Round. Marked P2. 1.05mg: Oval. Marked P3. 2.1mg: Oval. Marked P4. 3.15mg: Oval. Marked P5. **Store:** Original pack; protect (moisture).

Miramel Tablets (Clonmel) B. GMS.
Price, (30) 0.088mg, €3.96. (100) 0.18mg, €26.30. 0.7mg, €105.40.
Tablet (base), pramipexole dihydrochloride monohydrate 0.088mg, 0.18mg, 0.7mg. White (off-white). 0.088mg: Round. 0.18mg: Oval scored*. 0.7mg: Round scored*. *(divisible into equal halves).

Oprymea Tablets, Prolonged/R (Krka) B. GMS.
Price, 0.088mg (30) €3.74; 0.18mg (100) €24.82; 0.7mg (100) €99.50. Prolonged/R (30) 0.26mg, €11.61; 0.52mg, €26.04; 1.05mg, €42.80; 2.1mg, €75.52. 3.15mg €101.95.
Standard/R tablet (base), pramipexole dihydrochloride monohydrate 0.088mg, 0.18mg, 0.7mg. White. 0.088mg: Round. Marked P6. 0.18mg: Oval scored*. Marked P7 either side of score. 0.7mg: Round scored*. Marked P9 either side of score. *(divisible into equal halves).
Prolonged/R (base), as above 0.26mg, 0.52mg, 1.05mg, 2.1mg, 3.15mg. White (almost) round. 0.26mg: Marked P1. 0.52mg: Marked P2. 1.05mg: Marked P3. 2.1mg: Marked P4. 3.15mg: Marked P5; 315 on reverse.

Pramipexole Accord Tablets (Accord) B. GMS.
Price, (30) 0.088mg, €3.74. (100) 0.18mg, €24.82; 0.35mg, €49.92; 0.7mg, €99.49.
Standard/R tablet (base), pramipexole dihydrochloride monohydrate 0.088mg, 0.18mg, 0.35mg, 0.7mg. White (off-white) round. 0.088mg: Marked I1. 0.18mg: Scored. Marked I2. 0.35mg: Marked I3 scored (divisible into equal halves). 0.7mg: Scored. Marked I4.

Pramipexole Mylan 0.088mg (Gerard) B. GMS.
Price, (30) €3.96.
Standard/R tablet (base), pramipexole dihydrochloride monohydrate. White (off-white) round flat. Marked M, PX1.

Prapexin Prolonged/R Tablets (Rowex) B. GMS.
Price, (30) 1.05mg, €42.80; 2.1mg, €75.52.
Prolonged/R tablet (base), as above 1.05mg, 2.1mg. White (nearly) cylindrical. 10.5mg: Marked 105. 2.1mg: Marked 210.

Ropinirole

ATC Code: N04BC04. **Sport:** Permitted.
Driving: Somnolence/sudden sleep episodes.
Indications: Treatment, Parkinson's Disease.

Dose: Adult: STANDARD/R, initially 0.75mg/day (week 1); titrate in 0.75mg/day increments to 1.5mg/day (week 2), 2.25mg/day (week 3) and 3mg/day (week 4) then increase at weekly increments of 1.5-3mg/day. Usually 3-9mg/day; max 24mg/day. Oral in 3 divided doses preferably with food. Adjunctive, levodopa dose may be gradually reduced according to response.
PROLONGED/R, initially 2mg once daily (week 1); titrate to 4mg once daily (from week 2); insufficient control, increase by 2mg/week intervals to 8mg/day; max. 24mg/day. Adjunctive, may be possible to reduce levodopa. Switch from Standard/R to Prolonged/R, see manufacturers Full Prescribing Information.

Elderly: Over 65 years, clearance reduced; titrate carefully, monitor tolerability.

Renal Impairment: CrCl (mL/min) below 30, without regular dialysis, contraindicated. ESRD, on dialysis, initially 0.25mg 3-times daily; max. 18mg/day; no supplemental dose required after dialysis.

Hepatic Impairment: Contraindicated.

Interactions: Effect of Other Drugs on Ropinirole: Plasma levels increased: Oestrogens (high dose) ; ciprofloxacin, enoxacin, fluvoxamine.

Effect of Ropinirole on Other Drugs: Vitamin K antagonists: Monitor INR.

SP: Somnolence, episodes of sudden sleep, especially with Parkinson's disease (advise patient); consider dose reduction or discontinue. Patients with major psychotic disorders, use only if benefit outweighs risk. Monitor, BP especially at initiation (hypotension), development of impulse control disorders. Modutab releases medication over 24-hours; rapid GI transit may result in incomplete medication release and medication residue being passed in stool.

Pregnancy, Lactation: Pregnancy, not recommended unless benefit outweighs risk. Lactation, not recommended, may inhibit lactation.

ADR: Very common, somnolence, syncope, nausea, dyskinesia*. Common, hallucinations, confusion, dizziness including vertigo, sudden sleep onset, constipation, heartburn, vomiting, abdominal pain, oedema peripheral (including leg oedema), postural hypotension*. *(adjunctive treatment).

Notes: See 3.5.1 Dopaminergics Used In Parkinson's Disease.

ReQuip 0.25mg, 1mg, 2mg, 5mg, Modutab (GSK) B. GMS.
Price, (84) 0.25mg, €13.06. 1mg, €30.10. 2mg, €51.74. 5mg, €114.62. Modutab (21) 2mg, €28.62. (84) 2mg, €57.24. 4mg, €103.86. 8mg, €202.92.
Tablet, ropinirole HCl. Pentagonal f/c. 0.25mg: White. 1mg: Green. 2mg: Pink. 5mg: Blue. Lactose. **Store:** Below 25 deg C.
Prolonged/R tablet, as above. Cap-shaped f/c. Marked GS. 2mg: Pink. Marked 3V2. 4mg: Light brown. Marked WXG. 8mg: Red. Marked 5CC. Lactose, mannitol. **Store:** As above; original pack to protect (light).

Rolpryna SR 2mg, 4mg, 8mg (Krka) B. GMS.
Price, 2mg (21) €20.00; (84) €63.21. (84) 4mg, €114.38. 8mg, €210.52.
Prolonged/R tablet, ropinirole HCl. Oval. 2mg: Pink. 4mg: Light off-brown. 8mg: Brownish-red. Lactose.

Rotigotine

ATC Code: N04BC09. **Sport:** Permitted.
Driving: Somnolence, sudden sleep episodes, impaired alertness.
Indications: Treatment, Parkinson's disease. Restless Legs Syndrome (RLS).

Dose: Adult, Elderly: Parkinson's Disease, early stages, initially 2mg/24-hours; increase in weekly increments of 2mg/24-hours to effective dose; max. 8mg/24-hours; late stages, initially 4mg/24-hours increasing in weekly increments to effective dose; max. 16mg/24-hours (above 8mg/24-hours, use multiple patches). Withdraw gradually by 2mg/24-hour every other day.
Restless Legs Syndrome, initiate at 1mg/24-hours; based

124

on response increase weekly by 1mg/24-hours; max. 3mg/24-hours; review 6-monthly. Withdraw gradually by 1mg/24-hour every other day. Apply patch once daily, approx. same time each day; remains on skin for 24-hours then replace at different site.

Child: Safety/efficacy not established. No recommendation for RLS.

Renal Impairment: Acute worsening function, accumulation may occur.

Hepatic Impairment: Severe, caution lower rotigotine clearance. Worsening impairment, consider dose reduction.

CI: MRI or cardioversion.

Interactions: Effect of Other Drugs on Rotigotine: *Additive effects*: Other sedating medication, ALCOHOL.

SP: Compulsive disorders, hallucinations (see pramipexole above). Abnormal thinking and behaviour. Visual abnormalities, monitor. External heat should not be applied to the area of the patch. Application site reactions, rotate site daily; patch backing contains aluminium; remove if undergoing MRI or cardioversion (skin burns). Patients with severe cardiovascular disease, ask about symptoms of syncope and pre-syncope.

Pregnancy, Lactation: Pregnancy, not for use; women of childbearing potential to use effective contraception. Lactation, discontinue, may inhibit lactation.

ADR: *Very common*, headache, nausea, application site reactions.

Notes: See 3.5.1 Dopaminergics Used In Parkinson's Disease.

Neupro Transdermal *(UCB)* A. GMS.
Price, (28) 1mg, €94.99. 2mg, €86.73. 3mg, €119.70. 4mg, €111.73. 6mg, €135.95. 8mg, €157.31.
Transdermal patch, rotigotine. Thin matrix-type square with rounded edges containing 3 layers. Marked with name/strength/24-hours. Metabisulphite.

Tetrabenazine

ATC Code: N07XX06. **Sport:** Permitted.
Driving: Drowsiness.
Indications: Control of movement disorders including Huntington's chorea, hemiballismus, senile chorea.

Dose: Adult: Initially 12.5-25mg 3-times daily; titrate in 12.5-25mg increments at 3-4 day intervals to max. 200mg/day or until not tolerated (sedation, Parkinsonism, depression).

Elderly: Parkinson-like reactions could be dose-limiting.

Child: Not recommended.

Renal Impairment: Caution.

Hepatic Impairment: Mild/moderate, initially half dose; up-titrate slower. Severe, caution.

CI: Hypokinetic-rigid-syndrome (Parkinsonism), depression, phaeochromocytoma, prolactin-dependent tumours (pituitary, breast cancer).

Interactions: Effect of Other Drugs on Tetrabenazine: *Co-admin contraindicated*: Reserpine (action blocked), MAOIs (or within 2 weeks of admin). *Co-admin caution*: Drugs prolonging QTc (antipsychotics including chlorpromazine, thioridazine, antibiotics including gatifloxacin, moxifloxacin, Class I and III antiarrhythmics including quinidine, procainamide, amiodarone, sotalol), congenital long QT syndromes, cardiac arrhythmia history, CYP2D6 inhibitors (fluoxetine, paroxetine, terbinafine, moclobemide, quinidine) (consider tetrabenazine dose reduction). *Co-admin not recommended*: TCADs, ALCOHOL, opioids, beta-blockers, antihypertensives, hypnotics, neuroleptics.

Effect of Tetrabenazine on Other Drugs: Levodopa: *Effect altered*.

SP: Rarely NMS (mental changes, rigidity, hyperthermia, autonomic dysfunction, elevated CPK levels); withdraw immediately.

Pregnancy, Lactation: Pregnancy, not recommended. Lactation, contraindicated.

ADR: *Very common*, drowsiness, depression, parkinsonism.

Notes: See 3.5.1 Dopaminergics Used In Parkinson's Disease.

Nitoman 25mg *(Lundbeck)* B. GMS.
Price, (112) €121.02.
Tablet, tetrabenazine. Yellowish (buff) round scored. Marked CL25. Lactose.

3.5.2 - Levodopa

In This Chapter: *Co-Beneldopa, Co-Careldopa, Co-Careldopa/Entacapone combination.*

Class Effects
Driving: See Notes below.

Pharmacology: Levodopa (abbreviated LD), a dopamine precursor, is decarboxylated to form dopamine, which penetrates the blood-brain barrier supplying dopamine directly to the brain. Levodopa is usually combined with a peripheral decarboxylase inhibitor, benserazide or carbidopa (abbreviated CD). This maintains the levodopa dose as low as possible to minimise adverse events.

CI: Narrow-angle glaucoma, severe psychoses, suspicious undiagnosed skin lesions or malignant melanoma, severe endocrine, renal, hepatic or cardiac disorders (HF, arrhythmia, acute stroke). Conditions where adrenergics are contraindicated including phaeochromocytoma, hyperthyroidism, Cushing's syndrome.

Interactions: Effect of Other Drugs on Levodopa Combinations: *Co-admin contraindicated (or within 2 weeks of withdrawal)*: Non-selective MAOIs except selective MAO-B inhibitors (selegiline, rasagiline) and selective MAO-A inhibitors (moclobemide) which are not contraindicated; still may be associated with severe orthostatic hypotension. *Co-admin not recommended*: Dopamine-depleting agents (reserpine, tetrabenazine). *Decreased bioavailability*: Ferrous (sulfate, gluconate) (chelate formation). *Increased bioavailability*: COMT inhibitors (tolcapone, entacapone). *Mutual reduced therapeutic effect*: Dopamine receptor antagonists (phenothiazines, butyrophenones including haloperidol, risperidone, metoclopramide; thioxanthenes (flupentixol, zuclopenthixol), tetrabenazine, reserpine, isoniazid, benzodiazepines, papaverine. *Increase levodopa adverse events*: Amantadine.

Effect of Levodopa Combinations on Other Drugs: Antihypertensives: *Increased hypotensive response*.

SP: Caution, ischaemic heart disease, severe cardiovascular or pulmonary disease, bronchial asthma, renal, hepatic or endocrine disease, history of peptic ulcer, MI with residual atrial, nodal or ventricular arrhythmias, psychiatric disturbances (depression, convulsions). Somnolence, sudden onset sleep episodes (rarely); note (driving). Dyskinesias. Abrupt withdrawal, NMS. Anaesthesia, continue therapy as long as fluids and medication can be taken by mouth. Monitor, hepatic, haemopoietic, renal, cardiovascular function. LD interferes with diagnostic laboratory tests (glucose, ketone bodies, catecholamines in urine; glucose, uric acid in blood). Inhibits response to protirelin in thyroid function tests. False positive Coombe's tests. *Impulse control disorders*, see Notes below. Depression can be part of the clinical picture of Parkinson's disease and RLS; monitor for psychological changes and depression with or without suicidal ideation.

Pregnancy, Lactation: Pregnancy, lactation, not recommended. Women of childbearing potential to ensure adequate contraception.

Notes: See 3.6 Parkinson's Disease, RLS.

Co-Beneldopa (Benserazide, Levodopa)

ATC Code: N04BA02. **Sport:** Permitted.
Driving: Somnolence, sudden sleep episode, impaired alertness.
Indications: Management, Parkinson's Disease. Prolonged/R formulations are used for fluctuations in response to conventional levodopa (LD), alleviation of nocturnal symptoms and early morning akinesia.

Dose: Adult: *Previously levodopa (LD) untreated*, initially 62.5mg (50/12.5) 3 or 4-times daily; advanced disease, 125mg (100/25) 3-times daily; titrate by 125mg once or twice weekly, range 4-8x125mg tabs OR 2-4x250mg caps

3.5.2 Levodopa

daily in divided doses; usually 6x125mg tabs daily; rarely, 10x125mg tabs or 5x250mg caps* daily.
Previous treatment or previously levodopa treated, discontinue levodopa, and commence combination (LD, benserazide) on next day. Initial dose calculated as follows: *Number of levodopa 125mg/benserazide 25mg tabs = Number of 500mg levodopa tabs minus one.* Uptitrate as for previously untreated.
Previous LD + decarboxylase inhibitor combination, 12 hours after discontinuation of previous therapy, initially 62.5mg 3 or 4-times daily. Uptitrate as above. *CAPS, 250mg (200/50) only for maintenance once optimal dose determined. Oral, with or immediately after meals.
Elderly: *Previously levodopa untreated,* initiate with 62.5mg once or twice daily, increasing by 1x 62.5mg tab every 3-4 days.
Child: Under 25 years, not recommended (skeletal development must be complete).
Interactions: Effect of Other Drugs on Co-Beneldopa: *Co-admin caution:* Opioids, drugs interfering with central amine mechanisms (metoclopramide, amphetamines). *Increased absorption:* Metoclopramide. *Increased cardiovascular side effects:* Other sympathomimetics. *Increased bioavailability:* Domperidone.
SP: Monitor, IOP (regularly), cardiac function (initiation, then regularly), blood count (periodically), diabetics. Orthostatic hypotension especially at initiation or dose titration. Madopar may induce dopamine dysregulation syndrome resulting in excessive use of the product. If a general anaesthetic is needed, continue normal regimen as close to surgery as possible; except halothane, discontinue 12-48 hours before surgical intervention (BP fluctuations and/or arrhythmias); emergency surgery, avoid halothane. Caution, osteomalacia, sympathomimetic treatment (bronchial asthma), hypotension (with antihypertensives). Rapid mobilisation, caution injury risk.
ADR: *Unknown frequency,* haemolytic anaemia, leucopenia, thrombocytopenia, decreased appetite, a wide range of psychiatric, CNS and GI disorders, arrhythmias, orthostatic hypotension, altered LFTs, pruritus, rash, RLS, increased blood urea, chromaturia.
Notes: See 3.5.2 Levodopa.

Madopar Caps, Dispersible Tabs *(Roche)* B. GMS.
Price, (100) caps 250mg, €17.83. Disp tabs (100) 62.5mg, €10.37. 125mg, €13.63.
Capsules, levodopa/benserazide HCl 250mg. Opaque light-brown/powder blue. Marked Roche.
Dispersible tablet, as above 50/12.5, 100/25. Round white scored (facilitates breaking). Marked Roche/strength.

Co-Careldopa (Carbidopa, Levodopa)

ATC Code: N04BA02. **Sport:** Permitted.
Driving: Major influence; dizziness, orthostatic hypotension, somnolence, sudden sleep episode.
Indications: Treatment Parkinson's disease. Advanced levodopa-responsive disease with severe motor fluctuations and hyper-/dyskinesia (unsatisfactory result with available combinations) *(Duodopa).*
Dose: Adult: STANDARD/R *Sinemet,* best initiated with 1 tab of *Sinemet Plus* (*CD25mg/LD100mg) 3-times daily (provides CD75mg/day); increase by 1 tab daily or every other day as needed or until a dose equiv. to 8 tabs/day of *Sinemet Plus* is reached. Can use *Sinemet* 12.5mg/50mg or 10mg/100mg for dose titration, initiating with 1 tab 3 or 4 times a day; this may not provide optimal carbidopa (provide at least CD70-100mg/day for optimal inhibition of extra-cerebral LD decarboxylation). Max. CD/LD 200mg/2g per day (about CD3mg/kg, LD30mg/kg) in a 70kg patient.
Switch from previous combinations (LD/decarboxylase inhibitor), discontinue LD 12 hours (24 hours for slow-release) before starting *Sinemet* at a dose providing the same amount of LD.
PROLONGED/R, *Sinemet* CR (50mg/200mg), Half CR (25mg/100mg), oral tabs to be taken whole to maintain Prolonged/R properties; do not crush, chew or halve. Contain CD/LD in 1:4 ratio. *Current combinations* (LD/decarboxylase inhibitor), substitute initially at amount providing max. 10% more LD/day when dose is above 900mg/day; prolong dosing interval by 30-50% ranging from 4-12 hours; dose providing up to 30% more LD may be needed (Half CR is used to facilitate 100mg titration steps). LD must be discontinued at least 8 hours before commencing *Sinemet* CR. Mild/moderate disease, initially one CR tab twice daily. *Not* LD-treated, mild/moderate disease, initially one CR tab twice daily. Initially max. LD600mg/day minimum 6-hourly.
Duodopa, continuous intestinal admin. Morning dose (bolus admin by pump), LD100-200mg (5-10mL); max. LD300mg (15mL). Continuous maintenance dose, adjust in 2mg/hour (0.1mL/hour) steps. *CD (carbidopa); LD (levodopa); tab strength quoted as CD/LD.
Child: Under 18 years, not recommended *(Sinemet).* No relevant indication *(Duodopa).*
Renal Impairment: Severe, titrate dose with caution.
Hepatic Impairment: As for Renal above.
Interactions: Effect of Other Drugs on Co-Careldopa: *Loss of Antiparkinsonian effect:* Phenothiazine, butyrophenones (haloperidol). *Hypertension, dyskinesia:* TCADs. *Levodopa effect reversed:* Phenytoin, papaverine. *Severe orthostatic hypotension risk:* Selegiline. *Absorption impaired:* High protein diets.
SP: Drug-induced extrapyramidal reactions, not recommended. Mental changes, depression with suicidal tendencies, other serious antisocial behaviour, monitor. Current psychosis, history of convulsions, caution. *Intestinal admin,* precautions, see manufacturers Full Prescribing Information. Complications include bezoar, ileus, implant site erosion/ulcer, intestinal (haemorrhage, ischaemia, obstruction, perforation), intussusception, pancreatitis, peritonitis, pneumoperitoneum, wound infection.
ADR: Summary, *most common,* dyskinesias including choreiform, dystonic, other involuntary movements, nausea. Muscle twitching and blepharospasm (early signs to consider dosage reduction); *frequent,* hallucinations, confusion, dizziness, chorea, dry mouth.
Notes: See 3.5.2 Levodopa.

Sinemet, Plus, CR, Half CR *(MSD)* B. GMS.
Price, (90) 12.5/50mg, €9.29. (100) 10/100mg, €8.63; 25/250mg, €18.91; Plus 25/100mg, €12.56. (60) CR 50/200mg, €15.41; CR/Half 25/100mg, €9.66.
Standard/R tablet, carbidopa (mg)/levodopa (mg) 12.5/50, 10/100, Plus 25/100, 25/250mg. Round (except 12.5/50). 12.5/50: Yellow oval scored (facilitates breaking). Marked 520. 10/100: Light blue. Marked 647. Plus 25/100: Yellow. Marked 650. 25/250: Light blue. Marked 654.
Prolonged/R tablet (CR, Half CR), as above 50/200, 25/100. 50/200 (CR): Peach scored*. Marked 521. 25/100 (Half CR): Pink. Marked 601. Oval scored*. *(not intended to facilitate breaking).
Duodopa Intestinal Gel *(AbbVie)* B. HOS.
Price, (7) €724.58 (PTW).
Intestinal gel, levodopa, carbidopa monohydrate (mg) 20/5 per mL. White (slightly yellow). **Store:** Refrigerate.

Co-Careldopa (carbidopa, levodopa), Entacapone

ATC Code: N04BA03. **Sport:** Permitted.
Driving: Dizziness, symptomatic orthostatism, somnolence, sudden sleep episode.
Indications: Treatment, Parkinson's disease and 'end-of-dose' motor fluctuations not stabilised on levodopa/dopa decarboxylase (DDC) inhibitor treatment.
Dose: Adult, Elderly: *Transfer from Standard/R LD/DDC inhibitor (carbidopa or benserazide) + entacapone,* directly in equal doses; if individual component doses are not equal to fixed combination, initiate with closest LEVODOPA daily dose. If treatment is with LD/benserazide combination, discontinue night before starting fixed combination, initially with dose providing the same amount of LEVODOPA or slightly more (5-10%).
Transfer, no current entacapone treatment, corresponding doses to current treatment. Dyskinesias or dose above LD 800mg/day, recommend entacapone introduced separately before switch to fixed combination. Oral, whole with/without food; max. entacapone 2000mg/day.
Child: Under 18 years, not recommended.

126

Renal Impairment: Severe/dialysis, caution.

Hepatic Impairment: Mild/moderate, caution, consider dose reduction. Severe, not recommended.

Interactions: Effect of Other Drugs on Levodopa, Carbidopa, Entacapone Combination: *Co-admin not recommended*: Non-selective monoamine oxidase (MAO-A, MAO-B) inhibitors (phenelzine, tranylcypromine), selective MAO-A, MAO-B inhibitors. *Co-admin caution*: TCADs, noradrenaline reuptake inhibitors (desipramine, maprotiline, venlafaxine), COMT metabolised drugs (paroxetine).

Effect of Levodopa, Carbidopa, Entacapone Combination on Other Drugs: Selegiline: *Co-admin (max. dose 10mg)*. Warfarin: *Monitor*.

SP: Dyskinesias, rhabdomyolysis, NMS. Progressive anorexia, asthenia, weight loss, evaluate (general medical, LFTs). Prolonged or persistent diarrhoea with entacapone, may be sign of colitis, discontinue.

ADR: Summary, *most frequent*, dyskinesias, GI symptoms (nausea, diarrhoea), pain (muscle, musculoskeletal, connective tissue), chromaturia; *serious*, GI haemorrhage (uncommon), angioedema (rare).

Notes: See 3.5.2 Levodopa. See Co-Careldopa above. See 3.5.4 COMT Inhibitors (entacapone).

Stalevo Tablets *(Orion)* B. GMS.
Price, (100) all strengths, €77.87.
Tablet, levodopa/carbidopa/entacapone, 50/12.5, 75/18.75, 100/25, 125/31.25, 175/43.75, 200/50 all with entacapone 200mg. Brownish/greyish-red f/c. Marked LCE and **levodopa** strength. 50/12.5/200: Round. 150/37.5/200: Elongated elliptical. Other strengths: Oval. *Sucrose*.

Sastravi Tablets *(TEVA)* B. GMS.
Price, (100) 50/12.5/200, €44.14; all other strengths, €44.50.
Tablet, levodopa/carbidopa/entacapone, 50/12.5/200, 75/18.5/200, 100/25/200, 125/31.25/200, 175/43.75/200, 200/50/200. Brownish-red oval f/c. Marked LEC and **levodopa** strength. Soya lecithin. **Store:** Below 30 deg C.

3.5.3 - Selective MAOIs

In This Chapter: *Rasagiline, selegiline.*

Class Effects

Driving: See Notes below.

CI: Children under 18 years, not recommended.

Interactions: Effect of Other Drugs on selective MAOIs: *Co-admin not recommended, severe hypotension risk*: Non-selective MAOIs, pethidine. *Serious reactions*, co-admin not recommended*: Fluoxetine, fluvoxamine (commence selegiline minimum 5 weeks after discontinuation), other SSRIs (sertraline, paroxetine), SNRIs (venlafaxine). *Hypertensive reaction*: Other sympathomimetics (nasal and oral decongestants or cold medications containing ephedrine or pseudoephedrine). *Severe CNS toxicity, caution*: TCADs, amitriptyline, protriptyline. *(diaphoresis, flushing, ataxia, tremor, hyperthermia, hyper/hypotension, seizures, palpitation, dizziness, mental changes including agitation, confusion, hallucinations progressing to delirium and coma).

SP: Impulse control disorders, see Notes below.

Pregnancy, Lactation: Not recommended.

Notes: See 3.6 Parkinson's Disease, RLS (driving, impulse control disorders). See 3.3.2 MAOIs.

Rasagiline

ATC Code: N04BD02. **Sport:** Permitted.
Driving: Caution until effect known.

Indications: Treatment, idiopathic Parkinson's disease as monotherapy (without levodopa) or adjunctive (with levodopa) in patients with 'end of dose' fluctuations.

Dose: Adult, Elderly: Initially 1mg once daily with or without levodopa. *Admin*, oral, with or without food; can be used safely without dietary tyramine restrictions.

Child: Not recommended; lack of safety/efficacy data.

Renal Impairment: No dose adjustment.

Hepatic Impairment: Mild, caution (initiation). Moderate, avoid. Severe, contraindicated. Progression from mild to moderate hepatic impairment, discontinue.

Interactions: Effect of Other Drugs on Rasagiline: *Co-admin contraindicated*: Other MAOIs, St John's Wort, pethidine (allow 14-day interval). *Co-admin not recommended*: Dextromethorphan. *Co-admin avoid*: Fluoxetine, fluvoxamine (minimum 5-week interval between stopping fluoxetine and starting rasagiline; minimum 14 days between stopping rasagiline and starting fluoxetine or fluvoxamine). *Plasma levels increased*: Ciprofloxacin. *Plasma levels decreased*: Cigarette smoking. *Increased oral clearance*: Entacapone.

Effect of Rasagiline on Other Drugs: Levodopa (consider dose reduction): *Effect potentiated*.

SP: Hypotensive effects (levodopa co-admin). Skin lesion, specialist evaluation (melanoma risk).

Pregnancy, Lactation: Caution.

ADR: *Common*, hallucinations, neck pain, vertigo/balance disorder. Monotherapy, *very common*, headache. Adjunctive, *very common*, dyskinesia.

Notes: See 3.5.3 Selective MAOIs. See 3.5.2 Levodopa.

Azilect 1mg *(TEVA)* B. GMS.
Price, (28) €93.87.
Tablet, rasagiline mesilate. White (off-white) round flat. Marked GIL and 1. *Mannitol*.

Rasagiline Accord 1mg *(Accord)* B. GMS.
Price, (28) €37.55.
Tablet, rasagiline tartrate. White (off-white) round.

Rasagiline Clonmel 1mg *(Clonmel)* B. GMS.
Price, (30) €37.55.
Tablet, rasagiline tartrate. White (off-white) oblong. Marked R9SE; 1 on reverse.

Rasagiline HCS 1mg *(Krka)* B. GMS.
Price, (30) €37.55.
Tablet, rasagiline tartrate. White (almost) round; darker spots visible.

Rasagiline Mylan 1mg *(Gerard)* B. GMS.
Price, (30) €37.55.
Tablet, rasagiline tartrate. White round.

Rasagiline Rowex 1mg *(Rowex)* B. GMS.
Price, (30) €40.23.
Tablet, rasagiline tartrate. White (off-white) round.

Selegiline

ATC Code: N04BD01. **Sport:** Prohibited (in-competition).
Driving: Dizziness.

Indications: Treatment, Parkinson's disease, or symptomatic parkinsonism where disease is not controlled by conventional therapy or where 'on-off' symptoms develop at max. levodopa dose.

Dose: Adult, Elderly: 5-10mg daily, alone or adjunctive. Single dose in morning OR divided taken at breakfast and lunch. Adjunctive, reduce levodopa dose by average 30%.

Renal Impairment: Severe, caution.

Hepatic Impairment: As for Renal above.

CI: Active duodenal or gastric ulcer. Take into account contraindications for levodopa when co-prescribed.

Interactions: Effect of Other Drugs on Selegiline: *Co-admin contraindicated*: Sympathomimetics, pethidine, SSRIs, SNRIs. *Caution*: General anaesthesia, dopamine. *Avoid*: ALCOHOL. *Tyramine hypersensitivity risk, dietary restrictions*: MAO-A inhibitors (moclobemide). *CNS and cardiovascular disorders with co-admin*: MAOIs. *Increased bioavailability*: Oral contraceptives (gestodene/ethinyl oestradiol or levonorgestrel/ethinyl oestradiol).

SP: Caution, labile hypertension, arrhythmias, severe angina pectoris, severe liver of kidney dysfunction, peptic or duodenal ulcer, psychosis. At higher doses than recommended (10mg), selegiline may lose its MAO-B selectivity and hypertension risk rises. Selegiline potentiates effect of levodopa; addition of selegiline to levodopa may cause involuntary movements and/or agitation. Consider levodopa dose reduction to about 30% when in combination with selegiline.

ADR: *Common*, sleeping disorders, confusion, hallucinations, abnormal movements (dyskinesias), vertigo, dizziness, headache, bradycardia, nausea, transient ALAT rise, mild increase in liver enzymes.

Notes: See 3.5.3 Selective MAOIs, 3.5.2 Levodopa.

Eldepryl 5mg *(Orion)* B. GMS.
Price, (100) €37.35.
Tablet, selegiline HCl. White (almost) round u/c scored. *Mannitol*.

3.5.4 Reversible COMT Inhibitors

3.5.4 - Reversible COMT Inhibitors

In This Chapter: *Entacapone, tolcapone.*

Class Effects

Driving: See Notes below.

CI: Children under 18 years. Liver impairment, phaeochromocytoma, NMS and/or non-traumatic rhabdomyolysis.

Interactions: Effect of Other Drugs on COMT Inhibitors: *Co-admin not recommended:* Non-selective monoamine oxidase (MAO-A and MAO-B) inhibitors (phenelzine, tranylcypromine), selective MAO-A inhibitors plus a selective MAO-B inhibitor and entacapone. *Co-admin caution:* MAO-A inhibitors, TCADs, noradrenaline reuptake inhibitors (desipramine, maprotiline, venlafaxine), drugs metabolised by COMT (rimiterole, isoprenaline, adrenaline, noradrenaline, dopamine, dobutamine, alphamethyldopa, apomorphine, paroxetine), selegiline (max. dose 10mg). *Decreased bioavailability:* Iron (iron preparations should be taken 2-3 hours apart).

Effect of COMT Inhibitors on Other Drugs: Warfarin: *Monitor.*

SP: Rhabdomyolysis secondary to severe dyskinesias, NMS; always adjunctive to levodopa. Increased levodopa bioavailability, increased dopaminergic side effects, adjust levodopa dose. Orthostatic hypotension. Dyskinesias. Somnolence, episodes of sudden sleep onset. Diarrhoea, progressive anorexia, asthenia, excessive weight decrease (over short time), evaluate liver function. Impulse control disorders, see Notes below.

Pregnancy, Lactation: Not recommended.

ADR: Insomnia, hallucinations, confusion, paroniria; agitation, dyskinesias, aggravated parkinsonism, dizziness, dystonia, hyperkinesia, nausea, diarrhoea, abdominal pain, dry mouth, constipation, vomiting; anorexia, altered LFTs, erythematous or maculopapular rash, urine discolouration, fatigue, sweating, injury (falls).

Notes: See 3.6 Parkinson's Disease, RLS.

Entacapone

ATC Code: N04BX02. **Sport:** Permitted.
Driving: Dizziness, orthostatism, somnolence, sudden sleep episode.

Indications: Adjunctive, to levodopa/decarboxylase inhibitor combinations in Parkinson's disease with end-of-dose motor fluctuations.

Dose: Adult, Elderly: Initially 200mg with each levodopa/decarboxylase dose; max. 2g entacapone daily. *Admin,* oral, with or without food.

Renal Impairment: Dialysis, longer dosing interval.

SP: Ischaemic heart disease, caution. Prolonged or persistent diarrhoea may be sign of colitis, discontinue. Urine may be discoloured reddish-brown.

ADR: Summary, *most frequent,* dopaminergic effects, GI (nausea, vomiting, abdominal pain, constipation, diarrhoea).

Notes: See 3.5.4 Reversible COMT Inhibitors.

Comtess 200mg *(Orion)* B. GMS.
Price, (100) €82.04.
Tablet, entacapone. Brownish-orange oval f/c. Marked COMT. *Soya lecithin.* **Store:** No special conditions.
Entacapone Niche 200mg *(Niche)* B. GMS.
Price, (100) €32.81.
Tablet, entacapone. Brown cap-shaped f/c. Marked 70. *Lactose.*
Store: No special conditions.

Tolcapone

ATC Code: N04BX01. **Sport:** Permitted.
Driving: Somnolence, sudden sleep episode (with levodopa).

Indications: Adjunctive, to levodopa/decarboxylase inhibitor combinations in Parkinson's disease with end-of-dose motor fluctuations. Use tolcapone second-line adjunctive (due to hepatotoxicity).

Dose: Adult, Elderly: 100mg 3-times daily. Admin first dose with first levodopa dose; then subsequent doses 6-12 hours later. Max. 200mg 3-times. *Admin,* swallow whole (bitter taste) with or without food.

Child: No relevant indication; not recommended.

Renal Impairment: CrCl (mL/min) 30 and above, no adjustment; below 30, caution.

Hepatic Impairment: Contraindicated (liver disease, increased liver enzymes).

CI: Severe dyskinesia, neuroleptic malignant syndrome

SP: Potentially fatal acute liver injury risk; liver injury most often 1-6 months after initiation; females at higher risk. Do not initiate if LFTs abnormal. Monitor liver function every 2 weeks (year 1), then every 4 weeks (next 6 months), then 8-weekly. ALT and/or AST above ULN, or signs/symptoms of hepatic failure, discontinue immediately; may be at increased risk if re-introduced.

Pregnancy, Lactation: Pregnancy, if benefit outweighs risk. Lactation, not recommended.

ADR: See Notes below.

Notes: See 3.5.4 Reversible COMT Inhibitors.

Tasmar 100mg *(Meda)* B. GMS.
Price, (100) €125.45.
Tablet, tolcapone. Light-yellow hexagonal f/c. Marked Tasmar/strength. *Lactose.* **Store:** No special conditions.

3.5.5 - Antimuscarinics

In This Chapter: *Biperiden, procyclidine.*

Class Effects

Driving: See Notes below.

SP: Introduce and withdraw gradually. Impulse control disorders, see Notes below.

Pregnancy, Lactation: If benefit outweighs risk. Lactation, no data.

Notes: See 3.6 Parkinson's Disease, RLS.

Biperiden

ATC Code: N04AA02. **Sport:** Permitted.
Driving: Drowsiness.

Indications: Management, Parkinsonian syndromes to counteract muscular rigidity and tremor, drug-induced extrapyramidal symptoms (early dyskinesia, akathisia, parkinsonism).

Dose: Adult: *Parkinson's Disease, normal release,* initially 1mg twice daily; titrate by 2mg/day to max. 16mg/day; *retard,* 4-8mg, max. 12mg daily. Admin in divided doses with first dose in the morning.

Drug-induced movement disorders, normal release, 1-4mg 1-4 times daily. Oral, in divided doses throughout the day; *retard* tabs to be taken whole with some liquid with or without meals.

Elderly: Caution, especially with organic brain disease.

Child: *Drug-induced movement disorders, normal release,* 3-15 years, 1-2mg 1-3 times daily.

CI: Untreated narrow-angle glaucoma, mechanical GI tract stenoses, paralytic ileus, megacolon, prostatic adenoma, diseases predisposing to tachycardia.

Interactions: Effect of Other Drugs on Biperiden: *Co-admin not recommended:* ALCOHOL. *CNS and peripheral side effects potentiated:* Anticholinergic psychotropic drugs, antihistamines, antiparkinsonian drugs, antispasmodics. *Anticholinergic effect potentiated (especially AV conduction):* Quinidine. *Dyskinesia potentiated:* Levodopa. *Generalised choriec movements:* Co-careldopa.

Effect of Biperiden on Other Drugs: Neuroleptics: Induced tardive dyskinesia intensified. Metoclopramide: *Effect attenuated.*

SP: Thyrotoxicosis, cardiac failure, tachycardia, prostatic adenoma, increased tendency to convulsions.

ADR: Side effects occur particularly at beginning of treatment and if dose is increased too quickly. Only rare, very rare side effects reported.

Notes: See 3.5.5 Antimuscarinics.

Akineton 2mg, Retard 4mg *(Lab Farma)* B. GMS.
Price, (100) 2mg, €5.92. Retard 4mg, €11.10.
Tablet, biperiden HCl. Round biplanar white scored. *Lactose.*
Prolonged/R tablet, as above. Oblong yellowish scored. *Lactose.*

Procyclidine

ATC Code: N04AA04. **Sport:** Permitted.
Driving: Blurred vision, dizziness, confusion, disorientation.
Indications: Parkinson's disease, idiopathic (paralysis agitans), postencephalitic, arteriosclerotic. Symptoms responding well include rigidity, akinesia, tremor, speech and writing difficulties, gait, sialorrhoea and drooling, sweating, oculogyric crises, depressed mood. Control of extra-pyramidal symptoms induced by neuroleptics including pseudo-Parkinsonism, acute dystonic reactions, akathisia.

Dose: Adult: *Parkinson's disease,* initially 2.5mg 3-times daily*; titrate by 2.5mg/day to optimum; max. 30mg/day; up to 60mg/day has been used. Addition of a fourth dose before retiring has beneficial in some patients. May be combined with levodopa or amantadine if not controlled on monotherapy.
Neuroleptic-induced extrapyramidal effects, initiate and titrate as for Parkinson's disease; usually max. 20mg/day. *Admin,* with food (better tolerated). *(mean plasma elimination half-life sufficient to allow twice daily dosing if more convenient).

Elderly: May be more susceptible to anticholinergic effects; reduced dose may be required; especially those vulnerable to CNS disturbances (confusion, impaired cognitive function and memory, disorientation, hallucinations).

Child: Safety/efficacy not established.

Renal Impairment: Exercise care.

Hepatic Impairment: As for Renal above.

CI: Tardive dyskinesia.

Interactions: Effect of Other Drugs on Procyclidine: *Increased anticholinergic effects:* Amantadine, antihistamines, phenothiazines, butyrophenones (haloperidol), antidepressants, MAOIs. *Effect reduced:* Tacrine. *Hyperpyrexia:* Phenothiazine + high environmental temperature and humidity. *Plasma levels increased:* Paroxetine.

Effect of Procyclidine on Other Drugs: Ketoconazole: *Absorption reduced.* Levodopa: *Efficacy reduced (increased gastric emptying time; enhanced gastric degradation). Quinidine:* Vagolytic effects potentiated.

SP: Caution, elderly, patients with glaucoma predisposition, existing narrow-angle glaucoma, GI obstruction (pyloric stenosis, paralytic ileus), prostatic hypertrophy, tachycardia (thyrotoxicosis), tardive dyskinesia. Potential for abuse. Hyperpyrexia. Introduce dose gradually; avoid sudden withdrawal. Patients with mental disorders may experience precipitation of a psychotic episode when procyclidine is used to treat the extrapyramidal side effects of neuroleptics.

Pregnancy, Lactation: If benefit outweighs risk.

ADR: *Common,* blurred vision, dry mouth, constipation, urinary retention. Dizziness, mental confusion impaired cognition and memory, disorientation, anxiety, agitation, hallucinations at high doses.

Notes: See 3.5.5 Antimuscarinics.

> **Kemadrin 5mg** *(Aspen)* B. GMS.
> *Price,* (100) €7.29.
> *Tablet,* procyclidine HCl. White round scored (divisible into equal halves). Marked KT and 05. *Lactose, sodium 0.5mg.*

3.6 - Multiple Sclerosis, Motor Neurone Disease

3.6.1 - Multiple Sclerosis (MS)

In This Chapter: *Alemtuzumab, dimethyl fumarate, fampridine, fingolimod, glatiramer, interferon (beta-1a, beta-1b), natalizumab, peginterferon beta-1a, teriflunomide.*

Class Effects

CI: Hypersensitivity to any member of the class. Children, not recommended unless otherwise specified.

SP: Increased infection risk (including opportunistic) with all immunosuppressants; inform patients to report infection symptoms. May be increased risk of progressive multifocal leukoencephalopathy (PML) (opportunistic infection caused by the JC virus; fatal or severe disability). *Interferon-beta,* nephrotic syndrome with different underlying nephropathies reported; monitor for signs/symptoms (oedema, proteinuria, impaired renal function). Thrombotic microangiopathy, manifested as thrombotic thrombocytopenic purpura (TTP) or haemolytic uraemic syndrome (HUS), (including fatal). Elevated hepatic transaminases, hepatitis, autoimmune hepatitis, severe hepatic failure, serious hypersensitivity reactions, injection-site reactions (necrosis; rotate site), decreased peripheral blood counts. Laboratory abnormalities associated with interferons, monitor (blood counts and chemistry, LFTs, thyroid function). PAH (various time points; up to several years after starting treatment).

Notes: See manufacturers Full Prescribing Information.

Alemtuzumab

ATC Code: L04AA34. **Sport:** Permitted.
Driving: Dizziness.
Indications: Relapsing remitting MS (adults with active disease).

Dose: Adult, Elderly: Initial course, 12mg/day by IV infusion on 5 consecutive days (total 60mg). Second, 12mg/day on 3 consecutive days (total 36mg) admin 12 months after initial course. Dilute for infusion over approx. 4 hours. Pre-treatment, see SP below. *Elderly,* over 55 years, no data.

Child: Under 10 years, no relevant use; 10-18 years, no safety/efficacy data.

Renal Impairment: No data.

Hepatic Impairment: As for Renal above.

CI: HIV infection.

SP: *Pre-treat* with corticosteroids prior to admin on each of days 1-3 (any treatment course) + antihistamines + antipyretics; start oral prophylaxis for herpes infection on day 1 (each treatment course) continuing for 1 month after treatment. Hypersensitivity and/or anaphylactic reactions; resuscitation facilities to be available. Supply patients with Patient Alert Card and Patient Guide. Not for use in inactive disease. Formation of antibodies and increased risk of autoimmune-mediated conditions (immune thrombocytopenic purpura, thyroid disorders, nephropathies). Conduct complete blood counts, serum creatinine, thyroid function prior to initiation, then monthly for 48 months after last infusion (thyroid function every 3 months). Infusion-associated reactions (IARs) mainly due to cytokine release. Caution, initiation with pre-existing and/or on-going malignancy. Vaccination, laboratory monitoring, see manufacturers Full Prescribing Information.

Pregnancy, Lactation: Pregnancy, if benefit outweighs risk. Thyroid disease a special risk; untreated hypothyroidism increases risk for miscarriage and foetal effects (mental retardation, dwarfism). Women of childbearing potential to ensure adequate contraception*. Stop breastfeeding*. *(during and for 4 months following last infusion).

ADR: *Very common,* upper RTI, UTI, lymphopenia, leucopenia, headache, flushing, nausea, urticaria, rash, pruritus, pyrexia, fatigue.

Notes: See 3.6.1 Multiple Sclerosis (MS).

> ▼ **Lemtrada Parenteral 12mg** *(Genzyme)* A.
> *Price,* (1) €7504.00 (PTW).
> *Infusion,* alemtuzumab 10mg/mL. Clear colourless (slightly-yellow) conc for soln. Produced by rDNA technology. **Store:** Refrigerate; do not freeze.

Dimethyl Fumarate

ATC Code: N07XX09. **Sport:** Pending.
Driving: No data available.
Indications: Treatment, relapsing remitting MS.

Dose: Adult, Elderly: Initially 120mg twice daily; increase after 7 days to 240mg twice daily. Temporary reduction to 120mg twice daily may reduce flushing, GI adverse events; resume 240mg twice daily within 1 month. *Admin,* with food (improved) tolerability; do not crush, divide, dissolve, suck or chew capsule or contents (microtablet enteric-coating prevents gut irritation).

3.6.1   Multiple Sclerosis (MS)

Child: Age 10-18 years, safety/efficacy not established; under 10 years, no relevant use.

Renal Impairment: Severe, caution.

Hepatic Impairment: Severe, caution.

Interactions: Effect of Other Drugs on Dimethyl Fumarate: Co-admin (only exceptional cases): Live vaccines. Avoid co-admin: Other fumaric acid derivatives. Increased potential renal adverse events: Nephrotoxic agents (aminoglycosides, diuretics, NSAIDs, lithium). Increased GI adverse events: Undiluted strong alcoholic drinks (large quantities).

SP: Decreased lymphocytes; caution with low lymphocyte counts. Monitor, complete blood count, renal and hepatic function, baseline MRI (before initiation; as part of PML vigilance); blood counts after 6 months, renal and hepatic function after 3 and 6 months; then all parameters every 6-12 months. Caution, active GI disease. Flushing, may be severe (hypersensitivity or anaphylactoid reaction). Serious infection, consider suspending treatment; advise patients to report symptoms; PML reported (with severe and prolonged lymphopenia), see Notes below.

Pregnancy, Lactation: Pregnancy and women of childbearing potential not using contraception, not recommended; use only if clearly needed and benefit outweighs risk. Interaction with oral contraceptives not demonstrated; consider non-hormonal contraception. Lactation, stop breastfeeding or stop drug.

ADR: Summary, most common, flushing, GI events (diarrhoea, nausea, abdominal pain).

Notes: See 3.6.1 Multiple Sclerosis (MS).

▼ **Tecfidera 120mg, 240mg** (Biogen Idec) A. HT.
Price, (14) 120mg, €227.03; (56) 240mg, €1197.15.
Gastro-resistant capsule, dimethyl fumarate. Marked BG-12 and strength. 120mg: Green/white. 240mg: Green.

Fampridine

ATC Code: N07XX07. **Sport:** Pending.
Driving: Moderate influence; dizziness.

Indications: Improvement of walking, adults with MS with walking disability (EDSS 4-7).

Dose: Adult: 10mg twice daily (12 hours apart; morning and evening). Admin, with food; swallow whole; do not divide, crush, dissolve, suck or chew; do not admin more frequently or at higher dose. Prescribe initially for 2 weeks as clinical benefit usually identified within 2 weeks; no benefit, discontinue.

Elderly: Assess renal function before initiation; monitor.

Child: Under 18 years, no safety/efficacy data.

Renal Impairment: CrCl (mL/min) below 80, contraindicated. Monitor all patients, see Elderly above. Estimate CrCl using the Cockcroft-Gault formula.

CI: Seizure (current, prior history).

Interactions: Effect of Other Drugs on Fampridine: Co-admin contraindicated: Other fampridine-containing medicinals (4-aminopyridine), OCT2 inhibitors (cimetidine). Co-admin caution: OCT2 substrates (carvedilol, propranolol, metformin).

SP: Increases seizure risk; caution with factors lowering seizure threshold; if seizure experienced, discontinue. Hypersensitivity reactions (usually during first week); anaphylactic or other serious allergic reactions, discontinue; do not restart. Caution, cardiovascular symptoms (conduction disorders), increased (incidence of dizziness, balance disorder, risk of falls). Increased infection rate (cannot exclude impaired immune function).

Pregnancy, Lactation: Pregnancy, avoid. Lactation, not recommended.

ADR: Mostly, neurological (seizure, insomnia, anxiety, balance disorder, dizziness, paraesthesia, tremor, headache, asthenia); highest incidence, UTI.

Notes: See 3.6.1 Multiple Sclerosis (MS).

▼ **Fampyra 10mg** (Biogen Idec) A. GMS.
Price, (56), €157.85.
Prolonged/R tablet, fampridine. Off-white f/c oval. Marked A10.
NOTE: Only reimbursed if (consultant initiated, patients satisfy responder protocol).

Fingolimod

ATC Code: L04AA27. **Sport:** Permitted.
Driving: No or negligible effect; dizziness, drowsiness (initiation); observe for 6 hours (bradyarrhythmia).

Indications: Single disease modifying therapy in: Highly active relapsing remitting MS despite DMARD treatment; rapidly evolving severe relapsing remitting MS.

Dose: Adult, Elderly: 0.5mg/day with first-dose monitoring. Admin, oral, once daily with or without food. Switch, directly from beta interferon or glatiramer if no treatment-related abnormalities (cytopenia); directly from natalizumab, caution (natalizumab long half-life). Elderly, over 65 years, caution.

Child: Not recommended.

Hepatic Impairment: Mild/moderate, caution. Severe, contraindicated.

CI: Opportunistic infection risk (immunocompromised), severe active infection (hepatitis, TB), malignancy.

Interactions: Effect of Other Drugs on Fingolimod: Co-admin not recommended (only if benefit outweighs risk): Antiarrhythmics Class Ia (quinidine, disopyramide), Class III (amiodarone, sotalol), beta-blockers, other substances decreasing heart rate (verapamil, diltiazem, ivabradine, digoxin, anticholinesteratic agents, pilocarpine) (additive effect on heart rate); other antineoplastic, immunosuppressive or immune-modulation therapy (additive immune system effects), St John's Wort. Co-admin caution: Switch from long-acting therapies (natalizumab, teriflunomide, mitoxantrone), CYP3A4 inhibitors (protease inhibitors, azole antifungals, macrolides e.g. clarithromycin, telithromycin), CYP3A4 inducers (rifampicin, phenobarbital, phenytoin, efavirenz). Co-admin avoid: Medicinals prolonging QTc interval, live attenuated vaccines.

SP: Use not recommended, AV block, sick-sinus syndrome, sino-atrial heart block, significant QT prolongation, symptomatic bradycardia, syncope, ischaemic heart disease, cerebrovascular disease, MI (history), CHF, cardiac arrest, uncontrolled hypertension, severe sleep apnoea. Bradyarrhythmia, observe for 6 hours for bradycardia signs/symptoms. Measure (all patients) ECG, BP before and 6 hours after first dose. T-wave inversion reported. Before initiation, complete blood counts (then periodically); antibody testing for VZV (full course vaccination with varicella vaccine recommended for antibody-negative patients), recent (within last 6 months) transaminases, bilirubin levels to be available. Severe active infection, e.g. viral hepatitis, delay initiation. Discontinuation, elimination may take up to 2 months. Skin evaluation (initiation, yearly), basal cell carcinoma reported. Baseline MRI to be available (within 3 months) as reference; lesions suggestive of PML present, if PML suspected, suspend until PML excluded; PML can occur in the presence of a JCV infection. Macular oedema, with or without visual symptoms, increased risk in diabetics (regular ophthalmological examinations); if develops discontinue. Elevated liver transaminases (monitor at months 1, 3, 6, 9 and 12); significant liver injury, discontinue. Caution, severe respiratory disease, pulmonary fibrosis, COPD. Treatment of relapses with short-course corticosteroids not associated with increased infection rate. Cryptococcal meningitis reported.

Pregnancy, Lactation: Pregnancy, exclude before initiation. Women of childbearing potential to ensure adequate contraception during and for up to 2 months after discontinuation (serious risk to foetus; counsel patient). Lactation, not recommended.

ADR: Summary, most frequent, influenza, sinusitis, headache, diarrhoea, back pain, increased hepatic enzymes, cough; most serious, infection, macular oedema, transient AV block (at initiation).

Notes: See 3.6.1 Multiple Sclerosis (MS).

▼ **GILENYA 0.5mg** (Novartis) A. HT.
Price, (28) €1764.65.
Capsule, fingolimod HCl. Opaque hard bright yellow/white. Marked FTY 0.5mg with 2 radial bands. Mannitol. **Store:** Below 25 deg C; original pack to protect (moisture).

Glatiramer

ATC Code: L03AX13. **Sport:** Permitted.
Driving: Unlikely to impair.
Indications: Treatment, relapsing forms of MS (primary or secondary progressive MS, not indicated).
Dose: Adult, Elderly: Initially 20mg once daily. *Admin*, SC injection at a different site each day (abdomen, arms, hips, thighs).
Child: Age 12-18 years, as for Adult above. Under 12 years, not recommended.
Renal Impairment: Monitor.
Interactions: Effect of Other Drugs on Glatiramer: *Co-admin, monitor*: Protein-bound substances.
SP: Not for IV or IM admin. Warn patient of Post-Injection Reaction. Admin under neurologist supervision. Pre-existing cardiac disorders.
Pregnancy, Lactation: Not recommended. Lactation, if benefit outweighs risk. Advise adequate contraception.
ADR: *Very common*, infection, influenza, anxiety, depression, headache, vasodilatation, dyspnoea, nausea, rash, arthralgia, back pain, asthenia, chest pain, injection-site reactions (majority of patients), pain.
Notes: See 3.6.1 Multiple Sclerosis (MS).

Copaxone Parenteral 20mg, 40mg *(TEVA)* A. HT.
Price, (PFS) 20mg/mL (28), 40mg/mL (12), €916.33.
Injection, glatiramer acetate 20(40)mg/mL. Clear soln (PFS).
Store: Refrigerate; do not freeze.

Interferon, Peginterferon Beta-1a

ATC Code: L03AB07. **Sport:** Permitted.
Driving: CNS-related (dizziness).
Indications: Treatment, relapsing remitting MS *(all brands)*; single demyelinating event and at high risk of developing MS *(Avonex, Rebif)*.
Dose: Adult, Elderly: *Avonex*, initiate with quarter-dose increments per week to 30mcg/week (week 4) OR initiate with half-dose increments. Recommend 30mcg once weekly. *Admin*, IM; vary injection site each week.
Plegridy, initially 63mcg (dose 1, day 0; orange pen), then 94mcg (dose 2, day 14; blue pen), then 125mcg (full dose) (dose 3, day 28; grey pen), then 125mcg every 2 weeks. *Admin*, SC injection; remove from refrigerator; allow to warm to room temperature before injection. *Elderly*, safety/efficacy not established.
Rebif, initially 8.8mcg 3-times weekly (week 1, 2), 22mcg 3-times weekly (weeks 3, 4), then 44mcg 3-times weekly (week 5 onwards). First demyelinating event, 44mcg SC 3-times weekly.
Initially titrate dose to reduce incidence and/or severity of flu-like symptoms. Adjunctive anti-inflammatories, analgesics and/or antipyretics advised prior to and for 24 hours after admin.
Child: *Avonex*, age 12-16 years, no dose recommendation; under 12 years*. *Plegridy*, age 0-18 years*. *Rebif*, age 2-17 years, receiving 22mcg or 44mcg 3-times weekly, safety profile similar to adults; under 2 years, not recommended. *(safety/efficacy not established).
Renal Impairment: Severe, caution.
Hepatic Impairment: As for Renal above.
CI: Hypersensitivity to natural or recombinant interferon beta, severe depressive disorders and/or suicidal ideation.
Interactions: Effect of Other Drugs on Interferon beta-1a: *Co-admin caution*: Drugs with narrow therapeutic index and metabolised by hepatic cytochrome P450 (antiepileptics, some antidepressants).
SP: Caution, depression, mood disorders, suicidal ideation, consider discontinuing. Progressive MS development, discontinue. Advise patient of most common adverse events (flu-like syndrome). Caution, pre-existing seizure disorder, severe myelosuppression. Hepatic injury (usually within first 6 months), cardiac disease (angina, CHF, arrhythmia), monitor. Antibody development, reduced efficacy.
Pregnancy, Lactation: Pregnancy and initiation during pregnancy, contraindicated. Abortifacient potential, warn

patient; advise adequate contraception. Lactation, stop breastfeeding or stop drug.
ADR: Summary, *highest incidence*, flu-like symptoms (myalgia, fever, chills, sweating, asthenia, headache, nausea), injection-site reactions.
Notes: See 3.6.1 Multiple Sclerosis (MS).

Avonex Parenteral *(Biogen Idec)* A. HT.
Price, 30mcg/0.5mL: (4) PFP, €870.50; PFS, €894.62. PFP (12) €2862.80.
Injection, interferon beta-1a 30mcg/0.5mL. Clear colourless soln.
Store: Refrigerate; do not freeze; store at room temperature (max. 1 week).
▼ **Plegridy Parenteral** *(Biogen Idec)* A. HT.
Price, starter pack (1x 63mcg, 1x 94mcg), €780.36; 125mcg PFP (2), €890.76.
Injection, peginterferon beta-1a initiation pack (63mcg, 94mcg), 125mg soln. *Essentially sodium-free.* NOTE: Potency should not be compared to another pegylated or non-pegylated protein of same therapeutic class.
Rebif Parenteral *(Merck Serono)* A. HT.
Price, multidose pack (4) 22mcg, €810.39 (PFP) and €786.35. Multidose (4) 22mcg, €858.94; 44mcg, €1041.59. PFP (12) 22mcg, €896.11; 44mcg, €1051.86. PFS (12) 22mcg, €858.26; 44mcg, €1026.51; initiation pack (2) €650.93.
Injection, interferon beta-1a 8.8mcg, 22mcg, 44mcg. PFP or cartridge. Clear (opalescent) soln. Benzyl alcohol.

Interferon Beta-1b

ATC Code: L03AB08. **Sport:** Permitted.
Driving: CNS-related events may influence.
Indications: Treatment, single demyelinating event with active inflammatory process (needing IV corticosteroids, high risk of developing MS). Relapsing remitting MS (2 or more relapses in last 2 years). Secondary progressive MS with active disease.
Dose: Adult, Elderly: MS, relapsing-remitting, secondary progressive, 250mcg (8 million IU) by SC injection every other day. Initially 62.5mcg SC every other day; increase slowly to 250mcg.
Child: Adolescents 12-16 years, as for Adult above.
CI: Decompensated liver disease.
Interactions: Effect of Other Drugs on Interferon beta-1b: *Co-admin not recommended (insufficient data)*: Immunomodulators (other than corticoids or ACTH). *Co-admin caution*: Drugs affecting haemopoiesis.
SP: Pancreatitis, associated with hypertriglyceridaemia. Myelosuppression, anaemia, thrombocytopenia, caution. Admin of cytokines with pre-existing monoclonal gammopathy, associated with systemic capillary leak syndrome (shock-like symptoms, fatality).
ADR: *Very common*, arthralgia.
Notes: See 3.6.1 Multiple Sclerosis (MS). See Interferon beta-1a above.

Betaferon Parenteral 300mcg *(Bayer)* A. HT.
Price, 250mcg/mL (15) 3mL, €791.06.
Injection, interferon beta-1b 250mcg/mL (8 million IU/mL). Sterile white (off-white) powder; solvent for soln. **Store:** Below 25 deg C; do not freeze.

Natalizumab

ATC Code: L04AA23. **Sport:** Permitted.
Driving: Dizziness.
Indications: Single disease modifying therapy (DMT) in highly active relapsing remitting MS in patients with: Highly active disease despite DMT treatment; rapidly evolving severe relapsing MS (2 or more relapses in 1 year, 1 or more Gadolinium enhancing lesions or significant T2 lesion load).
Dose: Adult: 300mg once every 4 weeks. *Admin*, IV infusion over 1 hour (rate approx. 2mL/min); observe for 1 hour (hypersensitivity); not for bolus use.
Elderly: Over 65, not recommended.
Child: Under 18 years, contraindicated.
CI: PML, opportunistic infection (including immunocompromised), active malignancy (except cutaneous basal cell carcinoma).
Interactions: Effect of Other Drugs on Natalizumab: *Co-admin contraindicated*: Other DMTs. *Co-admin*, immunosuppressants, antineoplastics: current or prior

131

3.6.2 Motor Neurone Disease (MND)

therapy (mitoxantrone, cyclophosphamide), beta-interferons, glatiramer acetate.

SP: Patients to carry Patient Alert Card; counsel (importance of uninterrupted dosing). Resources to manage hypersensitivity and MRI to be available; if hypersensitivity occurs, discontinue. Ensure immunocompetent before initiation. Spontaneous serious liver injury (any time during treatment); if significant, discontinue. MRI scan before initiation, then yearly. Anaemia, haemolytic anaemia (rare), reported.

Opportunistic infections (especially with Crohn's disease), or antibody development, discontinue. PML, see Notes below. Increased PML risk with (anti-JCV antibodies, treatment beyond 2 years, prior immunosuppressants). Monitor for worsening neurological symptoms; evaluate (MRI). PML, JCV or GCN suspected, discontinue until excluded (see CI). Anti-JCV antibody negative, still at PML risk (new JCV infection, fluctuating antibody status, false negative test result). Increased encephalitis and meningitis risk due to herpes simplex and varicella zoster viruses; serious, life-threatening (fatal) cases reported; if diagnosed, discontinue. JCV also caused granule cell neuronopathy (GCN) with symptoms similar to PML (cerebellar syndrome). Re-inform patients of PML risk after 2 years.

Immune reconstitution Inflammatory Syndrome (IRIS) almost always occurs with discontinuation; can lead to serious neurological complications (fatal).

NOTE: Natalizumab remains in the blood for approx. 12 weeks after last dose. Prescribing physicians must ensure familiarity with Physician Information and Management Guidelines.

Pregnancy, Lactation: Pregnancy, evaluate risk/benefit; monitor newborns exposed during third trimester (haematological abnormalities). Consider discontinuing if pregnancy occurs on treatment. Lactation, stop drug or stop breastfeeding.

ADR: Summary, *highest incidence*, dizziness, nausea, urticaria, rigors associated with infusions.

Notes: See 3.6.1 Multiple Sclerosis (MS).

▼ **Tysabri Parenteral 300mg** *(Biogen Idec)* A. HOS.
Price, (1) €1581.08 (PTW).
Infusion, natalizumab conc (20mg/mL; dilute to infusion 2.6mg/mL). Recombinant humanised anti-alpha4-integrin antibody produced by rDNA technology. Colourless clear (slightly opalescent) conc for soln. *Sodium 52mg/vial.* **Store:** Refrigerate; do not freeze.

Teriflunomide

ATC Code: L04AA31. **Sport:** Permitted.
Driving: No or negligible effect; dizziness.
Indications: Relapsing remitting MS in adults.
Dose: Adult, Elderly: 14mg once daily. *Admin,* swallow whole with water with/without food. *Elderly,* caution.
Child: Under 10 years, no relevant use; 10-18 years, no safety/efficacy data.
Renal Impairment: Severe undergoing dialysis, contraindicated.
Hepatic Impairment: Severe, contraindicated.
CI: Severe (immunodeficiency states, active infection, hypoproteinaemia e.g. nephrotic syndrome), significant (bone marrow impairment, anaemia, leucopenia, neutropenia, thrombocytopenia).
Interactions: Effect of Other Drugs on Teriflunomide: *Co-admin not recommended:* Leflunomide; colestyramine, activated charcoal (unless accelerated elimination needed). *Co-admin avoid:* Live vaccines. *Co-admin caution:* Plasma levels decreased (rifampicin, carbamazepine, phenobarbital, phenytoin, St John's Wort).
Effect of Teriflunomide on Other Drugs: CYP2C8 substrates (repaglinide, paclitaxel, pioglitazone, rosiglitazone), OAT3 substrates (cefaclor, benzylpenicillin, ciprofloxacin, indomethacin, ketoprofen, furosemide, cimetidine, methotrexate, zidovudine), BCRP substrates (methotrexate, topotecan, sulfasalazine, daunorubicin, doxorubicin), OATP substrates (simvastatin, atorvastatin, pravastatin, methotrexate, nateglinide, repaglinide, rifampicin): *Caution, increased exposure.* CYP1A2 substrates (caffeine, duloxetine, alosetron, theophylline,

tizanidine): *Caution, reduced exposure/efficacy.* Warfarin: *Monitor INR.* Rosuvastatin: *Recommend 50% dose reduction.*

SP: Assess before initiation, monitor during treatment (BP, ALT/SGPT, full blood count, differential white count, platelets); elevated BP, haematological effects, hepatic effects*. Caution, substantial alcohol use. Highly protein bound, caution hypoproteinaemia. Interstitial lung disease/skin reactions (DRESS) reported; severe skin reaction reported (with teriflunomide). Peripheral neuropathy. Accelerated elimination procedure*. Caution, switching from natalizumab (half-life 2-3 months) or fingolimod (6-weeks clearance) to teriflunomide; switch from teriflunomide (interval of 5 half-lives; 3.5 months) to other therapy, caution concomitant exposure, additive effects. *See manufacturers Full Prescribing Information.

Pregnancy, Lactation: Contraindicated. Women of childbearing potential to ensure adequate contraception during treatment and after (as long as teriflunomide plasma conc above 0.02mg/L).

ADR: Summary, *most common*, diarrhoea, nausea, alopecia, increased ALT.

Notes: See 3.6.1 Multiple Sclerosis (MS).

▼ **AUBAGIO 14mg** *(Genzyme)* A. HT.
Price, (28) €944.24.
Tablet, teriflunomide. Pale-blue f/c pentagonal. Marked with logo and strength. *Lactose.* **Store:** No special conditions.

3.6.2 - Motor Neurone Disease (MND)

In This Chapter: *Riluzole.*

Class Effects

CI: Hypersensitivity to any member of the class.
Notes: See manufacturers Full Prescribing Information.

Riluzole

ATC Code: N07XX02. **Sport:** Permitted.
Driving: Dizziness, vertigo.
Indications: To extend life or time to mechanical ventilation in amyotrophic lateral sclerosis (ALS).
Dose: Adult, Elderly: 50mg orally 12-hourly.
Child: Not recommended.
Renal Impairment: Not recommended.
Hepatic Impairment: Hepatic disease or baseline transaminases above 3xULN.
Interactions: Effect of Other Drugs on Riluzole: *Decreased elimination:* CYP1A2 inhibitors (caffeine, diclofenac, diazepam, nicergoline, clomipramine, imipramine, fluvoxamine, phenacetin, theophylline, amitriptyline, quinolones). *Increased elimination:* CYP1A2 inducers (cigarette smoke, charcoal-broiled food, rifampicin, omeprazole).
SP: Liver impairment, caution/monitor. Neutropenia, advise patient to report febrile illness. Interstitial lung disease, discontinue; if respiratory symptoms develop (dry cough, dyspnoea), perform chest radiography.
Pregnancy, Lactation: Contraindicated.
ADR: Summary, *most common*, asthenia, nausea, abnormal LFTs.
Notes: See 3.6.2 Motor Neurone Disease (MND).

Rilutek 50mg *(SANOFI)* A. HT.
Price, (56) €180.90.
Tablet, riluzole. Cap-shaped white f/c. Marked RPR 202.

3.7 - Dementia

Class Effects

Driving: Moderate to severe Alzheimer's disease may impair driving ability.

SP: Therapy with these drugs should occur under specialist supervision and only initiated if a caregiver is available to regularly monitor drug intake.

3.7.1 - Cholinesterase Inhibitors

In This Chapter: *Donepezil, galantamine, rivastigmine.*

132

Class Effects

Indications: Symptomatic treatment of mild to moderately severe Alzheimer's dementia *(donepezil, galantamine, rivastigmine)*, dementia in patients with idiopathic Parkinson's disease *(rivastigmine)*.

CI: Hypersensitivity to any member of the class. Use in children.

Interactions: Effect of Other Drugs on Cholinesterase Inhibitors: *Effect exaggerated*: Succinylcholine-type muscle relaxants (during anaesthesia). *Co-admin not recommended*: Other acetylcholinesterase inhibitors, cholinergic agonists or antagonists. *Metabolism inhibited*: Ketoconazole, quinidine, itraconazole, erythromycin, fluoxetine (not rivastigmine in healthy volunteers). *Plasma levels reduced*: Rifampicin, phenytoin, carbamazepine, ALCOHOL. *Synergism*: Succinylcholine, other neuromuscular blockers, cholinergic agonists, beta blockers.

SP: Cholinesterase inhibitors may exaggerate succinylcholine-type muscle relaxation during anaesthesia. Cardiovascular conditions, caution, vagotonic effects (bradycardia) especially with sick sinus syndrome or other supraventricular cardiac conduction disturbances (SA or AV block); syncope and seizures, investigate possible heart block or long sinusal pauses. GI conditions (ulcer risk). May cause bladder outflow obstruction. Cholinomimetics may cause generalised convulsions, worsening of Parkinsonian symptoms, Neuroleptic Malignant Syndrome (NMS). Caution, asthma, obstructive pulmonary disease.

Pregnancy, Lactation: Pregnancy, lactation, use not recommended unless otherwise specified.

Notes: See 3.7 Dementia.

Donepezil

ATC Code: N06DA02. **Sport:** Permitted.
Driving: Minor or moderate influence; fatigue, dizziness, muscle cramp.

Indications: Mild to moderately severe Alzheimer's dementia.

Dose: Adult, Elderly: Initially 5mg/day for minimum 1 month to allow steady-state conc and assess clinical response; if needed titrate to max. 10mg/day. *Admin*, oral once daily in evening just before bedtime.

Hepatic Impairment: Mild/moderate, titrate with caution. Severe, no data.

CI: Hypersensitivity to piperidine derivatives.

SP: Rhabdomyolysis reported to occur independently of NMS and in association with donepezil initiation or dose increase.

Pregnancy, Lactation: Pregnancy, should not be used unless clearly necessary/contraindicated.

ADR: Summary, *most common*, diarrhoea, muscle cramps, fatigue, nausea, vomiting, insomnia.

Notes: See 3.9. Cholinesterase Inhibitors.

Interchangeability: Same strengths of all brands of donepezil film-coated (f/c) tabs and orodispersible tabs listed below are deemed interchangeable.

Reference Price: (28) 5mg, €9.24. 10mg, €13.44.

Aricept 5mg, 10mg *(Pfizer)* A. GMS.
Price, (28) 5mg, €34.03. 10mg, €47.71.
Tablet, donepezil HCl. Round f/c. Marked Aricept and strength. 5mg: White. 10mg: Yellow. *Lactose.*

Aripil 5mg, 10mg *(Gerard)* A. GMS.
Price, (28) 5mg, €8.40. 10mg, €12.04.
Tablet, donepezil HCl. White round f/c. Marked DL/strength; G on reverse. *Lactose.*

Donecept 5mg, 10mg *(Accord)* A. GMS.
Price, (28) 5mg, €8.40. 10mg, €12.04. (100) 5mg, €30.00. 10mg €43.00.
Tablet, donepezil HCl. Round f/c. Marked DZ/strength. 5mg: White. 10mg: Pale-yellow. *Lactose.*

Donepezil (Accord) 5mg, 10mg *(Accord)* A. GMS.
Price, (28) 5mg, €8.40. 10mg, €12.04.
Tablet, donepezil HCl. Round. Marked with strength. 5mg: White (off-white). 10mg: Yellow. *Lactose.*

Donepezil (Wockhardt) 5mg, 10mg *(Pinewood)* A. GMS.
Price, (28) 5mg, €8.40. 10mg, €12.04.
Tablet, donepezil HCl. Round f/c. Marked W one side. 5mg: White. Marked 3II. 10mg: Yellow. Marked 3I2. *Lactose.*

Cholinesterase Inhibitors   3.7.1

Donepezil Bluefish 5mg, 10mg *(Bluefish)* A. GMS.
Price, (28) 5mg, €8.40. 10mg, €12.04.
Tablet, donepezil hydrochloride monohydrate. Round f/c. Marked with strength. 5mg: White (off-white). 10mg: Yellow. *Lactose.*

Donepezil Krka 5mg, 10mg *(Krka)* A. GMS.
Price, (28) 5mg, €8.40. 10mg, €12.04.
Tablet, donepezil HCl. Rounded f/c. 5mg: White (nearly white). 10mg: Yellowish-brown. *Lactose.*

Donepezil TEVA 5mg, 10mg *(TEVA)* A. GMS.
Price, (28) 5mg, €8.40. 10mg, €12.04.
Tablet, donepezil HCl. Round f/c. Marked DN and strength. 5mg: White (off-white). 10mg: Yellow. *Lactose.*

Donesyn 5mg, 10mg *(Clonmel)* A. GMS.
Price, (28) 5mg, €8.40. 10mg, €12.04.
Tablet, donepezil HCl. Round f/c. Marked D9EI; strength on reverse. 5mg: White. 10mg: Yellow. *Lactose.*

Dozept 5mg, 10mg *(Rowex)* A. GMS.
Price, (28) 5mg, €8.40. 10mg, €12.04.
Tablet, donepezil HCl. Round f/c. 5mg: White. 10mg: Yellow scored (divisible into equal halves). *Lactose, soya lecithin.*

Galantamine

ATC Code: N06DA04. **Sport:** Permitted.
Driving: Dizziness, somnolence.

Indications: Mild to moderately severe Alzheimer's dementia adequately confirmed according to current guidelines.

Dose: Adult, Elderly: STANDARD/R, initially 8mg/day for 4 weeks; maintenance 16mg/day for at least 4 weeks; if needed titrate to 24mg/day; not tolerated reduce to 16mg/day. *Admin*, in 2 divided doses with morning and evening meals; ensure adequate fluid intake.

PROLONGED/R, as for Standard/R except dosed once daily in morning with food; swallow whole, do not crush or chew.

Renal Impairment: CrCl (mL/min) below 9, contraindicated. Significant renal AND hepatic impairment, contraindicated.

Hepatic Impairment: Moderate, *Standard/R*, initially 4mg/day in morning for 1 week; titrate to 8mg/day in 2 divided doses for 4 weeks; max. 8mg twice daily. *Prolonged/R*, initially 8mg once every other day in morning, for 1 week; then 8mg once daily for 4 weeks; max. 16mg/day. Severe, contraindicated. See Renal above.

SP: Patients treated with CYP2D6 or CYP3A4 inhibitors, consider dose reductions. Serious skin reaction reported (Stevens-Johnson syndrome, acute generalised exanthematous pustulosis); discontinue.

ADR: *Very common*, vomiting, nausea.

Notes: See 3.9. Cholinesterase Inhibitors.

Reminyl 8mg, 12mg, XL, Oral Soln *(Shire)* A. GMS.
Price, 8mg (56) €87.13. 12mg (56) €107.69; (168) €323.07. XL (28) 8mg, €35.08. 16mg, €43.57. 24mg, €53.85. Soln (100mL) €98.99.
Standard/R tablet, galantamine hydrobromide. Round f/c. Marked Janssen; G/strength on reverse. 8mg: Pink. 12mg: Orange-brown. *Lactose.* **Store:** No special conditions.
Prolonged/R Capsule (XL), as above 8mg, 16mg, 24mg. Hard gelatin opaque containing white (off-white) pellets. Marked G/strength. 8mg: White. 16mg: Pink. 24mg: Caramel. *Sucrose.* **Store:** Below 30 deg C.
Oral soln, as above 4mg/mL. Clear colourless. *Parabens.* **Store:** Do not freeze.

Galsya SR 8mg, 16mg, 24mg *(Krka)* A. GMS.
Price, (28) 8mg, €28.07. 16mg, €34.86. 24mg, €43.08.
Prolonged/R Capsule (SR), galantamine hydrobromide. Contain white oval prolonged/R tablet cores. Marked G and strength. 8mg: white; contains 1 core. 16mg: Pink; contains 2 cores. 24mg: Orange/pink; contains 3 cores.

Rivastigmine

ATC Code: N06DA03. **Sport:** Permitted.
Driving: Caution.

Indications: Mild to moderately severe dementia of Alzheimer's or Parkinson's disease.

Dose: Adult, Elderly: ORAL, initially 3mg/day; increase at 2-week intervals to 6mg/day, then 9mg/day, then 12mg/day; maintenance 6mg/day to max. 12mg/day. Several days treatment interruption, re-initiate at 3mg/day. *Admin*, in 2 divided doses with meals; caps to be swallowed whole.

TRANSDERMAL, initiate with 4.6mg/24-hour (9mg); after

3.7.2 Memantine

minimum 4 weeks, titrate to 9.5mg/24-hour (18mg); maintenance 9.5mg/24-hour.

Switch from oral to transdermal, oral 3-6mg/day, switch to 4.6mg/24-hour patch; oral 9-12mg/day, switch to 9.5mg/24-hour patch. Apply to clean, dry, hairless intact healthy skin once daily; upper or lower back, upper arm or chest in place that will not be rubbed by tight clothing.

Renal Impairment: Clinically significant impairment, more dose-dependent adverse reactions.

Hepatic Impairment: As for Renal above. Severe, close monitoring required.

CI: Carbamate hypersensitivity (transdermal patch).

Interactions: Effect of Rivastigmine on Other Drugs: Substances with butyrylcholinesterase-mediated metabolism: *May inhibit.*

SP: Avoid contact with eyes (transdermal patch). Body weight under 50kg, risk of more adverse events. May cause bradycardia; constitutes a risk factor for Torsade de Pointes, especially with risk factors.

ADR: Summary, *most common*, GI reactions including nausea, vomiting (females more susceptible). *Very common*, anorexia, dizziness, diarrhoea. Transdermal, *most frequent*, application-site reactions.

Notes: See 3.9. Cholinesterase Inhibitors.

Exelon Capsules, Transdermal *(Novartis)* A. GMS.
Price, (56) 1.5mg, €39.23. All other strengths, €40.32. Transdermal (30) 4.6mg, €59.37. 9.5mg, €63.95.
Capsules, rivastigmine hydrogen tartrate 1.5mg, 3mg, 4.5mg, 6mg. Contain off-white (slightly yellow) powder. Marked Exelon/strength. 1.5mg: Yellow. 3mg: Orange. 4.5mg: Red. 6mg: Red/orange.
Transdermal patch, rivastigmine 4.6mg (9.5mg)/24 hours. Thin matrix 3-layers. Marked Exelon/strength/24-hours.

Nimvastid Capsules *(Krka)* A. GMS.
Price, (56) 1.5mg, €31.38. All other strengths, €32.26.
Capsules, rivastigmine hydrogen tartrate 1.5mg, 3mg, 4.5mg, 6mg. Contain white (almost) powder. 1.5mg: Yellow. 3mg: Orange. 4.5mg: Brownish-red. 6mg: Brownish-red/orange.

Rivastigmine Actavis Capsules *(Accord)* A. GMS.
Price, (56) 1.5mg, €31.37; 3mg, €32.26; 4.5mg, 6mg, €32.26.
Capsules, rivastigmine hydrogen tartrate 1.5mg, 3mg, 4.5mg, 6mg. Contain off-white (slightly yellow) powder. Marked RIV/strength. 1.5mg: Yellow. 3mg: Orange. 4.5mg: Red. 6mg: Red/orange. **Store:** Below 25 deg C.

Rivastigmine Sandoz Capsules *(Rowex)* A. GMS.
Price, (56) 1.5mg, €31.38. All other strengths, €32.26.
Capsules, rivastigmine hydrogen tartrate 1.5mg, 3mg, 4.5mg, 6mg. Contain off-white (slightly yellow) powder. Marked RIV/strength. 1.5mg: Yellow. 3mg: Orange. 4.5mg: Red. 6mg: Red/orange.

3.7.2 - Memantine

In This Chapter: *Memantine.*

Class Effects
Notes: See 3.7 Dementia.

Memantine

ATC Code: N06DX01. **Sport:** Permitted.
Driving: Caution (especially outpatients).
Indications: Moderate to severe Alzheimer's dementia.

Dose: Adult, Elderly: Initially 5mg/day as single dose in morning for week 1 (day 1-7); titrate to 10mg/day for week 2 (day 8-14), then 15mg/day for week 3 (day 15-21); from week 4, maintenance 20mg/day. Oral once daily; same time each day with or without food. Oral soln, each pump activation delivers 5mg of memantine; not to be pumped directly into mouth; dose onto a spoon or into a glass of water using pump or pipette.

Child: No data available.

Renal Impairment: CrCl (mL/min) 30-49, 10mg/day; if tolerated after 7 days, titrate to 20mg/day; CrCl 5-29, 10mg/day.

Hepatic Impairment: No adjustment; severe, not recommended.

Interactions: Effect of Other Drugs on Memantine: *Co-admin not recommended, pharmacotoxic psychosis risk*: NMDA-antagonists (amantadine, ketamine, dextromethorphan). *Co-admin caution*: Phenytoin.

Increased plasma levels: Cimetidine, ranitidine, procainamide, quinidine, quinine, nicotine. *Plasma levels decreased*: Hydrochlorothiazide.

Effect of Memantine on Other Drugs: L-dopa, dopaminergic agonists, anticholinergic: *Effect enhanced*. Barbiturates, neuroleptics: *Effect reduced*. Antispasmodics, dantrolene, baclofen: *Effects modified, consider dose adjustment*.

SP: Epilepsy, convulsions. Factors raising urinary pH (drastic dietary changes, ingestion of alkalising gastric buffers, renal tubulary acidosis, severe UTI with Proteus bacteria), monitor. Recent MI, uncompensated CHF, uncontrolled hypertension, monitor.

Pregnancy, Lactation: Pregnancy, if benefit outweighs risk. Lactation, not recommended.

ADR: Summary, *most frequent*, dizziness, headache, constipation, somnolence, hypertension.

Notes: See 3.7.2 Memantine.

Interchangeability: Same strengths of all brands of memantine film-coated (f/c) tabs and oral soln 10mg/mL (5mg pump actuation) are deemed interchangeable.

Reference Price: 10mg (56) €16.80; 20mg (28) €16.80. Oral soln 1mg/mL (100mL) €60.70.

Ebixa 10mg, Oral Soln Pump Actuation *(Lundbeck)* A. GMS.
Price, 10mg (28), €17.16; (56), €34.31. Oral Soln Pump (50mL) €75.87. (100mL) €151.75.
Tablet, memantine HCl. Pale-yellow (yellow) oval scored (divisible into equal halves). Marked 10; MM on reverse. **Store:** No special conditions.
Oral soln, as above 5mg/0.5mL. Clear colourless (light-yellowish).
Sorbitol; potassium 0.5mg/mL. **Store:** Below 30 deg C; store and transport in vertical position.

Marixino 10mg *(Krka)* A. GMS.
Price, (28) €6.72; (56) €13.44.
Tablet, memantine HCl. White oval f/c scored (divisible into equal halves). *Lactose.*

Memantine 10mg *(Pinewood)* A. GMS.
Price, (28) €6.72; (56) €13.44.
Tablet, memantine HCl. White (off-white) f/c cap-shaped scored (divisible into equal doses). Marked M 12.

Memantine Accord 10mg, 20mg *(Accord)* A. GMS.
Price, 10mg (28), €6.72; (56) €13.44. 20mg (28), €13.44.
Tablet, memantine HCl. Oblong scored (divisible into equal halves). Marked MT and strength. 10mg: White. 20mg: Pale-red to grey-red. *Lactose.*

Memantine Clonmel 10mg, Oral Soln *(Clonmel)* A. GMS.
Price, 10mg (28), €6.72; (56) €13.44. Oral Soln Pump 10mg/mL (50mL) €30.35. (100mL) €60.70.
Tablet, memantine HCl. White slim through middle f/c scored both sides (divisible into equal doses). Marked 10.
Oral soln, as above 5mg/0.5mL. Clear colourless (light-yellowish). *Sorbitol; potassium 0.5mg/mL.*

Memantine LEK 10mg *(Rowex)* A. GMS.
Price, (28) €6.72; (56) €13.44.
Tablet, memantine HCl. Yellow oval f/c scored (divisible into equal halves).

Memantine Mylan 10mg, Oral Soln *(Gerard)* A. GMS.
Price, (28) €6.72; (56) €13.44. Oral Soln Pump (50mL) €30.35; (100mL) €60.70.
Tablets, memantine HCl. Dark-yellow f/c oblong scored (divisible into equal halves). Marked ME and 10. **Store:** No special conditions.
Oral soln, as above 5mg/0.5mL actuation. Clear colourless (light-yellowish). *Sorbitol; potassium 0.5mg/mL.* **Store:** Store and transport in vertical position.

Memantine Ratiopharm 10mg *(TEVA)* A. GMS.
Price, (28) €6.72.
Tablet, memantine HCl. White cap-shaped f/c scored (divisible into equal halves). Marked M10. *Lactose, soya lecithin.*

Nemdatine 10mg *(Accord)* A. GMS.
Price, (28) €6.72; (56) €13.44.
Tablet, memantine HCl. White cap-shaped f/c scored (divisible into equal halves). Marked M10. *Lactose.*

3.8 - Nausea and Vomiting, Vertigo, Motion Sickness

Class Effects
Antispasmodics may also be used, see Notes below.
CI: Hypersensitivity to any member of the class.
Notes: See 1.2 Antispasmodics.

3.8.1 - Meniere's Disease

In This Chapter: *Betahistine.*

Betahistine

ATC Code: N07CA01. **Sport:** Permitted.
Driving: Unlikely to impair at recommended dose; drowsiness.
Indications: Treatment of vertigo, tinnitus, hearing loss, nausea (associated with Meniere's Disease).
Dose: Adult, Elderly: Initially 8-16mg 3-times daily preferably with food.
Child: Under 18 years, not recommended.
CI: Phaeochromocytoma.
Interactions: Effect of Other Drugs on Betahistine: Co-admin caution: MAOIs including subtype B (selegiline). *Interaction theoretically possible:* Antihistamines. *Interaction case report:* Ethanol, pyrimethamine, dapsone, salbutamol.
SP: Caution, peptic ulcer (dyspepsia with betahistine), bronchial asthma (monitor carefully during therapy); urticaria, rashes, allergic rhinitis (may be aggravated).
Pregnancy, Lactation: Pregnancy, caution; use only if clearly necessary. Lactation, avoid; weigh benefit/risk.
ADR: *Common*, headache, nausea, dyspepsia.
Notes: See 3.8.1 Meniere's Disease.
Interchangeability: Same strengths of all brands of betahistine tabs listed below are deemed interchangeable.

Serc 8mg, 16mg *(BGP)* B. GMS.
Price, 8mg (120) €6.30. 16mg (84) €8.80.
Tablet, betahistine dihydrochloride. White (almost) round. 8mg: Flat. Marked 256. 16mg: Scored (divisible into equal doses). Marked 267. **Store:** No special temperature conditions; original pack.

Betahistine 8mg, 16mg *(Accord)* B. GMS.
Price, (84) 8mg, €4.08. 16mg, €8.15.
Tablet, betahistine dihydrochloride. White round flat. 8mg: Scored (facilitates breaking). Marked BE. 16mg: Scored (divisible into equal halves). Marked BF. *Lactose.*

By-Vertin 8mg, 16mg *(Fannin)* B. GMS.
Price, 8mg (120) €6.16. 16mg (84) €8.62.
Tablet, betahistine HCl. Biplanar. Marked B/strength. 16mg: Scored. *Lactose.*

Vertigon 8mg, 16mg *(Rowex)* B. GMS.
Price, (84) 8mg, €4.32. 16mg, €8.62.
Tablet, betahistine dihydrochloride. White flat round. Marked BH/strength; G on reverse. *Mannitol.*

3.8.2 - Neurokinin Receptor Antagonists

In This Chapter: *Aprepitant, fosaprepitant.*

Class Effects

Indications: Adjunctive, prevention, acute and delayed nausea and vomiting associated with highly emetogenic cisplatin-based cancer chemotherapy; moderately emetogenic cancer chemotherapy.

Aprepitant

ATC Code: A04AD12. **Sport:** Permitted.
Driving: Minor influence; dizziness, fatigue.
Indications: Adjunctive, prevention of nausea and vomiting associated with highly and moderately emetogenic chemotherapy (age 12 and above).
Dose: Adult, Elderly: *Highly emetogenic* chemotherapy, 125mg orally (day 1), then 80mg once daily (days 2 and 3). *Admin*, 1 hour prior to chemotherapy (day 1) and (days 2 and 3) in the morning. Swallow caps whole with or without food. Oral for 3 days with oral dexamethasone 12mg (day 1), 30 minutes prior to chemotherapy and then 8mg (days 2, 3 and 4) and 5-HT3 antagonist standard dose (day 1). *Admin*, with or without food; cap to be swallowed whole.
Moderately emetogenic chemotherapy, as above except that oral dexamethasone is admin as 12mg (only day 1).
Child: Age 12 years and over, recommended, 125mg orally (day 1), then 80mg once daily (days 2 and 3). *Admin*, 1 hour prior to chemotherapy (day 1) and (days 2 and 3) in the morning; oral for 3 days. If a corticosteroid (dexamethasone) is co-admin, reduce corticosteroid dose

to 50% of usual dose. For dose of 5-HT3 antagonist, see Full Prescribing Information.
Hepatic Impairment: Moderate, limited data; severe, caution.
Interactions: Effect of Other Drugs on Aprepitant: *Increased plasma levels:* Co-admin contraindicated, CYP3A4 inhibitors (pimozide, terfenadine, astemizole, cisapride); co-admin caution (ketoconazole, itraconazole, voriconazole, posaconazole, clarithromycin, telithromycin, nefazodone, protease inhibitors), CYP3A4 substrates with narrow therapeutic window (ciclosporin, tacrolimus, sirolimus, everolimus, alfentanil, ergot alkaloid derivatives, fentanyl quinidine). *Plasma levels decreased:* Co-admin avoid, CYP3A4 inducers (rifampicin, phenytoin, carbamazepine, phenobarbital); co-admin not recommended, St John's Wort.
Effect of Aprepitant on Other Drugs: CYP3A4 substrates (pimozide, terfenadine, astemizole, cisapride): *Increased plasma levels, co-admin contraindicated.* CYP2C9 substrates (warfarin, tolbutamide, phenytoin): *Plasma levels decreased.* Dexamethasone: *Reduce dose by 50%.* Methylprednisolone: *Reduce IV dose by 25%, oral dose by 50%.* Etoposide, vinorelbine, docetaxel, paclitaxel, ifosfamide: *Caution, monitor.* Midazolam, other benzodiazepines metabolised by CYP3A4 (alprazolam, triazolam), ergot alkaloids and derivatives: *Increase plasma levels, caution.* Oral contraceptives: *Reduced Efficacy.* Irinotecan: *Caution, increased toxicity.*
SP: See Interactions above.
Pregnancy, Lactation: Pregnancy, only if clearly necessary. Efficacy of hormonal contraceptives may be reduced; ensure alternate adequate contraception during and for two months after treatment. Lactation, not recommended.
ADR: Summary, *most common* (highly emetogenic chemotherapy), hiccups, increased ALT, dyspepsia, constipation, headache, decreased appetite; moderately emetogenic chemotherapy, fatigue; paediatric patients, hiccups, flushing.
Notes: See 3.8.2 Neurokinin Receptor Antagonists.

Emend 80mg, 125mg *(MSD)* A. GMS.
Price, 125mg (5) €109.64. (1) 2-day pack (2x 80mg), €42.41. 3-day pack (1x 125mg, 2x 80mg), €60.21.
Capsule, aprepitant. Hard opaque. Marked with strength. 80mg: White/white. Marked 461. 125mg: White/pink. Marked 462. *Sucrose.*

Fosaprepitant

ATC Code: A04AD12. **Sport:** Permitted.
Driving: Dizziness, fatigue.
Dose: Adult, Elderly: 150mg infusion over 20-30 minutes (day 1), approx. 30 minutes prior to chemotherapy, with dexamethasone 12mg/day (day 1), 30 minutes prior to chemotherapy), 8mg/day (day 2, morning), 8mg twice daily (day 3 and 4, morning, evening) and a 5-HT3 antagonist standard dose (day 1). Not for admin by IM, SC or bolus IV injection.
Child: Safety and efficacy not established; no dose recommendation.
SP: If immediate hypersensitivity reactions (during or soon after infusion) occur, not recommended to re-initiate.
ADR: See Notes below.
Notes: See Aprepitant above.

Ivemend Parenteral 150mg *(MSD)* A. HOS.
Price, (1) 150mg, €60.91.
Infusion, fosaprepitant dimeglumine 1mg/mL. White (off-white) amorphous powder for soln. *Lactose.* **Store:** Refrigerate.

3.8.3 - Antihistamines, Antispasmodics

In This Chapter: *Cinnarizine, cyclizine, promethazine.*

Cinnarizine (motion sickness)

ATC Code: N07CA02. **Sport:** Permitted.
Driving: Caution.
Indications: Motion sickness.
Dose: Adult, Elderly: 30mg 2 hours before travelling; then 15mg 8-hourly during journey. Oral, after food.
Child: Age 5-12 years, half adult dose.

3.8.4   5-HT3 Antagonists

Interactions: Effect of Cinnarizine on Other Drugs: CNS depressants, TCads, ALCOHOL: *Increased sedative effect, caution.*

SP: Epigastric discomfort, hypotensive patients. Parkinson's disease, only if benefit outweighs risk. May cause somnolence.

Pregnancy, Lactation: Not recommended.

ADR: Somnolence, GI disturbances, headache, dry mouth, weight gain, perspiration, allergic reactions. Lichen planus, lupus-like symptoms, cholestatic jaundice, rare. Aggravation or appearance of extrapyramidal symptoms (with or without depressive feelings), especially in elderly.

Notes: See 2.2.5 Peripheral Vascular Disorders (brand *Stugeron*).

Cyclizine

ATC Code: RO6AE03. **Sport:** Permitted.

Driving: Caution with ALCOHOL and other CNS depressants.

Indications: Adults, prevention and treatment, nausea and vomiting of motion sickness; caused by narcotic analgesics and general anaesthetics post-operative (PONV); associated with radiotherapy (especially for breast cancer). Relief of vomiting and vertigo associated with Meniere's disease, other vestibular disturbances.

Dose: Adult, Elderly: ORAL, motion sickness, initially 50mg; may be repeated up to 3-times daily. *Admin,* 1-2 hours before departure.

PARENTERAL, 50mg IM or IV up to 3-times daily. For prevention of PONV, admin by slow IV 20 minutes before anticipated end of surgery.

Child: ORAL, age 6-12 years, initially 25mg up to 3-times daily. PARENTERAL, not for use.

CI: Acute alcohol intoxication.

Interactions: Effect of Other Drugs on Cyclizine: *Additive effect:* ALCOHOL, other CNS depressants (hypnotics, tranquillisers, anaesthetics, antipsychotics, barbiturates).

Effect of Cyclizine on Other Drugs: Pethidine: *Enhanced soporific effect.* Other anticholinergics: *Side effects enhanced due to anticholinergic activity of cyclizine.* Other muscarinics: *Additive effect with atropine, some antidepressants (TCads, MAOIs).* Opioid analgesics: *Haemodynamic benefits may be counteracted.*

SP: Cyclizine, IV at half recommended dose increases lower oesophageal sphincter tone, reducing regurgitation and aspiration of gastric contents if admin to patients undergoing emergency surgery, before induction of general anaesthesia. Porphyria, avoid. *Caution*, glaucoma, urinary retention, obstructive GI disease, hepatic disease, phaeochromocytoma, hypertension, epilepsy, prostatic hypertrophy (monitor). severe HF or acute MI (decreased cardiac output with increased heart rate, mean arterial pressure, pulmonary wedge pressure); euphoric/hallucinatory effects; antiemetic effect may increase ALCOHOL toxicity; transient paralysis (IV) (underlying neuromuscular disease/epilepsy). May mask warning signs of damage caused by ototoxic drugs (aminoglycosides).

NOTE: In some countries the brand *Valoid* (oral), available without prescription has led to misuse. May produce a state of disorientated exhilaration associated with hallucinations. Co-admin with large amounts of alcohol is particularly dangerous (anti-emetic effect of cyclizine may increase alcohol toxicity). Cyclizine is a recognised drug of dependence. Often associated with concurrent opiate use. Withdrawal of cyclizine in such subjects can cause nausea, increase in pain (opiates used for analgesia), aggression and craving.

Pregnancy, Lactation: Not recommended.

ADR: Altered haematological profile, hypersensitivity reactions; psychiatric (disorientation, restlessness, agitation, nervousness, euphoria, insomnia, hallucinations), CNS (somnolence, drowsiness, in-coordination, headache, dystonia, dyskinesia, extrapyramidal motor disturbances, tremor, convulsions, dizziness, decreased consciousness, transient speech disorder, paraesthesia, generalised chorea); blurred vision, oculogyration, tinnitus; tachycardia, palpitations,

arrhythmias, hyper/hypotension, bronchospasm, apnoea, dry mouth, constipation, increased gastric reflux, nausea, vomiting, diarrhoea, stomach pain, loss of appetite, hepatobiliary disorders; urticaria, rash, pruritus, angioedema, allergic reactions, photosensitivity; twitching, muscle spasm, asthenia, malaise. Parenteral, injection-site reactions. Rapid IV admin can lead to symptoms of overdose.

Notes: See 3.8.3 Antihistamines.

Valoid 50mg, Parenteral (Concordia) B. GMS.
Price, 50mg (100) €9.89. Injection (5) €4.84.
Tablet, cyclizine HCl. White u/c scored (divisible into equal doses).
Marked T4A. *Lactose.* **Store:** Below 25 deg C.
Injection, cyclizine lactate 50mg/mL. Clear colourless soln. **Store:** Below 25 deg C; protect from direct sunlight.

3.8.4 - 5-HT3 Antagonists

In This Chapter: *Granisetron, ondansetron, netupitant (palonosetron combination), palonosetron.*

Class Effects

Interactions: Effect of Other Drugs on 5-HT3 Antagonists: *Serotonin syndrome:* Other serotonergics (SSRIs, SNRIs).

SP: Constipation; signs of constipation or sub-acute intestinal obstruction, monitor. Serotonin syndrome used as monotherapy or combination with other serotonergics, see Interactions above. May be associated with arrhythmias or ECG abnormalities. Caution, QT-prolongation risk with medicinals increasing QT-interval, history of QT-prolongation, electrolyte abnormalities, CHF, bradyarrhythmia, conduction disturbances; correct hypo-(kalaemia, magnesaemia) prior to admin.

Pregnancy, Lactation: Pregnancy, if benefit outweighs risk unless otherwise specified. Lactation, not recommended.

ADR: Insomnia, headache, constipation, diarrhoea, elevated transaminases.

Granisetron

ATC Code: A04AA02. **Sport:** Permitted.
Driving: Unlikely to impair.

Indications: Prevention and treatment, acute (as well as delayed) nausea and vomiting associated with cytotoxic chemotherapy and/or radiotherapy. Post-operative nausea and vomiting (PONV).

Dose: Adult, Elderly: ORAL, *chemo/radiotherapy*, first dose within 1 hour before chemotherapy then 2mg/day in 1-2 divided doses (up to 1 week; with dexamethasone up to 20mg once daily).

PARENTERAL, *chemo/radiotherapy*, treatment and prevention (acute and delayed nausea), 1-3mg as slow IV injection or as IV infusion over 5 minutes prior to chemotherapy. Treatment, further maintenance doses 10 minutes apart; max. 9mg over 24 hours (with dexamethasone 8-20mg IV before OR 250mg methylprednisolone before and after chemotherapy).

PONV, prevention and treatment, 1mg (1mg/mL formulation) diluted in 5mL by slow IV injection over 30 seconds as single dose, completed prior to anaesthesia. Max. 3mg in 24 hours. Dilute 3mg/3mL formulation infusion in 15mL infusion fluid as IV bolus over 30 seconds or diluted in 20-50mL infusion fluid and admin over 5 minutes.

Child: PARENTERAL, *cytostatic chemotherapy*, single dose of 10-40mcg/kg (up to 3mg diluted in 10-30mL infusion fluid) by IV infusion over 5 minutes prior to start of cytostatic therapy; 1 additional dose may be admin within 24-hour period if required; not less than 10 minutes after initial infusion.

Hepatic Impairment: Caution.

ADR: Summary, *most frequent*, headache, constipation.

Notes: See 3.8.4 5-HT3 Antagonists.

Kytril 1mg, 2mg (Roche) A. GMS.
Price, 1mg (10) €48.88. 2mg (5) €57.47.
Tablet, granisetron HCl. White (almost-white) triangular f/c. Marked K/strength. *Lactose, essentially sodium-free.* **Store:** No special conditions.

136

Kytril Parenteral *(Roche)* A. HOS.
Price, 1mg/mL (5) 1mL, €55.88; 3mL, €90.34 (PTW).
Infusion or injection, granisetron HCl 1mg/mL, 3mg/3mL. Clear colourless liquid. *Essentially sodium-free.* **Store:** Outer carton; protect (light).
Granisetron TEVA Parenteral *(TEVA)* A.
Price, 1mg/1mL, €55.09. 3mg/3mL, €140.32.
Infusion or injection, granisetron HCl 1mg/mL, 3mg/3mL. Sterile clear colourless. *Sodium 3.5mg/mL.*

Ondansetron

ATC Code: A04AA01. **Sport:** Permitted.
Driving: Unlikely to impair.
Indications: Management (adults, children from 6 months), nausea and vomiting associated with cytotoxic chemotherapy and radiotherapy (all formulations). Post-operative nausea and vomiting (PONV), *prevention,* adults, children (age 6 months to 17 years) (oral, IV); *treatment,* adults (oral, IV); children (age 1 month to 17 years) (IV).

Dose: Adult: *Chemo/radiotherapy* induced nausea and vomiting, 8mg orally OR 16mg supp rectally 1-2 hours before treatment OR 8mg by slow IV injection (not less than 30 seconds) OR slow IV infusion (over 15 minutes) or IM injection immediately before treatment; followed by 8mg orally twice daily (12-hourly) for max. 5 days or 16mg orally daily rectally for up to 3 days.
Highly emetogenic chemotherapy, single dose 24mg orally OR 16mg supp rectally with oral dexamethasone 12mg, 1-2 hours before chemotherapy; continue with 8mg orally twice daily up to 5 days (rectal for up to 3 days). Alternately 8mg as single slow IV injection (not less than 30 seconds) or short IV infusion over 15 minutes or IM injection immediately before chemotherapy (above 8mg up to max. 16mg admin only by IV infusion over minimum 15 minutes), then 2 further doses of 8mg by slow IV injection or IM 4-hours apart or by constant IV infusion at rate 1mg/hour for up to 24 hours. Efficacy may be enhanced by addition of single 20mg IV dexamethasone admin prior to chemotherapy.
PONV, prevention, 16mg orally 1 hour prior to anaesthesia or 4mg IM or slow IV injection admin at induction of anaesthesia. Established PONV, single 4mg IM or slow IV injection.
Elderly: *Chemo/radiotherapy* induced nausea and vomiting, age 65-74 years, as for Adult; 75 years and older, initially 8mg (max), diluted in 50-100mL 0.9% Sodium Chloride Injection, infused over 15 minutes; initial dose may be followed by 2 further IV doses of 8mg infused over 15 minutes, 4-hours apart. PONV, limited experience.
Child: *Chemo/radiotherapy,* age 6 months to 17 years, dose can be calculated by body surface are (BSA) or weight:
Dosing by BSA, 5mg/m2 IV as single dose immediately before chemotherapy, max. 8mg; commence oral after 12-hours as follows, (BSA under 0.6m2), 2mg OR (BSA 0.6-1.2m2), 4mg (day 1), then the same dose twice daily for up to 5 days (days 2-6).
Dosing by bodyweight, 0.15mg/kg IV as single dose immediately before chemotherapy (max. 8mg); then up to 3 doses of 0.15mg/kg 4-hourly (day 1), then either 2mg (10kg and under) or 4mg (over 10kg) orally 12-hourly for up to 5 days (days 2-6).
PONV prevention, age 1 month to 17 years, admin prior to or after induction of anaesthesia; slow IV injection over 30 seconds at 0.1mg/kg; max. 4mg. PONV treatment, as for prevention; no data for treatment of children under 2 years of age. Supps not recommended for use in children.
Hepatic Impairment: Moderate or severe, max. 8mg/day (clearance significantly reduced; serum half-life significantly prolonged).
Interactions: Effect of Other Drugs on Ondansetron: *Co-admin contraindicated:* Apomorphine (profound hypotension, loss of consciousness). *Co-admin caution:* Drugs either prolonging QT-interval or causing electrolyte disturbances; serotonergics (SSRIs, SNRIs), serotonin syndrome risk. *Plasma levels decreased:* Phenytoin, carbamazepine, rifampicin. *Increased arrhythmia risk:* Cardiotoxic drugs (anthracyclines e.g. doxorubicin, daunorubicin, trastuzumab), antibiotics (erythromycin,

ketoconazole), antiarrhythmics (amiodarone), beta-blockers (atenolol, timolol).
Effect of Ondansetron on Other Drugs: Tramadol: *Reduced analgesic effect.*
SP: Dose-dependent prolonged QT-interval; Torsades de Pointes; avoid in patients with (congenital long QT syndrome, electrolyte disturbances, CHF, bradyarrhythmias, cardiac rhythm or conduction disturbances, treated with antiarrhythmics or beta-blockers). Correct hypo- (kalaemia, magnesaemia) before initiation. Use with hepatotoxic chemotherapy, monitor hepatic function.
NOTE: When calculating paediatric dose on mg/kg basis (admin 3 doses at 4-hourly intervals), the total daily dose will be higher than if 1 single dose of 5mg/m2 followed by an oral dose is given.
Pregnancy, Lactation: Not recommended.
ADR: *Very common,* headache.
Notes: See 3.8.4 5-HT3 Antagonists.
Zofran 4mg, 8mg, Zydis *(Novartis)* A. GMS.
Price, 4mg (30) €69.87. 8mg (10) €34.64; (30) €103.90. Zydis (10) 4mg, €40.58. 8mg, €49.26.
Tablet, ondansetron hydrochloride dihydrate. Yellow oval f/c. 4mg: Marked GXET3. 8mg: Marked GXET5. *Lactose.*
OroDisp tab (Zydis), ondansetron 4mg, 8mg. Oral lyophilisate. White round. *Aspartame, parabens.*
Zofran Supps, Syrup *(Novartis)* A. GMS.
Price, supps 16mg (1) €12.08. Syrup (50mL) €44.07.
Supp, ondansetron 16mg. White smooth torpedo-shaped.
Oral soln, ondansetron hydrochloride dihydrate 4mg/5mL. Clear colourless (light-yellow) liquid; strawberry odour. *Sorbitol.*
Zofran Parenteral *(Novartis)* A.
Price, (5) 8mg/4mL, €71.26; 4mg/2mL, €49.90 (PTW).
Injection or infusion, ondansetron hydrochloride dihydrate 4mg/2mL, 8mg/4mL. Clear colourless soln.
Emizof 4mg, 8mg *(Gerard)* A. GMS.
Price, 4mg (30) €68.47. 8mg (10) €33.94.
Tablet, ondansetron hydrochloride dihydrate. Pale-yellow round f/c. 4mg: Marked 41. 8mg: Marked 42. *Lactose.*
Ondansetron Parenteral *(Accord)* A.
Price, (5) 2mL, €8.48. 4mL, €16.96.
Injection or infusion, ondansetron hydrochloride dihydrate 2mg/mL (2mL, 4mL). Clear colourless soln. *Sodium 3.62mg/mL.*
Ondansetron Parenteral *(Gerard)* A.
Price, (5) 2mL, €44.00. 4mL, €68.00.
Injection or infusion, ondansetron hydrochloride dihydrate 2mg/mL. Clear colourless soln. *Sodium 3.6mg/mL.*
Ondansetron 4mg, 8mg *(TEVA)* A. GMS.
Price, 4mg (30) €68.47. 8mg (10) €33.94.
Tablet, ondansetron HCl. Yellow oblong f/c. Marked with strength. 8mg: Scored. *Lactose.*
Ondansetron 4mg, 8mg *(Rowex)* A. GMS.
Price, 4mg (30) €68.47. 8mg (10) €33.94. 8mg (30) €101.82
Tablet, ondansetron hydrochloride dihydrate. Oval f/c. Marked O; strength on reverse. *Lactose.*
Ondansetron Parenteral *(Rowex)* A.
Price, not published by company.
Injection or infusion, ondansetron hydrochloride dihydrate 2mg/mL. Clear colourless soln.
Ondran 4mg, 8mg *(Pinewood)* A. GMS.
Price, (10) 4mg, €22.82. 8mg, €33.94.
Tablet, ondansetron. Yellow round. Marked 41 (4mg), 42 (8mg).
Ondran Parenteral *(Pinewood)* A.
Price, not published by company.
Injection, ondansetron hydrochloride dihydrate 22mg/mL. Soln.

Netupitant, Palonosetron

ATC Code: A04AA55. **Sport:** Permitted.
Driving: Moderate influence; dizziness, somnolence, fatigue.
Indications: Prevention of acute or delayed nausea and vomiting associated with moderately emetogenic or highly emetogenic cisplatin-based cancer chemotherapy.
Dose: Adult, Elderly: One capsule approx. 1 hour prior to start of each chemotherapy cycle; if co-admin, reduce the recommended oral dexamethasone dose by approx. 50%. *Elderly,* no adjustment; over 75 years, caution (long half-life; limited experience). *Admin,* with or without food; swallow whole.
Child: Safety and efficacy not established.
Renal Impairment: ESRD on dialysis, avoid (no data).

3.8.5   Propulsives

Hepatic Impairment: Severe, caution (increased netupitant exposure).

Interactions: Effect of Other Drugs Palonosetron, Netupitant: *Netupitant plasma levels affected:* CYP3A4 inhibitors or inducers. *Co-admin caution:* Strong CYP3A4 inhibitors (ketoconazole), digoxin, other P-gp substrates (dabigatran, colchicine). *Co-admin avoid:* Strong CYP3A4 inhibitors (rifampicin).

Effect of Palonosetron, Netupitant on Other Drugs: CYP3A4 substrates (docetaxel, irinotecan, other chemotherapeutic agents; chemotherapeutics needing CYP3A4 activation): *Increased exposure; efficacy affected for those needing CYP3A4 activation*.* Oral dexamethasone: *Increased dexamethasone exposure*; reduce dexamethasone dose by approx. 50%.* Midazolam, alprazolam, triazolam: *Consider potential effects of increased plasma levels.* *(due to netupitant).

Pregnancy, Lactation: Pregnancy, contraindicated; exclude before initiation; women of childbearing potential should not be pregnant or become pregnant during treatment; ensure effective contraception during and for one month after treatment. Lactation, discontinue during and for 1 month after treatment.

ADR: Summary, *common*, headache, constipation, fatigue.

Notes: See 3.8.4 5-HT3 Antagonists. See Palonosetron below.

▼ **Akynzeo 300/0.5** *(Chugai)* A.
Price, not published by company.
Capsule, netupitant 300mg, palonosetron HCl 0.5mg. Hard opaque white/caramel filled with 3 tabs and 1 soft cap. Marked HE1. *Sorbitol, sucrose.*

Palonosetron

ATC Code: A04AA05. **Sport:** Permitted.
Driving: Dizziness, somnolence, fatigue.
Indications: Nausea and vomiting associated with moderately and highly emetogenic chemotherapy.

Dose: Adult, Elderly: 250mcg as single IV bolus injection over 30 seconds approx. 30 minutes before start of chemotherapy with adjunctive corticosteroids if needed.

Child: Under 18 years, not recommended.

ADR: *Common*, headache, dizziness, constipation, diarrhoea.

Notes: See 3.8.4 5-HT3 Antagonists.

Aloxi Parenteral *(Fannin)* A.
Price, not published by company.
Injection, palonosetron HCl 250mcg/5mL. Clear colourless soln.

3.8.5 - Propulsives

In This Chapter: *Domperidone, metoclopramide.*

Class Effects
CI: Hypersensitivity to any member of the class.

Domperidone

ATC Code: A03FA03. **Sport:** Permitted.
Driving: Dizziness, somnolence observed.
Indications: Relief of symptoms of nausea and vomiting.

Dose: Adult: Under 12 years, under 35kg, not recommended. Age 12 years and older, weight 35kg or more, 10mg (1 tab or 10mL oral susp) orally up to 3-times daily; max. 30mg/day. *Admin*, before meals; if taken after food absorption may be delayed. OroDisp tab dissolves rapidly in mouth with saliva; can be taken with or without water.

Elderly: Age over 60 years, consult healthcare professional.

Child: TABS, over 12 years and over 35kg, as for Adult; under 35kg, due to need for accurate dosing, tablets are unsuitable.

ORAL SOLN, under age 12 years, weighing less than 35kg, 0.25mg/kg per intake at 4-6 hourly intervals up to 3-times daily; max. 0.75mg/kg/day. *Admin*, before food, see Adult above.

Renal Impairment: Severe (review regularly), elimination half-life prolonged; for repeated admin, reduce dose frequency to once or twice daily; dose may need to be reduced.

Hepatic Impairment: Mild, no dose modification; moderate/severe, contraindicated.

CI: Prolactin-releasing pituitary tumour (prolactinoma). Known existing prolonged cardiac conduction intervals (particularly QTc), significant electrolyte disturbances, underlying cardiac disease (CHF). When gastric motility stimulation could be harmful (GI haemorrhage, mechanical obstruction, perforation).

Interactions: Effect of Other Drugs on Domperidone: *Co-admin contraindicated:* All QTc-prolonging drugs (Torsades de Pointes risk) including antiarrhythmics Class I (disopyramide, hydroquinidine, quinidine), Class III (amiodarone, dofetilide, dronedarone, ibutilide, sotalol), antipsychotics (haloperidol, pimozide, sertindole), antidepressants (citalopram, escitalopram), erythromycin, levofloxacin, moxifloxacin, spiramycin, pentamidine, fluconazole, halofantrine, lumefantrine, cisapride, dolasetron, prucalopride, mequitazine, mizolastine, toremifene, vandetanib, vincamine, bepridil, diphemanil, methadone; potent CYP3A4 inhibitors, regardless of their QT prolonging effects, including (protease inhibitors (ritonavir, saquinavir, telaprevir), systemic azole antifungals (itraconazole, ketoconazole, posaconazole, voriconazole), macrolides (clarithromycin, telithromycin). *Co-admin not recommended:* Moderate CYP3A4 inhibitors (diltiazem, verapamil, some macrolides).

Effect of Domperidone on Other Drugs: Sustained release or enteric coated drugs: *Adjust dose due to increased gastric motility.* Dopaminergic agonists (bromocriptine, L-dopa): *Peripheral effects suppressed, central effects not antagonised.* Levodopa: *Plasma levels increased (no dose adjustment needed.*

SP: Use lowest effective dose for shortest duration to control nausea and vomiting (adults and children). Associated with QT interval prolongation (caution, electrolyte disturbances, underlying cardiac disease) and increased risk of serious ventricular arrhythmia, sudden cardiac death; at higher risk (over age 60 years, dose over 30mg/day, co-admin with QT-prolonging drugs or CYP3A4 inhibitors). Neurological effects, rare (risk higher in young children as metabolic functions and blood brain barrier are not fully developed in first months of life).

Pregnancy, Lactation: Pregnancy, if benefit outweighs risk. Lactation, stop breastfeeding or stop drug.

ADR: *Common*, dry mouth.

Notes: See 3.8.5 Propulsives.

Interchangeability: Same strengths of all domperidone f/c tabs and oral susp listed below are deemed interchangeable. Exception, *Motilium Fastmelts.*

▼ **Motilium Rx 10mg, Oral Susp** *(McNeil)* OTC. GMS.
Price, (100) €3.91. Susp (200mL) €2.25.
Tablet, domperidone. White (cream) round f/c. *Lactose.* **Store:** Below 30 deg C; do not refrigerate or freeze; original pack to protect (light).
Oral susp, as above 1mg/mL. White homogenous. **Store:** As above.

▼ **Motilium Fastmelts 10mg** *(McNeil)* OTC.
Price, not published by company.
OroDisp tablet, domperidone. White (off-white) round. *Aspartame.* **Store:** Below 25 deg C; original pack.

▼ **Domerid 10mg** *(Rowex)* B. GMS.
Price, (100) €3.82.
Tablet, domperidone maleate. White round. Marked Dm10.

Metoclopramide

ATC Code: A03FA01. **Sport:** Permitted.
Driving: Moderate influence; drowsiness, dizziness, dyskinesia, dystonia (may affect vision).
Indications: *Oral, parenteral*, prevention, delayed nausea and vomiting of chemotherapy (CINV)* and/or radiotherapy (RINV). Symptomatic treatment, nausea and vomiting including acute migraine induced. *Parenteral*, treatment of established post-operative nausea and vomiting (PONV)*. *(second-line in children).

Dose: Adult: TABS (all indications), 10mg up to 3-times daily (minimum 6-hour dose interval even if vomiting or dose rejection); max. 30mg or 0.5mg/day; max. 5 days. PARENTERAL, all indications except PONV, as for TABS above (shortest possible duration). Prevention of PONV, a single 10mg dose. *Admin*, slow bolus IV (at least 3 minutes) or IM.

138

Elderly: Consider dose reduction based on renal, hepatic function, overall frailty.

Child: TABS, CINV (age 15-18 years and over 60kg), 0.1-0.15mg/kg up to 3-times daily; max. 0.5mg/kg in 24 hours OR as for Adult above. Under 60kg or under 15 years, tabs not suitable.

PARENTERAL, all indications (age 1-18 years), 0.1-0.15mg/kg repeated up to 3-times daily by IV route (slow bolus over minimum 3 minutes); max. 0.25mg/kg in 24 hours; (age 1-3 years; 10-14kg), 1mg*; (age 3-5 years; 15-19kg), 2mg*; (age 5-9 years; 20-29kg), 2.5mg; (age 9-18 years; 30-60kg), 5mg*; (age 15-18 years; over 60kg), as for Adult above. Established PONV, max. 48 hours; nausea and vomiting of chemotherapy, max. 5 days. Under 1 year, contraindicated (oral, parenteral). *(up to 3-times daily).

Renal Impairment: CrCl (mL/min) 15-60, reduce dose by 50%; 15 and below, reduce dose by 75%.

Hepatic Impairment: Severe, reduce dose by 50%.

CI: Phaeochromocytoma (risk of severe hypertension episodes). Epilepsy (frequency, severity of seizures increased), neuroleptic or metoclopramide-induced tardive dyskinesia (or history of), Parkinson's disease. Methaemoglobinaemia or NADH cytochrome-b5 deficiency. GI haemorrhage, mechanical obstruction or perforation.

Interactions: Effect of Other Drugs on Metoclopramide: *Co-admin contraindicated:* Levodopa, dopaminergic agonists. *Co-admin avoid:* ALCOHOL. *Mutual antagonism:* Anticholinergics, morphine derivatives. *Increased serotonin syndrome risk:* SSRIs. *Increased metoclopramide exposure:* Strong CYP2D6 inhibitors (fluoxetine, paroxetine).

Effect of Metoclopramide on Other Drugs: CNS depressants (morphine derivatives, anxiolytics, sedative H1 antihistamines, sedative antidepressants, barbiturates, clonidine): *Sedative effects potentiated.* Neuroleptics: *Additive effect (extrapyramidal disorders).* Digoxin: *Decreased bioavailability.* Ciclosporin: *Increased bioavailability.* Mivacurium, suxamethonium: *Prolonged duration of neuromuscular block.*

SP: Extrapyramidal disorders may occur, especially (children, young adults, high doses); discontinue immediately (may require symptomatic treatment). May exacerbate Parkinson's Diseases. Potentially irreversible tardive dyskinesia especially in elderly (prolonged treatment). *Reported,* NMS (discontinue). methaemoglobinaemia. *Caution,* use with underlying neurological conditions; co-admin with other centrally acting drugs; history of atopy (including asthma) or porphyria, sick sinus syndrome. Not for use during first 3-4 days following surgery (pyloroplasty, gut anastomosis). Serious cardiovascular adverse events (circulatory collapse, severe bradycardia, cardiac arrest, QT prolongation), especially with IV admin. May cause elevated serum prolactin levels.

Pregnancy, Lactation: Pregnancy, can be used if clinically needed; use at end of pregnancy, cannot exclude extrapyramidal syndrome in newborn; avoid (if used monitor neonate). Lactation, not recommended.

ADR: *Very common,* somnolence; *common,* diarrhoea, asthenia, extrapyramidal disorders (see SP above), Parkinsonism, akathisia, depression, hypotension (IV).

Notes: See 3.8.5 Propulsives.

> **Maxolon 10mg** *(Concordia)* B. GMS.
> *Price,* (84) €6.87.
> *Tablet,* metoclopramide HCl. White (off-white) round scored (divisible into equal halves). Marked Maxolon. *Lactose.*
> **Metoclopramide Parenteral 5mg/mL** *(Concordia)* A.
> *Price,* 2mL (10) 10mg/2mL, €2.75 (PTW).
> *Injection,* metoclopramide HCl. Clear colourless soln. *Sodium metabisulphite.*

3.8.6 - Droperidol

In This Chapter: *Droperidol.*

Class Effects
CI: Hypersensitivity to any member of the class.

Droperidol
ATC Code: N05AD08. **Sport:** Permitted.
Driving: Major influence; patients should not drive for 24 hours after admin.

Indications: Prevention and treatment, post-operative nausea and vomiting (PONV) (adults) and second line in children/adolescents (age 2-18 years). Prevention of nausea and vomiting induced by morphine (and derivatives) during post-operative patient controlled analgesia (PCA) (adults).

Dose: Adult: PONV, 0.625-1.2mg (0.25-0.5mL); may be repeated 6-houly as needed. *Admin,* 30 minutes before anticipated end of surgery.
Prevention, PCA-associated nausea and vomiting, 15-50mcg droperidol per mg of morphine; max. 5mg droperidol per day.

Elderly: Reduce dose. PONV, 0.625mg (0.25mL) admin as for Adult above. PCA, no data.

Child: PONV, age 2-18 years, 10-50mcg/kg up to max. 1.25mg admin as for Adult above. Under 2 years, not recommended. PCA, not indicated.

Renal Impairment: As for Elderly above.

Hepatic Impairment: As for Elderly above.

CI: Butyrophenone hypersensitivity, prolonged QT interval (congenital, history), co-admin of medicinals prolonging QT interval), hypo- (kalaemia, magnesaemia), bradycardia (below 55 bpm), treatment leading to bradycardia, phaeochromocytoma, comatose states, Parkinson's Disease, severe depression.

Interactions: Effect of Other Drugs on Droperidol: *Co-admin contraindicated:* Medicinals known to cause Torsades de Pointes through QT-prolongation (Class II and III antiarrhythmics, macrolides, fluoroquinolones, antihistamines, certain antipsychotics, anti-malarials, cisapride, domperidone, methadone, pentamiline). *Co-admin avoid:* Metoclopramide (may increase extrapyramidal symptoms), ALCOHOL. *Caution:* Medicinals causing electrolyte imbalance (potassium-wasting diuretics, laxatives, glucocorticoids); strong CYP1A2 (ciprofloxacin, ticlopidine) and CYP3A4 (diltiazem, erythromycin, fluconazole, indinavir, itraconazole, ketoconazole, nefazodone, nelfinavir, ritonavir, saquinavir, verapamil) inhibitors or both (cimetidine, mibefradil) (decreased metabolism, prolonged pharmacological action). *CNS depression enhanced:* Other CNS depressants.

Effect of Droperidol on Other Drugs: Sedatives (barbiturates, benzodiazepines, morphine derivatives): *Action may be potentiated.* Dopamine agonists (bromocriptine, lisuride, L-dopa): *Action may be inhibited.*

SP: Individualise dose; consider (age, body weight, other medicinals, anaesthesia type, surgical procedure). Caution, patients with epilepsy or conditions predisposing to epilepsy or convulsions. Hyperthermia, discontinue (may be sign of malignant syndrome). Patients with history of alcohol abuse or recent high intakes, assess thoroughly before admin. Mild to moderate hypotension, occasionally (reflex) tachycardia observed; if hypotension persists, consider possible hypovolaemia. Risk factors for cardiac arrhythmia, evaluate carefully prior to admin (history of significant cardiac disease, family history of sudden death, renal failure particularly on chronic dialysis, COPD and respiratory failure, risk factors for electrolyte disturbances). Perform continuous pulse oximetry with identified or suspected ventricular arrhythmia; continue for 30 minutes following single IV admin.

Pregnancy, Lactation: Pregnancy, not recommended; in late pregnancy, if administered, monitor newborn neurological function. Lactation, limit droperidol to single admin; repeat admin not recommended.

ADR: Summary, *most frequent,* drowsiness, sedation; *less frequent,* hypotension, cardiac arrhythmias, NMS, movement disorders (dyskinesias), anxiety, agitation.

Notes: See 3.8.6 Droperidol.

> **Xomolix Parenteral** *(KyowaKirin)* A.
> *Price,* not published by company.
> *Injection,* droperidol 2.5mg/mL. Clear colourless soln free from particles. *Essentially sodium-free.*

3.9 - CNS Stimulants, Treatment of ADHD

In This Chapter: *Atomoxetine, caffeine, guanfacine, lisdexamfetamine, methylphenidate, modafinil.*

Class Effects

CI: Hypersensitivity to any member of the class.

SP: Only for initiation by a specialist in treatment of ADHD (atomoxetine, lisdexamfetamine, methylphenidate). Pre-treatment screening, cardiovascular status (BP, heart rate); comprehensive history (co-medication, medical or psychiatric disorders, family history of cardiac/unexplained death, pre-treatment height, weight). Ongoing monitoring (growth, psychiatric, cardiovascular) status. Record BP and pulse on centile chart (each dose adjustment, then 6-monthly); height, weight, appetite, psychiatric status 6-monthly. Monitor, increased pulse and/or increased BP, orthostatic hypotension (caution, hypertension), tachycardia, cardio- or cerebrovascular disease, QT-prolongation, hypotensive conditions, HF, recent MI); pre-existing structural cardiac abnormalities, sudden death (children, adolescents). Misuse associated with sudden death, serious cardiovascular adverse events. *Suicide-related* behaviour (attempts, ideation), treatment emergent psychotic/manic symptoms (hallucinations, delusional thinking, mania; agitation in children and adolescents without history of psychotic illness or mania), consider discontinuation; hostility (aggression, oppositional behaviour, anger; signs of worsening or emotional lability), monitor. Epilepsy, increased seizure risk. *Clinical evaluation* for tics and Tourette's syndrome before initiation of stimulant medications. Moderate reduced weight gain, slight growth retardation. Adolescents whose symptoms persist into adulthood and have shown clear benefit from treatment, may continue treatment into adulthood.

Pregnancy, Lactation: Pregnancy, not recommended; use only if benefit outweighs risk. Women of child-bearing age, ensure adequate contraception. Lactation, not recommended/avoid.

Notes: See manufacturers Full Prescribing Information.

Atomoxetine

ATC Code: N06BA09. **Sport:** Permitted.
Driving: Minor influence; fatigue, somnolence, dizziness.

Indications: Part of a comprehensive treatment programme for Attention Deficit Hyperactivity Disorder (ADHD) (children over 6 years, adolescents, adults).

Dose: Adult, Elderly: Initially 40mg/day for 7 days then titrate to maintenance 80mg to max. 100mg/day. *Admin,* as single daily dose in morning with or without food, or twice daily (morning, late afternoon/early evening). *Elderly,* over 65 years, not evaluated.

Child: Over *70kg,* initially 40mg/day; titrate after 7 days to maintenance 80mg/day; max. 100mg/day; *up to 70kg,* initially 0.5mg/kg; after 7 days titrate to maintenance 1.2mg/kg/day. Admin, as for Adult above.

Using oral soln, *starting dose* (16-19kg), 2mL/day; (20-28kg), 3mL/day; 29-35kg), 4mL/day; (36-44kg), 5mL/day; (45-51kg), 6mL/day; (52-59kg), 7mL/day; (60-67kg), 8mL/day; (68-69kg), 9mL/day; (70kg and above), 10mL/day. Not recommended to mix oral soln in food or water; may prevent full dose being taken or could negatively affect taste.

Renal Impairment: May exacerbate hypertension in ESRD.

Hepatic Impairment: Moderate, reduce to 50% of usual dose. Severe, reduce to 25% of usual dose.

CI: Narrow angle glaucoma, phaeochromocytoma, severe cardiovascular or cerebrovascular disorders.

Interactions: Effect of Other Drugs on Atomoxetine: *Co-admin not recommended:* MAOIs (or within 2 weeks). *Caution, additive effects:* Drugs affecting noradrenaline (imipramine, venlafaxine, mirtazapine, pseudoephedrine, phenylephrine). *Co-admin caution:* Antihypertensives, pressor agents, medication increasing BP (salbutamol). *Slower titration, final lower dosage required:* CYP2D6 inhibitors (SSRIs including fluoxetine, paroxetine;

quinidine, terbinafine). *QT-prolongation risk:* QT-prolonging drugs (neuroleptics, Class IA, III antiarrhythmics, moxifloxacin, erythromycin, methadone, mefloquine, TCADs, lithium, cisapride), drugs causing electrolyte imbalance (thiazides), CYP2D6 inhibitors. *Seizure risk:* Drugs lowering seizure threshold (TCADs or SSRIs, neuroleptics, phenothiazines or butyrophenone, mefloquine, chloroquine, bupropion, tramadol).

Effect of Atomoxetine on Other Drugs: Salbutamol or other beta-2-agonists (oral, parenteral, high-dose nebulised): *Action on cardiovascular system potentiated (monitor heart rate, BP).*

SP: Diagnosis according to current DSM criteria or ICD guidelines. Re-evaluate after 1 year. Allergic reactions (rash, angioedema, urticaria, anaphylaxis). Jaundice, liver injury, discontinue; do not restart. See Notes below. Patients developing symptoms (suggestive of cardiac disease, palpitations, exertional chest pain, unexplained syncope, dyspnoea) to undergo specialist cardiac evaluation. Caution, QT-prolongation.

Pregnancy, Lactation: Pregnancy, if benefit outweighs risk. Lactation, avoid.

ADR: *Very common, children/adolescents,* decreased appetite, headache, somnolence, abdominal pain, vomiting, nausea, increased BP/heart rate; *adults,* decreased appetite, insomnia, headache, dry mouth, nausea, increased BP/heart rate.

Notes: See 3.9 CNS Stimulants, Treatment of ADHD.

Strattera Caps, Oral Soln *(Lilly)* A. GMS.
Price, (7) 10mg, €20.50; 25mg, €20.86. (28) 10mg, €77.98; 18mg, €70.11; 25mg, €81.83; 40mg, €72.90; 60mg, €83.73; 80mg, €106.28; 100mg, €110.57. Oral soln (3x 100mL), €119.86.
Capsule, atomoxetine HCl 10mg, 18mg, 25mg, 40mg, 60mg, 80mg, 100mg. Opaque. Marked Lilly/strength. 10mg: White. 18mg: Gold/white. 25mg: Blue/white. 40mg: Blue. 60mg: Blue/gold. 80mg: Brown/white. 100mg: Brown. Marked 3227 (10mg), 3238 (18mg), 3228 (25mg), 3229 (40mg), 3239 (60mg), 3250 (80mg), 3251 (100mg).
Oral soln, as above. Clear colourless. *Sorbitol.*

Caffeine Citrate

ATC Code: N06BC01. **Sport:** Not applicable.
Driving: Not applicable.

Indications: Treatment, primary apnoea of premature newborn.

Dose: Adult, Elderly: Not applicable.

Child: Initially, loading dose 20mg/kg caffeine citrate (over 30 minutes)*; after 24-hours, maintenance 5mg/kg (over 10 minutes)* OR oral via nasogastric tube, every 24 hours. Preterm infants, insufficient response to loading dose above, second loading dose max. 10-20mg/kg may be admin after 24 hours. Consider higher maintenance of 10mg/kg if insufficient response, taking into account potential for accumulation of caffeine due to long half-life in preterm newborns. *Slow IV infusion by controlled IV infusion pump or metered device or oral. NOTE: Dose should always be expressed as *caffeine citrate.*

Renal Impairment: Limited experience, caution; frequency of adverse events may be higher (very premature infants with renal/hepatic impairment). Increased accumulation; reduce daily maintenance dose; adjust according to plasma caffeine measurements.

Hepatic Impairment: See Renal above; monitor plasma levels, adjust dose.

Interactions: Effect of Other Drugs on Caffeine Citrate: *Co-admin not recommended:* Theophylline (inter-conversion with caffeine). *Co-admin, consider dose reduction:* Cimetidine, ketoconazole. *Co-admin, consider dose increase:* Phenobarbital, phenytoin. *Increased necrotising enterocolitis risk:* H2-antagonists, PPIs. *Monitor cardiac rhythm, BP with co-admin:* Doxapram.

SP: For admin only in a neonatal intensive care unit. Exclude other causes of apnoea (CNS disorders, primary lung disease, anaemia, sepsis, metabolic disturbances, cardiovascular abnormalities, obstructive apnoea) prior to initiation. Measure baseline caffeine levels before initiation (especially if mothers have ingested large quantities of caffeine prior to delivery, infants previously treated with theophylline).

Caution, consider dose adjustment in risk situations (very premature infants particularly when receiving parenteral nutrition, infants with hepatic/renal impairment, seizure disorders, known cardiovascular disease, medicinals interfering with caffeine metabolism, mothers consuming caffeine while breastfeeding). Necrotising enterocolitis, monitor. Increased metabolism may result in higher energy and nutritional requirements. Fluid and electrolyte disturbances.

Pregnancy, Lactation: Caffeine is excreted in breast milk; readily crosses placenta into foetal circulation. Breastfeeding mothers should not ingest caffeine-containing (food, beverages, medicinals) while neonates treated with caffeine citrate.

ADR: Summary, CNS stimulation (convulsion, irritability, restlessness, jitteriness), cardiac effects (tachycardia, arrhythmia, hypertension, increased stroke volume), metabolic disorders (hyperglycaemia), infusion-site phlebitis/inflammation.

Notes: See 3.9 CNS Stimulants, Treatment of ADHD.
Peyona Infusion and Oral Soln *(Chiesi)* A.
Price, not published by company.
Infusion or oral soln, caffeine citrate 20mg/1mL (equiv. to caffeine base 10mg/mL). Clear colourless aqueous soln. pH 4.7.

Guanfacine
ATC Code: C02AC02. **Sport:** Pending.
Driving: Moderate to severe influence; dizziness, somnolence, syncope.
Indications: Treatment, attention deficit disorder (ADHD), age 6-17 (stimulants not suitable/tolerated or ineffective).
Dose: Adult, Elderly: For use age 6-17 years.
Child: 1mg once daily; increase by max. 1mg per week; maintenance range 0.05-0.12mg/kg/day depending on response and tolerability. Under 6 years, safety/efficacy not established. *Admin,* oral morning or evening; swallow tablets whole; do not crush, chew or break (increases guanfacine release rate); with or without food; do not admin with a high fat meal (increased exposure) or grapefruit juice. See Interactions, SP and Notes below.
Renal Impairment: GFR (mL/min) 29-15 and below 15 (ESRD) or requiring dialysis, may require dose adjustment.
Hepatic Impairment: May require dose adjustment.
Interactions: Effect of Other Drugs on Guanfacine: *Dose adjustment recommended*: Moderate/strong CYP3A4/5 inhibitors (ketoconazole, grapefruit juice) (50% guanfacine reduction); strong enzyme inducers (re-titrate to increase dose up to max. daily dose of 7mg). *Co-admin caution*: Medicinals reducing BP or heart rate (increased syncope risk) (advise patients to drink plenty of fluid). *Additive effect*: Drugs causing sedation, hypotension, QT-prolongation; CNS depressants (ALCOHOL, sedatives, hypnotics, benzodiazepines, barbiturates, antipsychotics). See Notes below.
Effect of Guanfacine on Other Drugs: Valproic acid, metformin: *Increased concentrations.*
SP: *Screen pre-treatment* for increased risk for somnolence, sedation, hypotension, bradycardia, QT-prolongation arrhythmia, weight increase or obesity; establish cardiovascular status (BP, heart rate), co-medication, co-morbidity (psychiatric, medical), family history; record pre-treatment height, weight and BMI. Caution, patients with these risk factors. *Monitor* every 3 months during year 1 (somnolence, sedation, hypotension, bradycardia, weight increase), then 6-monthly. *Down titration, discontinuation,* monitor BP, pulse. Emergent suicidal ideation or behaviour, evaluate.
Pregnancy, Lactation: Pregnancy and women of child bearing potential not using contraception, not recommended. Lactation, stop drug or stop breastfeeding.
ADR: Summary, *most frequent,* somnolence*, headache, fatigue, upper abdominal pain, sedation*; *serious, common,* hypotension, weight increase, bradycardia, syncope. *(start of treatment; may last for 2-3 weeks or longer).

Notes: See Manufacturers Full Prescribing Information. See 3.9 CNS Stimulants, Treatment of ADHD.
▼ **Intuniv 1mg, 2mg, 3mg, 4mg** *(Shire)* A. GMS.
Price, (28) 1mg, €74.11; 2mg, €77.36; 3mg, €86.62; 4mg, €100.71.
Prolonged/R Tablet, guanfacine HCl. Marked with strength in MG; 503 on reverse. 1mg: White (off-white) round. 2mg: White (off-white) oval. 3mg: Green round. 4mg: Green oblong. *Lactose.*

Lisdexamfetamine
ATC Code: L06BA12. **Sport:** Prohibited (in-competition).
Driving: Dizziness, drowsiness, visual disturbances (accommodation difficulty, diplopia, blurred vision).
Indications: Part of a comprehensive treatment programme for Attention Deficit Hyperactivity Disorder (ADHD) (children over 6 years, adolescents) (response to previous methylphenidate clinically inadequate).
Dose: Adult: See Child below.
Child: Age 6 years and older, initially 30mg once daily in morning; increase by 20mg at approx. weekly intervals to max. 70mg/day. Always use lowest effective dose. Paradoxal symptom aggravation, reduce dose or discontinue. *Admin,* swallow whole with or without food; capsule may be opened and contents dissolved in water or orange juice or mixed with soft food (yoghurt).
Renal Impairment: Dose reduction may be needed.
CI: Hyperthyroidism or thyrotoxicosis, agitated states, symptomatic cardiovascular disease, advanced arteriosclerosis, moderate or severe hypertension, glaucoma.
Interactions: Effect of Other Drugs on Lisdexamfetamine: *Co-admin contraindicated*: MAOIs (or within 2 weeks). *Co-admin caution*: Other sympathomimetics. *Increased urinary excretion, decreased half-life*: Urinary acidifiers. *Decreased urinary excretion, increased half-life*: Urinary alkalinisers (sodium bicarbonate, thiazides). *Reduced amphetamine effect*: Chlorpromazine, haloperidol, lithium. *Serotonin syndrome*: SSRIs, SNRIs.
Effect of Lisdexamfetamine on Other Drugs: Antihypertensives, guanethidine: *Decreased efficacy.* Narcotic analgesics: *Effect potentiated.*
SP: Cardiomyopathy (chronic use). See Notes below. May interfere with urinary steroid determinations.
Pregnancy, Lactation: Pregnancy, only if benefit outweighs risk. Lactation, not recommended.
ADR: Summary, *very common* (all age groups), decreased appetite, insomnia, dry mouth, headache, weight decreased.
Notes: See 3.9 CNS Stimulants, Treatment of ADHD.
▼ **Tyvense 30mg, 50mg, 70mg** *(Shire)* A. GMS.
Price, (28) 30mg, €73.48. 50mg, €84.67. 70mg, €100.33.
Capsule, lisdexamfetamine dimesylate. Opaque hard. Marked with strength and S489. 30mg: White/pink. 50mg: White/blue. 70mg: Blue/pink.

Methylphenidate
ATC Code: N06BA04. **Sport:** Prohibited (in-competition).
Driving: Dizziness, drowsiness, visual disturbances. See SP below.
Indications: Part of a comprehensive treatment programme for Attention Deficit Hyperactivity Disorder (ADHD) (children over 6 years, adolescents).
Dose: Adult, Elderly: Generally not for initiation/use.
Child: STANDARD/R, initially 5mg once or twice daily (breakfast, lunch); titrate by 5-10mg/day (weekly); max. 40-60mg. *Admin,* divided doses; last dose minimum 4 hours before bedtime.
PROLONGED/R, *Concerta XL,* increase by 18mg/day; max. 54mg/day. New patients, initially 18mg/day* or lower dose of short-acting. Current users, switch (Standard/R TO Prolonged/R), 5mg 3-times daily TO 18mg/day*; 10mg 3-times daily TO 36mg/day*; 15mg 3-times daily to 54mg/day*. Paradoxical symptom aggravation or adverse events, reduce dose or discontinue. *(once daily).
Equasym XL, initially, as for Standard/R above. Current users, switch to milligram (mg) equiv. of Prolonged/R; max. 60mg/day. Initiate under specialist care.

3.9 CNS Stimulants, Treatment of ADHD

Medikinet MR, initially as for Standard/R above. Consists of immediate-release component (50%) and Modified/R component (50%) (maintains treatment through afternoon without midday dose). *Switch*, as for *Equasym* above.

Ritalin LA, switch (Standard/R to Prolonged/R), 10mg twice daily TO 20mg/day*; 15mg 3-times daily TO 30mg/day*; 20mg twice daily TO 40mg/day*. *(once daily).

Prolonged/R should be used when, if taken in the morning, an effect lasting through day into evening is required (do not take too late; may cause sleep disturbance). *Admin*, oral, once daily with or without food. NOTE: *Medikinet* MUST be taken with food; swallow tabs/caps whole with liquid; do not crush, break or chew. Cap contents may be sprinkled over small amount of soft food; admin immediately.

CI: Marked anxiety, tension, Tourette's syndrome and motor tics, glaucoma, hyperthyroidism or thyrotoxicosis, phaeochromocytoma. Drug dependence or alcoholism; severe depression, anorexia nervosa, psychotic symptoms, schizophrenia, aggression, suicidal tendency. Episodic (Type I) Bipolar (affective) disorder; pre-existing cardiovascular disorders (severe hypertension, HF, arterial occlusive disease, congenital heart disease, cardiomyopathies, MI, life-threatening arrhythmias, channelopathies, angina pectoris) unless paediatric cardiac advice obtained; pre-existing cerebrovascular disorders (cerebral aneurysm, vascular abnormalities).

Interactions: Effect of Other Drugs on Methylphenidate: *Co-admin contraindicated*: MAOIs (or within 2 weeks), antipsychotics (counteracting mechanism). *Co-admin caution*: Drugs with narrow therapeutic window. *Co-admin not recommended (increased CNS adverse events)*: ALCOHOL. *Hypertension risk*: Vasopressor agents, halogenated anaesthetics (sudden BP increase risk; do not use methylphenidate on day of surgery). *Urinary clearance* changed*: Urinary acidifiers (increased*); urinary alkalinisers (decreased*). *Long-term safety not evaluated*: Alpha-2-agonists (clonidine).

Effect of Methylphenidate on Other Drugs: Coumarin anticoagulants, anticonvulsants (phenobarbitone, phenytoin, primidone), phenylbutazone, TCADs: *Metabolism inhibited; adjust dose, monitor.* Guanethidine, antihypertensives: *Antihypertensive effect decreased.*

SP: *Driving*, visual disturbance (accommodation difficulties, blurred vision); ability to drive likely affected; may be an offence to drive while under the influence of this medicine.

Symptoms of behaviour disturbance, thought disorder exacerbated in psychotic patients. Caution, drug dependence, alcohol abuse, conditions compromised by increased BP or heart rate. Monitor, FBC, platelets (prolonged therapy). Priapism reported usually with treatment regimen change; seek medical advice. Supervise withdrawal carefully; may unmask depression, chronic over-activity. May induce false positive lab tests for amphetamines. With acute (psychosis, mania, suicidality), treat/control before ADHD treatment considered. Aggressive or hostile behaviour, titrate up or down or interrupt treatment. See Notes below.

Concerta XL, pre-existing severe GI narrowing, dysphagia, swallowing difficulties; advise patient tab shell may appear in faeces.

Pregnancy, Lactation: Pregnancy, contraindicated unless postponing treatment is greater risk to pregnancy; neonatal cardiorespiratory toxicity (foetal tachycardia, respiratory distress). Lactation, stop drug or stop breastfeeding; excreted into breast milk.

ADR: *Very common*, insomnia, nervousness, headache. Attempted suicide, see SP above.

Notes: See 3.9 CNS Stimulants, Treatment of ADHD.

Concerta XL 18mg, 27mg, 36mg *(Janssen-Cilag)* CD. GMS.
Price, (30) 18mg, €20.21. 27mg, €23.36. 36mg, €27.51.
Prolonged/R tablet, methylphenidate HCl. Cap-shaped. Marked alza/strength. 18mg: Yellow. 27mg: Grey. 36mg: White. *Lactose*.

Store: Below 30 deg C; bottle tightly closed to protect (moisture).
Equasym XL 10mg, 20mg, 30mg *(Shire)* CD. GMS.
Price, (30) 10mg, €17.24. 20mg, €20.67. 30mg, €33.76.
Prolonged/R capsule, methylphenidate HCl. Hard opaque. Marked S544/strength. 10mg: Dark-green/white. 20mg: Blue/white. 30mg: Reddish-brown/white. *Sucrose*.
Medikinet 5mg, 10mg, 20mg, MR *(Flynn)* CD. GMS.
Price, (30) 5mg, €3.30. 10mg, €4.92. 20mg, €11.43. MR (30) 5mg, €12.85. 10mg, €17.03. 20mg, €30.32. 30mg, €39.23. 40mg, €51.65.
Standard/R tablet, methylphenidate HCl. White round scored (divisible into equal halves). 5mg: Marked D. 10mg: Marked M. 20mg: Marked L. *Lactose*.
Modified/R capsule (MR), as above 5mg, 10mg, 20mg, 30mg, 40mg. Opaque hard; contain white and blue pellets. 5mg: White. 10mg: White/mauve. 20mg: Mauve. 30mg, 40mg: Dark-violet/light-grey. *Sucrose*.
Ritalin 10mg, LA 20mg, 30mg, 40mg *(Novartis)* CD. GMS.
Price, (30) 10mg, €5.73. LA (30) 20mg, €27.70. 30mg, €35.40. 40mg, €49.38.
Standard/R tablet, methylphenidate HCl 10mg. White round flat scored (facilitates breaking; does not divide into equal doses). Marked CG; AB on reverse. *Lactose*. **Store:** Below 25 deg C; original pack to protect (moisture).
Prolonged/R capsule (LA), as above. Hard gelatin opaque. Marked NVR and R/strength. 20mg: White. 30mg: Yellow. 40mg: Light brown. *Sucrose*. **Store:** Below 30 deg C; bottle tightly closed to protect (moisture).

Modafinil

ATC Code: N06BA07. **Sport:** Prohibited (in-competition).
Driving: Level of wakefulness may not be normal; assess level of sleepiness; blurred vision, dizziness.

Indications: Excessive sleepiness associated with narcolepsy with or without cataplexy.

Dose: Adult: Initially 200mg/day; insufficient response, increase up to 400mg/day. Single daily dose (morning) or as 2 doses (morning, noon). *Admin*, swallow tabs whole.

Elderly: Over 65 years, initially 100mg/day.

Child: Under 18 years, not recommended.

Hepatic Impairment: Severe, reduce dose by half.

CI: Uncontrolled moderate to severe hypertension, cardiac arrhythmia.

Interactions: Effect of Other Drugs on Modafinil: *Plasma levels decreased*: Anticonvulsants (carbamazepine, phenobarbital).

Effect of Modafinil on Other Drugs: Phenytoin, warfarin: *Decreased clearance (monitor)*. Oral contraceptives: *Effectiveness reduced*. TCADs, diazepam, propranolol, omeprazole: *Dosage reduction*. Ciclosporin, HIV-protease inhibitors, buspirone, triazolam, midazolam, calcium channel blockers, statins: *Plasma levels decreased*.

SP: Serious rash (including Stevens-Johnson Syndrome, toxic epidermal necrosis, DRESS); first sign of rash, discontinue and do not re-start. Multi-organ hypersensitivity, psychiatric symptoms, discontinue (caution, psychiatric disorders including psychosis, depression, mania, major anxiety, agitation, insomnia, substance abuse). Onset or worsening of anxiety, psychotic or manic symptoms, hostile or aggressive behaviour. Caution, co-morbid bipolar disorder. Suicide-related behaviour including attempt, ideation.

Hypertensive patients, monitor BP, heart rate; underlying conditions, associated cardiovascular pathology, monitor. LVH or cor pulmonale, mitral valve prolapse (ischaemic ECG changes chest pain, arrhythmia), not recommended. Advise patients to maintain good sleep hygiene; insomnia, caution. Caution, admin with history of alcohol, drug, illicit substance abuse; low potential for dependence but cannot be excluded.

ADR: *Very common*, headache.

Notes: See 3.9 CNS Stimulants, Treatment of ADHD.

Provigil 100mg, 200mg *(TEVA)* A. GMS.
Price, (30) 100mg, €58.53. 200mg, €117.13.
Tablet, modafinil. White (off-white) cap-shaped. Marked with strength. *Lactose*.
Prosentio 100mg, 200mg *(Clonmel)* A. GMS.
Price, (30) 100mg, €23.41. 200mg, €46.85.
Tablet, modafinil. White (off-white) cap-shaped. Marked M; 100 MG on reverse. *Lactose*.

4

Analgesics, Anti-Inflammatories, Musculoskeletal Disorders

4.1 - Migraine

Class Effects
Prochlorperazine is also indicated for migraine management, see Notes below.

CI: Hypersensitivity to any member of the class.

SP: A definite migraine diagnosis should be made. Before treating acute attacks exclude other neurological conditions. Prolonged use or overuse of any type of painkiller for headaches or migraine can make them worse. Consider Medication Overuse Headache (MOH) if frequent or daily headaches despite (or because of) regular headache medication use.

Notes: See 4.2.1 Non-Opioid Analgesics, 4.4.2 NSAIDS (Non-Selective) and 3.2.1 Phenothiazines (prochlorperazine).

4.1.1 - Analgesics, Anti-Emetics

In This Chapter: *Paracetamol metoclopramide combination.*

Class Effects
Buclizine, codeine phosphate, paracetamol combination is also used for migraine *(Migraleve)*. Codeine-containing products, see Notes below (codeine).

Notes: See 4.1 Migraine. See 4.2.1 Non-Opioid Analgesics (codeine combinations).

Paracetamol, Metoclopramide
ATC Code: N02BE51. **Sport:** Permitted.
Driving: Caution.

Indications: Management, symptoms (pain, nausea, vomiting) associated with a migraine attack.

Dose: Adult, Elderly: 2 tabs at first warning of attack; may repeat to max. 6 tabs in 24 hours. Young adults (18-20 years), max. 5 tabs in 24 hours (max. metoclopramide 0.5mg/kg).

Child: Age 1-18 years, not recommended; under 1 year, contraindicated (increased pyramidal disorder risk).

Renal Impairment: CrCl (mL/min) 11-60, reduce daily dose by 50%; below 15, reduce daily dose by 75%.

Hepatic Impairment: Severe, reduce dose by 50%.

CI: GI haemorrhage, mechanical obstruction or perforation (stimulation of GI motility is a risk); immediate post-op (up to 3-4 days) following pyloroplasty or gut anastomosis;

history of neuroleptic or metoclopramide-induced tardive dyskinesia; confirmed epilepsy (benzamides may decrease epileptic threshold; increase seizure frequency and severity); phaeochromocytoma (risk of severe hypertensive episodes); Parkinson's disease; (history of) methaemoglobinaemia with metoclopramide or NADH cytochrome-b5 reductase deficiency.

Interactions: Effect of Other Drugs on Paracetamol, Metoclopramide Combination: *Mutual antagonism**: Levodopa, dopaminergics (co-admin contraindicated); anticholinergics, morphine derivatives. *Sedative effects potentiated**: ALCOHOL, CNS depressants (morphine derivatives, hypnotics, anxiolytics, sedative H1-antihistamines, sedative antidepressants, barbiturates, clonidine). *Increased clearance rate of paracetamol*: Oral contraceptives. *Paracetamol absorption speed increased*: Domperidone. *Paracetamol absorption speed decreased*: Colestyramine. *Co-admin**: Drugs with potential central stimulant effects (MAOIs, sympathomimetics) effect modified, dose may need adjustment. *Additive effect* (extrapyramidal effects)*: Neuroleptics. *(metoclopramide).

Effect of Paracetamol, Metoclopramide on Other Drugs: Paracetamol: *Chloramphenicol (elimination half-life increased), warfarin, other coumarins (anticoagulant effect enhanced; increased bleeding risk).* Metoclopramide: *Digoxin, ciclosporin (increased bioavailability; monitor plasma levels).*

SP: Severe-cutaneous reactions (including life threatening), Stevens-Johnson syndrome, toxic epidermal necrolysis (reported with paracetamol); advise patient (progressive skin rash with blisters or mucosal lesions); discontinue. Vomiting with rejection of dose, wait specified interval before re-admin to avoid overdose. Renal or severe hepatic impairment, consider dose reduction (loss of conjugation, increased extrapyramidal effect risk). Parkinson's disease, careful risk-benefit (symptoms may be exacerbated). Extrapyramidal disorders, caution. Epileptic threshold may be decreased. Metoclopramide may induce Torsade de Pointes, (caution).

Pregnancy, Lactation: Pregnancy, if judged necessary by physician. Lactation, stop breastfeeding or stop drug.

ADR: Extrapyramidal symptoms (incidence greater in children, young adults with metoclopramide above 0.5mg/kg/day); tardive dyskinesia (incidence greater neuroleptic co-admin); drowsiness, restlessness, decreased level of consciousness, increased muscle tone, anxiety, depression, hallucination, confusion (higher metoclopramide doses), suicidal ideation, NMS; diarrhoea, haematological disorders, hyperprolactinaemia associated amenorrhea, galactorrhoea, gynaecomastia, hypersensitivity (anaphylaxis), asthenia, skin rash, hypotension, bradycardia, heart block (especially IV).

Notes: See 3.8.5 Propulsives (metoclopramide).

Paramax 500/5 Tablets *(SANOFI)* B. GMS.
Price, (14) €1.56.
Tablet, paracetamol, metoclopramide HCl 500/5mg. White round scored (facilitates breaking). Marked Paramax.

4.1.2 - Acute Migraine, 5HT1-Agonists

In This Chapter: *Almotriptan, eletriptan, frovatriptan, naratriptan, sumatriptan, zolmitriptan.*

Class Effects
CI: Migraine prophylaxis. Use in children and adolescents under 18 years. Elderly, over 65 years unless otherwise stated. Confirmed CAD (previous MI, angina pectoris, confirmed silent ischaemia), signs/symptoms of ischaemic heart disease or Prinzmetal's angina (drug class associated with coronary vasospasm). Hypertension (moderate to severe, uncontrolled or untreated mild or moderate). CVA or TIA, peripheral vascular disease, severe hepatic impairment.

Interactions: Effect of Other Drugs on 5HT1-Agonists: *Co-admin caution*: Ergotamine and derivatives (including methysergide) (co-admin contraindicated); 5-HT 1B/1D agonists, triptans (co-admin avoid); allow 6-hour interval after 5HT1-agonist admin before ergotamine; allow 24-

4.1.2 Acute Migraine, 5HT1-Agonists

hour interval after ergotamine admin before 5HT1-agonist. Co-admin caution (serotonin syndrome risk): St John's Wort; SSRIs (fluoxetine, paroxetine, sertraline), SNRIs (venlafaxine, duloxetine), MAOIs, triptans.

SP: Admin as early as possible after headache onset; are effective if taken at a later stage. Do not exceed dose. Use only if there is a clear diagnosis of migraine. Caution, high cardiovascular risk, postmenopausal women, males over 40, other risk factors for CHD e.g. uncontrolled hypertension, hypercholesterolaemia, obesity, diabetes, smoking, family history of cardiovascular disease (evaluate for cardiac disease); cerebral and/or subarachnoid haemorrhage, stroke, other cerebrovascular events reported (CVA, TIA). Serotonin Syndrome, potentially life-threatening; altered mental status (agitation, hallucinations, coma), autonomic instability (tachycardia, labile BP, hyperthermia), neuromuscular abnormalities (hyperreflexia, in-coordination) and/or GI symptoms (nausea, vomiting, diarrhoea). Medication overuse headaches, see Notes below.

Pregnancy, Lactation: Caution, pregnancy, use only if clearly needed; lactation, minimise infant exposure by avoiding breastfeeding for 24 hours post-treatment.

Notes: See 4.1 Migraine.

Almotriptan

ATC Code: N02CC05. **Sport:** Permitted.
Driving: Somnolence.

Indications: Treatment, acute migraine.

Dose: Adult, Elderly: Age 18-65 years, initially 12.5mg; a second dose can be taken if symptoms reappear within 24 hours; minimum 2-hour interval between doses. Max. 25mg in 24 hours. Elderly, over 65 years, caution. Admin, with liquid, with or without food.

Renal Impairment: Severe, max. 12.5mg in 24 hours.

SP: Caution, sulfonamide hypersensitivity. Coronary vasospasm, MI, transient chest pain, tightness. Mild, transient BP increase; especially elderly.

Pregnancy, Lactation: Animal studies do not indicate direct or indirect harmful effects.

ADR: Common, dizziness, somnolence, nausea, vomiting, fatigue.

Notes: See 4.1.2 Acute Migraine, 5HT1-Agonists.

Almogran 12.5mg (Almirall) B. GMS.
Price, (3) €12.23. (6) €20.90. (9) €35.28.
Tablet, almotriptan D,L-hydrogen malate equiv. to almotriptan 12.5mg. White round f/c. Marked A. Mannitol.

Eletriptan

ATC Code: N02CC06. **Sport:** Permitted.
Driving: Caution.

Indications: Acute treatment, headache phase of migraine with or without aura.

Dose: Adult, Elderly: Age 18 years and over, initially 40mg; if headache recurs within 24 hours, a second dose of same strength may be taken; minimum interval 2 hours. No response after first dose, do not take a second dose. Efficacy not obtained with 40mg, max. 80mg may be used in subsequent attacks. Elderly, over 65 years, not recommended. Swallow whole with water.

Renal Impairment: Mild to moderate, initially 20mg; max. 40mg. Severe, contraindicated.

Hepatic Impairment: Severe, contraindicated.

CI: Significant arrhythmias, heart failure.

Interactions: Effect of Other Drugs on Eletriptan: Co-admin not recommended: Potent CYP3A4 inhibitors (ketoconazole itraconazole, erythromycin, clarithromycin, josamycin, ritonavir, indinavir, nelfinavir).

SP: Not for treatment of headache related to stroke, aneurysm rupture; cerebrovascular vasoconstriction may be harmful. Increased BP especially with renal impairment and the elderly.

ADR: Summary, most common, asthenia, somnolence, nausea and dizziness.

Notes: See 4.1.2 Acute Migraine, 5HT1-Agonists.

Relpax 40mg (Pfizer) B. GMS.
Price, (6) €22.26.
Tablet, eletriptan hydrobromide. Round orange f/c. Marked REP 40; Pfizer on reverse. Lactose, Sunset Yellow.

Frovatriptan

ATC Code: N02CC07. **Sport:** Permitted.
Driving: Caution.

Indications: Treatment, acute migraine.

Dose: Adult: Initially 2.5mg; if migraine recurs, a second dose may be taken after minimum interval of 2 hours; max. 5mg/day. Tabs to be swallowed whole with water.

Interactions: Effect of Other Drugs on Frovatriptan: Co-admin not recommended: MAOIs. Co-admin caution: SSRIs (citalopram, fluoxetine, fluvoxamine, paroxetine, sertraline), potential hypertension, coronary vasoconstriction, serotonin syndrome risk; methylergometrine, hypertension, coronary artery constriction risk. Plasma levels increased: Fluvoxamine, oral contraceptives.

SP: Hypersensitivity reactions (cutaneous, angioedema, anaphylaxis); if serious, discontinue and do not re-admin.

ADR: Summary, most common, dizziness, fatigue, paraesthesia, headache, vascular flushing.

Notes: See 4.1.2 Acute Migraine, 5HT1-Agonists.

Frovex 2.5mg (A.Menarini) B. GMS.
Price, (2) €6.87. (6) €19.01.
Tablet, frovatriptan succinate monohydrate equiv. to frovatriptan 2.5mg. Round white f/c. Marked m; 2.5 on reverse. Lactose.

Naratriptan

ATC Code: N02CC02. **Sport:** Permitted.
Driving: Drowsiness.

Indications: Treatment, acute migraine.

Dose: Adult, Elderly: Age 18 years and over, initially 2.5mg; if migraine recurs, a second dose may be taken after minimum of 4 hours; max. 5mg in any 24-hour period. Elderly, over 65 years, not recommended. Admin, swallow tabs whole with water.

Renal Impairment: Mild/moderate, max. 2.5mg/day. Severe, contraindicated.

Hepatic Impairment: As for Renal above.

SP: Transient, chest pain or tightness may occur (may be intense and involve throat); if thought to be ischaemic heart disease, discontinue. Sulfonamide hypersensitivity.

ADR: Common, nausea, vomiting, sensation of heat, malaise/fatigue. See SP above.

Notes: See 4.1.2 Acute Migraine, 5HT1-Agonists.

Naraverg 2.5mg (TEVA) B. GMS.
Price, (6) €27.77. (12) €55.54.
Tablet, naratriptan HCl. Green round f/c. Marked NT 2.5. Lactose.

Sumatriptan

ATC Code: N02CC01. **Sport:** Permitted.
Driving: Caution.

Indications: Treatment, acute migraine with or without aura. Menstrual associated migraine.

Dose: Adult: ORAL, usually 50mg as single dose; 100mg may be required. If patient responded to first dose but symptoms recur, 1 or 2 additional doses may be given in next 24 hours; max. 300mg in 24 hours; minimum dose interval of 2 hours. If patient does not respond to first dose, a second dose should not be taken for the same attack (treat with paracetamol, aspirin or NSAIDs). Swallow tabs whole with water; swallowing difficulties, Imigran Ftab may be dispersed in small amount of water before admin; bitter taste.

NASAL SPRAY, 18 years and over (not for prophylactic use), optimum 20mg admin into 1 nostril (10mg may be effective in some patients). Subsequent dosing as for oral; max. 4x10mg nasal sprays in 24 hours (2x 20mg doses). If no response to first dose, a second dose should not be taken for same attack.

Elderly: Over 65 years, not recommended.

Child: NASAL SPRAY, adolescents (12-17 years), on specialist recommendation. 10mg admin into 1 nostril; if there is response to first dose but symptoms recur, a second dose may be admin in next 24 hours; minimum 2 hours between doses; max. 2x 10mg sprays in 24 hours. If patient does not respond to first dose, a second dose should not be taken for same attack (treat with paracetamol, aspirin or NSAIDs). Under 12 years, not recommended.

ORAL, under 17 years, not recommended.

Renal Impairment: Caution.

Hepatic Impairment: Caution. Severe, not recommended.

CI: Seizures, risk factors lowering seizure threshold, caution. Known hypersensitivity to sulfonamides.

Interactions: Effect of Other Drugs on Sumatriptan: Co-admin contraindicated: MAOIs (or within 2 weeks), MAOI + SSRIs in combination, ergotamine preparations (allow 24-hour interval following ergotamine; allow 6-hour interval following sumatriptan use).

SP: Do not exceed dose. Transient, symptoms of chest pain or tightness (may be intense and involve the throat), increases in BP and peripheral vascular resistance (caution, hypertensives).

Pregnancy, Lactation: Not recommended.

ADR: *Very common,* dysgeusia, unpleasant taste (spray). *Parenteral,* transient injection-site reactions.

Notes: See 4.1.2 Acute Migraine, 5HT1-Agonists.

Imigran Ftab 50mg, 100mg, Nasal Spray *(GSK)* B. GMS.
Price, 50mg (2) €8.02; (6) €20.46. 100mg (2) €11.26; (6) €30.03. Spray 10mg (2) €11.16; (6) €33.47. 20mg (2) €15.92; (6) €47.75.
Tablet, sumatriptan succinate equiv. to sumatriptan 50mg or 100mg. Triangular f/c. Marked with strength. 50mg: Pink. Marked GS 1YM. 100mg: White. Marked GS YE7.
Nasal spray, as above. 10mg or 20mg/0.1mL soln in nasal applicator. Clear pale (dark yellow) buffered.
Sumatran 50mg, 100mg *(Rowex)* B. GMS.
Price, 50mg (2) €4.22; (6) €12.66. 100mg (2) €7.44; (6) €22.32.
Tablet, sumatriptan succinate. Oblong scored both sides. 50mg: Pink. 100mg: White (off-white). *Lactose.*
Sumatriptan (Accord) 50mg, 100mg *(Accord)* B. GMS.
Price, (6) 50mg, €12.66. 100mg, €22.32.
Tablet, sumatriptan succinate. Cap-shaped f/c. 50mg: Pink. 100mg: White (off-white). *Lactose.*

Zolmitriptan

ATC Code: N02CC03. **Sport:** Permitted.
Driving: Caution.
Indications: Treatment, acute migraine.

Dose: Adult: Initially 2.5mg; if symptoms recur within 24 hours, a second dose may be taken after minimum 2 hours. Relief not achieved with 2.5mg, consider 5mg for subsequent attacks; max. (10mg/day; 2 doses in 24 hours). *Admin,* swallow tabs whole with water. Orodispersible tablet rapidly dissolves when placed on tongue; swallow with saliva.

Renal Impairment: CrCl (mL/min) below 15, not recommended.

Hepatic Impairment: Severe, max. 5mg in 24 hours.

Interactions: Effect of Other Drugs on Zolmitriptan: Plasma levels increased *(max. dose zolmitriptan 5mg in 24 hours):* Moclobemide (dose over 300mg/day, co-admin not recommended); cimetidine, other CYP1A2 inhibitors (fluvoxamine, quinolones).

SP: Symptomatic Wolff-Parkinson-White syndrome or arrhythmias associated with cardiac accessory conduction pathways, not recommended.

ADR: *Common,* abdominal pain, dry mouth, nausea, vomiting, dysphagia, muscle weakness, myalgia, abnormal or disturbed sensation, dizziness, headache, hyperaesthesia, paraesthesia, somnolence, warm sensation, palpitations, asthenia; heaviness, tightness, pain or pressure in throat, neck, limbs or chest.

Notes: See 4.1.2 Acute Migraine, 5HT1-Agonists.

Zomig 2.5mg, Rapimelt 2.5mg *(AstraZeneca)* B. GMS.
Price, 2.5mg (3) €7.89. (6) €15.80. Rapimelt (2) €5.27. (6) €15.80.
Tablet, zolmitriptan. Yellow f/c. Marked Z. *Lactose.* **Store:** Below 30 deg C.

OroDisp tablet (Rapimelt), as above. Round white u/c. Marked Z. *Aspartame.* **Store:** As above.
Zolmitriptan Actavis 2.5mg OroDisp *(Accord)* B. GMS.
Price, (2) €4.21. (6) €12.64.
OroDisp tablet, zolmitriptan. White round flat. *Aspartame.*

4.1.3 - Migraine Prophylaxis

In This Chapter: *Clonidine, flunarizine.*

Class Effects
A number of different drug classes are also indicated for migraine prophylaxis, see Notes below.

Notes: See 2.1.7 Beta-Blockers (metoprolol, propranolol). See 3.1.6 Miscellaneous Antiepileptics (topiramate).

Clonidine (migraine prophylaxis)

ATC Code: N02CX02. **Sport:** Permitted.
Driving: Dizziness, sedation, accommodation disorder.
Indications: Prophylaxis, migraine or recurrent vascular headache. Menopausal flushing.

Dose: Adult, Elderly: Initially 50mcg twice daily; titrate after 2 weeks to 75mcg twice daily.

Child: Under 18 years, not recommended. Off-label use with methylphenidate in ADHD, serious adverse reactions (including death) reported.

Renal Impairment: Caution; monitor blood pressure.

CI: Severe bradyarrhythmia (sick-sinus syndrome, AV block of second or third degree).

Interactions: Effect of Other Drugs on Clonidine: *Alpha 2-receptor effects antagonised:* Alpha 2-receptor blockers. *Bradycardia or dysrhythmia (AV-block):* Beta-blockers, cardiac glycosides. *PVD risk:* Beta-blockers. *Orthostatic hypotension risk:* TCADs, neuroleptics (with alpha-receptor blocking properties). *Effect antagonised:* TCADs. *Effect potentiated:* Tranquilisers, hypnotics, ALCOHOL.
Effect of Clonidine on Other Drugs: Antihypertensives, vasodilators, diuretics: *Increased hypotensive effect.*

SP: *Caution,* cerebrovascular disease, coronary insufficiency, HF, occlusive PVD (Raynaud's disease), constipation, depression, antihypertensive co-admin. Pre-existing conduction abnormalities (bradycardia, arrhythmia). Decreased lacrimation (warn contact lens users). Sudden discontinuation after prolonged high dose treatment (restlessness, palpitations, rapid BP rise, nervousness, tremor, headache, nausea); reduce over 2-4 days; counsel patient not to discontinue without medical advice.

Pregnancy, Lactation: *Pregnancy,* not for use unless considered essential (benefit outweighs risk), especially first trimester. Passes placental barrier and may lower foetal heart rate. Monitor mother and child. *Lactation,* not recommended.

ADR: *Very common,* dizziness, sedation, orthostatic hypotension, dry mouth.

Notes: See 2.1.5 Centrally Acting Antihypertensives (clonidine).

Dixarit 25mcg *(Boehringer)* B. GMS.
Price, (112) €2.55.
Tablet, clonidine HCl. Blue s/c. *Lactose, sucrose.*

Flunarizine

ATC Code: N07CA03. **Sport:** Permitted.
Driving: Somnolence.
Indications: Migraine prophylaxis.

Dose: Adult, Elderly: Age 18 years and over, initially 10mg at night (age 18-64 years) or 5mg at night (elderly, age 65 years and older). Maintenance, same daily dose; interrupt by 2 successive drug-free days every week. Even if prophylactic maintenance successful, interrupt after 6 months; only re-initiated if patient relapses. If depressive, extrapyramidal adverse events develop OR no improvement after 2 months, discontinue.

Child: Under 18 years, not recommended.

CI: Current depressive illness, Parkinson's Disease, other extrapyramidal disorders.

4.2 Analgesia

Interactions: Effect of Other Drugs on Flunarizine: *Galactorrhoea:* Oral contraceptives. *Excessive sedation:* ALCOHOL, hypnotics, tranquillisers.

Effect of Flunarizine on Other Drugs: Antihypertensives: *Adjust dose.*

SP: May cause extrapyramidal and depressive symptoms and reveal Parkinsonism, (especially elderly), monitor; if detected, discontinue. Do not exceed recommended dose. Females with a history of depressive illness, at risk of depression (chronic treatment). Fatigue may increase progressively, discontinue or initiate at lower dose.

Pregnancy, Lactation: Pregnancy, avoid. Lactation, stop breastfeeding or stop drug.

ADR: *Very common,* weight increase.

> **Sibelium 5mg** *(Janssen-Cilag)* B. GMS.
> *Price,* (20) €2.60.
> *Tablet,* flunarizine dihydrochloride equiv. to flunarizine 5mg. White oblong. Marked J-C; Fl 5 on reverse. *Lactose.*

4.2 - Analgesia

Class Effects
Carbamazepine is used for deafferentation pain, see Notes below.

Notes: See 3.1.5 Carboxamides (carbamazepine).

4.2.1 - Non-Opioid Analgesics

In This Chapter: *Acetylsalicylic acid (aspirin), paracetamol. Combinations include caffeine, diphenhydramine, hyoscine.*

Class Effects
Acetylsalicylic acid (aspirin), an analgesic, antipyretic and anti-inflammatory, is also used as an antiplatelet, see Notes below.

CI: Hypersensitivity to any member of the class.

SP: Simple analgesia, take non-prescription products only when necessary; avoid prolonged use except with medical supervision. Use minimum effective dose for shortest duration to minimise undesirable effects. Before co-admin with other drugs, consult doctor or pharmacist. No improvement within 24 hours, seek medical advice. Elderly, always use lowest possible dose for shortest duration; particularly susceptible to adverse effects of NSAIDs.

Pregnancy, Lactation: *Caffeine,* appears in breast milk; irritability and poor sleeping patterns in infants reported.

ADR: *Caffeine,* nausea (GI irritation), insomnia, restlessness (CNS stimulation).

Notes: See 4.4.2 NSAIDs, Non-Selective. See 2.6.7 Non-Steroidal Antiplatelets (aspirin).

Acetylsalicylic Acid (aspirin) (analgesia)
ATC Code: N02BA01. **Sport:** Permitted.
Driving: Unlikely to impair.

Indications: Analgesic for symptomatic relief of mild to moderate pain (headache, toothache, neuralgia, menstrual pain), upper RTI, influenza (pyrexia, cold and flu, sore throat, feverish colds).

Dose: Adult: *Analgesia,* 300-900mg 3 or 4-times daily; range 4-8g in divided doses.

Child: Under 16 years, contraindicated.

Renal Impairment: Caution.

Hepatic Impairment: Caution.

CI: Aspirin/NSAID hypersensitivity (bronchospasm, rhinitis, urticaria). Active peptic ulceration, coagulation deficiency disorder (haemophilia).

Interactions: Effect of Other Drugs on Acetylsalicylic Acid: *Co-admin not recommended:* Warfarin, heparin, other NSAIDs, antacids (cause premature drug release with E/C aspirin). *Nephrotoxicity risk increased:* Diuretics. *Reduced metabolism/elimination:* Probenecid. *Increased absorption rate (no special precautions):* Metoclopramide. *Increased GI bleeding/ulceration risk:* Corticosteroids, nicorandil.

Effect of Acetylsalicylic Acid on Other Drugs: Antihypertensives, diuretics: *Reduced effect.* Cardiac glycosides: *Increased cardiac failure risk, reduced GFR, increased plasma levels.* Lithium, methotrexate: *Decreased excretion.* Ciclosporin: *Increased nephrotoxicity risk.* Corticosteroids: *Increased GI bleeding risk.* Aminoglycosides: *Reduced renal function, decreased elimination, increased plasma levels.* Oral hypoglycaemic agents: *Metabolism inhibited, prolonged half-life, increased hypoglycaemia risk.* Phenytoin, valproate: *Effect enhanced, no special precautions.* Spironolactone: *Natriuretic effect decreased.* Probenecid, sulphinpyrazone: *Uricosuric effect inhibited.* Warfarin, heparin: *Co-admin not recommended, anticoagulant effect enhanced.* Uricosurics: *Effect inhibited.* Oral hypoglycaemics (sulfonylureas): *Metabolism inhibited, prolonged half-life, increased hypoglycaemia risk.*

SP: Possible association between aspirin and Reye's syndrome (children); rare disease, affecting brain and liver (can be fatal). Aspirin should not be given to children and adolescents aged under 16 years unless specifically indicated. Ibuprofen may inhibit effect of low dose aspirin on platelet aggregation; no firm data for regular ibuprofen use; occasional use, no likely effect. Caution, cardiac impairment; peptic ulceration, inflammatory bowel disease, coagulation abnormalities (aspirin may induce GI haemorrhage). Hypertension, monitor. See ADR below.

Pregnancy, Lactation: Caution in pregnancy; has ability to alter platelet function with risk of haemorrhage in infants. Prolonged pregnancy and labour, with increased bleeding before and after delivery, decreased birth weight and increased rate of stillbirth reported with high blood salicylate levels. High doses there may be premature closure of the ductus arteriosus and possible kernicterus or persistent pulmonary hypertension in the newborn. Analgesic doses of aspirin should be avoided during the last trimester of pregnancy. Lactation, is secreted in breast milk; risk of Reye's syndrome in infant; may impair platelet function in infant; generally not recommended.

ADR: Precipitation of bronchospasm, rhinitis or urticaria or asthma attacks induced; nausea, diarrhoea, vomiting, GI blood loss (anaemia), GI ulceration, perforation, major haemorrhage, increased transaminases, kidney dysfunction, urate kidney stone, severe skin reactions, tinnitus.

Notes: See 4.2.1 Non-Opioid Analgesics.

> **Nu-Seals 300mg** *(Alliance)* B. GMS.D.
> *Price,* (100) €5.03.
> *Tablet,* acetylsalicylic acid. White g/r. Marked with strength.

Paracetamol (analgesia)
ATC Code: N02BE01. **Sport:** Permitted.
Driving: No or negligible effect.

Indications: *Paracetamol* is used for relief of mild to moderate pain (osteoarthritis), post-operative; mild to moderate pain/fever in babies and children from age 3 months, post-operative; supps are used if oral not suitable (nausea, vomiting).

Paracetamol IV, is used short-term for moderate pain (following surgery), treatment of fever, when urgent need to treat pain or hyperthermia, other routes not possible.

Dose: Adult: ORAL, tablets 500mg, usually 500mg to 1g 3-4 times daily (4-6 hourly); max. 3g daily *(Paracetamol Actavis)* or 4g in 24 hours. Max. 1g as single dose *(Paralief).*

RECTAL, *Paracetamol Supps* (Phoenix, Ricesteele), 1x or 2x 500mg supps 6-hourly. *Tipol Supps,* age 12 years and older (above 43kg), 1x or 2x 500mg supps (500-1000mg)* OR 1x 1g supp*; max. 4g/24-hours.*Admin as single dose, or at dosing intervals of at least 6-hours. Insert deep into rectum after bowel movement.

PARENTERAL, dosing based on weight, *(Perfalgan 50mL* vial), 10kg and under, 7.5mg/kg per admin (max. 30mg/kg/day); 10-33kg, 15mg/kg per admin (max. 60mg/kg/day not exceeding 2g). *(Perfalgan 100mL* vial/bag, *Paracetamol Actavis),* 33-50kg, 15mg/kg per admin (max. 60mg/kg/day not exceeding 3g); over 50kg (with hepatotoxicity risk), 1g per admin (max. 3g/day); over 50kg (no hepatotoxicity risk), 1g per admin (max. 4g/day).

Caution, dosing errors, see SP below. Minimum 4-hour

intervals; max. 4 doses in 24 hours. IV infusion over 15 minutes.

Elderly: Clearance and plasma half-life longer.

Child: ORAL SUSP *(120mg/5mL)*, all dosed 4-times in 24 hours, age 3-6 months, 60mg; 6-24 months, 120mg; 2-4 years, 180mg; 4-6 years, 240mg; 8-10 years, 360mg; 10-12 years, 420mg. Post-vaccination fever (age 2-3 months), 1x 60mg dose (if needed after 4-6 hours as second 60mL dose can be given); max. 2 doses.

ORAL SUSP *(250mg/5mL)*, all dosed 4-times in 24 hours, age 6-8 years, 250mg; 8-10 years, 375mg; 10-12 years, 500mg. Over 12 years, as for Adult above.

ORAL TABS, 60mg/kg in 4-6 divided doses OR 15mg/kg 6-hourly OR 10mg/kg 4-hourly. Age 8-11 years (26-34kg), 250mg 4-hourly OR 500mg 6-hourly; max. 1.5g/day; 11-12 years (34-43kg), 500mg 6-hourly; max. 2g/day; 12-15 years (43-50kg), 500mg 4-hourly; max. 2.5g/day.

RECTAL, all admin 6-hourly, *Paracetamol (Phoenix)*, *Paralink* supps, age 3-12 months, 1x 80mg or 90mg (half 180mg); age 1-3 years, 1x 125mg or 1x 180mg; age 3-6 years, 1x 250 or 270mg (1.5x 180mg); age 6-12 years, 1x 500mg; over 12 years, as for Adult above. *Tipol Supps*, age 6-7 months (7kg) 1x 125mg supp*; max 375mg/24-hours. Age 7 months to 2 years (8-12kg), 1x 125mg supp*; max. 500mg/24-hours. Age 2-4 years (13-15kg), 1x 250mg supp*; max. 750mg/24-hours. Age 4-8 years (16-25kg), 1x 250mg supp*; max. 1g/24-hours. Age 8-11 years (26-32kg), 1x 500mg supp*; max. 1.5g/24-hours. Age 11-12 years (33-43kg), 1x 500mg supp*; max 2g/24-hours. Age 12 years and older, see Adult above. *Admin as single dose, or at dosing intervals of at least 6-hours. Insert high into rectum after bowel movement.

PARENTERAL, IV infusion over 15 minutes; minimum 4-hourly. See Adult above. Pre-term newborn infants, no data.

Renal Impairment: CrCl (mL/min) below 30, increase dosing interval to 6-hourly; below 10, increase dosing interval to 8-hourly. Rectal, as for Hepatic below.

Hepatic Impairment: Caution. Severe hepatocellular insufficiency, Gilbert's syndrome, chronic alcoholism and/or malnutrition (low hepatic glutathione reserves), dehydration, max. 3g/day (IV) or 2g/day (oral). Rectal, reduce dose or reduce dosing interval.

CI: Hypersensitivity to paracetamol or pro-drug (propacetamol). Not for use under 6 years unless otherwise specified (paediatric formulations are available for children from age 3 months).

Interactions: Effect of Other Drugs on Paracetamol: *Absorption reduced*: Colestyramine (allow 1-hour dosing interval). *Absorption increased*: Metoclopramide, domperidone. *Reduced metabolism, prolonged plasma half-life*: Barbiturates, TCADs, ALCOHOL. *Increased first pass metabolism or clearance*: Anticonvulsants, oral contraceptives (chronic ingestion). *Increased hepatotoxicity (of overdose)*: ALCOHOL. *Reduced clearance, (consider dose reduction) IV)*: Probenecid (inhibits paracetamol conjugation with glucuronic acid). *Elimination half-life prolonged (IV)*: Salicylamide.

Effect of Paracetamol on Other Drugs: Warfarin: *Potentiation (regular daily high dose paracetamol use).* Chloramphenicol: *Plasma levels increased.* Enzyme inducers (rifampicin, carbamazepine, phenobarbital, phenytoin, primidone): *Plasma-paracetamol conc halved (considered to be an indication for antidote treatment).*

SP: NOTE: Caution, to avoid dosing errors due to confusion between milligram (mg) and millilitre (mL) (which could result in accidental overdose and death), when writing prescriptions, include both the total dose in mg and the total dose in volume. For non-prescription medications, patients should consult doctor/pharmacist if taking other paracetamol-containing medications.

Paracetamol dependence. Chronic (alcoholism, malnutrition; low hepatic glutathione reserves), dehydration. Doses exceeding recommended (serious liver damage risk; clinical signs and symptoms usually after 2 days, and peak 4-6 days after admin).

Caution, with renal and hepatic impairment. Overdose hazard greater with non-cirrhotic alcoholic liver disease.

Advise patients not to take other paracetamol or propacetamol-containing products and not to consume large amounts of alcohol (severe liver damage may occur). Overdose, seek immediate medical advice (liver damage risk). Severe-cutaneous adverse reactions reported (Stevens-Johnson syndrome, toxic epidermal necrolysis).

Pregnancy, Lactation: Studies in human pregnancy have shown no ill effects at recommended dosage; patients to follow medical advice. Frequent use (daily or most days) in late pregnancy may be associated with increased risk of persistent wheezing in the infant. Epidemiological evidence exists of safety of paracetamol in human pregnancy; use if benefit outweighs risk. Lactation, available data does not contraindicate; may be used at recommended dose.

ADR: Side effects at therapeutic doses are rare but hypersensitivity (skin rash) may occur; most adverse reactions relate to overdose (hepatotoxicity, renal toxicity). Thrombocytopenia purpura, methaemoglobinaemia, agranulocytosis, hepatobiliary disorders.

Notes: See 4.2.1 Non-Opioid Analgesics.

Paracetamol Supps *(Phoenix)* OTC. GMS.
Price, (10) 80mg, €4.41. 125mg, €4.75. 250mg, €4.97.
Supps, paracetamol 80mg, 125mg, 250mg, 500mg. White torpedo-shaped.
Paracetamol Actavis 500mg *(Accord)* B. GMS.D.
Price, (100) €1.40.
Tablet, paracetamol. Cap-shaped f/c white scored (divisible into equal halves). Marked Pinex 500; A and L on reverse.
Paracetamol Actavis Parenteral *(Accord)* A.
Price, not provided by company.
Infusion, 10mg/mL (100mL). Clear slightly yellowish soln. *Sodium 0.076mg/mL.*
Paralief 500mg *(Clonmel)* OTC. GMS.D.
Price, (100) €1.40.
Tablet, paracetamol. White cap-shaped scored. Marked 293; logo on reverse.
Paralink Supps 180mg, 500mg *(Ricesteele)* OTC. GMS.D.
Price, (10) 180mg, €4.77. 500mg, €5.81.
Supps, paracetamol 180mg, 500mg. White.
Perfalgan Parenteral 10mg/mL *(BMS)* A.
Price, 100mL (12) 10mg/mL, €54.73.
Infusion, paracetamol. Clear slightly yellowish soln. *Sodium 0.04mg/mL.*
Tipol Supps, Max. Supps *(Carysfort)* OTC. GMS.
Price, (10) 125mg, €4.51; 250mg, €4.72; 500mg, €5.49; Max. 1000mg, €9.90.
Supp, paracetamol. White (ivory) odourless torpedo-shaped.

4.2.2 - Opioid Analgesics

In This Chapter: *Buprenorphine, codeine phosphate, fentanyl, hydromorphone, meptazinol, morphine (sulfate, tartrate), oxycodone, pethidine, tapentadol, tramadol (and combination).*

Class Effects

Driving: Opioids have the potential to cause sedation or altered reactions, depending on dose, susceptibility, other CNS depressants including ALCOHOL, not recommended to drive or operate machinery if affected.

Opioids are also used in anaesthesia; *buprenorphine* and *methadone* are used as substitution treatment for major opioid drug dependence; *codeine, dihydrocodeine* are used for mild to moderate pain relief; higher codeine doses (15mg, 30mg) are used for more severe pain. See Notes below.

CI: Hypersensitivity to any member of the class. Children not recommended unless otherwise specified. Acute respiratory depression; raised intracranial pressure, head injury, coma; phaeochromocytoma (some opioids can induce endogenous histamine release and stimulate catecholamine release); use during acute asthma exacerbations.

NOTE: Codeine-containing medicines should only be used in children over age 12 years to treat acute moderate pain, and only if pain cannot be relieved by other pain killers (paracetamol or ibuprofen alone); it should not be used in children under 12 years because of the risk of opioid toxicity due to variable and unpredictable metabolism of codeine to morphine. Codeine is contraindicated in patients under

4.2.2   Opioid Analgesics

18 years for pain relief following tonsillectomy and/or adenoidectomy for Obstructive Sleep Apnoea Syndrome (OSAS) due to increased risk of developing serious and life-threatening adverse reactions (loss of consciousness, respiratory depression). Codeine is contraindicated in patients of any age known to be CYP2D6 ultra-rapid metabolisers. Always use the lowest effective dose for the shortest period of time; limit treatment duration to 3 days. See SP and Pregnancy, Lactation below.

Interactions: Effect of Other Drugs on Opioids: *Co-admin avoid (contraindication with some brands)*: MAOIs (or admin within previous 14 days) (hypertensive crisis). *Co-admin caution*: Mixed agonist/antagonist opioid analgesics (buprenorphine, nalbuphine, pentazocine, nalbuphine). *Severe hypotension risk*: Phenothiazines, certain anaesthetics. *Effect enhanced*: Other CNS depressants (other opioids, tranquillisers, sedatives, hypnotics). *Concentration (of morphine, active metabolite of codeine) reduced*: Quinidine. *Increased respiratory depression risk/sedation risk*: Centrally acting muscle relaxants, CNS depressants (sedatives or hypnotics, phenothiazines, benzodiazepines, other tranquillisers, ALCOHOL).

SP: *Codeine* is not recommended in children with neuromuscular disorders, severe cardiac or respiratory conditions, upper respiratory or lung infections, multiple trauma or extensive surgical procedures; symptoms of morphine toxicity may be increased.

Caution, consider dose reduction, increased sensitivity to central/GI effects with hypothyroidism, renal disease, chronic hepatic disease, impaired respiratory function/depression (may be associated with neuromuscular disorders), severe cardiac or respiratory conditions (COPD), upper respiratory or lung infections, multiple trauma, extensive surgery, elderly/debilitated, children, Addison's disease. *Caution*, history of allergic reactions to opiates (hypersensitivity, anaphylactic reactions); raised intracranial pressure, head injury, convulsive disorders, seizures (may lower seizure threshold), acute alcohol intoxication, shock, impaired consciousness, adrenocortical insufficiency, asthma (acute exacerbations, not recommended; controlled asthma, caution), prostatic hypertrophy, hypotension, if unable to maintain homeostatic BP (depleted blood volume, hypovolaemia), previous or pre-existing bradyarrhythmias; inflammatory or obstructive bowel disorders (opioids increase tone, decrease propulsive contractions of GI smooth muscle; constipation); post-operative, use only when bowel function is normal; use within 24 hours post-operative (caution); hypothyroidism. Patients undergoing cordotomy (other pain relieving surgical procedures) should not receive opioids for 1-dose interval before surgery then adjust dose to new post-operative requirement. Deafness associated with long-term use of codeine + paracetamol combination. Overdose, seek immediate medical advice (delayed serious liver damage due to paracetamol).

Dependence, withdrawal (all opioids), recognised abuse and addiction potential (especially prolonged use); withdrawal syndrome on abrupt withdrawal or admin of narcotic antagonist (abstinence syndrome). Always withdraw slowly. Tolerance.

Transdermal, not recommended immediate post-op analgesia or where there is a narrow therapeutic index or rapidly varying analgesic requirement; not for acute pain.

Pregnancy, Lactation: Pregnancy, (towards end) can cause respiratory depression in neonate even with short-term admin; long-term use during pregnancy, risk of neonatal withdrawal symptoms. Lactation, not recommended.

NOTE: *Codeine* is contraindicated for use in pregnancy or lactation. Nursing mothers who are ultra-rapid codeine metabolisers, higher than expected serum and breast milk morphine levels can occur. Morphine toxicity in babies can cause excessive somnolence, hypotonia, miosis, difficulty breastfeeding or breathing. Severe cases respiratory depression and death can occur; naloxone may be appropriate to reverse effects. Many codeine-containing analgesics are available without prescription. Use the

148

lowest effective dose, for shortest possible time. Advise nursing mothers to monitor infant.

ADR: Respiratory depression (higher doses). Bradycardia, tachycardia, palpitations, orthostatic hypotension, hypothermia, raised intracranial pressure, headache, restlessness, vertigo, mood changes, hallucinations, muscle rigidity, dizziness, dry mouth, biliary spasm, decreased libido/potency, micturition difficulties, ureteric spasm, antidiuretic effect, hyperhidrosis, facial flushing, miosis, asthenia. See SP above. *Codeine*, dizziness, drowsiness, nausea, vomiting, constipation, urinary retention, light-headedness, confusion, euphoria, dysphoria, miosis, bradycardia, abdominal pain (rarely codeine-induced pancreatitis reported with history of cholecystectomy), allergic reactions, pruritus.

Notes: Paracetamol combinations, see 4.2.1 Non-Opioid Analgesics (paracetamol). See also 14.1.2 Opioids In Anaesthesia and 15.3.3 Opiate Dependence (buprenorphine, methadone).

Buprenorphine (analgesia)

ATC Code: N02AE01. **Sport:** Prohibited (in-competition). May cause positive reaction to sports doping control tests.
Driving: Drowsiness especially with ALCOHOL, other CNS depressants.

Indications: Moderate to severe pain, including cancer pain, not responding to non-opioids/only adequately managed with opioids; not indicated for acute or post-operative pain.

Dose: Adult, Elderly: *BuTrans*, initially (including when converting from opioids), 5mcg/hour patch; titrate after 3 days to larger patch or combination (max. 2) patches if needed; replace every 7 days.

TransTec, no previous analgesics or WHO Step-I or II analgesic, initially 35mcg/hour patch; replace every 96 hours. Apply patch to intact skin on upper outer arm, upper chest/back or side of chest; avoid scarred skin. Initially, use additional short-acting analgesics until efficacy attained.

Hepatic Impairment: Caution. Severe, not recommended.

CI: Acute alcoholism or delirium tremens, use during acute asthma attack, myasthenia gravis. Opioid-dependent patients, narcotic withdrawal treatment.

Interactions: Effect of Other Drugs on Buprenorphine: *Plasma levels increased*: CYP3A4 inhibitors (ketoconazole, gestodene, troleandomycin, ritonavir, indinavir, saquinavir). *Increased clearance*: CYP3A4 inducers (phenobarbital, carbamazepine, phenytoin, rifampicin). *Decreased hepatic elimination*: Drugs reducing hepatic blood flow (halothane). *Respiratory depression potentiated*: Benzodiazepines. *Increased CNS depressant effect*: Other opioid derivatives (analgesics, antitussives containing morphine, dextropropoxyphene, codeine, dextromethorphan, noscapine), certain antidepressants, sedative H1-receptor antagonists, ALCOHOL, anxiolytics, neuroleptics, clonidine.

SP: Intracranial lesions. Lower dependence liability than pure agonists; limited euphorigenic effects. If withdrawal occurs, usually mild.

Pregnancy, Lactation: Not recommended.

ADR: *Serious*, respiratory depression, especially with other CNS depressants, hypotension; *very common*, headache, dizziness, somnolence, constipation, dry mouth, nausea, vomiting, pruritus, erythema, application site reaction.

Notes: See 4.2.2 Opioid Analgesics.

BuTrans Transdermal *(Mundipharma)* CD. GMS.
Price, (2) 5mcg €10.48. (4) 10mcg €33.77; 15mcg €56.03; 20mcg (4) €60.99.
Transdermal patch, buprenorphine 7-day patches. Beige. Marked with name/strength. 5mcg and 20mcg/hour: Square. 10mcg and 15mcg/hour: Rectangular. **Store:** Below 25 deg C.
Transtec Transdermal *(Mundipharma)* CD. GMS.
Price, (4) 35mcg, €22.13. 52.5mcg, €33.10. 70mcg, €43.54.
Transdermal patch, buprenorphine. 72-hour patches. Skin-coloured. Marked with name/strength, buprenorphine/strength.

Codeine Phosphate (analgesia)

ATC Code: N02AA59. **Sport:** Permitted.
Driving: Sedation, dizziness.

Indications: Treatment, acute moderate pain not relieved by other analgesics (paracetamol, ibuprofen), patients older than 12 years. There are a number of non-prescription products available as antitussives for non-productive cough.

Dose: Adult, Elderly: 30mg repeated 6-hourly as needed; max 240mg/day; duration 3 days, then seek medical advice. *Elderly*, reduced dose may be needed (metabolism, elimination of opioids is slower).

Child: Age 12-18 years, 30-60mg every 6 hours when needed (based on 0.5-1mg/kg body weight); max. 240mg. Under 12 years, contraindicated.

Renal Impairment: Caution.

Hepatic Impairment: Failure, contraindicated.

CI: See Notes below.

Interactions: Effect of Other Drugs on Codeine Phosphate: *Co-admin contraindicated*: MAOIs (within 14 days). *Sedative effect enhanced*: ALCOHOL, other CNS depressants.

SP: In inflammatory bowel disease codeine reduces peristalsis, increases tone and segmentation in the bowel and can raise colonic pressure; caution, use in diverticulitis, acute colitis, diarrhoea (pseudomembranous colitis associated), after bowel surgery. Avoid, in biliary disorders, gall bladder disease, gall stones (may cause biliary obstruction), GI or urinary tract surgery, prostatic hypertrophy. Codeine is partially metabolised by CYP2D6; if deficient or completely lacking this enzyme, adequate analgesic effect will not be obtained. Ultra-rapid metabolisers, increased risk of opioid toxicity even at low doses (nausea, vomiting, constipation, lack of appetite, somnolence, circulatory and respiratory depression). See Notes below.

Pregnancy, Lactation: See Notes below.

ADR: See Notes below.

Notes: See 4.2.2 Opioid Analgesics.

Codant 30mg *(Concordia)* A. GMS.
Price, (100) €10.51.
Tablet, codeine phosphate. White round. *Lactose*. **Store:** Below 25 deg C; original pack; protect (light).

Codeine Phosphate, Paracetamol

ATC Code: N02BE51/N02AA59. **Sport:** Permitted.
Driving: Drowsiness, dizziness, sedation.

Indications: Relief, mild, moderate to severe acute pain (adults, children over 12 years only if not relieved by other analgesics alone e.g. paracetamol, ibuprofen).

Dose: Adult, Elderly: Age 12 years and over, all strengths/combinations, 1-2 caps, tabs or effervescent tabs 4-6 hourly; max. 8 tabs (4g paracetamol, 240mg codeine) in 24 hours. *Admin*, dissolve effervescent tabs in glass of water. Do not take codeine-containing products for more than 3 days without medical advice. *Elderly*, consider dose reduction.

Child: Age 12 years and over, as for Adult *except*, age 12-18 years: *Kapake*, 1 tab 6-hourly; max. 4 tabs in 24-hour period; *Solpadol*, 1-2 tabs 6-hourly; max. 8 tabs in 24-hour period; *Tylex*, 30-60mg codeine 6-hourly; max. 240mg codeine/day (based on 0.5-1mg/kg bodyweight). Under 12 years, codeine not recommended (risk of opioid toxicity due to variable and unpredictable metabolism); brand *Codipar* not recommended under 18 years. See Contraindications (CI) below.

Renal Impairment: Severe, contraindicated. OTC products, advise patient to seek medical advice. *Kapake*, caution.

Hepatic Impairment: As for Renal above. Underlying liver or alcoholic liver disease, increased risk of paracetamol-related liver damage.

CI: High dose codeine phosphate, see Notes below (morphine sulfate). Acute asthma. Acute alcohol intoxication *(Kapake)*. Age under 18 years and under 12 years, see Notes below (opioid analgesics).

SP: Avoid excessive caffeine intake. Inflammatory or obstructive bowel disorders, acute abdominal conditions, history of cholecystectomy (acute pancreatitis risk), consult doctor before use. Rarely *serious* skin reactions; blood dyscrasias (thrombocytopenia, agranulocytosis) with paracetamol.

Pregnancy, Lactation: Caffeine may have stimulating effect on infant. Codeine, see Notes below (opioid analgesics).

ADR: Increased risk of caffeine-related adverse events when combined with dietary caffeine.

Notes: See Class Effects 4.2.2 Opioid Analgesics. More information, see Codeine Phosphate above and Morphine Sulphate below. See 4.2.1 Non-Opioid Analgesics (paracetamol).

Codipar 15/500 Caps, Effervescent *(Concordia)* A. GMS.
Price, (100) caps, €8.78; effervescent, €9.13.
Effervescent tablet, codeine phosphate 15mg, paracetamol 500mg. Flat round white. *Sorbitol; sodium 379mg/tab.*
Capsule, as above. Hard red/white; contains white powder.

Kapake 15/500, 30/500 *(Galen)* A. GMS.
Price, (100) 15/500, €8.42; 30/500, €7.37.
Tablet, codeine phosphate, paracetamol 15(30)/500. White oblong u/c scored (facilitates breaking). 15/500: Marked K1. 30/500: Marked Kapake.

Maxilief 8/500 Effervescent *(Clonmel)* OTC. GMS.D.
Price, (60) €6.99.
Effervescent tablet, codeine phosphate 8mg, paracetamol 500mg, caffeine 30mg. Flat white scored (facilitates breaking). *Sorbitol*

Solpadeine 8/500 Caps, Soluble Caps *(Chefaro)* OTC. GMS.
Price, caps (32) €2.58. Eff (60) €7.43.
Capsule, codeine phosphate hemihydrate 8mg, paracetamol 500mg, caffeine 30mg. Hard gelatin opaque red/white. Marked Solpadeine on both halves or plain on both halves.
Effervescent tablet (Soluble), as above. Flat white scored (divisible into equal halves). *Sorbitol, sodium 427mg/tab.*
NOTE: Solpadeine tabs are not reimbursed.

Solpadol 30/500 Tabs, Effervescent *(SANOFI)* A. GMS.
Price, (100) caplets, €8.06. Eff, €9.99.
Effervescent tablet, codeine phosphate hemihydrate 30mg, paracetamol 500mg. White scored. *Sorbitol, sodium 388mg.*
Store: Below 25 deg C; original pack.
Tablet (caplet), as above. White (off-white) cap-shaped. Marked Solpadol. **Store:** Below 25 deg C; original pack.

Tylex 30/500 Caps, Effervescent *(UCB)* A. GMS.
Price, (100) caps 100, €9.07. Eff 100, €9.96.
Effervescent tablet, codeine phosphate hemihydrate 30mg, paracetamol 500mg. Round white (off-white). *Sodium 326.6mg/tabs, aspartame.*
Capsule, as above. Hard gelatin white/red. Marked C30. *Sodium metabisulphite.*

Fentanyl (analgesia)

ATC Code: N02AB03. **Sport:** Prohibited (in-competition).
Driving: May impair mental and/or physical ability.

Indications: Breakthrough pain, management of exacerbation, of otherwise controlled persistent pain, already receiving maintenance opioids for chronic cancer pain. Intractable chronic pain requiring opioids, including severe in children. *Maintenance opioid therapy*, patients taking at least 60mg/day oral morphine, 25mcg/hour fentanyl transdermal, 30mg/day oxycodone, 8mg/day oral hydromorphone or equi-analgesic dose of another opioid for a week or longer.

Dose: Adult: OROMUCOSAL, *Actiq*, initially, 200mcg over 15 minutes; adequate analgesia not obtained repeat with same strength; max. 2 units for any individual pain episode. Maintenance, max. 4 units/day. More than 4 episodes of breakthrough pain/day over 4 consecutive days or more, re-evaluate dose of long-acting opioid for persistent pain. Place in mouth against cheek, move around to maximise mucosal exposure; suck, do not chew; use water to moisten buccal mucosa with dry mouth.

BUCCAL, SUBLINGUAL (both brands), initially 100mcg. If switching from other fentanyl products, the switch must NOT be on a 1:1 basis; individual titration needed. Inadequate analgesia after 30 minutes, admin a second tab of same strength. Admin, *Effentora (buccal)*, do not suck, chew or swallow; should remain in buccal cavity for 30 minutes*. *Abstral (sublingual)*, admin under tongue at deepest part; do not suck, chew or swallow; allow to

149

4.2.2 Opioid Analgesics

completely dissolve in sublingual cavity*. *Do not take food and/or drink in this time.

NASAL SPRAY, *Instanyl*, initially 50mcg in 1 nostril titrating up through 50, 100 and 200mcg; inadequate analgesia, re-dose at same strength, earliest after 10 minutes; patients should wait 4 hours (exceptionally 2 hours) before treating another breakthrough pain episode. Before using for first time, prime spray until a fine mist appears (usually 3-4 sprays).

TRANSDERMAL, *opioid naive*, titrate with low dose opioids to equi-analgesic dose, then transdermal 12-25mcg/hour starting with 12mcg/hour; *opioid tolerant*, base dose on previous 24-hour analgesic need; titrate by 12mcg or 25mcg/hour to lowest effective dose. Apply to non-irritated, non-irradiated, non-hairy skin; wear continuously for 72 hours.

When converting from other opioids determine analgesic need over last 24-hours; convert to equivalent oral morphine dose; base fentanyl dose on daily oral morphine (stabilised on oral morphine, conversion ratio of oral morphine to transdermal fentanyl approx. equal to 150:1) or (highly opioid tolerant, conversion ratio of oral morphine to transdermal fentanyl approx. equal to 100:1). If dose exceeds 300mcg/hour, consider additional or alternative analgesia. Discontinuation, may take 17 hours or more for serum conc to decrease by 50%; discontinue gradually to prevent withdrawal.

Elderly: TRANSDERMAL, observe for signs of fentanyl toxicity, reduce dose. BUCCAL, SUBLINGUAL, titrate with caution. See Renal below.

Child: TRANSDERMAL, opioid-tolerant, age 2-16 years (already receiving at least 30mg oral morphine equivalents per day), oral morphine 30-44mg/day, use 12mcg/hour; oral morphine 45-134mg/day use 25mcg/hour. Caution, choice of application site (upper back; reduced risk of accidental ingestion). Age 16 years and above, as for Adult above.

Renal Impairment: Moderate or severe, caution; consider dose reduction. Observe for signs of fentanyl toxicity.

Hepatic Impairment: As for Renal above.

CI: Severe, respiratory depression or obstructive lung conditions, CNS impairment. Transdermal, hypersensitivity to patch, use in acute or post-operative pain (dose titration not possible and possibility of serious or life-threatening hypoventilation). Buccal/nasal spray, no maintenance opioid therapy (increased respiratory depression risk). Nasal spray, previous facial radiotherapy, recurrent epistaxis (opioid naive patients). Brands indicated for breakthrough pain are not for use for other acute pain (post-operative, headache, migraine).

Interactions: Effect of Other Drugs on Fentanyl: *Co-admin not recommended (nasal delivery):* Oxymetazoline, other nasally admin treatments. *Increased bioavailability, decreased clearance, increased or prolonged opioid effect:* Strong CYP3A4 inhibitors including macrolides (erythromycin, clarithromycin, troleandomycin), azole antifungals (ketoconazole, itraconazole), ritonavir, nelfinavir; moderate CYP3A4 inhibitors including amprenavir, aprepitant, verapamil, diltiazem, erythromycin, fluconazole, fosamprenavir, amiodarone, grapefruit juice. *Additive depressant effect:* Other opioids, sedatives or hypnotics, general anaesthetics, phenothiazines, tranquillisers, skeletal muscle relaxants, sedating antihistamines, ALCOHOL. *Serotonin Syndrome risk (potentially life-threatening):* Other serotonergics (SSRIs, SNRIs), drugs impairing serotonin metabolism (MAOI). *Withdrawal symptoms may be precipitated by co-admin:* Opioid antagonists (naloxone), mixed agonist/antagonists (pentazocine, butorphanol, buprenorphine, nalbuphine) (*brands Actiq, Instanyl*).

SP: Serious adverse events, monitor patient for minimum 24 hours after fentanyl discontinuation (serum fentanyl levels decline gradually; are reduced by about 50% after 17 hours; range 13-22 hours). *Caution*, opioid-naive (respiratory depression risk), intracranial CO_2 retention, bradycardia especially IV (caution with bradyarrhythmias), hypovolaemia, hypotension, chronic pulmonary disease, non-epileptic (myo) clonic reactions, serotonin syndrome,

if suspected, discontinue. *Extreme caution*, increased intracranial pressure. Use for breakthrough pain, discontinue immediately if patient no longer has breakthrough pain episodes; maintain persistent background pain treatment as prescribed.

Oromucosal, recommend normal oral hygiene to avoid tooth damage. Caution, accidental child exposure; keep lozenges out of reach and sight of children.

Transdermal, fever (or exposure to external heat), monitor for opioid side effects (increased body temp. may increase fentanyl delivery rate). Not possible to ensure interchangeability; when changing brand of fentanyl transdermal, counsel patient. Do not cut or use damaged patches. Accidental transfer of patch to skin of non-patch wearer (especially child) may result in opioid overdose.

Nasal spray, recurrent epistaxis episodes or nasal discomfort, consider alternative.

Pregnancy, Lactation: Pregnancy, use only if clearly necessary; neonatal withdrawal syndrome reported in newborn following chronic maternal use. Delivery, not recommended; passes through the placenta (foetal respiratory depression risk). Lactation, not recommended; passes into breast milk; may cause sedation or respiratory depression in newborn/infant. Do not restart breastfeeding until minimum 48 hours after last admin (*Effentora Buccal, Instanyl*, 5 days).

ADR: *Very common*, somnolence, dizziness, headache, nausea, vomiting, constipation. *Actiq*, application site reactions. *Durogesic DTrans*, adverse event profile in children, similar to adults; neonatal withdrawal, see Pregnancy, Lactation above.

Notes: See 4.2.2 Opioid Analgesics.

Abstral Sublingual *(KyowaKirin)* CD. GMS.
Price, all strengths (10) €64.51. (30) €189.66.
Sublingual tablet, fentanyl citrate 1, 2, 3, 4, 6, 8 (hundred)mcg. White. 100mcg: Round. 200mcg: Oval. 300mcg: Triangular. 400mcg: Diamond-shaped. 600mcg: D-shaped. 800mcg: Cap-shaped. *Mannitol*.

Actiq Oral Lozenge *(TEVA)* CD. GMS.
Price, all strengths (3 units) €25.03. (30 units) €262.69.
Oral lozenge with integral applicator, fentanyl citrate 2, 4, 6, 8, 12, 16 (hundred)mcg. White (off-white) compressed powder drug matrix attached to plastic applicator. Marked dosage strength. *Dextrans; glucose 1.89g/dosage unit*.

Durogesic DTrans Transdermal *(Janssen-Cilag)* CD. GMS.
Price, all strengths, (5 patches) 12mcg, €10.91. 25mcg, €16.15. 50mcg, €29.72. 75mcg, €43.09. 100mcg, €52.64.
Transdermal patch, fentanyl. Rectangular clear with sticky back. Marked Durogesic/strength (mcg) fentanyl/hour.

Effentora Buccal *(TEVA)* CD. GMS.
Price, all strengths (4) €25.79. (28) €180.53.
Buccal tablet, fentanyl citrate 1, 2, 4, 6, 8 (hundred)mcg. Round. Marked C. 100mcg: Marked 1. 200mcg: Marked 2. 400mcg: Marked 4. 600mcg: Marked 6. 800mcg: Marked 8. *Mannitol; sodium 8mg/100mcg tab, 16mg/tab (other strengths)*.

Fentadur Transdermal *(Aribamed)* CD. GMS.
Price, (5 patches) 12mcg, €13.33. 25mcg, €36.40. 50mcg, €67.99. 75mcg, €94.76. 100mcg, €116.79.
Transdermal patch, fentanyl. Rectangular tan. Marked Fentanyl and strength.

Fental Matrix Transdermal *(Rowex)* CD. GMS.
Price, (5 patches) 25mcg, €15.42. 50mcg, €28.80. 75mcg, €40.15. 100mcg, €49.50.
Transdermal patch, fentanyl. Transparent rounded oblong. Soya-bean oil.

Instanyl Nasal Spray *(Takeda)* CD. GMS.
Price, (1) (10 dose) 50mcg, €78.34; 100mcg, €80.37; 200mcg, €80.33. (20-dose) 50mcg, €156.67; 100mcg, €160.73; 200mcg, €160.67. HOS: SDU (6) 50mcg, 200mcg, €53.95; 100mcg, €53.77 (PTW).
Nasal spray, fentanyl citrate 50, 100, 200mcg/dose. Clear colourless soln. **Store:** Upright. Blister in outer carton. Below 30 deg C.

Matrifen Transdermal *(Takeda)* CD. GMS.
Price, (5 patches) 12mcg, €9.62. 25mcg, €15.79. 50mcg, €26.86. 75mcg, €38.86. 100mcg, €56.97.
Transdermal patch, fentanyl 12, 25, 50, 75, 100mcg. Rectangular translucent. Marked name, active substance/strength.

Hydromorphone

ATC Code: N02AA03. **Sport:** Prohibited (in-competition).
Driving: May impair especially with other CNS depressants.
Indications: Severe pain, intractable pain.

Dose: Adult: STANDARD/R, initially 1.3mg or 2.6mg 4-hourly; if needed titrate alone or in combination with Prolonged/R formulation. PROLONGED/R (SR), initially 4mg 12-hourly. NOTE: 1.3mg hydromorphone has efficacy equiv. to 10mg morphine sulfate (oral); 4mg of hydromorphone HCl has efficacy equivalent to 30mg morphine sulfate (oral).

Elderly: Consider dose reduction.

Child: Under 12 years, not recommended.

Renal Impairment: May require lower doses to achieve pain control.

Hepatic Impairment: As for Renal above.

CI: Severe chronic obstructive airways disease, coma, acute abdomen, paralytic ileus. Prolonged/R not recommended for pre-operative use or within first 24 hours post-operative.

Interactions: Effect of Other Drugs on Hydromorphone: CNS depressant effects enhanced: Tranquillisers, anaesthetics (barbiturates), hypnotics and sedatives, neuroleptics, barbiturates, antidepressants, antihistaminic drugs, other opioids, ALCOHOL.

SP: Respiratory depression is major risk of opioids, caution (delirium tremens, toxic psychosis, hypotension with hypovolaemia, diseases of biliary tract, biliary or ureteric colic, pancreatitis, obstructive and inflammatory bowel disorders, chronic obstructive airways disease, reduced respiratory reserve, elderly). Cross tolerance with other opioids. Abuse profile similar to other strong opioid agonists. Possibility of development of paralytic ileus, first 24-hours post-operative (not recommended).

Pregnancy, Lactation: Pregnancy and/or labour, should not be used (impaired uterine contractility, neonatal respiratory depression risk). Prolonged use can result in neonatal withdrawal syndrome.

ADR: Very common, dizziness, somnolence, constipation, nausea.

Notes: See 4.2.2 Opioid Analgesics.

Palladone 1.3mg, 2.6mg, SR (Mundipharma) CD. GMS. Price, (56) 1.3mg, €9.27. 2.6mg, €18.54. SR (56) 2mg, €17.13. 4mg, (28.11. 8mg, €54.82. 16mg, €103.05. 24mg, €148.40. Standard/R capsule, hydromorphone HCl. Caps contain white (off-white) spherical pellets. Marked HNR/strength. 1.3mg: Clear/opaque orange. 2.6mg: Clear/opaque red. Lactose. Store: Below 25 deg C.
Prolonged/R capsule, as above (SR) 2mg, 4mg, 8mg, 16mg, 24mg. Caps contain white (off-white) spherical pellets. Marked HCR/strength. 2mg: Opaque white/yellow. 4mg: Clear/opaque pale-blue. 8mg: Clear/opaque pink. 16mg: Clear/opaque brown. 24mg: Clear/opaque dark blue. Lactose. Store: As above.

Meptazinol

ATC Code: N02AX05. **Sport:** Permitted.
Driving: Dizziness, drowsiness.
Indications: Oral, short-term relief of moderate pain. Parenteral, moderate to severe pain, including post-operative, obstetric and renal colic pain.

Dose: Adult, Elderly: ORAL, 200mg 3-6 hourly as required; usually 200mg 4-hourly.
PARENTERAL, 75-100mg IM; may be repeated 2-4 hourly. Obstetric pain, 100-150mg orally according to weight (approx. 2mg/kg) OR 50-100mg by slow IV injection. May be repeated 2-4 hourly as needed.

Child: Under 12 years, not recommended.

Renal Impairment: Reduce dose. Renal failure, parenteral not recommended.

Hepatic Impairment: As for Renal above.

CI: Acute alcoholism, paralytic ileus risk. Injection, intrathecal or epidural routes.

Interactions: Effect of Other Drugs on Meptazinol: Co-admin contraindicated: MAOIs (or within two weeks of admin; including moclobemide). Increased sedation: TCADs, anxiolytics, hypnotics. Enhanced sedative and hypotensive effects: Antipsychotics, ALCOHOL. Plasma levels increased: Antivirals, cimetidine. GI side effects antagonised: Metoclopramide, domperidone.

Effect of Meptazinol on Other Drugs: Quinolones (ciprofloxacin): Plasma levels decreased.

SP: Compromised respiratory system.

Pregnancy, Lactation: Pregnancy (apart from labour) and lactation, only if considered essential by physician.

ADR: Very common, dizziness, headache, vertigo, somnolence, drowsiness, abdominal pain, constipation, diarrhoea, dyspepsia, nausea, vomiting, increased sweating, rash.

Notes: See 4.2.2 Opioid Analgesics.

Meptid 200mg, Parenteral (Almirall) A. GMS.
Price, (100) €26.08. 112, €29.21. Injection (10) €22.83.
Tablet, meptazinol HCl. Oval orange f/c. Marked MPL 023. Sunset Yellow.
Injection, as above 100mg/mL. Clear colourless soln free from particulate matter. Glucose.

Morphine Sulfate

ATC Code: N02AA01. **Sport:** Prohibited (in-competition).
Driving: Likely to impair; enhanced with ALCOHOL or CNS depressants; may modify reaction time (depending on dose).
Indications: Moderate to severe pain (including cancer pain, not responding to non-opioids or only adequately managed with opioids); severe pain, intractable pain.

Dose: Adult: ORAL, MST, severe pain uncontrolled on weaker opioids, initially 30mg 12-hourly; titrate by 30-50% increments as needed; under 70kg, 20mg 12-hourly; over 70kg, 30mg 12-hourly. First 24 hours post-operative or until normal bowel function has returned, not recommended. Admin, swallow tabs whole; do not chew. Susp, mix contents of sachet with 10mL water or sprinkle on soft food (yoghurt); do not chew, crush or break granules (rapid morphine release; absorption of potentially fatal dose).
Oramorph, 10-20mg 4-hourly; max. 120mg/day.
Sevredol, 1 tab 4-hourly. Switch from parenteral morphine, increase oral dose by up to 100%.
PARENTERAL, (10mg, 30mg and 60mg/mL strengths), 10-15mg (SC or IM) 4-hourly if needed. Admin, IV; 4-10mg diluted in 4-5mL water for injection admin over 4-5 minutes.
EPIDURAL, (1mg/5mL strength), initially 5mg in the lumbar region or 2-4mg over 24 hours to start an epidural infusion; may be increased to 2mg daily. Incidence of early and late respiratory depression increased if admin in thoracic region.
INTRATHECAL, (1mg/5mL strength), 0.2-1mg as single injection in lumbar area; do not be repeat. Dose depends on (pain severity, previous analgesic requirement).

Elderly: Caution, consider dose reduction; titrate to provide optimal relief.

Child: ORAL, MST, severe cancer pain, initially 0.2-0.8mg/kg 12-hourly; under 1 year not recommended.
Oramorph, age 13-18 years, 5-20mg*; max. 120mg/day. Age 6-12 years, 5-10mg*; max. 60mg/day. Age 1-5 years, 5mg*; max. 30mg/day. Under 1 year not recommended. *(every 4 hours).
Sevredol, age 3-5 years, 5mg; 6-12 years, 5-10mg every 4 hours; under 3 years, not recommended.
PARENTERAL, from age 1 year, 0.1-0.2mg/kg SC or IM every 4 hours as needed; max. 15mg/dose. Strength 1mg/5mL is for epidural or intrathecal admin; not for use in children.

Renal Impairment: Moderate/severe, caution (parenteral not recommended); severe/prolonged respiratory depression with renal impairment due to accumulation of active metabolite (morphine-6-glucuronide); consider dose reduction. Chronic conditions, consider dose reduction.

Hepatic Impairment: Severe, not recommended (may precipitate coma). Chronic conditions, reduce dose.

CI: Paralytic ileus, 'acute abdomen', obstructive airways disease, delayed gastric emptying, acute (hepatic disease, alcoholism). Epidural or intrathecal route contraindicated if (infection presence at injection site, anticoagulant therapy, bleeding diathesis, drug therapy/medical condition which would contraindicate epidural/intrathecal technique).

Interactions: Effect of Other Drugs on Morphine: Metabolism inhibited: Cimetidine. Plasma levels increased: Ritonavir. Anticholinergic adverse events potentiated:

151

4.2.2 Opioid Analgesics

Medicinals blocking acetylcholine action (antihistamines, anti-Parkinson's drugs, anti-emetics). *Increased opioid adverse events*: Voriconazole, gabapentin.

Effect of Morphine on Other Drugs: Tranquillisers, general anaesthetics, hypnotics, sedatives, ALCOHOL, muscle relaxants, antihypertensives, TCADs, antipsychotics, gabapentin: *Effects enhanced*. Esmolol: *Plasma levels increased*. Domperidone, metoclopramide: *Effects antagonised*. Mexiletine: *Absorption delayed*.

SP: Hyperalgesia (will not respond to further morphine dose increase), especially at high doses. *Parenteral*, repeated intrathecal admin, not recommended; hospital/hospice use only. NOTE: Bioequivalence between different brands of controlled release morphine is not established; do not change without retitration and clinical assessment.

Pregnancy, Lactation: Rapidly crossed the placental barrier; not for use during pregnancy and labour or in premature delivery*. Lactation, not recommended; is excreted in breast milk*. (*may cause respiratory depression in neonate/newborn). See Notes below.

ADR: *Most common*, nausea, abdominal pain, vomiting, constipation, drowsiness, disorientation, dizziness, confusion, insomnia, headache, palpitations, hallucinations, bronchospasm, colic, urticaria, pruritus. *Parenteral, most serious*, respiratory depression.

Notes: See 4.2.2 Opioid Analgesics.

MST Continus, Oral Susp *(Mundipharma)* CD. GMS.
Price, (60) 5mg, €3.96. 10mg, €8.21. 15mg, €13.73. 30mg, €23.17. 60mg, €41.68. 100mg, €64.08. Susp (30 sachets) 20mg €21.66. 30mg €27.64. 60mg, €47.15.
Prolonged/R tablet, morphine sulfate 5mg, 10mg, 15mg, 30mg, 60mg, 100mg. f/c. Marked with logo; strength on reverse. 5mg: White. 10mg: Golden brown. 15mg: Green. 30mg: Purple. 60mg: Orange. 100mg: Grey. *Lactose (not 100mg), cetostearyl alcohol, Sunset Yellow (30mg, 60mg)*. **Store:** Below 25 deg C; original pack. *Sachets (Prolonged/R granules for oral susp)*, as above 20mg, 30mg, 60mg. Pink granules. *Ponceau 4R*. **Store:** Below 25 deg C.

Oramorph Oral Soln, Conc *(Boehringer)* CD. GMS.
Price, 10mg/5mL (GMS): 100mL, €2.39; 300mL, €6.87; 500mL, €10.72. 20mg/1mL (GMS): 30mL, €6.28; 120mL, €24.59. Conc 20mg/mL (HOS): 30mL, €5.82; 120mL, €22.77 (PTW).
Oral soln, morphine sulfate 10mg/5mL, 20mg/1mL (conc). 10mg: Clear colourless. *Parabens, ethanol, sucrose*. 20mg: Clear red; with calibrated pipette; sugar-free. *Amaranth*.

Sevredol 10mg, 20mg, 50mg *(Mundipharma)* CD. GMS.
Price, (56) 10mg, €8.29. 20mg, €16.59. 50mg, €35.34.
Tablet, morphine sulfate. Cap-shaped scored f/c. Marked IR left of score; strength on right. 10mg: Blue. 20mg: Pink. 50mg: Pale-green. *Lactose. Sunset Yellow E110 (20mg)*.

Morphine Sulphate Parenteral *(Concordia)* CD.
Price, (10) 10mg, €3.88. 30mg, €13.59. 60mg, €26.55 (PTW).
Injection, morphine sulfate (10mg, 30mg, 60mg per mL). Clear colourless (almost colourless) sterile soln. *Metabisulphite*.

Morphine Tartrate, Cyclizine

ATC Code: N02AA51. **Sport:** Prohibited (in-competition).
Driving: Orthostatic hypotension, dizziness, sedation. CNS depression.

Indications: Relief, moderate to severe pain (medical, surgical conditions) where reduction of nausea and vomiting associated with morphine is required.

Dose: Adult: Usually 10-20mg SC, IM or IV; additional doses not more frequently than 4-hourly; not more than 3 doses max. 150mg cyclizine tartrate in 24 hours. With IV use, inject slowly over 4-5 minutes with patient in recumbent position.

Elderly: Reduce dose; titrate to provide optimal pain relief (may have increased duration, decreased clearance, increased half-life, increased sensitivity to adverse effects).

Child: Age 6-12 years, 5-10mg as max. single dose; age 1-5 years, 2.5-5mg as max. single dose.

Renal Impairment: Moderate/severe, not for use; severe and prolonged respiratory depression due to active metabolite accumulation.

Hepatic Impairment: Severe, not recommended as may precipitate coma.

CI: Acute alcohol intoxication (antiemetic properties of cyclizine may increase alcohol toxicity).

Interactions: Effect of Cyclizine on Other Drugs: Anticholinergics: *Enhanced side effects*. Pethidine: *Soporific effect enhanced*.

SP: Cyclizine may precipitate incipient glaucoma; caution, obstructive GI disease. Morphine may lower seizure threshold in epilepsy. Use IV route with caution (all patients), especially with underlying neuromuscular disorders (paralysis).

ADR: *Cyclizine*, urticaria, drug rash, drowsiness/sedation, dry mouth, nose and throat, blurred vision, tachycardia, hypertension, urinary retention, constipation, restlessness, nervousness, insomnia, apnoea auditory and visual hallucinations (particularly at high doses). See SP above.

Notes: See 4.2.2 Opioid Analgesics. See Morphine Sulfate above. See 3.8.3 Antihistamines, Antispasmodics (cyclizine).

Cyclimorph Parenteral *(Concordia)* CD. GMS.
Price, (5) 10mg/mL, €7.25. 15mg/mL, €7.52.
Injection, morphine tartrate, cyclizine tartrate 10/50 and 15/50. Clear (slightly coloured) soln. *Sodium metabisulphite; essentially sodium-free*.

Oxycodone

ATC Code: N02AA05. **Sport:** Prohibited (in-competition).
Driving: May modify patient reactions depending on dose/susceptibility.

Indications: Treatment, severe pain managed only with opioid analgesics.

Dose: Adult, Elderly: ORAL, *OxyContin*, debilitated elderly, opioid naive, severe pain, initially 10mg 12-hourly; if needed titrate after 24 hours in 25-50% increments; escape medication needed more than twice daily; increased oxycodone dose needed. Non-malignant pain, usually 160mg/day; cancer-related pain, titrate to dose achieving pain relief unless limited by side effects. NOTE: Dose 60mg or more may cause fatal respiratory depression in opioid naive patients. *Admin*, 12-hourly; swallow tabs whole; do not break, chew or crush (may lead to rapid release/absorption and potentially fatal dose).

OxyNorm, Oxycodone Actavis, debilitated elderly, opioid naive, severe pain, initially 5mg every 4-6 hours; if needed increase daily by 25-50%. Non-malignant pain, cancer-related pain, as for OxyContin. Disperse OroDisp tab in mouth before swallowing; swallow caps whole with water.

Dancex SR, Reltebon Prolonged/R, 10mg 12-hourly; initiate at 5mg may minimise side effect incidence. Titrate every 1-2 days until stable twice daily dose achieved usually in one-third of daily dose increments. *Admin*, fixed schedule with or without food with liquid; swallow whole, do not chew.

PARENTERAL, *OxyNorm*, 1-10mg IV bolus slowly over 1-2 minutes (minimum 4-hourly) or infuse initially 2mg/hour. PCA admin bolus 0.03mg/kg with minimum lock-out time of 5 minutes. SC bolus, initially admin 5mg, repeat 4-hourly. SC infusion, initially 7.5mg/day (opioid naive).

Switch from oral morphine, 10-13mg oral oxycodone is equiv. to 20mg oral morphine. *Switch* from oral oxycodone to parenteral, 2mg oral oxycodone equiv. to 1mg parenteral.

Child: Under 20 years, not recommended. *Dancex SR, Oxycodone Actavis, Reltebon*, under 12 years, not recommended.

Renal Impairment: Initiate conservatively, recommend reducing adult starting dose by 50%; titrate cautiously.

Hepatic Impairment: Acute disease, contraindicated. Severe, as for Renal above.

CI: Any situation where opioids are contra-indicated (severe respiratory depression with hypoxia, hypercarbia; head injury, paralytic ileus, acute abdomen, delayed gastric emptying, severe chronic obstructive lung disease, severe bronchial asthma, cor pulmonale).

Interactions: Effect of Other Drugs on Oxycodone: *Metabolism inhibited, increased exposure*: CYP2D6 inhibitors (quinidine; may be observed with fluoxetine, paroxetine; also increase metabolite noroxycodone), CYP3A4 inhibitors or substrates (may inhibit) (cimetidine, erythromycin, ketoconazole, voriconazole).

Effect of Oxycodone on Other Drugs: Phenothiazines, TCADs, anaesthetics, hypnotics, sedatives, ALCOHOL, muscle relaxants, antihypertensives, SSRIs, other opioids, neuroleptics: *Effects potentiated (CNS depression)*; *caution*. Coumarins: *Clinically relevant INR changes*. Anticholinergics: *Increased anticholinergic adverse effects*.

SP: Caution (consider dose reduction), opioid dependency, toxic psychosis, delirium tremens, hypovolaemia, disease of biliary tract, biliary or ureteric colic, pancreatitis, obstructive or inflammatory bowel disorders, chronic obstructive airways disease, reduced respiratory reserve, severely impaired respiratory function, debilitated; caution, post abdominal surgery until bowel function normal; not recommended pre-operatively or within 12-24 hours post-surgery. Paralytic ileus, discontinue. Tolerance; cross-tolerance with other opioids. Dependence with prolonged use; withdraw gradually. Abuse profile similar to other strong opioids. Abuse of oral dosage form by parenteral admin (local tissue necrosis, infection, pulmonary granuloma, increased endocarditis and valvular heart injury risk; may be fatal). Change to other analgesics, re-titrate carefully. Alcohol, avoid co-admin.

Parenteral, caution pre- or intra-operative and within 24 hours post-op; increased risk (ileus, respiratory depression).

Pregnancy, Lactation: See Notes below.

ADR: *Very common*, somnolence, dizziness, headache, constipation, nausea, vomiting, pruritus.

Notes: See 4.2.2 Opioid Analgesics. See Morphine Sulfate above.

OxyContin Prolonged/R Tablets *(Mundipharma)* CD. GMS.
Price, (28) 5mg, €6.79. (56) 10mg, €10.96. 20mg, €21.91. 40mg, €43.12. 80mg, €79.38.
Prolonged/R tablet, oxycodone HCl. Round. Marked OC; strength on reverse. 5mg: Light-blue. 10mg: White. 20mg: Pink. 40mg: Yellow. 80mg: Green. *Lactose.*

OxyNorm Caps, Dispersa *(Mundipharma)* CD. GMS.
Price, caps (56) 5mg, €5.98. 10mg, €16.69. 20mg, €33.37. Dispersa (28) 5mg, €5.98. 10mg, €16.69. 20mg, €33.36.
Capsule, oxycodone HCl. Hard. Marked ONR/strength. 5mg: Orange/beige. *Sunset Yellow.* 10mg: White/beige. 20mg: Pink/beige.
OroDisp tablet (Dispersa), as above. White (off-white) round flat. Marked O; strength on reverse. *Aspartame, sucrose.*

OxyNorm Parenteral, Oral Soln *(Mundipharma)* CD. GMS.
Price, injection (5) (10mg/mL) 1mL, €7.81. 2mL, €12.91. (50mg/mL) 1mL, €39.20. Oral Soln 1mg/mL (250mL) €11.79; conc 10mg/mL (120mL) €56.99.
Injection or infusion, oxycodone HCl 10mg/mL, 50mg/mL (45mg base). Clear colourless (pale-yellow) soln. *Sodium 2.78mg/mL; 50mg/mL 0.998mg/mL.*
Oral concentrate, as above 10mg/mL. Clear orange conc. *Benzoate, Sunset Yellow.*
Oral solution, as above 1mg/mL. Clear colourless (straw-coloured). *Benzoate.*

Dancex SR Tablets *(Rowex)* CD. GMS.
Price, (28) 5mg, €5.43. (56) 10mg, €8.77. 20mg, €17.53. 40mg, €34.51. 80mg, €63.51.
Prolonged/R tablet, oxycodone HCl 5mg, 10mg, 20mg, 40mg, 80mg. Round. 5mg: Blue. 10mg: White. 20mg: Pink. 40mg: Yellow. 80mg: Green. *Lactose.*

Oxycodone Actavis 5mg, 10mg, 20mg *(TEVA)* CD. GMS.
Price, (56) 5mg, €4.78. 10mg, €13.35. 20mg, €25.13.
Capsule, oxycodone HCl. Hard. Marked OXY and strength. 5mg: Dark-pink/brown. 10mg: White/brown. 20mg: Light-pink/brown. **Store:** Below 30 deg C.

Reltebon Prolonged/R Tablets *(TEVA)* CD. GMS.
Price, (28) 5mg, €5.43. (56) 10mg, €8.77. 20mg, €17.53. 40mg, €34.51. 80mg, €63.51.
Prolonged/R tablet, oxycodone HCl 5mg, 10mg, 20mg, 40mg, 80mg. Round. Marked OX and strength. 5mg: Blue. 10mg: White. 20mg: Pink. 40mg: Yellow. 80mg: Green. *Lactose.* **Store:** Blisters below 25 deg C.

Oxycodone, Naloxone

ATC Code: N02AA05, V03AB15. **Sport:** Prohibited (in-competition).
Driving: May impair especially with other CNS depressants.
Indications: Treatment, severe pain (managed only with opioids). Second-line treatment, severe idiopathic Restless Legs Syndrome (RLS) (patients suffering from RLS for at least 6 months).
Dose: Adult: *Analgesia, opioid naive*, initially 10mg/5mg 12-hourly, max. 80mg/40mg; *already receiving opioids*, higher starting dose may be needed; max. 160mg/80mg

---

Opioid Analgesics   4.2.2

per day. Consider supplemental prolonged/R oxycodone (max. 400mg/day Prolonged/R oxycodone). Consider immediate release 'rescue' medication for breakthrough pain; more than two 'rescues' needed per day, consider dose increase in 5mg/2.5mg (or 10mg/5mg if needed) increments twice daily every 1-2 days.
RLS, initially 5mg/2.5mg 12-hourly increasing weekly; mean 20mg/10mg in clinical trials; up to max. 60mg/30mg. Both indications, admin on fixed time schedule; swallow whole; do not break, chew or crush.
Child: Under 18 years, no data.
Renal Impairment: Caution.
Hepatic Impairment: Mild, caution. Moderate/severe, contraindicated.
CI: Severe respiratory depression with hypoxia and/or hypercapnia, severe (COPD, bronchial asthma), cor pulmonale, non-opioid induced paralytic ileus. Indication RLS, opioid abuse.
SP: Naloxone counteracts opioid-induced constipation by blocking oxycodone action at opioid receptors locally in gut. Diarrhoea (possible effect of naloxone). Respiratory depression. Not for treatment of withdrawal. Prolonged/R tab matrix may be visible in stool.
Pregnancy, Lactation: See Notes below.
ADR: *Common*, decreased or loss of appetite, insomnia, dizziness, headache, somnolence, vertigo, hot flush, abdominal pain, constipation, diarrhoea, dry mouth, dyspepsia, vomiting, nausea, flatulence, pruritus, skin reactions, hyperhidrosis, asthenia, fatigue.
Notes: See 4.2.2 Opioid Analgesics. See Oxycodone above.

Targin Prolonged/R Tablets *(Mundipharma)* CD. GMS.
Price, (56) 5/2.5mg, €18.14. 10/5mg, €36.29. 15/7.5mg, €54.43. 20/10mg, €72.58. 30/15mg, €108.86. 40/20mg, €145.15. 60/30mg, €217.73. 80/40mg, €290.30.
Prolonged/R tablet, oxycodone HCl/naloxone HCl. Oblong f/c. Marked OXN/strength. *Lactose.* 5/2.5mg: Blue. 10/5mg: White. 20/10mg: Pink. 40/20mg: Yellow. **Store:** Below 25 deg C; original pack to protect (light). 15/7.5mg: Grey. 30/15mg: Brown. **Store:** Below 25 deg C. 60/30mg: Red. 80/40mg: Brown. **Store:** No special conditions.

Pethidine

ATC Code: N02AB02. **Sport:** Prohibited (in-competition).
Driving: Drowsiness, impaired cognitive function.
Indications: Moderate, severe pain (including cancer pain), not responding to non-opioids or only adequately managed with opioids. Adjunct to anaesthesia, pre-operative including labour, sole IV analgesic in surgical procedures, respiratory depressant/analgesic with prolonged assisted ventilation, neuroleptanalgesia (with neuroleptics).
Dose: Adult: *Pain*, 25-100mg IM or SC OR 25-50mg by slow IV, 4-hourly. *Obstetric analgesia*, 50-100mg IM or SC; repeat after 1-3 hours if needed; max. 400mg in 24 hours. *Pre-anaesthesia*, 25-100mg IM or SC about 1 hour before surgery. Adjunct to nitrous oxide-oxygen anaesthesia, 10-25mg by slow IV route.
Elderly: Initially max. 25mg.
Child: 0.5-2mg/kg 4-hourly IM for pain or 1 hour before surgery. Neonates, premature infants, see SP below.
Renal Impairment: Extreme caution, reduce dose.
Hepatic Impairment: As for Renal above.
Interactions: Effect of Other Drugs on Pethidine: *Co-admin not recommended*: Selegiline. *Severe hypotension*: Phenothiazines, depleted blood volume. *Neurotoxicity*: Anticholinergics. *Plasma levels increased*: Cimetidine, ritonavir. *Increased hepatic metabolism*: Phenytoin.
SP: Neonates, premature infants, elderly, debilitated, hypothyroidism, adrenocortical insufficiency, shock, prostatic hypertrophy, renal or hepatic impairment, biliary tract disorder, extreme caution, reduce dose. Convulsions with excessive doses.
Pregnancy, Lactation: Prior to labour, not recommended; use during labour, respiratory depression risk in newborn.
ADR: *Very common*, nausea, vomiting, light-headedness, dizziness, sedation, respiratory depression, sweating, hypotension.

4.2.2 Opioid Analgesics

Notes: See 4.2.2 Opioid Analgesics.

Pethidine Parenteral 50mg/mL *(Concordia)* CD.
Price, (10) 1mL, €2.62. 2mL, €3.21.
Injection, pethidine HCl. Clear colourless sterile soln.

Tapentadol

ATC Code: N02AX06. **Sport:** Permitted.
Driving: Major influence may affect CNS functions; caution with ALCOHOL or tranquilisers.
Indications: Management of pain, moderate/severe acute (Standard/R, oral soln), severe chronic (Prolonged/R).
Dose: Adult: STANDARD/R (tab, oral soln 20mg/1mL), 50mg every 4-6 hours; on first day, additional 50mg can be taken 1 hour after initial dose if pain control not achieved. Doses above 700mg/day (day 1) and 600mg/day (maintenance) not recommended. Admin tabs with sufficient liquid, with or without food. Oral soln can be taken undiluted or diluted in water or any non-alcoholic drink; measure using supplied oral syringe; can be admin via enteral tubes. For acute pain management; if longer-term treatment required, consider Prolonged/R.
PROLONGED/R (SR), opioid naive, initially 50mg twice daily; taking opioids, higher doses may be required. Daily dose above SR 500mg, not recommended. Not to be divided or chewed; to be taken whole with sufficient liquid with/without food.
Elderly: As for Renal/Hepatic function.
Child: Under 18 years, not recommended.
Renal Impairment: Severe, not recommended.
Hepatic Impairment: Moderate, caution; initiate at lowest strength (50mg) 8-hourly (Standard/R) or 24-hourly (Prolonged/R); max. 150mg/day. Severe, not recommended.
CI: Acute intoxication (alcohol, hypnotics, centrally acting analgesics, psychotropics), significant respiratory depression (where no resuscitative equipment), acute bronchial asthma or hypercapnia, suspected paralytic ileus.
Interactions: Effect of Other Drugs on Tapentadol: Co-admin caution: Strong enzyme inducers (rifampicin, phenobarbital, St John's Wort). Co-admin, possible increased systemic exposure: Strong inhibitors of UGT1A6, UGT1A9, UGT2B7 isoforms. Serotonin syndrome risk with co-admin: SSRIs.
SP: May cause spasm of sphincter of Oddi; caution with biliary tract disease including pancreatitis.
Pregnancy, Lactation: See Notes below.
ADR: Summary, *most frequent,* GI disorders, CNS (nausea, vomiting, somnolence, dizziness, headache).
Notes: See 4.2.2 Opioid Analgesics.

Palexia, SR, Oral Soln *(Grunenthal)* CD. GMS.
Price, tabs 50mg (28) €15.88; (56) €31.75. 75mg (28) €21.40; (56) €42.56. 100mg (28) €31.75. Prolonged/R SR 50mg (28) €15.88; (56) €31.75. (56) 100mg, €63.50. 150mg, €95.26. 200mg, €127.01. 250mg, €158.76. Oral soln 200mL, €45.36.
Standard/R tablet, tapentadol HCl 50mg, 75mg, 100mg. Round f/c. Marked with logo. 50mg: White. Marked H6. 75mg: Pale-yellow. Marked H7. 100mg: Pale-pink. Marked H8. *Lactose.*
Prolonged/R tablet, as above (SR) 50mg, 100mg, 150mg, 200mg, 250mg. Oblong f/c. Marked with logo. 50mg: White. Marked H1. 100mg: Pale-yellow. Marked H2. 150mg: Pale-pink. Marked H3. 200mg: Pale-orange. Marked H4. 250mg: Brownish-red. Marked H5. *Lactose.*
Oral soln, as above 20mg/1mL. Clear colourless.

Tramadol

ATC Code: N02AX02. **Sport:** Permitted.
Driving: Somnolence, dizziness; especially with ALCOHOL, other psychotropics.
Indications: Treatment, moderate to severe pain.
Dose: Adult: ORAL, STANDARD/R (50mg, 100mg), age 12 years and over, *acute* pain, initially 100mg, then 50-100mg every 4-6 hours; *chronic* pain, initially 50mg then titrate according to severity. Max. 400mg in 24 hours except in special circumstances.
PROLONGED/R, **SR**, initially 50-100mg twice daily, titrate to range 100-200mg twice daily if needed; max. 400mg/day. *Admin,* dissolve sachet contents or effervescent tabs in water. PROLONGED/R, **XL**, 1 tab daily

at 24-hour intervals; titrate up if needed. *Admin,* swallow tabs or caps whole; don not crush or chew. Administered only for as long as absolutely necessary.
PARENTERAL, initial bolus 100mg IM or slow IV injection; then 50-100mg every 4-6 hours; max. 400mg/day; duration, short and intermittent to avoid dependence. *Zydol* injection may also be admin SC or diluted for admin by infusion or patient-controlled analgesia (PCA); up to 600mg/day has been tolerated (for PCA, initially 100mg bolus; then 20mg increments; minimum interval or lock-out of 5 minutes between doses).
Elderly: Over 75 years, elimination may be prolonged; consider dose interval increase.
Child: ORAL, over 12 years as for Adult; under 12 years, not recommended. PARENTERAL, age above 1 year, 1-2mg/kg as single dose; repeat dose, max. 8mg/kg/day or 400mg/day whichever is lower.
Renal Impairment: As for Elderly above.
Hepatic Impairment: As for Elderly above.
CI: Acute intoxication (alcohol, hypnotics, analgesics, opioids, psychotropics), uncontrolled epilepsy, use for narcotic withdrawal.
Interactions: Effect of Other Drugs on Tramadol: Co-admin contraindicated: MAOIs or within 14 days of admin. Plasma levels possibly increased: Cimetidine. Plasma levels decreased (decreased analgesic efficacy; shorter duration of action): Carbamazepine. Serotonin Syndrome risk: SSRIs, SNRIs, triptans, MAOIs, mirtazapine, TCADs. Increased requirement (post-operative pain): 5-HT3 antagonists (ondansetron). Analgesic effect may be reduced (withdrawal); contraindicated (Tramake): Mixed agonists/antagonists (buprenorphine, nalbuphine, pentazocine).
Effect of Tramadol on Other Drugs: SSRIs, TCADs, antipsychotics, other medicinals potentially lowering seizure threshold (bupropion, mirtazapine, tetrahydrocannabinol): Increased convulsion potential. Coumarins, warfarin: Increased INR, bleeding risk.
SP: Not a suitable substitute in opioid dependence (cannot suppress morphine withdrawal symptoms); at therapeutic doses, withdrawal symptoms reported. Drowsiness, convulsions (especially at high doses), increased seizure risk (caution, epileptics or susceptible to seizures). Biliary tract disorders. Anaesthesia (avoid). Unsuitable for intra-operative analgesia; increased awareness experienced.
Pregnancy, Lactation: See Notes below. May be used during labour (may induce changes in neonatal respiratory rate).
ADR: *Very common,* dizziness, nausea, vomiting *(Tramake); common,* headache, somnolence, constipation, dry mouth, vomiting, hyperhidrosis, fatigue.
Notes: See 4.2.2 Opioid Analgesics.
Interchangeability: Same strengths of all brands of tramadol capsules/tablets and Prolonged/R capsules/tablets are deemed interchangeable.

Zydol 50mg, SR *(Grunenthal)* A. GMS.D*.
Price, 50mg* (100) €7.00. SR (60) 50mg, €4.94; 100mg, €8.65; 150mg, €13.48; 200mg, €17.96.
Standard/R capsule, tramadol HCl. Yellow/yellow shiny.
Prolonged/R tablet (SR), tramadol HCl 50mg, 100mg, 150mg, 200mg. Marked with logo. SR: 50mg: Pale-yellow. Marked T0. 100mg: White. Marked T1. 150mg: Peach. Marked T2. 200mg: Brownish-orange. Marked T3. *Lactose.*
Zydol Parenteral *(Grunenthal)* A. GMS.
Price, 50mg (5) €4.04.
Soln for injection or infusion, tramadol HCl 50mg/mL. Clear colourless. *Sodium 0.7mg/mL.*
Tradol 50mg, Effervescent 50mg, SR *(Rowex)* A. GMS.D*.
Price, (100) 50mg*, €7.00. Effervescent (30) 50mg*, €5.95. SR (60) 100mg, €8.65. 150mg, €13.48. 200mg, €17.96.
Capsule, tramadol HCl. Yellow/green. **Store:** Below 25 deg C.
Effervescent tablet, as above. White round flat scored; orange odour. *Lactose.* **Store:** As above; tightly closed to protect (moisture).
Prolonged/R tablets (SR), as above 100mg, 150mg, 200mg. Round flat Prolonged/R bi-layered green. Marked TR and strength. **Store:** Below 25 deg C.

Tradol Parenteral *(Rowex)* A. GMS.
Price, 50mg/mL (5) 2mL, €2.70.
Injection or infusion, tramadol HCl 50mg/mL. Clear colourless soln. *Sodium less than 1mmoL/mL.* **Store:** Below 25 deg C.
Tramadol (Actavis) 50mg *(Accord)* A. GMS.D.
Price, (100) €7.00.
Capsule, tramadol. Hard gelatin dark green/yellow. Marked TK. **Store:** Original pack to protect (light).
Tramake 50mg, 100mg *(Galen)* A. GMS.D*.
Price, 50mg* (100) €7.00. 100mg (60) €18.41.
Tablet, tramadol HCl. White u/c. 50mg: Marked T50. 100mg: Marked TRAMAKE 100. *Lactose.* **Store:** Below 25 deg C.
Tramapine 50mg *(Pinewood)* A. GMS.D.
Price, 50mg (100) €7.00.
Capsule, tramadol HCl. Green/yellow. *Lactose.* **Store:** Below 25 deg C; original pack.
Xymel SR, SR 100mg *(Clonmel)* A. GMS.D*.
Price, 50mg* (100) €7.00. SR 100mg (60) €8.65.
Capsule, tramadol HCl. Green/yellow. Marked TRA50.
Prolonged/R tablet, as above. White round f/c.

Tramadol, Paracetamol

ATC Code: N02AX52. **Sport:** Permitted.
Driving: Drowsiness, dizziness; enhanced by alcohol, other CNS depressants.

Indications: Treatment, moderate to severe pain when a combination is needed.

Dose: Adult: Age 12 years and over, initially 2 tabs (equiv. to tramadol 75mg, paracetamol 650mg); additional doses as needed 6-hourly; max 8 tabs (equiv. to 300mg tramadol, 2600mg paracetamol) per day. *Admin,* swallow f/c tabs whole with liquid; do not break or chew; dissolve effervescent tabs in glass of water.

Elderly: Over 75 years, elimination may be prolonged; consider extending dosing interval.

Child: Under 12 years, not recommended.

Renal Impairment: As for Elderly above. CrCl (mL/min) below 10, not recommended.

Hepatic Impairment: As for Elderly above; severe, not recommended (paracetamol component).

SP: Severe respiratory insufficiency, not recommended. Do not use other paracetamol or tramadol products concurrently. Non-cirrhotic alcoholic liver disease, caution (paracetamol overdose).

Pregnancy, Lactation: Not recommended.

ADR: Summary, *most common,* nausea, dizziness, somnolence.

Notes: See 4.2.2 Opioid Analgesics and Tramadol above. See 4.2.1 Non-Opioid Analgesics (paracetamol).

Interchangeability: Same strengths of all brands of tramadol/paracetamol f/c tablets are deemed interchangeable.

Ixprim Tabs, Effervescent *(Grunenthal)* A. GMS.
Price, (60) 37.5/325mg, €10.01. Eff, €9.98.
Tablet, tramadol 37.5mg, paracetamol 325mg. Pale-yellow f/c. Marked with logo; T5 on reverse.
Effervescent tablet, as above. Off-white (slightly rosy coloured) with some coloured speckles; round flat. *Sunset Yellow.*
Tradol Plus 37.5/325mg *(Rowex)* A. GMS.
Price, (60) 37.5/325mg, €5.70.
Tablet, tramadol 37.5mg, paracetamol 325mg. White elongated scored (not intended for breaking). **Store:** No special conditions.
Tramadol/Paracetamol KRKA Tabs *(Krka)* GMS.
Price, (60) 37.5/325mg, €4.00.
Tablet, tramadol 37.5mg, paracetamol 325mg. Yellow-brown oval f/c. **Store:** No special conditions.
Tramadol/Paracetamol TEVA Tabs *(TEVA)* A. GMS.
Price, (60) 37.5/325mg, €4.01.
Tablet, tramadol 37.5mg, paracetamol 325mg. Peach cap-shaped f/c. Marked T37.5 one side; A325 on reverse. **Store:** No special conditions.
Xymel Comp 37.5/325mg *(Clonmel)* A. GMS.
Price, (60) 37.5/325mg, €4.01.
Tablet, tramadol 37.5mg, paracetamol 325mg. Light-yellow oblong f/c. **Store:** No special conditions.

4.2.3 - Other Analgesics

In This Chapter: *Methoxyflurane, ziconotide.*

Other Analgesics   4.2.3

Class Effects
Included are inhalation and intrathecal analgesics.

CI: Hypersensitivity to any member of the class.

Methoxyflurane

ATC Code: N02BG09. **Sport:** Permitted.
Driving: Minor influence; dizziness, somnolence, drowsiness.

Indications: Emergency relief, moderate to severe pain (conscious adults with trauma and associated pain).

Dose: Adult, Elderly: 1x 3mL vial to be vapourised in a *Penthrox* inhaler; on finishing the 3mL dose, another 3mL may be used; max. 6mL in one admin. Use lowest effective dose to provide analgesia. Onset of pain relief after 6-10 inhalations. Continuous inhalation provides analgesia for 25-30 minutes. *Admin,* on consecutive days not recommended; max. 15mL per week.

Elderly: Use lowest effective dose.

Child: Under 18 years, not recommended.

Renal Impairment: Clinically significant, contraindicated. May cause nephrotoxicity at high doses; nephrotoxicity related to rate of metabolism. Known risk factors for renal disease, use lowest effective dose.

Hepatic Impairment: Increased exposure with hepatic impairment can cause toxicity. Underlying hepatic conditions, caution. See Contraindications (CI) below. Previous exposure, especially less than 3-month interval, may increase hepatic injury potential.

CI: Use as anaesthetic agent. Hypersensitivity to fluorinated anaesthetics. Malignant hyperthermia (known, susceptible to, history of). Liver damage after previous methoxyflurane or halogenated anaesthetic. Altered level of consciousness (head injury, drugs, alcohol). Clinically evident cardiovascular instability, respiratory depression.

Interactions: Effect of Other Drugs on Methoxyflurane: *Increased nephrotoxicity risk:* Increased rate of metabolism with hepatic enzyme inducers (ALCOHOL, isoniazid, phenobarbital, rifampicin), genetic variations (fast metaboliser status), potentially nephrotoxic agents (tetracyclines, gentamicin, colistin, polymyxin B, amphotericin B, contrast agents). *Additive CNS depression:* Opioids, sedatives, hypnotics, general anaesthetics, phenothiazines, tranquillisers, skeletal muscle relaxants, sedating antihistamines, ALCOHOL. There are no interactions when used at analgesic dose (3-6mL). *Avoid:* Sevoflurane anaesthesia following methoxyflurane analgesia (raised serum fluoride levels/nephrotoxicity).

SP: Older people with hypotension and bradycardia, caution due to possible reduced BP. CNS effects (sedation, euphoria, amnesia, ability to concentrate, altered sensorimotor co-ordination, changed mood); can be risk factor for potential abuse. Regular exposure to methoxyflurane may be an occupational hazard. Not appropriate for relief of: Breakthrough pain/exacerbations (chronic pain); trauma-related pain in closely repeated episodes (same patient).

Pregnancy, Lactation: Pregnancy, exercise care especially first trimester. Lactation, caution.

ADR: Summary, *most common non-serious,* dizziness, somnolence; *serious,* dose-related nephrotoxicity (large doses over prolonged periods during general anaesthesia); methoxyflurane is no longer used for anaesthesia.

Notes: See Class Effects 14.1.4 Inhalation Anaesthetics (isoflurane, sevoflurane).

▼ **PENTHROX Inhalation** *(Galen)* A.
Price, (1) 3mL, €23.05 (PTW).
Inhalation vapour liquid, methoxyflurane 99.9%. Clear almost colourless volatile liquid; fruity odour. **Store:** No special conditions.

Ziconotide

ATC Code: N02BG08. **Sport:** Permitted.
Driving: Not applicable.

Indications: Treatment, severe chronic pain requiring intrathecal analgesia.

Dose: Adult, Elderly: Initially 2.4mcg/day; titrate up by up to 2.4mcg/day; max. 21.6mcg/day; minimum interval of 24-hours between increases. Continuous infusion via intrathecal catheter capable of delivering accurate infusion volume.

Child: Under 18 years, not recommended.

Renal Impairment: Caution.

Hepatic Impairment: As for Renal above.

Interactions: Effect of Other Drugs on Ziconotide: *Co-admin not recommended:* Intrathecal chemotherapy. *Co-admin caution:* Systemic chemotherapy, intrathecal morphine. *Increased somnolence:* Systemic baclofen, clonidine, bupivacaine, propofol.

SP: Treatment under direction of physicians experienced in intrathecal drug admin. Recommend neuropsychiatric evaluation before and after starting intrathecal ziconotide. *Long-term treatment,* systemic chemotherapy, caution. Serious infection risk (meningitis, may be life-threatening). Lower catheter tip placement (lumbar) may reduce neurological adverse events. Monitor CPK levels (myopathy, rhabdomyolysis). Potential for severe allergic reactions. Cognitive and neuropsychiatric disturbances (particularly confusion). Depressed levels of consciousness, discontinue; do not reintroduce. May cause or worsen depression with suicide risk.

Pregnancy, Lactation: If benefit outweighs risk.

ADR: Summary, *most common,* dizziness, nausea, nystagmus, confusional state, abnormal gait, memory impairment, blurred vision, headache, asthenia, vomiting, somnolence.

Notes: See 4.2.1 Non-Opioid Analgesics.

Prialt Intrathecal 100mcg/mL *(Eisai)* A.
Price, (1) 1mL, €399.16. 5mL, €1995.80.
Intrathecal infusion, ziconotide acetate. Clear colourless soln.
Store: Refrigerate; do no freeze; protect (light).

4.3 - Neuromuscular Disorders

4.3.1 - Skeletal Muscle Relaxants

In This Chapter: *Baclofen, botulinum toxin, dantrolene, tizanidine.*

Class Effects

Diazepam is also used to treat muscle spasm. Dantrolene IV is indicated for the treatment of malignant hyperthermia

CI: Hypersensitivity of any member of class.

Notes: See 3.3.5 Benzodiazepine Anxiolytics (diazepam). See manufacturers Full Prescribing Information.

Baclofen

ATC Code: M03BX01. **Sport:** Permitted.
Driving: Dizziness, sedation, somnolence, visual impairment; caution when spasticity is needed to sustain upright posture and balance in locomotion.

Indications: Relief of voluntary muscle spasticity associated with MS, spinal cord lesions (syringomelia, MND, transverse myelitis), Adults, spasticity of cerebral origin (meningitis, cerebral palsy, traumatic head injury, cerebrovascular accident) *(both brands).* Paediatric (0-18 years), symptomatic treatment of spasticity of cerebral origin (infantile cerebral palsy, CVA, neoplastic or degenerative brain disease) *(Lioresal).*

Dose: Adult: Initially 15mg/day in 2-4 divided doses; increase cautiously by 15mg/day at 3-day intervals; sensitive patients, initiate at 5-10mg, increase more gradually. Optimum range 30-80mg/day (usually 60mg/day); max. 100mg/day unless hospitalised. Hospital use, 100-120mg may be required. No effect within 6 weeks at max. recommended dose, decide whether to continue. Spastic states of cerebral origin, initiate and titrate with caution. *Admin,* oral with food or a little liquid; milk beverage (especially with nausea). NOTE: Liquid and tabs are bioequivalent.

Elderly: Side effect more common especially at initiation. Initiate at low dose under careful medical supervision.

Child: Age 0-18 years, 0.3mg/kg/day in 2-4 divided doses (preferably 4 divided doses); titrate cautiously at 1-2 week intervals; maintenance range 0.75-2mg/kg. Under 33kg, tablets not suitable.

Renal Impairment: Impaired function, chronic haemodialysis, 5mg/day. ESRD, use only if benefit outweighs risk. Haemodialysis effectively removes baclofen (alleviates clinical symptoms of overdose).

CI: Pulmonary insufficiency.

Interactions: Effect of Other Drugs on Baclofen: *Increased risk (sedation, respiratory depression):* Other CNS drugs, other muscle relaxants (tizanidine), synthetic opiates, ALCOHOL. *Caution, increased (CNS depression, hypotensive effect):* MAOIs (mutual dose reduction may be required), morphine, intrathecal baclofen. *Effect potentiated:* TCADs. *Increased hypotensive effect:* Anti-hypertensives. *Reduced excretion, increased toxicity:* Drugs which may produce renal insufficiency (ibuprofen). *Mental confusion, hallucinations, nausea, agitation:* Parkinson's treated with levodopa/carbidopa.

Effect of Baclofen on Other Drugs: Insulin and/or oral hypoglycaemic agents: *Dose adjustment may be required.* Lithium: *Aggravation of hyperkinetic symptoms.* Fentanyl-induced anaesthesia: *Prolongation.*

SP: Psychiatric and nervous system disorders (porphyria, alcoholism, hypertension, psychotic disorders, schizophrenia, depressive or manic disorders, confusional states, Parkinson's disease); epilepsy (history of convulsions), may be exacerbated (caution). Use with caution in patients with peptic ulcer, cerebrovascular disease, respiratory, renal or hepatic impairment, sphincter hypertonia (may experience acute urinary retention). *Discontinue* gradually over 1-2 weeks; abrupt withdrawal (anxiety, confusional states, hallucinations, psychotic, manic or paranoid states, convulsions including status epilepticus, dyskinesia, tachycardia, hyperthermia, rebound aggravation of spasticity). Rarely elevated serum SGOT, ALP, glucose. Paradoxical increased spasticity. Excess muscular hypotonia. Upright posture, see Driving above.

Pregnancy, Lactation: Pregnancy, if benefit outweighs risk; crosses placental barrier. Lactation, at therapeutic dose, passes into breast milk in small quantities; no undesirable effect on infant expected.

ADR: Unwanted effects occur mainly (at treatment initiation, too rapid dose increase, at large doses, elderly). If nausea persist following dose reduction, ingested with food or a milk beverage. Lowering of convulsion threshold; convulsions may occur, particularly in epileptics. Certain patients, increased muscle spasticity (paradoxical reaction). History of psychiatric illness, cerebrovascular disorders (stroke), older patients, adverse events may be more serious.

Notes: See 4.3.1 Skeletal Muscle Relaxants.

Lioresal 10mg, Oral Soln *(Novartis)* B. GMS.
Price, 10mg (100) €5.77. Soln 5mg/5mL 300mL, €7.80.
Tablet, baclofen. Round flat white (faintly yellowish) scored (divisible into equal halves). Marked CG and KJ. Wheat starch.
Oral soln, as above 5mg/5mL. Clear colourless (faintly yellow) slightly viscous; raspberry odour. *Parabens; sodium 1.62mg/mL.*
Baclopar 10mg *(Gerard)* B. GMS.
Price, (100) €5.65.
Tablet, baclofen. White flat scored (divisible into equal halves). Marked BN and 10; G on reverse. *Lactose.*

Botulinum Toxin Type A

ATC Code: M03AX01. **Sport:** Permitted.
Driving: Asthenia, muscle weakness, visual disturbances.
Indications: *BOTOX,* focal spasticity associated with dynamic equinus foot deformity in paediatric cerebral palsy patients (age 2 years and over); of wrist and hand, ankle in adult post stroke; blepharospasm, hemifacial spasm; cervical dystonia; chronic migraine. Idiopathic overactive bladder, neurogenic detrusor overactivity. Severe primary hyperhidrosis of the axillae. *Dysport,* focal spasticity affecting upper limbs (fingers, wrist, elbow) (adults), dynamic equinus foot in cerebral palsy patients (age 2 and older); spasmodic torticollis, blepharospasm, hemifacial spasm; severe primary hyperhidrosis of the axillae. *Azzalure, Vistabel,* temporary improvement of appearance of facial lines when severity has important psychological impact on adult patient. *Xeomin,* blepharospasm, cervical

dystonia (spasmodic torticollis), post-stroke spasticity of upper limb (flexed wrist, clenched fist).

Dose: Adult: NOTE: Botulinum toxin units are not interchangeable. For dilutions, recommended needle size, method of admin and dose distribution amongst muscle groups, see Notes below.

AZZALURE, glabellar lines, 50 Speywood units (SU) divided into 5 injection sites (10 SU per site). Lateral canthal lines, 30 SU (60 SU for both sides) divided into 3 injection sites of 10 SU each.

BOTOX, blepharospasm, hemifacial spasm, initially 1.25-2.5 Units at 3 sites; max. 100 Units every 12 weeks. *Cervical dystonia,* range 140-280 Units; max 50 Units at any 1 site; total 300 Units at any 1 sitting. *Paediatric cerebral palsy, hemiplegia,* initially 4 Units/kg body weight in affected limb; diplegia, initially 6 Units/kg divided between affected limbs; max. 200 Units. *Focal limb spasticity,* lower (stroke), 75 Units at 3 sites; upper (stroke), flexor digitorum profundus and sublimis, 15-50 Units; flexor carpi radialis, 15-60 Units; flexor carpi ulnaris, 10-50 Units; adductor pollicis, flexor pollicis longus, 20 Units (all in 1-2 sites). *Axillary hyperhidrosis,* 50 Units intradermally approx. 1-2cm apart. *Overactive bladder (OAB),* use intravesical instillation of diluted local anaesthetic prior to injection, with or without sedation; 100 Units as 5 Unit injections across 20 sites in detrusor. Urinary incontinence due to neurogenic detrusor overactivity, local anaesthetic (as for OAB) or general anaesthetic; 200 Units as 6.7 Units across 30 sites in detrusor. *Chronic migraine* (under neurologist supervision), 155-195 Units IM as 5 Units in 31-39 sites; divided across 7 specific head/neck muscle areas.

DYSPORT, focal spasticity of upper limb, tailor dose*; max. 1000 units (U) at any treatment session. Distribute among flexor carpi radialis and ulnaris (1-2 injections each), 100-200U; flexor digitorum profundus and superficialis (1-2 injections each), flexor pollicis longus (1 injection), 100-200U; adductor pollicis (1 injection), 25-50U; brachialis, biceps brachii (as 1-2 injections) 200-400U; brachioradialis (1- 2 injections) and pronator teres (as 1 injection), 100-200U. Repeat at minimum 12 weeks. *Dynamic equinus foot* deformity paediatric cerebral palsy (age 2 years and older), tailor dose*; per treatment session, max. 15 units/kg (unilateral lower limb) OR 30 units/kg (bilateral). Total dose per session, max. 1000 units or 30 units/kg (whichever lower) divided between affected spastic muscles of lower limb(s) if possible across more than 1 injection site in any single muscle. Repeat at minimum 12 weeks; majority of patients range 16-22 weeks. *Admin,* IM injection. *Spasmodic torticollis,* initially 500 units as a divided dose admin into the 2 or 3 most active neck muscles; range 250 units to max. 1000 units; may be repeated every 16 weeks. *Blepharospasm, hemifacial spasm,* 40 units per eye; 80 units may be used; max. 120 units per eye. *Axillary hyperhidrosis,* 100 units per axilla, up to max. 200 units per axilla for subsequent injections; minimum every 12 weeks. *(size, number/location of muscles involved, spasticity severity, local muscle weakness, response to previous treatment).

VISTABEL, glabellar lines, max. 4 U into max. 5 injection sites; max. 3-monthly intervals. Crow's Feet Lines, max. 4 U into max. 3 injection sites per side (6 sites, total 24 U).

XEOMIN, blepharospasm, initially 1.25-2.5 Units per injection site; max. 25 U per eye; max. 100 Units every 12 weeks. *Spasmodic torticollis,* total dose max. 200 U; up to 300 U may be given; max. 50 U per injection site. *Post-stroke spasticity,* 170-400 U depending on patient need; max. 400 U per session.

Elderly: Use lowest effective dose with longest clinically indicated interval between injections; significant medical history and concomitant medication, caution.

Child: *BOTOX,* see Adult above. Not recommended, under 2 years (focal spasticity of paediatric cerebral palsy), under 12 years (blepharospasm, hemifacial spasm, cervical dystonia, primary hyperhidrosis*), under 18 years (upper/lower limb spasticity associated with stroke, chronic migraine, overactive bladder, detrusor overactivity). *Limited experience in adolescents 12-17 years.

Dysport, see Adult above. Not recommended, under 2 years (cerebral palsy).

Azzalure, Vistabel, under 18 years, not recommended. *Xeomin,* under 17 years not recommended.

CI: Infection at proposed injection site. Use in urinary incontinence/bladder dysfunction (UTI, acute urinary retention, catheterisation post-treatment not possible). Myasthenia gravis, Eaton Lambert Syndrome *(Vistabel, Xeomin),* see SP below.

Interactions: Effect of Other Drugs on Botulinum Toxin Type A: *Effect potentiated:* Neuromuscular blockers, depolarising (succinylcholine), non-depolarising (tubocurarine derivatives) lincosamides, polymyxins, quinidine, magnesium sulfate, anticholinesterases; aminoglycosides, spectinomycin.

SP: Do not exceed recommended dose and/or frequency; use lowest effective dose to minimise excessive muscle weakness. Support measures to be available (anaphylaxis); hypersensitivity reactions, antibody formation.

Caution, dysphagia, pneumopathy and/or significant debility, asthenia. Injection site inflammation; excessive weakness or atrophy; treatment of amyotrophic lateral sclerosis or disorders with peripheral neuromuscular dysfunction; injection into vulnerable anatomic structures or blood vessels. *Extreme caution,* subclinical or clinical evidence of defective neuromuscular transmission (myasthenia gravis) or Eaton Lambert Syndrome with peripheral neuropathic diseases or underlying neurological disorders.

Blepharospasm, reduced blinking leading to corneal exposure, persistent epithelial defect, corneal ulceration (especially with VII nerve disorders), ecchymosis; caution angle closure glaucoma. *Cervical dystonia* patients, inform of possibility of dysphagia, potential for aspiration, dyspnoea, occasional need for tube feeding. Autonomic dysreflexia. *Spasmodic torticollis,* adult post-stroke spasticity, use usually restricted to hospital specialist units. Chronic medication overuse headache, no data.

BOTOX, not for use for focal spasticity of ankle (post-stroke) if muscle tone reduction is not expected to result in improved function (walking) or improved symptoms (pain) or to facilitate care (increased fall risk).

Pregnancy, Lactation: Pregnancy, women of child-bearing potential not using contraception, only if clearly necessary and benefit outweighs risk; some brands are not recommended. Lactation, not recommended.

ADR: Most frequent, *Azzalure,* headache, injection-site reactions (both indications); eyelid oedema (lateral canthal lines); *other brands,* generalised muscle weakness, flu-like syndrome, injection-site reactions. See SP above, Notes below.

Notes: See 4.3.1 Skeletal Muscle Relaxants.

Azzalure Parenteral *(Galderma)* A.
Price, not published by company.
Injection, Clostridium botulinum toxin type A, 125 Speywood units per vial. White powder for soln. **Store:** Refrigerate; do not freeze.

BOTOX Parenteral *(Allergan)* A. HOS.
Price, (1) Units (U): 50 U, €123.41; 100 U, €191.80; 200 U, €411.38 (PTW).
Injection, Clostridium botulinum toxin type A, 100 Allergan units (U)/vial. Powder for soln. **Store:** Refrigerate or freeze.

Dysport Parenteral *(Ipsen)* A.
Price, 500 units (2), not published by company.
Injection, Clostridium botulinum type A toxin-haemagglutinin complex 500 Units. White lyophilised powder for soln. **Store:** Refrigerate; do not freeze.

Vistabel Parenteral *(Allergan)* A.
Price, not published by company (50-unit vial).
Injection, Clostridium botulinum toxin type A, 4 Allergan units per 0.1mL. White powder for soln. *Essentially sodium-free.* **Store:** Refrigerate.

Xeomin Parenteral *(Merz)* A.
Price, 50 units, €110.00; 100 units, €195.00 (PTW).
Injection, Clostridium botulinum toxin type A, 100 LD50 units/vial. White powder for soln. **Store:** Below 25 deg C.

Botulinum Toxin Type B

ATC Code: M03AX01. **Sport:** Permitted.
Driving: Muscle weakness, blurred vision, eyelid ptosis.
Indications: Treatment of cervical dystonia (torticollis).

4.3.2 Drugs Enhancing Neuromuscular Transmission

Dose: Adult, Elderly: Initially 10000 units divided between the 2-4 most affected muscles. IM injection only.

Child: Under 18 years, not recommended.

CI: Other neuromuscular disease (ALS, peripheral neuropathy, neuromuscular junctional disorders,(myasthenia gravis, Lambert-Eaton Syndrome).

SP: Bleeding disorders, anticoagulant therapy. Children (unapproved use) and patients with underlying neuromuscular disorders (swallowing disorders), at increase adverse event risk. Respiratory difficulties, choking, new or worsening dysphagia, seek medical advice.

Pregnancy, Lactation: Pregnancy, only if clinical condition requires this treatment. Lactation, not recommended.

ADR: Dry mouth, worsening of torticollis from baseline, injection site pain, neck pain, dysphagia, dyspepsia, voice alteration, myasthenia, taste perversion.

Notes: See Botulinum Toxin Type A above.

NeuroBloc Parenteral (Eisai) A. HOS.
Price, (1) 2500 U/mL, €179.47. 5000 U/mL: 1mL, €180.57; 2mL, €260.31 (PTW).
Injection, botulinum toxin type B. Clear colourless (light-yellow) soln. **Store:** Refrigerate; do not freeze. Can be stored below 25 deg C for max. 3 months then discarded.

Dantrolene

ATC Code: M03CA01. **Sport:** Permitted.
Driving: Not recommended.

Indications: Treatment, chronic severe spasticity resulting from stroke, MS, spinal cord injury, cerebral palsy. Malignant hyperthermia (MH).

Dose: Adult, Elderly: ORAL, initially 25mg/day (week 1), then 25mg twice daily (week 2 and 3), then 25mg 3-times daily (week 4 and 5), then 25mg 4-times daily (week 6) then 100mg 4-times daily (week 7). Maintain each dose level for 7 days; max. 400mg/day. No benefit after 45 days, discontinue.

PARENTERAL, continuous rapid IV push starting at minimum 1mg/kg and continuing until symptoms subside or max. dose is reached (10mg/kg).

Child: ORAL, over 5 years, initially 0.5mg/kg twice daily (week 1), then 1mg/kg twice daily (week 2), then 2mg/kg twice daily (week 3), then 2mg/kg 3-times daily (week 4), then 3mg/kg (week 5), then 3mg/kg 4-times daily (week 6). PARENTERAL, as for Adult above.

Hepatic Impairment: See SP below.

CI: Where spasticity is utilised to sustain upright posture and balance in locomotion; obtain or maintain increased function (oral).

Interactions: Effect of Other Drugs on Dantrolene: *Enhanced hepatotoxicity:* Other hepatotoxic drugs, oestrogen. *Caution:* Tranquilisers, ALCOHOL. *Co-admin of IV not recommended:* Calcium channel blockers.

Effect of Dantrolene on Other Drugs: Vecuronium-induced blockade: *Potentiated by IV dantrolene.*

SP: Oral, cardiovascular or respiratory disease, caution. Fatal and non-fatal hepatic disorders. Hepatotoxicity, signs or symptoms (discoloured faeces, generalised pruritus, jaundice, anorexia, nausea, vomiting), risk factors include dose (above 400mg/day), duration (most frequently reported between 2-12 months), females, over 30 years, history of liver disease, co-admin with other hepatotoxic therapy, elderly. Exclude liver disease before initiation.

Parenteral, in management of MH, not a substitute for supportive measures. Advise patients that decrease in grip strength, weakness of leg muscles, light-headedness can be expected post-op. When mannitol is used to prevent/treat renal complications of hyperthermia, mannitol content of Dantrium vial to be taken into account (3000mg mannitol per 20mg dantrolene sodium).

Pregnancy, Lactation: Oral, not recommended. Parenteral, if benefit outweighs risk. Dantrolene crosses the placenta. Lactation, if benefit outweighs risk; detected in human milk at low conc (below 2mcg/mL) during repeated IV admin over 3 days.

ADR: *Common,* anorexia, mental (depression, confusion) (oral), seizure, disturbances (visual, speech), headache, drowsiness, dizziness, pericarditis, pleural effusion with eosinophilia, respiratory depression, nausea, vomiting, abdominal pain, diarrhoea (may be severe and require temporary withdrawal) (oral), hepatotoxicity, abnormal LFTs, acne-like rash, skin eruptions, chills, fever, weakness, fatigue, general malaise. IV, local injection-site reactions, thrombophlebitis. See manufacturers Full Prescribing Information.

Notes: See 4.3.1 Skeletal Muscle Relaxants.

Dantrium 25mg, 100mg (Norgine) B. GMS.
Price, (100) 25mg, €19.97. 100mg, €52.44.
Capsule, dantrolene sodium. 25mg: White/orange. 100mg: White/green. *Lactose.* **Store:** Below 30 deg C.

Dantrium Parenteral (Norgine) A.
Price, not published by company.
Injection, dantrolene sodium 0.33mg/mL. Pale orange (yellow) powder for soln. **Store:** Below 25 deg C; do not refrigerate or freeze reconstituted soln.

Tizanidine

ATC Code: M03BX02. **Sport:** Permitted.
Driving: Drowsiness, dizziness.

Indications: Spasticity associated with multiple sclerosis or spinal cord injury or disease.

Dose: Adult: Initially 2mg, titrating at half-weekly intervals by 2mg increments; max. 12mg in any single dose; max. 36mg/day although usually dose exceeding 24mg not needed; efficacy achieved at 8mg and above. Oral, in divided doses up to 3-4 times daily. Max. effect seen within 2-3 hours of dosing; relatively short duration of action.

Elderly: If benefit outweighs risk.

Child: Under 18 years, not recommended.

Renal Impairment: CrCl (mL/min) below 25, initially 2mg once daily. Titrate slowly in max. 2mg increments to effective dose.

Hepatic Impairment: Significant, contraindicated.

Interactions: Effect of Other Drugs on Tizanidine: *Co-admin contraindicated:* CYP450 1A2 inhibitors (fluvoxamine), fluoroquinolones (ciprofloxacin). *Co-admin caution:* Drugs increasing QT-interval, antiarrhythmics (amiodarone, mexiletine, propafenone), cimetidine, fluoroquinolones (enoxacin, norfloxacin), ticlopidine, oral contraceptives. *Increased sedation:* ALCOHOL, other sedatives. *Clearance may be reduced:* Oral contraceptives.

Effect of Tizanidine on Other Drugs: Antihypertensives (including diuretics): *Effect potentiated.* Beta-adrenoceptor blocking drugs, digoxin: *May potentiate hypotension or bradycardia.*

SP: Increased plasma levels, overdose symptoms (QTc prolongation). Hypotension (loss of consciousness, circulatory collapse). Sudden withdrawal (rebound hypertension, tachycardia); do not stop abruptly. Hepatic dysfunction; exclude pre-existing liver disease before commencing treatment; failure reported. Symptoms of liver dysfunction (unexplained nausea, anorexia, tiredness), monitor; hepatitis or jaundice appears, discontinue.

Pregnancy, Lactation: If benefit outweighs risk.

ADR: *Common,* bradycardia, tachycardia, drowsiness, fatigue, dizziness, dry mouth, nausea, GI disturbances, reduced BP, rebound hypertension.

Notes: See 4.3.1 Skeletal Muscle Relaxants.

Zanaflex 2mg, 4mg (TEVA) A. GMS.
Price, (120) 2mg, €33.84. 4mg, €46.93.
Tablet, tizanidine HCl. White (off-white) round flat cross-scored (facilitates breaking). Marked A. 2mg: Marked 592. 4mg: Marked 594. *Lactose.*

Tizanidine 2mg, 4mg (Niche) A. GMS.
Price, (120) 2mg, €33.16. 4mg, €45.99.
Tablet, tizanidine HCl. White round. 2mg: Marked N 62. 4mg: Scored (divisible into equal halves). Marked N 63. *Lactose.*

4.3.2 - Drugs Enhancing Neuromuscular Transmission

In This Chapter: *Pyridostigmine.*

Class Effects
CI: Hypersensitivity to any member of the class.

Pyridostigmine (myasthenia gravis)

ATC Code: N07AA02. **Sport:** Permitted.
Driving: Caution.
Indications: Myasthenia gravis.
Dose: Adult, Elderly: 300-1200mg/day in divided doses.
Child: Neonates, 5-10mg 4-hourly; under 6 years, initially 30mg; age 6-12 years, initially 60mg; titrate by 15-30mg/day increments until control.
Renal Impairment: Caution, reduce dose.
CI: Obstruction (intestinal, urinary).
Interactions: Effect of Other Drugs on Pyridostigmine: *Effect diminished*: Antibiotics (aminoglycosides, polymyxins, clindamycin) chloroquine, lithium, procainamide, propranolol, quinidine.
Effect of Pyridostigmine on Other Drugs: Non-depolarising muscle relaxants: *Effect antagonised.* Suxamethonium: *Effect Enhanced.*
SP: Parkinson's Disease, epilepsy, cardiac disease, vagotonia, asthma.
Pregnancy, Lactation: Pregnancy, if benefit outweighs risk. Lactation, caution.
ADR: Nausea, increased salivation, diarrhoea, colic.
Notes: See 4.3.2 Drugs Enhancing Neuromuscular Transmission.

> **Mestinon 60mg** *(Meda)* B. GMS.
> *Price,* (200) €58.15.
> *Tablet,* pyridostigmine bromide. White quarter-scored. Marked ICN. *Lactose.*

4.4 - Rheumatic Disease, Anti-Inflammatories, Gout

4.4.1 - Drugs Suppressing Rheumatic Disease Process

In This Chapter: *Selective immunosuppressants (abatacept, apremilast, leflunomide), calcineurin inhibitors (ciclosporin), interleukin inhibitors (anakinra, ixekizumab, secukinumab, tocilizumab, ustekinumab), TNF-inhibitors (adalimumab, certolizumab, etanercept, golimumab, infliximab), antimalarials (hydroxychloroquine), antimetabolites (methotrexate).*

Class Effects

CI: Hypersensitivity to any member of the class. Immunosuppressives are not for use in presence of (or risk of) severe, active, uncontrolled infection (sepsis, opportunistic infections, tuberculosis).
Interactions: Effect of Other Drugs on Immunosuppressives: *Co-admin not recommended*: Live vaccines, other therapeutic infectious agents (BCG bladder instillation for cancer treatment).
SP: Generally specialist supervision required. In immunosuppressed patients, avoid use of live-attenuated vaccine (medicinals affecting immune system may reduce effectiveness of immunisations). *Infections*, increased predisposition (opportunistic infections); severe and/or life-threatening; may be localised or disseminated; symptoms (e.g. fever) may be masked. With TNF-inhibitors, interleukin inhibitors, increased susceptibility to serious infections (TB, sepsis/pneumonia, invasive fungal, parasitic, other opportunistic; may be fatal). Hepatitis B reactivation in chronic carriers; worsening of hepatitis C; evaluate for HBV infection before, during, after use. Exposure to TB or endemic mycoses, evaluate risk/benefit prior to initiation. Monitor for signs of infection before, during, after treatment (e.g. certolizumab has long half-life). Suspect invasive fungal infection if a serious systemic illness develops.
Do not initiate, presence of active infection; symptoms suggestive of TB (persistent cough, wasting or weight loss, low grade fever), advise patient to seek medical advice. Chronic infection, conditions predisposing to infection (diverticulitis, diabetes, interstitial lung disease), caution.

Immunosuppressants all have potential to increase malignancy risk. Regular skin examination. Malignancies, including fatal, reported (children, adolescents, young adults) with TNF-inhibitors; lymphomas approx. half of cases; also leukaemia; melanoma and Merkel cell carcinoma. Caution, COPD (increased malignancy risk; mostly lung or head and neck), CNS demyelinating disorders reported with TNF-inhibitors. Pancytopenia, leucopenia, neutropenia, thrombocytopenia. Vasculitis associated with TNF-inhibitors. Progressive multifocal leucoencephalopathy (PML).
In order to improve traceability of biologicals, the brand name and the batch number should be clearly noted in the patient file.
Pregnancy, Lactation: May cross placenta; infants may be at increased infection risk; admin of live vaccines to infants exposed during pregnancy, not recommended for a specified period following last exposure of mother (see individual molecules below).
Notes: Conventional drugs used to treat psoriasis, see 10.5 Eczema, Psoriasis, Scalp Disorders. Other antimetabolites used to treat malignancy, see 13.1.3 Anti-Metabolites.

Abatacept

ATC Code: L04AA24. **Sport:** Permitted.
Driving: Negligible effect (dizziness, reduced visual acuity reported).
Indications: Treatment (with methotrexate), moderate/severe rheumatoid arthritis (RA) (responded to previous therapy); highly active progressive RA (no previous methotrexate) *(both formulations)*; Polyarticular Juvenile Idiopathic Arthritis (JIA) in children, if insufficient response to other DMARDs including at least one TNF-inhibitor *(IV infusion only)*.
Dose: Adult: *IV INFUSION,* RA, initially 500mg (under 60kg), 750mg (60-100kg), 1000mg (over 100kg) by IV infusion over 30 minutes. Following initial dose, admin at 2 and 4 weeks after first infusion, then every 4 weeks (approx. 10mg/kg).
SC INJECTION, may be initiated with or without IV loading dose. 125mg weekly by SC injection regardless of weight. If single IV loading use is admin before SC, the first 125mg SC injection should be admin within a day of IV infusion then weekly. Rotate injection sites.
Elderly: Over 65 years, higher infection and/or malignancy incidence.
Child: *IV INFUSION,* JIA age 6-17 years (below 75kg), 10mg/kg based on body weight; (75kg or more), as for Adult, max. 1000mg. Under 6 years, not recommended. Under 18 years, SC injection not recommended. *Admin,* as for Adult above.
Interactions: Effect of Other Drugs on Abatacept: *Co-admin not recommended*: TNF-inhibitors, anakinra, rituximab; immunosuppressives or immunomodulators (effects on immune system potentiated); live vaccinations.
SP: Allergic reactions (anaphylaxis, anaphylactoid reaction) after first infusion (life-threatening); permanently discontinue. Serious infections (sepsis, pneumonia; fatal); discontinue. Screen for viral hepatitis. May receive concurrent vaccinations except live vaccines. Periodic skin examinations recommended, especially with skin cancer risk.
Pregnancy, Lactation: Pregnancy, use only if clearly necessary; women of childbearing potential to ensure adequate contraception. Admin of live vaccines to infants, not recommended for 14 weeks following last exposure of mother (see below). Lactation, not recommended; withhold breastfeeding for up to 14 weeks after last dose.
ADR: Summary, *most frequent*, headache, nausea, upper RTI (including sinusitis). See SP above.
Notes: See 4.4.1 Drugs Suppressing Rheumatic Disease Process.

> **Orencia Parenteral** *(BMS)* A. HT.
> *Price,* (4) 125mg PFS (Clickject) and PFS, €976.32. HOS: (1) 250mg, €340.66 (PTW).
> *Infusion,* abatacept 250mg. White (off-white) powder (whole or

4.4.1 Drugs Suppressing Rheumatic Disease Process

fragmented cake) for soln. *Sodium 0.375mmoL/vial.* **Store:** Refrigerate; original pack to protect (light).
Injection, abatacept 125mg PFS. Clear colourless (pale-yellow) soln. *Sodium 0.322mg/PFS.* **Store:** As above; do not freeze.

Adalimumab

ATC Code: L04AB04. **Sport:** Permitted.
Driving: Vertigo, visual impairment.

Indications: *Adults,* rheumatoid arthritis (RA)* (moderate to severe; severe, active and progressive). Ankylosing spondylitis. Severe axial spondyloarthritis without radiographic evidence of ankylosing spondylitis. Psoriatic arthritis. Psoriasis (moderate to severe chronic plaque in candidates for systemic therapy). Hidradenitis suppurativa. Crohn's disease (moderate to severe). Ulcerative colitis (moderate to severe active). Non-infectious intermediate, posterior and panuveitis (corticosteroids inadequate or inappropriate). *Paediatric,* polyarticular juvenile idiopathic arthritis (JIA)* (from age 2 years). Enthesitis-related arthritis (from age 6 years). Paediatric plaque psoriasis (from age 4 years). Paediatric Crohn's disease (moderate to severe, active) (from age 6 years). *(monotherapy or with methotrexate).

Dose: Adult, Elderly: *RA (with methotrexate), ankylosing spondylitis, axial spondyloarthritis,* 40mg every OTHER week as single SC injection; RA monotherapy, may need to increase to 40mg every week. Clinical response usually within 12 weeks.

Psoriasis, initially 80mg, then 40mg every OTHER week starting 1 week after initial dose. After 16 weeks, patients with adequate response may benefit from 40mg every week; no response in 16 weeks, reconsider continued therapy. *Hidradenitis suppurativa,* initially 160mg* (day 1), then 80mg (2x 40mg injections in single day) (day 15) then 2 weeks later (day 29) continue with 40mg every week. No response in 12 weeks, reconsider continued treatment.

Crohn's disease, 80mg (week 0), 40mg (week 2); more rapid response, consider 160mg (week 0)*; 80mg (week 2). After induction, 40mg every other week; no response by week 4, may benefit with continued maintenance through week 12. *Ulcerative colitis,* 160mg (week 0)*, 80mg (week 2) then 40mg every other week. Clinical response usually in 2-8 weeks. *Uveitis,* initially 80mg, then 40mg every other week starting 1 week after initial dose (combination with corticosteroids and/or other non-biologic immunomodulators). Evaluate long-term treatment yearly.

Admin, by SC injection. Patients to carry alert card. *(as 4 SC injections in 1 day or 2 SC injections per day for 2 consecutive days).

Child: *Polyarticular JIA* (age 2-12 years), 24mg/m2 BSA every other week SC; max. 20mg (age 2 to under 4 years); max. 40mg (age 4-12 years); age 13-17 years, 40mg SC every other week regardless of BSA.

Enthesitis-related arthritis (age 6 years and over), 24mg/m2 BSA to max. single dose of 40mg SC every other week.

Paediatric Crohn's disease (age 6 years and over), under 40kg, 40mg (week 0) then 20mg (week 2); if more rapid response needed, as for weight above 40kg with higher risk for adverse events with higher induction dose; after induction 20mg SC every other week. Weight 40kg and above, 80mg (week 0) admin as 2x SC injection in 1 day, then 40mg (week 2); after induction 40mg SC every other week.

Paediatric plaque psoriasis (age 4 years and over), 0.8mg/kg (max. 40mg) SC weekly (dose 1 and 2), then every other week.

CI: Moderate to severe heart failure (NYHA class III/IV).

Interactions: Effect of Other Drugs on Adalimumab: *Co-admin not recommended*: Anakinra, abatacept, other TNF-antagonists. *Increased (antibody formation; clearance), reduced efficacy*: Admin **without** methotrexate.

SP: *Infections,* see Notes below; monitor before, during and for up to 5 months after treatment (active or latent TB). Hepatitis B reactivation. Serious allergic reactions (anaphylaxis). Cannot exclude lymphomas, other malignancies. New onset or exacerbation of CNS

demyelinating disorders (MS, optic neuritis, peripheral demyelinating disease including Guillain-Barre syndrome), caution; if these disorders develop, consider discontinuation. Worsening of CHF. Antibody formation (lupus-like syndrome), discontinue. Surgery, limited data; note long half-life.

Pregnancy, Lactation: Pregnancy, not recommended; women of childbearing potential to ensure adequate contraception* Lactation, not recommended*. *(during and for at least 5 months after treatment).

ADR: Summary, *most common*, infections (nasopharyngitis, upper RTI, sinusitis), injection-site reactions (erythema, itching, haemorrhage, pain, swelling), headache, musculoskeletal pain; *serious*, fatal, life-threatening infections (sepsis, opportunistic infections, TB), HBV reactivation, malignancies (leukaemia, lymphoma, HSTCL); haematological, neurological, autoimmune reactions.

Notes: See 4.4.1 Drugs Suppressing Rheumatic Disease Process.

> **Humira Parenteral 40mg** *(AbbVie)* A. HT.
> *Price,* (2) 40mg/0.4mL, (PFS) €1071.66; (PFP) €1079.95. Paed Soln 40mg/0.8mL vial (2) €1093.45.
> *Injection,* adalimumab. Clear soln. PFP/PFS (0.4mL), vial (0.8mL).
> **Store:** Refrigerate; do not freeze. PFP/PFS may be stored below 25 deg C (max. 14 days).

Apremilast

ATC Code: L04AA32. **Sport:** Permitted.
Driving: No or negligible effect.

Indications: Treatment, active psoriatic arthritis (monotherapy or combination), inadequate response or intolerant to previous DMARD; severe plaque psoriasis (failed or intolerant to previous systemic therapy e.g. ciclosporin, methotrexate or PUVA).

Dose: Adult, Elderly: Initial titration, 10mg (morning) (day 1), 10mg (morning), 10mg evening (day 2), 10mg morning, 20mg evening (day 3), 20mg morning, 20mg evening (day 4), 20mg morning, 30mg evening (day 5), then 30mg twice daily (morning, evening; 12-hourly) from day 6 onwards. *Admin,* swallow tabs whole with or without food.

Child: Age 0-17 years, safety/efficacy not established.

Renal Impairment: CrCl (mL/min) below 30, reduce dose to 30mg/day; use only morning schedule for initial titration see Adult, Elderly above.

Hepatic Impairment: No adjustment.

Interactions: Effect of Other Drugs on Apremilast: *Co-admin not recommended (reduced exposure)*: CYP3A4 inducers (rifampicin, phenobarbital, carbamazepine, phenytoin, St John's Wort).

SP: Increased psychiatric disorder risk (insomnia, depression); suicidal ideation and behaviour (including suicide) observed (with or without depression history). Counsel to report behaviour or mood changes. New or worsening psychiatric symptoms or suicidal ideation, discontinue.

Pregnancy, Lactation: Pregnancy, contraindicated; exclude before initiation. Women of childbearing potential to ensure adequate contraception. Lactation, not for use; risk to infant cannot be excluded.

ADR: Summary, *most common*, diarrhoea, nausea, upper respiratory tract infections, headache, tension headache.

Notes: See 4.4.1 Drugs Suppressing Rheumatic Disease Process.

> ▼ **Otezla 10mg, 20mg, 30mg** *(Celgene)* A. HT.
> *Price,* 14-day initiation pack: 4x10mg, 4x20mg, 19x30mg, €365.95. (56) 30mg, €759.00.
> *Tablet,* apremilast. Diamond-shaped f/c. Marked APR and strength. **Store:** Below 30 deg C.

Anakinra

ATC Code: L04AC03. **Sport:** Permitted.
Driving: Unlikely to impair.

Indications: Treatment (with methotrexate), rheumatoid arthritis (RA) (inadequate response to methotrexate alone). Treatment, Cryopyrin-Associated Periodic Syndromes (CAPS) (8 months and older; 10kg or above).

Drugs Suppressing Rheumatic Disease Process   4.4.1

Dose: Adult, Elderly: *RA*, recommended 100mg once daily by SC injection at approx. same time each day.
CAPS, initial and maintenance, 1-2mg/kg/day by SC injection; severe, increase to 3-4mg/kg/day; max. 8mg/kg/day. Therapeutic response (reduction in clinical symptoms, inflammatory serum markers).
Child: *RA*, under 18 years, not recommended. *CAPS*, age 8 months and older, body weight 10kg or above, as for Adult; under 8 months, no data.
Renal Impairment: CrCl (mL/min) 30-50, caution; below 30, contraindicated.
Hepatic Impairment: Severe, caution.
CI: Hypersensitivity to *E. coli* derived proteins. Not for initiation in neutropenia.
Interactions: Effect of Other Drugs on Anakinra: *Co-admin not recommended*: Other TNF antagonists, live vaccines. *Higher Incidence (serious infections, neutropenia)*: Etanercept.
SP: *Infections*, see Notes below. Alternate injection site to avoid discomfort. Allergic reactions (maculopapular, urticaria); severe, discontinue. Hepatic events reported mainly with predisposing factors. Neutropenia, monitor; assess neutrophil count before initiation. Use with pre-existing malignancy, not recommended. Elderly, caution. Neutralising antibodies (incidence higher in children).
Pregnancy, Lactation: Pregnancy, not recommended. Women of childbearing potential to ensure adequate contraception. Lactation, stop breastfeeding.
ADR: *Very common*, headache, injection site reaction, increased blood cholesterol; *common*, serious infection, neutropenia, thrombocytopenia.
Notes: See 4.4.1 Drugs Suppressing Rheumatic Disease Process.

Kineret Parenteral 100mg *(SOBI)* A. HT.
Price, (28) €947.47.
Injection, anakinra 100mg/0.67mL (graduated PFS). Clear colourless (white) soln; may contain translucent (white) amorphous particles.

Certolizumab

ATC Code: L04AB05. **Sport:** Permitted.
Driving: Vertigo, visual impairment, fatigue.
Indications: Treatment (with methotrexate), moderate to severe active rheumatoid arthritis (RA), psoriatic arthritis; monotherapy (intolerant to methotrexate or continued methotrexate inappropriate). Severe axial spondyloarthritis (ankylosing spondylitis, axial spondyloarthritis without radiographic evidence of ankylosing spondylitis).
Dose: Adult, Elderly: Loading dose, 400mg (2x SC injections of 200mg each) at weeks 0, 2 and 4 (rheumatoid or psoriatic arthritis, continue methotrexate). Maintenance, (RA, axial spondyloarthritis, psoriatic arthritis), 200mg every 2 weeks or 400mg every 4 weeks once clinical response confirmed (RA, continue methotrexate). *Elderly*, higher infection incidence. *Admin*, SC injection only (thigh, abdomen). Patients may self inject where appropriate.
Child: Under 18 years, no data.
Renal Impairment: No dose recommendation.
Hepatic Impairment: As for Renal above.
CI: Moderate/severe HF (NYHA III/IV).
Interactions: Effect of Other Drugs on Certolizumab: *Co-admin not recommended*: Anakinra, abatacept.
SP: Supply patients with special alert card. Interferes with certain coagulation assays. Hepatosplenic T-cell lymphoma reported. Patients may self-inject with proper training.
Pregnancy, Lactation: Pregnancy, not recommended; women of childbearing potential to ensure adequate contraception during and for minimum 5 months after last admin. Do not admin live vaccines to infants for 5 months following last admin of drug to mother (see Notes below). Lactation, stop breastfeeding or stop drug.
ADR: *Common*, bacterial/viral infection, eosinophilic disorders, leucopenia, neutropenia, lymphopenia, headache including migraine, sensory abnormalities, hypertension, nausea, hepatitis, elevated hepatic

enzymes, rash, pyrexia, pain, asthenia, pruritus, injection site reaction.
Notes: See 4.4.1 Drugs Suppressing Rheumatic Disease Process.

Cimzia Parenteral 200mg/mL *(UCB)* A. HT.
Price, PFS/PFP, 200mg/mL (2mL) (1) €981.64.
Injection (PFS, PFP Autoclick), certolizumab pegol. Recombinant humanised antibody Fab fragment. Clear opalescent colourless (yellow) soln; pH 4.7. *Store:* Refrigerate; do not freeze; protect (light).

Ciclosporin (systemic)

ATC Code: L04AD01. **Sport:** Permitted.
Driving: Unlikely to impair.
Indications: *Transplant*, prevention, graft rejection following kidney, liver, heart, combined heart-lung, lung, pancreas or bone-marrow transplantation; treatment, transplant rejection. Prophylaxis of graft-versus-host disease (GVHD); treatment of established GVHD. *Non-transplantation*, severe psoriasis, atopic dermatitis (conventional treatment ineffective or inappropriate), severe active RA (slow-acting anti-rheumatics inappropriate or ineffective). Endogenous uveitis, active sight-threatening intermediate or posterior, non-infectious (conventional treatment failed or not tolerated). Behcet uveitis with repeated inflammatory attacks involving retina. Nephrotic Syndrome, with steroid-dependent and -resistant nephrotic syndrome due to glomerular disease; to induce remission and for maintenance including steroid-induced remission (allowing steroid withdrawal).
Dose: Adult: ORAL, TRANSPLANT, initiate 4-12 hours before transplantation; 10-15mg/kg body weight as single or 2 divided doses. Continue at 10-15mg/kg/day for 1-2 weeks post-op (oral or IV) reducing gradually to 2-6mg/kg/day (oral). Co-admin with other immunosuppressants, initiate at 3-6mg/kg/day. *Bone marrow transplant, prevention and treatment of GVHD*, initiate with IV (see below) OR 12.5-15mg/kg/day orally starting 1 day before transplantation, then 12.5mg/kg/day for 3-6 months.
NON-TRANSPLANT, *psoriasis**, 2.5mg/kg/day; no improvement after 1 month, titrate gradually to max. 5mg/kg; if rapid improvement required, initiate at 5mg/kg/day. *RA*, initially 3mg/kg/day for 6 weeks; if needed titrate gradually to max. 5mg/kg. *Endogenous uveitis**, 5mg/kg/day; refractory may need 7mg/kg/day; maintenance, max. 5mg/kg/day. *Nephrotic syndrome**, 5mg/kg/day. *Atopic dermatitis*, initially 2.5mg/kg/day; titrate after 2 weeks to max. 5mg/kg/day; severe, initiate at 5mg/kg/day. Soft gelatin caps to be taken with mouthful of water. Oral soln, dilute immediately before admin; can be taken with water. Do not take with grapefruit juice.
PARENTERAL, IV dose is approx. one third of corresponding oral dose; switch to oral as soon as possible. Solid organ transplant, initiate within 12 hours before surgery, 10-15mg/kg in 2 divided doses. Bone marrow transplantation, prevention, treatment of GVHD, 3-5mg/kg/day IV starting day before transplantation and continuing for up to 2 weeks until oral maintenance, see above. NOTE: Bioavailability is not equivalent for all oral brands; switch from oral *Sandimmun* to oral *Neoral*, may result in increased ciclosporin exposure. *(remission induction)
Elderly: Monitor renal function.
Child: *Nephrotic syndrome*, remission induction max. 6mg/kg/day in 2 divided doses; *transplant*, reduce dose.
Renal Impairment: Nephrotic syndrome, impaired renal function, initiate at max. 2.5mg/kg/day.
Hepatic Impairment: Consider dose adjustment.
CI: Psoriatic, atopic dermatitis and RA patients with abnormal renal function, uncontrolled hypertension, malignancy (other than of skin in atopic dermatitis).
Interactions: Effect of Other Drugs on Ciclosporin: *Co-admin avoid*: Live attenuated vaccines. *Caution*: Aminoglycosides, amphotericin B, ciprofloxacin, melphalan, trimethoprim, vancomycin, NSAIDs (diclofenac, naproxen, sulindac), H2-antagonists (cimetidine, ranitidine), methotrexate, lercanidipine. *Plasma levels increased*: Azole antifungals (ketoconazole, fluconazole, itraconazole, voriconazole), macrolides (erythromycin,

161

4.4.1 Drugs Suppressing Rheumatic Disease Process

azithromycin, clarithromycin), oral contraceptives, calcium channel blockers (diltiazem, nicardipine, verapamil), doxycycline, propafenone, lipid solutions, methylprednisolone (high dose), metoclopramide, danazol, allopurinol, amiodarone, protease inhibitors, cholic acid derivatives, oral contraceptives, imatinib. *Plasma levels decreased:* Phenytoin, carbamazepine, oxcarbazepine, barbiturates, rifampicin, nafcillin, sulphadiazine, probucol, octreotide, orlistat, ticlopine, sulfinpyrazone, terbinafine, bosentan. *Marked plasma and whole blood levels decreased:* IV (not oral) sulfadimidine and trimethoprim, St John's Wort (co-admin not recommended). *Increased nephrotoxicity risk:* NSAIDs, tacrolimus (avoid). *Increased muscular toxicity (muscle pains, weakness):* Colchicine. *Increased gingival hyperplasia:* Nifedipine. *Hyperkalaemia risk:* Potassium (-sparing diuretics, supplements, - containing medications, high dietary intake). *Increased bioavailability:* Grapefruit juice, fat rich meal.

Effect of Ciclosporin on Other Drugs: Prednisolone: *Reduced clearance.* Diclofenac, sirolimus, everolimus: *Increased plasma levels.* Lovastatin, simvastatin, atorvastatin, pravastatin; fluvastatin (rarely): *Increased myotoxicity potential (rhabdomyolysis).* Digoxin, colchicine, prednisolone, statins: *Clearance reduced.*

SP: *Monitor,* renal and/or hepatic function, hyperkalaemia, hyperuricaemia, BP (antihypertensives if needed), blood lipids; enhanced magnesium clearance. Parenteral, hypersensitivity reactions (castor oil), observe for minimum 30 minutes after infusion. *Additional precautions,* potential skin malignancy risk (avoid excessive unprotected sun exposure, concomitant ultraviolet B irradiation or PUVA photochemotherapy). Clear active herpes simplex infections before initiation. Nephrotic syndrome, malignancy (including Hodgkin's lymphoma); monitor serum creatinine. Lower extremity pain (part of Calcineurin-Inhibitor Induced Pain Syndrome).

Pregnancy, Lactation: Pregnancy, if benefit outweighs risk. Lactation, not recommended.

ADR: *Very common,* hyperlipidaemia, tremor, headache, hypertension, renal dysfunction.

Notes: See 4.4.1 Drugs Suppressing Rheumatic Disease Process.

Neoral 25mg, 50mg, 100mg, Oral Soln *(Novartis)* B. HT.
Price, caps (30) 25mg, €21.49. 50mg, €41.37. 100mg, €79.38. Oral soln 100mg/mL (50mL) €128.31.
Soft capsule, ciclosporin. Oval. Marked NVR; strength on reverse. 25mg, 100mg: Blue/grey. 50mg: Yellow/white. *Castor oil, macrogolglycerol hydroxystearate, ethanol.*
Conc for oral soln, as above 100mg/mL. Clear yellow (faintly-yellow, brownish-yellow) liquid. *Ethanol, macrogolglycerol hydroxystearate, castor oil.*

Sandimmun Capsules, Oral Soln *(Novartis)* B. HT.
Price, caps (30) 25mg, €26.63. 50mg, €49.36. 100mg, €96.85. Oral soln 100mg/mL (50mL) €150.47.
Capsule, ciclosporin 25mg, 50mg, 100mg. Soft gelatin; contains oleaginous liquid; clear or with white precipitate. 25mg, 100mg: Dusty-pink. 50mg: Yellow. *Ethanol, sorbitol.*
Conc for oral soln, as above 100mg/mL. Yellow (brownish-yellow) clear liquid or with a small amount of fine sediment. *Ethanol.*

Sandimmun Parenteral *(Novartis)* A. HT.
Price, (10) €23.28.
Infusion, ciclosporin 50mg/mL. Clear brown-yellow oleaginous conc. *Ethanol, macrogolglycerol ricinoleate (castor oil).*

Etanercept

ATC Code: L04AB01. **Sport:** Permitted.
Driving: Unlikely to impair.

Indications: Treatment, *rheumatoid arthritis* (RA), moderate to severe active (monotherapy or with methotrexate); severe active, progressive (no previous methotrexate); *psoriatic arthritis,* active or progressive; *axial spondyloarthritis,* severe active ankylosing spondylitis; severe non-radiographic axial spondyloarthritis; *plaque psoriasis,* moderate to severe. *Juvenile Idiopathic Arthritis* (JIA), treatment, polyarthritis, extended oligoarthritis (children), psoriatic arthritis (adolescents); *paediatric plaque psoriasis,* chronic, severe; enthesitis-related arthritis (adolescents).

Dose: Adult, Elderly: *RA,* psoriatic arthritis, ankylosing

spondylitis, non-radiographic axial spondyloarthritis, 25mg twice weekly OR 50mg once weekly.
Plaque psoriasis, as for RA OR 50mg twice weekly (12 weeks), then 25mg twice weekly or 50mg once weekly until remission (up to 24 weeks). *Admin,* SC injection.
Child: *JIA,* age 2 years and over, 0.4mg/kg (max. 25mg/dose) SC, twice weekly (3-4 day dose interval) OR 0.8mg/kg (up to max. 50mg/dose) SC once weekly. Age 18 years and over, as for Adult above.
Paediatric plaque psoriasis, age 6 years and over, 0.8mg/kg (max. 50mg/dose) once weekly (up to 24 weeks). NOTE: 10mg vial strength more appropriate for children below 25kg. *Benepali* is only available as 50mg PFS/PFP; not possible for admin to paediatric patients requiring less than a full 50mg dose; if a dose other than a full 50mg is required, *Benepali* should not be used.

Hepatic Impairment: Sepsis (risk of), active infections.

Interactions: Effect of Other Drugs on Etanercept: Co-admin not recommended: Anakinra (increased infection risk), abatacept (increased adverse event incidence). Co-admin caution: Sulfasalazine.

SP: *Infection,* see Notes below; new (monitor), serious (discontinue), hepatitis C (caution). Allergic reactions (angioedema, urticaria; serious or anaphylactic), discontinue. Malignancies e.g. breast and/or lung carcinoma, lymphoma, leukaemia. Autoantibody formation. Pancytopenia, aplastic anaemia; signs and symptoms of blood dyscrasias or infection (persistent fever, sore throat, bruising, bleeding, paleness), advise patient to seek medical advice. CHF (including new onset), caution. Not effective treatment for Wegener's granulomatosis. Interstitial lung disease. NOTE: Supply patients with a Patient Alert Card.

Pregnancy, Lactation: Not recommended (crosses placenta; infants may be at risk of infection; admin of live vaccines to infants for 16 weeks after last dose of mother, not recommended). Women of childbearing potential to ensure adequate contraception during and for 3 weeks after treatment discontinuation. Lactation, stop drug or stop breastfeeding.

ADR: *Summary, most common,* injection-site reactions (pain, swelling, itching, reddening, bleeding at puncture site), infections (upper respiratory, bronchitis, bladder, skin, viral), allergic reactions, autoantibody development, itching, fever. *Serious,* infections (fatal, life-threatening, sepsis), malignancies (breast, lung, skin, lymphoma); haematological, neurological and autoimmune reactions (pancytopenia, aplastic anaemia), central and peripheral demyelinating events, lupus, vasculitis.

Notes: See 4.4.1 Drugs Suppressing Rheumatic Disease Process.

Enbrel, Paed Parenteral *(Pfizer)* A. HT.
Price, (4) 25mg injection, €506.17; PFS, €495.20. 50mg PFS/PFP, €810.37. Paediatric (4): Powder/solvent for injection 10mg, €202.59; PFS 25mg, €524.12.
Injection, etanercept 25mg, 50mg, paed 10mg. Vial: White powder. Clear colourless solvent for soln. PFS: Clear colourless (pale-yellow) soln. **Store:** Refrigerate; do not freeze; outside of refrigerator below 25 deg C (max. 4 weeks), then discard.

▼ **Benepali Parenteral 50mg** *(Biogen Idec)* A. HT.
Price, (4) PFP/PFS, €709.06.
Injection, etanercept. Clear colourless (pale-yellow) soln. **Store:** Refrigerate; do not freeze; outside of refrigerator below 25 deg C (max. 4 weeks), then discard.

Golimumab

ATC Code: L04AB06. **Sport:** Permitted.
Driving: Dizziness.

Indications: Treatment, rheumatoid arthritis*, moderate-severe, active; severe, active, progressive (no previous methotrexate). Psoriatic arthritis, active and progressive (monotherapy or*). Ankylosing spondylitis, severe active. Severe non-radiographic axial spondyloarthritis. Ulcerative colitis, moderate to severe active. *(with methotrexate).

Dose: Adult, Elderly: Age 18 years and over, *rheumatoid arthritis* (with methotrexate), *psoriatic arthritis, ankylosing spondylitis* (monotherapy) and *non-radiographic axial spondyloarthritis,* 50mg once monthly. Bodyweight above 100kg, consider 100mg once monthly.

162

Drugs Suppressing Rheumatic Disease Process   4.4.1

Ulcerative colitis, initially 200mg, then 100mg (week 2), followed by either 50mg every 4 weeks (80kg or under) OR 100mg every 4 weeks (80kg and over). *Admin*, by SC injection, on same date each month; multiple injections, admin at different body sites.

CI: Moderate or severe HF (NYHA class III/IV).

Interactions: Effect of Other Drugs on Golimumab: *Co-admin not recommended*: Anakinra (serious infection risk, neutropenia), abatacept and other biologicals (increased infection risk).

SP: *Infection, melanoma*, see Notes below; chronic/recurrent, infection (caution); serious or sepsis (discontinue). Hepatitis B reactivation. Cases of active TB have occurred; monitor. Worsening CHF/increased mortality due to CHF (some cases fatal); mild HF (NYHA Class I/II), caution. CNS demyelinating disorders (MS, peripheral demyelinating disorders), discontinue. Use post-surgery (including arthroplasty), limited data. Autoimmune processes (suggestive of lupus-like syndrome), discontinue. Pancytopenia, leucopenia, neutropenia, aplastic anaemia, thrombocytopenia. Serious hypersensitivity reactions (anaphylaxis).

Pregnancy, Lactation: Pregnancy, not recommended; use only if clearly necessary. Live vaccine admin not recommended to infants for 6 months following last injection to mother during pregnancy (see Notes below). Lactation, not recommended for and minimum 6 months after treatment.

ADR: Summary, *most common*, upper respiratory tract infection; *most serious*, infections (sepsis, pneumonia, TB, invasive fungal and opportunistic infections), demyelinating disorders, HBV reactivation, CHF, autoimmune (lupus-like syndrome), haematologic reactions, serious systemic hypersensitivity (anaphylactic reaction), vasculitis, lymphoma and leukaemia.

Notes: See 4.4.1 Drugs Suppressing Rheumatic Disease Process.

Simponi Parenteral *(MSD)* A. HT.
Price, (1) 50mg/0.5mL (PFP, PFS) and 100mg/1mL (PFP), €1085.40.
Injection, golimumab 50mg/0.5mL (PFS, PFP), 100mg/1mL (PFP). Human monoclonal antibody (murine). Clear (slightly opalescent) colourless (light-yellow) soln. *Natural dry rubber (needle cover), sorbitol.* **Store:** In outer carton; refrigerate; do not freeze.

Hydroxychloroquine

ATC Code: P01BA02. **Sport:** Permitted.
Driving: Impaired visual accommodation/blurred vision.
Indications: Treatment, rheumatoid arthritis, discoid and SLE, dermatological conditions caused or aggravated by sunlight (adults); juvenile idiopathic arthritis, discoid and SLE (children).

Dose: Adult, Elderly: 6.5mg/kg/day (calculate from ideal body weight, not actual body weight); either 200mg or 400mg*/day. Light-sensitive treatment, give only during periods of max. exposure to light. *Admin*, tabs with a meal or glass of milk; use minimum effective dose. *(not for use in adults with ideal body weight below 62kg).

Child: Max. 6.5mg/kg/day based on ideal body weight; 200mg tab not suitable in children under 31kg. Under 6 years, under 35kg, contraindicated.

CI: Pre-existing maculopathy of the eye.

Interactions: Effect of Other Drugs on Hydroxychloroquine: *Co-admin avoid*: Oculotoxic or haemotoxic drugs. *Effect potentiated*: Aminoglycosides. *Increased plasma levels*: Cimetidine. *Reduced absorption*: Antacids (allow 4-hours between dosing).

Effect of Hydroxychloroquine on Other Drugs: Digoxin: *Plasma levels increased (monitor)*. Neostigmine, pyridostigmine: *Effect antagonised*. Intradermal human diploid-cell rabies vaccine: *Reduction of antibody response to primary immunisation*. Insulin, antidiabetic drugs: *Enhanced effects*.

SP: All patients to have ophthalmological examination, before treatment and every 12 months; more frequently if (daily dose exceeding 6.5mg/kg lean body weight, renal impairment, visual acuity below 6/8, cumulative dose

above 200g, over 65 years); retinal toxicity usually dose-related. Pigmentary abnormality, visual field defect, accommodation difficulty, discontinue. Caution, co-admin with drugs causing adverse ocular or skin reactions, hepatic or renal disease, severe GI or neurological or blood disorders, sensitivity to quinine, G-6-PD deficiency, porphyria cutanea tarda, psoriasis. Bone marrow depression (periodic blood counts). Young children particularly sensitive to toxic effects of 4-aminoquinolines; keep out of reach of children. Long-term therapy (examine skeletal muscle function periodically); weakness, discontinue. Cardiomyopathy (fatal) reported (monitor); if develops, discontinue.

Pregnancy, Lactation: Pregnancy, if considered essential; crosses placenta. Lactation, is excreted in human milk; careful consideration to use as infants are extremely sensitive to toxic effects of 4-aminoquinolines.

ADR: *Very common*, abdominal pain, nausea.

Notes: See 4.4.1 Drugs Suppressing Rheumatic Disease Process.

Plaquenil 200mg *(SANOFI)* B. GMS.
Price, (60) €6.25.
Tablet, hydroxychloroquine sulfate. White f/c. Marked HCQ; strength on reverse. *Lactose.*

Infliximab

ATC Code: L04AB02. **Sport:** Permitted.
Driving: Dizziness.
Indications: Rheumatoid arthritis (RA) (with methotrexate), active; moderate to severe active and progressive. Ankylosing spondylitis, severe active. Psoriasis, moderate to severe. Adjunctive or monotherapy, psoriatic arthritis, active and progressive. Monotherapy, Crohn's disease including paediatric, severe active; fistulising active. Moderate to severe ulcerative colitis.

Dose: Adult: *RA* (with methotrexate), initially 3mg/kg; then 3mg/kg at 2 and 6 weeks; then every 8 weeks. Inadequate or response lost within 12 weeks, titrate up by approx. 1.5mg/kg to max. 7.5mg/kg every 8 weeks OR 3mg/kg every 4 weeks. Re-admin, see Ulcerative Colitis.
Crohn's disease, moderate to severely active, initially 5mg/kg; then 5mg/kg at 2 and 6 weeks; then every 8 weeks OR *re-admin* 5mg/kg if signs of disease recur within 16 weeks following last infusion, followed by 5mg/kg every 8 weeks. Fistulising, active, no response after first three doses, discontinue; if there is response, additional 5mg/kg every 8 weeks OR *re-admin* as above.
Ulcerative colitis, psoriatic arthritis, psoriasis, initially 5mg/kg; then 5mg/kg at 2 and 6 weeks; then every 8 weeks.
Ankylosing spondylitis, initially 5mg/kg; then 5mg/kg at 2 and 6 weeks; then 5mg/kg at 6-8 weeks; no response after 6 weeks, discontinue; no additional treatment should be given.
Admin by IV infusion over 2 hours. Monitor for 1-2 hours post-infusion for acute infusion-related reactions (emergency equipment to be available); consider pre-treatment with antihistamine, hydrocortisone and/or paracetamol); slow infusion rate to reduce risk.

Elderly: Age 65 years and over, increased serious infection incidence.

Child: Crohn's disease, ulcerative colitis, age 6-17 years, 5mg/kg by IV infusion over 2 hours; then additional 5mg/kg at 2 and 6 weeks, then every 8 weeks. Other indications, under 18 years, not recommended.

CI: Moderate or severe HF (NYHA class III/IV), murine protein hypersensitivity.

Interactions: Effect of Other Drugs on Infliximab: *Co-admin not recommended*: Anakinra, abatacept (serious infections), other biologicals; live vaccines.

SP: Infusion-related reactions (anaphylactic shock, delayed hypersensitivity); antibody development. Fistulising Crohn's disease with acute suppurative fistulas, exclude abscess. Hepatitis B (HBV) reactivation; monitor (screen before initiating). Cases of active tuberculosis reported (monitor during and after treatment for latent TB). Jaundice, non-infectious hepatitis, liver failure. Autoimmune

163

4.4.1 Drugs Suppressing Rheumatic Disease Process

processes (lupus-like syndrome). Neurological (optic neuritis, seizure, CNS demyelinating disorders including MS; peripheral demyelinating disorders including Guillain-Barre syndrome); pre-existing/recent onset demyelinating disorders, assess benefit/risk; discontinue. Malignancies, lymphoproliferative disorders (lymphoma; caution heavy smokers); conduct periodic cervical cancer screening in women including over 60 years. Psoriasis, extensive immunosuppressant therapy or prolonged PUVA treatment, HF (NYHA class I/II), caution. Surgical procedures, monitor for infection. Patients to be supplied with special alert card. *Infection*, see Notes below.

Pregnancy, Lactation: Pregnancy, not recommended; crosses placenta, detected up to 6 months in serum of infants born to women treated during pregnancy. In infants exposed in utero to infliximab, fatal outcome due to disseminated Bacillus Calmette Guerin (BCG) infection reported following admin of BCG vaccine after birth. Recommended to wait at least a six months following birth before admin of live vaccines to these infants. Women of childbearing potential, ensure adequate contraception*. Lactation, not recommended*. *(during treatment and for at least 6 months after discontinuation).

ADR: Summary, *most common*, upper RTI; *most serious*, HBV reactivation, CHF, serious infections (sepsis, opportunistic, TB), delayed hypersensitivity reactions, haematologic reactions, systemic lupus erythematosus, lupus-like syndrome, demyelinating disorders, hepatobiliary events, lymphoma, HSTCL, leukaemia, Merkel cell carcinoma, melanoma, paediatric malignancy, sarcoidosis, sarcoid-like reaction, intestinal or perianal abscess (in Crohn's disease), serious infusion reactions.

Notes: See 4.4.1 Drugs Suppressing Rheumatic Disease Process. See 1.6 Chronic Bowel Disorders for other drugs used for Crohn's disease and ulcerative colitis.

Remicade Parenteral *(MSD)* A. HOS.
Price, (1) 100mg, €469.50 (PTW).
Infusion, infliximab 100mg. Powder for conc for soln.

Ixekizumab

ATC Code: L04AC13. **Sport:** Permitted.
Driving: No or negligible effect.
Indications: Treatment, moderate to severe plaque psoriasis (adults, candidates for systemic therapy).

Dose: Adult: 160mg (2x 80mg injections) at Week 0; then 80mg at Weeks 2, 4, 6, 8, 10 and 12; then maintenance 80mg every 4 weeks. No response after 16-20 weeks, consider discontinuing. *Admin*, by SC injection alternating sites; avoid areas of skin showing psoriasis; do not shake the soln/syringe.

Elderly: Age 75 years and older, limited data.

Child: Age 6-18 years, safety/efficacy not established; under 6 years, no relevant use.

Renal Impairment: Not studied, no dose recommendation.

Hepatic Impairment: As for Renal above.

CI: Serious hypersensitivity.

Interactions: Effect of Ixekizumab on Other Drugs: CYP450 substrates with narrow therapeutic index (warfarin): *Therapeutic monitoring with ixekizumab initiation*

SP: Increased rate of infections (upper respiratory tract, oral candidiasis, conjunctivitis, tinea infections). Serious hypersensitivity reactions (angioedema, urticaria, urticaria, dyspnoea, high antibody titres); serious hypersensitivity, discontinue immediately. Crohn's disease (exacerbations), ulcerative colitis.

Pregnancy, Lactation: Pregnancy, avoid; women of childbearing potential to ensure effective contraception during and for minimum 10 weeks after treatment. Lactation, stop breastfeeding or stop drug.

ADR: Summary, *most frequent*, injection-site reactions, upper respiratory infections (nasopharyngitis).

Notes: See 4.4.1 Drugs Suppressing Rheumatic Disease Process.

▼ **Taltz Parenteral 80mg/mL** *(Lilly)* A. HT.
Price, 1mL (1) €1114.56; (2) €2229.12.
Injection, ixekizumab. Recombinant humanised monoclonal

antibody. Clear colourless (slightly yellow) soln (PFS, PFP). **Store:** Refrigerate; do not freeze; unrefrigerated below 30 deg C (max. 5 days).

Leflunomide

ATC Code: L04AA13. **Sport:** Permitted.
Driving: Dizziness.

Indications: Active, rheumatoid arthritis, psoriatic arthritis.

Dose: Adult, Elderly: Loading dose, 100mg/day for 3 days. Maintenance, *rheumatoid arthritis*, 10-20mg/day; *psoriatic arthritis*, 20mg/day. Monitor ALT (SGPT) and FBC (differential WBC, platelets) before initiation, every 2 weeks during first 6 months, then every 8 weeks. *Admin*, once daily; swallow tabs whole with water, with or without food.

Child: Under 18 years, not recommended.

Renal Impairment: Moderate to severe, contraindicated.

Hepatic Impairment: Contraindicated.

CI: Hypersensitivity (previous Stevens-Johnson syndrome, toxic epidermal necrolysis, erythema multiforme). Severe immunodeficiency (AIDS), significantly impaired bone marrow function, significant anaemia, leucopenia, neutropenia or thrombocytopenia due to causes other than RA or psoriatic arthritis, serious infection, hypoproteinaemia (nephrotic syndrome).

Interactions: Effect of Other Drugs on Leflunomide: *Co-admin not recommended*: Live attenuated vaccines, other hepatotoxic or haematotoxic DMARDs (methotrexate). *Co-admin caution*: Drugs metabolised by CYP2C9 (phenytoin, phenprocoumon, warfarin, tolbutamide; not NSAIDs), ALCOHOL. *Rapid, significantly decreased plasma levels*: Colestyramine, activated charcoal.

SP: *Caution*, active metabolite has long half-life (1-4 weeks), consider (switching treatment); serious (hepatotoxicity, haematotoxicity, allergic reactions) even after treatment cessation*. *Severe liver injury* including fatal; check ALT, full blood counts before initiation, every 2 weeks (first 6 months), then every 8 weeks; elevated ALT 2-3xULN, consider dose reduction, monitor weekly; avoid alcohol. Metabolite is highly protein bound, increased plasma levels with hypoproteinaemia. Haematological risk increased with pre-existing anaemia, leucopenia, and/or thrombocytopenia, impaired bone marrow function, consider washout; severe reactions (pancytopenia), discontinue*. *Skin reactions*, ulcerative stomatitis, Stevens Johnson Syndrome, toxic epidermal necrosis, DRESS, discontinue*; re-exposure contraindicated. Interstitial lung disease (cough, dyspnoea), pulmonary hypertension, peripheral neuropathy. Monitor BP before initiation, then periodically. *Infection*, see Notes below. *See manufacturers Full Prescribing Information.

Pregnancy, Lactation: Pregnancy, contraindicated (leflunomide active metabolite suspected to cause serious birth defects). Women of childbearing potential, ensure adequate contraception during and up to 2 years after treatment or up to 11 days* after treatment. Procreation (men); advise of possible male-mediated foetal toxicity; ensure reliable contraception during treatment*. Lactation, contraindicated. *See manufacturers Full Prescribing Information (washout procedure).

ADR: Summary, *most frequent*, increased BP, leucopenia, paraesthesia, headache, dizziness, diarrhoea, nausea, vomiting, oral mucosal disorders, abdominal pain, increased hair loss, eczema, rash, pruritus, dry skin, tenosynovitis, CPK increased, anorexia, weight loss (insignificant), asthenia, mild allergic reactions, elevated liver parameters.

Notes: See 4.4.1 Drugs Suppressing Rheumatic Disease Process.

Arava 10mg, 20mg *(SANOFI)* A. GMS.
Price, (30) 10mg, €42.96. 20mg, €50.70.
Tablet, leflunomide. f/c. 10mg: White (almost) round. 20mg: Yellowish (ochre) triangular. 10mg: Marked ZBN. 20mg: Marked ZBO. Lactose.

Methotrexate

ATC Code: L04AX03. **Sport:** Permitted.
Driving: Caution.

Indications: Adults, (2.5mg) severe active, classical or

Drugs Suppressing Rheumatic Disease Process   4.4.1

definite rheumatoid arthritis (RA)*; (2.5mg, 10mg), severe uncontrolled psoriasis* (all brands). Polyarthritic forms of severe active juvenile idiopathic arthritis (JIA) (NSAIDs inadequate) (Nordimet). Treatment, wide range of neoplastic disease (Accord, Concordia, Hospira Parenteral). *(not controlled or intolerant to other treatment).

Dose: Adult: WARNING: Methotrexate for treatment of rheumatic or skin disease must only be taken ONCE WEEKLY.

ORAL, RA, initially 7.5-15mg ONCE WEEKLY; dose can be admin in 3 divided doses (2.5mg 12-hourly for 3 days as a course) ONCE WEEKLY. Max 20mg once weekly. Psoriasis, 10-25mg (some licences state 7.5-15mg) ONCE WEEKLY; adjust based on response. Max. 25mg/week. Admin, once weekly on same day; prescriber may specify admin day on prescription.

ORAL, wide variety of neoplastic diseases e.g. Burkitt's lymphoma 15mg/m2/day for 5 days. As cytostatic, doses up to 30mg/m2 possible.

PARENTERAL, RA (SC, IM or IV), initially 7.5mg once weekly; titrate by 2.5mg/week to max. 25mg/week (range 10-25mg/week).

Antineoplastic chemotherapy, ALL (examples), 3.3mg/m2/day (combination) (4-6 weeks); 2.5mg/kg every 2 weeks; 30mg/m2/week maintenance, 20mg/m2 (combination) once weekly. Choriocarcinoma, trophoblastic disease, 15-30mg/m2 IM (5 days); repeat 3-5 times as needed; 1 or more weeks between courses. Non-Hodgkin's Lymphoma, Stage III, 0.625-2.5mg/kg/day as part of polychemotherapy and 90-900mg/m2 IV infusion followed by calcium folinate. Head and neck cancer, monotherapy, 40-60mg/m2 once weekly IV bolus; 240-1080mg/m2 IV infusion with calcium folinate rescue (metastatic or recurrent tumours). Breast cancer, 40mg/m2 IV (days 1 and 8 of cycle) in combination. IV 10-60mg/m2 also used in combination (advanced breast cancer). Osteosarcoma, high-dose 12g/m2; can be increased to 15g/m2 in combination.

Before initiation, admin test dose, 5-10mg (parenteral) or 2.5-5mg (oral) 1 week prior to therapy. IM, IV (bolus injection or infusion), intrathecal, intra-arterial routes. Dose based on bodyweight and BSA; except intrathecal, max. 15mg. Doses above 100mg, usually admin by IV infusion over max. 24 hours. Folate admin can mask B12 deficiency.

Elderly: Caution, consider dose reduction (possible reduced hepatic/renal function, lower folate reserves).

Child: Safety and efficacy only established in cancer therapy. ALL, 1000-5000mg/m2 IV with subsequent folinic acid. Oral up to 20mg/m2/week uses with IV and intrathecal CNS prophylaxis as maintenance.

Renal Impairment: Caution, CrCl (mL/min) 20-50 (some licences state 30-59), use 50% of dose; significantly impaired function or under 20 (some licences state 30), must not be used/contraindicated.

Hepatic Impairment: Extreme caution/contraindicated (especially significant impairment or with current/previous liver disease especially if due to alcohol).

CI: Alcoholism, alcoholic liver disease, fibrosis, cirrhosis, recent or active hepatitis. Severe acute or chronic infections, immunodeficiency. Bone marrow hypoplasia, haematological impairment, anaemia, leucopenia, thrombocytopenia. Mouth, GI infections.

Interactions: Effect of Other Drugs on Methotrexate: Co-admin not recommended: Live attenuated vaccines. Increased toxicity: Salicylates, NSAIDs (high dose, fatal methotrexate toxicity; lower dose, caution), sulfonamides, phenylbutazone, diuretics, hypoglycaemics, diphenylhydantoins, tetracyclines, chloramphenicol, p-aminobenzoic acid, acidic anti-inflammatories, folate deficiency states. Increased nephrotoxicity: Nephrotoxic drugs, chemotherapeutics e.g. cisplatin. Increased hepatotoxicity: Hepatotoxic agents (ALCOHOL, leflunomide, azathioprine, sulfasalazine, retinoids). Reduced renal tubular transport: Probenecid, penicillin, PPIs (omeprazole). Caution: Folate antagonists (co-trimoxazole), drugs with anti-folate potential (nitric oxide, trimethoprim).

Altered response: Vitamin preparations containing folic acid or derivatives. Reduced efficacy, intrathecal route: Calcium folinate (high doses). Increased plasma levels: Acitretin after ingestion with alcohol; etretinate formation. Decreased intestinal absorption: Tetracycline, chloramphenicol, non-absorbable broad spectrum antibiotics.

Effect of Methotrexate on Other Drugs: Theophylline, mercaptopurine: Reduced clearance, monitor levels.

SP: Before initiation or re-admin, complete haematological analysis, urinalysis, renal function tests, LFTs, plasma determinations (monitor).

Caution, haematological depression, peptic ulcer, ulcerative colitis/stomatitis, diarrhoea, debility, young children, elderly; malignancy and pre-existing haematopoietic impairment; neoplastic disease (use only if benefit outweighs risk of severe myelosuppression).

Extreme caution, impaired renal function; death reported in malignancy treatment; use only in life-threatening neoplastic disease. Pleural effusions, ascites (drain before treatment); diarrhoea, ulcerative stomatitis, interrupt treatment; haemorrhagic enteritis and death from intestinal perforation may occur; vomiting resulting in dehydration, discontinue; severe, occasionally fatal; Stevens-Johnson Syndrome, toxic epidermal necrolysis, erythema multiforme. Hepatotoxicity, liver fibrosis, cirrhosis; liver enzyme elevation. Systemic toxicity (cardiovascular). Malignant lymphoma (discontinue), folate deficiency, acute or chronic interstitial pneumonia (associated with blood eosinophilia), potentially fatal opportunistic infections (Pneumocystis carinii pneumonia), tumour lysis syndrome. See ADR below.

Pregnancy, Lactation: Pregnancy, contraindicated; neoplastic disease, not recommended unless benefit outweighs risk (may cause foetal death embryotoxicity, abortion, teratogenic effects). Both partners to ensure adequate contraception. Avoid conception for minimum 3 months post methotrexate treatment. Lactation, contraindicated.

ADR: Most common, bone marrow suppression, mucosal damage, leucopenia, nausea, other GI disorders, malaise, abnormal fatigue, chills, fever, dizziness, reduced immunity to infection. Most serious, bone marrow suppression, toxicity (pulmonary, hepatic, renal, neuro), thromboembolic events, anaphylactic shock, Stevens-Johnson syndrome.

Notes: See 4.4.1 Drugs Suppressing Rheumatic Disease Process.

Interchangeability: Same strengths of all brands of methotrexate tablets are deemed interchangeable.

Methotrexate (Accord) 2.5mg, 10mg (Accord) A. GMS.
Price, (28) 2.5mg, €3.76. (100) 2.5mg, €13.11; 10mg, €44.67. Tablet, methotrexate. Yellow u/c. 2.5mg: Round. 10mg: Cap-shaped scored. Lactose. **Store:** Original pack to protect (light).

Methotrexate (Concordia) 2.5mg (Concordia) A. GMS.
Price, (28) €3.76.
Tablet, methotrexate sodium. Round yellow scored. Marked M above score, 1 below; 2.5 on reverse. Lactose. **Store:** Below 25 deg C; original pack to protect (light).

Methotrexate (Hospira) Tabs, Parenteral (Hospira) A. GMS.
Price, (100) 2.5mg, €13.11. 10mg, €44.67. Injection (5) 2.5mg/mL, €27.54. 25mg/mL, €32.93.
Tablet, methotrexate 2.5mg, 10mg. Round yellow. Marked M and strength. Lactose. **Store:** Outer carton to protect (light). Injection, as above 2.5(25, 100)mg/mL. Clear yellow soln. NOTE: Parenteral not suitable for intrathecal use. **Store:** Below 25 deg C; do not freeze; container in outer carton.

Methotrexate Orion 2.5mg, 10mg (Orion) A. GMS.
Price, 2.5mg (28) €3.76. 10mg (100) €43.15.
Tablet, methotrexate. Yellow round u/c. Marked M and strength. 10mg: Scored (divisible into equal halves). Lactose. **Store:** Outer carton to protect (light).

Metoject Parenteral (Fannin) A. GMS.
Price, (1) 10mg/mL, 1mL, €16.70; 1.5mL, €19.28; 2mL, €22.47; 2.5mL, €24.39. 50mg/mL: 0.15mL, €14.72; 0.2mL, €15.89; 0.3mL, €18.61; 0.4mL, €21.93. 0.5mL, €25.84.
Injection, methotrexate 10(50)mg/mL. Clear yellow soln in PFS. **Store:** Below 25 deg C; PFS in outer carton to protect (light).

165

4.4.1　Drugs Suppressing Rheumatic Disease Process

Nordimet Parenteral *(Nordic)* A. GMS
Price, PFP (1) 7.5mg, €13.25; 10mg, €14.30; 12.5mg, €16.68; 15mg, €16.75; 17.5mg, €19.36; 20mg, €19.74; 22.5mg, €23.22; 25mg, €23.25.
Injection (PFP), methotrexate 25mg/mL (7.5mg, 10mg, 12.5mg, 15mg, 17.5mg, 20mg, 22.5mg, 25mg). Clear yellow soln. **Store:** Below 25 deg C; outer carton to protect (light).

Secukinumab

ATC Code: L04AC10. **Sport:** Permitted.
Driving: No or negligible effect.
Indications: Treatment (adults), moderate to severe plaque psoriasis; active psoriatic arthritis (alone or combination with methotrexate) when response to DMARDs inadequate; ankylosing spondylitis (adequate response to conventional therapy).

Dose: Adult, Elderly: *Plaque psoriasis, psoriatic arthritis (with plaque psoriasis or anti-TNR inadequate responders),* 300mg (as 2x 150mg SC injections) at weeks 0, 1, 2 and 3 then monthly starting at week 4. *Other psoriatic arthritis patients, ankylosing spondylitis,* 150mg SC at weeks 0, 1, 2 and 3, then monthly from week 4. No response in 16 weeks, consider discontinuing.

Child: Under 18 years, no safety/efficacy data.

Renal Impairment: No dose recommendation.

Hepatic Impairment: As for Renal above.

Interactions: Effect of Secukinumab on Other Drugs: CYP450 substrates with narrow therapeutic index (warfarin): *Therapeutic monitoring required.*

SP: Crohn's diseases, caution; exacerbations, including serious, observed. Rare anaphylactic reactions. Combination with immunosuppressants (including biologicals or phototherapy), not evaluated.

Pregnancy, Lactation: Pregnancy, avoid; women of childbearing potential to use effective contraception during and for at least 20 weeks after treatment. Lactation, stop breastfeeding or stop drug.

ADR: Summary, *most frequent,* upper respiratory tract infections (nasopharyngitis, rhinitis).

Notes: See 4.4.1 Drugs Suppressing Rheumatic Disease Process.

▼ **Cosentyx Parenteral 150mg** *(Novartis)* A. HT.
Price, PFP (1) €565.60; (2) €1204.49.
Injection (PFP), secukinumab recombinant 150mg/mL. Clear colourless (slightly yellow) in SensoReady pen. **Store:** Refrigerate; do not freeze; original pack to protect (light).

Tocilizumab

ATC Code: L04AC07. **Sport:** Permitted.
Driving: Caution.
Indications: Treatment (with methotrexate)*, (adults) severe active and progressive rheumatoid arthritis (RA) (no previous methotrexate); moderate to severe active RA (previous DMARD or TNF antagonist). Treatment, (child) active systemic juvenile idiopathic arthritis (sJIA)* OR polyarticular juvenile idiopathic arthritis (pJIA)*. *(as monotherapy if methotrexate intolerant or inappropriate).

Dose: Adult, Elderly: IV INFUSION, *RA,* 8mg/kg over 1 hour once every 4 weeks; weight above 100kg, dose above 800mg per infusion, not recommended.
SC INJECTION, 162mg once every week.

Child: Age 2 years and older, *sJIA,* weight 30kg or more, 8mg/kg by IV infusion once every 2 weeks; under 30kg, 12mg/kg every 2 weeks, *pJIA,* weight 30kg or more, 8mg/kg once every 4 weeks; under 30kg, 10mg/kg every 2 weeks. Under 18 years, SC injection not recommended.

Renal Impairment: Moderate/severe, no data, monitor.

Hepatic Impairment: No dose recommendation.

Interactions: Effect of Other Drugs on Tocilizumab: Co-admin not recommended: Other TNF antagonists, other biologicals, live vaccines. *Caution, monitor:* Starting/stopping tocilizumab, patients taking medicinals which are individually adjusted and metabolised via CYP3A4, 1A2, 2C9, 2C19 (atorvastatin, calcium channel blockers, theophylline, warfarin, phenprocoumon, phenytoin, ciclosporin, benzodiazepines); monitor (consider dose increase to maintain therapeutic effect);

effect of tocilizumab on CYP450 enzyme activity may persist for several weeks after discontinuation (long elimination half-life).

Effect of Tocilizumab on Other Drugs: Simvastatin: *Plasma levels decreased.*

SP: Hypersensitivity reactions (more severe, potentially fatal if occurred with previous infusion); anaphylactic, serious hypersensitivity, or infusion related reactions, permanently discontinue. GI perforation, diverticulitis complications (generalised purulent peritonitis, fistula, abscess). Combination (methotrexate), elevated transaminases, caution (hepatic disease or impairment; elevated ALT or AST above 1.5xULN); baseline ALT/AST above 1.5xULN, not recommended. Decreased neutrophils, platelets; elevated lipids (usually respond to lipid-lowering agents). Demyelinating disorders, caution. Increased malignancy risk; cardiovascular risk factors (hyper-tension, lipidaemia). Viral reactivation (HBV). Issue all patients with a Patient Alert Card.

Pregnancy, Lactation: Pregnancy, use only if clearly necessary. Women of childbearing potential to ensure effective contraception during and up to 3 months after treatment. Lactation, stop breastfeeding or stop drug.

ADR: Summary, *most common,* upper RTI, nasopharyngitis, headache, hypertension, increased ALT; *most serious,* serious infections, diverticulitis complications, hypersensitivity reactions.

Notes: See 4.4.1 Drugs Suppressing Rheumatic Disease Process.

RoActemra Parenteral *(Roche)* A. HT.
Price, PFS 162mg (4), €1090.57. HOS: 80mg/4mL, €138.87. 200mg/10mL, €347.61. 400mg/20mL, €694.01 (PTW).
Infusion, tocilizumab 20mg/mL. Clear (opalescent) colourless (pale-yellow) sterile conc for soln. *Sodium 2.21mg (4.43mg; 8.85mg) per 80mg (200mg; 400mg) vial.* **Store:** Refrigerate; do not freeze.
Injection (SC), as above 162mg. Colourless (slightly-yellow) soln. **Store:** Refrigerate; do not freeze.

Ustekinumab

ATC Code: L04AC05. **Sport:** Permitted.
Driving: No or negligible effect.
Indications: Treatment, moderate to severe plaque psoriasis in patients aged 12 years and over, who have failed to respond, contraindicated or intolerant to other systemic therapies (ciclosporin, methotrexate, PUVA; psoralens and ultraviolet A). Psoriatic arthritis (active).

Dose: Adult, Elderly: Initially 45mg, then 45mg after 4 weeks; then every 12 weeks. Body weight above 100kg, 90mg initially, and maintenance as above. SC injection (avoid areas of skin showing psoriasis). No response up to 28 weeks treatment, consider discontinuation.

Child: Age 12 years and older, admin at weeks 0 and 4, then every 12 weeks; under 60kg, 0.75mg/kg; 60-100kg, 45mg; over 100kg, 90mg. See Adult above.

SP: Serious hypersensitivity reactions several days after treatment in some cases (anaphylaxis, angioedema), discontinue. Serious skin conditions (erythrodermic psoriasis, exfoliative dermatitis).

Pregnancy, Lactation: Pregnancy, avoid. Women of childbearing potential and males to ensure adequate contraception*. Lactation, stop breast feeding or stop drug* (risk/benefit). *during and for 15 weeks after treatment.

ADR: Summary, *most common,* nasopharyngitis, headache, upper respiratory tract infection; *most serious,* hypersensitivity reactions including anaphylaxis.

Notes: See 4.4.1 Drugs Suppressing Rheumatic Disease Process.

Stelara Parenteral *(Janssen-Cilag)* A. HT.
Price, (1) 45mg/0.5mL (inj) €3196.71; (PFS) €3160.74. (1) 90mg/mL (PFS) €3211.48.
Injection, ustekinumab 45mg/0.5mL, 90mg/1mL. Human IgG1k monoclonal antibody to interleukin (IL)-12/23 recombinant. Clear (slightly opalescent) colourless (light-yellow) soln in PFS. *Dry rubber (needle cover).* **Store:** Refrigerate; do not freeze; outer carton; protect (light).

4.4.2 - Non-Steroidal Anti-Inflammatories (NSAIDs), (Non-Selective)

In This Chapter: *Benzydamine, capsaicin, dexketoprofen, diclofenac, diclofenac and combinations (misoprostol), etofenamate, felbinac, ibuprofen, ketoprofen, lornoxicam, mefenamic acid, meloxicam, nabumetone, naproxen and combinations (esomeprazole), piroxicam.*

Class Effects
Driving: No or negligible effect; if dizziness, drowsiness, fatigue, vertigo, visual disturbances or other CNS effects are experienced while taking NSAIDs, refrain from driving or operating machinery; unlikely with topicals unless extensive systemic absorption.

CI: Not for use in children unless otherwise specified and suitable paediatric formulations are available.

GI ulceration (chronic dyspepsia that might be indicative of ulceration), bleeding, perforation (present or related to previous NSAID therapy); disorders predisposing to bleeding (ulcerative colitis, Crohn's disease, GI cancers, diverticulitis); active peptic/GI ulcer or haemorrhage, inflammatory disorders or coagulation or bleeding disorders.

Hypersensitivity, serious allergic reaction especially cutaneous (erythema multiforme, Stevens-Johnson syndrome, toxic epidermal necrolysis), previous skin reaction (regardless of severity) following NSAIDs or other medication. Photosensitivity. Asthma, bronchospasm, acute rhinitis, nasal polyps, angioedema, urticaria, other allergic-type reactions (after taking aspirin/acetylsalicylic acid or NSAIDs including COX-2 inhibitors).

Moderate to severe CHF (NYHA II-IV), ischaemic heart disease, severe cardiac, renal or hepatic impairment, bleeding disorders including cerebrovascular, peripheral arterial disease, coagulation disorders or other active bleeding. See SP and Interactions below. Severe dehydration.

Treatment of pain after coronary artery bypass graft (CABG) surgery *(mefenamic acid, diclofenac sodium + misoprostol, meloxicam).*

Interactions: Effect of Other Drugs on NSAIDs: *Co-admin contraindicated:* Other NSAIDs (including COX-2 inhibitors), salicylates at anti-inflammatory or analgesic doses (1g or more as single intake or 3g/day or more). *Increased GI toxicity, bleeding risk:* Corticosteroids. *Increased haemorrhage risk (especially GI):* Heparin, oral anticoagulants (warfarin) (co-admin only with medical supervision), antiplatelets (aspirin), SSRIs. *Plasma levels increased:* Probenecid. *Hyperkalaemia risk, monitor:* Potassium-sparing diuretics, ciclosporin, tacrolimus, trimethoprim, potassium salts, ACEIs, AIIAs, other NSAIDs, heparin. *Increased renal failure risk:* Tenofovir disoproxil fumarate.

Effect of NSAIDs on Other Drugs: Lithium, pemetrexed (decreased excretion), digoxin (monitor): *Increased plasma levels.* Methotrexate (especially above 15mg/week): *Increased haematological toxicity.* Hydantoins, sulfonamides: *Increased toxic effects.* Diuretics, ACEIs, AIIAs: *Effect reduced; with compromised renal function (dehydration, elderly) co-admin may result in further deterioration; ensure adequate hydration.* Pentoxifylline, thrombolytics, ginkgo biloba: *Increased bleeding risk.* Zidovudine: *Increased red cell toxicity, severe anaemia.* Sulfonylureas, other antidiabetics: *Increased or decreased hypoglycaemic effect.* Beta-blockers, ACEIs, diuretics: *Hypotensive effect reduced.* Ciclosporin, tacrolimus: *Increased nephrotoxicity.* Quinolones: *Convulsions, caution.* Mifepristone: *Effect reduced; allow 8-12 day dosing interval.* Aminoglycosides: *Reduced renal function; decreased excretion.*

SP: NOTE: To minimise undesirable effects, use lowest effective dose for shortest possible duration, especially *elderly* and *children*, frail or low body weight or with risk factors for cardiovascular events. Elderly more prone to adverse events especially with long-term use (consider risk/benefit).

Allergic reactions (anaphylactic, anaphylactoid) can occur; may precipitate bronchospasm (with previous history). With asthma, chronic (rhinitis, sinusitis) and/or nasal polyps, higher risk of allergy to aspirin and/or NSAIDS. May mask signs/symptoms of infection.

GI/hepatic, GI bleeding ulceration or perforation (may be fatal); if occurs, withdraw NSAID. Caution, symptoms or history of gastric or intestinal ulceration, bleeding or perforation (increased frequency in elderly), GI toxicity history, co-medication (see Interactions above), ulcerative colitis or Crohn's disease. High bleeding/ulceration risk, consider combination (PPI or misoprostol). Hepatic impairment, close supervision; prolonged use, monitor function regularly.

Impaired cardiac or renal function, hypertension and/or mild to moderate CHF, elderly, co-medication, volume depletion (caution); fluid retention, oedema reported. Monitor renal function (especially with prolonged use); impairment risk if dehydrated (especially children, adolescents); ensure adequate hydration. High doses may be associated with increased arterial thrombotic event (MI, stroke) risk. Treat after careful consideration with uncontrolled hypertension, CHF, ischaemic heart disease, peripheral arterial disease, cerebrovascular disease, cardiovascular risk factors (hypertension, hyperlipidaemia, diabetes mellitus, smoking). May inhibit platelet aggregation; monitor blood counts. Hyperkalaemia with underlying diabetes, renal failure, co-admin of agents causing hyperkalaemia).

Special precautions (readiness for emergency) with asthma, seasonal allergic rhinitis, nasal polyps, COPD, chronic respiratory infection, Quincke's oedema, urticaria; also with allergies to other substances.

Meloxicam, piroxicam, tenoxicam, life-threatening cutaneous reactions, Stevens-Johnson syndrome (SJS), toxic epidermal necrolysis (TEN); advise patients of signs/symptoms, monitor; if signs/symptoms occur (progressive skin rash with blisters or mucosal lesions), discontinue. If SJS or TEN has occurred, do not re-start at any time.

PARENTERAL, local (pain, induration). TOPICAL, usually well tolerated. Local allergic skin reactions (exanthema, erosion, erythema, eczema, ulceration), photosensitivity (avoid exposure to direct sunlight). Prolonged or excessive use, possible systemic side effects. Caution, avoid contact with eyes and mucous membranes; wash hands after use unless treatment site. Do not apply to broken or irritated skin, open wounds, diseased skin areas (usually contain alcohol). Generally not for use with occlusion, in presence of local infection, or co-admin with other topicals.

Pregnancy, Lactation: Contraindicated in third trimester, unless otherwise specified; may result in premature closure of ductus arteriosus or uterine inertia. Lactation, not recommended. Inhibition of prostaglandin synthesis may adversely affect pregnancy (prolonged bleeding in mother and child at end of pregnancy) and/or embryo and or foetal development (cardiopulmonary and renal toxicity).

Topical, if use is deemed necessary during first and second trimester, do not apply to large areas of skin (above 600cm2 body surface) OR use long-term (systemic absorption risk). Third trimester, contraindicated.

Notes: See 4.2.1 Non-Opioid Analgesics (acetylsalicylic acid, ibuprofen/codeine phosphate).

Benzydamine (musculoskeletal)
ATC Code: M02AA05. **Sport:** Permitted.
Driving: Unlikely to impair.
Indications: Musculo-skeletal pain (myalgia, bursitis, rheumatism) and trauma (soft tissue injuries, sprains, strains, contusions, after-effects of fractures).
Dose: Adult, Elderly: Apply and massage lightly up to 3-times daily; severe conditions, up to 6-times daily.
SP: Not for application to eyes or mucosal surfaces.
ADR: Photosensitivity, skin reactions, anaphylactic reactions (frequency unknown).
Notes: See 4.4.2 NSAIDS (Non-Selective).

167

4.4.2 Non-Steroidal Anti-Inflammatories (NSAIDs), (Non-Selective)

Difflam 3% Cream *(Meda)* OTC. GMS.
Price, (50g) €5.75.
Topical cream, benzydamine HCl 3% w/w. Ivory-white homogenous perfumed. *Parabens, cetyl alcohol, propylene glycol.*

Capsaicin

ATC Code: N01BX04. **Sport:** Permitted.
Driving: No or negligible effect.
Indications: Post-herpetic neuralgia (following *Herpes zoster* infection; after open lesions have healed). Painful diabetic peripheral polyneuropathy *(Axsain).* Symptomatic relief, pain associated with osteoarthritis *(Zacin).* Peripheral neuropathic pain *(Qutenza).*

Dose: Adult, Elderly: TOPICAL CREAM, apply small amount of cream (pea-sized) to affected area 3-4 times daily; rub in gently; leave no residue on surface; wash off after 30 minutes. *Axsain,* painful diabetic peripheral polyneuropathy, under consultant supervision; duration, 8 weeks.

CUTANEOUS PATCH, apply to most painful areas (max. 4 patches) to intact, non-irritated, dry skin. Leave in place for 30 minutes (feet e.g. HIV-associated neuropathy, painful diabetic peripheral neuropathy) OR 60 minutes (other areas e.g. post-herpetic neuralgia). Repeat every 90 days, as needed for persistence or return of pain. Area can be pre-treated with local anaesthetic (area and 1-2cm surround) or oral analgesic admin to reduce application-related discomfort.

Child: Under 18 years, no safety/efficacy data.

Renal Impairment: No dose adjustment.

Hepatic Impairment: As for Renal above.

SP: Apply to dry intact skin. Application site reactions (burning, pain, erythema). Avoid inhalation of vapours; well ventilated treatment area. *Cream,* avoid hot bath or shower just after application. Skin irritation. Transient irritation of mucous membranes of eyes, respiratory tract; asthma exacerbation. Not for use under tight bandages. *Patches,* wear nitrile gloves when handling. Do not apply above hairline of scalp and/or close to mucous membranes. Diabetic peripheral neuropathy, carefully examine feet before each application for skin lesions (underlying neuropathy, vascular insufficiency). Reduced sensory function reported; caution (reduced sensation in feet, increased risk for sensory changes). Pain after application, use local cooling or oral analgesics (short-acting opioids); severe pain, examine for chemical burn. Exposure to skin not for treatment, apply cleansing gel (1 minute), wipe off with dry gauze; wash with soap and water; flush eyes or mucous membranes with water; shortness of breath, provide appropriate medical care. Monitor BP during treatment (diabetics with CAD, hypertension, cardiovascular autonomic neuropathy).

Pregnancy, Lactation: Pregnancy, caution (unlikely to affect). Lactation, discontinue breastfeeding.

ADR: *Cream,* skin irritation, transient burning on application. See SP above. *Patch, most commonly,* transient local application site burning, pain, erythema, pruritus.

Notes: See 4.4.2 NSAIDS (Non-Selective).

Axsain Cream *(TEVA)* B. GMS.
Price, (45g) €17.52.
Topical cream, capsaicin 0.075% w/w. Smooth white. *Benzyl, cetyl alcohol.*
Qutenza 179mg Patch *(Grunenthal)* B.
Price, not published by company.
Cutaneous patch, capsaicin 179mg/patch (640mcg/cm2). Adhesive side with active substance and outer surface backing layer. Marked 'capsaicin 8%'. Cleansing gel 50g tube. *Butylhydroxyanisole.* Store: Flat; below 25 deg C; original pack.
Zacin Cream *(TEVA)* B. GMS.
Price, (45g) €17.52.
Topical cream, capsaicin 0.025% w/w. Smooth white. *Cetyl alcohol.*

Dexketoprofen

ATC Code: M01AE17. **Sport:** Permitted.
Driving: Dizziness, visual disturbance, drowsiness.
Indications: Mild to moderate musculoskeletal, dental pain; dysmenorrhoea. Parenteral, for moderate to severe, acute pain post-op, in renal colic and low back pain.

Dose: Adult: ORAL, usually 12.5mg every 4-6 hours OR 25mg 8-hourly; max. 75mg/day. *Admin,* absorption delayed if taken with food; acute pain, admin 30 minutes before food (granules 15 minutes). Swallow whole with one glass of water.

PARENTERAL, 50mg every 8-12 hours; 6-hourly if needed; max. 150mg/day. IM (slow, deep into muscle) or IV slow infusion over 10-30 minutes OR bolus over minimum 15 seconds.

Elderly: Initiate at 50mg/day total dose.

Child: Safety/efficacy not established.

Renal Impairment: CrCl (mL/min), 60-90, 50mg/day total dose; 59 and below, not recommended.

Hepatic Impairment: Mild/moderate, 50mg/day total dose. Severe, not recommended.

CI: Photoallergic or phototoxic reactions with ketoprofen or fibrates, severe dehydration.

SP: Exclude oesophagitis, gastritis and/or peptic ulceration. *Caution,* haematopoietic disorders, SLE, mixed connective tissue disease, impaired cardiac function, conditions predisposing to fluid retention, congenital disorder of porphyrin metabolism, dehydration, directly after major surgery.

ADR: *Common,* nausea and/or vomiting, abdominal pain, diarrhoea, dyspepsia. Parenteral, injection site pain, reaction (inflammation, bruising, haemorrhage).

Notes: See 4.4.2 NSAIDS (Non-Selective).

Keral 25mg, Granules 25mg *(A.Menarini)* B. GMS.D.
Price, 25mg (50) €6.81. Sachets (20) €4.41.
Tablet, dexketoprofen trometamol. White round f/c scored (divisible into equal halves).
Granules, as above. Lemon-yellow for oral soln. *Sucrose.*
Keral Parenteral *(A.Menarini)* A.
Price, (50) €13.87.
Injection or infusion, dexketoprofen trometamol. Clear colourless soln. pH (7-8). *Ethanol, sodium 4mg/mL.*
Dexketoprofen Rowex 25mg *(Rowex)* B. GMS.D.
Price, (50) €5.45.
Tablet, dexketoprofen trometamol. White cylindrical-shaped scored (divisible in equal halves). Marked DT2.

Diclofenac Potassium

ATC Code: M01AB06. **Sport:** Permitted.
Driving: Dizziness, vertigo, somnolence, visual disturbance.
Indications: Acute pain and inflammation (post-trauma, musculoskeletal, post-operative). Dysmenorrhoea. Migraine. Acute gout. Painful syndromes of vertebral column. Non-articular rheumatism. Adjuvant, severe painful inflammatory infections of ear, nose or throat.

Dose: Adult: *Pain,* acute, 100-150mg/day; milder pain, 75-100mg/day usually sufficient admin in 2-3 divided doses. *Migraine,* initially 50mg at first sign of attack; insufficient pain relief, after 2 hours admin further 50mg; then 50mg doses may be taken every 4-6 hours; max. 200mg/day. *Primary dysmenorrhoea,* initially 50-100mg; titrate to max. 200mg/day. *Admin,* swallow tabs whole with liquid with or after food; total daily dose in 2-3 divided doses.

Elderly: Increased risk of adverse reactions.

Child: Over 14 years, 75-100mg/day in 2 or 3 divided doses; max. 150mg/day. Migraine, use not established. Under 14 years, tabs not recommended.

Renal Impairment: Mild/moderate, caution (no dose recommendations). Severe, contraindicated.

Hepatic Impairment: As for Renal above.

Interactions: Effect of Other Drugs on Diclofenac Potassium: *Co-admin caution, increased exposure:* Potent CYP2C9 inhibitors (sulfinpyrazone, voriconazole); moderate CYP2C9 inhibitors (fluconazole, miconazole, amiodarone)

Effect of Diclofenac Potassium on Other Drugs: Digoxin, phenytoin: *Plasma levels increased, monitor.*

SP: Abnormal LFTs, signs and symptoms of liver disease (eosinophilia, rash), discontinue; hepatitis (without prodromal symptoms), hepatic porphyria (triggered).

ADR: *Common*, (oral) headache, dizziness, vertigo, nausea, vomiting, diarrhoea, dyspepsia, abdominal pain, flatulence, decreased appetite, increased transaminases, rash.

Notes: See 4.4.2 NSAIDS (Non-Selective).

Interchangeability: Same strengths of all brands of diclofenac potassium film-coated (f/c) tabs listed below are deemed interchangeable.

> **Cataflam 50mg** *(Novartis)* B. GMS.D.
> *Price,* (30) €1.67.
> *Tablet,* diclofenac potassium. Round s/c. Reddish-brown. *Sucrose.*
> **Kyflam 50mg** *(Accord)* B. GMS.D.
> *Price,* (56) €3.29.
> *Tablet,* diclofenac potassium. Round reddish-brown f/c. *Soya lecithin.*

Diclofenac Sodium (musculoskeletal)

ATC Code: M02AA15. **Sport:** Permitted.
Driving: Dizziness, vertigo, somnolence, visual disturbance.

Indications: *Oral,* relief of all grades of pain and inflammation (arthritic conditions, musculoskeletal disorders, trauma). Dysmenorrhoea. Juvenile chronic arthritis. Inflammatory infections (ear, nose, throat). *Parenteral,* acute conditions (renal colic, gout, trauma, fractures); post-operative pain in hospital setting *(IV infusion).* *Topical,* localised forms of rheumatism (soft tissue, degenerative rheumatism).

Dose: Adult: ORAL, STANDARD/R, 75-150mg/day in divided doses; max. 150mg/day.
PROLONGED/R, 75-100mg/day; max. 150mg/day. Swallow all gastro-resistant dosage forms whole with water; preferably with or after food.
RECTAL, insert 1 supp into the rectum at night.
PARENTERAL (IM), 75mg IM once or twice daily (deep intragluteal into upper quadrant); max. 2 days; continue with oral or rectal. Severe cases (renal colic) 1x75mg amp IM; 1 further amp after 30 minutes if needed.
IV INFUSION, 1 amp (75mg) diluted in minimum 100-500mL normal saline; admin over 30 minutes; if needed admin second dose 4-6 hours after first infusion; max. 150mg in any 24 hours; max. 2 doses given IV. NOT for bolus IV injection.
TOPICAL, *gel,* rub 2-4g gently into skin 3-4 times daily; *spray gel,* spray onto skin of affected site; 4-5 pump strokes 3-times daily; max. 15 pump strokes per day. Smooth gently into skin; allow to dry before dressing. Combination dosage forms may be used (tabs, supps).

Elderly: Use lowest effective dose.

Child: ORAL, STANDARD/R, age 9 years or over (min 35kg body weight), 2mg/kg/day in 3 divided doses depending on severity *(Difene)*; over 1 year, 0.5-2mg/kg/day in 2-3 divided doses; for juvenile rheumatoid arthritis, 3mg/kg/day in divided doses can be used; max. 150mg/day *(Voltarol)*. Prolonged/R formulations and supps not recommended for use in children.
TOPICAL, PARENTERAL, age 14 years and over, as for Adult; if needed for more than 7 days, consult medical advice. Under 14 years, contraindicated. Topical not to be used with occlusion.

Renal Impairment: Mild/moderate, caution (no dose recommendations). Severe, contraindicated.

Hepatic Impairment: As for Renal above.

SP: See Notes below (diclofenac potassium).

ADR: See Notes below (diclofenac potassium).

Notes: See Diclofenac Potassium above. See 4.4.2 NSAIDS (Non-Selective).

Interchangeability: Same strengths of all brands of diclofenac sodium Standard/R tabs, Prolonged/R tabs, Modified/R capsules, suppositories, topical gel (1%, 3%) listed below are deemed interchangeable. See 10.1.6 Photodamage, Actinic Keratosis. Topical gel (4%) is not deemed interchangeable.

> **Voltarol Tabs, Retard, Supps** *(Novartis)* B. GMS.D*.
> *Price,* Standard/R tabs 25mg* (100) €2.51. 50mg* (50) €2.94. Retard (30) 75mg*, €3.33. 100mg, €4.57. Supps (10) Paed 12.5mg, €0.52.
> *Tablets,* diclofenac sodium. Standard/R tablets, 25mg, 50mg, Prolonged/R (Retard) 75mg, 100mg. *Standard/R:* 25mg, 50mg:

Round g/r. 25mg: Yellow. Marked Geigy; Voltarol 25 on reverse. 50mg: Light-brown. Marked CG; GT on reverse. *Lactose.* *Prolonged/R (Retard):* f/c. 75mg: Pale pink triangular. Marked CG; ID on reverse. 100mg: Pale-red. Marked CGC; CG on reverse. *Cetyl alcohol, sucrose.*
Supps, as above 12.5mg. Yellowish-white torpedo-shaped.
> **Voltarol Emulgel P** *(Novartis Consumer)* OTC.
> *Price,* 30g, €5.15; 50g, €7.02; 100g, €10.82.
> *Topical gel (Emulgel),* diclofenac diethylammonium equiv. to diclofenac 1% w/w. White perfumed homogenous non-greasy emulsion in aqueous gel. *Propylene glycol, benzyl benzoate.*
> **Diclac Tablets, Retard, Supps, Topical** *(Rowex)* B. GMS.D*.
> *Price,* Standard/R* (100) 25mg, €3.50. 50mg, €8.23. Retard* 75mg (60) €6.65. 100mg (30) €4.48. Supps* 100mg (10) €1.05. Gel 50g, €1.76.
> *Tablet,* diclofenac sodium 25mg, 50mg, (Retard) 75mg, 100mg. 25mg, 50mg: Yellowish-brown g/r. 75mg Prolonged Release: Round flat two-layered pink/white. 100mg Retard: White round. *Lactose.*
> *Supps,* as above 100mg.
> *Topical gel,* as above 1% w/w. Slightly yellow emulsion with alcoholic smell.
> **Diclac Parenteral** *(Rowex)* A. GMS.D.
> *Price,* 25mg/mL (10 x 3mL) €8.10.
> *Injection,* diclofenac sodium 25mg/mL. Colourless (slightly yellow) soln. *Benzyl alcohol.*
> **Difene Caps, Dual/R, Supps, Topical** *(Astellas)* B. GMS.D*.
> *Price,* Standard/R* caps (56) 25mg, €1.26. 50mg, €3.06. Dual/R SR* 75mg (56) €7.47. 100mg (28) €5.21. Supps* 100mg (10) €0.97. Gel 50g, €1.18. Spray Gel 25g, €6.53.
> *Capsule (Dual/R),* diclofenac sodium 25mg, 50mg, (Dual Release) 75mg, 100mg. Opaque blue/transparent hard contains white (cream-colour) pellets. Standard/R 25mg, 50mg: g/r. Marked D/strength. *Sucrose.* Dual Release 75mg, 100mg: Contains 25mg pellets g/r and 50mg (75mg) Prolonged/R pellets. Marked DstrengthM. **Store:** Below 25 deg C.
> *Supps,* as above 100mg. White torpedo-shaped. **Store:** Below 25 deg C.
> *Topical gel (1%),* cutaneous spray gel (4%), as above. Slightly turbid colourless; isopropyl alcohol odour (gel). Golden-yellow transparent; peppermint odour (gel-like consistency after admin) (spray gel). *Propylene glycol.*

Diclofenac Sodium, Misoprostol

ATC Code: M01AB55. **Sport:** Permitted.
Driving: Dizziness, other CNS disturbances.

Indications: Where the NSAID diclofenac is required in combination with misoprostol. Diclofenac (osteoarthritis, rheumatoid arthritis); misoprostol (prophylaxis of NSAID-induced gastric and duodenal ulceration required).

Dose: Adult, Elderly: 1 tab 2-3 times daily. *Admin,* swallow tabs whole; do not chew; take with food. *Elderly,* monitor.

SP: Caution with renal, cardiac or hepatic impairment, and in elderly (monitor). Exceptional use, advanced (cardiac or renal failure, liver disease), severe dehydration; close monitoring.

Pregnancy, Lactation: Pregnancy and women planning pregnancy, contraindicated; exclude before initiation (misoprostol induces uterine contractions; associated with abortion, premature birth, foetal death). Women of childbearing potential, ensure adequate contraception. If pregnancy suspected, discontinue. Lactation, not recommended; both components excreted in breast milk. See Notes below.

ADR: *Very common,* abdominal pain, diarrhoea, nausea, dyspepsia.

Notes: See Diclofenac Sodium above. See 4.4.2 NSAIDS (Non-Selective) and 1.3.3 Prostaglandin Analogues (misoprostol).

Interchangeability: Same strengths of all brands of diclofenac sodium/misoprostol Modified/R tabs are deemed interchangeable (includes parallel imports).

> **Arthrotec 50mg, 75mg** *(Pfizer)* A. GMS.
> *Price,* (60) 16.97. 75mg, €21.57.
> *Modified/R tablet,* diclofenac sodium core g/r (mg), misoprostol outer (mcg). White round. Marked Searle. 50/200: Marked 1411; four A's on reverse. 75/200: Marked A and 75; 1421 on reverse. *Lactose.* **Store:** Below 25 deg C; original pack.

4.4.2 Non-Steroidal Anti-Inflammatories (NSAIDs), (Non-Selective)

Etofenamate

ATC Code: M02AA06. **Sport:** Permitted.
Driving: Unlikely to impair.
Indications: Inflammatory disorders of the musculoskeletal system.
Dose: Adult, Elderly: Rub 5-10cm strip of gel in gently up to 4 times daily.
Notes: See 4.4.2 NSAIDS (Non-Selective).

Etoflam Gel *(Phoenix)* B. GMS.
Price, (100g) €9.14.
Topical gel, etofenamate 5% w/w. Nearly transparent yellowish. Alcohol.

Felbinac

ATC Code: M02AA08. **Sport:** Permitted.
Driving: Unlikely to impair.
Indications: Pain and inflammation associated with musculoskeletal conditions (soft tissue trauma, extra-articular rheumatism, rheumatic or non-serious arthritic conditions).
Dose: Adult, Elderly: Rub 1g gel (approximately 2.5cm) lightly into affected area 2-4 times daily; max. 25g/day regardless of number of affected areas.
ADR: *Very common,* paraesthesia, mild local irritation, dermatitis, pruritus.
Notes: See 4.4.2 NSAIDS (Non-Selective).

Traxam Gel *(Concordia)* B. GMS.
Price, (100g) €11.03.
Topical gel, felbinac 3% w/w. Clear smooth non-greasy.

Ibuprofen

ATC Code: M01AE01, M02AA13 (topical). **Sport:** Permitted.
Driving: Dizziness, drowsiness, fatigue, visual disturbance.
Indications: Mild to moderate pain and fever (dysmenorrhoea, headache, colds and flu). Pain and inflammation (rheumatoid arthritis, including juvenile RA or Still's disease, other musculoskeletal disorders, dental pain, post-operative pain). Analgesic, mild to moderate pain, pyrexia in children (paediatric formulations). Topical symptomatic treatment of musculoskeletal disorders.
Dose: Adult, Elderly: ORAL, STANDARD/R, 1200-1800mg/day; max. 2400mg; maintenance 600-1200mg/day in divided doses. *Admin,* tabs with plenty of water, swallow whole; do not crush or chew; with or after food. *Brufen* may be taken on an empty stomach to achieve faster onset of action; recommended that patients with sensitive stomach take ibuprofen with food.
TOPICAL, apply gel up to 3-times daily massaging gently.
Child: ORAL, STANDARD/R, usually 20mg/kg/day; juvenile rheumatoid arthritis, increase to 40mg/kg in severe cases; under 30kg, max. 500mg/day using paed suspension.
PAED SUSPENSION, age 3-6 months (weight under 5kg), 5mg/kg 3-times daily; age 6-12 months, 50mg 3-times daily; age 1-2 years, 50mg 3-4 times daily; age 3-7 years, 100mg 3-4 times daily; age 8-12 years, 200mg 3-4 times daily (usually 20mg/kg/day); over 12 years, as for Adult above. Admin with or after food.
PAED SUPPOSITORY, age 8-12 months (7.5-10kg), insert 1x 75mg supp 6-hourly; max. 225mg/day; age 12 month to 3 years (10-15kg), 1x 75mg supp 6-hourly; max. 300mg/day. Max. duration 4 days then consult medical advice. Insert deep into rectum after bowel movement.
TOPICAL, over 12-14 years, as for Adult above.
Renal Impairment: Adjust dosage.
Hepatic Impairment: As for Renal above. Severe, contraindicated.
SP: Oral ibuprofen may inhibit effect of low dose acetylsalicylic acid on platelet aggregation (co-admin); no firm conclusion for regular ibuprofen use; no clinically relevant effect likely for occasional ibuprofen use. Transient burning in mouth with susp or if tabs are chewed. Aseptic meningitis rarely reported. See notes below.
ADR: *Most common,* GI adverse events. Supps may cause local irritation, secretion of bloody mucous, painful defaecation.

Notes: See 4.4.2 NSAIDS (Non-Selective).

Brufen Tabs, Retard, Paed Susp *(BGP)* B. GMS.D*.
Price, tabs (60) 400mg*, €1.78. 600mg*, €5.82. Retard 800mg*, €7.89. Susp (200mL) €2.06.
Tablet, ibuprofen 400mg, 600mg. White pillow-shaped f/c. *Lactose.* **Store:** Below 25 deg C; original pack to protect (moisture).
Prolonged/R tablet, as above 800mg (Retard). White pillow-shaped f/c. *Lactose.* **Store:** As above.
Oral susp, as above 100mg/5mL. Orange coloured/flavoured, syrup-like. *Parabens, sucrose, sorbitol,* Sunset Yellow. **Store:** No special conditions.

Buplex Rx 200mg, 400mg, 600mg *(TEVA)* B. GMS.D.
Price, (100) 200mg, €3.63. 400mg, €2.80. 600mg, €4.45.
Tablet, ibuprofen. White oval f/c scored (divisible into equal halves).

Fenopine 200mg, 400mg, 600mg *(Pinewood)* B. GMS.D.
Price, 200mg (100) €3.63; (500) €18.17. 400mg (100) €2.91; (500) €14.55. 600mg (100) €4.62.
Tablet, ibuprofen. Pink f/c. Marked IBU/strength. 200mg, 400mg: Round. 600mg: Cap-shaped.

Ibugel 5% *(Dermal)* B. GMS.
Price, (100g) €7.61.
Topical gel, ibuprofen 5% w/w (50mg/g). Non-greasy fragrance-free clear aqueous-alcoholic. *Propylene glycol.*

Melfen 200mg, 400mg *(Clonmel)* B. GMS.D.
Price, 200mg (100) €3.01. 400mg (100) €2.91; (500) €15.22.
Tablet, ibuprofen. Bright-pink s/c. Marked with logo. 200mg: Marked 178. 400mg: Marked 179.

Phorpain Gel *(Concordia)* OTC. GMS.
Price, (100g) €4.07.
Topical gel, ibuprofen 5% w/w. Clear colourless smooth.

Tefin Supps 75mg, 150mg *(Carysfort)* OTC. GMS.
Price, (10) 75mg, €4.55; 150mg, €5.91.
Supps, ibuprofen. White odourless torpedo-shaped.

Ketoprofen

ATC Code: M02AA10. **Sport:** Permitted.
Driving: Somnolence, dizziness, convulsions.
Indications: Pain and inflammation associated with rheumatoid conditions, gout, non-infectious arthropathy, acute articular and periarticular disorders, sciatica, painful musculoskeletal disorders, dysmenorrhoea. Topical local pain relief of rheumatism and musculoskeletal disorders.
Dose: Adult, Elderly: SYSTEMIC, 100-200mg as a single dose with food.
TOPICAL, apply 5-10cm gel (push pump dispenser 3-6 times) to affected area 2-3 times daily; rub gel in well to ensure local absorption.
Child: SYSTEMIC, safety/efficacy not established. TOPICAL, under 12 years, not recommended.
CI: Fenofibrate, acetylsalicylic acid hypersensitivity. Recent proctitis. Eczema, acne, skin infection. See Notes below.
SP: *Topical,* do not expose treated areas to direct sunlight, including solarium, during treatment or following 2 weeks; protect from sunlight. Wash hands thoroughly after each application. Not for use under occlusive bandage. Skin reaction, discontinue.
ADR: *Topical,* localised skin reactions which may spread beyond application area; severe reactions (bullous or phlyctenular eczema); *systemic, common,* dyspepsia, nausea, abdominal pain, vomiting.
Notes: See 4.4.2 NSAIDS (Non-Selective).

Fastum Gel *(A.Menarini)* B. GMS.
Price, (100g) €6.69.
Topical gel, ketoprofen 2.5% w/w. Colourless non-greasy non-staining; aromatic fragrance. *Ethanol.*

Oruvail 200mg *(SANOFI)* B. GMS.
Price, (28) €10.04.
Prolonged/R capsule, ketoprofen. Hard gelatin transparent-pink/opaque-white contains off-white (cream) spherical pellets. Marked name/strength. *Sucrose.* **Store:** Below 25 deg C.

Lornoxicam

ATC Code: M01AC05. **Sport:** Permitted.
Driving: Dizziness, sleepiness.
Indications: Short-term relief, mild to moderate pain; pain and inflammation in osteoarthritis (OA) and rheumatoid arthritis (RA).
Dose: Adult: *Pain,* including acute, 8-16mg/day in 2 or 3 divided doses; max. 16mg/day.
OA, RA, initially 12mg/day in 2 or 3 divided doses;

maintenance, max. 16mg/day. Oral with a sufficient quantity of liquid. Delayed absorption with food; if quick onset required, take without food.

Elderly: Caution, GI adverse events less well tolerated.

Child: Under 18 years, no data.

Renal Impairment: Mild/moderate, max. 12mg/day in 2 or 3 divided doses. Severe, contraindicated.

Hepatic Impairment: Moderate to severe, as for Renal above.

Interactions: Effect of Other Drugs on Lornoxicam: *Plasma levels increased*: Cimetidine.

ADR: *Common*, mild transient headache, dizziness, nausea, abdominal pain, dyspepsia, diarrhoea, vomiting.

Xefo 8mg, Rapid 8mg *(Takeda)* B. GMS.
Price, (30) 8mg, €5.80. Rapid 8mg, €6.77.
Tablet, lornoxicam. White (yellowish) f/c. 8mg: Oblong. Marked L08. Rapid 8mg: Round. *Lactose*.

Mefenamic Acid

ATC Code: M01AG01. **Sport:** Permitted.
Driving: Dizziness, drowsiness, fatigue, visual disturbance.
Indications: Anti-inflammatory analgesic for symptomatic relief of rheumatic, musculoskeletal, arthritic disorders (rheumatoid arthritis, Still's Disease, osteoarthritis), trauma, headache, dental pain, post-operative or post-partum. Management of primary dysmenorrhoea, dysfunctional menorrhagia, premenstrual syndrome. Control of pyrexia in children.

Dose: Adult, Elderly: Age 12 years and older, 1500mg/day in divided doses, with or after food. *Elderly*, caution, use lowest dose.

Child: Under 12 years, not recommended.

Interactions: Effect of Other Drugs on Mefenamic Acid: *Caution, increased plasma levels (reduced metabolic clearance)*: Known/suspected poor CYP2C9 metabolisers (based on previous history/experience with other CYP2C9 substrates).

Effect of Mefenamic Acid on Other Drugs: Zidovudine: *Increased haematological toxicity risk*.

SP: Prolonged use, monitor liver function; rash, blood dyscrasias, diarrhoea, discontinue. See Notes below.

ADR: GI side-effects most frequent reported (diarrhoea, usually dose related).

Notes: See 4.4.2 NSAIDS (Non-Selective).

Ponstan 250mg, Forte 500mg *(Chemidex)* B. GMS.D.
Price, 250mg (100) €6.15; (500) €27.66. 500mg (100) €11.22.
Capsule, mefenamic acid. Ivory/blue. Marked with name/strength. *Lactose*.
Tablet, as above (Forte). Yellow f/c. *Lactose, Sunset Yellow*.
Mefac 250mg *(Rowex)* B. GMS.D.
Price, (100) €3.79.
Capsule, mefenamic acid. Blue/white. Marked with name/strength *Lactose*

Meloxicam

ATC Code: M01AC06. **Sport:** Permitted.
Driving: Visual disturbances (blurred vision), other CNS disturbances, dizziness, drowsiness, vertigo.
Indications: Symptomatic, short-term, osteoarthrosis exacerbations; long-term, rheumatoid arthritis (RA), ankylosing spondylitis.
Dose: Adult: Osteoarthrosis exacerbations, 7.5mg/day; if needed titrate to max. 15mg/day.
RA, ankylosing spondylitis, 15mg/day; according to response, reduce to 7.5mg/day; max. 15mg/day. Admin as a single dose with water during meal.
Elderly: *RA, ankylosing spondylitis*, long-term, 7.5mg/day.
Child: Under 15-16 years, not recommended/contraindicated.
Renal Impairment: Mild/moderate, no adjustment; if receiving pemetrexed, interrupt meloxicam at least 5 days prior to, on day of, and 2 days after pemetrexed admin. Severe, ESRD on dialysis, max. 7.5mg/day. Severe, non-dialysed, contraindicated.
Hepatic Impairment: Severe, contraindicated.
Interactions: Effect of Other Drugs on Meloxicam:

Reduced elimination: Colestyramine. *Caution, increased GI adverse reaction risk*: Deferasirox.

SP: Not for relief of acute pain. Skin rash, see Notes below.

ADR: *Very common*, GI disorders (dyspepsia, nausea, vomiting, abdominal pain, constipation, flatulence, diarrhoea).

Notes: See 4.4.2 NSAIDS (Non-Selective).

Mobic 7.5mg, 15mg *(Boehringer)* B. GMS.
Price, (30) 7.5mg, €1.36. 15mg, €1.91.
Tablet, meloxicam. Light-yellow round scored (facilitates breaking). Marked with company logo. 7.5mg: Marked 59D/59D. 15mg: Marked 77C/77C. *Lactose*.
Areloger 7.5mg, 15mg *(Gerard)* B. GMS.
Price, (30) 7.5mg, €1.36. 15mg, €1.91.
Tablet, meloxicam. Pale-yellow round scored (7.5mg: To facilitate breaking; 15mg: Divisible into equal doses). *Lactose*.
Melcam 7.5mg, 15mg *(Rowex)* B. GMS.
Price, (30) 7.5mg, €1.36. 15mg, €1.91.
Tablet, meloxicam. Pale-yellow round scored (facilitates breaking). *Lactose*.
Mobiglan 7.5mg, 15mg *(Niche)* B. GMS.
Price, (30) 7.5mg, €1.36. 15mg, €1.91.
Tablet, meloxicam. Light-yellow round. Marked B. 7.5mg: Marked 18. 15mg: Marked 19.

Nabumetone

ATC Code: M01AX01. **Sport:** Permitted.
Driving: No or negligible effect.
Indications: Symptomatic relief of, various arthritic conditions, gout, acute musculoskeletal disorders.
Dose: Adult, Elderly: 1g as single dose at night time; severe/persistent symptoms, acute exacerbations, admin additional 500mg-1g in morning. Acute conditions (sports injuries) admin 1g (loading dose); max. 2g/day. *Elderly*, max. 1g/day.
Child: Not recommended.
ADR: *Most common*, GI adverse events.
Notes: See 4.4.2 NSAIDS (Non-Selective).

Relifex 500mg, 1g *(Meda)* B. GMS.
Price, 500mg (56) €20.10. 1g (30) €14.79.
Tablet, nabumetone. f/c. 500mg: Dark red. Marked Relifex; strength on reverse. 1g: White (off-white) scored (divisible into equal halves).

Naproxen

ATC Code: M01AE02. **Sport:** Permitted.
Driving: Drowsiness, dizziness, vertigo, insomnia, depression.
Indications: Age 16 years and over, see Dose below.
Dose: Adult, Elderly: *Rheumatoid arthritis, osteoarthritis, ankylosing spondylitis*, usually 500mg-1g/day in 2 divided doses (12-hour interval).
Acute gout, initially 750mg then 250mg 8-hourly until attack has passed.
Acute musculoskeletal disorders, dysmenorrhoea, initially 500mg then 250mg every 6-8 hours; max. daily dose after first day of 1250mg. Swallow tabs whole; do not crush or chew.
Child: Under 16 years, not recommended.
Renal Impairment: Caution, monitor and ensure adequate hydration. CrCl (mL/min) below 30, not recommended.
Hepatic Impairment: Use lowest effective dose.
CI: Cross-sensitivity; severe anaphylactic-like reactions reported.
SP: May interfere with some tests laboratory tests; temporarily discontinue for 48 hours before adrenal function and other affected tests.
ADR: *Most common*, GI adverse events.
Notes: See 4.4.2 NSAIDS (Non-Selective).
Interchangeability: Same strengths of all naproxen/esomeprazole modified-release tabs listed below are deemed interchangeable (includes parallel imports).

Naprosyn EC 250mg, 500mg *(Roche)* B. GMS.
Price, (56) 250mg, €3.37. 500mg, €6.75.
Tablet, naproxen. White f/c, g/r. Marked NPR EC/strength. 250mg: Round. 500mg: Cap-shaped.

171

4.4.3 Non-Steroidal Anti-Inflammatories (NSAids), (Selective)

Naproxen, Esomeprazole

ATC Code: M01AE52. **Sport:** Permitted.
Driving: Minor influence; dizziness.

Indications: Symptomatic treatment, osteoarthritis, rheumatoid arthritis, ankylosing spondylitis at risk for NSAID-associated gastric and/or duodenal ulcers and lower NSAID doses insufficient.

Dose: Adult: Recommended, 1 tab (500mg/20mg) twice daily. May be used to treat 'flares'; not for acute conditions (dental pain) due to enteric coat. Swallow whole with water 30 minutes before food; do not split, chew or crush.

Elderly: When max. naproxen 1000mg not appropriate, use non-fixed combination.

Child: Under 18 years, no data.

Renal Impairment: Mild/moderate, caution (monitor); consider reduction in total naproxen daily dose, then as for Elderly above. CrCl (mL/min) below 30, contraindicated.

Hepatic Impairment: As for Renal above. Severe, contraindicated.

Interactions: Effect of Other Drugs on Naproxen, Esomeprazole Combination: Co-admin contraindicated: Atazanavir, nelfinavir. Co-admin caution: Ciclosporin. Co-admin discourage: Clopidogrel. Altered absorption: Drugs dependent on gastric acidity (ketoconazole, itraconazole).

Effect of Naproxen, Esomeprazole Combination on Other Drugs: Tacrolimus: Monitor tacrolimus levels and renal function.

SP: Porphyria, rigorous benefit/risk ratio. Serious skin reactions (naproxen), subacute cutaneous lupus erythematosus (SCLE) (esomeprazole); mixed connective tissue disease (increased aseptic meningitis risk). Treatment of 1 year or more, regular surveillance. Visual change or disturbance, examine. Hepatorenal syndrome. Increased Chromogranin A (CgA) levels may interfere with neuroendocrine tumour investigation; stop treatment at least 5 days before CgA measurements.

ADR: Very common, dyspepsia.

Notes: See 4.4.2 NSAIDS (Non-Selective). See 1.3.2 PPIs (esomeprazole).

Interchangeability: Same strengths of all brands of naproxen/esomeprazole Modified/R tabs are deemed interchangeable (includes parallel imports).

VIMOVO 500mg/20mg (AstraZeneca) B. GMS.
Price, (60) €19.00.
Modified/R tablet, naproxen 500mg, esomeprazole magnesium trihydrate 20mg. Oval yellow; containing g/r naproxen and f/c esomeprazole. Marked 500/20. Parabens. **Store:** Below 30 deg C; original pack.

Piroxicam

ATC Code: M01AC01. **Sport:** Permitted.
Driving: Not relevant

Indications: Topical management of pain, inflammation, associated with osteoarthritis, acute musculoskeletal disorders, localised forms of soft tissue rheumatism.

Dose: Adult: Apply 1g gel of topical gel (approx. 3cm) to affected area 2-4 times daily.

Elderly: See SP below.

Child: Contraindicated.

Renal Impairment: Caution.

Hepatic Impairment: Caution

SP: Do not use occlusive dressings. Elderly more prone to adverse events, use lowest dose. May prolong bleeding time and decrease platelet aggregation. Life-threatening cutaneous reactions, Stevens-Johnson syndrome (SJS), toxic epidermal necrolysis (TEN) reported; signs or symptoms of SJS or TEN, discontinue; do not re-start.

Pregnancy, Lactation: Pregnancy, avoid. Lactation, not recommended.

ADR: Local irritation, rash, possibly photosensitivity; severe cutaneous reactions (SJS, TEN), rare; contact dermatitis, eczema. Mild, transient skin discolouration and staining of clothing when gel is not rubbed in completely.

Notes: See 4.4.2 NSAIDS (Non-Selective).

Feldene Gel (Pfizer) B. GMS.
Price, (60g) €4.75.
Topical gel, piroxicam 5mg/g. Clear pale-yellow. Propylene glycol.

4.4.3 - Non-Steroidal Anti-Inflammatories (NSAids), (Selective)

In This Chapter: Celecoxib, etoricoxib, parecoxib.

Class Effects

CI: Hypersensitivity to any member of the class. Not for use in children under 18 years unless otherwise specified. Asthma, acute rhinitis, nasal polyps, angioedema, urticaria or other allergic reactions after taking acetylsalicylic acid or NSAIDs including COX-2 inhibitors. Active peptic ulceration, GI bleeding. Inflammatory bowel disease. Severe hepatic dysfunction (serum albumin less than 25g/L). Renal dysfunction, CrCl (mL/min) below 30, CHF, ischaemic heart disease and/or cerebrovascular disease. Treatment, of pain after coronary artery bypass graft (CABG) surgery (parecoxib).

Interactions: Effect of COX-2 Inhibitors on Other Drugs: See Notes below.

SP: Decision to prescribe selective COX-2 inhibitors should be based on assessment of individual patient overall risk. NOT a substitute for acetylsalicylic acid (aspirin) for prophylaxis of cardiovascular thrombo-embolic diseases. Caution, risk factors for: GI complications (other NSAID, aspirin, glucocorticoid, SSRI use; alcohol ingestion; elderly, prior history of GI disease; upper GI complications (PUBs); cardiovascular or thromboembolic events (hypertension, hyperlipidaemia, diabetes mellitus, smoking; PAD), initiate with careful consideration. Increased incidence of stroke, MI (long-term use). With compromised renal perfusion, COX-2 inhibitors may reduce prostaglandin formation, reduce renal blood flow, impaired renal function. Fluid retention, oedema (caution, history of cardiac failure, LVD, hypertension, pre-existing oedema; evidence of deterioration, discontinue). Exfoliative dermatitis, Stevens-Johnson syndrome, toxic epidermal necrolysis; some fatal reported with parecoxib/valdecoxib. Anaphylaxis, angioedema. May mask fever or other signs of inflammation.

Pregnancy, Lactation: Contraindicated. Women of childbearing age to ensure adequate contraception. The use of any drug known to inhibit cyclo-oxygenase/prostaglandin synthesis, not recommended in women attempting to conceive.

ADR: Use for shortest duration at lowest effective dose to minimise adverse events, especially in elderly. Cardiovascular risk increases with dose, duration of exposure.

Notes: See 4.4.2 NSAIDS (Non-Selective).

Celecoxib

ATC Code: M01AH01. **Sport:** Permitted.
Driving: Dizziness, vertigo, somnolence.

Indications: Symptomatic relief in osteoarthritis, rheumatoid arthritis, ankylosing spondylitis.

Dose: Adult: Usually 200mg/day in osteoarthritis, in 1-2 divided doses and in rheumatoid arthritis, in 2 divided doses; increase to max. 200mg twice daily if needed.
Ankylosing spondylitis, initially 200mg/day in 1-2 divided doses; if needed increase to max. 400mg/day in 1-2 divided doses. CYP2C9 poor metabolisers, consider dose reduction to half recommended dose. If no benefit in 2 weeks, consider alternatives. Admin, with or without food. Swallowing difficulties, contents of Celebrex, Celecoxib Rowex capsule can be added to applesauce, rice gruel, yoghurt or mashed banana and ingested immediately with 240mL water; applesauce, rice gruel or yoghurt, stable for up to 6 hours refrigerated; mashed banana should be ingested immediately.

Elderly: Over 65 years, as for Adult; caution, under 50kg.

Renal Impairment: Mild/moderate, caution. CrCl (mL/min) below 30, contraindicated.

Hepatic Impairment: Moderate (serum albumin 25-

172

35g/L), half recommended dose. Experience limited to cirrhotic patients. Severe (serum albumin below 25g/L), contraindicated.

CI: Sulfonamide hypersensitivity.

Interactions: Effect of Other Drugs on Celecoxib: *Plasma levels increased (use half recommended dose):* Fluconazole. *Plasma levels decreased:* CYP2C9 inducers (rifampicin, carbamazepine, barbiturates).

Effect of Celecoxib on Other Drugs:

SP: Hypersensitivity; increased risk with sulfonamide allergy. Severe hepatic reactions reported.

ADR: *Very common,* hypertension.

Notes: See 4.4.3 NSAIDs (Selective).

> **Celebrex 100mg, 200mg** *(Pfizer)* B. GMS.
> *Price,* 100mg (60) €14.50; (100) €24.17. 200mg (30) €14.50; (100) €48.34.
> *Capsule,* celecoxib. Hard opaque white. Marked 7767/strength. 100mg: 2 blue bands. 200mg: 2 gold bands. *Lactose.* **Store:** Below 30 deg C.
> **Celecoxib Actavis 100mg, 200mg** *(Accord)* B. GMS.
> *Price,* (60) 100mg, €10.74; (30) 200mg €10.72.
> *Capsule,* celecoxib. Hard opaque white. Marked C90X-strength. 100mg: Two blue bands. 200mg: Yellow band. *Lactose.* **Store:** No special conditions.
> **Celecoxib Krka 100mg, 200mg** *(Krka)* B. GMS.
> *Price,* (60) 100mg, (30) 200mg €10.74.
> *Capsule,* celecoxib. Hard; contain white (almost) granulate. 100mg: White. 200mg: Brownish-yellow. *Lactose.* **Store:** Below 25 deg C.
> **Celecoxib Rowex 100mg, 200mg** *(Rowex)* B. GMS.
> *Price,* (60) 100mg, €10.74; (30) 200mg, €10.72.
> *Capsule,* celecoxib. Hard; contains white (slightly yellowish) pellets. 100mg: White/blue. 200mg: White/orange. *Lactose.* **Store:** No special conditions.

Etoricoxib

ATC Code: M01AH05. **Sport:** Permitted.
Driving: Dizziness, vertigo, somnolence.

Indications: Symptomatic relief in osteoarthritis (OA), rheumatoid arthritis (RA), ankylosing spondylitis (AS); pain and inflammation (acute gouty arthritis). Moderate pain (dental surgery).

Dose: Adult, Elderly: Age 16 years and over, *OA,* 30mg/day; increase to max. 60mg/day if needed; *RA, AS,* 60mg/day; increase to max. 90mg/day if needed; *dental pain,* 90mg/day (max. 3 days); *acute gouty arthritis,* max. 120mg/day (max. 8 days). *Admin,* oral once daily with or without food; onset of action may be faster without food; consider if rapid symptomatic relief required. *Elderly,* caution.

Child: Under 16 years, contraindicated.

Renal Impairment: CrCl (mL/min) below 30, contraindicated.

Hepatic Impairment: Mild, max. 60mg once daily. Moderate, max. 30mg once daily. Severe, contraindicated.

CI: Uncontrolled hypertension (persistently above 140/90mmHg).

Interactions: Effect of Other Drugs on Etoricoxib: Co-admin not recommended (plasma levels decreased): Rifampicin.

Effect of Etoricoxib on Other Drugs: Oral contraceptives (containing ethinyl oestradiol), HRT (conjugated oestrogens): *Plasma levels increased; increased adverse event risk.* Digoxin: *Digoxin toxicity risk, monitor.* Drugs metabolised by human sulfotransferases (oral salbutamol, minoxidil): *Increased plasma levels.*

SP: Associated with more frequent and severe hypertension than other NSAIDs and selective COX-2 inhibitors especially at high doses; monitor BP. Liver dysfunction, abnormal LFTs, monitor. Caution, initiating treatment if dehydrated; rehydrate first.

ADR: *Very common,* abdominal pain.

Notes: See 4.4.3 NSAIDs (Selective).

> **Arcoxia 30mg, 60mg, 90mg, 120mg** *(Grunenthal)* B. GMS.
> *Price,* (28) 30mg, €21.57; 60mg, €26.60; 90mg, €29.13; 120mg, €30.61. 90mg (5) €5.18. 120mg (7) €7.66;
> *Tablet,* etoricoxib. Apple-shaped f/c. 60mg, 90mg, 120mg: Marked ARCOXIA/strength. 30mg: Blue-green. Marked 101; ACX 30 on reverse. 60mg: Dark-green. Marked 200. 90mg: White.

Marked 202. 120mg: Pale-green. Marked 204. *Lactose.* **Store:** Original pack, tightly closed to protect (moisture).

> **Etoricoxib Krka Tablets** *(Krka)* B. GMS.
> *Price,* (28) 30mg, €8.63; 60mg, €10.64; 90mg, €11.65; 120mg, €12.25.
> *Tablet,* etoricoxib 30mg, 60mg, 90mg, 120mg. Round f/c 30mg: White (almost white). 60mg: Brownish-yellow. Marked 60. 90mg: Pink. Marked 90. 120mg: Brownish-red scored (not intended for breaking). **Store:** No special conditions.
> **Etoricoxib (Rowex) Tablets** *(Rowex)* B. GMS.
> *Price,* (28) 30mg, €8.63; 60mg, €10.64; 90mg, €11.65; 120mg, €12.25.
> *Tablet,* etoricoxib 30mg, 60mg, 90mg, 120mg. Round f/c. 30mg: Blue-green. 60mg: Dark-green. 90mg: White. 120mg: Pale-green. *Lactose.* **Store:** No special conditions.
> **Etoricoxib TEVA Tablets** *(TEVA)* B. GMS.
> *Price,* (28) 30mg, €8.63; 60mg, €10.64; 90mg, €11.65; 120mg, €12.25.
> *Tablet,* etoricoxib 30mg, 60mg, 90mg, 120mg. Round f/c. Marked with strength. 30mg: Blue. 60mg: Dark-green. 90mg: White. 120mg: Pale-green. **Store:** Original pack to protect (light).

Parecoxib

ATC Code: M01AH04. **Sport:** Permitted.
Driving: Caution.

Indications: Short-term treatment, post-operative pain.

Dose: Adult: Initially 40mg, then 20-40mg every 6-12 hours; max. 80mg/day. Admin IV (bolus may be given rapidly directly into vein or existing IV line) or IM (slow admin deeply into muscle). See SP below.

Elderly: Under 50kg, initiate with half adult dose; max. 40mg/day. See SP below.

Renal Impairment: Severe or with predisposition to fluid retention, initiate at lowest recommended dose.

Hepatic Impairment: Moderate, introduce with caution at half adult dose; max. 40mg/day. Severe, contraindicated.

CI: Sulfonamide hypersensitivity.

Interactions: Effect of Other Drugs on Parecoxib (active metabolite valdecoxib): *Plasma levels increased (reduce dose):* Fluconazole.

Effect of Parecoxib (active metabolite valdecoxib) on Other Drugs: CYP2D6 substrates (dextromethorphan) with narrow therapeutic margin (flecainide, propafenone, metoprolol): *Plasma levels increased.* CYP2C19 substrates (phenytoin, diazepam, imipramine): *Caution.*

SP: Limited data for use longer than 3 days. Can be used with opioid analgesics. Caution, initiation of treatment in dehydration; rehydrate first.

Pregnancy, Lactation: Trimesters (1, 2), use if benefit outweighs risk. Trimester (3), contraindicated (suspected to cause serious birth defects). May cause premature closure of ductus arteriosus or uterine inertia. Use trimesters (2, 3) may cause foetal renal dysfunction; may result in reduction of amniotic fluid volume or oligohydramnios in severe cases. Lactation, not for use. Use during labour, no data.

ADR: Summary, *most common,* nausea; *most serious (uncommonly to rarely),* cardiovascular events e.g. MI, severe hypotension; hypersensitivity events e.g. anaphylaxis, angioedema, severe skin reactions.

Notes: See 4.4.3 NSAIDs (Selective).

> **Dynastat Parenteral 40mg** *(Pfizer)* A. HOS.
> *Price,* (10) €68.30 (PTW).
> *Injection,* parecoxib sodium 20mg/mL. White (off-white) powder for soln. Clear colourless solvent. *Reconstituted with NaCl 0.9% soln, 20mg (40mg) vial contains 0.22 mmoL (0.44) sodium.* **Store:** No special conditions.

4.4.4 - Osteoarthritis, Soft Tissue Disorders

In This Chapter: *Glucosamine, hyaluronic acid.*

Class Effects

CI: Hypersensitivity to any member of the class. Use in children not recommended.

Glucosamine

ATC Code: M01AX05. **Sport:** Permitted.
Driving: Headache, somnolence, visual disturbances.
Indications: Symptomatic relief of mild to moderate osteoarthritis of knee as diagnosed by a doctor.
Dose: Adult, Elderly: Either 400mg or 500mg 3-times daily OR 1x or 2x 750mg tabs twice daily OR 1x 1500mg sachet once daily; max. 1200-1500mg/day. Swallow caps/tabs whole with water; dissolve contents of sachet in water; take with food.
Renal Impairment: Caution, under medical supervision.
Hepatic Impairment: As for Renal above.
CI: Shellfish allergy (glucosamine derived from shellfish), phenylketonurics.
Interactions: Effect of Glucosamine on Other Drugs: Coumarin anticoagulants (warfarin): *Effect enhanced (monitor coagulation parameters).* Tetracyclines: *Absorption enhanced.* Hypoglycaemics: *Caution.*
SP: Diabetics, impaired glucose tolerance, monitor blood sugar periodically; consider hypoglycaemic dose adjustment (including insulin). Cholesterol, monitor. Caution, asthmatics. If symptoms deteriorate after use, seek medical advice.
Pregnancy, Lactation: Not for use during pregnancy. Lactation, not recommended.
ADR: Summary, *most common,* nausea, abdominal pain, dyspepsia, flatulence, constipation, diarrhoea. Potential severe allergic reactions.
Notes: See 4.4.4. Osteoarthritis, Soft Tissue Disorders.

Dona 500mg, Sachets 1500mg *(Meda)* OTC.
Price, 500mg (90) sachets (30) €5.95
Sachet, glucosamine sulfate sodium chloride. White crystalline odourless powder for oral soln. *Aspartame, sodium* 384mg/sachet, sorbitol.
Capsule, as above. Hard gelatin snap-fit red/red. Marked ROTTA. *128mg sodium/cap.*
Arthrimel 750mg *(Phoenix)* OTC.
Price, (60) €11.33 (PTW).
Tablet, glucosamine sulfate sodium chloride equiv. to 750mg glucosamine sulfate. Oblong off-white f/c. *Lactose, sodium 75.9mg/tab.*
Glucosamine P/Nord 400mg *(Pharma Nord)* B.
Price, (90) €12.23.
Capsule, glucosamine hemisulfate 506mg equiv. to 400mg glucosamine. White hard gelatin. *Potassium 87mg/cap.*

Hyaluronic Acid (musculoskeletal)

ATC Code: M09AX01. **Sport:** Permitted.
Driving: Unlikely to impair.
Indications: Sustained pain relief in osteoarthritis of knee.
Dose: Adult, Elderly: Contents of 1 prefilled syringe (20mg/2mL) injected into the affected joint once weekly; total 5 injections; can be repeated at 6-monthly intervals. For intra-articular injection only.
CI: Avian protein hypersensitivity; injection site infection.
Interactions: Effect of Other Drugs on Hyaluronic Acid: *Not recommended:* Simultaneous admin or mixture with other intra-articular injection. *Co-admin not recommended (precipitation risk):* Quaternary ammonium salts.
SP: Remove joint effusion prior to injection. Inflammation, evaluate treatment initiation; following injection, do not overburden joint.
Pregnancy, Lactation: If benefit outweighs risk. Woman of child bearing potential to seek medical advice regarding continued use if intending pregnancy or pregnancy suspected.
ADR: Pain, swelling, heat redness at injection site, allergic reactions.
Notes: See 4.4.4. Osteoarthritis, Soft Tissue Disorders.

Hyalgan Parenteral 20mg/2mL *(Fidia)* A. GMS.
Price, (1) €41.06.
Intra-articular injection, hyaluronic acid sodium. Sterile soln.

4.4.5 - Gout, Cytotoxic Hyperuricaemia

In This Chapter: *Allopurinol, febuxostat, rasburicase.*

Class Effects

NSAIDs are used in acute gout attacks; aspirin is not indicated. Uricosurics are not for treatment of acute gout; correct hyperuricaemia with long-term treatment. Allopurinol and febuxostat, reduce uric acid formation from purines. Colchicine, used for acute gout is not licensed in Ireland.
CI: Hypersensitivity to any member of the class.
SP: Allopurinol, febuxostat used in *acute gouty attacks,* initiate after acute attack has completely subsided (may precipitate further attacks); advisable to admin anti-inflammatory or colchicine prophylactically for at least 1 month; acute attacks (flares) where allopurinol or febuxostat is being admin, continue treatment at same dosage and treat acute attack concurrently.
Notes: See 4.4.2 NSAIDS (Non-Selective) and 4.4.3 NSAIDs (Selective).

Allopurinol

ATC Code: M04AA01. **Sport:** Permitted.
Driving: Somnolence, vertigo, ataxia.
Indications: Reduction of urate/uric acid formation in conditions where deposition has already occurred (gouty arthritis, skin tophi, nephrolithiasis) or is a clinical risk (treatment of malignancy potentially leading to acute uric acid nephropathy); urate/uric acid deposition may occur are with idiopathic gout, uric acid lithiasis, acute uric acid nephropathy, neoplastic and myeloproliferative disease with high cell turnover rates (spontaneous or after cytotoxic therapy), certain enzyme disorders. Management of 2,8-dihydroxyadenine (2,8-DHA) renal stones. Management of recurrent mixed calcium oxalate renal stones in the presence of hyperuricosuria.
Dose: Adult: Initially 100mg/day. If serum urate response unsatisfactory increase (mild conditions) to 100-200mg/day; (moderately severe) to 300-600mg/day; (severe) to 700-900mg/day. Above 300mg/day, admin in divided doses; max. 300mg for any 1 dose. *Admin,* oral, with or after food.
Elderly: Use lowest possible dose; consider renal function.
Child: Under 15 years, 10-20mg/kg/day; max. 400mg/day admin in 3 divided doses.
Renal Impairment: CrCl (mL/min) 10-20, 100-200mg/day; below 10, 100mg/day or longer dose intervals (every 2 or 3 days); severe insufficiency, advisable to use less than 100mg/day or single doses of 100mg at longer intervals. maintain plasma oxipurinol levels below 100mcg/L (15.2mg/L). Removed by dialysis; with 2-3 times weekly dialysis consider 300-400mg after each dialysis with none in-between.
Hepatic Impairment: Reduce dose, monitor.
Interactions: Effect of Other Drugs on Allopurinol: *Co-admin not recommended:* Didanosine (consider didanosine dose reduction). *Accelerated excretion, reduced efficacy:* Probenecid, salicylates (large doses). *Increased skin rash incidence:* Ampicillin, amoxicillin (use alternative), captopril (especially with CRF). *Increased hypersensitivity risk:* Diuretics (thiazides), ACEIs. *Increased serum urate:* Furosemide.
Effect of Allopurinol on Other Drugs: 6-Mercaptopurine, azathioprine: *Activity prolonged; admin one-quarter of usual dose.* Vidarabine (adenine arabinoside): *Plasma half-life increased.* Chlorpropamide: *Prolonged hypoglycaemic activity (especially with renal impairment).* Coumarin anticoagulants, warfarin, theophylline: *Monitor levels.* Ciclosporin: *Possible enhanced toxicity.*
SP: Allopurinol treatment should not be started until an acute gout attack has completely subsided. Xanthine deposition, ensure adequate hydration. Impaction of uric acid renal stones, adequate allopurinol therapy will dissolve large uric acid renal pelvic stones; remote possibility of impaction in ureter. Treatment of high urate turnover conditions e.g. neoplasia, Lesch-Nyhan syndrome, it is advisable to correct existing hyperuricaemia and/or hyperuricosuria with allopurinol before starting cytotoxic therapy. NOTE: Hypersensitivity reactions including maculopapular exanthema, hypersensitivity syndrome (DRESS), Stevens-Johnson Syndrome (SJS), toxic epidermal necrolysis (TEN); if occur, withdraw immediately, with DRESS, SJS or TEN do not rechallenge. Increased

hypersensitivity risk with chronic renal impairment. HLA-B*5801 allele presence associated with hypersensitivity risk. Increased TSH values observed (long-term treatment).

Pregnancy, Lactation: Pregnancy, use only when no safer alternative and disease carries risk for mother/unborn child. Lactation, excreted in breast milk but no data concerning effects on breast-fed baby; stop drug or stop breastfeeding.

ADR: *Common*, rash; *uncommon*, hypersensitivity reactions, nausea, vomiting, diarrhoea, asymptomatic increased LFTs.

Notes: See 4.4.5. Gout, Cytotoxic Hyperuricaemia.

Zyloric 100mg, 300mg *(Aspen)* B. GMS.
Price, 100mg (100) €5.23. 300mg (28) €4.06.
Tablet, allopurinol. White (off-white) round scored. 100mg: Marked Z1. 300mg: Marked Z3. **Store:** Below 25 deg C; original pack.

Allopurinol (Actavis) 100mg, 300mg *(Accord)* B. GMS.
Price, (28) 100mg, €1.43. 300mg, €2.69.
Tablet, allopurinol. allopurinol. White round u/c. Marked C. 100mg: Marked AD on either side of score. 300mg: Marked AG either side of score. *Lactose.*

Allopurinol TEVA 100mg, 300mg *(TEVA)* B. GMS.
Price, (100) 100mg, €4.91. 300mg, €11.45.
Tablet, allopurinol. White round. 100mg: Marked 4K1. 300mg: Marked 2K1. *Lactose.*

Alopur 100mg, 300mg *(Rowex)* B. GMS.
Price, (100) 100mg, €5.12. 300mg, €14.21.
Tablet, Scored (divisible into equal doses). 100mg: White round. 300mg: White (off-white) oblong.

Purinol 100mg, 300mg *(Pinewood)* B. GMS.
Price, (100) 100mg, €5.12. 300mg, €14.21.
Tablet, allopurinol. White. Marked AP/strength; R on reverse.

Tipuric 100mg, 300mg *(Clonmel)* B. GMS.
Price, (100) 100mg, €5.12. 300mg, €14.21.
Tablet, allopurinol. White. Marked with logo. 100mg: Marked 230. 300mg: Marked 242.

Febuxostat

ATC Code: M04AA03. **Sport:** Permitted.
Driving: Somnolence, dizziness, paraesthesia, blurred vision.
Indications: Treatment, chronic hyperuricaemia (urate deposition has already occurred). Prevention and treatment, hyperuricaemia in adults undergoing chemotherapy for haematologic malignancies at intermediate to high risk of Tumour Lysis Syndrome (TLS).
Dose: Adult, Elderly: *Gout,* 80mg/day; consider 120mg/day if serum uric acid above 6mg/dL after 2-4 weeks. Flare prophylaxis recommended for 6 months.
TLS, 120mg/day starting 2 days before cytotoxic therapy; continue for minimum 7 days; may be prolonged up to 9 days depending on chemotherapy duration. *Admin,* once daily with or without food.
Child: Under 18 years, not recommended.
Renal Impairment: CrCl (mL/min) below 30, safety/efficacy not evaluated.
Hepatic Impairment: *Gout,* mild impairment 80mg/day; moderate, limited data; severe, efficacy/safety not evaluated. *TLS,* no adjustment; severe, no data.
Interactions: Effect of Other Drugs on Febuxostat: *Co-admin not recommended*: Mercaptopurine, azathioprine (consider dose reduction). *Theoretical increased exposure*: Glucuronidation inhibitors (UGT enzyme inhibitors) (NSAIDs, probenecid). *Decreased exposure*: UGT inducers
Effect of Febuxostat on Other Drugs: Theophylline *Febuxostat 80mg can be co-admin with theophylline without risk of increasing theophylline plasma levels; 120mg, no data.* Warfarin: *INR and Factor VII activity not affected (febuxostat 80mg or 120mg).*
SP: Ischaemic heart disease, CHF, patients where urate formation greatly increased (malignant disease, Lesch-Nyhan syndrome), organ transplant recipients, use not recommended. Patients at risk of TLS to under cardiac monitoring. Monitor LFTs prior to initiation, then periodically based on clinical judgement. Altered thyroid function. Serious hypersensitivity reactions, see Notes below (allopurinol).
Pregnancy, Lactation: Should not be used.
ADR: Summary, *most common*, gout flares, headache, diarrhoea, nausea, rash, abnormal LFTs, oedema; *serious*, hypersensitivity.

Notes: See 4.4.5 Gout, Cytotoxic Hyperuricaemia. See Allopurinol above.

Adenuric 80mg, 120mg *(A.Menarini)* B. GMS.
Price, (28) 80mg, €27.29. 120mg, €27.85.
Tablet, febuxostat. Pale-yellow (yellow) cap-shaped f/c. Marked with strength. *Lactose.*

Rasburicase

ATC Code: V03AF07. **Sport:** Permitted.
Driving: Not applicable.
Indications: Treatment and prophylaxis, acute hyperuricaemia to prevent acute renal failure with chemotherapy initiation for haematological malignancy.
Dose: Adult, Elderly: Initially 0.2mg/kg/day once daily as 30-minute IV infusion in 50mL 0.9% NaCl soln immediately prior to and during chemotherapy initiation for up to 7 days.
Child: As for Adult above.
CI: Cellular metabolic disorders causing haemolytic anaemia (G-6-PD deficiency).
Interactions: Effect of Other Drugs on Rasburicase: *Co-admin (no data)*: Allopurinol.
SP: Allergic-like reactions, severe hypersensitivity (anaphylaxis); caution, atopic allergies (history). Methaemoglobinaemia, haemolysis, discontinue. Specialist supervision.
Pregnancy, Lactation: Pregnancy, and lactation, not recommended; not known if excreted in human milk.
ADR: Summary, *most common*, nausea, vomiting, headache, fever, diarrhoea; *common*, allergic reactions (rash, urticaria).
Notes: See 4.4.5. Gout, Cytotoxic Hyperuricaemia.

Fasturtec Parenteral *(SANOFI)* A.
Price, (3) 1.5mg/mL, €194.40.
Infusion, rasburicase 1.5mg/mL. Powder/solvent for conc for soln.

4.5 - Neuropathic Pain

In This Chapter: *Duloxetine, gabapentin, lidocaine, pregabalin.*

Class Effects
Duloxetine, gabapentin and pregabalin are also used to treat neuropathic pain and are discussed under indications outlined in Notes below.
CI: Hypersensitivity to any member of class.
Notes: See 3.3.3 SSRIs, SNRIs (antidepressants; duloxetine) and 3.1.3 GABAergic Drugs (epilepsy; gabapentin, pregabalin).

Lidocaine (neuropathic pain)

ATC Code: N01BB02. **Sport:** Permitted.
Driving: Unlikely to affect.
Indications: Symptomatic relief, neuropathic pain associated with post-herpetic neuralgia (PHN).
Dose: Adult, Elderly: Cover painful area with plaster once daily for up to 12 hours (max.) within 24-hour period i.e. 12-hour plaster-free interval; max. 3 plasters for use at same time. Apply to intact dry non-irritated skin after shingles healing. Evaluate after 2-4 weeks; no response, discontinue and weigh benefit/risk.
Child: Under 18 years, no data.
Renal Impairment: Severe, caution.
Hepatic Impairment: As for Renal above.
Interactions: Effect of Other Drugs on Lidocaine (topical): *Co-admin caution (additive systemic effects)*: Class I antiarrhythmics (tocainide, mexiletine), other local anaesthetics.
SP: Not for use on inflamed or broken skin, mucous membranes. Avoid contact with eyes. Severe cardiac impairment, caution.
Pregnancy, Lactation: Pregnancy, only if clearly necessary. Lactation, only very low levels expected in breast milk.
ADR: *Very common*, mild skin reactions.
Notes: See 14.2 Local anaesthetics (lidocaine).

Versatis 5% Medicated Plaster *(Grunenthal)* A. GMS.
Price, (30) €93.96.
Medicated plaster, lidocaine 5% w/w (700mg). White hydrogel containing adhesive material. *Parabens, propylene glycol.*

175

5

Respiratory, Allergic Disorders

5.1 - Asthma, COPD

Class Effects
Bronchodilators include sympathomimetic beta agonists (adrenoreceptor agonists), antimuscarinics (anticholinergics), xanthines and corticosteroids.

CI: Hypersensitivity to any member of the class.

SP: In severe or unstable asthma bronchodilators should be used as 'add on' therapy. Regular medical assessment required; death may occur in severe asthma (constant symptoms, frequent exacerbations, limited physical capacity; PEF values below 60% predicted at baseline with above 30% variability, usually not returning entirely to normal after a bronchodilator; requirement for high dose inhaled or oral corticosteroid therapy). Sudden worsening of symptoms may require increased corticosteroids; urgent medical supervision. *Always* instruct patient on correct inhaler usage. *Paradoxical bronchospasm* can occur with inhaled medicines; may be life-threatening; if occurs, discontinue treatment immediately; substitute with alternative.

Combinations, generally not indicated first-line. If dosing other than available in the fixed-combination inhaler is required, use doses of the individual inhalers. Use lowest effective dose at which asthma control is maintained. Long-acting bronchodilators are not for use in treating acute asthma or acute COPD exacerbation.

5.1.1 - Adrenoreceptor (Beta-2) Agonist Bronchodilators

In This Chapter: *Formoterol, indacaterol, olodaterol, salbutamol, salmeterol, terbutaline.*

Class Effects
Driving: Generally these drugs have no influence on ability to drive; at higher doses, treatment initiation, or with ALCOHOL, ability may be affected. Dizziness, transient muscle cramps, tremor, caution.

Sport: All beta-2 agonists are prohibited except inhaled salbutamol (max. 1600mcg over 24-hours; max. 800mcg every 12 hours), inhaled formoterol (max. 54mcg over 24-hours), inhaled salmeterol (max. 200mcg over 24-hours). Higher doses or other beta-2 agonists, the TUE Policy applies.

Pharmacology: Long-acting selective beta-2-agonists (formoterol, indacaterol, olodaterol, salmeterol, vilanterol); intermediate (terbutaline); short-acting (salbutamol). They may be used in combination with muscarinic anticholinergics (e.g. glycopyrronium, ipratropium, umeclidinium), see Notes below.

Indications: Not for use in children unless otherwise stated; no relevant use for treatment of COPD in children.

Interactions: Effect of Other Drugs on Beta-2 Agonists: *Co-admin not recommended*: Effect mutually antagonised by beta-blockers (including eye drops) especially non-selective (propranolol); other anticholinergics. *Co-admin avoid*: Other selective and non-selective beta-2 agonists, halothane anaesthetics, other halogenated anaesthetics (caution). *Hypokalaemia (increased cardiac arrhythmia risk; digoxin toxicity risk)*: Xanthine derivatives, corticosteroids, diuretics, digoxin. *Hyperglycaemia*: Corticosteroids, antidiabetic therapy (may need dose adjustment).

SP: Sudden and progressive asthma deterioration can be potentially life-threatening; consider increasing steroid therapy. COPD, re-evaluate regimen. Long-acting beta-2-agonists, not indicated for acute bronchospasm (rescue); usually used as 'add-on' therapy to maintenance with inhaled corticosteroids. If prophylaxis for exercise-induced bronchoconstriction is required several times every week despite adequate maintenance (corticosteroids, long-acting beta-2-agonists), reassess management.

Beta-2-agonist treatment, should be adjunctive to regular inhaled or oral corticosteroids, and/or sodium cromoglicate. Increasing use may be sign of worsening asthma, reassess therapy. Myocardial ischaemia rarely associated with beta-agonists; underlying severe heart disease, advise patient to seek medical advice (chest pain, worsening heart disease). Not for use in hypertrophic cardiomyopathy (positive inotropic effect). Dyspnoea, chest pain, investigate, respiratory or cardiac origin. Tocolysis, caution; cardiorespiratory function, ECG monitoring. May increase pulse rate, BP, ECG changes. *Hyperglycaemia*, ketoacidosis found in diabetic pregnant women after beta-2-stimulants; consider insulin dose adjustment. Monitor, blood glucose (hyperglycaemic effect), serum potassium (blood glucose). Thyrotoxicosis, caution. Lactic acidosis reported with high dose of parenteral and nebulised short-acting beta-agonist therapy, mainly treatment of acute asthma exacerbation. Potentially serious hypokalaemia may result with high dose beta-2 adrenoreceptor agonists.

Pregnancy, Lactation: Pregnancy, if benefit outweighs risk; avoid if possible. May inhibit labour (relaxant effect on uterine smooth muscle). Lactation, caution; passes into breast milk in small amounts; stop breast feeding or stop drug.

ADR: Hypo-, hyperkalaemia, hyperglycaemia, headache, tremor, nervousness, palpitations, tachycardia, myocardial ischaemia, oropharyngeal irritation with inhalation, muscle cramp, myalgia, nausea, vomiting, hypersensitivity reactions, angioedema, urticaria, pruritus, exanthema.

Notes: See Class Effects 5.1 Asthma, COPD. For combinations, see 5.1.3 Adrenoreceptor (Beta-2) Agonist, Antimuscarinic Combinations.

Formoterol

ATC Code: R03AC13. **Sport:** Restricted. See Notes below.
Driving: No or negligible effect.
Indications: Prophylaxis, treatment of bronchoconstriction, as 'add-on' therapy in asthma induced by allergens, cold air, exercise, reversible or irreversible COPD.

Dose: Adult, Elderly: *Foradil,* asthma, COPD, maintenance, 12-24mcg twice daily, morning, evening; max. 48mcg/day. Prophylaxis, exercise or allergen induced, 12mcg inhaled 15 minutes prior to exercise or exposure; severe bronchospasm, 24mcg.

Oxis Turbohaler, asthma, acute symptom relief, 6-12mcg. Regular use, 6-12mcg twice daily; up to 36mcg once or twice daily, max. 72mcg inhalations in 24 hours; max. 36mcg on any single occasion. Prophylaxis, exercise induced, 12mcg before exercise. COPD, regular use, 12mcg once or twice daily; max. 24mcg; symptom relief, max. 48mcg; max. 24mcg on any single occasion.

Admin, by inhalation; capsules are not to be swallowed.

Child: *Foradil,* age 6-12 years, asthma, 12mcg twice daily, morning and evening; max. 24mcg/day (not for acute use); prophylaxis, as for Adult; max. 12mcg.

Oxis Turbohaler, age 6 years and over, asthma, acute

symptom relief, 6-12mcg; regular use, 12mcg twice daily; max. 48mcg in 24 hours; max. 12mcg on any single occasion. Prophylaxis, exercise induced, 6-12mcg before exercise. Admin see Adult above.

Hepatic Impairment: Severe liver cirrhosis, increased exposure may be expected.

Interactions: Effect of Other Drugs on Formoterol: *Increased ventricular arrhythmia risk*: Drugs prolonging QT-interval, quinidine, disopyramide, procainamide, phenothiazines, antihistamines, MAOIs, macrolides, TCAds. *Adverse events potentiated*: Other sympathomimetics (beta-2-agonists, ephedrine). *Increased arrhythmia risk*: Anaesthesia (halogenated hydrocarbons). *Bronchodilatory effect enhanced*: Anticholinergics. *Hypokalaemic effects potentiated*: Xanthine derivatives, steroids, diuretics (hypokalaemia may increase cardiac arrhythmia susceptibility with digitalis). *Effect antagonised/weakened*: Beta-adrenergic blockers (including eye drops); co-admin only if compelling reasons.

SP: Caution, ischaemic heart disease, cardiac arrhythmias (especially third-degree AV block), severe cardiac decompensation, idiopathic subvalvular aortic stenosis, hypertrophic obstructive cardiomyopathy, QT-prolongation, thyrotoxicosis, phaeochromocytoma, severe hypertension, aneurysm, tachyarrhythmia, severe heart failure. Do not exceed max. daily dose.

ADR: *Common*, headache, tremor, palpitations; serious asthma exacerbations (children age 5-12 years) *(Foradil)*.

Notes: See 5.1.1 Adrenoreceptor Agonist Bronchodilators.

Foradil Aerolizer 12mcg *(Novartis)* B. GMS.
Price, inhaler (60 caps) €22.42.
Inhalation powder (capsule), formoterol fumarate dihydrate. Colourless transparent contains powder. Marked CG, FXF. *Lactose*.

Oxis Turbohaler 6mcg, 12mcg *(AstraZeneca)* B. GMS.
Price, (60-dose) 6mcg, €16.55. 12mcg, €20.11.
Inhalation powder (capsule), formoterol fumarate dihydrate. Metered dose; white inhalation powder. *Lactose*.

Indacaterol

ATC Code: R03AC18. **Sport:** Prohibited.
Driving: No or negligible effect.

Indications: Maintenance bronchodilator treatment (adults) with COPD.

Dose: Adult, Elderly: 150mg inhaled once daily; max. 300mg once daily (provides addition benefit with breathlessness, especially in severe COPD). Remove caps from blister immediately before use; do not swallow; admin by inhalation using Onbrez Breezhaler.

Hepatic Impairment: Severe, no data.

SP: Not for use in asthma.

ADR: Summary, *most common*, nasopharyngitis, upper RTI, cough, headache, muscle spasm.

Notes: See 5.1.1 Adrenoreceptor Agonist Bronchodilators.

Onbrez Breezhaler 150mcg, 300mcg *(Novartis)* B. GMS.
Price, (30) 150mcg, €31.53. 300mcg, €34.15.
Inhalation powder (capsule), indacaterol maleate. Transparent uncoloured capsule; contains white powder. Marked IDL/strength and logo. *Lactose*.

Olodaterol

ATC Code: R03AC19. **Sport:** Prohibited.
Driving: Dizziness.

Indications: Maintenance bronchodilator treatment (adults) with COPD.

Dose: Adult, Elderly: 5mcg given as 2 puffs once daily at same time of day.

Renal Impairment: Severe, limited data.

Hepatic Impairment: Severe, no data.

Interactions: Effect of Other Drugs on Olodaterol: *May potentiate action on cardiovascular system*: MAOIs, TCADs, other drugs prolonging QTc interval.

SP: Not for use in asthma.

ADR: *Uncommon*, nasopharyngitis, dizziness, rash.

Notes: See 5.1.1 Adrenoreceptor Agonist Bronchodilators.

▼ **Striverdi Respimat** *(Boehringer)* B. GMS.
Price, (60-dose), €28.49.
Inhalation soln, olodaterol HCl 2.5mcg/puff. Clear colourless.

Salbutamol

ATC Code: R03AC02. **Sport:** Restricted. See Notes below.
Driving: No or negligible effect.

Indications: *Inhalation, oral*, treatment and prevention of bronchospasm; provides short-acting bronchodilation in reversible airway obstruction due to asthma, COPD (chronic bronchitis, emphysema). In asthmatics, may be used to relieve symptoms when they occur and prevent them prior to known trigger. *Parenteral*, severe bronchospasm (asthma, bronchitis, status asthmaticus). Short-term management, uncomplicated premature labour. To arrest between 22 and 37 weeks gestation if no contraindication to tocolytic therapy.

Dose: Adult: ORAL, 4-8mg 3-4 times daily (10-20mL oral soln).

INHALATION, *soln or powder*, 100-200mcg as needed in bronchospasm or before exercise or allergen exposure. Chronic treatment, 200mcg up to 4-times daily; max. 800mcg in 24 hours.

WET INHALATION, *nebules*, initially 2.5mg; increase to 5mg up to 4-times daily if needed; max. 40mg/day under strict medical supervision in hospital for severe airways obstruction.

PARENTERAL (age 12 years and over), *bronchospasm, status asthmaticus*, initially 5mcg per minute (3-20mcg/min generally adequate).

Premature labour (or to control contractions or counteract overdosage of oxytocics), initially 10mcg/min (10-45mcg/min generally adequate). Once uterine contractions have ceased, maintain infusion at same level for 1 hour then reduce by 50% decrements 6-hourly.

Elderly: ORAL, initially 2mg three or four times daily.

Child: ORAL (age 2-6 years), 1-2mg (2.5-5mL soln) 3 or 4-times daily; age 6-12 years, 2mg (5mL soln) 3 or 4-times daily; over 12 years, 2-4mg (5-10mL soln) 3 or 4-times daily.

INHALATION, *inhalation soln or powder* (4-11 years) acute use, 100mcg inhalation as single minimum starting dose, increasing to 200mcg if needed as a single dose; chronic use (under 12 years), using spacer device, initially 100mcg, if needed increasing to 200mcg 4-times daily; max 800mcg in 24-hours.

WET INHALATION, *nebules* (age 4-11 years), initially 2.5mg; may be increased to 5mg repeated 4-times daily; other pharmaceutical forms may be preferable for children under 4 years; under 18 months, efficacy uncertain.

PARENTERAL, under 12 years, no dose recommendation.

CI: Non-IV salbutamol formulations must not be used to arrest uncomplicated premature labour or threatened abortion.

Interactions: Effect of Other Drugs on Salbutamol: *Co-admin not recommended*: Non-selective beta-blockers (propranolol). *Co-admin caution*: Guanethidine, reserpine, methyldopa, TCADs, anaesthetics (chloroform, cyclopropane, halothane, other halogenated agents).

Effect of Salbutamol on Other Drugs: *Oxytocics*: *Effect inhibited (IV salbutamol)*.

SP: Should not be only or main treatment in severe or unstable asthma. Failure to respond quickly or fully rescue or previously effective inhaled dose fails to give relief for at least 3 hours, seek medical advice. Prostatic enlargement, caution micturition difficulties. Inhalers, therapeutic effect may be decreased when canister is cold. Nebulisers, caution not to let fluid or mist enter eyes. *Use during labour*, maternal BP may fall during infusion, effect greater on diastolic BP. Foetal heart rate, increased by up to 20 bpm. Assess maternal cardiovascular status with known heart disease.

Pregnancy, Lactation: Maternal pulmonary oedema, myocardial ischaemia reported during or following treatment of premature labour with beta-2-agonists; monitor (fluid balance, cardio-respiratory function including ECG). Signs of pulmonary oedema, myocardial ischaemia, discontinue. Congenital abnormalities following

5.1.2 Antimuscarinic Bronchodilators

intrauterine exposure (cleft palate, limb defects, cardiac disorders) (rare); some mothers were taking multiple medications.

ADR: *Common*, tremor, headache, tachycardia, nausea, sweating, restlessness, dizziness; taste alteration, mouth/throat irritation (inhaled); electrolyte disturbances, tachycardia, palpitations, decreased diastolic pressure, hypotension (parenteral).

Notes: See 5.1.1 Adrenoreceptor Agonist Bronchodilators.

Ventolin Diskus, Evohaler, Nebules *(GSK)* B. GMS.
Price, Diskus 200mcg (60) €4.48. Evohaler 100mcg (200) €3.20. Nebules (20) 2.5mg, €1.40. 5mg, €2.67.
Inhaler, salbutamol sulfate. *Diskus 200mcg*: White inhalation powder. *Lactose*. Evohaler: CFC-free metered dose aerosol.
Nebuliser soln (nebules), as above 2.5mg (5mg)/2.5mL. Clear colourless (pale-yellow) sterile isotonic aqueous.

Ventolin Oral Soln *(GSK)* B. GMS.
Price, (150mL) €0.92.
Oral soln, salbutamol sulfate 2mg/5mL. Clear colourless (pale straw-coloured). *Benzoate, sodium 5.61mg/5mL.*

Ventolin Parenteral 500mcg *(GSK)* A. GMS.
Price, 0.5mg/mL: 1mL injection (5) €2.66; 5mL infusion (10) €38.62.
Injection, salbutamol sulfate (0.5mg/mL) or infusion (1mg/mL). Clear colourless (pale straw-coloured) sterile aqueous soln. **Store:** Below 30 deg C; outer carton to protect (light).

Novolizer Salbutamol *(Meda)* B. GMS.
Price, 100mcg (200-dose) €8.90. Refill €6.44.
Inhalation powder, salbutamol sulfate 100mcg.

Salamol CFC-Free, Easi-Breathe *(TEVA)* B. GMS.
Price, 100mcg (200-dose) CFC-Free, €2.96. Easi-Breathe, €7.95.
Inhaler (pressurised) CFC-free, salbutamol 100mcg. Metered. *Ethanol.*

Salbul Pressurised Inhalation *(Rowex)* B. GMS.
Price, 100mcg (200-dose) €3.01.
Pressurised inhalation susp, salbutamol sulphate 100mcg/dose. White susp.

Salbutamol CFC-Free Inhaler *(Fannin)* B. GMS.
Price, 100mcg (200-dose) €3.00.
Pressurised inhalation susp, salbutamol sulphate.

Steri-Neb Salamol *(TEVA)* B. GMS.
Price, (20) 2.5mg, €1.77. 5mg, €6.38.
Inhalation soln, salbutamol sulfate 2.5mg (5mg)/5mL.

Salmeterol

ATC Code: R03AC12. **Sport:** Restricted. See Notes below.
Driving: No studies performed.

Indications: Regular bronchodilator in reversible airways obstruction due to asthma, chronic bronchitis, emphysema, COPD; prevention of night-time symptoms and/or day-time fluctuations before exercise, unavoidable allergen challenge. Prevention of exercise-induced asthma. Not indicated for acute symptoms due to slower onset of action.

Dose: Adult, Elderly: Asthma, COPD, chronic bronchitis, 2x 25mcg inhalations (blister) twice daily; severe obstruction, up to max. 4 inhalations (100mcg) twice daily.

Child: *Serevent*, asthma, age 4 years and older, 2x 25mcg inhalations twice daily. *Salmeterol Neolab*, under 12 years, not recommended.

Interactions: Effect of Other Drugs on Salmeterol: *Increased systemic exposure (may cause QTc-interval prolongation, palpitations)*, avoid co-admin: Ketoconazole.

SP: Not for first-line asthma treatment or treatment of acute symptoms. Do not initiate during acute severe exacerbations or worsening or deteriorating asthma. Caution, patients with thyrotoxicosis.

ADR: *Common*, headache, tremor, palpitations, muscle cramp.

Notes: See 5.1.1 Adrenoreceptor Agonist Bronchodilators.

Serevent Evohaler 25mcg, Diskus *(GSK)* B. GMS.
Price, Evohaler 25mcg (120-dose) €27.85. Diskus 50mcg (60) €24.80.
Inhalation, salmeterol xinafoate. *Evohaler 25mcg*: Pressurised inhalation susp. *Diskus 50mcg*: Inhalation powder. *Lactose*.

Salmeterol Neolab 25mcg *(Fannin)* B. GMS.
Price, 25mcg (120-dose) €26.37.
Pressurised inhalation, salmeterol xinafoate 25mcg/metered-dose. White susp.

Terbutaline

ATC Code: R03AC03. **Sport:** Prohibited.
Driving: None stated.

Indications: Relief and prevention bronchospasm in bronchial asthma, other bronchopulmonary disorders *(inhalation, parenteral)*. Short-term management of uncomplicated premature labour; to arrest labour between 22 and 37 weeks gestation in patients with no medical or obstetric contraindication to tocolytic therapy *(parenteral)*.

Dose: Adult, Elderly: INHALATION, 1 inhalation (0.5mg) as needed; max. 4 in 24 hours; rinse mouth after use. PARENTERAL, *bronchodilation*, SC or IM injection or slow IV bolus, 0.25-0.5mg up to 4-times daily; continuous infusion, 1.5-2.5mg at rate 10-20 drops (0.5-1mL)/min for 8-10 hours.
Uncomplicated premature labour, initially 5mcg/min for first 20 minutes; increase by 2.5mcg/min at 20 minute intervals until contractions stop; usually 10mcg/min; max. 20mcg/min; if successful, continue infusion for 1 hour, then decrease by 2.5mcg/min every 20 minutes to lowest dose suppressing contractions. Avoid if maternal heart rate above 120 beats/min.

Child: INHALATION, as for Adult above. PARENTERAL, SC, IM, slow IV bolus, age 2-15 years, 0.01mg/kg; max. 0.3mg total.

CI: *Parenteral (premature labour)*, gestational age under 22 weeks, pre-existing or significant risk factors for ischaemic heart disease, threatened abortion during first and second trimester, conditions where prolonged labour is hazardous (severe toxaemia, intra-uterine infection, vaginal bleeding resulting from placenta praevia, eclampsia, or severe pre-eclampsia, placental abruption, cord compression). Intrauterine foetal death, known lethal (congenital or chromosomal) malformation. Pre-existing medical conditions (pulmonary hypertension, hypertrophic obstructive cardiomyopathy, obstruction of left ventricular outflow tract including aortic stenosis).

Interactions: Effect of Other Drugs on Terbutaline: *Caution*: Other sympathomimetics. *Possible interaction*: MAOIs, TCADs.

SP: Careful control of hydration essential to avoid risk of maternal pulmonary oedema. Use with caution in tocolysis; supervise cardiorespiratory function, perform ECG monitoring throughout treatment. Monitor (BP, heart rate, ECG, electrolyte/fluid balance, glucose and lactate levels especially with diabetics, potassium). Myocardial ischaemia (chest pain, ECG changes), discontinue; not for use with risk factors for heart disease (tachyarrhythmias, HF, valvular heart disease). Caution, hyperthyroidism. Respiratory indications, chest pain or other symptoms of worsening heart disease, advise patient to seek medical advice; assess symptoms (dyspnoea, chest pain) as may be either respiratory or cardiac. Potentially serious hypokalaemia. Lactic acidosis reported with high doses.

Pregnancy, Lactation: Pregnancy, caution first trimester. Lactation, does pass into breast milk; effect on infant unlikely at therapeutic doses.

ADR: Inhaled, *very common*, tremor, headache. Parenteral, *very common*, tachycardia, tremor, headache, nausea.

Notes: See 5.1.1 Adrenoreceptor Agonist Bronchodilators.

Bricanyl Turbohaler *(AstraZeneca)* B. GMS.
Price, (100-dose) 500mcg, €5.82.
Inhalation powder, terbutaline sulfate 500mcg/dose. White (off-white) spherical particles which break into powder (breath-actuated, metered). **Store:** Below 30 deg C.

Bricanyl Parenteral *(AstraZeneca)* A. GMS.
Price, 0.5mg/mL (5) €1.74.
Injection, terbutaline sulfate 0.5mg/mL. Clear aqueous. *Less than 1mmoL/mL sodium.* **Store:** Below 25 deg C; protect from light.

5.1.2 - Antimuscarinic Bronchodilators

In This Chapter: Aclidinium, glycopyrronium, ipratropium, tiotropium, umeclidinium.

Class Effects

Driving: Generally these drugs have no influence on ability to drive; at higher doses, treatment initiation, or with

ALCOHOL, ability may be affected. Dizziness, transient muscle cramps, tremor, caution.

Antimuscarinics are also called anticholinergics. They may be used in combination with beta-2-agonists (formoterol, vilanterol, olodaterol), see Notes below.

Indications: Not for use in children unless otherwise stated; no relevant use for medicinals indicated for treatment of COPD.

CI: Hypersensitivity to any member of the class.

SP: Caution, anticholinergic effects (narrow-angle glaucoma, seek specialist advice; prostatic hyperplasia, bladder-outflow obstruction, urinary retention; MI, unstable angina, arrhythmia, HF, cardiovascular safety profile in line with anticholinergic effects). Dry mouth; dental caries (long term use). Avoid contact of drug powder with eyes, ocular complications (narrow-angle glaucoma, eye pain or discomfort, temporary blurred of vision, visual halos or coloured images in association with red eyes from conjunctival congestion and corneal oedema). As with all inhaled medicines, paradoxical bronchospasm may occur; may be life-threatening (discontinue).

Pregnancy, Lactation: Pregnancy, if benefit outweighs risk. Lactation, stop breastfeeding or stop drug.

Notes: See Class Effects 5.1 Asthma, COPD. For combinations, see 5.1.3 Adrenoreceptor (Beta-2) Agonist, Antimuscarinic Combinations.

Aclidinium

ATC Code: R03BB05. **Sport:** Permitted.
Driving: Headache, blurred vision, dizziness may influence.
Indications: Maintenance bronchodilator treatment (adults) with COPD.
Dose: Adult, Elderly: One inhalation (322mcg) twice daily.
Child: No relevant use.
Renal Impairment: No adjustment.
Hepatic Impairment: As for Renal above.
Pregnancy, Lactation: Pregnancy, if benefit outweighs risk. Lactation, stop breastfeeding or stop drug.
ADR: *Common*, sinusitis, nasopharyngitis, headache, cough, diarrhoea, nausea.
Notes: See 5.1.2 Antimuscarinic Bronchodilators.

▼ **Eklira Genuair 322** *(A.Menarini)* B. GMS.
Price, (60-dose) €33.76.
Inhalation powder, aclidinium bromide 322mcg/dose. White (almost) powder. Lactose. **Store:** Inhaler inside pouch until use.

Glycopyrronium (bronchospasm)

ATC Code: R03BB06. **Sport:** Permitted.
Driving: No or negligible effect.
Indications: Maintenance bronchodilator to relieve symptoms of COPD.
Dose: Adult, Elderly: Inhalation of contents of 1 cap once daily using inhaler. *Admin*, same time each day; do not swallow.
Renal Impairment: Severe, ESRD, if benefit outweighs risk.
SP: Immediate hypersensitivity reactions, discontinue.
Pregnancy, Lactation: See Notes below.
ADR: *Common*, nasopharyngitis, insomnia, headache, dry mouth, UTI.
Notes: See 5.1.2 Antimuscarinic Bronchodilators.

▼ **Seebri Breezhaler** *(Novartis)* B. GMS.
Price, caps 44mcg (30) €33.52.
Inhalation powder, glycopyrronium bromide 44mcg/dose. Hard cap transparent orange; contains white powder. Marked GPL50 and logo. Lactose.

Ipratropium (bronchospasm)

ATC Code: R03BB01. **Sport:** Permitted.
Driving: Caution; dizziness, accommodation disorder, mydriasis, blurred vision.
Indications: Maintenance, bronchospasm associated with asthma, COPD; adjunctive with inhaled beta-2-agonists, acute and chronic asthma, acute bronchospasm associated with COPD.
Dose: Adult, Elderly: INHALER (20mcg/puff), usually 20-40mcg 3-4 times daily; 80mcg at a time might be needed for max. benefit.

Antimuscarinic Bronchodilators   5.1.2

NEBULISER (250mcg/mL), 500mcg 3-4 times daily. Acute bronchospasm, 500mcg, repeat until patient is stable. Above 2mg, only under medical supervision.
Child: INHALER (20mcg/puff), age 6-12 years, usually 20-40mcg 3-times daily; under 6 years, 20mcg 3-times daily.
NEBULISER (250mcg/mL), under 12 years, 250mcg up to max. 1mg/day; acute bronchospasm, repeat until patient is stable. Above 1mg/day, only under medical supervision. Over 3 years, 100-500mcg up to 3-times daily. Under 6 years, with medical supervision *(Atrovent UDV)*.
Interactions: Effect of Other Drugs on Ipratropium: *Enhanced effect*: Beta-adrenergics, xanthines. Co-admin *(increased glaucoma risk with narrow-angle glaucoma history)*: Beta-2-agonists. Chronic co-admin *not recommended*: Other anticholinergics.
SP: Immediate hypersensitivity reactions; urticaria, rash, angioedema, bronchospasm, oropharyngeal oedema, anaphylaxis. Cystic fibrosis, caution GI motility disturbances. Chronic co-admin with anticholinergics, not recommended. NOTE: UDVs and disodium cromoglicate inhalation solns containing benzalkonium chloride are not for co-admin in same nebuliser (precipitation may occur).
Pregnancy, Lactation: Pregnancy, no data. Lactation, if benefit outweighs risk.
ADR: *Most frequent*, headache, throat irritation, cough, dry mouth, GI motility disorders (constipation, diarrhoea, vomiting), nausea, dizziness.
Notes: See 5.1.2 Antimuscarinic Bronchodilators.

Atrovent CFC-Free Inhaler, UDV *(Boehringer)* B. GMS.
Price, inhaler €2.67. UDVs 250mcg: 1mL and 2mL (20) €4.16; (60) €12.47.
Inhaler, ipratropium bromide monohydrate 20mcg/metered dose. Pressurised inhalation soln CFC-free. Clear colourless liquid. **Store:** Below 25 deg C; outer carton; do not expose to temp above 50 deg C.
Nebuliser soln (UDVs), as above 250mcg/1mL, 500mcg/2mL. Clear colourless aqueous soln. **Store:** Below 25 deg C; outer carton to protect (light).
Steri-Neb Ipratropium *(TEVA)* B. GMS.
Price, 250mcg/mL (20) 1mL, €1.86. 2mL, €4.50.
Nebuliser soln, ipratropium bromide.

Tiotropium

ATC Code: R03BB04. **Sport:** Permitted.
Driving: Dizziness, blurred vision, headache.
Indications: Maintenance bronchodilator to relieve symptoms of COPD *(HandiHaler, Respimat, Braltus)*. Add-on maintenance bronchodilator treatment, adults with asthma currently treated with combination (inhaled corticosteroids + long-acting beta-2-agonists) with 1 or more severe exacerbations (previous year) *(Respimat)*.
Dose: Adult, Elderly: 18mcg once daily *(HandiHaler)*, 5mcg (2 puffs) *Respimat* OR inhalation of contents of 1 cap (10mcg) once daily. *Admin*, same time of day; caps not for oral use.
Child: COPD, no relevant use; asthma, safety and efficacy not established.
Renal Impairment: CrCl (mL/min) 50 or less, if benefit outweighs risk. Severe, no data.
CI: Hypersensitivity (atropine or derivatives).
Interactions: Effect of Other Drugs on Tiotropium: Co-admin not recommended: Other anticholinergics.
SP: *Respimat*, not for initial treatment (acute episodes of bronchospasm i.e. rescue) or first-line monotherapy (asthma). Immediate hypersensitivity may occur after admin. Do not exceed dose. Increased anticholinergic effects with increasing age. Use not recommended in cystic fibrosis; may increase signs and symptoms (serious adverse events, pulmonary exacerbations, respiratory tract infections). Caution, recent MI, unstable/life-threatening cardiac arrhythmia, HF (NYHA Class II or IV). Avoid getting drug powder in eyes.
Pregnancy, Lactation: Pregnancy, avoid. Lactation, not recommended.
ADR: Anticholinergic effects include *common*, dry mouth; *serious*, glaucoma, constipation, intestinal obstruction (ileus paralytic, urinary retention).
Notes: See 5.1.2 Antimuscarinic Bronchodilators.

5.1.3 Adrenoreceptor (Beta-2) Agonist, Antimuscarinic Combinations

Spiriva, Respimat *(Boehringer)* A. GMS.
Price, HandiHaler 18mcg, €34.78. Respimat Inhaler Soln 2.5mcg, €33.27
Inhalation powder, tiotropium bromide monohydrate 18mcg (HandiHaler); delivered dose 10mcg tiotropium. Hard capsule light-green. Marked TI 01 and logo. *Lactose.* **Store:** Below 25 deg C; do not freeze.
Inhalation soln, tiotropium bromide monohydrate 2.5mcg/puff (Respimat). Clear colourless. *Benzalkonium chloride.* **Store:** Do not freeze.
Braltus 10mcg *(TEVA)* A. GMS.
Price, (30) €31.24.
Inhalation powder (capsule), tiotropium hydrobromide 10mcg/dose (Zonda inhaler). Hard cap colourless transparent; contains white powder. *Lactose.*

Umeclidinium

ATC Code: R03BB07. **Sport:** Permitted.
Driving: No or negligible effect.
Indications: Maintenance bronchodilator (adults) with COPD.
Dose: Adult, Elderly: 1 inhalation once daily (max.) at same time of day each day. The 'discard by' date is 6 weeks after the date of opening the tray.
Hepatic Impairment: Severe, caution.
Interactions: Effect of Other Drugs on Umeclidinium: *Co-admin not recommended*: Other long-acting muscarinic antagonists.
SP: Not for use in asthma or relief of acute symptoms.
Pregnancy, Lactation: See Notes below.
ADR: *Common*, nasopharyngitis, upper RTI, UTI, sinusitis, pharyngitis, headache, tachycardia, cough.
Notes: See 5.1.2 Antimuscarinic Bronchodilators.
▼ **Incruse 55** *(GSK)* B. GMS.
Price, (30-dose), €32.02.
Inhalation powder, umeclidinium bromide 55mcg. White pre-dispensed. *Lactose.* **Store:** Below 30 deg C; if refrigerated, return to room temperature before use.

5.1.3 - Adrenoreceptor (Beta-2) Agonist, Antimuscarinic Combinations

Class Effects
Corticosteroid combinations, see Notes below.
Driving, Sport: See Notes below (beta-2 agonist bronchodilators).
Notes: See Class Effects for each component, 5.1.1 Adrenoreceptor (Beta-2) Agonist Bronchodilators and 5.1.2 Antimuscarinic Bronchodilators. Corticosteroid combinations, see 5.2 Respiratory Corticosteroids.

Aclidinium, Formoterol

ATC Code: R03AL05. **Sport:** Restricted. See Notes below.
Driving: Blurred vision, dizziness.
Indications: Maintenance bronchodilator treatment (adults) with COPD.
Dose: Adult, Elderly: 1 inhalation (340/12mcg) twice daily.
Interactions: Effect of Formoterol Component on Other Drugs: See Notes below (formoterol).
SP: Not for use in asthma or acute bronchospasm. *Caution*, severe cardiovascular disorders including MI (previous 6 months), unstable angina, newly diagnosed arrhythmia (previous 3 months), heart failure NYHA Class II or IV requiring hospitalisation; convulsive disorders, thyrotoxicosis, phaeochromocytoma. Due to beta-2-adrenergics, increased (pulse, BP), ECG changes, QT-prolongation (discontinue), hyper/hypoglycaemia (at high doses). Beta-2-adrenergic effects (formoterol) and anticholinergic effects, see Notes below.
Pregnancy, Lactation: Use if benefit outweighs risk.
ADR: Summary, *most frequent*, nasopharyngitis, headache.
Notes: See 5.1.3 Adrenoreceptor (Beta-2) Agonist, Antimuscarinic Combinations.
▼ **Brimica Genuair 340/12** *(A.Menarini)* B. GMS.
Price, (60-dose) €45.36.
Inhalation powder, aclidinium bromide 340mcg, formoterol 12mcg per dose. White (almost) powder. *Lactose.* **Store:** Inside sealed pouch; no special temperature conditions.

Indacaterol, Glycopyrronium

ATC Code: R03AL04. **Sport:** Prohibited.
Driving: No or negligible effect; dizziness.
Indications: Maintenance bronchodilator (adults) with COPD.
Dose: Adult, Elderly: Content of 1 cap (max.) inhaled once daily using Ultibro Breezhaler. Do not swallow caps.
Renal Impairment: Severe or ESRD requiring dialysis, use if benefit outweighs risk.
Hepatic Impairment: Severe, caution.
SP: Anticholinergic effects of glycopyrronium; narrow-angle glaucoma, urinary retention, cardiovascular disorders (CAD, acute MI, arrhythmias, hypertension), caution. Immediate hypersensitivity reactions (angioedema, urticaria, skin rash), discontinue.
ADR: Summary, *most common*, cough, nasopharyngitis, headache.
Notes: See 5.1.3 Adrenoreceptor (Beta-2) Agonist, Antimuscarinic Combinations.
▼ **Ultibro Breezhaler 85/43** *(Novartis)* B. GMS.
Price, (30) €48.70.
Inhalation powder (capsule), indacaterol maleate 85mcg, glycopyrronium 43mcg per dose. Transparent cap containing white (almost) powder. Marked IGP110.50 and company logo. *Lactose.*

Ipratropium, Salbutamol

ATC Code: R03AK04. **Sport:** Restricted. See notes below.
Driving: Dizziness, accommodation disorder, mydriasis, blurred vision.
Indications: Bronchospasm associated with COPD (adults, regular combination treatment needed).
Dose: Adult, Elderly: NEBULISER, 1 vial nebulised 3-4 times daily (dilute only with sterile sodium chloride 0.9%). Initiate and administer under medical supervision (e.g. hospital setting).
Child: Age 12 years and over, as for Adult above.
Renal Impairment: Caution, no data.
Hepatic Impairment: As for Renal above.
CI: Hypertrophic obstructive cardiomyopathy, tachyarrhythmia, atropine hypersensitivity.
SP: Chronic co-admin with other anticholinergics, not recommended.
Pregnancy, Lactation: Pregnancy, if benefit outweighs risk. Lactation, caution.
ADR: No commonly reported adverse events.
Notes: See 5.1.3 Adrenoreceptor (Beta-2) Agonist, Antimuscarinic Combinations.
Ipramol Steri-Neb 0.5/2.5mg *(TEVA)* B. GMS.
Price, 0.5/2.5mg (2.5mL) (20) €3.80. (60) €8.90.
Nebuliser soln, ipratropium bromide monohydrate, salbutamol sulfate 0.5/2.5mg per 2.5mL. Colourless soln.

Tiotropium, Olodaterol

ATC Code: R03AL06. **Sport:** Prohibited.
Driving: Dizziness, blurred vision.
Indications: Maintenance bronchodilator (adults) with COPD.
Dose: Adult, Elderly: 2 puffs (tiotropium 5mcg, olodaterol 5mcg) by inhalation, once daily at same time of day.
Renal Impairment: CrCl (mL/min) 50 or less, if benefit outweighs risk. Severe, no data.
Hepatic Impairment: Severe, no data.
SP: Not for acute use.
Pregnancy, Lactation: Pregnancy, avoid. Lactation, stop breastfeeding or stop drug.
ADR: *Common*, dry mouth.
Notes: See 5.1.3 Adrenoreceptor (Beta-2) Agonist, Antimuscarinic Combinations.
▼ **Spiolto Respimat** *(Boehringer)* B. GMS.
Price, (30-dose), 2.5/2.5mcg, €45.36.
Inhalation soln, tiotropium bromide monohydrate, olodaterol HCl 2.5mcg/2.5mcg per puff. Clear colourless soln. **Store:** Do not freeze.

Umeclidinium, Vilanterol

ATC Code: R03AL03. **Sport:** Prohibited.
Driving: No or negligible effect.
Indications: Maintenance bronchodilator in COPD.
Dose: Adult, Elderly: 1 inhalation once daily (max.) at same time of day. The 'discard by' date is 6 weeks after date of opening the tray.
Child: No relevant use.
Hepatic Impairment: Severe, caution.
Interactions: Effect of Other Drugs on Umeclidinium, Vilanterol: *Co-admin caution:* CYP3A4 inhibitors (ketoconazole, clarithromycin, itraconazole, ritonavir, telithromycin; increased vilanterol exposure), methylxanthines, steroids, diuretics (hypokalaemia potentiated). *Co-admin not recommended:* Other long acting (muscarinic antagonists, beta-2-adrenergic agonists). *Co-admin avoid:* Beta-blockers.
SP: Not for use in asthma, acute bronchospasm episodes.
Pregnancy, Lactation: Pregnancy, use if benefit outweighs risk. Lactation, stop breastfeeding or stop drug.
ADR: Summary, *most frequent,* nasopharyngitis.
Notes: See 5.1.3 Adrenoreceptor (Beta-2) Agonist, Antimuscarinic Combinations.

▼ **Anoro 55/22 Inhalation** *(GSK)* B. GMS.
Price, (30-dose) €43.15.
Inhalation powder, umeclidinium bromide, vilanterol trifenatate 55/22mcg per delivered dose. White pre-dispensed. *Lactose.*
Store: Below 30 deg C; if refrigerated, return to room temperature before use.

5.1.4 - Xanthines

In This Chapter: *Aminophylline, theophylline.*

Class Effects
Interactions: Effect of Other Drugs on Xanthines: *Co-admin avoid:* Fluvoxamine (if not possible, halve theophylline dose; monitor). *Reduced elimination, reduce dose:* Allopurinol, carbimazole, cimetidine, quinolones (monitor theophylline levels), macrolides, corticosteroids, calcium channel blockers, disulfiram, fluconazole, frusemide, interferon, isoniazid, isoprenaline, methotrexate, mexiletine, nizatidine, propafenone, propranolol, oxpentifylline, ofloxacin, thiabendazole, ticlopidine, rofecoxib, viloxazine, zileuton, influenzae and BCG-vaccines, oral contraceptives; other factors including viral infection, liver disease, HF, fever. *Increased elimination, increase dose:* Aminoglutethimide, carbamazepine, lithium, moricizine, phenytoin, rifampicin, primidone, sulphinpyrazone, barbiturates, St John's Wort *(Hypericum perforatum),* ritonavir, smoking, ALCOHOL consumption. *Effect potentiated:* Influenza vaccine, beta-adrenergic agonists, glucagon, other xanthines, adrenaline, ephedrine.
Effect of Xanthines on Other Drugs: *Beta-2-agonists, steroids, diuretics: Hypokalaemia caused by these drugs might be potentiated, monitor. Phenytoin: Steady state levels decreased. Lithium: Monitor lithium levels. Halothane: Serious cardiac arrhythmia with theophylline.*
SP: NOTE: Different Prolonged/R xanthine products may have different bioequivalence; re-titrate when changing. Hypokalaemia risk, monitor. Cardiac disease; severe adverse events (cramps, convulsions, supraventricular tachycardia) at high serum conc; discontinue. Insomnia, caution.
Pregnancy, Lactation: Only if considered essential by physician. Theophylline crosses placenta and enters breast milk; use in second and third trimesters only with strict benefit risk assessment.
Notes: See 5.1 Asthma, COPD.

Aminophylline

ATC Code: R03DA05. **Sport:** Permitted.
Driving: No or negligible effect.
Indications: Treatment and prophylaxis, bronchospasm and inflammation associated with asthma, emphysema,

chronic bronchitis. Adults, cardiac asthma, left ventricular or CHF. Not first drug of choice in asthma in children.
Dose: Adult, Elderly: ORAL, usual maintenance 225mg twice daily; titrate to higher dose as needed. Plasma theophylline conc should be ideally maintained at 5-12mcg/mL (5mcg/mL is probably the lower level of clinical effectiveness; significant adverse reactions usually seen at levels above 20mcg/mL). Consider plasma theophylline monitoring with (higher doses, co-morbidities with impaired clearance; medication reducing theophylline clearance). *Admin,* swallow tabs whole, do not chew.
PARENTERAL, *loading dose,* not receiving xanthines, initially 6mg/kg at max. rate 25mg/min over 20-30 minutes; already receiving xanthines, reduce dose to 3.1mg/kg and admin slowly (will increase serum level by about 5mcg/mL); serum level range, 10-20mcg/mL. *Maintenance,* healthy non-smoking adults, 0.7mg/kg/hour (first 12-hours), then 0.5mg/kg/hour; CHF or with liver failure, 0.5mg/kg/hour (first 12 hours), then 0.1-0.2mg/kg/hour. Young adult smokers, see Child below.
Child: ORAL (age 6 years and above), usual maintenance 10mg/kg twice daily; some children with chronic asthma may tolerate 11-18mg/kg twice daily. Rapid clearance observed in children decreases towards adult values in late teens. Under 6 years (22kg), not recommended; under 6 months, contraindicated. Calculate mg/kg dose on basis of lean (ideal) body weight. Ideal concentrations, see Adult above.
PARENTERAL, *loading dose,* not currently receiving xanthines, age 1-9 years, 3-6mg/kg over 30 minutes; *maintenance,* 0.9mg/kg/hour for first 12 hours. Age 6-16 and young adult smokers, 1mg/kg/hour (first 12 hours), then 0.8mg/kg/hour. Under 1 year, not recommended.
CI: Hypersensitivity to ethylenediamine or allergic to theophylline, caffeine, theobromine (parenteral). Porphyria.
Interactions: Effect of Other Drugs on Aminophylline: *Co-admin contraindicated in children under 6 years (increased toxicity):* Ephedrine. *Plasma levels altered:* Thyroid disease or associated treatment. *Effect potentiated:* Beta-adrenergic agonists, glucagon, other xanthines, hypokalaemia (beta- agonists, steroids, diuretics, hypoxia). *Increased clearance (consider dose increase):* Aminoglutethimide, carbamazepine, isoprenaline, phenytoin, rifampicin, sulphinpyrazone, barbiturates, ritonavir, St John's Wort, smoking, alcohol consumption. *Reduced clearance (consider dose decrease):* Aciclovir, allopurinol, carbimazole, cimetidine, clarithromycin, diltiazem, disulfiram, erythromycin, fluconazole, interferon, isoniazid, methotrexate, mexiletine, nizatidine, pentoxifylline, propafenone, propranolol, thiabendazole, verapamil, oral contraceptives; ciprofloxacin, enoxacin (possibly); fluvoxamine (avoid).
Effect of Aminophylline on Other Drugs: Adenosine receptor agonists (adenosine, regadenoson, dipyridamole) (effect inhibited), benzodiazepines (sedatory effect opposed), halothane (reduced arrhythmia occurrence), lomustine (thrombocytopenia), lithium (increased urinary clearance): *Caution with co-admin.* Phenytoin: *Steady state level decreased.*
SP: Mood change, effects on level of cerebral function (children; especially if dose exceeded). Acute episodes, IV admin required. Monitor serum levels, consider dose reduction in elderly with (cardiac/hepatic disease, exacerbation of lung disease, hypothyroidism, fever, viral infections). Caution, peptic ulcer, cardiac arrhythmias, seizures, elderly males with urinary tract obstruction (urinary retention risk), severe asthma. *Parenteral,* monitor serum theophylline levels; maintain in range 10-20mcg/mL. Aminophylline may prolong seizures or cause multiple seizures (proconvulsant effect); admin of aminophylline solely to terminate a seizure induced by regadenoson (adenosine receptor agonist), not recommended.
Pregnancy, Lactation: If benefit outweighs risk.
ADR: *Unknown frequency,* anaphylactic/toid reactions, hypersensitivity, hyperuricaemia, agitation, anxiety, insomnia, sleep disorder, convulsions, dizziness,

5.1.5 Other Drugs Used In Obstructive Airway Disease

headache, tremor, tachycardia (atrial, sinus), palpitations, abdominal pain, diarrhoea, gastric irritation, GORD, nausea, vomiting, pruritus, rash, diuresis, urinary retention; (parenteral), (parenteral), GI irritation, CNS stimulation, effects on cardiovascular system; hypotension, arrhythmias, convulsions may follow IV injection (if injected too rapidly); sudden deaths reported. Severe toxicity may occur without preceding milder symptoms.

Notes: See 5.1.4 Xanthines.

Phyllocontin Continus *(Mundipharma)* B. GMS.
Price, 225mg (56) €2.92.
Prolonged/R tablet, aminophylline hydrate 225mg. Pale-yellow f/c round. Marked logo; SA on reverse. **Store:** Below 25 deg C.
Aminophylline Parenteral 250mg *(Concordia)* A. GMS.
Price, 250mg/10mL (10) €5.30.
Injection, aminophylline hydrate. Clear colourless soln. **Store:** Below 25 deg C; outer carton to protect (light).

Theophylline

ATC Code: R03DA04. **Sport:** Permitted.
Driving: Unlikely to impair.

Indications: *Both brands,* treatment and prophylaxis of bronchospasm and inflammation associated with asthma, chronic bronchitis, emphysema. *Uniphyllin* (adults), cardiac asthma, left ventricular or CHF. Theophylline should not be first drug of choice in treatment of asthma in children.

Dose: Adult: *Uniphyllin Continus,* asthma, 200mg 12-hourly; severe, 300-400mg 12-hourly; emphysema, chronic bronchitis, LV failure, CHF, weight 70kg and over, initially 200-300mg 12-hourly (week 1), then 400mg 12-hourly; under 70kg initially 200mg 12-hourly (week 1), then 300mg 12-hourly. *Elderly,* may require dose reduction. Tabs not to be broken, crushed or chewed as this may lead to rapid theophylline release with potential for toxicity.

Zepholin SR, begin treatment in evening and increase slowly over 2-3 days. Body weight 60-70kg, non-smokers, theophylline 11-13mg/kg/day (660-910mg/day); smokers, theophylline 18mg/kg/day (1080-1260mg/day). *Admin,* oral; swallow caps whole after meals with plenty of fluid. Divide daily dose between morning (breakfast) and evening (shortly before bed). In case of adipose patients, use normal weight.

Elderly: Clearance decelerated.

Child: Age 6 years and over, *Uniphyllin Continus,* asthma, 200mg 12-hourly; if needed and tolerated 300mg 12-hourly. *Zepholin SR,* age 6-8 years (20-25kg), theophylline 24mg/kg/day/day (480-600mg/day); age 8-12 years (25-40kg), 20mg/kg/day (500-800mg/day); age 12-16 years (40-60kg), 18mg/kg/day (720-1080mg/day). *Admin,* see Adult above. *Both brands,* under 6 years, not recommended; under 6 months, contraindicated.

Renal Impairment: Severe, an accumulation of theophylline metabolites may occur. Severe, not recommended *(Zepholin).*

Hepatic Impairment: Clearance often reduced with impaired liver function. *Zepholin,* as for Renal above. Cystic fibrosis, lower dose may be required.

CI: Co-admin with electroconvulsive therapy (ECT), not recommended. Recent MI, acute tachycardiac arrhythmia *(Zepholin).*

SP: *Caution,* elderly males with pre-existing partial outflow obstruction (prostatic enlargement), urinary retention risk; peptic ulcer, hyperthyroidism, severe hypertension, epilepsy (may become uncontrolled; history of seizures, use alternative), unstable angina, history of tachycardiac arrhythmia, hypertrophic obstructive cardiac myopathy, porphyria, alcohol consumption. Dose above 100mg/day, insufficient effect at recommended dose or presence of adverse events, regular theophylline level monitoring required. Fever decreases theophylline clearance, consider dose reduction to avoid intoxication. Use in older, polymorbid, critically ill and/or intensive medically treated patients associated with increased risk for intoxication; control by therapeutic drug monitoring (TDM). In patients receiving electroconvulsive therapy, caution as may prolong seizures.

ADR: *Common,* headache, nausea.

Notes: See 5.1.4 Xanthines.

Uniphyllin Continus Tablets *(Mundipharma)* B. GMS.
Price, (56) 200mg, €4.03. 300mg, €6.52. 400mg, €8.19.
Prolonged/R tablet, theophylline monohydrate 200mg, 300mg, 400mg. White cap-shaped. Marked U/strength. 400mg: Marked Uniphyllin; logo on reverse. *Cetostearyl alcohol.*
Zepholin SR 100mg, 200mg, 350mg *(Astellas)* B. GMS.
Price, (56) 100mg, €1.49. 200mg, €2.34. 350mg, €8.35.
Prolonged/R capsule, theophylline. Hard opaque/transparent contains white pellets. Marked TH/strength. 100mg: Blue/white. 200mg, 350mg, 500mg: Green/green.

5.1.5 - Other Drugs Used In Obstructive Airway Disease

In This Chapter: *Alpha1-proteinase inhibitor, omalizumab, pirfenidone, roflumilast.*

Class Effects
CI: Hypersensitivity to any member of the class.
Notes: See 5.1 Asthma, COPD.

Alpha1-proteinase inhibitor

ATC Code: B02AB02. **Sport:** Permitted.
Driving: Caution.

Indications: Long-term augmentation therapy in alpha1-proteinase inhibitor deficiency with moderate airflow obstruction (FEV1 35-60%).

Dose: Adult, Elderly: Usually, 60mg active ingredient/kg body weight once weekly (75kg patient) as short-term infusion maintaining serum alpha1-proteinase inhibitor level constantly over 80mg/dL. *Admin,* by slow IV infusion, rate max. 0.08mL/kg/min.

Child: Under 18 years, not recommended.

CI: Selective IgA deficiency with known IgA antibodies.

SP: Severe hypersensitivity (BP fall below 90mmHg, dyspnoea, anaphylaxis shock), discontinue. CHF, caution, circulatory overload. Consider hepatitis A and B vaccination. Record batch for tracing. Recommend smoking cessation.

Pregnancy, Lactation: Pregnancy, caution. Lactation, stop drug or stop breastfeeding.

ADR: *Uncommon,* chills, fever, flu-like symptoms, chest pain, urticaria, dizziness, headache, dyspnoea, rash, nausea, joint pain/arthralgia.

Notes: See 5.1.5 Other Drugs Used In Obstructive Airway Disease.

Prolastin Parenteral *(Caragen)* A.
Price, not published by company.
Infusion, alpha1-proteinase inhibitor (human) 1000mg. White (beige) powder and solvent for soln. *Sodium 4.8mmoL/vial.* **Store:** Below 25 deg C; do not freeze; once prepared do not refrigerate.

Omalizumab

ATC Code: R03DX05. **Sport:** Permitted.
Driving: Dizziness, fatigue, faintness, drowsiness.

Indications: Add-on therapy to improve asthma control, age 6 years and above with convincing IgE mediated asthma (positive skin test or *in vitro* reactivity to a perennial aeroallergen and reduced lung function as well as frequent daytime symptoms or night-time awakenings and multiple severe asthma exacerbations) *(both strengths).* Add-on therapy, chronic spontaneous urticaria (12 years and above) with inadequate response to H1-antihistamine treatment *(150mg).*

Dose: Adult, Elderly: *Allergic asthma,* dose and frequency determined by baseline IgE (IU/mL) and body weight (kg); range 75-600mg in 1-4 SC injections may be needed for each admin; max. 600mg every 2 weeks. IgE below 76 IU/mL, less likely to benefit. Not for IV or IM admin.
Chronic spontaneous urticaria, 300mg by SC injection every 4 weeks; periodically reassess need for continued therapy; long-term treatment beyond 6 months, limited data.

Child: As for Adult above. Safety/efficacy not established, allergic asthma, under 6 years; chronic spontaneous urticaria, under 12 years.

Renal Impairment: Caution.

182

Hepatic Impairment: As for Renal above.

Interactions: Effect of Omalizumab on Other Drugs: Drugs used to treat helminthic, other parasitic infections: *Efficacy may be reduced (indirectly)*.

SP: Determine baseline IgE levels before initiating. Assess after 16 weeks. After initiation, abrupt discontinuation of systemic or inhaled corticosteroids, not recommended. *Allergic reactions (Type I)*, local or systemic (anaphylaxis, anaphylactic shock; usually within 2 hours; history of anaphylaxis may be a risk factor); antibody development. *Serum sickness*, delayed Type III reactions seen 1-5 days after admin. Churg-Strauss syndrome and hypereosinophilic syndrome (severe asthma). Parasitic infections (helminthic infection, caution).

Pregnancy, Lactation: Pregnancy, only if clearly necessary; crosses placental barrier. Lactation, not recommended.

ADR: Summary, *most common* (age 12 years and older), headache, injection-site pain, swelling, erythema, pruritus; (age 6-12 years), headache, pyrexia, upper abdominal pain.

Notes: See 5.1.5 Other Drugs Used In Obstructive Airway Disease.

Xolair Parenteral 75mg, 150mg *(Novartis)* A. HOS.
Price, (1) PFS 75mg, €178.85. 150mg, €340.94.
Injection, omalizumab. Humanised monoclonal antibody. Clear (slightly opalescent) colourless (pale brownish-yellow) soln (PFS). *Natural rubber latex needle cover.* **Store:** Refrigerate; do not freeze.

Pirfenidone

ATC Code: L04AX05. **Sport:** Pending.
Driving: Moderate influence: dizziness, fatigue.

Indications: Treatment, mild to moderate Idiopathic Pulmonary Fibrosis (IPF).

Dose: Adult, Elderly: Initially, 1 cap (267mg) 3-times daily (days 1-7), then 2 caps 3-times daily (days 8-14), then 3 caps 3-times daily (day 15 onwards). Maintenance, 3 caps 3-times daily (2403mg/day). *Admin*, swallow caps whole with water; with food to reduce nausea, dizziness.

Child: No relevant use.

Renal Impairment: CrCl (mL/min) below 30 or ESRD requiring dialysis, contraindicated.

Hepatic Impairment: Mild/moderate, caution; severe or end-stage liver disease, contraindicated.

CI: Angioedema (history of).

Interactions: Effect of Pirfenidone on Other Drugs: *Co-admin contraindicated*: Fluvoxamine. *Increased exposure*: Strong CYP1A2 inhibitors (enoxacin), reduce pirfenidone dose to 801mg/day; moderate CYP1A2 inhibitors (ciprofloxacin at dose 750mg twice daily); reduce pirfenidone dose to 1602mg/day; other moderate CYP1A2 inhibitors (ciprofloxacin at dose 250-500mg once or twice daily; amiodarone, propafenone). Caution if CYP1A2 inhibitors are co-admin with other CYP inhibitors such as CYP2C9 (amiodarone, fluconazole), 2C19 (chloramphenicol), 2D6 (fluoxetine, paroxetine). *Plasma levels decreased*: Cigarette smoking, omeprazole, rifampicin.

SP: Monitor ALT, AST, bilirubin prior to initiation, at monthly intervals for first 6 months and then 3-monthly (rare elevations reported). Photosensitivity reaction; avoid exposure to direct sunlight (including sun lamps); use sunblock. Reported, dizziness, fatigue, weight loss, angioedema (some serious; discontinue).

Pregnancy, Lactation: Pregnancy, avoid. Lactation, stop breastfeeding or stop drug.

ADR: Summary, *most frequent*, nausea, rash, diarrhoea, fatigue, dyspepsia, anorexia, headache, photosensitivity reaction.

Notes: See 5.1.5 Other Drugs Used In Obstructive Airway Disease.

▼ **Esbriet 267mg** *(Roche)* A. HT.
Price, 14-day starter kit, €632.88. (252) €2471.23.
Capsules, pirfenidone. Opaque white*/white*; contains white (pale-yellow) powder. Marked PFD 267mg. *(off-white). **Store:** Below 30 deg C.

Roflumilast

ATC Code: R03DX07. **Sport:** Pending.
Driving: No influence.

Indications: Maintenance treatment, severe COPD (FEV1 post-bronchodilator below 50% predicted) associated with chronic bronchitis with frequent exacerbations as 'add on' to bronchodilator therapy.

Dose: Adult, Elderly: 500mcg (1 tab) once daily; may need to be taken for several weeks to achieve effect.

Child: No relevant use.

Hepatic Impairment: Mild, caution; moderate/severe, contraindicated.

Interactions: Effect of Other Drugs on Roflumilast: *Co-admin not recommended*: CYP3A4 strong inducers (phenobarbital, carbamazepine, phenytoin; efficacy reduced), immunosuppressives (methotrexate, azathioprine, infliximab, etanercept, oral corticosteroids used long-term), theophylline. *Increased exposure, persistent intolerability*: Enoxacin, cimetidine, fluvoxamine.

SP: Not for use as 'rescue' for relief of acute bronchospasm, in severe immunological diseases, severe acute infectious diseases, cancers (except basal cell carcinoma), patients treated with immunosuppressives, CHF (NYHA III, IV), history of depression. Limited experience with latent infections. Weight decrease, monitor bodyweight of underweight patients at each visit. Patients with baseline body weight under 60kg or 75 years and older, may have higher risk of sleep disorders (insomnia). Increased risk of psychiatric disorders (insomnia, anxiety, nervousness, depression); rarely suicidal ideation and behaviour. Persistent intolerability, reassess.

Pregnancy, Lactation: Pregnancy, not recommended. Women of childbearing potential to ensure adequate contraception. Lactation, not recommended.

ADR: Summary, *most common*, diarrhoea, decreased weight, headache, nausea, abdominal pain. See SP above.

Notes: See 5.1.5 Other Drugs Used In Obstructive Airway Disease.

▼ **Daxas 500mcg** *(Takeda)* B.
Price, not published by company (30).
Tablet, roflumilast. Yellow D-shaped f/c. Marked D. *Lactose*.

5.1.6 - Devices, Nebuliser Diluents

Class Effects

Included are paediatric spacer devices and nebuliser diluents.

Babyhaler *(GSK)* OTC. GMS.
Price, (1) €15.62.
Paediatric spacer device, for use with Ventolin and Becotide Inhalers. 350mL device for babies and very young children aged 1 year and older with asthma (with face mask and 2 spare valves).

Steri-Neb Saline *(TEVA)* OTC. GMS.
Price, (20) €4.16.
Nebuliser diluent, sodium chloride 0.9%. Single dose unit preservative free.

Volumatic *(GSK)* OTC. GMS.
Price, (1) €3.34.
Reservoir chamber device, 2-piece, 750mL for aerosol actuator.

5.2 - Respiratory Corticosteroids and Combinations

In This Chapter: *Beclometasone, budesonide, ciclesonide, fluticasone, mometasone.*

Class Effects

Sport: Use of corticosteroids and beta-2 agonists (combinations) in sport, see Notes below.

Pharmacology: Inhaled corticosteroids may be used in combination with either antimuscarinic or beta-2 agonist bronchodilators, see Notes below.

CI: Hypersensitivity to any member of the class.

Interactions: Effect of Other Drugs on Inhaled Corticosteroids: *Increased risk of systemic effects*: Cobicistat. See Notes below.

SP: *Inhaled corticosteroids*, instruct patient regarding

5.2 Respiratory Corticosteroids and Combinations

proper inhaler use; to use regularly even when asymptomatic. To minimise risk of oropharyngeal candida, rinse mouth after inhalation. Paradoxical bronchospasm with inhaled medicines. Caution, active or latent TB and viral, bacterial or fungal infections (eye, mouth, respiratory tract); bacterial infections, consider antibiotics. Pulmonary TB, use inhaled steroid only if TB is treated. Not indicated for treatment of acute asthma attack, dyspnoea or status asthmaticus. Increasing bronchodilator use (short-acting inhaled beta-2-agonists), to relieve symptoms may indicate deteriorating asthma control (less effective, more inhalations needed), reassess; consider increased inhaled dose or oral corticosteroids. Do not stop high-dose inhaled steroids abruptly. Always use lowest dose. Increased pneumonia (including requiring hospitalisation) incidence in COPD patients using inhaled corticosteroids; risk factors (current smoking, older age, low BMI, severe COPD).

Systemic effects of inhaled corticosteroids may occur used high doses for prolonged periods e.g. adrenal suppression, growth retardation in children (monitor height) and adolescents, decreased bone mineral density, cataracts, glaucoma. Above 1500mcg/day may induce adrenal suppression. Ensure systemic steroid cover in stress situations or elective surgery. See Notes below.

Transfer to inhaled steroids from prolonged use or high dose of systemic steroids, caution (impaired adrenocortical function recovery is slow). Patient should be in stable phase. Withdraw systemic steroids gradually. During withdrawal, non-specific feeling of being unwell may occur. Replacement of systemic steroids with inhaled may unmask allergic rhinitis, eczema. Massive mucous secretion in respiratory tract, de-obstruct; follow with short course of oral steroids. NOTE: Transfer from oral steroids with impaired adrenocortical function, a steroid warning card to be carried indicating that supplementary systemic steroids may be needed during stress periods (worsening asthma attacks, chest infections, major intercurrent illness, surgery, trauma). Fluticasone furoate 100mcg once daily approx. equiv. to fluticasone propionate 250mcg twice daily. See Notes below (corticosteroids).

Pregnancy, Lactation: Pregnancy, if benefit outweighs risk; if glucocorticoid treatment unavoidable, use inhaled glucocorticoids with lower systemic effect. Lactation, if benefit to mother outweighs risk to child; plasma levels following inhaled corticosteroids are likely to be low.

ADR: Candidiasis of mouth/throat, hoarseness; See SP above. Paradoxical bronchospasm after dosing, discontinue. Possible systemic effects. Hypersensitivity reactions (rash, urticaria, pruritus, erythema, oedema of the eyes, face, lips and throat). Nervousness, restlessness, depression, behavioural disturbances. Contusion/bruising. Pneumonia reported in COPD patients following inhaled corticosteroid admin. See SP above. Combinations, see Notes below.

Notes: For systemic corticosteroid effects, see Class Effects 11.1.1 Glucocorticoids. Combinations, see 5.1.1 Adrenoceptor (Beta-2) Agonist Bronchodilators and/or 5.1.2 Antimuscarinic Bronchodilators.

Beclometasone (bronchospasm)

ATC Code: R03BA01. **Sport:** Permitted.
Driving: Unlikely to impair.
Indications: Prophylaxis and management, mild to severe asthma; management, chronic asthma.
Dose: Adult, Elderly: Beclazone, 100mcg inhaled 3-4 times daily OR 150-200mcg twice daily; severe, up to 600-800mcg/day.

Becotide Evohaler, mild asthma, 200-600mcg/day; moderate, 600-1000mcg/day; severe, 1000-2000mcg/day. Admin, in divided doses.

Qvar, mild to moderate asthma, 50-200mcg twice daily; severe, up to max. 400mcg twice daily.

Child: Beclazone, age 6-12 years, up to 100mcg 2-4 times daily; max. 400mcg. Severe, higher doses may be required.

Becotide Evohaler, over 4 years, up to 400mcg/day in divided doses.

Qvar, age 5-11 years, 50mcg twice daily.

Notes: See 5.2 Respiratory Corticosteroids.

Becotide Evohaler 50, 100, 250 (GSK) B. GMS.
Price, (200-dose) 50mcg, €3.05. 100mcg, €12.18. 250mcg, €15.57.
Inhaler, beclometasone dipropionate. Clear colourless soln in aluminium canister with valve. Ethanol (Evohaler). Store: Do not (refrigerate, freeze, expose to temp. above 50 deg C).
Beclazone Easi-Breathe, CFC-Free (TEVA) B. GMS.
Price, (200-dose) Easi-Breathe 50mcg, €5.58. 100mcg, €10.86. 200mcg, €21.09. 250mcg, €23.24. CFC-Free 50mcg, €5.36. 100mcg, €10.45. 200mcg, €21.09. 250mcg, €22.35.
Inhaler Easi-Breathe/CFC-Free, beclometasone dipropionate (mcg) 50, 100, 200, 250. Breath-actuated aerosol or inhaler.
Qvar CFC-Free (TEVA) B. GMS.
Price, (200-dose) 50mcg, €10.86. 100mcg, €23.24.
Inhaler, beclometasone dipropionate 50mcg, 100mcg. Aerosol.

Budesonide (bronchospasm)

ATC Code: R03BA02. **Sport:** Permitted.
Driving: No influence.
Indications: Turbohaler, bronchial asthma, COPD. Respules, Nebuliser Susp, persistent bronchial asthma (pressurised inhaler or dry powder formulation unsatisfactory); infants and children with acute croup (viral laryngotracheobronchitis or laryngitis subglottica) in which hospitalisation is indicated.

Dose: Adult, Elderly: Pulmicort Turbohaler, COPD, 400mcg twice daily. Bronchial asthma, range 200-1600mcg/day; mild/moderate, 200-800mcg/day in 1-2 divided doses; severe, up to 1600mcg/day in divided doses. If pressurised inhaler/dry powder unsatisfactory, use respules, in severe asthma, while reducing or discontinuing oral glucocorticosteroids, initially 1-2mg twice daily; maintenance, 0.5-1mg twice daily. See SP below.

Budesonide Teva Nebuliser Susp, 0.5-2mg/day by inhalation in 2 divided doses; increase if severe; maintenance, 0.5-2mg/day in divided doses; mild/moderate stable asthma and maintenance 0.25-1mg/day once daily.

Novolizer Budesonide, persistent asthma, 200-400mcg/day in evening or twice daily; max. 800mcg twice daily.

Child: Pulmicort Turbohaler, bronchial asthma, age 5 years and over, 200-800mcg/day, single or divided doses; max. 800mcg/day; under 5 years, may not be able to handle device properly. Respules, age 12 years and over, as for Adult; age 3 months to 12 years, initially 0.5-1mg twice daily in severe asthma and while reducing or discontinuing oral glucocorticosteroids; (2mg/day over limited periods); maintenance, 0.25-0.5mg twice daily.

Budesonide Teva Nebuliser Soln, age 6 months and above, 0.25-1mg/day; maintenance, 0.25-1mg; with oral steroids, consider initial dose up to 2mg/day; admin twice daily; over 12 years, as for Adult above.

Novolizer Budesonide, persistent asthma, age 6-12 years, 200mcg twice daily or 200-400mcg once daily; max. 400mcg twice daily.

Croup, using Respules or Budesonide Teva Nebuliser Soln, usually 2mg as single dose or as 2x 1mg doses at a 30-minute interval; repeat 12-hourly for max. 36 hours or until clinical improvement.

Hepatic Impairment: Severe, not recommended.
CI: Untreated local airways bacterial, fungal or viral infection, pulmonary TB.
Interactions: Effect of Other Drugs on Budesonide: Increased systemic exposure: CYP3A4 inhibitors (ketoconazole, itraconazole, protease inhibitors).
SP: Transfer from oral steroids, a high dose of Pulmicort is given in combination with previously used oral steroid dose for about 10 days; then gradually reduce oral steroids by 2.5mg prednisolone or equiv. each month to lowest possible dose.
Pregnancy, Lactation: Pregnancy, if benefit outweighs risk. Is excreted in breast milk; no effects on suckling child anticipated at therapeutic dose; can be used during breastfeeding. Maintenance with inhaled budesonide (200-400mcg twice daily) in asthmatic nursing women resulted in negligible systemic exposure to infant.

ADR: *Common*, oropharyngeal candidiasis, pneumonia (COPD patients), cough, hoarseness, throat irritation.

Notes: See 5.2 Respiratory Corticosteroids.

Pulmicort Turbohaler, Respules *(AstraZeneca)* B. GMS.
Price, Turbohaler 100mcg (200-dose) €15.50. 200mcg (100-dose) €12.51. 400mcg (50-dose) €13.20. Respules (20) 0.5mg, €17.20. 1mg, €24.82.
Inhalation powder (Turbohaler), budesonide 100, 200, 400. Breath-actuated metered dose. White (off-white) spherical granules (break into fine powder on inhalation). *Nebuliser soln (Respules),* as above 0.5mg, 1mg. White (off-white) single dose units.

Budesonide TEVA Pharma Nebuliser Susp *(TEVA)* B. GMS.
Price, (20) 0.5mg/2mL. 1mg/2mL, €19.86.
Nebuliser susp, budesonide 0.5(1)mg/2mL. White (off-white) susp.

Novolizer Budesonide *(Meda)* B. GMS.
Price, 200mcg (100-dose) €20.00. Refill €13.36. 400mcg (50-dose) €20.00.
Inhalation powder (refill), budesonide 200mcg, 400mcg. Breath actuated. *Lactose.* **Store:** Original pack; tightly closed; protect (moisture).

Budesonide, Formoterol

ATC Code: R03AK07. **Sport:** Restricted. See Notes below.
Driving: No or negligible effect.

Indications: Asthma, regular treatment, already controlled on inhaled corticosteroid + long acting beta-agonist (or combination) OR inadequate control with inhaled corticosteroids + 'as needed' ('as needed') short-acting beta-2-agonists. Severe COPD (FEV1 below 70% predicted normal), history of repeated exacerbations, significant symptoms despite regular long-acting bronchodilator therapy.

Dose: Adult, Elderly: *Symbicort, asthma* (strengths 100/6, 200/6), maintenance, 1-2 inhalations*; max. 4 inhalations*; maintenance and reliever therapy, 2 inhalations*; (strength 400/12), maintenance therapy only, 1 inhalation*; max. 2 inhalations*. Strength 100/6 not for use in severe asthma. COPD (strength 200/6), 2 inhalations*; (strength 400/12), 1-2 inhalations*. *(admin twice daily).

Bufomix, asthma (strengths 80/4.5, 160/4.5), maintenance 1-2 inhalations*; max. 4 inhalations*; maintenance and reliever therapy, 2 inhalations per day; either 1 in morning AND evening or 2 inhalations in morning OR evening; maintenance of 2 inhalations* (may be appropriate); take 1 additional inhalation as needed (max. 6 inhalations on any single occasion); (strength 320/9), maintenance only, 1 inhalation*; 2 inhalations* may be needed. Strength 80/4.5 not for use in severe asthma. COPD (strength 160/4.5), 2 inhalations* OR (strength 320/9), 1 inhalation*. *(admin twice daily).

DuoResp Spiromax, asthma (strength 160/4.5), maintenance, 1-2 inhalations*; max. 4 inhalations*; (strength 320/9), maintenance only, 1 inhalation*; max. 2 inhalations*; maintenance and reliever therapy (strength 160/4.5), 2 inhalations daily as single dose or in 2 divided doses (morning, evening); take 1 additional inhalation as needed; if symptoms persist, take an additional inhalation; max. 6 inhalations on any single occasion; 8 inhalations/day normally not needed; 12 inhalations/day can be used for a limited period. COPD (strength 160/4.5), 2 inhalations* OR (strength 320/9), 1 inhalation*. *(admin twice daily).

Child: *Symbicort, asthma* (strengths 100/6, 200/6), maintenance, age 12-17 years, as for Adult; (strength 100/6), age 6 years and over, 2 inhalations twice daily. Maintenance and reliever therapy, under 18 years, not recommended; (strength 400/12), age 12-17 years, 1 inhalation twice daily.

Bufomix, asthma (strengths 80/4.5, 160/4.5), maintenance only, age 12-17 years, 1-2 inhalations* OR (strength 320/9), 1 inhalation*. Age 6 years and older (strength 80/4.5), 2 inhalations*. Not recommended, 160/4.5, 320/9, under 12 years; 80/4.5, under 6 years. Maintenance and reliever therapy, under 18 years, not recommended *(admin twice daily).

Hepatic Impairment: Cirrhosis, increased exposure expected.

CI: Hypersensitivity to inhaled lactose.

Interactions: Effect of Other Drugs on Formoterol, Budesonide: *Co-admin avoid:* Itraconazole, ketoconazole, voriconazole, posaconazole, clarithromycin, telithromycin, nefazodone, ritonavir, HIV protease inhibitors, other potent CYP3A4 inhibitors (allow longest dosing interval possible). See SP below.

SP: Presence of potent CYP3A4 inhibitors, fixed combination (budesonide, formoterol), not recommended.

Pregnancy, Lactation: Use if benefit outweighs risk. Use lowest effective budesonide dose.

ADR: *Common*, Candida infections (oropharynx), headache, tremor, palpitations, throat irritation, coughing, hoarseness.

Notes: See 5.2 Respiratory Corticosteroids.

Symbicort Turbohaler *(AstraZeneca)* B. GMS.
Price, (120-dose) 100/6mcg, €38.53. 200/6mcg, €40.10. (60-dose) 400/12mcg, €38.13.
Inhalation powder, budesonide (mcg)/formoterol fumarate dihydrate (mcg) 400/12, 200/6, 100/6. Metered dose. *Lactose.* **Store:** Below 30 deg C.

Bufomix Easyhaler *(Orion)* B. GMS.
Price, (120-dose) 80mcg, 160mcg and (60-dose) 320mcg, €31.86.
Inhalation powder, budesonide (mcg)/formoterol fumarate dihydrate (mcg) 80/4.5, 160/4.5, 320/9. White (yellowish) in metered inhaler (Easyhaler). *Lactose.* **Store:** No special conditions.

DuoResp Spiromax *(TEVA)* B. GMS.
Price, 160mcg (120-dose) €37.58; 320mcg (60-dose), €36.85.
Inhalation powder, budesonide (mcg)/formoterol fumarate dihydrate (mcg) 160/4.5, 320/9. White powder. *Lactose.*

Ciclesonide

ATC Code: R03BA08. **Sport:** Permitted.
Driving: Unlikely to impair.

Indications: Persistent asthma.

Dose: Adult, Elderly: Initially, 160mcg once daily in evening (morning shown to be effective). Severe asthma and while reducing or discontinuing oral corticosteroids, up to 640mcg/day (320mcg twice daily) may be used. Symptom improvement within 24 hours. Once controlled, individualise dose; reduction to 80mcg once daily may be effective maintenance for some patients. Deteriorating control, consider increased anti-inflammatory treatment e.g. higher doses for a short period or oral corticosteroids.

Child: Under 12 years, not recommended.

Hepatic Impairment: Severe, no data.

Interactions: Effect of Other Drugs on Ciclesonide: *Plasma levels increased:* CYP3A4 inhibitors (ketoconazole, itraconazole, ritonavir, nelfinavir).

ADR: *Uncommon*, nausea, vomiting, bad taste, application site (reaction, dryness), oral fungal infection, headache, dysphonia, cough (after inhalation), paradoxical bronchospasm, eczema, rash.

Notes: See 5.2 Respiratory Corticosteroids.

Alvesco Inhaler 80mcg, 160mcg *(AstraZeneca)* A. GMS.
Price, (60-dose) 80mcg, €15.90. 160mcg, €19.97.
Pressurised inhalation soln, ciclesonide metered dose. Clear colourless. *Ethanol.* **Store:** No special conditions; pressurised container.

Fluticasone (bronchospasm)

ATC Code: R03BA05. **Sport:** Permitted.
Driving: Unlikely to impair.

Indications: Treatment and prevention, asthma, COPD.

Dose: Adult, Elderly: *Evohaler, Diskus, mild asthma*, 100-250mcg twice daily; moderate, 250-500mcg twice daily; severe, 500-1000mcg twice daily. COPD, 500mcg twice daily adjunctive to long-acting bronchodilators (only 250 and 500mcg devices suitable).

Nebules, prophylaxis, treatment of acute exacerbations, 500-2000mcg twice daily.

Child: *Evohaler, Diskus*, asthma, over 4 years, 50-100mcg twice daily adjusting according to individual response.

Nebules, age 4-16 years, acute exacerbations, 1000mcg twice daily.

Interactions: Effect of Other Drugs on Fluticasone:

5.2 Respiratory Corticosteroids and Combinations

Increased systemic exposure (caution): CYP3A4 inhibitors (ketoconazole; ritonavir, avoid).

SP: NOTE: Nebules are not for use alone in acute bronchospasm; intended for regular daily treatment and as anti-inflammatory therapy in acute asthma exacerbations.

Notes: See 5.2 Respiratory Corticosteroids.

Flixotide Evohaler, Diskus, Nebules *(GSK)* B. GMS.
Price, Evohaler 50mcg (120-dose) €8.85. 125mcg (60-dose) €9.15; (120-dose) €18.30. 250mcg (60-dose) €15.44; (120-dose) €30.88. Diskus (60-dose) 50mcg, €5.64. 100mcg, €9.01. 250mcg, €17.95. 500mcg, €29.78. Nebules (10) 0.5mg/2mL, €8.60. 2mg/2mL, €25.46.
Pressurised inhalation susp (Evohaler), fluticasone propionate 50, 125, 250. Metered dose. **Store:** Below 30 deg C; do not (refrigerate, freeze); original pack to protect (frost, direct sunlight). *Inhalation powder (Diskus),* as above 50, 100, 250, 500. Fine white (off-white) powder pre-dispensed *(Diskus)*. *Lactose.* **Store:** Below 30 deg C; dry place.
Nebuliser liquid, as above 0.5mg, 2mg. White opaque susp *(Nebules)*. **Store:** Below 30 deg C; original pack*; do not freeze; once removed from foil use within 28 days*. *(protect from light).

Fluticasone, Formoterol

ATC Code: R03AK11. **Sport:** Restricted. See Notes below.
Driving: No or negligible effect.

Indications: Regular asthma treatment already controlled (inhaled corticosteroid + long acting beta-agonist) or combination appropriate; inadequate control with inhaled corticosteroids and 'as required' short-acting beta-2-agonists OR already controlled (inhaled corticosteroid + long-acting beta-2-agonist).

Dose: Adult, Elderly: *Strength 50/5,* 2 inhalations twice daily. If asthma poorly controlled use (125/5) OR (250/10), 2 inhalations twice daily. Severe asthma, (50/5) not appropriate.

Child: Over 12 years, as for Adult; use only *strengths 50/5 or 125/5.* Under 12 years, not recommended.

Hepatic Impairment: Severe, increased exposure.

Interactions: Effect of Other Drugs on Fluticasone, Formoterol Combination: *Co-admin avoid:* Ritonavir, atazanavir, clarithromycin, indinavir, itraconazole, nelfinavir, saquinavir, ketoconazole, telithromycin.

SP: Contains sodium cromoglicate at non-pharmacological levels; patients should not discontinue cromoglicate-containing medications.

Pregnancy, Lactation: Pregnancy, not recommended unless benefit outweighs risk. Lactation, stop breastfeeding or stop drug.

ADR: See Notes below.

Notes: See 5.2 Respiratory Corticosteroids.

Flutiform Pressurised Inhalation *(Mundipharma)* B. GMS.
Price, (120-dose) 50/5, €25.03. 125/5, €35.34. 250/10, €53.44.
Inhalation susp, fluticasone propionate (mcg), formoterol fumarate dihydrate (mcg) 50(125)/5, 250/10. White (off-white) susp.

Fluticasone, Salmeterol

ATC Code: R03AK06. **Sport:** Restricted. See Notes below.
Driving: No or negligible effect.

Indications: Regular asthma* treatment already controlled on combination (inhaled corticosteroid + long acting beta-agonist) or where use of a combination is appropriate; inadequate control with inhaled corticosteroids and 'on-demand' short-acting beta-2-agonists. Symptomatic COPD treatment with FEV1 below 60% predicted normal and repeated exacerbations, with significant symptoms despite regular long-acting bronchodilator therapy. *(Aerivo, severe asthma).*

Dose: Adult, Elderly: *Seretide, inhaler,* (S) salmeterol 25mcg/(F) fluticasone 50mcg (125mcg, 250mcg), asthma, 2 inhalations of either (25/50) OR (25/125) OR (25/250) twice daily. *Inhalation powder (Diskus),* (S) 50mcg/(F) 100mcg (250mcg, 500mcg), asthma, 1 inhalation of either (50/100) OR (50/250) OR (50/500) twice daily; COPD, 1 inhalation (50/500) twice daily.

AirFluSal (age 12 years and older), asthma, 1 inhalation

(S) 50mcg/(F) 250mcg (50/250) or 1 inhalation (50/500) twice daily. COPD, 1 inhalation (50/500) twice daily.

Aerivio (age 18 years and older), asthma and COPD, 1 inhalation (S) 50mcg/(F) 500mcg twice daily.

Child: *Seretide,* age 4 years and older, *inhaler* salmeterol 25mcg, fluticasone 50mcg (25/50), 2 inhalations twice daily; *inhalation powder (Diskus)* salmeterol 50mcg/fluticasone 100mcg (50/100), 1 inhalation twice daily. Max. fluticasone 100mcg/day. Under 12 years, may have difficulty synchronising aerosol actuation with inspiration of breath.

AirFluSal, not for use in children under 12 years; *Aerivio,* under 18 years.

SP: Not for treatment of acute symptoms. Do not initiate: During exacerbation, worsening or acutely deteriorating asthma. After initiation, if symptoms remain uncontrolled or worsen, advise patient to seek medical advice. Do not stop abruptly. NOTE: Seretide 25/50mcg, not indicated for severe asthma.

Pregnancy, Lactation: Pregnancy, if benefit outweighs risk; use lowest effective fluticasone dose. Lactation, stop breastfeeding or stop drug.

ADR: *Very common,* headache, nasopharyngitis.

Notes: See 5.2 Respiratory Corticosteroids.

Seretide Evohaler, Diskus *(GSK)* B. GMS.
Price, Evohaler (120-dose) 50mcg, €25.06; 125mcg, €33.80; 250mcg, €43.76. Diskus (60-dose) 100mcg, €24.41. 250mcg, €31.65. 500mcg, €40.50.
Pressurised inhalation (Evohaler), salmeterol xinafoate 25mcg, fluticasone propionate 50, 125, 250mcg). White (off-white) susp. **Store:** Below 25 deg C; contains pressurised liquid.
Inhalation powder (Diskus) pre-dispensed, salmeterol 50mcg, fluticasone (100, 250, 500mcg). *Lactose.* **Store:** Below 30 deg C.
Aerivio Spiromax *(TEVA)* B. GMS.
Price, (60-dose) 50/500mcg, €33.85.
Inhalation powder, salmeterol xinafoate 50mcg, fluticasone propionate 500mcg. White powder. *Lactose.* **Store:** Below 25 deg C; keep mouthpiece cover closed.
AirFluSal Forspiro *(Rowex)* B. GMS.
Price, (60-dose) 50/250mcg, €31.67; 50/500mcg, €41.41.
Inhalation powder, salmeterol xinafoate 50mcg, fluticasone propionate 250(500)mcg. White homogenous pre-dispensed in blister. *Lactose.* **Store:** Below 25 deg C.

Fluticasone, Vilanterol

ATC Code: R03AK10. **Sport:** Prohibited.
Driving: No or negligible effect.

Indications: Regular treatment of asthma (combination appropriate; inadequate control with inhaled corticosteroids and 'as needed' inhaled short-acting beta-2 agonists). Symptomatic treatment of COPD (FEV1 below 70%) predicted normal post-bronchodilator (exacerbation history despite regular bronchodilator therapy).

Dose: Adult, Elderly: *Asthma* (age 12 years and over), initially 1 inhalation (92/22mcg) once daily; if inadequately controlled, increase to 1 inhalation (184/22mcg) for additional control. Use strength containing fluticasone dose for severity of disease.

COPD (age 18 years and over), 1 inhalation (92/22mcg) once daily; no additional benefit to use 184/22mcg combination. *Admin,* at same time each day.

Child: *Asthma,* under 12 years not recommended. No relevant use for COPD.

Hepatic Impairment: Increased systemic exposure to fluticasone furoate, caution. Moderate/severe, max. 92/22 per day.

Interactions: Effect of Other Drugs on Fluticasone, Vilanterol Combination: *Co-admin not recommended:* Other long-action beta-2 adrenergic agonists. *Co-admin caution (increased exposure):* Strong CYP3A4 inhibitors (ketoconazole, ritonavir). *Co-admin avoid (unless compelling reasons):* Beta-2 adrenergic blockers (selective and non-selective).

SP: Paradoxical bronchospasm. Increase in pneumonia incidence including needing hospitalisation in COPD patients. Caution, severe cardiovascular disease or rhythm abnormalities, thyrotoxicosis, uncorrected hypokalaemia, low serum potassium (arrhythmias).

Pregnancy, Lactation: Pregnancy, if benefit outweighs risk. Lactation, stop breastfeeding or stop drug.

ADR: Summary, *most common*, headache, nasopharyngitis.

Notes: See 5.2 Respiratory Corticosteroids.

▼ **Relvar Ellipta** *(GSK)* B. GMS.
Price, (30-dose) 92/22, €33.32; 184/22, €39.34.
Inhalation powder, fluticasone furoate, vilanterol trifenatate 92/22mcg, 184/22mcg. White pre-dispensed. *Lactose*. **Store:** Below 25 deg C; original pack to protect (moisture).

Mometasone (bronchospasm)

ATC Code: R03BA07. **Sport:** Permitted.
Driving: Unlikely to impair.

Indications: Persistent asthma *(200mcg, 400mcg)*. Treatment, prophylaxis, seasonal allergic or perennial allergic rhinitis; symptomatic treatment, nasal polyps.

Dose: Adult, Elderly: *Asthma (200mcg, 400mcg strengths)*, mild to moderate, initially 400mcg once daily in evening OR 200mcg twice daily; severe, 400mcg twice daily. Ensure patient in upright position when inhaling.

Allergic rhinitis (50mcg strength), 100mcg (2 actuations) in each nostril once daily; symptoms inadequately controlled, max 200mcg/day in each nostril; symptoms controlled, reduce to 50mcg/day in each nostril. Prophylaxis, initiate up to 4 weeks prior to start of pollen season.

Nasal polyposis (50mcg strength), 100mcg (2 actuations) in each nostril once daily; if inadequately controlled after 5-6 weeks increase to 100mcg in each nostril twice daily (total 400mcg); effective control, reduce to once daily.

Child: *Asthma (200mcg, 400mcg strengths)*, under 12 years, not recommended. *Allergic rhinitis (50mcg strength)*, ages 6-11 years, 50mcg in each nostril once daily (total 100mcg); under 6 years, not recommended; nasal polyposis, under 18 years, not recommended.

CI: Localised infection of nasal mucosa, nasal surgery/trauma.

Interactions: Effect of Other Drugs on Mometasone: *Systemic exposure increased*: CYP3A4 inhibitors (ketoconazole).

SP: Post-dose bronchospasm with increased wheezing, treat with fast-acting inhaled bronchodilator *(200mcg, 400mcg strengths)*. Unilateral polyps, polyps associated with cystic fibrosis, or if completely obstructing nasal cavities, not recommended *(50mcg strength)*.

Pregnancy, Lactation: Lactation, if benefit to mother greater than possible risk to child.

Notes: See 5.2 Respiratory Corticosteroids.

Asmanex Twisthaler 200, 400 *(MSD)* A. GMS.
Price, 200mcg (30-dose) €14.01; (60-dose) €20.58. 400mcg (30-dose) €21.84; (60-dose) €34.64.
Inhalation powder, mometasone furoate 200mcg, 400mcg. White (off-white) powder agglomerates. *Lactose*. **Store:** Below 30 deg C; do not (refrigerate, freeze).

Mometasone (Rowex) 50mcg *(Rowex)* A. GMS.
Price, 50mcg (140-dose) €4.00.
Nasal spray, mometasone furoate monohydrate 50mcg/dose White homogenous susp. *Benzalkonium chloride*.

In This Chapter: *Montelukast, zafirlukast.*

Class Effects
CI: Hypersensitivity to any member of the class.

SP: Not a substitute for inhaled or oral steroids. Caution, severe asthma when steroid reduction is being considered. Rarely, systemic eosinophilia, sometimes presenting with clinical features of systemic vasculitis, consistent with Churg-Strauss syndrome (eosinophilia, vasculitic rash, worsening pulmonary symptoms, cardiac complications and/or neuropathy); re-evaluate treatment regimen.

Montelukast

ATC Code: R03DC03. **Sport:** Permitted.
Driving: No or negligible effect (drowsiness, dizziness).

Indications: Add-on therapy, mild to moderate persistent asthma; alternative to low-dose inhaled corticosteroids in mild persistent asthma. Prophylaxis, exercise-induced bronchospasm. Symptomatic relief, seasonal allergic rhinitis.

Dose: Adult, Elderly: *Asthma, seasonal allergic rhinitis* (15 years and over), 10mg (f/c tab) in evening. *Admin*, f/c tabs with or without food.

Child: *Asthma*, age 6-14 years, 5mg*/day; age 2-5 years, 4mg*/day (evening); age 6 months to 5 years, 1 sachet (4mg)/day (evening). *Admin*, once daily. Chew tabs to be chewed before swallowing; admin 1 hour before or 2 hours after food. Granules, admin directly into mouth or mix with spoonful of soft food; may be taken with or without food; do not dissolve in liquid for admin. Under 15 years, 10mg (f/c tab) not indicated; under 2 years, safety/efficacy not established (4mg*). *(chew tab).

Hepatic Impairment: Severe, no data.

Interactions: Effect of Other Drugs on Montelukast: *Co-admin caution, especially children (exposure decreased)*: CYP3A4, 2C8, 2C9 inducers (phenytoin, phenobarbital, rifampicin). *Potential increased adverse reactions (increased exposure)*: Gemfibrozil.

Effect of Montelukast on Other Drugs: Paclitaxel, rosiglitazone, repaglinide: *Co-admin, caution (metabolism inhibited)*.

SP: Not for use in acute asthma attacks. Add-on therapy to inhaled corticosteroids, do not abruptly substitute montelukast for inhaled corticosteroids. Aspirin-sensitive patients, avoid aspirin, other NSAIDs.

Pregnancy, Lactation: Use only if clearly essential.

ADR: *Common*, headache, abdominal pain.

Notes: See Class Effects 5.3.2 Leukotriene Receptor Antagonists.

Interchangeability: Same strengths of all brands of montelukast f/c tabs 10mg, chewable tabs (4mg, 5mg) and granules (4mg) listed below are deemed interchangeable.

Reference Price: (28) 10mg f/c tab, chewable 5mg, 4mg, €7.56. Granules (28 sachets) 4mg, €13.69.

Singulair 10mg, Paed Chew, Granules *(MSD)* B. GMS.
Price, (28) tabs/chew all strengths, €10.89. Grans 4mg, €17.79.
Tablet, montelukast sodium. Beige rounded square. Marked Singulair; MSD 117 on reverse. *Lactose*. **Store:** Original pack to protect (light, moisture).
Chewable tablet, as above 4mg, 5mg. Pink. Marked Singulair, MSD. *Aspartame*. 4mg: Oval. Marked 711. *Phenylalanine*. 5mg: Round. Marked 275. *Mannitol*. **Store:** As above.
Oral granules (sachet), as above 4mg. White coarse free-flowing. *Mannitol*. **Store:** Below 25 deg C; as above.

Montelair 10mg, Paed Chew *(Clonmel)* B. GMS.
Price, (28) chew 4mg, €5.61; chew 5mg, 10mg f/c, €6.16.
Tablet, montelukast sodium. Beige round. *Lactose*
Chewable tablet, as above 4mg, 5mg. Pink round. Marked M and strength. *Aspartame*.

Montelukast (Accord) 10mg, Paed Chew *(Accord)* B. GMS.
Price, (28) chew 4mg, €5.61; chew 5mg, 10mg f/c, €6.16.
Tablet, montelukast sodium. Beige rounded square. Marked M10. *Lactose*.
Chewable tablet, as above 4mg, 5mg. Pink mottled oval. Marked M and strength. *Aspartame*.

Montelukast (Krka) 10mg, Paed Chew *(Krka)* B. GMS.
Price, (28) chew 4mg, €5.61; chew 5mg, 10mg f/c, €6.16.
Tablet, montelukast sodium. Apricot-coloured round. *Lactose*.
Chewable tablet, as above 4mg, 5mg. Pink marbled round. Marked with strength. *Aspartame*.

Montelukast (Niche) 10mg, Paed Chew *(Niche)* B. GMS.
Price, (28) chew 4mg, €5.61; chew 5mg, 10mg f/c, €6.16.
Tablet, montelukast sodium. Apricot-coloured round. *Lactose*.
Chewable tablet, as above 4mg, 5mg. Pink marbled round. Marked with strength. *Aspartame*.

Montelukast (Rowex) 10mg, Paed Chew *(Rowex)* B. GMS.
Price, (28) chew 4mg, €5.61; chew 5mg, 10mg f/c, €6.16.
Tablet, montelukast sodium. Beige rounded-square. Marked X; 54 on reverse. *Lactose*.
Chewable tablet, as above 4mg, 5mg. Pink mottled oval. Marked X. 4mg: Marked 52. 5mg: Marked 53. *Aspartame, Allura Red*.

Montelukast Actavis 10mg, Paed Chew *(Accord)* B. GMS.
Price, (28) chew 4mg, €5.61; chew 5mg, 10mg f/c, €6.16.
Tablet, montelukast sodium. Beige square. Marked M. *Lactose.*
Chewable tablet, as above 4mg, 5mg. Pink mottled oval. Marked M and strength. *Lactose, aspartame.*
Montelukast Mylan 10mg, Paed Chew *(Gerard)* B. GMS.
Price, (28) chew 4mg, €5.61; chew 5mg, 10mg f/c, €6.16.
Tablet, montelukast sodium. Blue round. Marked MO over 10; M on reverse. *Sunset Yellow.* **Store:** No special conditions.
Chewable tablet (paed), as above 4mg, 5mg. White (off-white) oval. Marked M. 4mg: Marked MS1. 5mg: Marked MS2. *Aspartame.* **Store:** Original pack to protect (light, moisture).
Montelukast TEVA Tab, Paed Chew, Sachets *(TEVA)* B. GMS.
Price, (28) chew 4mg, €5.61; chew 5mg, 10mg f/c, €6.16; granules 4mg (28) €12.32.
Tablet, montelukast sodium 10mg. Beige round f/c. Marked 93; 7426 on reverse. *Lactose.*
Chewable tablet, as above 4mg, 5mg. Pink mottled triangular-shaped. Marked 93 and 7424. *Aspartame.*
Oral granules in sachet, as above 4mg. White (off-white).

Zafirlukast

ATC Code: R03DC01. **Sport:** Permitted.
      Driving: Unlikely to impair.
Indications: Asthma, prophylaxis and chronic treatment, age 12 years and older.
Dose: Adult: Initial, maintenance, 20mg twice daily; titrate to max. 40mg twice daily if needed. Swallow whole with water; should not be taken with food.
Elderly: Over 65 years, clearance reduced. Initiate as for adult; adjust according to clinical response.
Child: Under 12 years, not recommended.
Renal Impairment: Mild to severe, no dosing recommendations, caution.
Hepatic Impairment: Contraindicated, including hepatic cirrhosis.
Interactions: Effect of Zafirlukast on Other Drugs: Warfarin: *Monitor prothrombin time.*
SP: Serum transaminase elevation; early evidence of hepatotoxicity (hepatocellular injury, fulminant hepatitis, liver failure), monitor.
Pregnancy, Lactation: Pregnancy, if benefit outweighs risk. Lactation, not recommended.
ADR: *Very common,* infection.
Notes: See 5.3.2 Leukotriene Receptor Antagonists.
      Accolate 20mg *(AstraZeneca)* B. GMS.
      Price, (56) €21.11.
      Tablet, zafirlukast. White round intagliated f/c. Marked Accolate/strength. *Lactose.*

5.4 - Other Respiratory System Products

In This Chapter: *Doxapram, ivacaftor, ivacaftor/lumacaftor, poractant.*

Class Effects
These drugs are used in specialised units and under the care of specialised physicians. Always consult the manufacturers Full Prescribing Information.
CI: Hypersensitivity to any member of the class.

Doxapram

ATC Code: R07AB01. **Sport:** Prohibited (in-competition).
      Driving: No or negligible effect.
Indications: Ventilatory stimulant following anaesthesia to stimulate ventilation post-op (aid to reduce pulmonary complications, to permit use of effective dose narcotic analgesics without problems of ventilatory depression).
Dose: Adult, Elderly: 1-1.5mg/kg by IV (only) injection over minimum 30 seconds; may be repeated at 1-hour intervals if needed.
Child: Not recommended.
Renal Impairment: No data.
Hepatic Impairment: Caution, metabolised in liver.
CI: Severe hypertension, status asthmaticus, CAD, epilepsy and other convulsive disorders, cerebral oedema, CVA, hyperthyroidism/thyrotoxicosis, physical obstruction of respiratory tract, head injury, pulmonary embolism.
Interactions: Effect of Other Drugs on Doxapram: *Effect*

enhanced: MAOIs. *Increased CNS stimulation with co-admin*: Aminophylline, theophylline.
SP: Admin with oxygen (severe irreversible airway obstruction or decreased lung compliance); use with beta-adrenoceptor bronchodilators (bronchoconstriction). Caution, admin with sympathomimetics (additive pressor effect). Anaesthetics sensitising myocardium to catecholamines (halothane, cyclopropane, enflurane), delay initiation for 10 minutes following end of anaesthesia. May mask residual effects of curare-type muscle relaxants. See Interactions above. Sudden hypertension or dyspnoea, discontinue. Caution, hypermetabolic states (phaeochromocytoma). Monitor BP and deep tendon reflexes to prevent overdose. Do not use with mechanical ventilation. May induce vomiting; ensure airway protection. Hypertension, impaired cardiac reserve, caution.
Pregnancy, Lactation: Pregnancy, use only if compelling reason. Lactation, caution.
ADR: Increased BP, arrhythmias, sinus tachycardia, bradycardia, extrasystoles, chest pain/tightness, dyspnoea, cough, bronchospasm, laryngospasm, nausea, vomiting, urinary retention, urinary bladder stimulation (spontaneous voiding). *Off license use,* in preterm neonates and infants (neurodevelopmental delay, significant QT-interval prolongation with AV block, blood in stools, abdominal distension, necrotising enterocolitis, multiple gastric perforations, early teeth eruption of lower central incisors).
Notes: See 5.4 Other Respiratory System Products.
      Doxapram Parenteral 20mg/mL *(Concordia)* A.
      Price, 5mL (5) €14.70 (PTW).
      Injection, doxapram HCl. Clear colourless soln. **Store:** Below 25 deg C; do not refrigerate.

Ivacaftor

ATC Code: R07AX02. **Sport:** Pending.
      Driving: Minor influence; dizziness.
Indications: Treatment, cystic fibrosis (CF) age 6 years and older and weighing 25kg or more (tabs) or children age 2 years and older and under 25kg (granules) with 1 of the following gating (class III) CFTR gene mutations (G551D, G1244E, G1349D, G178R, G551S, S1251N, S1255P, S549N, S549R); also CF patients age 18 years and older CFTR gene mutation (R117H) (tabs).
Dose: Adult, Elderly: TABS, recommended (age 6 years and older and 25kg or more), 150mg 12-hourly with fat-containing food (300mg/day); avoid grapefruit or Seville oranges; swallow tablets whole; do not break, chew or dissolve.
CYP3A4 inhibitors: Reduce dose to 150mg TWICE WEEKLY with co-admin with strong CYP3A4 inhibitors (ketoconazole, itraconazole, posaconazole, voriconazole, telithromycin, clarithromycin). Reduce dose to 150mg ONCE DAILY with moderate CYP3A4 inhibitors (fluconazole, erythromycin). *Elderly,* over 65 years, no adjustment.
Child: TABS, over 6 years and over 25kg, as for Adult; under 18 years with R117H mutation, efficacy not established.
GRANULES, age 2 years and older, under 14kg, 50mg 12-hourly* (100mg/day); 14kg to under 25kg, 75mg 12-hourly* (150mg/day); 25kg and over, see Adult above. *(with fat-containing food). Under 2 years, no data. *Admin,* by mixing each sachet of granules with 5mL of age-appropriate soft food or liquid; should be consumed immediately. See Adult above.
Reduce dose to 50mg (under 14kg) OR 75mg (14kg to under 25kg) TWICE WEEKLY with co-admin with strong CYP3A4 inhibitors (ketoconazole, itraconazole, posaconazole, voriconazole, telithromycin, clarithromycin). Reduce dose as above but admin ONCE DAILY with co-admin moderate CYP3A4 inhibitors (fluconazole, erythromycin).
Renal Impairment: Mild/moderate, no adjustment. CrCl (mL/min) below 30 or ESRD, caution.
Hepatic Impairment: Moderate, reduce dose to 150mg once daily (adults); 50mg once daily (children* under 14kg); 75mg once daily (children* 14kg to under 25kg). Severe, not recommended unless benefit outweighs risk; use dose as above but dosed every other day. *(age 2 years and older).

Interactions: Effect of Other Drugs on Ivacaftor: *Increased exposure*: CYP3A4 inhibitors (see Dose). *Avoid*: Grapefruit, Seville oranges. *Reduced exposure (reduced ivacaftor efficacy)*: Strong CYP3A4 inhibitors (rifampicin, rifabutin, phenobarbital, carbamazepine, phenytoin, St John's Wort); weak/moderate CYP3A4 inhibitors (dexamethasone, high-dose prednisone).

Effect of Ivacaftor on Other Drugs: CYP3A4 and/or P-gp substrates (alprazolam, diazepam, triazolam; digoxin, ciclosporin, tacrolimus): *Increased or prolonged effect; caution and monitor.* Warfarin: *Monitor INR.*

SP: Confirm presence of 1 gating (class III) mutations (see Indications above) in at least 1 allele of CFTR gene before initiation; use not recommended in patients without gene. Moderate transaminase elevations, monitor LFTs before initiation, every 3 months during year 1, then annually. Use in transplanted patients, not recommended. Cases of non-congenital lens opacities without impact on vision reported (children up to age 12), recommend ophthalmic examinations in children before initiation.

Pregnancy, Lactation: Pregnancy, use only if clearly needed. Lactation, if benefit outweighs risk.

ADR: Summary, *most common* (all ages), nasal congestion, upper respiratory infection, bacteria in sputum, elevated transaminases; (age 6 years and older), headache, oropharyngeal pain, abdominal pain, nasopharyngitis, diarrhoea, dizziness, rash; *serious*, abdominal pain, elevated transaminases.

Notes: See 5.4 Other Respiratory System Products.

▼ **Kalydeco 150mg, Granules** *(Vertex)* A. HT.
Price, tabs, granules (56) €18000.00.
Tablet, ivacaftor. Light-blue cap-shaped f/c. Marked V150. *Lactose*. **Store:** Below 30 deg C.
Granules (sachet), as above 50mg, 75mg. White (off-white). *Lactose*. **Store:** As above.

Ivacaftor, Lumacaftor

ATC Code: R07AX30. **Sport:** Pending.
Driving: No or negligible effect. Ivacaftor may cause dizziness.
Indications: Treatment, cystic fibrosis (CF) in patients 12 years and older who are homozygous for the F508del mutation in the CFTR gene.

Dose: Adult: Age 12 years and older, recommended 2 tabs (lumacaftor 200mg/ivacaftor 125mg) every 12 hours. Total daily dose lumacaftor 800mg/ivacaftor 500mg.
CYP3A4 inhibitors: No adjustment when initiated in patients currently on *Orkambi*. When initiating *Orkambi* in patients taking strong CYP3A4 inhibitors (clarithromycin, telithromycin, itraconazole, ketoconazole, posaconazole, voriconazole)*, reduce *Orkambi* dose to 1 tab daily (lumacaftor 200mg/ivacaftor 125mg) for first week, then recommended dose. *Monitor closely for breakthrough infection as exposure may be reduced. *Admin*, orally with fat-containing food just before or just after dosing. Swallow tabs whole; do not chew, break or dissolve.
Elderly: Age 65 years and older, safety/efficacy not evaluated.
Child: Under 12 years, safety/efficacy not established.
Renal Impairment: Mild/moderate, no adjustment. CrCl (mL/min) below 30 or ESRD, caution.
Hepatic Impairment: Mild, no adjustment; moderate, reduce dose to 2 tabs (morning) and 1 tab (evening). Severe, caution (weigh risk/benefit); max. daily dose 1 tab (morning), 1 tab (evening) (lumacaftor 400mg/ivacaftor 250mg/day).
Interactions: Effect of Other Drugs on Ivacaftor, Lumacaftor Combination: *Increased exposure*: CYP3A4 inhibitors (see Dose). *Co-admin not recommended*: Carbamazepine, phenobarbital, phenytoin (exposure of both substances decreased), St John's Wort. See Notes below (ivacaftor).
Effect of Ivacaftor, Lumacaftor Combination on Other Drugs: Montelukast, clarithromycin, telithromycin, erythromycin, fluconazole, ibuprofen, rifabutin, rifampicin, rifapentine, midazolam, triazolam, hormonal contraceptives, immunosuppressants used after organ transplant (ciclosporin, everolimus, sirolimus, tacrolimus), esomeprazole, lansoprazole, omeprazole, citalopram, escitalopram, sertraline, bupropion, methylprednisolone,

prednisone, repaglinide: *Possible decreased exposure, decreased efficacy.* Fexofenadine, dabigatran, digoxin, warfarin, ranitidine: *Exposure increased or decreased.*

SP: *Orkambi* is not effective in CF patients who are heterozygous for the F508del mutation in the CFTR gene and not for use in CF patients who have a gating (Class III) mutation in the CFTR gene. Respiratory events (chest discomfort, dyspnoea, abnormal respiration) were common during initiation. Additional monitoring if FEV1 is below 40. Not advisable to initiate during pulmonary exacerbation. Increased blood pressure observed, monitor. Advanced liver disease, caution; weigh benefit/risk; monitor closely. Assess liver function (ALT, AST, bilirubin) before initiation, every 3 months (year 1) then annually. Significant AST or ALT elevation with/without elevated bilirubin, discontinue until abnormalities resolve then weigh risk/benefit. Cases of non-congenital lens opacities without impact on vision reported; baseline and follow-up ophthalmological examinations recommended in paediatric patients. Use in transplant patients not recommended.

Pregnancy, Lactation: Pregnancy, avoid. Lactation, stop drug or stop breastfeeding.

ADR: Summary, *most common*, dyspnoea, diarrhoea, nausea; *serious*, hepatobiliary events (elevated transaminases, cholestatic hepatitis, hepatic encephalopathy).

Notes: See Ivacaftor above. See 5.4 Other Respiratory System Products.

▼ **Orkambi 200/125** *(Vertex)* A. HT.
Price, (112) €12144.00.
Tablet, lumacaftor/ivacaftor 200/125mg. Pink oval f/c. Marked 2V125. **Store:** No special conditions.

Poractant alfa

ATC Code: R07AA02. **Sport:** Permitted.
Driving: Not applicable.
Indications: Treatment, respiratory distress syndrome (RDS) or hyaline membrane disease (newborn premature infants 700g or more). Prophylaxis, premature infants (24-31 weeks gestational age) at RDS risk or evidence of surfactant deficiency.
Dose: Adult, Elderly: Paediatric use only.
Child: RESCUE, initially 100-200mg/kg body weight; up to 2 further 100mg/kg doses at 12-hourly intervals if needed; max. total dose 300-400mg/kg.
PROPHYLAXIS, 100-200mg/kg as single dose within 15 minutes after birth; then a further 100mg/kg 6-12 hours after first dose and then after further 12 hours if still intubated; max. as for rescue. *Admin*, by endotracheopulmonary route; via endotracheal tube by disconnecting baby from ventilator, or without disconnecting baby from ventilator, or in delivery room before mechanical ventilation started, or in spontaneous breathing preterm infants using Less Invasive Surfactant Admin with a thin catheter (LISA).
Renal Impairment: Safety/efficacy not evaluation.
Hepatic Impairment: As for Renal above.
SP: Admin by experienced personnel trained in management of preterm infants. Stabilise general condition of baby (correct acidosis, hypotension, anaemia, hypoglycaemia, hypothermia). Increased frequency (bradycardia, apnoea, reduced oxygen saturation) with LISA technique.
ADR: Sepsis, haemorrhage (intracranial, pulmonary), bradycardia, hypotension, bronchopulmonary dysplasia, pneumothorax, hyperoxia, cyanosis neonatal, apnoea, decreased oxygen saturation, abnormal ECG, endotracheal intubation complication.
Notes: See 5.4 Other Respiratory System Products.

Curosurf Endotracheopulmonary Instillation *(Chiesi)* A. HOS.
Price, 120mg/1.5mL. €443.93. 240mg/3mL. €847.17.
Endotracheopulmonary instillation susp, poractant alfa (porcine lung phospholipid) 80mg/mL. White (yellow) sterile susp. **Store:** Refrigerate. Unopened unused vials that have warmed to room temp can be returned to refrigerated storage within 24 hours for future use (only once).

5.5 Mucolytics

5.5 - Mucolytics

In This Chapter: *Bromhexine, carbocisteine, dornase alfa, erdosteine.*

Class Effects
CI: Hypersensitivity to any member of the class.

Bromhexine

ATC Code: R05CB02. **Sport:** Permitted.
Driving: Unlikely to impair.
Indications: Mucolytic; management of mucoid secretions associated with bronchitis, bronchiectasis, sinusitis.
Dose: Adult, Elderly: Oral 8mg 3-times daily; up to 12mg 4-times daily.
Child: Age 5-12 years, 4mg 4-times daily; 2-5 years, 4mg twice daily.
SP: Caution, existing or history of peptic ulceration. Severe skin reactions (erythema multiforme, Stevens-Johnson syndrome, toxic epidermal necrolysis, acute generalised exanthematous pustulosis) reported; signs or symptoms of progressive skin rash, discontinue immediately.
Pregnancy, Lactation: Caution, first trimester not recommended; crosses placental barrier. Lactation, not recommended; passes into breast milk.
ADR: *Uncommon,* diarrhoea, nausea, vomiting, hypersensitivity, rash.
Notes: See 5.5 Mucolytics.

> **Bisolvon Oral Soln** *(SANOFI)* OTC. GMS.
> *Price,* (250mL) €1.79.
> *Oral soln,* bromhexine 4mg/5mL. Colourless faintly opalescent slightly viscous; fruity fresh odour. *Maltitol liquid.* **Store:** Original pack.

Carbocisteine

ATC Code: R05CB03. **Sport:** Permitted.
Driving: Unlikely to impair.
Indications: Mucolytic. Adjunctive, respiratory tract disorders characterised by excessive or viscous mucous.
Dose: Adult, Elderly: *Syrup 250mg/5mL,* 750mg 3-times daily; satisfactory response, reduce to 500mg 3-times daily. *Mucodyne Caps 375mg,* 750mg 3-times daily; reduce to 375mg 4-times daily.
Child: *Syrup* (250mg/5mL), age 6-12 years, 250mg 2-3 times daily; 2-5 years, 125mg 2-3 times daily; or 20mg/kg in divided doses using paediatric syrup.
CI: Active peptic ulceration.
Interactions: Effect of Other Drugs on Carbocisteine: *Carbocisteine precipitation from solution*: Pholcodine linctus.
SP: Caution, elderly, gastroduodenal ulcers, concomitant medication known to cause GI bleeding. Because of possible effect on mucous glands of stomach, history of peptic ulceration, caution.
Pregnancy, Lactation: If benefit outweighs risk.
ADR: Nausea, GI upset, vomiting, GI bleeding, headache, allergic skin reactions, anaphylactic reactions, fixed drug eruption.
Notes: See 5.5 Mucolytics.

> **Exputex 250mg/5mL** *(Phoenix)* OTC. GMS.
> *Price,* (100mL) €1.35. (300mL) €3.37.
> *Oral soln,* carbocisteine. Viscous orange-coloured; condensed milk/orange odour. *Sodium 100mg/15mL dose, parabens, Sunset Yellow, ethanol.*
> **Mucodyne 375mg Caps** *(SANOFI)* OTC. GMS.
> *Price,* (120) €16.01.
> *Capsule,* carbocisteine. Hard opaque yellow; contain white (almost) powder. Marked Mucodyne 375.
> **Viscolex Syrup 250mg/5mL** *(Pinewood)* OTC. GMS.
> *Price,* (100mL) €1.32. (250mL) €2.74.
> *Oral syrup,* carbocisteine. Clear yellow; orange odour/flavour. *Sodium 37.7mg/5mL, parabens, Sunset Yellow, ethanol.*

Dornase alfa

ATC Code: R05CB13. **Sport:** Permitted.
Driving: Unlikely to impair.
Indications: Management of cystic fibrosis, FVC above 40% of predicted, to improve pulmonary function.
Dose: Adult, Elderly: 2.5mg (2500 U) deoxyribonuclease I by inhalation once daily; over 21 years may benefit from twice daily dose. Advise patients to take medication every day without a break; continue with regular medical care including chest physiotherapy.
Child: Under 5 years, not recommended.
SP: RTI exacerbation, continue admin.
Pregnancy, Lactation: Pregnancy, caution, safety/efficacy not established. Lactation, caution; no measurable conc expected in human milk.
ADR: Conjunctivitis, dysphonia, dyspnoea, pharyngitis, laryngitis, rhinitis (non-infectious), dyspepsia, rash, urticaria, chest pain, pleuritic/non-cardiac; pyrexia, decreased pulmonary function tests.
Notes: See 5.5 Mucolytics.

> **Pulmozyme 2500 U/2.5mL** *(Roche)* A. HT.
> *Price,* amps (6) €140.27.
> *Nebuliser soln,* dornase alfa 2500 U (2.5mg) per 2.5mL. Phosphorylated glycosylated recombinant protein human deoxyribonuclease 1. **Store:** Refrigerate; outer carton to protect (light); stability not affected (single 24 hours below 30 deg C).

Erdosteine

ATC Code: R05CB15. **Sport:** Permitted.
Driving: Unlikely to impair.
Indications: Expectorant. Treatment, acute exacerbations of chronic bronchitis.
Dose: Adult, Elderly: 300mg twice daily; max. 10 days. **Admin,** swallow whole with glass of water.
Child: Under 18 years, not recommended.
Renal Impairment: CrCl (mL/min) below 25, not recommended.
Hepatic Impairment: Mild, max. 300mg/day. Severe, not recommended.
CI: Active peptic ulcer.
Pregnancy, Lactation: Not recommended.
ADR: Headache, cold, dyspnoea, taste alterations, nausea, vomiting, diarrhoea, epigastric pain, angioedema, urticaria, erythema, eczema, oedema.
Notes: See 5.5 Mucolytics.

> **Erdotin 300mg** *(Galen)* A. GMS.
> *Price,* (20) €7.19.
> *Capsule,* erdosteine. Hard green/yellow.

5.6 - Cough, Cold and Flu

In This Chapter: *Combinations of sedating antihistamines (diphenhydramine, triprolidine), sympathomimetic decongestants (pseudoephedrine) and cough suppressants (codeine phosphate, dihydrocodeine, dextromethorphan, pholcodine).*

Class Effects
Methoxyphenamine is PROHIBITED for use in sport.
Interactions: Effect of Cold and Flu Preparations On Other Drugs: Preparations containing sedating antihistamines: Anticholinergics (psychotropics, atropine): *Effect potentiated (tachycardia, mouth dryness, urinary retention, headache).* ALCOHOL, barbiturates, sedatives and hypnotics, opioid analgesics, antipsychotics: *Effect potentiated.*
SP: Do not exceed stated dose; if symptoms persist for more than 5 days or worsen consult doctor. Caution, patients taking other cough/cold medication(s). *Sympathomimetics* (including pseudoephedrine), ensure no co-admin by several routes (orally, topically). *Sedating antihistamines,* narrow-angle glaucoma, prostatic hypertrophy. May act as a cerebral stimulant in children (insomnia, nervousness, hyperpyrexia, tremors, epileptiform convulsions); do not leave children on

treatment unattended. *Opioid analgesics,* constipation, drug or alcohol addiction; physical and psychological dependence resulting in withdrawal (restlessness, irritability) when stopped. *Cough suppressants, decongestants,* use under medical supervision for persistent or chronic cough (smoking, asthma, emphysema, excessive secretions).

Pregnancy, Lactation: If benefit outweighs risk.

ADR: *Sedating antihistamines,* drowsiness, dizziness, GI disturbance; dry (mouth, nose, throat); urination difficulty, blurred vision, hypersensitivity reactions (skin rash, bronchospasm, angioedema, anaphylaxis).

Notes: See 4.2.2 Opioid Analgesics (codeine phosphate). See 5.7.1 Sedating Antihistamines.

Dihydrocodeine (cough)

ATC Code: N02AA08. **Sport:** Permitted.
Driving: Caution.
Indications: Management of non-productive cough.

Dose: Adult, Elderly: 10-30mg (tabs) OR 5-10mL (syrup) OR 14-20 drops up to 3-times daily.

Child: Age 12 years and over, as for Adult; age 6-12 years, 2.5-5mL syrup or 6-12 drops up to 3-times daily. Under 6 years (syrup, drops) or under 12 years (tabs), contraindicated.

Renal Impairment: Chronic, reduce dose.

Hepatic Impairment: As for Renal above.

CI: Respiratory depression, obstructive airways disease, opiate addiction, elevated intracranial pressure, hypotension, hypovolaemia. Long-term admin in chronic constipation.

Interactions: Effect of Other Drugs on Dihydrocodeine: *Caution:* MAOIs (or within 2 weeks).

SP: Not for admin during asthma attack or if likely. Hypothyroidism, reduce dose. Alcohol, avoid.

ADR: Constipation, nausea, vomiting, headache, vertigo.

Notes: See 5.6 Cough, Cold, Flu. See also 4.2.2 Opioid Analgesics.

Paracodin 10mg, Syrup, Drops *(Teofarma)* A. GMS.
Price, tabs 10mg (20) €3.13. Drops, syrup, not reimbursed.
Tablet, dihydrocodeine hydrogen tartrate. Round off-white. *Lactose.*
Oral syrup, as above 12.1mg/5mL. Clear colourless (faintly yellow); cherry flavour. *Sucrose.*
Oral drops, dihydrocodeine hydrorhodanide 0.5mg/drop. Clear brown soln.

Pseudoephedrine

ATC Code: R01BA02. **Sport:** Prohibited (in-competition; urine conc above 150mcg/mL).
Driving: No or negligible effect.
Indications: Symptomatic relief of nasal congestion (allergic rhinitis, vasomotor rhinitis, common cold, influenza).

Dose: Adult, Elderly: 60mg (1 tab or 10mL) every 4-6 hours, up to 4-times daily.

Child: Age 6-12 years, 5mL syrup every 4-6 hours, up to 4-times daily; max. 20mL. Age 12 years and over, as for Adult above.

Renal Impairment: Severe, caution.

Hepatic Impairment: As for Renal above.

CI: Hypertension, acute ischaemic heart disease, thyrotoxicosis, glaucoma, urinary retention, at risk for respiratory failure.

Interactions: Effect of Other Drugs on Pseudoephedrine: *Co-admin contraindicated:* MAOIs (within preceding 2 weeks), other sympathomimetics, furazolidone. *Co-admin caution:* Antihypertensives, TCADs, other sympathomimetics (decongestants, appetite suppressants, amphetamine-like psychostimulants). *Antihypertensive action reversed:* Bretylium, bethanidine, guanethidine, reserpine, debrisoquine, methyldopa, alpha- and beta-blockers. *Ventricular arrhythmias provoked or worsened:* Chloroform, cyclopropane, halothane, enflurane, isoflurane.

SP: Insomnia, nervousness, hyperpyrexia, tremor, epileptiform convulsions. May increase blood sugar level.

Pregnancy, Lactation: Pregnancy, caution, use if benefit outweighs risk. Lactation, effect on breast-fed infant not known.

ADR: CNS excitation (sleep disturbances, hallucinations), skin rash, urinary retention, cardiovascular (increased heart rate, tachycardia, palpitations).

Notes: See 5.6 Cough, Cold, Flu.

Non-Drowsy Sudafed Tabs, Syrup *(McNeil)* OTC.
Price, not published by company. 60mg (12, 24).
Tablet, pseudoephedrine HCl 60mg. Reddish-brown round f/c. Marked Sudafed. *Lactose.*
Syrup, as above 30mg/5mL. Clear red; raspberry odour/taste. *Parabens, Ponceau 4R.*

5.7 - Anti-Allergic Drugs

5.7.1 - Sedating Antihistamines

In This Chapter: *Chlorphenamine, hydroxyzine, promethazine.*

Class Effects

Indications: Generally used for symptomatic relief of allergic conditions (rhinitis, conjunctivitis), cough and symptoms of the common cold (often in combination), pruritic skin conditions as well as severe allergic conditions.

CI: Hypersensitivity to any member of the class. Hepatic or renal dysfunction, epilepsy, Parkinson's disease, hypothyroidism, phaeochromocytoma, myasthenia gravis, prostatic hypertrophy, glaucoma, agranulocytosis associated with phenothiazines, coma especially if associated with other CNS depressants, concomitant haemotoxic drugs (some products list these as a Special Warning, see SP below).

Interactions: Effect of Other Drugs on Sedating Antihistamines: *Co-admin not recommended (avoid):* MAOIs (or within 2 weeks of admin).

Effect of Sedating Antihistamines on Other Drugs: CNS depressants (ALCOHOL, barbiturates, sedatives, hypnotics, anxiolytics, opioid analgesics, antipsychotics): *Enhanced sedative effect.* Anticholinergics (atropine, some psychotropics): *Effect potentiated (tachycardia, dry mouth, GI disturbance, dyskinesia, colic, urinary retention, headache).* Ototoxics (aminoglycosides): *Ototoxicity masked.*

SP: May act as cerebral stimulant especially in children (insomnia, nervousness, hyperpyrexia, tremors, epileptiform convulsions); do not leave children unattended. Caution, epilepsy, prostatic hypertrophy, glaucoma, hepatic or renal impairment; bronchitis, bronchiectasis, asthma (thickened lung secretions), thyrotoxicosis, raised IOP, severe hypertension, cardiovascular disease, coronary insufficiency (caution hypotension, especially elderly). Prolonged use, jaundice, blood dyscrasias, monitor. Children, elderly more prone to neurological anticholinergic effects.

Pregnancy, Lactation: Pregnancy, if benefit outweighs risk. Lactation, not recommended.

ADR: Extrapyramidal disorders, depression, sedation ranging from drowsiness to deep sleep, lassitude, dizziness, incoordination, headache, psychomotor impairment, convulsions, tremor, sleep disturbances, inability to concentrate. Thickened respiratory tract secretions, blurred vision, urinary retention, dry mouth, nausea, vomiting, diarrhoea, epigastric pain, abdominal pain, constipation, dyspepsia, anorexia, rash, bronchospasm, angioedema, exfoliative dermatitis, photosensitivity, urticaria, agranulocytosis, leucopenia, haemolytic anaemia, thrombocytopenia, increased sweating, palpitation, tachycardia, arrhythmia, hypotension, ECG changes, hepatitis, jaundice. Paradoxical excitation in children. Confusional psychosis in elderly. Effects of alcohol increased.

Notes: See 3.2.1 Phenothiazines, 5.6 Cough, Cold and Flu.

191

5.7.2 Non-Sedating Antihistamines

Chlorphenamine

ATC Code: R06AB04. **Sport:** Permitted.
Driving: Drowsiness.
Indications: Acute allergic reactions.
Dose: Adult, Elderly: ORAL, 4mg every 4-6 hours; max. 24mg in 24 hours (elderly max. 12mg).
PARENTERAL, 10-20mg; max 40mg in 24 hours. *Admin,* SC, IM or IV slowly over 1 minute to avoid (hypotension, CNS stimulation).
Child: ORAL, age 6-12 years, 0.1mg/kg or 2mg every 4-6 hours; max. 12mg in 24 hours.
PARENTERAL, age 1 month to 1 year, 0.25mg/kg; age 1-5 years, 2.5-5mg OR 0.2mg/kg; age 6-12 years, 5-10mg OR 0.2mg/kg; age 12-18 years, 10-20mg OR 0.2mg/kg.
CI: Pre-coma states.
Interactions: Effect of Other Drugs on Chlorphenamine: *Co-admin contraindicated:* MAOIs.
Effect of Chlorphenamine on Other Drugs: Phenytoin: *May inhibit metabolism leading to toxicity.*
Pregnancy, Lactation: Use during third trimester may result in reaction in newborn or premature neonates.
ADR: Children more likely to experience neurological anticholinergic effects; paradoxical excitation (agitation).
Notes: See 5.7.1 Sedating Antihistamines.

> **Chlorphenamine Parenteral 10mg/mL** *(KyowaKirin)* A.
> *Price,* 10mg/1mL (5) €18.93.
> *Injection,* chlorphenamine maleate. Clear colourless soln. **Store:** Below 25 deg C; outer carton; protect (light).
> **Piriton 4mg** *(GSK Consumer)* OTC.
> *Price,* not published by company.
> *Tablet,* chlorphenamine maleate. Yellow round scored (divisible in equal halves). Marked P. *Lactose.*

Hydroxyzine

ATC Code: N05BB01. **Sport:** Permitted.
Driving: Tiredness, dizziness, sedation, visual disturbances especially at higher doses and/or with alcohol or sedative drugs.
Indications: Management, anxiety and tension states, psychomotor agitation, acute stress (allergic states, minor surgery). Treatment, allergic pruritus (chronic urticaria; atopic, contact or histamine-related pruritus).
Dose: Adult: Adults and children over 40kg (max. 100mg/day), *pruritus,* initially 25mg before resting, then up to 25mg 3-4 times daily; *anxiety,* 50mg/day as 12.5mg (morning and midday), 25mg at night; up to max. 100mg/day can be used.
Elderly: Initiate with half adult dose due to prolonged action; max. 50mg/day. Use not recommended because of decreased elimination and increased risk of adverse reactions (anticholinergic effects).
Child: From 12 months, up to 40kg, max. 2mg/kg/day; over 40kg, as for Adult above, max. 100mg/day. Symptomatic treatment of pruritus, 1-2mg/kg/day in divided doses.
Renal Impairment: Moderate to severe, reduce dose due to decreased excretion of metabolite cetirizine.
Hepatic Impairment: Reduce dose by 33%.
CI: Hypersensitivity to cetirizine, other piperazine derivatives, aminophylline, ethylenediamine. Porphyria, pre-existing prolonged QT-interval or known risk factors (cardiovascular disease, electrolyte imbalance, family history of sudden cardiac death, significant bradycardia).
Interactions: Effect of Other Drugs on Hydroxyzine: *Co-admin contraindicated:* Drugs prolonging QT-interval or inducing Torsade de Pointes including antiarrhythmics Class IA (quinidine, disopyramide), Class III (amiodarone, sotalol), some antihistamines, antipsychotics (haloperidol), antidepressants (citalopram, escitalopram), mefloquine, erythromycin, levofloxacin, moxifloxacin, pentamidine, prucalopride, toremifene, vandetanib, methadone. *Co-admin caution:* Drugs causing bradycardia or inducing hypokalaemia. *Plasma levels increased:* Potent liver enzyme inhibitors, cimetidine.
Effect of Hydroxyzine on Other Drugs: Adrenaline, phenytoin, anticholinesterases, betahistine: *Effect antagonised.*

SP: Convulsions, especially children. Avoid use with alcohol. Arrhythmias, caution. Cases of prolonged QT-intervals and Torsade de Pointes (usually with other risk factors); signs or symptoms of arrhythmias, discontinue immediately.
Pregnancy, Lactation: Contraindicated.
ADR: Summary, mainly related to (CNS depressant or paradoxical CNS stimulation effects, anticholinergic activity, hypersensitivity reactions).
Notes: See 5.7.1 Sedating Antihistamines.

> **Ucerax 25mg, Syrup 10mg/5mL** *(UCB)* B. GMS.
> *Price,* 25mg (25) €1.41. Syrup 200mL, €2.02.
> *Tablet,* hydroxyzine HCl. White oblong f/c scored (divisible into equal halves). *Lactose.*
> *Oral syrup,* as above. Clear colourless (slightly yellowish); odour, taste (menthol, hazelnut). *Ethanol, sucrose.*

Promethazine

ATC Code: R06AD02. **Sport:** Permitted.
Driving: Caution.
Indications: Allergic conditions and reactions. Anti-emetic. Tranquiliser.
Dose: Adult, Elderly: Usually 25-75mg as single oral daily dose at bedtime or in 3 divided doses.
Child: Using oral soln, age 6-12 years as tranquiliser, 25mg at bedtime. Other indications, age 2-5 years, 5-15mg once daily; 5-10 years, 10-25mg once daily. When 2 doses are required in 24 hours, use lower dose.
CI: Pre-coma states, blood dyscrasias.
Interactions: Effect of Promethazine on Other Drugs: Antihypertensives: *Adjust dose (hypotension).* Anticonvulsants: *Adjust dose (convulsion threshold lowered).* Hepatotoxic drugs: *Increased toxicity.* Photosensitising drugs (tetracyclines): *Additive effect.*
SP: Not for use in children under 2 years, potential fatal respiratory depression risk. Body temperature drop, caution elderly. May delay early diagnosis of intestinal obstruction or increased intracranial pressure by suppressing vomiting. May mask signs of ototoxicity caused by ototoxic drugs (salicylates). NMS. Children or adolescents with signs or symptoms of Reye's Syndrome, avoid. Risk of drug abuse (risk greater with drug abuse history).
Pregnancy, Lactation: If benefit outweighs risk; 2 weeks prior to delivery, not recommended (irritability and excitement in neonate). Lactation, not recommended.
ADR: See Notes below.
Notes: See 5.7.1 Sedating Antihistamines and 3.2.1 Phenothiazines.

> **Phenergan 25mg, Oral Soln** *(SANOFI)* OTC. GMS.D.
> *Price,* tabs (56) €1.91. Oral soln, not published by company (non-GMS/D).
> *Tablet,* promethazine HCl. Pale-blue round f/c. Marked PN25.
> *Oral soln,* as above 5mg/5mL. Clear bright golden; orange odour. *Maltitol, sulphite, benzoate.*

5.7.2 - Non-Sedating Antihistamines

In This Chapter: Bilastine, cetirizine, desloratadine, fexofenadine, levocetirizine, loratadine, ketotifen, sodium cromoglicate.

Class Effects

CI: Hypersensitivity to any member of the class.
SP: Antihistamines (class) associated with tachycardia, palpitations (patients with cardiovascular disease or history of). Response to allergy skin tests are inhibited by antihistamines; a wash-out (3 days) is needed.
Notes: See also 5.7.1 Sedating Antihistamines.

Bilastine

ATC Code: R06AX29. **Sport:** Permitted.
Driving: Drowsiness.
Indications: Allergic rhino-conjunctivitis (seasonal, perennial), urticaria.
Dose: Adult: 20mg once daily. Oral 1 hour before or 2 hours after food.
Elderly: Over 65 years, caution.

Child: Under 12 years, no data.

Interactions: Effect of Other Drugs on Bilastine: *Bioavailability decreased*: Food, grapefruit (and other) juices. *Plasma levels decreased*: Ritonavir, rifampicin. *Severe renal impairment, increased plasma levels with co-admin (avoid)*: P-glycoprotein inhibitors (ketoconazole, erythromycin, ciclosporin, ritonavir, diltiazem).

Pregnancy, Lactation: Pregnancy, avoid. Lactation, stop breastfeeding or stop drug.

ADR: *Common*, somnolence, headache.

Notes: See 5.7.2 Non-Sedating Antihistamines.

Drynol 20mg *(A.Menarini)* B. GMS.
Price, (30) €7.45.
Tablet, bilastine. Oval white scored (facilitates breaking). **Store:** No specific conditions.

Cetirizine

ATC Code: R06AE07. **Sport:** Permitted.
Driving: Unlikely to impair at usual dose; reduced alertness, impaired performance with alcohol/other CNS depressants.

Indications: Relief of, nasal and ocular symptoms of seasonal and perennial allergic rhinitis; symptoms of chronic idiopathic urticaria. Senile pruritus *(Zirpine)*.

Dose: Adult: Age 12 years and over, 10mg once daily (1 tab or 10mL oral soln). *Admin*, swallow tabs with glass of liquid; tabs can be swallowed as such.

Elderly: As for Renal below.

Child: Age 6-12 years, 5mg twice daily (half tab or 5mL oral soln); age 2-6* years, 2.5mg (2.5mL oral soln) twice daily. *(tablet formulation not suitable).

Renal Impairment: CrCl (mL/min) 50 and above, 10mg once daily; 30-49, 5mg once daily; below 30, 5mg once every 2 days; below 10 (ESRD/dialysis), contraindicated; not effectively removed by dialysis.

Hepatic Impairment: Only hepatic, no adjustment. Hepatic and renal impairment, as for CrCl (mL/min) 49 and below.

CI: Hydroxyzine hypersensitivity.

SP: No clinically significant interaction with ALCOHOL (blood level 0.5g/L; caution is recommended). May increase risk of urinary retention; caution with risk factors (spinal cord lesion, prostatic hyperplasia). Caution, epilepsy, patients at risk of convulsions. Absorption rate (not extent) may be decreased if taken with food. Pruritus and/or urticaria may occur on discontinuation; usually resolve when treatment is restarted.

Pregnancy, Lactation: Pregnancy, lactation, caution; passes into breast milk.

ADR: Summary, *minor* CNS effects (somnolence, fatigue, dizziness, headache). Paradoxical CNS stimulation. Isolated cases (micturition difficulty, eye accommodation disorders, dry mouth).

Notes: See 5.7.2 Non-Sedating Antihistamines.

Interchangeability: Same strengths of all cetirizine 10mg f/c tabs listed below are deemed interchangeable.

Zirtek 10mg *(UCB)* OTC. GMS.
Price, (30) €2.05.
Tablet, cetirizine dihydrochloride. White oblong f/c scored (divisible into equal doses). Marked with Y-Y logo. *Lactose*.

Zirtek Oral Soln *(UCB)* OTC.
Price, (200mL) €11.87.
Oral soln, cetirizine dihydrochloride 1mg/mL. Clear colourless liquid. *Sorbitol, parabens*.

Cetrine 10mg *(Rowex)* B. GMS.
Price, (30) €2.05.
Tablet, cetirizine dihydrochloride. White oblong f/c scored (divisible into equal halves). *Lactose*.

Histek 10mg *(Fannin)* B. GMS.
Price, (30) €2.05.
Tablet, cetirizine dihydrochloride. White (almost) oval f/c scored (divisible into equal halves). Marked C; J and E on reverse. *Lactose*.

Zirpine 10mg *(Pinewood)* B. GMS.
Price, (30) €2.05.
Tablet, cetirizine dihydrochloride. White f/c scored. Marked AG.

Zirtene 10mg *(Gerard)* B. GMS.
Price, (30) €2.05.
Tablet, cetirizine dihydrochloride. White cap-shaped f/c scored (facilitates breaking). Marked CZ and 10; G on reverse. *Lactose*.

Desloratadine

ATC Code: R06AX27. **Sport:** Permitted.
Driving: No or negligible effect.

Indications: Allergic rhinitis, urticaria.

Dose: Adult, Elderly: Age 12 years and over, 5mg/day. Oral, once daily, with or without food.

Child: Age 6-11 years, 2.5mg/day (5mL oral soln); 1-5 years, 1.25mg/day (2.5mL oral soln). Admin once daily. Under 1 year, no data. Most cases of rhinitis below 2 years is usually of infectious origin; no data to support treatment with desloratadine.

Renal Impairment: Severe, caution.

SP: Cases of alcohol intolerance and intoxication reported (with ALCOHOL).

Pregnancy, Lactation: Pregnancy, avoid as precautionary measure. Lactation, stop breastfeeding or stop drug.

ADR: *Common*, headache, dry mouth, fatigue; *children*, headache.

Notes: See 5.7.2 Non-Sedating Antihistamines.

Neoclarityn 5mg, Syrup *(MSD)* B. GMS.
Price, 5mg (30) €5.59. Syr 100mL, €5.28. 150mL, €6.72.
Tablet, desloratadine. Blue f/c. Marked with logo. *Lactose*.
Oral soln, as above 0.5mg/mL. *Sucrose, sorbitol*.

Dasselta 5mg *(Krka)* B. GMS.
Price, (30) €4.47.
Tablet, desloratadine. Light-blue round f/c. *Lactose*.

Deslor 5mg, Oral Soln *(Rowex)* B. GMS.
Price, (30) €4.47. Oral soln (100mL) €3.23.
Tablet, desloratadine. Round f/c light-blue. Marked 5.
Oral soln, as above 0.5mg/mL. Clear colourless. *Sorbitol*.

Desloratadine Actavis 5mg *(Accord)* B. GMS.
Price, (30) €4.47.
Tablet, desloratadine. Blue round f/c. Marked LT.

Desloratadine Ratiopharm 5mg *(TEVA)* B. GMS.
Price, (30) €4.47.
Tablet, desloratadine. Blue round f/c. *Lactose*.

Efestad 5mg *(Clonmel)* B. GMS.
Price, (30) €4.47.
Tablet, desloratadine. Round f/c blue. *Isomalt*.

Fexofenadine

ATC Code: R06AX26. **Sport:** Permitted.
Driving: Unlikely to impair.

Indications: Age 12 years and over, seasonal allergic rhinitis *(120mg)*. Chronic idiopathic urticaria *(180mg)*.

Dose: Adult, Elderly: Allergic rhinitis, 120mg/day; urticaria, 180mg/day. *Admin*, once daily before food. *Elderly*, caution.

Child: Under 12 years, not recommended.

Renal Impairment: Caution.

Hepatic Impairment: Caution.

Interactions: Effect of Other Drugs on Fexofenadine: *Plasma levels increased*: Erythromycin, ketoconazole. *Reduced bioavailability*: Aluminium or magnesium hydroxide gels (admin 2 hours apart).

SP: Fexofenadine is an active metabolite of terfenadine.

Pregnancy, Lactation: Pregnancy, use only if clearly necessary. Lactation, not recommended.

ADR: *Common*, headache, drowsiness, dizziness, nausea.

Notes: See 5.7.2 Non-Sedating Antihistamines.

Telfast 120mg, 180mg *(SANOFI)* B. GMS.
Price, (30) 120mg, €5.05. 180mg, €6.57.
Tablet, fexofenadine HCl. Peach modified cap-shaped f/c. Marked e. 120mg: Marked 012. 180mg: Marked 018.

Fexofenadine 120mg, 180mg *(Niche)* B. GMS.
Price, (30) 120mg, €4.04. 180mg, €5.26.
Tablet, fexofenadine HCl. Oblong f/c. 120mg: Peach. 180mg: Yellow scored (facilitates breaking).

Levocetirizine

ATC Code: R06AE09. **Sport:** Permitted.
Driving: Somnolence, fatigue, asthenia.

Indications: Allergic rhinitis. Urticaria.

Dose: Adult: Age 12 years and above, 5mg once daily. *Admin*, swallow tabs whole with liquid, with or without food. Oral soln to be measured with oral syringe provided and poured into a spoon or glass of water.

5.7.3   Other Drugs Used In Allergic Disorders

Elderly: As for Renal below.

Child: Age 6-12 years, 5mg once daily; age 2-6 years, 1.25mg twice daily; over 12 years, as for Adult above. Under 2 years, insufficient data.

Renal Impairment: Adult, CrCl (mL/min) 50 and above, 5mg daily; 30-49, 5mg every 2 days; below 30, 5mg every 3 days; below 10, ESRD/dialysis, contraindicated.

CI: Hypersensitivity to hydroxyzine or piperazine derivatives.

Interactions: Effect of Other Drugs on Levocetirizine: *Caution*: ALCOHOL, other CNS depressants.

SP: Caution, concurrent alcohol intake (additional reduction in alertness, impaired performance); predisposing factors e.g. spinal cord lesion, prostatic hyperplasia as levocetirizine may increase urinary retention risk.

Pregnancy, Lactation: Pregnancy, use may be considered if necessary. Lactation, caution.

ADR: *Common*, headache, somnolence, dry mouth, fatigue.

Notes: See Cetirizine above. See 5.7.2 Non-Sedating Antihistamines.

Interchangeability: Same strengths of all levocetirizine f/c tabs listed below are deemed interchangeable.

Xyzal 5mg, Oral Soln, Drops *(UCB)* B. GMS.
Price, 5mg (30) €5.42. Soln 200mL, €5.81. Drops 20mL, €9.74.
Tablet, levocetirizine dihydrochloride. White (off-white) oval f/c. Marked with Y logo. *Lactose*. **Store:** No specific conditions.
Oral soln, as above 0.5mg/mL, drops 5mg/mL. Clear colourless. *Parabens, maltitol.* **Store:** As above. Protect drops from light.

Levocetirizine Glenmark 5mg *(Rowex)* B. GMS.
Price, (30) €4.34.
Tablet, levocetirizine dihydrochloride. White oval scored (divisible into equal halves). Marked G either side of score. *Lactose*.

Levocetirizine Krka 5mg *(Krka)* B. GMS.
Price, (30) €4.34.
Tablet, levocetirizine dihydrochloride. White round f/c. *Lactose*.

Rinozal 5mg *(Clonmel)* B. GMS.
Price, (30) €4.34.
Tablet, levocetirizine dihydrochloride. White (off-white) oval f/c. Marked L9CZ; 5 on reverse. *Lactose*.

Loratadine

ATC Code: R06AX13. **Sport:** Permitted.
Driving: Drowsiness (very rarely).

Indications: Allergic rhinitis, chronic idiopathic urticaria.

Dose: Adult, Elderly: Age 12 years and over, 10mg once daily with or without food.

Child: Age 2-12 years, over 30kg, 10mg once daily; under 30kg, 5mg* once daily Under 2 years, safety/efficacy not established. *10mg f/c tablet not suitable unless divisible into equal halves (brand *Lorat*)

Hepatic Impairment: Severe, initially 10mg every other day (adults, children over 30kg); under 30kg, 5mg every other day. See Child above.

Interactions: Effect of Other Drugs on Loratadine: *Increased plasma levels (no clinical significance)*: Ketoconazole, erythromycin, cimetidine. *Plasma levels (potentially) elevated*: CYP3A4 or CYP2D6 inhibitors.

Pregnancy, Lactation: Pregnancy, avoid. Lactation, not recommended.

ADR: *Summary, most frequent*, somnolence, headache, increased appetite, insomnia.

Notes: See 5.7.2 Non-Sedating Antihistamines.

Clarityn 10mg *(Bayer)* OTC.
Price, (7) €3.99; (30) €9.99.
Tablet, loratadine. White (off-white) oval scored (facilitates breaking). Marked with logo and strength. *Lactose*.

Lorat 10mg *(Rowex)* B. GMS.
Price, (30) €8.49.
Tablet, loratadine. White oval scored (divisible into equal halves). Marked LT10. *Lactose*.

Histaclar 10mg *(Gerard)* B. GMS.
Price, (30) €8.93.
Tablet, loratadine. White round f/c scored (divisible into equal halves). Marked LR 10. *Lactose*.

5.7.3 - Other Drugs Used In Allergic Disorders

In This Chapter: *Allergen extracts (grass pollen), ketotifen.*

Class Effects
CI: Hypersensitivity to any member of the class.
Notes: See 5.7 Anti-Allergic Drugs.

Allergen Extract (Grass Pollen)

ATC Code: V01AA02. **Sport:** Permitted.
Driving: Unlikely to impair.

Indications: Disease-modifying treatment, grass pollen induced rhinitis and conjunctivitis.

Dose: Adult: *Grazax*, 1 oral lyophilisate daily. Place under tongue to disperse; avoid swallowing for 1 minute; do not take food or drink for following 5 minutes. Duration, 3 years.
Oralair, initiation, 1x 100 IR (day 1), 2x 100 IR (day 2), 1x 300 IR (days 3-30); continue with 1x 300 IR daily until end of pollen season. Place under tongue until completely dissolved (at least 1 minute), then swallow; morning preferably on empty stomach. See SP below.

Elderly: No data, over 65 years *(Grazax)*, over 50 years *(Oralair)*.

Child: Age 5 years and older, as for Adult above.

CI: Malignancy, systemic immune system diseases, inflammatory conditions of oral cavity including oral lichen planus with ulcerations, severe oral mycosis, uncontrolled or severe asthma.

Interactions: Effect of Other Drugs on Allergen Extract (Grass Pollen): *Increased tolerance to immunotherapy*: Symptomatic anti-allergics (antihistamines, corticosteroids, mast cell stabilisers) *(Grazax)*.

SP: Admin first dose under medical supervision; monitor for 20-30 minutes; initiate 4 months prior to expected start of grass pollen season; continue throughout season; no relevant improvement during first pollen season, no indication to continue. Oral surgery including dental extraction, stop treatment for 7 days to allow healing. *Allergic reactions*, local, significant, treat with anti-allergics. Systemic, flushing, intensive itching of palms of hands, soles of feet, nettle rash, heat, general discomfort, agitation/anxiety; angioedema, swallowing difficulty, breathing difficulty, voice changes, feeling of fullness in throat; discontinue, seek medical advice. Severe, treat with adrenaline. Simultaneous vaccination, no data; evaluate general condition of patient.

Pregnancy, Lactation: Pregnancy, do not initiate; if pregnancy occurs during treatment, evaluate patient condition; pre-existing asthma, close supervision. Lactation, no effects on infant anticipated.

ADR: *Very common*, ear pruritus, throat irritation, sneezing, oral oedema/pruritus. See SP above.

Notes: See 5.7.3 Other Drugs Used In Allergic Disorders.

Grazax 75000 SQ-T *(ALK-Abello)* B. GMS.
Price, (30) €81.00
Oral lyophilisate, standardised allergen extract of grass pollen from Timothy *(Phleum pratense)* 75000 SQ-T. White (off-white). Marked with image.

Oralair Sublingual 100IR, 300IR *(Stallergenes)* B. GMS.
Price, initiation pack (3 x 100IR and 28 x 300IR tabs) €83.68. Tabs 300IR (30) €85.68. (90) €257.04.
Sublingual tablet, standardised allergen extract of grass pollen from Cocksfoot, Sweet vernal grass, rye grass, meadow grass, Timothy 100IR*, 300IR*. Slightly speckled white (beige). Marked with strength. *Lactose*. *Index of Reactivity.

Ketotifen (systemic)

ATC Code: R06AX17. **Sport:** Permitted.
Driving: Caution.

Indications: Prophylaxis, bronchial asthma. Treatment, allergic rhinitis, conjunctivitis.

Dose: Adult, Elderly: 1mg twice daily with food; titrate to 2mg twice daily if needed; if known to be easily sedated, initially 0.5-1mg at night (first few days).

Child: Age 2-3 years, 0.05mg/kg body weight twice daily (morning, evening); over 3 years, 1mg twice daily. With food.

194

Interactions: Effect of Other Drugs on Ketotifen: *Co-admin avoid*: Oral antidiabetic agents.

Effect of Ketotifen on Other Drugs: Sedatives, hypnotics, antihistamines, ALCOHOL: *Effect potentiated*.

SP: Asthma exacerbation, continue existing treatment for minimum 2 weeks after starting ketotifen; especially systemic corticosteroids. Discontinue over 2-4 weeks; asthma symptoms may recur. Infection, treat with specific antibiotic. Caution, may lower seizure threshold.

Pregnancy, Lactation: Not recommended.

ADR: Drowsiness, dry mouth, slight dizziness, CNS stimulation, weight gain, cystitis, rarely severe skin reaction (erythema multiforme, Stevens-Johnson Syndrome).

Notes: See 5.7.2 Non-Sedating Antihistamines.

> **Zaditen 1mg, Oral Soln** *(CD Pharma)* B. GMS.
> *Price*, 1mg (60) €10.71. Soln 300mL, €11.75.
> *Tablet*, ketotifen hydrogen fumarate equiv. to 1mg ketotifen base. White round flat scored. Marked HI. *Lactose.*
> *Oral soln*, as above 1mg/5mL. Clear colourless; strawberry odour. *Maltitol, parabens, ethanol.*

5.8 - Allergic Emergencies

In This Chapter: *Adrenaline, C1 inhibitor, icatibant.*

Class Effects

When using adrenaline for an allergic emergency, clearly inform patient/carer that after use they should: Call for immediate medical assistance, ask for an ambulance and state 'anaphylaxis' (even if symptoms appear to be improving); conscious patients to lie flat with feet elevated but to sit up if they have breathing difficulties; unconscious patients to be placed on their side in the recovery position; patient should if possible remain with another person until medical assistance arrives.

CI: Hypersensitivity to any member of the class.

Adrenaline (epinephrine) (allergy)

ATC Code: C01CA30. **Sport:** Prohibited (in-competition). **Driving:** Not recommended (symptoms of anaphylaxis).

Indications: Treatment, allergic emergencies (anaphylaxis) due to food (peanuts), drugs, insect bites or stings, other allergens, exercise-induced or idiopathic.

Dose: Adult, Elderly: 300mcg by IM injection on first signs or symptoms of anaphylaxis (*Emerade*, 300-500mcg); no improvement or deterioration, admin second injection after 5-15 minutes. Larger adults may need more than 1 injection; weight 15-30kg, use 150mcg. Effective range 0.005-0.01mg/kg but higher doses may be needed. *Admin*, IM into the anterolateral thigh; NOT for injection into buttock. Recommended, patients prescribed 2 pens to be carried at all times.

Child: Weight 15-30kg, use 150mcg as for Adult; over 30kg, as for Adult; effective range 0.005-0.01mg/kg (higher doses may be needed). Under 15kg, not recommended unless life-threatening and medical supervision. *Admin*, see Adult above.

CI: No absolute contraindications for use during allergic emergency.

Interactions: Effect of Other Drugs on Adrenaline: *Effect potentiated*: TCADs. *Increased risk (adrenaline-induced ventricular arrhythmias, acute pulmonary oedema if hypoxia present)*: Halothane. *Severe hypertension, bradycardia*: Non-selective beta-blockers (propranolol). *Bronchodilating effect inhibited*: Propranolol. *Increased arrhythmia risk*: Digoxin, quinidine.

Effect of Adrenaline on Other Drugs: Hypoglycaemic agents: *Loss of control due to adrenaline-induced hyperglycaemia (even at low doses).*

SP: Ensure patients understand indication for use and correct admin method. Caution, patients with heart disease, diabetes, hyperthyroidism, hypertension, elderly. Elderly, psychoneurosis, long-standing bronchial asthma (severe anaphylactic reaction risk), emphysema. Patients with thick subcutaneous fat layer, risk of adrenaline not reaching muscle tissue; suboptimal effect. See also CI above.

Pregnancy, Lactation: Pregnancy, if benefit outweighs risk.

Lactation, unlikely to affect nursing infant (poor oral bioavailability, short half-life).

ADR: Cardiovascular (tachycardia, hypertension), undesirable CNS effects.

Notes: See 5.8 Allergic Emergencies.

> **Anapen, Junior Parenteral** *(Lincoln)* B. GMS.
> *Price*, 300mcg and Junior 150mcg, (1) €35.41, (2), €58.26.
> *Injection*, adrenaline (0.3mL), 300mcg, Junior 150mcg Auto-Injector. Clear colourless soln practically free from particles. *Sodium metabisulphite, sodium chloride.* **Store:** Below 25 deg C.
>
> **Emerade 150mcg, 300mcg** *(Bausch&Lomb)* A. GMS.
> *Price*, both strengths (1), €36.15.
> *Injection*, adrenaline 1mg/mL. Clear colourless soln (PFP). *Sodium chloride, sodium meta-bisulphite, disodium edetate.* **Store:** Below 25 deg C; do not freeze.
>
> **Epipen, Junior Parenteral** *(Meda)* B. GMS.
> *Price*, 300mcg and Junior (150mcg) (1) €32.35 (2) €64.69
> *Injection*, adrenaline (0.3mL), 300mcg, Junior 150mcg. Clear colourless soln (PFP). *Metabisulphite, sodium chloride 1.8mg/dose.* **Store:** Do not (refrigerate, freeze).
>
> **Jext Parenteral 300mcg, 150mcg** *(ALK-Abello)* B. GMS.
> *Price*, (both strengths) €35.41.
> *Injection*, adrenaline tartrate. Clear colourless soln (PFP). *Sodium metabisulphite, sodium chloride less than 23mg/dose.* **Store:** Do not freeze.

C1 Inhibitor (human)

ATC Code: B06AC01. **Sport:** Permitted. **Driving:** Minor influence.

Indications: Treatment and pre-procedure prevention of angioedema attacks in patients with hereditary angioedema (HAE). Routine prevention in patients with severe and recurrent attacks of HAE who are intolerant to or insufficiently protected by oral prevention or inadequately managed with repeated acute treatment.

Dose: Adult, Elderly: *Treatment*, 1000 Units IV (rate 1mL/min) at first sign of onset of attack; admin second dose of 1000 Units if inadequate response after 60 minutes (admin sooner if severe attack or treatment initiation delayed).

Prevention, routine prevention, 1000 Units IV every 3-4 days; adjust interval according to individual response. *Pre-procedure*, 1000 Units IV within 24 hours before medical, dental or surgical procedure.

Child: Adolescents (age 12-17 years), as for Adult above.

SP: Risk factors for thrombotic events (including in-dwelling catheters), monitor. Regular plasma-derived C1 inhibitor, consider Hepatitis A and B vaccination. Hypersensitivity.

Pregnancy, Lactation: Pregnancy, only if clearly indicated. Lactation, stop drug or stop breastfeeding.

ADR: *Common*, rash.

Notes: See 5.8 Allergic Emergencies.

> ▼ **Cinryze Parenteral** *(Shire)* A. HOS.
> *Price*, (1) €1391.22.
> *Injection*, C1 inhibitor (human) 500 Units/vial. White powder; clear colourless solvent for solution. *Sodium 11.5mg/vial.*

Icatibant

ATC Code: C01EB19. **Sport:** Permitted. **Driving:** Fatigue, lethargy, tiredness, somnolence, dizziness.

Indications: Acute attacks of hereditary angioedema (HAE), adults with C1-esterase-inhibitor deficiency.

Dose: Adult: 30mg as single SC injection; repeat after 6 hours if needed; a third dose may be given after further 6 hours; max. 3 doses in 24-hours. Admin slowly due to volume (3mL).

Elderly: Over 65 years, limited data.

SP: Laryngeal attack, seek medical advice. Acute ischaemic heart disease, unstable angina pectoris, following stroke, caution.

Pregnancy, Lactation: Pregnancy, use only if benefit outweighs risk. Lactation, do not breastfeed for 12 hours after treatment.

ADR: *Very common*, injection-site reactions.

Notes: See 5.8 Allergic Emergencies.

> **Firazyr 10mg/mL Parenteral** *(Shire)* A. HT.
> *Price*, (1) PFS (3mL), €1812.01.
> *Injection (PFS)*, icatibant acetate. Clear colourless liquid. **Store:** Below 25 deg C; do not freeze.

6

Ear, Nose, Oropharynx

Class Effects

Betamethasone *(Betnesol)* is used for inflammatory conditions of eye, ear, nose; and in combination with neomycin *(Betnesol-N)* when infection is present. Gentamicin *(Genticin)* is used for infections due to sensitive organism in eye, ear.

CI: Hypersensitivity to any member of the class.

SP: For respiratory corticosteroids, systemic effects of topically applied corticosteroids, see Notes below.

Notes: See 7.2 Anti-Infective Eye Preparations (gentamicin), 7.3 Ophthalmic Corticosteroids and Anti-Inflammatories (betamethasone and neomycin combination) and 5.2 Respiratory Corticosteroids. For corticosteroid systemic effects, see 11.1.1 Glucocorticoids.

6.1 - Ear

Class Effects

CI: Hypersensitivity to any member of the class. Perforated ear drum.

SP: *Aminoglycosides,* with topical application into middle ear, theoretical risk of irreversible, partial or total deafness (high doses; children, infants); systemic admin or absorption from topical application to open wounds or damaged skin, irreversible partial or total deafness (dose related; enhanced by renal and/or hepatic failure; elderly). *Corticosteroids,* avoid prolonged use (possible adrenal suppression in infants due to systemic absorption; growth retardation in children, monitor height). Cataract development. Not for use for 'red eyes' until definitive diagnosis. Mydriasis, ptosis, epithelial punctate keratitis. Systemic effects may occur with intranasal admin (high doses, prolonged use). *Combined antibacterial, corticosteroids,* prolonged use, superinfection risk; overgrowth of non-susceptible organisms, including fungi.

Notes: See Chapter 6 Ear, Nose, Oropharynx.

6.1.1 - Anti-Infectives, Anti-Inflammatories

In This Chapter: *Ciprofloxacin, Gentamicin (combination).*

Ciprofloxacin (ear)

ATC Code: S02AA07. **Sport:** Permitted.
Driving: Unlikely to effect.

Indications: Acute otitis externa (specialist ENT supervision).

Dose: Adult, Elderly: Instil 4 drops into ear canal twice daily; if using otowick, double dose for first-admin only.

Child: Age 1 year and over, instil 3 drops into ear canal twice daily; otowick, double dose for first-admin only.

Renal Impairment: Not recommended.

Hepatic Impairment: As for Renal above.

SP: For otic use only. Skin rash, other signs of hypersensitivity, discontinue immediately; serious anaphylactic reactions, immediate emergency treatment. Avoid excessive sunlight. Superinfection risk. Tendon inflammation, discontinue. Systemic effect, see Notes below (quinolones).

Pregnancy, Lactation: Pregnancy, use if only if benefit outweighs risk. Lactation, caution.

ADR: *Uncommon,* headache, ear (pain, congestion, pruritus), otorrhoea, tinnitus, dermatitis, pyrexia.

Notes: See 6.1 Ear and 9.1.5 Quinolones.

Ciloxan Ear Drops *(Novartis)* A. GMS.
Price, 3mg/mL (5mL) €4.75.
Ear drops, ciprofloxacin HCl 3mg/mL. Clear colourless (pale-yellow). *Benzalkonium chloride.* **Store:** Do not (refrigerate, freeze).

Hydrocortisone, Gentamicin

ATC Code: S02CA03. **Sport:** Permitted.
Driving: Unlikely to impair.

Indications: Treatment, eczema and infection of outer ear (otitis externa). Prophylaxis, following trauma. Post-operative, surgery to infected mastoid cavities.

Dose: Adult, Elderly: Instil 2-4 drops 3-4 times a day and at night OR wicks medicated with *Gentisone HC* drops may be placed in external ear or mastoid cavity.

Child: As for Adult above.

CI: Perforated ear drum, myasthenia gravis.

SP: Cross-sensitivity with other aminoglycosides. Severe infection, use adjunctive to systemic antibiotics.

Pregnancy, Lactation: If benefit outweighs risk.

ADR: Local sensitivity, ototoxicity, vestibular disorder, hearing loss, irritation, burning sensation, stinging, pruritus, dermatitis.

Notes: See 6.1 Ear and 7.2 Anti-Infective Eye Preparations (gentamicin).

Gentisone HC Ear Drops *(Concordia)* A. GMS.
Price, (10mL) €5.00.
Ear drops, hydrocortisone acetate 1%, gentamicin base 0.3% w/v. White odourless susp. *Benzalkonium chloride.* **Store:** Below 25 deg C; do not (freeze, mix with other liquids).

6.1.2 - Wax Removal, Ear Pain

In This Chapter: *Choline salicylate, glycerol combination.*

Class Effects

CI: Perforated ear drum.

Notes: See 6.1 Ear.

Choline Salicylate, Glycerol

ATC Code: S02DC. **Sport:** Permitted.
Driving: Unlikely to impair.

Indications: Removal of ear wax. Pain of otitis media, otitis externa, furuncles and other local inflammation.

Dose: Adult, Elderly: Fill affected external auditory canal with drops; plug with cotton wool soaked in ear drops; instil every 3-4 hours.

CI: Salicylate hypersensitivity.

SP: If using other medication, consult medical advice.

Pregnancy, Lactation: Can be used.

Notes: See 6.1.2 Wax Removal.

Audax Ear Drops *(SSL)* OTC. GMS.
Price, (10mL) €1.74.
Ear drops, choline salicylate 20%, glycerol 12.6% w/v. Faintly tan soln; characteristic odour.

6.2 - Nose

6.2.1 - Rhinitis

In This Chapter: *Azelastine and fluticasone combination, beclometasone, budesonide, fluticasone, ipratropium, mometasone, triamcinolone.*

Class Effects

CI: Hypersensitivity to any member of the class.

SP: Regular use essential. Avoid prolonged use of nasally inhaled corticosteroids at high doses (systemic effects). Caution transferring from systemic steroids; may be adrenal insufficiency for a number of months until recovery of HPA axis function; pre-existing allergic conditions may be unmasked. Inhibitory effect on wound healing, recent nasal septal ulcers, nasal surgery or trauma, use with caution until fully healed. Glaucoma and/or cataracts. For systemic effects of topical corticosteroids, see Notes below.

ADR: Nasal irritation, sneezing, stinging, dryness with all nasal sprays.

Notes: See Chapter 6 Ear, Nose, Oropharynx. For systemic corticosteroid effects, see 11.1.1 Glucocorticoids.

Azelastine

ATC Code: R01AC03. **Sport:** Permitted.
Driving: Caution.

Indications: Perennial and seasonal allergic rhinitis.

Dose: Adult, Elderly: 1 spray into each nostril twice daily. Moderate/severe rhinitis (with nasal blockage), increase to 2 sprays in each nostril twice daily.

Child: Age 5-12 years, 1 spray into each nostril twice daily.

Pregnancy, Lactation: Minimal systemic exposure expected; caution as with all medicines.

ADR: *Common*, bitter taste.

Notes: See 6.2.1 Rhinitis.

Rhinolast Spray *(Meda)* B. GMS.
Price, (20mL) €14.66.
Nasal spray, azelastine HCl 0.1% w/v (140mcg/spray). Clear colourless aqueous soln.

Azelastine, Fluticasone

ATC Code: R01AD58. **Sport:** Permitted.
Driving: Fatigue, weariness, exhaustion, dizziness or weakness may occur. Alcohol may enhance this effect.

Indications: Relief, symptoms of moderate to severe seasonal and perennial allergic rhinitis if monotherapy is insufficient.

Dose: Adult, Elderly: 1 spray in each nostril morning and evening. Regular use essential; suitable for long-term use.

Child: Age 12 years and older, as for adult; under 12 years, safety/efficacy not established.

Pregnancy, Lactation: If benefit outweighs risk.

ADR: *Very common*, epistaxis.

Notes: See Azelastine above, Fluticasone (rhinitis) below.

Dymista Nasal Spray *(Meda)* B. GMS.
Price, (1) €21.33
Nasal spray, azelastine HCl 1000mcg, fluticasone propionate 365mcg (125mcg/50mcg per actuation). White homogenous suspension. *Benzalkonium chloride*. **Store:** Do not (refrigerate, freeze).

Beclometasone (rhinitis)

ATC Code: R01AD01. **Sport:** Permitted.
Driving: Unlikely to impair.

Indications: Prophylaxis, treatment of perennial and seasonal allergic and vasomotor rhinitis.

Dose: Adult, Elderly: 2 sprays in each nostril twice daily OR 1 spray in each nostril 3-4 times daily; max. 8 sprays/day.

Child: Under 6, not recommended.

SP: Local monilial infection. Sneezing following use.

Pregnancy, Lactation: If benefit outweighs risk.

ADR: Rash, urticaria, pruritus, erythema, oedema of eyes, face, lips and throat, anaphylactoid or anaphylactic reactions, bronchospasm, unpleasant taste and/or smell, glaucoma, raised IOP, cataract, epistaxis, nasal/throat dryness/irritation, nasal septal perforation.

Notes: See 6.2.1 Rhinitis and 5.2 Respiratory Corticosteroids (betamethasone).

Nasobec 50mcg *(TEVA)* B. GMS.
Price, (200-dose) 50mcg/spray, €2.41.
Nasal spray, beclometasone dipropionate. Aqueous.

Budesonide (rhinitis)

ATC Code: R01AD05. **Sport:** Permitted.
Driving: Unlikely to impair.

Indications: Rhinitis (seasonal, perennial, vasomotor). Treatment, nasal polyps.

Dose: Adult, Elderly: *Rhinitis*, 2 sprays (400mcg) in each nostril in morning OR 1 spray (200mcg) in each nostril morning and evening; effect achieved, reduce to 1 spray in each nostril once daily.
Nasal polyps, 1 spray (200mcg) in each nostril morning and evening.

Child: Not recommended.

Pregnancy, Lactation: Pregnancy, *Rhinocort* can be used. Lactation, is excreted into breast milk; no effect on child anticipated at therapeutic dose.

ADR: *Common*, haemorrhagic secretion and epistaxis, sneezing, stinging, dryness.

Notes: See 6.2.1 Rhinitis and 5.2 Respiratory Corticosteroids (budesonide).

Rhinocort Turbohaler 100mcg *(AstraZeneca)* B. GMS.
Price, (200-dose) €21.11.
Nasal powder (metered dose inhaler), budesonide 100mcg/dose. White (off-white) granules.

Fluticasone (rhinitis)

ATC Code: F01AD08. **Sport:** Permitted.
Driving: No or negligible effect.

Indications: Prophylaxis, treatment of seasonal allergic rhinitis, hay fever, perennial rhinitis.

Dose: Adult, Elderly: Initially, 2 sprays into each nostril in morning; 2 sprays twice daily might be needed; max. 4 sprays/day in each nostril. Adequate control, reduce to lowest dose for effective control.

Child: *Nasofan*, age 4-11 years, 1 spray in each nostril once daily; if needed 1 spray twice daily.
Avamys, age 6-11 years, initially 1 spray in each nostril once daily; max. 2 sprays/day in each nostril; once controlled, reduce to lowest effective dose. Age 12 years and over, as for Adult above; under 6 years, no dose recommendation.

Renal Impairment: No adjustment.

Hepatic Impairment: No adjustment.

6.2.2   Nasal Staphylococci

Interactions: Effect of Other Drugs on Fluticasone: *Co-admin not recommended (increased systemic exposure):* Ritonavir. *Caution:* Potent CYP3A4 inhibitors (ketoconazole).

SP: Local monilial infections. Several days to get full benefit. Potential systemic effects.

Pregnancy, Lactation: Pregnancy, if benefit outweighs risk. Lactation, only if benefit to mother greater than risk to child.

ADR: Summary, *most common*, epistaxis, nasal ulceration, headache; *most serious*, hypersensitivity reactions including anaphylaxis.

Notes: See 6.2 Nose and 5.2 Respiratory Corticosteroids (fluticasone).

> **Avamys 27.5mcg Spray** *(GSK)* B. GMS.
> *Price,* (120-dose) €8.81.
> *Nasal spray, fluticasone furoate. White susp. Benzalkonium chloride.* **Store:** Do not (refrigerate, freeze).
> **Nasofan Aqueous 50mcg** *(TEVA)* B. GMS.
> *Price,* (120-dose) €4.28.
> *Nasal spray, fluticasone propionate. White opaque aqueous susp (metered-dose). Benzalkonium chloride.*

Ipratropium (rhinitis)

ATC Code: R01AX03. **Sport:** Permitted.
Driving: Caution.

Indications: Symptomatic relief of rhinorrhoea, allergic, non-allergic.

Dose: Adult, Elderly: 2 sprays in each nostril 2-3 times daily.

Child: Under 12 years, not recommended.

Interactions: Effect of Other Drugs on Ipratropium: *Co-admin not recommended*: Other anticholinergics including orally inhaled.

SP: Narrow-angle glaucoma, prostatic hypertrophy, bladder outflow obstruction. Avoid contact with eyes. Caution, cystic fibrosis. Hypersensitivity reactions including urticaria, angioedema, rash, bronchospasm, oropharyngeal oedema, anaphylaxis. Mydriasis, increased IOP, glaucoma, eye pain.

Pregnancy, Lactation: Pregnancy, if benefit outweighs risk. Lactation, caution.

ADR: Nasal drying/epistaxis/irritation, pharyngitis, sinusitis, headache, nausea, blurred vision, increased heart rate, palpitation, urinary retention, GI motility disturbance, allergic reactions, see SP above.

Notes: See 6.2.1 Rhinitis and 5.1.2 Antimuscarinic Bronchodilators (ipratropium).

> **Rinatec Nasal Spray 21mcg** *(SANOFI)* B. GMS.
> *Price,* (180-dose) €5.30.
> *Nasal spray, ipratropium bromide. Clear colourless (almost colourless) soln. Benzalkonium chloride.* **Store:** Below 25 deg C.

Mometasone (rhinitis)

ATC Code: R01AD09. **Sport:** Permitted.
Driving: Unlikely to impair.

Indications: Treatment, symptoms of seasonal or perennial allergic rhinitis, nasal polyps.

Dose: Adult, Elderly: *Allergic rhinitis,* age 12 years and older, 2 sprays (50mcg/spray) in each nostril once daily (total 200mcg); if needed max. 4 sprays in each nostril once daily (total 400mcg). When controlled reduce to 1 spray in each nostril once daily.

Nasal polyposis, age 18 years and over, as for allergic rhinitis; use lowest dose effective dose; no improvement after 5-6 weeks, discontinue.

Child: *Allergic rhinitis,* age 3-11 years, 1 spray (50mcg) in

each nostril once daily (total 100mcg); under 3 years, no data.

SP: Initiate some days before start of pollen season in patients with allergic rhinitis history.

Pregnancy, Lactation: If benefit outweighs risk.

ADR: *Very common,* epistaxis.

Notes: See 6.2.1 Rhinitis and 5.2 Respiratory Corticosteroids (mometasone).

> **Nasonex Spray 50mcg** *(MSD)* A. GMS.
> *Price,* (140-dose) €7.92.
> *Nasal spray, mometasone furoate 50mcg/spray. White (off-white) opaque susp. Benzalkonium chloride.* **Store:** Below 25 deg C; do not freeze.

Triamcinolone (rhinitis)

ATC Code: R01AD11. **Sport:** Permitted.
Driving: Unlikely to impair.

Indications: Allergic rhinitis (seasonal, perennial).

Dose: Adult, Elderly: 2 sprays (220mcg) in each nostril once daily; maintenance 1 spray in each nostril once daily.

Child: Age 6 years and over, 1 spray in each nostril once daily; max. 3 months.

SP: Reduction in growth velocity observed in children post-marketing.

Pregnancy, Lactation: If benefit outweighs risk.

ADR: *Common,* flu syndrome, pharyngitis, rhinitis, headache, bronchitis, epistaxis, cough, dyspepsia, tooth disorder.

Notes: See 6.2.1 Rhinitis.

> **Nasacort Nasal Spray** *(SANOFI)* A. GMS.
> *Price,* (120-dose) €10.50.
> *Nasal spray, triamcinolone acetonide 55mcg/dose. Unscented thixotropic aqueous susp. Benzalkonium chloride.*

6.2.2 - Nasal Staphylococci

In This Chapter: *Chlorhexidine/neomycin combination, mupirocin.*

Class Effects

CI: Hypersensitivity to any member of the class.

Chlorhexidine, Neomycin

ATC Code: D06AX04. **Sport:** Permitted.
Driving: Unlikely to impair.

Indications: Eradication of staphylococcal infections and carriage in the nose.

Dose: Adult, Elderly: *Prophylaxis,* use twice daily.

Eradication, 4-times daily for 10 days. Apply to inside of each nostril pressing sides of nose together to spread ointment.

SP: Avoid contact with eyes. No improvement or aggravation, discontinue. Caution, use in children, elderly or with impaired hearing.

ADR: Local irritation, skin sensitisation (prolonged use), anaphylactic reactions to chlorhexidine.

Notes: See Class Effects, Chapter 6 Ear, Nose, Oropharynx above.

> **Naseptin Nasal Cream** *(Alliance)* A. GMS.
> *Price,* (15g) €2.30.
> *Nasal cream, chlorhexidine dihydrochloride 0.1%, neomycin sulfate 0.5% (3250 IU/g) w/w. White non-greasy water-miscible. Cetostearyl alcohol.*

Mupirocin (nasal)

ATC Code: R01AX06. **Sport:** Permitted.
Driving: No or negligible effect.

Indications: Treatment, nasal carriage of staphylococci, including methicillin resistant *Staphylococcus aureus* (MRSA).

Dose: Adult, Elderly: Apply 2-3 times daily to inside of each nostril pressing sides of nose together to spread ointment; carriage should clear in 5-7 days.

SP: Avoid contact with eyes. Sensitisation reaction, severe local irritation, discontinue. Ointment is not suitable for ophthalmic use.

Pregnancy, Lactation: Pregnancy, insufficient data; animal studies do not indicate reproductive toxicity. Lactation, inadequate data.

ADR: *Uncommon*, nasal mucosa reactions.

Notes: See Class Effects, Chapter 6 Ear, Nose, Oropharynx above.

> **Bactroban Nasal Ointment** *(GSK)* A. GMS.
> *Price*, (3g) €6.60.
> *Nasal ointment*, mupirocin calcium equiv. to mupirocin 2% w/w (20mg/g). Smooth off-white. **Store:** Below 25 deg C.

6.3 - Oropharyngeal Preparations

In This Chapter: *Miconazole, nystatin.*

Class Effects
Systemic antifungals are also used in the treatment of oropharyngeal conditions. There are also a large number of preparations available without prescription.

CI: Hypersensitivity to any member of the class.

SP: For systemic effects of antifungals, see Notes below.

Notes: See 9.2 Antifungals.

Miconazole (oropharyngeal)

ATC Code: A01AB09. **Sport:** Permitted.
Driving: Unlikely to impair.

Indications: Management, fungal infections of oral cavity and GI tract (from age 4 months).

Dose: Adult, Elderly: *Oropharyngeal* candidosis, 2.5mL of gel applied 4-times daily; continue for 1 week after symptoms have disappeared; keep in mouth for as long as possible. Dental prostheses should be removed at night and brushed with gel.

GI candidosis, 20mg/kg/day in 4 divided doses; max. 250mg 4-times daily; continue for 1 week after symptoms have disappeared. One measuring spoon (provided) is equiv. to miconazole 124mg/5mL.

Child: *Oropharyngeal* candidosis, age 4-24 months, 1.25mL applied 4-times daily; 2 years and older, as for Adult above. Under 4 months or swallowing reflex not sufficiently developed, contraindicated.

Gastrointestinal candidosis, as for Adult above.

Hepatic Impairment: Not recommended.

CI: Imidazole hypersensitivity.

Interactions: Effect of Other Drugs on Miconazole: *Co-admin not recommended*: Drugs prolonging QT-interval, astemizole, cisapride, dofetilide, mizolastine, pimozide, quinidine, sertindole, terfenadine, ergot alkaloids and derivatives, HMG-CoA reductase inhibitors (simvastatin, lovastatin), triazolam, oral midazolam.

Effect of Miconazole on Other Drugs: Warfarin,

sulphonylureas, phenytoin, HIV protease inhibitors, antineoplastics (vinca alkaloids, busulphan, docetaxel), dihydropyridines, verapamil, immunosuppressives (ciclosporin, tacrolimus, sirolimus), carbamazepine, cilostazol, disopyramide, buspirone, alfentanil, sildenafil, alprazolam, brotizolam, midazolam IV, rifabutin, methylprednisolone, trimetrexate, ebastine, reboxetine: *Increased or prolonged therapeutic outcome.*

SP: Miconazole is effective against some Gram positive bacteria (*Streptococcus pyrogenes*, *Staphylococcus aureus* and *Erysipelothrix*). Severe hypersensitivity, discontinue. Infants, young children, caution that gel does not obstruct throat; divide dose into smaller portions for application; not to be applied to back of throat or to the nipple of a breast-feeding woman for admin to infant. Consider the variability of maturation of swallowing reflex in infants (especially 4-6 months). Serious skin reactions reported (toxic epidermal necrolysis, Stevens-Johnson syndrome).

Pregnancy, Lactation: Pregnancy, if benefit outweighs risk. Lactation, caution; not known if excreted in human milk.

ADR: Adults, *common*, nausea, abnormal product taste, oral discomfort, dry mouth, dysgeusia, vomiting. Paediatrics, *very common*, nausea, vomiting; *common*, regurgitation.

Notes: See 6.3 Oropharyngeal Preparations.

> **Daktarin Oral Gel** *(McNeil)* OTC. GMS.D.
> *Price*, (40g) €3.14.
> *Oral gel*, miconazole 124mg/5mL. White. Orange flavour. *Ethanol 96% 7.59mg/g.* **Store:** Below 30 deg C.

Nystatin (oropharyngeal)

ATC Code: A07AA02. **Sport:** Permitted.
Driving: Unlikely to impair.

Indications: Prevention and treatment, mycotic infections due to *Candida albicans*, affecting the oral cavity, oesophagus, intestinal tract.

Dose: Adult, Elderly: *Oral, intestinal candidiasis (prevention, treatment)*, 4-6mL 4-times daily; retain in mouth for several minutes before swallowing; if needed, increase dose; continue treatment for minimum 48 hours after clinical cure and/or normal cultures to avoid relapse; if signs/symptoms worsen or persist beyond 14 days, re-evaluate.

Child: *Prevention (oral candidiasis)*, neonates (birth to 1 month), 1mL*; infants (1 month - 2 years), 2mL*.

Prevention (intestinal candidiasis), neonates, infants (birth to 2 years) 1-2mL* admin with milk or other liquid. Dose can be increased if needed. Age over 2 years, both indications, as for Adult above. *Admin 4-times daily.

SP: Not for treatment of systemic mycoses. All potential infection sites to be treated simultaneously.

Pregnancy, Lactation: Pregnancy, if benefit outweighs risk. Lactation, caution.

ADR: Generally well tolerated. *Uncommon*, diarrhoea, abdominal discomfort, nausea, vomiting, rash.

Notes: See 6.3 Oropharyngeal Preparations.

> **Mycostatin Oral Susp (Ready Mixed)** *(BMS)* B. GMS.
> *Price*, (30mL) €1.95.
> *Oral susp*, nystatin 100000 units/mL. Light creamy yellow. *Ethanol, sucrose, parabens, sodium.*

199

7

Ophthalmology

Class Effects

Driving: Transient blurring of vision may occur on instillation of eye drops. Do not drive or operate hazardous machinery unless vision is clear. Some drops may cause local irritation.

CI: Hypersensitivity to any member of the class.

SP: Eye drops are not for injection; never inject subconjunctivally or directly introduce into the anterior chamber of eye. To avoid contamination or possible eye injury, do not touch tip of bottle or vial to any surface and avoid contact with eye. *Systemic absorption* may be reduced by closing eyelids for 1 minute following instillation or nasolacrimal occlusion (compressing lacrimal sac at medial canthus for a minute following instillation); blocking passage of drops via naso lacrimal duct to absorptive area of nasal and pharyngeal mucosa (especially advisable in children). If multiple topical ophthalmic drugs are used, instil different products 5-15 minutes apart; always instil ointment last. *Benzalkonium chloride* (preservative), remove contact lenses before instillation as may cause irritation, discolour soft lenses; reinsert after 15 minutes. *Phosphate-containing* eye-drops in patients with damaged corneas, cases of corneal calcification reported very rarely.

ADR: With all eye drops local eye irritation may occur.

7.1 - Glaucoma

Class Effects

A number of different classes of drugs are used in glaucoma management, either systemically or topically applied as eye drops or gel. The osmotic diuretic, mannitol, is also used for urgent reduction of intraocular pressure (IOP) and prior to surgery.

Notes: See Chapter 7 Ophthalmology and 2.9.3 Osmotic Diuretics (mannitol).

7.1.1 - Topical Beta-Blockers

In This Chapter: *Levobunolol, timolol.*

Class Effects

Driving: See Notes below (ophthalmology).

CI: Use in children. Sinus bradycardia, sick sinus syndrome, sino-atrial block, second and third degree AV block not controlled by pacemaker. Overt cardiac failure, cardiogenic shock. Reactive airway disease (bronchial asthma, severe COPD).

Interactions: Effect of Other Drugs on Topical Beta-Blockers: *Caution, additive effects*: Systemic beta-blockers, other systemic antihypertensives including calcium channel blockers, anti-arrhythmics, digitalis glycosides, parasympathomimetics or guanethidine, CYP2D6 co-admin (quinidine, fluoxetine, paroxetine).

Effect of Topical Beta-Blockers on Other Drugs: Adrenaline: *Response can be decreased.*

SP: Systemic absorption may occur; for systemic effects, see Notes below. Cardiovascular disease (coronary heart disease, Prinzmetal's angina, cardiac failure); observe for cardiac failure signs (if present, discontinue), check pulse rate. Severe peripheral circulatory disturbance (Raynaud's disease/syndrome), caution. Respiratory reactions (bronchospasm in asthmatics). Beta-blockers may mask signs/symptoms of acute hypoglycaemia, hyperthyroidism. Muscle weakness consistent with myasthenic symptoms. Choroidal detachment with aqueous suppressant therapy after filtration procedures. Effects of systemic beta-blockers may be exaggerated, when topical beta-blocker added; use of 2 topical beta-blockers not recommended. Severe renal impairment/dialysis, caution (hypotension). General anaesthesia, inform anaesthetist. Caution, use with restricted pulmonary function, myasthenia gravis, corneal disease (ophthalmic beta-blockers may induce eye dryness).

Pregnancy, Lactation: Pregnancy, if benefit outweighs risk; if used close to delivery, monitor neonatal heart rate/hypoglycaemia during first 3-5 days after birth. Lactation, not recommended; beta-blockers are excreted in breast milk.

ADR: *Local reactions* including irritation, burning, itching and pain, blurred vision, photophobia, xerosis, conjunctival hyperaemia, conjunctival discharge, conjunctivitis, blepharitis; diffuse superficial keratitis, decreased corneal sensitivity; refractory changes, diplopia, ptosis.

Systemic reactions including bradycardia, hypotension, syncope, heart block, CVA, cerebral ischaemia, CHF, palpitation, cardiac arrest; bronchospasm, dyspnoea; rash, headache, lassitude, vertigo, nausea, depression, asthenia.

Notes: See Class Effects Chapter 7 Ophthalmology above and 7.1 Glaucoma. Beta-blocker systemic effects, see 2.1.7 Beta Blockers.

Levobunolol

ATC Code: S01ED03. **Sport:** Prohibited (specific sports).
Driving: Transient blurring, fatigue, drowsiness.
Indications: Reduction of elevated IOP in ocular hypertension, chronic open-angle glaucoma.
Dose: Adult, Elderly: Instil 1 drop once or twice daily.
Renal Impairment: Caution.
Hepatic Impairment: As for Renal above.
ADR: Blepharo-conjunctivitis, decreased heart rate and BP, urticaria.
Notes: See 7.1.1 Topical Beta-Blockers.

Betagan 5mg/mL, Unit Dose *(Allergan)* B. GMS.
Price, 5mg/5mL (1) €2.84. (3) €14.99. UDV (30) €9.77.
Eye drops, levobunolol HCl. Clear colourless (brown) soln. *Benzalkonium chloride (drops); preservative-free (UDV).*

Timolol

ATC Code: S01ED01. **Sport:** Prohibited (specific sports).
Driving: Dizziness, visual disturbances.
Indications: Reduction of elevated IOP in ocular hypertension, chronic open-angle glaucoma *(both brands)*, (including aphakic patients), secondary glaucoma *(Timoptol)*.
Dose: Adult, Elderly: *Timoptol,* instil 1 drop (0.25%) twice daily; inadequate response, 1 drop (0.5%) twice daily; maintenance, 1 drop once daily. Provided IOP is maintained at satisfactory levels, once-a-day therapy can be considered.
Timofluid, instil 1 drop (1mg/g) once daily (morning). A single-dose contains enough get to treat both eyes; for single use only.
Child: *Timoptol,* only recommended for use in primary congenital and juvenile glaucoma for transitional period before surgery/other options. If benefit outweighs risk, use lowest conc once daily; if IOP not controlled, titrate carefully to max. 2 drops daily per affected eye.
CI: Reactive airway disease (bronchial asthma, severe COPD), sinus bradycardia, sick sinus syndrome, sino-atrial

block, second or third degree AV block (not pacemaker controlled), overt cardiac failure, cardiogenic shock. Severe circulatory disorders, Prinzmetal's angina, untreated phaeochromocytoma, hypotension, severe allergic rhinitis, Raynaud's disease, corneal disease *(both brands)*; untreated phaeochromocytoma, corneal dystrophies.

Interactions: Effect of Other Drugs on Timolol: *Co-admin contraindicated*: Floctafenine, sultopride. *Co-admin not recommended (caution)*: Amiodarone (conduction and/or myocardial contractility disorders), calcium antagonists (bradyarrhythmias, conduction disorders, cardiac failure). *Co-admin caution*: Reserpine (additive effect, hypotension), MAOIs; oral calcium channel blockers, cardiac glycosides (digitalis), Class I antiarrhythmics (conduction disturbances), clonidine and other centrally action antihypertensives (rebound hypertension; exacerbated by oral beta-blockers), insulin, oral antidiabetics (hypoglycaemia signs masked), general anaesthesia, lidocaine (IV), iodine contrast media. *Potentiated systemic beta-blockade (decreased heart rate, depression)*: CYP2D6 inhibitors (quinidine, SSRIs). *Mydriasis*: Epinephrine (adrenaline). *Increased plasma levels*: Cimetidine. *Ventricular arrhythmia risk (Torsades de Pointes)*: Amisulpride. *Increased bradycardia risk*: Parasympathomimetics. *Prolonged QT-interval*: Mefloquine.

Notes: See 7.1.1 Glaucoma, Topical Beta-Blockers.

Timoptol Eye Drops *(Santen)* B. GMS.
Price, (5mL) 0.25%, €3.03; 0.5%, €2.74.
Eye drops, timolol maleate 0.25%, 0.5% (5mL). Clear colourless (light-yellow) soln. *Benzalkonium chloride.*

Timofluid Eye Gel *(Thea Pharma)* B. GMS.
Price, 1mg/0.4g sachet (30) €6.07.
Eye gel, timolol maleate 1mg/g. Opalescent colourless (slightly yellow) gel in single-dose unit.

7.1.2 - Carbonic Anhydrase Inhibitors

In This Chapter: *Acetazolamide, brinzolamide, dorzolamide (sulfonamide derivatives) and beta-blocker combinations. Brinzolamide and brimonidine combination.*

Class Effects

Driving: Oral carbonic anhydrase inhibitors may impair ability to perform tasks requiring mental alertness and/or physical coordination. See Notes below (ophthalmology).

Sport: Beta-blocker combinations, see Notes below (beta-blockers).

CI: Sulfonamide hypersensitivity. *Combinations* with topical beta-blockers, sinus bradycardia, second and third degree AV block not controlled by pacemaker. Overt cardiac failure, cardiogenic shock. Reactive airway disease (bronchial asthma, severe COPD).

SP: Glaucoma (pseudoexfoliative, pigmentary). Narrow angle glaucoma, no data. Compromised cornea (diabetes, corneal dystrophies), monitor. Carbonic anhydrase inhibitors may affect corneal hydration; wearing contact lenses may increase risk for corneal damage. Preservatives, see Notes below (class effects).

ADR: *Sulfonamide-related, with systemic absorption,* fever, agranulocytosis, thrombocytopenia, thrombocytic purpura, leucopenia, aplastic anaemia, bone marrow depression, pancytopenia, rash (erythema multiforme, Stevens-Johnson Syndrome, toxic epidermal necrolysis), anaphylaxis, crystalluria, calculus formation, renal and ureteral colic, renal lesions, hepatic necrosis.

Notes: See Class Effects Chapter 7 Ophthalmology above and 7.1 Glaucoma. See 2.1.7 Beta-Blockers.

Acetazolamide

ATC Code: S01EC01. **Sport:** Prohibited.
Driving: Drowsiness, fatigue, myopia.
Indications: Glaucoma, chronic open-angle; secondary glaucoma; perioperatively, acute-angle closure glaucoma where surgery is delayed to lower IOP. Abnormal fluid retention. Adjunctive in epilepsy.
Dose: Adult: *Glaucoma,* PROLONGED/R 250mg, 1-2 caps daily; STANDARD/R, 250-1000mg/day in divided doses.

Carbonic Anhydrase Inhibitors   7.1.2

Fluid retention, diuresis, usually 250-375mg daily for 2 days, rest 1 day, and repeat, OR admin every other day. Fluid retention in PMS, 125-375mg/day as single dose.
Epilepsy, 250-1000mg/day in divided doses.
Elderly: Caution.
Child: STANDARD/R, *glaucoma,* 125-750mg/day. *Epilepsy,* children, 125-750mg/day; infants, 125mg/day. Divided doses.
Renal Impairment: Moderate to severe, *Prolonged/R,* use half dose OR increase to 12-hour dose interval. Severe, not recommended.
Hepatic Impairment: Significant impairment, hepatic cirrhosis, not recommended.
CI: Depressed sodium and/or potassium serum levels, adrenal gland failure, hyper-chloraemic acidosis. Chronic non-congestive angle-closure glaucoma (long-term admin).
Interactions: Effect of Other Drugs on Acetazolamide: *Co-admin not recommended*: Aspirin (severe acidosis, increased CNS toxicity), other carbonic anhydrase inhibitors (additive effects). *Co-admin, adjust dose*: Cardiac glycosides, antihypertensives.
Effect of Acetazolamide on Other Drugs: Folic acid antagonists, hypoglycaemics, oral anti-coagulants: *Effect potentiated.* Phenytoin, carbamazepine: *Increased plasma levels.* Anticonvulsants: *Severe osteomalacia.* Primidone: *Plasma levels decreased.*
SP: Increasing dose does not increase diuresis but may increase incidence of drowsiness and/or paraesthesia. Long-term use, caution; advise patient to report unusual skin rash (monitor blood counts/electrolytes). Pulmonary obstruction/emphysema, diabetes (acidosis risk). Elderly, potential urinary tract obstruction, disorders of electrolyte balance, caution. History of renal calculi, use if benefit outweighs risk. Suicide, suicidal ideation, see Notes below (antiepileptics).
Pregnancy, Lactation: Pregnancy, not recommended especially in first trimester. Lactation, caution.
ADR: *Short-term use,* paraesthesia, loss of appetite, taste disturbance, polyuria, flushing, thirst, headache, dizziness, fatigue, irritability, depression, reduced libido, drowsiness, confusion, photosensitivity. *Long-term use,* metabolic acidosis, electrolyte imbalance, transient myopia, GI (nausea, vomiting, diarrhoea). *Other,* urticaria, melaena, haematuria, glycosuria, impaired hearing, tinnitus, abnormal liver function, renal failure, hepatitis/cholestatic jaundice, flaccid paralysis, convulsions. Side effects similar to sulfonamides.
Notes: See 7.1.2 Carbonic Anhydrase Inhibitors. See 3.1 Antiepileptics.

Diamox 250mg, SR 250mg *(Concordia)* B. GMS.
Price, 250mg (112) €16.79. SR 250mg (30) €16.68.
Tablet, acetazolamide. White round quarter scored (divisible into equal halves). Marked FW and 147.
Modified/R capsule (SR), as above. Clear/orange; contains orange spherical pellets. Marked GS250. *Sunset Yellow.*

Brinzolamide

ATC Code: S01EC04. **Sport:** Permitted.
Driving: Blurred vision, visual disturbances.
Indications: Reduction of elevated IOP in ocular hypertension, open-angle glaucoma (monotherapy or adjunctive).
Dose: Adult, Elderly: Instil 1 drop twice daily; 3-times daily may be required.
Child: Under 18 years, not recommended.
Renal Impairment: CrCl (mL/min) below 30, hyperchloraemic acidosis, contraindicated.
Hepatic Impairment: Not recommended.
Interactions: Effect of Other Drugs on Brinzolamide: *Metabolism Inhibited*: Ketoconazole, itraconazole, clotrimazole, ritonavir, troleandomycin.
SP: Hypersensitivity reactions common to all sulphonamides; brinzolamide is a sulphonamide.
Pregnancy, Lactation: Pregnancy, women of childbearing potential not using contraception, not recommended. Lactation, stop drug or stop breastfeeding.

201

7.1.3 Prostaglandin Analogues

ADR: *Common*, dysgeusia, headache, blepharitis, blurred vision, eye irritation/pain, dry eye, discharge, pruritus, foreign body sensation, hyperaemia, dry mouth.

Notes: See 7.1.2 Carbonic Anhydrase Inhibitors.

Azopt Eye Drops *(Novartis)* B. GMS.
Price, (5mL) €5.43.
Eye drops, brinzolamide 10mg/mL. White (off-white) susp. *Benzalkonium chloride.* **Store:** No special conditions.
Brinzolamide Actavis Eye Drops *(Accord)* B. GMS.
Price, (5mL) €3.91.
Eye drops, brinzolamide 10mg/mL. White (off-white) susp. *Benzalkonium chloride.*
Brinzolamide Sandoz Eye Drops *(Rowex)* B. GMS.
Price, (5mL) €3.91.
Eye drops, brinzolamide 10mg/mL. White (off-white) susp. *Benzalkonium chloride.*

Brinzolamide, Brimonidine

ATC Code: S01EC54. **Sport:** Permitted.
Driving: Dizziness, fatigue, drowsiness; blurred vision.

Indications: Reduction of elevated IOP in ocular hypertension, open-angle glaucoma (monotherapy insufficient).

Dose: Adult, Elderly: Instil 1 drop twice daily.

Child: Age 2-17 years, safety/efficacy not established; under 2 years, contraindicated.

Hepatic Impairment: Caution.

Interactions: Effect of Other Drugs on Brinzolamide, Brimonidine Combination: *Co-admin contraindicated:* MAOIs, antidepressants affecting noradrenergic transmission (TCADs, mianserin). *Co-admin caution:* Antihypertensives, cardiac glycosides (BP reduction); alcohol, barbiturates, opiates, sedatives, anaesthetics (additive effects); chlorpromazine, methylphenidate, reserpine, SSRIs, SNRIs (affect circulating amines); adrenergic receptor agonists or antagonists (isoprenaline, prazosin); CYP3A4 inhibitors (ketoconazole, itraconazole, clotrimazole, ritonavir, troleandomycin).

SP: Small decreases in BP observed; caution with severe or unstable and uncontrolled cardiovascular disease. *Caution*, patients with depression, cerebral or coronary insufficiency, Raynaud's phenomenon, orthostatic hypotension, thromboangiitis obliterans.

Pregnancy, Lactation: Not recommended including women of childbearing potential not using contraception.

ADR: Summary, *most common*, ocular hyperaemia, ocular allergic type reactions, dysgeusia (bitter or unusual taste).

Notes: See Brinzolamide above. See 7.1.4 Sympathomimetics (brimonidine).

SIMBRINZA Eye Drops *(Novartis)* B. GMS.
Price, (5mL) €14.19.
Eye drops, brinzolamide, brimonidine tartrate 10mg/2mg per mL. White (off-white) susp. *Benzalkonium chloride.* **Store:** No special conditions.

Brinzolamide, Timolol

ATC Code: S01ED51. **Sport:** Prohibited (specific sports).
Driving: Blurred vision, visual disturbances.

Indications: Reduction of elevated IOP in ocular hypertension, open-angle glaucoma (monotherapy insufficient).

Dose: Adult, Elderly: Instil 1 drop twice daily.

Notes: See Brinzolamide above. See 7.1.1 Topical Beta-Blockers (timolol).

Azarga Eye Drops *(Novartis)* B. GMS.
Price, (5mL) €12.56.
Eye drops, brinzolamide 10mg/mL, timolol 5mg/mL. White (off-white) uniform susp. *Benzalkonium chloride.* **Store:** No special conditions.

Dorzolamide

ATC Code: S01EC03. **Sport:** Permitted.
Driving: Blurred vision.

Indications: Reduction of elevated IOP in ocular hypertension, open-angle glaucoma (monotherapy or adjunctive). Pseudoexfoliative glaucoma when beta-blocker monotherapy insufficient.

Dose: Adult, Elderly: Instil 1 drop 3-times daily. Adjunctive with beta-blocker, 1 drop twice daily.

Child: Limited data. Use 3-times daily dosing.

Renal Impairment: CrCl (mL/min) below 30, hyperchloraemic acidosis, not recommended.

Hepatic Impairment: Caution.

Interactions: Effect of Other Drugs on Dorzolamide: *Co-admin not recommended:* Oral carbonic anhydrase inhibitors, topical beta-adrenergic blockers.

SP: Allergic reactions, discontinue. Pre-existing chronic corneal defects and/or history of intra-ocular surgery, caution. CAD, withdraw gradually. Adverse events with systemic sulfonamides may occur including severe Stevens-Johnson syndrome, toxic epidermal necrolysis.

Pregnancy, Lactation: No data.

ADR: *Very common*, eye-burning/stinging, dysgeusia. See SP above.

Notes: See 7.1.2 Carbonic Anhydrase Inhibitors.

Trusopt, Preservative-Free Eye Drops *(Santen)* B. GMS.
Price, (2%) (60) 0.2mL, €28.61. (1) 5mL, €5.45.
Eye drops (multidose), dorzolamide HCl 20mg/mL (2%). Multidose: Slightly viscous aqueous soln. *Benzalkonium chloride.*
Store: Original pack to protect (light).
Eye drops (SDU), as above. Clear colourless slightly viscous. *Preservative-free.* **Store:** As above; below 30 deg; do not freeze.
Dorzolamide Actavis Eye Drops *(Accord)* B. GMS.
Price, (5mL) €4.36.
Eye drops, dorzolamide 20mg/mL. Isotonic buffered slightly viscous clear colourless aqueous soln. *Benzalkonium chloride.*

Dorzolamide, Timolol

ATC Code: S01ED51. **Sport:** Prohibited (specific sports).
Driving: Blurred vision.

Indications: Reduction of elevated IOP in ocular hypertension, open-angle glaucoma (monotherapy or adjunctive). Pseudoexfoliative glaucoma when beta-blocker monotherapy insufficient.

Dose: Adult, Elderly: Instil 1 drop twice daily.

Child: Age 2-6 years, limited data. Under 2 years, no data.

Hepatic Impairment: Caution.

ADR: *Very common*, burning, stinging, dysgeusia.

Notes: See Dorzolamide above. See 7.1.1 Topical Beta-Blockers (timolol).

COSOPT, Preservative-Free Eye Drops *(Santen)* B. GMS.
Price, (5mL) €9.08. UDV 0.2mL (60) €21.69.
Eye drops, dorzolamide HCl, timolol 20mg/5mg per mL (0.8mg/0.2mg per drop). Clear colourless (nearly colourless) slightly viscous soln. *Benzalkonium chloride (multidose); preservative-free (UDV).* **Store:** Below 30 deg C; do not freeze; original pack to protect (light).
Dorzolamide/Timolol Actavis Eye Drops *(Accord)* B. GMS.
Price, (5mL) €5.40.
Eye drops, dorzolamide HCl 20mg, timolol 5mg per mL. Clear colourless slightly viscous aqueous soln. *Benzalkonium chloride.*

7.1.3 - Prostaglandin Analogues

In This Chapter: *Bimatoprost, latanoprost, tafluprost, travoprost (and timolol combinations).*

Class Effects

Driving: See Notes below (ophthalmology).

CI: Hypersensitivity to any member of the class. Use in children unless otherwise stated. See Notes below (beta-blocker combinations).

Interactions: Effect of Other Drugs on Prostaglandin Analogues: *Co-admin not recommended:* Other prostaglandin analogues (paradoxical IOP elevations).

SP: Eyelash growth, darkening of eyelid or periocular skin, increased brown iris pigmentation may occur (permanent eye colour change likely), inform patient. Periorbital and lid changes (deepening of eyelid sulcus). *Inflammatory ocular conditions*, caution; glaucoma (angle-closure, open-angle in pseudophakic patients, pigmentary, pseudoexfoliative, neovascular, congenital), limited/no data. *Macular oedema* risk factors (aphakic patients with torn posterior lens capsule or anterior chamber lenses or at risk for cystoid macular oedema), iritis/uveitis, caution. Bacterial keratitis with multidose containers. *Beta-blocker combinations*, see Notes below (beta-blockers).

Pregnancy, Lactation: Pregnancy, should not be used. Women of childbearing potential to ensure adequate contraception. Lactation, not recommended.

ADR: See individual molecules below.

Notes: See Chapter 7 Ophthalmology, 7.1 Glaucoma. Beta-blocker combinations, see 7.1.1 Topical Beta-Blockers.

Bimatoprost

ATC Code: S01EE03. **Sport:** Permitted.
Driving: Transient blurred vision.
Indications: Reduction of elevated IOP in ocular hypertension and chronic open-angle glaucoma.
Dose: Adult, Elderly: Instil 1 drop (max.) once daily (evening).
Renal Impairment: Caution.
Hepatic Impairment: Moderate to severe, caution.
SP: *Caution*, respiratory impairment, COPD, asthma; heart block above first degree, uncontrolled CHF; cystoid macular oedema (with risk factors); bradycardia, hypotension; predisposing risk factors, aphakic or pseudophakic patients, torn posterior lens capsule. Significant ocular viral infection (herpes simplex). Potential for hair growth in areas where soln comes repeatedly in contact with skin surface; avoid soln running down cheek or other skin areas.
ADR: *Very common*, conjunctival hyperaemia.
Notes: See 7.1.3 Prostaglandin Analogues.

LUMIGAN Eye Drops *(Allergan)* A. GMS.
Price, (3mL) 0.01% (1) €14.00.
Eye drops (multidose), bimatoprost 0.1mg/mL. Colourless (slightly yellow) soln. *Benzalkonium chloride.*

Bimatoprost, Timolol

ATC Code: S01ED51. **Sport:** Prohibited (specific sports).
Driving: Transient blurred vision.
Indications: IOP reduction (adults) with open-angle glaucoma or ocular hypertension (monotherapy insufficient).
Dose: Adult, Elderly: Instil 1 drop once daily (morning or evening; same time each day).
Renal Impairment: Caution.
Hepatic Impairment: As for Renal above.
CI: Reactive airway disease (bronchial asthma, severe COPD), sinus bradycardia, sick sinus syndrome, sino-atrial block, second or third degree atrioventricular block not controlled with pacemaker, overt cardiac failure, cardiogenic shock.
SP: Choroidal detachment reported with aqueous suppressant therapy (timolol, acetazolamide) after filtration procedures.
ADR: Summary, *most common*, conjunctival hyperaemia.
Notes: See Bimatoprost above. See 7.1.1 Topical Beta-Blockers (timolol).

GANfort, SD Eye Drops *(Allergan)* A. GMS.
Price, (3mL) €17.33. SD 0.4mL (30) €20.81.
Eye drops, bimatoprost/timolol 0.3mg/5mg per 1mL. Colourless (slightly yellow) soln. *Benzalkonium chloride.* **Store:** No special conditions.
Single dose eye drops (SD), as above. Colourless (slightly yellow) soln. **Store:** In pouch to protect (light, moisture).

Latanoprost

ATC Code: S01EE01. **Sport:** Permitted.
Driving: Transient blurred vision.
Indications: Reduction of elevated IOP in ocular hypertension and chronic open-angle glaucoma.
Dose: Adult, Elderly: Instil 1 drop (max.) once daily (evening).
Child: As for Adult above. Preterm infants (below 36 weeks gestational age)/age under 1 year, no/limited data. See SP below. *Monopost Unidose*, no data.
SP: Asthmatics, caution. Perioperative with cataract surgery, limited data. Children age 0-3 years with Primary Congenital Glaucoma, surgery (trabeculotomy/goniotomy)

Prostaglandin Analogues   7.1.3

remains first-line treatment. Long-term safety in children not established.

ADR: *Very common*, increased iris pigmentation, conjunctival hyperaemia, eye irritation, eyelash and vellus hair changes. Safety profile in paediatrics similar to adults.
Notes: See 7.1.3 Prostaglandin Analogues.

Xalatan Eye Drops *(Pfizer)* A. GMS.
Price, (2.5mL) €9.24.
Eye drops, latanoprost 1.5mcg/drop. Clear colourless liquid. *Benzalkonium chloride.* **Store:** Below 25 deg C; outer carton; protect (light).
Latacris Eye Drops *(Merit)* A. GMS.
Price, (2.5mL) €7.66.
Eye drops, latanoprost 50mcg/mL (1.5mcg/drop). Clear colourless soln. *Benzalkonium chloride.*
Latanoprost Actavis Eye Drops *(Accord)* A. GMS.
Price, (2.5mL) €7.66.
Eye drops, latanoprost 50mcg/mL (1.5mcg/drop). Clear colourless liquid. *Benzalkonium chloride.*
Latop Eye Drops *(Rowex)* A. GMS.
Price, (2.5mL) €7.66.
Eye drops, latanoprost 50mcg/mL (1.5mcg/drop). Clear colourless soln. *Benzalkonium chloride.*
Monopost Unidose Eye Drops *(Thea Pharma)* A. GMS.
Price, 50mcg/mL SDU (30) €10.97.
Eye drops, latanoprost 50mcg/mL (1.5mcg/drop). Slightly yellow opalescent. *Hydrogenated castor oil.*
Zanopro Eye Drops *(Clonmel)* A. GMS.
Price, (2.5mL) €7.66.
Eye drops, latanoprost 50mcg/mL (1.5mcg/drop). Clear colourless. *Benzalkonium chloride.*

Latanoprost, Timolol

ATC Code: S01ED51. **Sport:** Prohibited (specific sports).
Driving: Transient blurred vision.
Indications: IOP reduction (adults) with open-angle glaucoma or ocular hypertension (monotherapy insufficient).
Dose: Adult, Elderly: Instil 1 drop once daily.
CI: Reactive airway disease (bronchial asthma, severe COPD), sinus bradycardia, sick sinus syndrome, sino-atrial block, second or third degree atrioventricular block not controlled with pacemaker, overt cardiac failure, cardiogenic shock.
ADR: *Very common*, increased iris pigmentation. *Common*, eye irritation/pain.
Notes: See Latanoprost above. See 7.1.1 Topical Beta-Blockers (timolol).

Xalacom Eye Drops *(Pfizer)* A. GMS.
Price, (2.5mL) €12.86.
Eye drops, latanoprost/timolol 50mcg/5mg per 1mL. Soln. *Benzalkonium chloride.*
Latanoprost/Timolol Actavis Eye Drops *(Accord)* A. GMS.
Price, (2.5mL) €10.29.
Eye drops, latanoprost/timolol 50mcg/5mg per 1mL. Clear colourless liquid. *Benzalkonium chloride.*
Latop-Comp Eye Drops *(Rowex)* A. GMS.
Price, (2.5mL) €10.29.
Eye drops, latanoprost/timolol 50mcg/5mg per 1mL. Colourless soln. *Benzalkonium chloride.*
Zanopro Plus Eye Drops *(Clonmel)* A. GMS.
Price, (2.5mL) €9.59.
Eye drops, latanoprost/timolol 50mcg/5mg per 1mL. Clear colourless liquid. *Benzalkonium chloride.*

Tafluprost

ATC Code: S01EE05. **Sport:** Permitted.
Driving: Transient blurred vision.
Indications: Reduction of elevated IOP in ocular hypertension and chronic open-angle glaucoma.
Dose: Adult, Elderly: Instil 1 drop max. once daily.
Renal Impairment: Caution, not studied.
Hepatic Impairment: As for Renal above.
SP: Severe asthma, caution.
ADR: *Common*, headache.
Notes: See 7.1.3 Prostaglandin Analogues.

Saflutan Eye Drops *(Santen)* B. GMS.
Price, UDV (30) €19.13.
Eye drops, tafluprost 15mcg/mL (0.45mcg/drop). Single dose clear colourless soln.

7.1.4　Sympathomimetics

Tafluprost, Timolol

ATC Code: S01ED51. **Sport:** Prohibited (specific sports).
Driving: Transient blurred vision.
Indications: IOP reduction (adults) with open-angle glaucoma or ocular hypertension (monotherapy insufficient).
Dose: Adult, Elderly: Instil 1 drop once daily; single use only; one container sufficient to treat both eyes.
Child: Under 18 years, not recommended.
Renal Impairment: Caution.
Hepatic Impairment: Caution.
ADR: *Most frequent,* conjunctival/ocular hyperaemia.
Notes: See Tafluprost above. See 7.1.1 Topical Beta-Blockers (timolol).

> **Taptiqom Eye Drops** *(Santen)* B. GMS.
> *Price,* (28) SDU, €21.84.
> *Eye drops,* tafluprost 4.5mcg, timolol maleate 1.5mg per 0.3mL single dose unit. Clear colourless soln.

Travoprost

ATC Code: S01EE04. **Sport:** Permitted.
Driving: Transient blurred vision.
Indications: Reduction of elevated IOP in ocular hypertension and chronic open-angle glaucoma.
Dose: Adult, Elderly: Instil 1 drop once daily.
Child: Age 2 months to 18 years, as for Adult above; 2 months -3 years, limited data; under 2 months, no data.
SP: Thyroid eye disease. Avoid contact with skin.
ADR: *Very common,* ocular hyperaemia.
Notes: See 7.1.3 Prostaglandin Analogues.

> **Travatan Eye Drops** *(Novartis)* A. GMS.
> *Price,* (2.5mL) €13.77.
> *Eye drops,* travoprost 40mcg/mL. Clear colourless soln. *Polyquaternium-1, propylene glycol, hydrogenated castor oil.* **Store:** No special conditions.

Travoprost, Timolol

ATC Code: S01ED51. **Sport:** Prohibited (specific sports).
Driving: Temporary blurred vision.
Indications: IOP reduction (adults) with open-angle glaucoma or ocular hypertension (monotherapy insufficient).
Dose: Adult, Elderly: Instil 1 drop (max.) once daily at same time of day.
ADR: *Common,* nervousness, dizziness, heart rate (irregular, decreased), increased/decreased blood pressure, bronchospasm, extremity pain.
Notes: See Travoprost above. See 7.1.1 Topical Beta-Blockers (timolol).

> **DuoTrav Eye Drops** *(Novartis)* A. GMS.
> *Price,* (2.5mL) €16.98.
> *Eye drops,* travoprost/timolol maleate 40mcg/5mg per mL. Clear colourless. *Polyquaternium-1, propylene glycol, castor oil.* **Store:** Below 30 deg C.

7.1.4 - Sympathomimetics

In This Chapter: *Apraclonidine, brimonidine, brimonidine/timolol combination.*

Class Effects

CI: Hypersensitivity to any member of the class.
SP: Caution, history of vasovagal attack, angina, severe cerebral or coronary insufficiency, recent MI, overt cardiac failure, hypertension, CVD (apoplexy), Parkinson's disease, Raynaud's disease, thromboangiitis obliterans, depression.
Notes: See Chapter 7 Ophthalmology and 7.1 Glaucoma.

Apraclonidine

ATC Code: S01EA03. **Sport:** Permitted.
Driving: Drowsiness.
Indications: Short-term, adjunctive, chronic glaucoma requiring additional IOP reduction.

Dose: Adult, Elderly: Instil 1 drop 3-times daily; max. duration 1 month.
Child: Under 12 years, not recommended.
Renal Impairment: Chronic failure, caution.
CI: Hypersensitivity to systemic clonidine. Severe, unstable or uncontrolled cardiovascular disease.
Interactions: Effect of Other Drugs on Apraclonidine: *Co-admin contraindicated:* MAOIs, sympathomimetics (systemic), TCADs. *Consider additive effect:* CNS depressants (ALCOHOL, barbiturates, opiates, sedatives, anaesthetics). *Caution:* Beta-blockers (ophthalmic and systemic), antihypertensives, cardiac glycosides.
SP: End-stage, if reduced vision occurs immediately after admin, discontinue. Avoid contact with soft contact lenses.
Pregnancy, Lactation: Pregnancy, no adequate data; potential risk unknown. Lactation, caution.
ADR: *Common,* ocular hyperaemia.
Notes: See 7.1.4 Sympathomimetics, 2.11 Centrally Acting Antihypertensives (clonidine).

> **Iopidine Eye Drops** *(Novartis)* B. GMS.
> *Price,* 0.5% (5mL) €12.47.
> *Eye drops,* apraclonidine HCl 5mg/mL. Colourless (pale-yellow). *Benzalkonium chloride.* **Store:** Below 25 deg C; outer carton.

Brimonidine (ophthalmic)

ATC Code: S01EA05. **Sport:** Permitted.
Driving: Fatigue and/or drowsiness, blurred and/or abnormal vision especially at night or in reduced lighting.
Indications: Reduction of elevated IOP ocular hypertension and chronic open-angle glaucoma.
Dose: Adult, Elderly: Instil 1 drop twice daily (12-hourly).
Child: Age 12-17 years, no data; under 12 years, not recommended; under 2 years, contraindicated.
Renal Impairment: Caution.
Hepatic Impairment: As for Renal above.
Interactions: Effect of Other Drugs on Brimonidine: *Co-admin contraindicated:* MAOIs, antidepressants affecting noradrenergic transmission (TCADs, mianserin). *Effects potentiated:* CNS depressants (ALCOHOL, barbiturates, opiates, sedatives, anaesthetics). *Co-admin caution:* Drugs affecting metabolism and uptake of circulating amines (chlorpromazine, methylphenidate, reserpine), antihypertensives, cardiac glycosides, adrenergic receptor agonists or antagonists (isoprenaline, prazosin).
SP: Children age 2-7 years and/or weighing 20kg and under, caution; monitor as high incidence and severity of somnolence. Allergic reactions, discontinue as delayed ocular hypersensitivity reactions with increased IOP reported. Orthostatic hypotension.
Pregnancy, Lactation: Pregnancy, if benefit outweighs risk; if administered up to time of delivery, monitor neonate during first days of life. Lactation, not recommended.
ADR: *Very common,* headache, drowsiness, oral dryness, fatigue.
Notes: See 7.1.4 Sympathomimetics.

> **Alphagan Eye Drops** *(Allergan)* B. GMS.
> *Price,* 0.2% (5mL) €8.58.
> *Eye drops,* brimonidine tartrate 2mg (1.3mg brimonidine)/mL. Clear greenish-yellow. *Benzalkonium chloride.*

Brimonidine, Timolol

ATC Code: S01ED51. **Sport:** Prohibited (specific sports).
Driving: Transient blurred vision, visual disturbance, fatigue and/or drowsiness
Indications: Reduction of elevated IOP ocular hypertension and chronic open-angle glaucoma (monotherapy insufficient).
Dose: Adult, Elderly: Instil 1 drop twice daily (12-hourly).
Child: Under 2 years, contraindicated; age 2-17 years, not recommended.
CI: Sinus bradycardia, sick sinus syndrome, sino-atrial block, second or third degree AV block not controlled with pacemaker, overt cardiac failure, cardiogenic shock.
SP: Cardiac reactions (timolol).
Notes: See Brimonidine above. See 7.1.1 Topical Beta-Blockers (timolol).

Combigan Eye Drops *(Allergan)* B. GMS.
Price, (5mL) €13.09.
Eye drops, brimonidine tartrate 2mg (1.3mg brimonidine), timolol 5mg per mL. *Benzalkonium chloride.*

7.1.5 - Miotics

In This Chapter: *Acetylcholine, pilocarpine.*

Class Effects
Driving: See Notes below.
CI: Hypersensitivity to any member of the class.
Notes: See Chapter 7 Ophthalmology and 7.1 Glaucoma.

Acetylcholine
ATC Code: S01EB09. **Sport:** Permitted.
Driving: Hospital use.
Indications: Cataract surgery, penetrating keratoplasty, iridectomy, other anterior segment surgery where rapid complete miosis is required.
Dose: Adult, Elderly: For intraocular irrigation during surgery, 0.5-2mL produces miosis lasting approx. 20 minutes; second application at surgeon discretion.
Interactions: Effect of Other Drugs on Acetylcholine: *Reports of being ineffective:* Topical NSAIDs.
SP: Obstructions to miosis, anterior or posterior synechiae may require surgery prior to admin. Should only be used for lens delivery in cataract surgery.
Pregnancy, Lactation: Should not be used.
ADR: Bradycardia, hypotension, flushing, breathing difficulties, sweating. Isolated cases of corneal oedema, clouding, decompensation.
Notes: See 7.1.5 Miotics.

> **Miochol-E Intraocular Irrigation** *(Bausch&Lomb)* A.
> *Price,* (2mL) €10.79.
> *Intraocular irrigation,* acetylcholine chloride 10mg/mL. White solid powder. Clear colourless solvent.

Pilocarpine (ophthalmic)
ATC Code: S01EB01. **Sport:** Permitted.
Driving: Transient blurred vision.
Indications: Emergency glaucoma treatment; miotic for reversing the action of weaker mydriatics.
Dose: Adult, Elderly: *Simple glaucoma,* 1-2 drops 3-times daily; *closed-angle,* 1-2 drops as required. *To reverse mydriasis,* 1-2 drops. *Miosis,* 1-2 drops.
Child: Concentrations of up to 2% may be safely used; no dose recommendation. Under 18 years, initiate at lowest available dose and concentration.
CI: Pupillary constriction undesirable such as acute iritis, anterior uveitis, secondary glaucoma.
Interactions: Effect of Other Drugs on Pilocarpine: *Co-admin not recommended:* Other miotics. *Effect antagonised:* Corticosteroids (topical, systemic), systemic anticholinergics, antihistamines, pethidine, sympathomimetics, TCADs.
SP: *Caution,* systemic absorption with inflamed eye, acute heart failure, bronchial asthma, peptic ulcer, hypertension, urinary tract obstruction, Parkinson's disease, corneal abrasions. With retinal disease, caution retinal detachment. Chronic glaucoma or long-term use, regularly monitor IOP. Patients with dark irises may need higher conc pilocarpine eye drops.
Pregnancy, Lactation: If benefit outweighs risk.
ADR: Brow and/or, headache, sweating, salivation, eye (burning, itching, blurred vision, ciliary spasm, conjunctival vascular congestion, induced myopia, sensitisation of lids and conjunctiva, reduced visual acuity in poor illumination, lens changes (chronic use), increased papillary block, retinal detachment, vitreous haemorrhage, lacrimation), bradycardia, hypotension, pulmonary oedema, bronchial spasm, nausea, vomiting, diarrhoea.
Notes: See 7.1.5 Miotics.

> **Minims Pilocarpine 2%** *(Bausch&Lomb)* B. GMS.
> *Price,* 2% (20) €6.40.
> *Eye drops,* pilocarpine nitrate. Single dose clear colourless sterile soln. *Preservative-free.* NOTE: Use with soft contact lenses, not recommended.

7.2 - Anti-Infective Eye Preparations

In This Chapter: *Aciclovir, azithromycin, cefuroxime, chloramphenicol, fusidic acid, gentamicin, ofloxacin.*

Class Effects
Driving, and use of preservative *(benzalkonium chloride),* see Notes below.
CI: Hypersensitivity to any member of the class.
SP: Avoid wearing contact lenses with bacterial ocular infection and during treatment. Severe infection, supplement with systemic treatment. Prolonged antibacterial use, caution (superinfection, emergence of resistant organisms). *Aminoglycosides,* may cause irreversible partial or total deafness when given systemically or when applied topically to open wounds or damaged skin; effect is dose-related, enhanced by renal and/or hepatic impairment; more likely in children, elderly. *Fluoroquinolones,* corneal perforation risk especially with corneal (epithelial defects, ulcers). Allergic reactions, discontinue (may be serious or fatal). Not for prophylaxis or treatment of gonococcal conjunctivitis including gonococcal ophthalmia neonatorum.
Notes: See Chapter 7 Ophthalmology. Systemic effects of topical anti-infectives, see Chapter 9 Infectious Diseases.

Aciclovir (ophthalmic)
ATC Code: S01AD03. **Sport:** Permitted.
Driving: Can affect visual ability.
Indications: Treatment, Herpes simplex keratitis.
Dose: Adult, Elderly: Place 1cm ointment inside the lower conjunctival sac 5 times daily at 4-hourly intervals; continue for at least 3 days after fully healed.
CI: Valaciclovir hypersensitivity.
Pregnancy, Lactation: If benefit outweighs risk.
ADR: Superficial punctate keratopathy, mild stinging, conjunctivitis, blepharitis; rarely hypersensitivity.
Notes: See 7.2 Anti-Infective Eye Preparations.

> **Zovirax Eye Ointment** *(GSK)* A. GMS.
> *Price,* (4.5g) €8.99.
> *Eye ointment,* aciclovir 3% w/w. White (off-white) soft homogenous.

Azithromycin (ophthalmic)
ATC Code: S01AA26. **Sport:** Permitted.
Driving: Transient blurred vision on instillation.
Indications: Conjunctivitis caused by susceptible strains (purulent bacterial conjunctivitis, trachomatous conjunctivitis) in children and adults.
Dose: Adult, Elderly: Instil 1 drop twice daily (morning, evening) for 3 days.
Child: Birth to 17 years, as for Adult above.
SP: Allergic reactions, discontinue. Not necessary to continue treatment beyond 3 days. Not for prophylactic treatment of bacterial conjunctivitis in newborn. Use with other eye drops, 15-minute interval between instillations.
Pregnancy, Lactation: Can be used.
ADR: *Very common,* ocular discomfort (pruritus, burning, stinging) on instillation.
Notes: See 7.2 Anti-Infective Eye Preparations.

> **Azyter Eye Drops** *(Thea Pharma)* A. GMS.
> *Price,* single dose (6) €6.11.
> *Eye drops,* azithromycin dihydrate (single dose). Clear colourless (slightly-yellow) oily liquid.

Cefuroxime (ophthalmic)
ATC Code: S01AA27. **Sport:** Permitted.
Driving: Not relevant.
Indications: Antibiotic prophylaxis of post-op endophthalmitis after cataract surgery.
Dose: Adult, Elderly: Recommended, 0.1mL of reconstituted soln. Do not inject more than recommended dose. For intracameral use by slow injection at end of cataract surgery.
Child: No data.
SP: Caution, penicillin/beta-lactam allergics. Risk for

resistant strains, consider alternative. Complicated cases and special patient groups, use if benefit outweighs risk.

Pregnancy, Lactation: Pregnancy, can be used as systemic exposure negligible. Lactation, can be used.

ADR: Very rarely, anaphylactic reaction.

Notes: See 7.2 Anti-Infective Eye Preparations.

Aprok Parenteral (Thea Pharma) A.
Price, not published by company.
Intracameral injection, cefuroxime sodium 50mg/vial. White (almost) powder for soln.

Chloramphenicol

ATC Code: S01AA01. **Sport:** Permitted.
Driving: Transient blurred vision on instillation.

Indications: Treatment, ocular infection due to sensitive organisms.

Dose: Adult, Elderly: Instil 1-2 drops or 1 ointment application 3-hourly (more frequently if needed); continue for minimum 48 hours after eye appears normal.

Child: As for Adult above; dose adjustment may be needed in newborns (reduced systemic elimination due to immature metabolism; risk of dose-related adverse effects). Max. duration 10-14 days.

SP: Caution, previous recent conjunctivitis, glaucoma, dry eye syndrome, eye surgery or laser treatment (last 6 months), concurrent other eye preparations, contact lens use.

Pregnancy, Lactation: If benefit outweighs risk.

ADR: Aplastic anaemia, bone marrow failure, anaphylactic reaction, burning sensation, angioedema, dermatitis, urticaria, stinging sensation, pyrexia.

Notes: See 7.2 Anti-Infective Eye Preparations.

Chloromycetin Redidrops (Concordia) A. GMS.
Price, Redidrops 0.5% (10mL) €2.43.
Eye drops, chloramphenicol 0.5%. Clear colourless sterile aqueous soln. Phenylmercuric nitrate. **Store:** Refrigerate.
Minims Chloramphenicol 0.5% (Bausch&Lomb) A. GMS.
Price, 0.5% (20) €6.64.
Eye drops, chloramphenicol. Clear colourless single dose. Preservative-free.

Fusidic Acid (ophthalmic)

ATC Code: S01AA13. **Sport:** Permitted.
Driving: Transient blurred vision on instillation.

Indications: Treatment, ocular infection due to sensitive organisms.

Dose: Adult, Elderly: Instil 1 drop 12-hourly.

SP: Microcrystalline fusidic acid may cause scratches in contact lens or cornea; contact lenses should not be worn.

Pregnancy, Lactation: Pregnancy, can be used if considered necessary. Lactation, no effects on suckling child anticipated, can be used.

ADR: Transient stinging, burning. Pruritus, rash, allergic reactions.

Notes: See 7.2 Anti-Infective Eye Preparations.

Fucithalmic Eye Drops (Concordia) A. GMS.
Price, (5g) €2.84.
Eye drops, fusidic acid hemihydrate. White (off-white) viscous susp. Benzalkonium chloride.

Gentamicin (eye, ear)

ATC Code: S01AA11. **Sport:** Permitted.
Driving: Transient blurred vision on instillation.

Indications: Treatment, superficial infection OR prophylaxis of infection in trauma of ear and eye.

Dose: Adult, Elderly: Eye, instil 1-2 drops up to 6-times daily; severe infection, initially 1-2 drops every 15-20 minutes, reducing frequency as infection is controlled. Ear, instil 2-3 drops 3-4 times daily and at night.

Child: As for Adult above.

CI: Perforated ear drum (use in otitis externa). Myasthenia gravis.

Interactions: Effect of Other Drugs on Gentamicin: Co-admin not recommended: Sulfacetamide. Co-admin caution: Other nephro or ototoxic drugs.

SP: Cross-sensitivity with other aminoglycosides.

Irreversible toxic effects may result from direct contact of gentamicin with middle and inner ear; not for use if integrity of ear drum cannot be guaranteed. Remove contact lenses during treatment for ocular infections.

Pregnancy, Lactation: If benefit outweighs risk.

ADR: Local sensitivity, blurred vision, eye irritation, burning/stinging sensation, eye pruritus, ototoxicity, vestibular disorders, hearing loss, dermatitis, nephrotoxicity (systemic), acute renal failure.

Notes: See 7.2 Anti-Infective Eye Preparations.

Genticin Eye/Ear Drops (Concordia) A. GMS.
Price, (10mL) €2.43.
Eye drops, gentamicin sulfate 0.3% w/v gentamicin base. Clear colourless liquid. Benzalkonium chloride.

Ofloxacin (ophthalmic)

ATC Code: S01AE01. **Sport:** Permitted.
Driving: Transient blurred vision on instillation.

Indications: Topical treatment of external ocular infections (conjunctivitis, keratoconjunctivitis) caused by ofloxacin-sensitive organisms.

Dose: Adult, Elderly: 1-2 drops 3-4 times daily; max. 10 days.

Child: Contraindicated for use in children or adolescents before epiphyseal closure.

CI: Use in children or adolescents before epiphyseal closure.

Interactions: Effect of Other Drugs on Ofloxacin: Caution: Drugs prolonging QT-interval (Class IA and III anti-arrhythmics, TCADs, macrolides, antipsychotics). Systemic absorption affected: Mineral antacids. Renal toxicity: Phenylpropionic acid derived NSAIDs.

SP: Allergic reactions, discontinue. Serious (fatal) anaphylactic or anaphylactoid reactions reported with systemic quinolones. Rhinopharyngeal passage risk. Neonates with ophthalmia neonatorum caused by Neisseria gonorrhoea or Chlamydia trachomatis, not recommended.
Caution, use with existent CNS disorders, epilepsy, hepatic or renal insufficiency, or severe dehydration. Photosensitivity reactions may occur. Evidence of CNS irritability reported (particularly elderly). Corneal perforation risk in patients with corneal epithelial defects or corneal ulcers. Risk factors for QT-prolongation (elderly and women more sensitive to QTc-prolonging medications).

Pregnancy, Lactation: Contraindicated.

ADR: Common, eye irritation, ocular discomfort.

Notes: See 7.2 Anti-Infective Eye Preparations. For systemic effects, see 9.1.5 Quinolones.

Exocin Eye Drops (Allergan) A. GMS.
Price, 0.3% (5mL) €2.79.
Eye drops, ofloxacin 0.3% w/v (3mg/mL). Clear pale (light yellow-green); visible particle practically-free. Benzalkonium chloride.

In This Chapter: Betamethasone (and neomycin combination), ciclosporin, dexamethasone (and framycetin, gramicidin combinations), ciclosporin, diclofenac, epinastine, fluorometholone, ketorolac, ketotifen, loteprednol, nepafenac, olopatadine, prednisolone, sodium cromoglicate.

Class Effects

Driving: See Notes below.

CI: Hypersensitivity to any member of the class. Corticosteroids, ocular viral infections (Herpes simplex, vaccinia, varicella), fungal, TB or mycobacterial infections, history of herpes simplex keratitis, purulent bacterial infections; nasal infection, pulmonary TB or following nasal surgery until healed. NSAIDs, asthma, urticaria, acute rhinitis precipitated by aspirin or other NSAIDs.

Interactions: Effect of Other Drugs on Ophthalmic Corticosteroids: Increased potential for corneal healing problems with co-admin: Topical NSAIDs.

SP: Corticosteroids, prolonged use may increase IOP

and/or glaucoma with damage to optic nerve, reduced visual acuity, visual field defects, increased incidence of lenticular opacities. Use for longer than 1 week only with medical supervision. May induce corneal perforation, especially with diseases causing thinning of cornea or sclera. Cataracts. Not for use for undiagnosed red eye; inappropriate use potentially blinding. May exacerbate severity or prolong course of viral eye infections. Acute purulent untreated infection of eye may be masked or activity enhanced. Persistent corneal ulceration, consider fungal infection. For systemic effects, see Notes below (glucocorticoids). *Combinations* (corticosteroid + antibiotic), exclude fungal or viral disease before use. Prolonged antibacterial use may lead to overgrowth of non-susceptible bacteria or fungi. Topical aminoglycoside hypersensitivity may occur; products containing neomycin sulphate, advise patient to consult doctor if ocular pain, redness, swelling or irritation worsens or persists; *serious* adverse reactions (neurotoxicity, ototoxicity, nephrotoxicity) have occurred with systemic neomycin or applied topically to open wounds or damaged skin. Nephrotoxic and neurotoxic reactions with systemic polymyxin B. For systemic effects of anti-infectives, see Notes below (infectious diseases).

Topical NSAIDs, may slow or delay wound healing. Use may result in keratitis; continued use may result in epithelial breakdown, corneal thinning, erosion, ulceration or perforation (may be sight threatening); epithelial breakdown, discontinue. Increased corneal event risk with complicated or repeat ocular surgeries, corneal denervation or epithelial defects, diabetes mellitus, ocular surface diseases, rheumatoid arthritis. Systemic effects of NSAIDS, see Notes below (NSAIDs)

Intravitreous injection can be associated with endophthalmitis (patient to report suggestive symptoms; eye pain, blurred vision), intraocular inflammation, increased IOP, retinal detachment. Eye drops are not for injection. With multiple medications, eye ointments should be administered last. Contact lens wear is not recommended during treatment of ocular inflammation.

Benzalkonium chloride, phosphate-containing eye-drops, see Notes below (Chapter 7 Ophthalmology).

Pregnancy, Lactation: *Pregnancy, corticosteroids,* foetal development abnormalities (cleft palate, intrauterine growth retardation) reported (animal use), avoid prolonged or extensive use; foetal ototoxicity risk (aminoglycosides). *Lactation,* systemic corticosteroids appear in human milk in quantities that could affect breastfed child; with topical instillation, systemic exposure is low.

ADR: Hypersensitivity reactions (irritation, burning, stinging, itching). *Corticosteroids,* increased IOP (optic nerve damage, reduced visual acuity, visual field defects). Prolonged use, formation of posterior subcapsular cataracts. Secondary ocular irritation.

Notes: See Class Effects, Chapter 7 Ophthalmology above, 11.1.1 Glucocorticoids, 4.4.2 NSAIDS (Non-Selective), 9.1 Antibacterials.

Betamethasone (eye, ear, nose)

ATC Code: S01BA06. **Sport:** Permitted.
Driving: Transient blurred vision on instillation.
Indications: Corticosteroid responsive inflammation of eye, ear and nose, without infection.
Dose: Adult, Elderly: *Drops,* EYE, instil 1-2 drops every 1-2 hours; EAR, instil 2-3 drops every 2-3 hours; NOSE, instil 2-3 drops into each nostril 2-3 times daily.
Ointment, EYE, introduce one quarter inch beneath lower lid 2-3 times daily and/or at night.
CI: Herpetic keratitis. Perforated ear drum.
SP: No response in 7 days, discontinue. Use lowest effective dose; following prolonged treatment (6-8 weeks) withdraw slowly.
ADR: Nasal irritation/dryness, sneezing, headache, light-headedness, urticaria, nausea, epistaxis, rebound congestion, bronchial asthma, perforation of nasal septum, anosmia, parosmia, taste disturbance.
Notes: See 7.3 Ophthalmic Corticosteroids.

Betnesol Eye, Ear, Nasal Drops *(Recipharm)* B. GMS.
Price, (10mL) €1.65.
Eye, ear, nose drops, betamethasone sodium phosphate 0.1% w/v. Colourless soln. *Benzalkonium chloride.* **Note:** A patient leaflet should be supplied with this product.

Betamethasone, Neomycin

ATC Code: S01CA05. **Sport:** Permitted.
Driving: Transient blurred vision on instillation.
Indications: Corticosteroid responsive inflammation requiring antibiotic prophylaxis.
Dose: Adult, Elderly: EYE, instil 1-2 drops up to 6-times daily. EAR, instil 2-3 drops 3-4 times daily. NOSE, instil 2-3 drops into each nostril 2-3 times daily.
Notes: See Betamethasone above. See 7.3 Ophthalmic Corticosteroids.

Betnesol-N Eye, Ear, Nasal Drops *(Recipharm)* A. GMS.D.
Price, (10mL) €1.68.
Eye, ear, nose drops, betamethasone sodium phosphate 0.1% w/v, neomycin sulfate 3500 IU per mL. *Benzalkonium chloride.*

Ciclosporin (ophthalmic)

ATC Code: S01AX18. **Sport:** Permitted.
Driving: Moderate influence; temporary blurred vision, other visual disturbances.
Indications: Treatment (adults) severe keratitis with dry eye disease not improved by tear substitutes.
Dose: Adult, Elderly: 1 drop once daily applied to affected eye(s) at bedtime. Assess response 6-monthly. Allow 15-minute dosing interval with other topical ophthalmics.
Child: Under 18 years, no relevant use.
CI: Active or suspected periocular infection.
SP: Ocular herpes, glaucoma, caution. Remove contact lenses before instillation at bedtime; may be reinserted in morning. Immunosuppressant (may affect host defences); possibly potentiated (with corticosteroids).
Pregnancy, Lactation: Pregnancy, not recommended unless benefit outweighs risk. Women of childbearing potential not using effective contraception, not recommended. Lactation, stop breastfeeding or stop drug.
ADR: *Most common,* eye (pain, irritation), lacrimation, ocular hyperaemia, eyelid erythema.
Notes: For systemic effects, see 4.4.1 Drugs Suppressing Rheumatic Disease Process.

IKERVIS Eye Drops 1mg/mL *(Santen)* A. GMS.
Price, (30) 0.3mL, €86.64.
Eye drops, ciclosporin. Milky white emulsion. *Cetalkonium chloride.* **Store:** Do not freeze.

Dexamethasone (ophthalmic)

ATC Code: S01BA01. **Sport:** Permitted.
Driving: No or negligible influence. Temporary reduced vision (intravitreal injection).
Indications: Non-infectious inflammatory eye conditions (anterior segment) *(Dexafree).* Allergic and inflammatory eye conditions *(Maxidex).* Treatment (adults) with, visual impairment due to diabetic macular oedema (DME) (pseudophakic or insufficiently responsive/unsuitable for non-corticosteroid therapy); macular oedema following either Branch (BRVO) or Central Retinal Vein Occlusion (CRVO); inflammation of posterior segment of eye presenting as non-infectious uveitis *(Ozurdex).*
Dose: Adult, Elderly: *Dexafree,* instil 1 drop 4-6 times daily; severe, initiate with 1 drop every hour; reduce to 4-hourly when favourable response observed (max. 14 days).
Maxidex, instil 1 drop every 30-60 minutes for 3-4 days or until satisfactory response.
Ozurdex, 1 implant admin intra-vitreally to affected eye; not recommended to treat both eyes concurrently. Retreatment, method of admin, see manufacturers Full Prescribing Information.
Child: *Dexafree*, Ozurdex,* no relevant use (DME, B/CRVO); uveitis*. *Maxidex,* under 2 years*. *(safety and efficacy not established).
Renal Impairment: Safety, efficacy not established.
Hepatic Impairment: As for Renal above.
CI: Ocular or periocular infection (active, suspected),

7.3   Ophthalmic Corticosteroids, Anti-Inflammatories, Antihistamines

herpes simplex keratitis; advanced uncontrolled glaucoma, aphakic eyes with rupture of posterior lens capsule, eyes with Anterior Chamber Intraocular Lens (ACIOL), iris or trans-scleral fixated intraocular lens and ruptured posterior lens capsule. Corticosteroid-induced ocular hypertension, perforation, ulceration, corneal injury.

Interactions: Effect of Other Drugs on Dexamethasone (ophthalmic): *Plasma levels may be increased:* Ritonavir.

SP: Ocular use only. Implant, caution with anti-coagulants or anti-platelets. Monitor for device migration.

Pregnancy, Lactation: Not recommended unless clearly necessary. Lactation, suggest stop treatment or stop breastfeeding; *Dexafree* use instead.

ADR: *Most common, Dexafree,* raised IOP; *Maxidex,* ocular discomfort; *Ozurdex,* raised IOP, cataract, conjunctival haemorrhage.

Notes: See 7.3 Ophthalmic Corticosteroids.

Dexafree 1mg/mL Drops *(Thea Pharma)* B. GMS.
Price, (30) SDU, €7.78.
Eye drops, dexamethasone sodium phosphate. Clear colourless (slightly-brown). *Preservative-free.*

Maxidex Eye Drops *(Novartis)* A. GMS.
Price, drops (5mL) €1.98. Ointment (3g) €2.47.
Eye drops, dexamethasone 0.1% w/v. White susp flocculates-free. *Benzalkonium chloride.* **Store:** Below 25 deg C; do not (refrigerate, freeze).

Ozurdex Intravitreal Implant *(Allergan)* A. HOS.
Price, (1) 700mcg, €996.14 (PTW).
Intravitreal implant, dexamethasone 700mcg. Disposable injection device containing implant.

Dexamethasone, Framycetin, Gramicidin

ATC Code: S01CA01. **Sport:** Permitted.
Driving: Transient blurred vision on instillation.
Indications: Otitis externa. Steroid responsive eye conditions, with antibiotic prophylaxis. Blepharitis.

Dose: Adult, Elderly: EAR, instil 2-3 drops 3-4 times daily. EYE, instil 1-2 drops up to 6-times daily. Duration max. 7 days.

Child: Infants, contraindicated.

CI: Herpetic keratitis. Perforated ear drum.

SP: Prolonged ocular use, delayed hypersensitivity including irritation, burning, stinging, itching, dermatitis. Risk of irreversible, partial or total deafness due to aminoglycoside; risk at high doses; small children or infants. Adrenal suppression in infants.

ADR: See Notes below.

Notes: See 7.3 Ophthalmic Corticosteroids.

Sofradex Eye/Ear Drops *(SANOFI)* A. GMS.
Price, (10mL) €5.24.
Ear/eye drops, dexamethasone 0.05%, framycetin sulfate 0.5%, gramicidin 0.005% w/v. Practically clear colourless (slightly green-yellow) aqueous soln.

Dexamethasone, Neomycin, Polymyxin B

ATC Code: S01CA01. **Sport:** Permitted.
Driving: Transient blurred vision on instillation.
Indications: Short-term treatment, steroid-responsive eye conditions requiring antibiotic prophylaxis after excluding fungal/viral disease.

Dose: Adult, Elderly: Instil 1-2 drops up to 6-times daily or more frequently if needed. Shake bottle well before use.

Child: As for Adult above.

Renal Impairment: Not studied.

Hepatic Impairment: Not studied.

SP: Signs of serious hypersensitivity, discontinue. Cushing's syndrome and/or adrenal suppression with systemic absorption; may occur with intensive or long-term continuous therapy in predisposed patients e.g. children, patients treated with ritonavir.

ADR: Summary, *most common,* ocular discomfort, keratitis, eye irritation.

Notes: See Sofradex above. See 7.3 Ophthalmic Corticosteroids.

Maxitrol 0.1% Eye Drops *(Novartis)* A. GMS.
Price, drops 0.1% (5mL) €2.32. Ointment (3.5g) €1.93.
Eye drops, dexamethasone 1mg, polymyxin B sulfate 6000 IU,

neomycin sulfate 3500 IU per mL. White (pale-yellow) opaque susp. *Benzalkonium chloride.* **Store:** Below 25 deg C. Original pack; do not (refrigerate, freeze).

Diclofenac Sodium (ophthalmic)

ATC Code: S01BC03. **Sport:** Permitted.
Driving: Blurred vision.

Indications: Pre- and post-operative prevention of post-surgery aphakic cystoid macular oedema with cataract lens extraction, intraocular lens implantation; post-operative inflammation in cataract surgery. Inhibition of intra-operative miosis. Non-infected inflammatory conditions of anterior segment of eye. Inflammation following trauma and non-penetrating injuries. Ocular pain, discomfort, corneal epithelial defects after excimer PRK surgery.

Dose: Adult, Elderly: *Pre-operative,* instil 1 drop 4-times during the 2 hours immediately before surgery; *post-operative,* instil 1 drop 4-times daily; up to 12 weeks; *post PRK* use, instil 1 drop twice within hour pre-operative, then 1 drop twice (5 minutes apart) immediately after surgery; then 1 drop every 2-5 hours while awake; up to 24 hours. *Other indications,* instil 1 drop 4-5 times daily.

Child: Experience limited to a few clinical trials in strabismus surgery.

CI: Asthma, urticaria, acute rhinitis precipitated by aspirin, other prostaglandin synthetase inhibitors. Intraocular use during surgical procedure.

ADR: Hypersensitivity, itching, reddening, photosensitivity, keratitis punctata, corneal epithelial discontinuity. Prolonged use, corneal ulcer or thinning. Dyspnoea, asthma exacerbation.

Notes: See 7.3 Ophthalmic Corticosteroids.

Voltarol Ophth Multidose 0.1% *(Thea Pharma)* B. GMS.
Price, (5mL) €4.07.
Eye drops, diclofenac sodium 0.1% w/v. Clear colourless soln. *Benzalkonium chloride.*

Epinastine

ATC Code: S01GX10. **Sport:** Permitted.
Driving: Transient blurred vision on instillation.

Indications: Seasonal allergic conjunctivitis.

Dose: Adult, Elderly: Instil 1 drop twice daily.

Child: Over 12 years, as for Adult above; age 3-12 years, limited data; under 3 years, no data.

SP: For topical use only.

Pregnancy, Lactation: Caution.

ADR: *Most common,* burning sensation in eye (mostly mild); no serious adverse reactions occurred.

Notes: See 7.3 Ophthalmic Corticosteroids.

Relestat Drops *(Allergan)* A. GMS.
Price, 0.5mg/mL (5mL) €7.59.
Eye drops, epinastine HCl 0.5mg/mL. Clear colourless sterile soln. *Benzalkonium chloride.*

Fluorometholone

ATC Code: S01CB05. **Sport:** Permitted.
Driving: Transient blurred vision on instillation.

Indications: Inflammation of the palpebral and bulbar conjunctiva, cornea, and anterior segment of the globe.

Dose: Adult, Elderly: Instil 1-2 drops 2-4 times daily; initial 24-48 hours frequency may be increased to 2 drops hourly.

Child: Over 2 years, as for Adult above.

SP: Undiagnosed red eye may be due to Herpes simplex; aggravated by corticosteroid; corneal ulceration, possible vision loss. Skin atrophy, striae, telangiectasia of facial skin.

Pregnancy, Lactation: Use only if clearly necessary.

ADR: *Common,* raised IOP.

Notes: See 7.3 Ophthalmic Corticosteroids.

FML Liquifilm 0.1% *(Allergan)* A. GMS.
Price, (5mL) €2.20.
Eye drops, fluorometholone 0.1% w/v (1mg/mL). White microfine susp. *Benzalkonium chloride.* **Store:** Below 25 deg C; do not (refrigerate, freeze).

Ketorolac

ATC Code: S01BC05. **Sport:** Permitted.
Driving: Transient blurred vision on instillation.
Indications: Inflammation following cataract surgery.
Dose: Adult, Elderly: Instil 1 drop 3-times daily starting 24 hours pre-operative; continue for 3-4 weeks. Use with other topical eye medication, leave 5-minute interval between admin.
CI: Acetylsalicylic acid, other NSAID sensitivity.
SP: Coagulation disorders, may mask signs of infection. Caution, concomitant NSAIDs, corticosteroids; corneal epithelial breakdown; may also delay wound healing.
Pregnancy, Lactation: Pregnancy, not recommended; women of childbearing potential to ensure adequate contraception. Lactation, not recommended.
ADR: *Very common*, eye irritation, burning sensation, eye pain, stinging.
Notes: See 7.3 Ophthalmic Corticosteroids.

> **Acular 0.5% Drops** *(Allergan)* B. GMS.
> *Price*, (5mL) €5.36.
> *Eye drops*, ketorolac trometamol 5mg/mL. Clear colourless (pale-yellow) aqueous soln. *Benzalkonium chloride.*

Ketotifen (ophthalmic)

ATC Code: S01GX08. **Sport:** Permitted.
Driving: Blurred vision, somnolence.
Indications: Seasonal allergic conjunctivitis.
Dose: Adult, Elderly: Instil 1 drop twice daily.
Child: 3 years and older, as for Adult above.
Pregnancy, Lactation: Pregnancy, caution. Lactation, can be used.
ADR: Punctate corneal epithelial erosion, dry eyes, eyelid disorder, conjunctivitis, eye pain, photophobia, subconjunctival haemorrhage. *Systemic*, headache, somnolence, skin rash, eczema, urticaria, dry mouth, allergic reaction. See Notes below (ketotifen).
Notes: See 7.3 Ophthalmic Corticosteroids. See 5.7.3 Other Drugs Used in Allergic Disorders (ketotifen).

> **Zaditen 0.25% Eye Drops** *(Thea Pharma)* B. GMS.
> *Price*, (5mL) €7.53.
> *Eye drops*, ketotifen hydrogen fumarate 0.25mg/mL. Clear colourless (faintly yellow) soln. *Benzalkonium chloride.*

Loteprednol

ATC Code: S01BA14. **Sport:** Permitted.
Driving: Transient blurred vision on instillation.
Indications: Post-operative inflammation following ocular surgery.
Dose: Adult, Elderly: 1-2 drops 4-times daily commencing 24 hours after surgery; duration max. 2 weeks.
Child: Not recommended.
Interactions: Effect of Loteprednol on Other Drugs: Ocular hypotensives: *Decreased hypotensive effect; increased IOP.*
SP: If used for 10 days or longer, monitor IOP.
Pregnancy, Lactation: Pregnancy, use only if clearly necessary. Lactation, contraindicated.
ADR: *Common*, corneal defect, eye discharge, discomfort, dry eye, epiphora, foreign body sensation, conjunctival hyperaemia, eye itching, instillation site burning, headache.
Notes: See 7.3 Ophthalmic Corticosteroids.

> **Lotemax 0.5% Drops** *(Bausch&Lomb)* A.
> *Price*, not published by company (GMS-pending).
> *Eye drops*, loteprednol etabonate 5mg/mL. Milky-white susp. *Benzalkonium chloride.*

Nepafenac

ATC Code: S01BC10. **Sport:** Pending.
Driving: Transient blurred vision on instillation.
Indications: Prevention and treatment, post-operative pain and inflammation following cataract surgery; reduction in risk, post-operative macular oedema with cataract surgery in diabetics.
Dose: Adult, Elderly: Instil 1 drop 3-times daily starting 1 day prior to surgery, continue on day of surgery with additional drop 30-120 minutes prior to surgery; then for up to 21 days post-operative (prevention and treatment, pain and inflammation) or up to 60 days (reduction in post-operative macular oedema risk).
Child: Under 18 years, not recommended.
Interactions: Effect of Other Drugs on Nepafenac: *Co-Admin Not Recommended*: Prostaglandin analogues.
SP: Do not inject or swallow. Avoid sunlight during treatment. Increased bleeding of ocular tissue in conjunction with ocular surgery, caution with known bleeding tendencies or medicinals prolonging bleeding time. Potential cross-sensitivity with aspirin, phenylacetic acid derivatives, NSAIDs.
Pregnancy, Lactation: Pregnancy, not recommended; not for use in women of childbearing potential not using contraception. Lactation, can be used.
ADR: Summary, *most common*, punctate keratitis, foreign body sensation, eyelid margin crusting.
Notes: See 7.3 Ophthalmic Corticosteroids.

> **NEVANAC 1mg/mL Drops** *(Novartis)* B.
> *Price*, 5mL, €20.00.
> *Eye drops*, nepafenac. Light-yellow (light-orange) susp. pH 7.4. *Benzalkonium chloride.* **Store:** Below 30 deg C.

Olopatadine

ATC Code: S01GX09. **Sport:** Permitted.
Driving: Transient blurred vision on instillation.
Indications: Seasonal allergic conjunctivitis.
Dose: Adult, Elderly: Instil 1 drop twice daily.
Child: Over 3 years, as for Adult above.
SP: Hypersensitivity, discontinue. Wait 10-15 minutes after instillation before inserting contact lenses; do not admin while wearing contact lenses.
Pregnancy, Lactation: Pregnancy, women of childbearing potential not using contraception, lactation, not recommended.
ADR: *Common*, headache, dysgeusia, eye pain/irritation, dry eye, abnormal sensation, nasal dryness, fatigue.
Notes: See 7.3 Ophthalmic Corticosteroids.

> **Opatanol 1mg/mL Drops** *(Novartis)* B. GMS.
> *Price*, 1mg/mL (5mL) €7.44.
> *Eye drops*, olopatadine HCl. Clear colourless soln. *Benzalkonium chloride.* **Store:** No special conditions.

Prednisolone (ophthalmic)

ATC Code: S01BA04. **Sport:** Permitted.
Driving: Transient blurred vision on instillation.
Indications: Non-infected inflammatory eye conditions.
Dose: Adult, Elderly: *Minims*, instil 1-2 drops as required. *Pred Mild/Forte*, instil 1-2 drops 2-4 times daily; initially 2 drops every hour if needed. Do not discontinue therapy prematurely.
Child: On medical advice.
Pregnancy, Lactation: Pregnancy, if benefit outweighs risk. Lactation, not recommended.
Notes: See 7.3 Ophthalmic Corticosteroids.

> **Minims Prednisolone 0.5%** *(Bausch&Lomb)* A. GMS.
> *Price*, (20) €7.48.
> *Eye drops*, prednisolone sodium phosphate. Clear colourless aqueous single dose. *Disodium edetate.* **Store:** Below 25 deg C; do not freeze.
> **Pred Mild 0.12%, Forte 1%** *(Allergan)* A. GMS.
> *Price*, (5mL) Mild, €1.72. Forte, €1.92.
> *Eye drops*, prednisolone acetate. Sterile off-white microfine susp. *Benzalkonium chloride.* **Store:** Below 25 deg C; do not (refrigerate, freeze).

Sodium Cromoglicate (ophthalmic)

ATC Code: S01GX01. **Sport:** Permitted.
Driving: Transient blurred vision on instillation.
Indications: Acute and chronic allergic conjunctivitis, hay fever, vernal keratoconjunctivitis.
Dose: Adult, Elderly: Instil 1-2 drops 4-times daily.
Pregnancy, Lactation: Use only with medical advice.
Notes: See 7.3 Ophthalmic Corticosteroids.

7.4 Ocular Lubricants

Opticrom 2% Eye Drops *(SANOFI)* OTC. GMS.
Price, (13.5mL) €7.00.
Eye drops, sodium cromoglicate. Clear colourless (pale-yellow) aqueous soln. *Benzalkonium chloride.*

Hay-Crom Aqueous 2% *(TEVA)* OTC. GMS.
Price, (13.5mL) €5.00.
Eye drops, sodium cromoglicate. *Benzalkonium chloride.*

Vividrin 2% Eye Drops, SDU *(Bausch&Lomb)* OTC. GMS.
Price, (13.5mL) Drops, €6.32. SDU (20) €3.06.
Eye drops, sodium cromoglicate. Multidose. *Benzalkonium chloride.* Single dose 0.5mL. *Preservative-free.*

7.4 - Ocular Lubricants

In This Chapter: *Acetylcysteine, carbomer, carmellose, hyaluronic acid (hyaluronate) and polyethylene glycol combination, hyetellose (hydroxyethylcellulose), hypromellose and dextran combination, paraffin ophthalmic ointment, polyvinyl alcohol, retinol (Vitamin A), sodium chloride, trehalose and hyaluronate combination.*

Class Effects

Driving, and use of preservative *(benzalkonium chloride),* see Notes below.

SP: Remove contact lenses before applying ocular lubricants; re-insert after 15 minutes. Admin other ocular medications after a 15-minute interval. If irritation persists or worsens or continued redness occurs, discontinue; consult medical advice.

Pregnancy, Lactation: Generally there is insufficient safety evidence; use if benefit outweighs risk.

ADR: Transient blurring of vision on instillation; eye irritation (burning, stinging, discomfort), increased lacrimation.

Notes: See Chapter 7 Ophthalmology.

Acetylcysteine (ophthalmic)

ATC Code: S01XA08. **Sport:** Permitted.
Driving: Transient blurred vision on instillation.
Indications: Dry eye syndromes (deficient tear secretion or impaired or abnormal mucous production).

Dose: Adult, Elderly: Instil 1-2 drops 3-4 times daily.

Notes: See 7.4 Ocular Lubricants.

Ilube 5% Eye Drops *(Moorfields)* A. GMS.
Price, (10mL) €5.31.
Eye drops, acetylcysteine 5% w/v. Clear colourless soln. *Benzalkonium chloride.*

Carbomer

ATC Code: S01XA20. **Sport:** Permitted.
Driving: Transient blurred vision on instillation.
Indications: Substitution of tear fluid in management of dry eye conditions (keratoconjunctivitis sicca, unstable tear film).

Dose: Adult, Elderly: Instil 1 drop 1-4 times daily depending on requirement; up to 5-times daily and at night before going to bed. Individual dosage regimen required.

Child: As for Adult above.

SP: Blurred vision which can last for up to 1 hour; vigorous blinking aids recovery.

ADR: Eye redness or irritation, keratitis, conjunctivitis.

Notes: See 7.4 Ocular Lubricants.

GelTears 0.2% Eye Gel *(Bausch&Lomb)* OTC. GMS.
Price, (10g) €2.89.
Eye gel, carbomer 0.2% w/w. Homogenous colourless gel. *Benzalkonium chloride.*

Liposic Eye Gel *(Bausch&Lomb)* OTC. GMS.
Price, (10g) €2.91.
Eye gel, carbomer 2mg/g. White turbid highly viscous. *Benzalkonium chloride.* **Store:** Below 25 deg C.

Liquivisc 2.5mg/g Eye Gel *(Thea Pharma)* OTC. GMS.
Price, (10g) €3.10.
Eye gel, carbomer 2.5mg/g. Slightly yellow opalescent. *Benzalkonium chloride.*

Vidisic 0.2% Eye Gel, SDU *(Bausch&Lomb)* OTC. GMS.
Price, (10g) Gel, €3.16. SDU (30) €8.69.
Eye gel, carbomer 0.2%. *Benzalkonium chloride (multidose); single 0.6mL (preservative-free).* **Store:** Below 30 deg C.

Xailin 0.2% Eye Gel *(Nicox)* OTC. GMS.
Price, 0.2% 10g, €2.89.
Eye gel, carbomer 0.2% w/w. Multidose. *Preservative-free.*

Carmellose

ATC Code: S01XA20. **Sport:** Permitted.
Driving: Transient blurred vision on instillation.
Indications: Dry eye syndromes (deficient tear secretion or impaired mucous production).

Dose: Adult, Elderly: *Celluvisc,* instil 2 drops as needed.
Xailin, instil 1 drop 2-4 times daily as needed. 1-2 drops can be applied directly to contact lens before application.

Child: As for Adult above.

SP: Irritation, pain, changes in vision or if condition worsens, discontinue.

Pregnancy, Lactation: Can be used *(Celluvisc)*; consult medical advice *(Xailin).*

Notes: See 7.4 Ocular Lubricants.

Celluvisc 0.5%, 1% SDU *(Allergan)* OTC. GMS.
Price, 1% 0.4mL (60) €13.60. 0.5% (30) €3.89.
Eye drops, carmellose sodium. Clear colourless (slightly yellow) viscous SDU.

Xailin Fresh 0.5% SDU *(Nicox)* OTC. GMS.
Price, 0.5% 0.4mL (30) €3.50.
Eye drops, carmellose sodium 0.5%. Preservative-free.

Hyaluronic Acid (ophthalmic)

ATC Code: S01KA01. **Sport:** Pending.
Driving: Transient blurred vision on instillation.
Indications: Persistent and severe dry eye syndrome and after surgical procedure.

Dose: Adult, Elderly: Instil 1 drop into conjunctival sac 3-4 times daily or as required.

Child: As for Adult above.

Notes: See 7.4 Ocular Lubricants.

HYLO-Tear, HYLO-Forte Eye Drops *(Scope)* OTC. GMS.
Price, (7.5mL) 0.1% (Tear), €6.16; 0.2% (Forte), €6.72.
Eye drops, hyaluronic acid 0.1% (Tear) or 0.2% (Forte) w/v. Soln.

Hyaluronic Acid (ophthalmic), Dexpanthenol

ATC Code: S01KA51. **Sport:** Pending.
Driving: Transient blurred vision on instillation.
Indications: Moistening and to aid healing in damaged or injured cornea (surgery) or dry eyes.

Dose: Adult, Elderly: Instil into eye(s) 3 times daily but can be used more often if there is serious discomfort.

Child: As for Adult above.

SP: Compatible with all types of contact lenses.

Pregnancy, Lactation: Can be used.

Notes: See 7.4 Ocular Lubricants.

HYLO-CARE Eye Drops *(Scope)* OTC. GMS.
Price, 7.5mL, €6.54.
Eye drops, hyaluronic acid 0.1%, dexpanthenol 2%. *Preservative and phosphate free.*

Hyaluronic Acid (ophthalmic), Polyethylene Glycol

ATC Code: S01KA51. **Sport:** Pending.
Driving: Transient blurred vision on instillation.
Indications: Relief from persistent dry irritated feeling eyes.

Dose: Adult, Elderly: Instil into eye(s) as required depending on symptom severity.

Notes: See 7.4 Ocular Lubricants.

blink intensive tears PLUS *(Abbott AMO)* OTC. GMS.
Price, (10mL), €6.35.
Liquid gel eye drops, hyaluronate sodium 0.38%, polyethylene glycol (400) 0.25%. High viscosity hypotonic soln. *Oxidative preservative*

Hyetellose (Hydroxyethylcellulose)

ATC Code: S01XA20. **Sport:** Permitted.
Driving: Transient blurred vision on instillation.
Indications: Dry eye syndromes (deficient tear secretion or impaired mucous production).

Dose: Adult, Elderly: Instil 1-2 drops 3-4 times daily or as needed.

Notes: See 7.4 Ocular Lubricants.

Minims Artificial Tears *(Bausch&Lomb)* OTC. GMS.
Price, (20) €7.07.
Eye drops, hyetellose 0.44%, sodium chloride 0.35% w/w. Sterile single use soln.

Hypromellose

ATC Code: S01XA20. **Sport:** Permitted.
Driving: Transient blurred vision on instillation.
Indications: Symptomatic treatment, dehydration of cornea and conjunctiva (dry eye) acting as lubricant, artificial tear. *(both brands).* Lubrication with rigid or gas permeable contact lenses.
Dose: Adult, Elderly: Instil 1 drop into conjunctival sac 3-5 times daily or as required.
Child: As for Adult above.
Interactions: Effect of Hypromellose on Other Drugs: Other topical ophthalmics: *Contact time prolonged.*
Notes: See 7.4 Ocular Lubricants.

Artelac, SDU *(Bausch&Lomb)* OTC. GMS.
Price, drops (10mL) €2.30. SDU 0.5mL (30) €5.59. (60) €9.59.
Eye drops, hypromellose 0.32%. Sterile. *Benzalkonium chloride (multidose); single (preservative-free).*
Hydromoor SDU *(Moorfields)* OTC. GMS.
Price, (30) 0.4mL, €4.32.
Eye drops, hypromellose 0.3% w/v. Sterile. *Preservative-free.*

Hypromellose, Dextran

ATC Code: S01XA20. **Sport:** Permitted.
Driving: Transient blurred vision on instillation.
Indications: Ocular lubricant, artificial tears.
Dose: Adult, Elderly: Instil 1-2 drops as required.
Child: As for Adult above.
Pregnancy, Lactation: Can be used.
Notes: See 7.4 Ocular Lubricants.

Tears Naturale *(Novartis)* OTC. GMS.
Price, (15mL) €2.20.
Eye drops, hypromellose 0.3%, dextran 70 0.1% w/v. Slightly viscous clear (almost clear). *Benzalkonium chloride.* **Store:** Below 25 deg C; do not refrigerate; container tightly closed.

Paraffin (ophthalmic)

ATC Code: S01XA20. **Sport:** Permitted.
Driving: Transient blurred vision on instillation.
Indications: Ocular lubricant.
Dose: Adult, Elderly: Instil a small amount of ointment as needed.
CI: Lanolin hypersensitivity.
Interactions: Effect of Ophthalmic Ointment on Other Drugs: Other topical ophthalmics: *Contact time prolonged.*
SP: Remove contact lenses before application; re-insert after 30 minutes.
Pregnancy, Lactation: No special precautions.
Notes: See 7.4 Ocular Lubricants.

LACRI-LUBE *(Allergan)* OTC. GMS.
Price, (3.5g) €2.43. (5g) €3.07.
Eye ointment, no specific active ingredient(s). Smooth homogenous off-white sterile. *Wool alcohols.*
Xailin Night Eye Ointment *(Nicox)* OTC. GMS.
Price, 5g, €2.76.
Lubricating eye ointment, soft paraffin 57.3%, white mineral oil 42.5%, lanolin alcohol 0.2% (w/w). Preservative-free.

Polyvinyl Alcohol

ATC Code: S01XA20. **Sport:** Permitted.
Driving: Transient blurred vision on instillation.
Indications: Dry eye syndromes (deficient tear secretion or impaired mucous production).
Dose: Adult, Elderly: Instil 1-2 drops as required.
Pregnancy, Lactation: No special precautions.
Notes: See 7.4 Ocular Lubricants.

Liquifilm Tears *(Allergan)* OTC. GMS.
Price, (15mL) €2.15.
Eye drops, polyvinyl alcohol 1.4%. Clear colourless soln (15mL). *Benzalkonium chloride.*

Retinol

ATC Code: S01XA02. **Sport:** Pending.
Driving: Transient blurred vision on instillation.
Indications: Symptomatic relief of burning, itching, dry eyes, foreign-body sensation.
Dose: Adult, Elderly: Instil 1 drop of ointment into conjunctival sac once daily before bedtime; max. twice daily; if more is required seek medical advice.
Child: As for Adult above.
SP: Apply about 30 minutes after other ophthalmic drugs. Not for use with contact lenses.
Notes: See 7.4 Ocular Lubricants.

VitA-POS Eye Ointment *(Scope)* OTC. GMS.
Price, (5g) €2.91.
Eye ointment, retinol palmitate 250 IU/g, vaseline, paraffin (liquid, light liquid), wool fat (lanolin).

Sodium Chloride

ATC Code: S01XA03. **Sport:** Permitted.
Driving: None known.
Indications: Topical ocular irrigation.
Dose: Adult, Elderly: Use adequate soln to irrigate eye.
Child: As for Adult above.

Minims Saline 0.9% *(Bausch&Lomb)* OTC.
Price, (20-dose) €6.98.
Eye drops, sodium chloride. Clear colourless sterile single use.

Trehalose, Hyaluronate

ATC Code: S01KA51. **Sport:** Permitted.
Driving: Transient blurred vision on instillation.
Indications: Treatment, moderate to severe dry eye syndrome (protects, hydrates, lubricates).
Dose: Adult, Elderly: Instil 1 drop into each eye 4-6 times daily. CAN be used when wearing contact lenses.
SP: Allow 10-minute interval between instillation of other eye products. Do not use if safety ring is damaged.
ADR: Mild eye irritation (unusual).
Notes: See 7.4 Ocular Lubricants.

THEALOZ DUO Eye Drops *(Thea Pharma)* OTC. GMS.
Price, 10mL, €6.75.
Eye drops, trehalose 3%, sodium hyaluronate 0.15%. Sterile hypotonic pH-neutral aqueous soln. *Preservative-free.*

7.5 - Anaesthetics, Mydriatics, Diagnostics

7.5.1 - Topical Anaesthetics

In This Chapter: *Oxybuprocaine, proxymetacaine, tetracaine.*

Class Effects
SP: Protect anaesthetised eye from foreign body contamination. Caution in inflamed eye as hyperaemia increases rate of systemic absorption. Prolonged use may result in corneal damage.
Notes: See Chapter 7 Ophthalmology.

Oxybuprocaine

ATC Code: S01HA02. **Sport:** Permitted.
Driving: Caution.
Indications: Topical ocular anaesthetic.
Dose: Adult, Elderly: *Tonometry,* 1 drop 1 minute before measuring. *Contact lens fitting,* instil 1 drop, then a second drop after 90 seconds. *Foreign body removal,* instil 3 drops at 90 second intervals.
Child: As for Adult above.
SP: Transient burning, stinging.
Notes: See 7.5.1 Topical Anaesthetics.

Minims Oxybuprocaine 0.4% *(Bausch&Lomb)* B.
Price, (20-dose) €6.98.
Eye drops, oxybuprocaine HCl (2mg/0.5mL). Single-use clear colourless sterile soln.

7.5.2 Mydriatics, Cycloplegics

Proxymetacaine

ATC Code: S01HA04. **Sport:** Permitted.
Driving: Transient blurred vision on instillation.
Indications: Topical ocular anaesthetic.
Dose: Adult, Elderly: *Deep anaesthesia,* 1 drop every 5-10 minutes (5-7 applications). *Suture removal,* 1-2 drops 2-3 minutes before removal. *Foreign body removal,* 1-2 drops prior to removal. *Tonometry,* 1-2 drops before measuring.
Child: As for Adult above.
CI: Use in premature babies.
SP: *Caution,* known allergies, cardiac disease, hyperthyroidism (increased sensitivity reaction risk). Not miscible with fluorescein which can be added after eye anaesthetised. Avoid rubbing, irritating chemicals or introduction of foreign bodies during anaesthesia.
Pregnancy, Lactation: Only if considered essential.
ADR: Rarely, pupillary dilatation or cycloplegic effects, irritation of conjunctiva, other toxic reactions, hyperallergic corneal reaction.
Notes: See 7.5.1 Topical Anaesthetics.
Minims Proxymetacaine 0.5% *(Bausch&Lomb)* A.
Price, (20-dose) €10.22.
Eye drops, proxymetacaine HCl. Clear colourless (pale-yellow) soln.

Tetracaine (ophthalmic)

ATC Code: S01HA03. **Sport:** Permitted.
Driving: Caution.
Indications: Topical ocular anaesthetic.
Dose: Adult, Elderly: Instil 1 drop or as required.
Child: As for Adult above.
CI: Patients being treated with sulfonamides. Premature babies, avoid.
Interactions: Effect of Other Drugs on Tetracaine: *Co-admin contraindicated*: Sulfonamides.
SP: Protect anaesthetised eye from dust/bacterial contamination. Inflamed eye, hyperaemia increases rate of systemic absorption though conjunctiva. Corneal damage with prolonged application.
Pregnancy, Lactation: Only if considered essential by physician.
ADR: Dermatitis, transient burning sensation, corneal punctate keratitis, oedema.
Notes: See 7.5.1 Topical Anaesthetics.
Minims Tetracaine 0.5%, 1% *(Bausch&Lomb)* A.
Price, 0.5%, 1%, (20-single doses) €7.71.
Eye drops, tetracaine. Clear colourless aqueous sterile SDU.

7.5.2 - Mydriatics, Cycloplegics

In This Chapter: *Anticholinergics (atropine, cyclopentolate, tropicamide), sympathomimetics (phenylephrine).*

Class Effects

CI: *Anticholinergics,* paralytic ileus, narrow-angle glaucoma, shallow anterior chamber.
SP: Caution, inflamed eye as hyperaemia increases systemic absorption. *Anticholinergics,* raised IOP, prostatic enlargement, coronary insufficiency. The effect of antimuscarinics may be enhanced by co-admin with other drugs with antimuscarinic properties (antihistamines, butyrophenones, phenothiazines, TCADs, amantadine). Systemic absorption, benzalkonium chloride, phosphate-containing eye drops, see Notes below.
Pregnancy, Lactation: If benefit outweighs risk; if considered essential.
ADR: *Local anticholinergics,* transient stinging, blurred vision, light sensitivity, photophobia with or without corneal staining. Prolonged admin, local irritation, hyperaemia, oedema, conjunctivitis.
Systemic anticholinergics, dry mouth, flushing, skin dryness, bradycardia followed by tachycardia (palpitations, arrhythmias), urinary (urgency, difficulty, retention), constipation, vomiting, dizziness, staggering. Rash (children), abdominal distention (infants). Psychotic

212

reactions, behavioural disturbances, cardio-respiratory collapse (caution, children).
Notes: See Chapter 7 Ophthalmology.

Atropine (ophthalmic)

ATC Code: S01FA01. **Sport:** Permitted.
Driving: Caution.
Indications: Pre-operative for ophthalmic surgery. Treatment, uveitis and refraction.
Dose: Adult, Elderly: *Uveitis,* instil 1 drop 2-3 times daily; *refraction,* instil 1 drop twice daily prior to examination.
Notes: See 7.5.2 Mydriatics, Cycloplegics.
Minims Atropine Sulphate 1% *(Bausch&Lomb)* B.
Price, (20-dose) €6.98.
Eye drops, atropine sulfate. Single-use clear colourless sterile soln.

Cyclopentolate

ATC Code: S01FA04. **Sport:** Permitted.
Driving: Blurred vision, difficulty focusing, sensitivity to light.
Indications: Topical mydriatic and cycloplegic. Pre-operative for ophthalmic surgery. Refraction and treatment of iritis and iridocyclitis *(Minims)*. Diagnostic for funduscopy and cycloplegic refraction. Pupil dilation in inflammatory conditions of iris and uveal tract *(Mydrilate)*.
Dose: Adult: *Minims Cyclopentolate, mydriasis,* instil 1 drop into eye; *refraction,* instil 1 drop (if needed repeat after 5 minutes); *iritis, iridocyclitis,* instil 1-2 drops every 6-8 hours. *Mydrilate,* instil 1 drop (0.5%) into eye (repeat after 15 minutes if needed), 40 minutes before examination; deeply pigmented eyes may require using 1% soln.
Child: *Minims Cyclopentolate,* use only at discretion of physician (3 months to 18 years); not recommended (under 3 months).
Mydrilate, refraction, under 6 years, 1 or 2 drops (1%), repeat after 15 minutes if needed; 6-16 years, 1 drop (1%), as for under 6 years; *uveitis, iritis, iridocyclitis,* at discretion of physician. Avoid use in first 3 months of life.
CI: Neonates (except with compelling need), paralytic ileus, narrow-angle glaucoma or shallow anterior chamber, geriatrics or predisposition to increased intraocular pressure. Children with organic brain syndromes (congenital or neuro- developmental abnormalities, especially predisposing to epileptic seizures).
SP: Systemic absorption may occur; more likely in infants. Remove contact lenses before instillation.
ADR: *Common,* local irritation.
Notes: See 7.5.2 Mydriatics, Cycloplegics.
Minims Cyclopentolate 1% *(Bausch&Lomb)* B. GMS.
Price, 1% (20-dose) €6.40.
Eye drops, cyclopentolate HCl. Single-use clear colourless sterile soln. **Store:** Below 25 deg C; do not freeze; original pack to protect (light).
Mydrilate 0.5%, 1% *(Intrapharm)* B. GMS.
Price, (5mL) 0.5% and 1%, €6.64.
Eye drops, cyclopentolate HCl. Clear colourless (almost colourless) soln. *Benzalkonium chloride.* **Store:** Refrigerate; do not freeze; original pack.

Phenylephrine (ophthalmic)

ATC Code: S01FB01. **Sport:** Permitted.
Driving: Caution; photophobia, blurred vision.
Indications: Mydriasis for diagnostic or therapeutic procedures.
Dose: Adult: Instil 1 drop to each eye; if needed, repeat only once, 1 hour after first drop. Recommend using a drop of topical anaesthetic a few minutes before phenylephrine instillation to prevent stinging.
Elderly: Use contraindicated because of increased systemic toxicity risk.
Child: As for Elderly above.
CI: Use of contact lenses. Cardiac disease, hypertension, aneurysms, thyrotoxicosis, long-standing insulin-dependent diabetes mellitus, tachycardia. Closed angle glaucoma; narrow angle prone to glaucoma precipitated by mydriatics.
Interactions: Effect of Other Drugs on Phenylephrine: *Co-admin contraindicated*: MAOIs (increased risk of adrenergic

events), TCADs (cardiac arrhythmia risk), antihypertensives (including beta-blockers) (action may be reversed).

Effect of Phenylephrine on Other Drugs: Cardiac glycosides, quinidine: *Cardiac arrhythmia risk.* Adrenergic blockers, phenothiazines: *Decreased effect.* General anaesthesia: *Caution.*

SP: *Caution,* in presence of diabetes, cerebral arteriosclerosis, long-standing bronchial asthma. Corneal clouding may occur if instilled when corneal epithelium is damaged or denuded.

ADR: Local side effects (eye irritation); systemic effects (serious cardiovascular reactions).

Notes: See 7.5.2 Mydriatics, Cycloplegics.

> **Minims Phenylephrine 2.5%, 10%** *(Bausch&Lomb)* B. GMS.
> *Price,* (20-dose) 10%, €7.48. Non-GMS, 2.5%, €8.15.
> *Eye drops,* phenylephrine HCl. Single dose clear colourless sterile soln.

Tropicamide

ATC Code: S01FA06. **Sport:** Permitted.
Driving: Caution.

Indications: Topical mydriatic and cycloplegic.

Dose: Adult, Elderly: Instil 1 drop; repeat after 5 minutes; if required repeat after 30 minutes.

Child: On medical advice.

Interactions: Effect of Other Drugs on Tropicamide: *Effect enhanced:* Amantadine, some antihistamines, butyrophenones (haloperidol), phenothiazines, TCADs.

ADR: Transient stinging, dry mouth, blurred vision.

Notes: See 7.5.2 Mydriatics, Cycloplegics.

> **Minims Tropicamide 0.5%, 1%** *(Bausch&Lomb)* A.
> *Price,* (20-dose) €8.15.
> *Eye drops,* tropicamide. Single-use clear colourless soln. **Store:** Below 25 deg C; do not freeze.

7.5.3 - Ophthalmic Diagnostics

In This Chapter: *Fluorescein and lidocaine combination.*

Class Effects
Pregnancy, Lactation: If benefit outweighs risk.
Notes: See Class Effects, Chapter 7 Ophthalmology.

Fluorescein

ATC Code: S01JA01. **Sport:** Permitted.
Driving: Caution.

Indications: Diagnostic examination of eye, fitting of hard contact lenses.

Dose: Adult, Elderly: Instil sufficient soln to stain damaged areas.

CI: Soft contact lenses. Amide-type anaesthetic hypersensitivity.

ADR: Allergic-type reactions, anaphylaxis.

Notes: See 7.5.3 Ophthalmic Diagnostics.

> **Minims Fluorescein 1%, 2%** *(Bausch&Lomb)* A. GMS.
> *Price,* 2% (20-dose) €6.40. 1%, not published by company (non-GMS).
> *Eye drops,* fluorescein sodium. Sterile clear aqueous orange-red single-use soln.

Fluorescein, Lidocaine

ATC Code: S01JA51. **Sport:** Permitted.
Driving: Caution.

Indications: Combined diagnostic stain and topical anaesthetic for measurement of IOP.

Dose: Adult, Elderly: Instil 1 or more drops as required.

Child: On medical advice.

CI: Hypersensitivity to amide-type local anaesthetics.

SP: Cornea may be damaged by prolonged application of anaesthetic eye drops; protect anaesthetised eye from dust and contamination.

Notes: See Fluorescein above. See 7.5.1 Topical Anaesthetics.

> **Minims Lidocaine, Fluorescein** *(Bausch&Lomb)* A.
> *Price,* (20-dose) €9.84.
> *Eye drops,* lidocaine HCl 4%, fluorescein sodium 0.25% w/v. Single-use sterile clear slightly (yellow, viscous) soln.

7.6 - Other Ophthalmologicals

In This Chapter: *Aflibercept, ocriplasmin, pegaptanib, ranibizumab, verteporfin.*

Class Effects

Driving: Intravitreal injection may be followed by temporary visual disturbances. Caution.

CI: Hypersensitivity to any member of the class. Use in children. Ocular or periocular infection, severe intraocular inflammation.

SP: *Intravitreal injection,* for admin by qualified ophthalmologist experienced in intravitreal injection technique. Associated with endophthalmitis, intraocular inflammation, rhegmatogenous retinal detachment, retinal tear, iatrogenic traumatic cataract. *Systemic events including non-ocular haemorrhage and arterial thromboembolic events reported following intravitreal injection of VEGF inhibitors. Monitor* for infection during week following injection (patient to report any symptoms of endophthalmitis or any other visual or ocular symptoms), intraocular inflammation, elevated IOP.

Notes: See Class Effects Chapter 7 Ophthalmology.

Aflibercept (ophthalmology)

ATC Code: S01LA05. **Sport:** Permitted.
Driving: Possible temporary visual disturbance.

Indications: Neovascular (wet) age-related macular degeneration (AMD); visual impairment due to macular oedema secondary to central retinal vein occlusion (branch or central RVO), visual impairment due to diabetic macular oedema (DME).

Dose: Adult, Elderly: *Wet AMD and DME,* 2mg by intravitreal injection per month for 3 consecutive doses (AMD) or 5 consecutive doses (DME); then 1 injection every 2 months; treatment interval may be extended after first 12 months.
CRVO, initially 2mg injection, then monthly (dose interval not shorter than 1 month); no improvement in visual/anatomic outcomes after first 3 injections, continued treatment not recommended.

SP: Potential for immunogenicity. Clinical signs of irreversible ischaemic visual function loss, treatment not recommended. See ADR below.

Pregnancy, Lactation: Pregnancy, if benefit outweighs risk. Women of childbearing potential to use effective contraception during and for minimum 3 months after last intravitreal injection. Lactation, not recommended.

ADR: Summary, *most frequent,* conjunctival haemorrhage, reduced visual acuity, eye pain, increased IOP*, vitreous detachment*/floaters, cataract*; *serious,* retinal detachment, endophthalmitis, increased IOP and *above.

Notes: See 7.6 Other Ophthalmologicals.

> ▼ **Eylea Parenteral** *(Bayer)* A.
> *Price,* not published by company.
> *Intravitreous injection,* aflibercept 40mg/mL (50 microlitres). Clear colourless (pale-yellow) soln. **Store:** Refrigerate; do not freeze; outer carton to protect (light).

Ocriplasmin

ATC Code: S01XA22. **Sport:** Pending.
Driving: Possible temporary visual disturbance.

Indications: Treatment, vitreomacular traction (VMT) (adults) including when associated with macular hole (diameter 400 microns or less).

Dose: Adult, Elderly: Recommended, 0.125mg (0.1mL diluted soln) by intravitreal injection to affected eye once as single dose (repeat admin not recommended); treatment of other eye concurrently or within 7 days of initial injection not recommended. Repeated admin to same eye not recommended (to monitor post-injection course e.g. decreased vision). Post-operative antibiotic drops may be admin at discretion of ophthalmologist.

Child: Under 18 years, no relevant use.

Renal Impairment: No adjustment.

Hepatic Impairment: As for Renal above.

7.6 Other Ophthalmologicals

Interactions: Effect of Other Drugs on Ocriplasmin: Co-admin no data: VEGF-inhibitors. Co-admin with other medicinals: Not recommended.

SP: Post-injection monitoring, following intravitreal injection, monitor for intraocular inflammation/infection, IOP elevation. Transient IOP elevation (transient blindness, non-perfusion of the optic nerve) seen within 60 minutes of injection. Instruct patients to report symptoms of intraocular inflammation or infection or any other visual or ocular symptoms.

Lens subluxation or phacodonesis (possible). Caution, non-proliferative diabetic retinopathy, history of uveitis (including active severe inflammation), significant eye trauma. Risk of new or enlarged macular holes (due to potential increased tractional forces). Risk for significant, but transient loss of visual acuity during first week after injection (monitor); night blindness.

Pregnancy, Lactation: Use only if benefit outweighs risk.

ADR: Very common, vitreous floaters, eye pain, conjunctival haemorrhage.

Notes: See 7.6 Other Ophthalmologicals.

▼ **Jetrea Parenteral** (Novartis) A.
Price, (1) €3099.00 (PTW).
Intravitreal injection, ocriplasmin 0.5mg/vial (0.125mg/0.1mL diluted). Clear colourless conc for soln. Store: Freeze (-20 deg C, +/- 5 deg C).

Pegaptanib

ATC Code: S01LA03. **Sport:** Permitted.
Driving: Possible temporary visual disturbance.
Indications: Treatment, neovascular (wet) age-related macular degeneration (AMD).

Dose: Adult, Elderly: Intravitreal injection only, 0.3mg every 6 weeks (9 injections per year). See SP below.

Child: Not recommended.

Renal Impairment: Severe, no data.

SP: Raised IOP following injection; monitor IOP and perfusion of optic nerve head. Immediate or delayed intravitreous haemorrhage. Endophthalmitis risk. After 2 consecutive injections, if no treatment benefit demonstrated at 12-week visit, consider discontinuation. Allergic reactions. NOTE: PFS is supplied with excess product volume.

Pregnancy, Lactation: Pregnancy, if benefit outweighs risk. Lactation, not recommended.

ADR: Very common, anterior chamber inflammation, eye pain, increased IOP, punctate keratitis, vitreous floaters, vitreous opacities.

Notes: See 7.6 Other Ophthalmologicals.

Macugen Parenteral (PharmaSwiss) A.
Price, 0.3mg (1) €640.00 (T).
Intravitreous injection, pegaptanib sodium 1.65mg. Clear colourless.

Ranibizumab

ATC Code: S01LA04. **Sport:** Permitted.
Driving: Possible temporary visual disturbance.
Indications: Treatment, neovascular (wet) age-related macular degeneration (AMD). Treatment of visual impairment due to diabetic macular oEdema (DME); macular oedema secondary to retinal vein occlusion (branch RVO or central RVO); choroidal neovascularisation (CNV) secondary to pathologic myopia (PM).

Dose: Adult: Single 0.5mg intravitreal injection, initially 1 per month until max. visual acuity achieved and/or no signs of disease activity. Wet AMD, DME, RVO, initially 3 or more consecutive monthly injections may be needed then treatment interval may be extended. Macular oedema secondary to BRVO with laser photocoagulation, admin Lucentis 30 minutes after laser. CNV secondary to PM, initiate with single injection; some patients may need 1-2 injections in year 1, some may need more frequent treatment.

Elderly: Over 75 years with DME, limited experience.

Child: Under 18 years, no data.

Interactions: Effect of Other Drugs on Ranibizumab: Co-admin not recommended: Other anti-VEGF agents (systemic or ocular).

SP: Only for intravitreal injection. Monitor IOP, optic nerve perfusion. Limited data on bilateral use do not suggest increased risk of systemic adverse events. Potential for immunogenicity. Not for co-admin with other anti-VEGF agents. Withhold dose, do not resume treatment earlier than next scheduled treatment if, decrease in best-corrected visual acuity (BCVA) of 30 letters or more, IOP 30mmHg or more, retinal break, subretinal haemorrhage, intraocular surgery within previous or next 28 days. Rhegmatogenous retinal detachment, discontinue. When initiating, caution in presence of risk factors for retinal pigment epithelial tears. Insufficient data regarding effect in patients with RVO presenting irreversible ischaemic visual function loss.

Pregnancy, Lactation: Not recommended. Women of childbearing potential to ensure adequate contraception; if planning pregnancy, wait for minimum 3 months after last dose before conceiving.

ADR: Summary, very common (non-ocular), nasopharyngitis, headache, arthralgia; (ocular) eye (pain, irritation, foreign body sensation, dryness, pruritus), ocular hyperaemia, increased IOP, vitritis, vitreous (detachment, floaters), haemorrhage (vitreous, conjunctival), visual disturbance, increased lacrimation, blepharitis.

Notes: See 7.6 Other Ophthalmologicals.

Lucentis Parenteral (Novartis) A. HOS.
Price, (1) PFS 1.65mg/0.165mL, €758.14 (PTW).
Single-use intravitreal injection, ranibizumab 10mg/mL. Clear colourless (pale-yellow) aqueous soln.

Verteporfin

ATC Code: S01LA01. **Sport:** Permitted.
Driving: Possible temporary visual disturbance.
Indications: AMD with predominantly classic subfoveal choroidal neovascularisation OR subfoveal choroidal neovascularisation secondary to pathologic myopia.

Dose: Adult, Elderly: 10-minute IV infusion, 6mg/m2 BSA (diluted in 30mL infusion soln) then light-activation at 15 minutes after start of infusion. Re-evaluate 3-monthly; recurrent CNV leakage, admin up to 4-times per year.

Hepatic Impairment: Moderate impairment or biliary obstruction, caution.

CI: Porphyria, severe hepatic impairment.

Interactions: Effect of Other Drugs on Verteporfin: Increased photosensitivity reactions: Photosensitising agents (tetracyclines, sulfonamides, phenothiazines, sulfonylurea, hypoglycaemic agents, thiazides, griseofulvin).

SP: Patients will be photosensitive for 48 hours after infusion; avoid exposure to direct sunlight, bright indoor lighting, tanning salons, light-emitting medical devices; UV sunscreens are NOT effective; ambient indoor light is safe; outdoors, use protective clothing, dark sunglasses. Severely decreased vision (4 lines or more) within 1-week post-treatment, do not re-treat until vision completely recovers (if benefit outweighs risk). Extravasation, especially if area exposed to light; severe pain, inflammation, swelling, blistering, discolouration, stop infusion immediately. Chest pain, vaso-vagal and/or hypersensitivity reactions related to Visudyne infusion; may include convulsions. Anaesthetised patients, caution.

Pregnancy, Lactation: Pregnancy, only if clearly necessary. Lactation, interrupt breastfeeding for 48 hours after admin; is excreted in human milk.

ADR: Most frequent, injection-site reactions (pain, oedema, inflammation, extravasation, rash, haemorrhage, discolouration), visual impairment (blurred, fuzzy vision, photopsia, reduced visual acuity and visual field defects, including scotoma and black spots).

Notes: See 7.6 Other Ophthalmologicals.

Visudyne Parenteral 15mg (Novartis) A. HOS.
Price, vial 15mg (1) €1087.43 (PTW).
Infusion, verteporfin. Dark-green (black) powder for soln.

8

Obstetrics, Gynaecology, Urological Disorders

8.1 - Obstetrics

Class Effects
CI: Hypersensitivity to any member of the class.

8.1.1 - Prostaglandins, Oxytocics

In This Chapter: *Dinoprostone, ergometrine, oxytocin.*

Class Effects
CI: Where prolonged contractions of uterus inappropriate such as history of C-section or major uterine surgery, cephalopelvic disproportion, foetal malpresentation, foetal distress, history of difficult labour and/or traumatic delivery, grand multiparae with over 5 previous term pregnancies, multiple gestation, engagement of head not taken place, either maternal or foetal benefit/risk ratio favours surgical intervention. Ruptured membranes. Pelvic inflammatory disease (PID). Placenta praevia, unexplained discharge and/or abnormal bleeding during this pregnancy.
SP: Increased post-partum disseminated intravascular coagulation risk (35 years or older, pregnancy complications, gestational age over 40 weeks) when labour is induced pharmacologically (dinoprostone, oxytocin).

Dinoprostone
ATC Code: G02AD02. **Sport:** Permitted.
Driving: Not applicable.
Indications: Induction of labour (absence of foetal and maternal contraindications).
Dose: Adult: VAGINAL GEL, *primigravida* with unfavourable induction features, initially 2mg (max. 4mg); *other patients,* 1mg (max. 3mg). Both groups, after 6 hours, admin 1mg (if uterine activity insufficient for progress of labour) OR 2mg (if minimal response to initial dose). Avoid admin into cervical canal.
PARENTERAL (IV) infusion at 0.25mcg/min for minimum 30 minutes; inadequate uterine response, increase to 0.5mcg/min and then 1mcg/min after 2 hours; up to 4mcg/min may be required. No response in first 12-24 hours, discontinue.
Renal Impairment: Contraindicated.
Hepatic Impairment: As for Renal above.
CI: Active cardiac, pulmonary disease.
Interactions: Effect of Other Drugs on Dinoprostone: *Co-admin not recommended:* Oxytocin (allow 6-hour dosing interval).
SP: Hospital use only in specialised obstetric units. Prevent contact with skin when handling. *Caution,* asthma, epilepsy, raised IOP or glaucoma, compromised

(cardiovascular, hepatic, renal) function, hypertension, compromised uteri. *Monitor,* uterine activity, foetal status, cervical dilation progression; hypertonic uterine contractility or tetanic uterine contraction, monitor continuously.
Pregnancy, Lactation: Pregnancy, at or near term any dose producing sustained increased uterine tone may decrease uterine blood flow, putting the embryo or foetus at risk. Lactation, prostaglandins are excreted in breast milk.
ADR: *Most common,* vomiting, nausea, diarrhoea. *Rare, noteworthy* hypersensitivity (anaphylaxis reaction/shock, anaphylactoid reaction); uterine rupture, cardiac arrest. Increased post-partum DIC risk where labour is pharmacologically induced.
Notes: See 8.1.1 Prostaglandins, Oxytocics.

Prostin E2 Vaginal Gel, Parenteral *(Pfizer)* C.
Price, vaginal gel (3g) 1mg, €19.57. 2mg, €21.56.
Vaginal gel, dinoprostone 1mg, 2mg. Translucent thixotropic.
Infusion, as above 1mg/mL. Clear colourless conc for soln; particulate free. *Anhydrous ethanol 591.7mg/amp.*

Ergometrine, Oxytocin
ATC Code: G02AB03. **Sport:** Permitted.
Driving: Not applicable.
Indications: Active management, third stage of labour or following birth of placenta, to prevent postpartum haemorrhage.
Dose: Adult: *Third stage labour,* active management, 1mL admin to mother following delivery of the baby anterior shoulder or immediately after delivery of baby.
Postpartum haemorrhage, prevention and treatment, 1mL admin to mother following expulsion of placenta or when bleeding occurs. IM recommended (IV limited to severe haemorrhage).
Renal Impairment: Mild, moderate, caution. Severe, not recommended.
Hepatic Impairment: As for Renal above.
CI: Pregnancy and labour, induction, stages prior to anterior shoulder delivery. Severe, hypertension including pre-eclamptic toxaemia, eclampsia, occlusive vascular disorders, severe cardiac disorders, sepsis.
Interactions: Effect of Other Drugs on Oxytocin, Ergometrine Combination: *Uterotonic effect decreased:* Halothane anaesthesia. *Co-admin avoid:* CYP3A4 inhibitors including macrolides (troleandomycin, erythromycin, clarithromycin), HIV protease inhibitors or reverse transcriptase inhibitors (ritonavir, indinavir, nelfinavir, delavirdine), azole antifungals (ketoconazole, itraconazole, voriconazole). *Ergometrine effect may be reduced:* CYP3A4 inducers (nevirapine, rifampicin).
Effect of Oxytocin, Ergometrine Combination on Other Drugs: Vasoconstrictors, prostaglandins, other ergot alkaloids, triptans, sympathomimetics, beta-blockers: *Vasopressor effects enhanced.* Glyceryl trinitrate, other antianginals: *Effect reduced.*
SP: IV route, caution. Breech presentation, admin after delivery is complete; multiple births, admin after last child delivered. Caution, hypertension (mild, moderate), malnutrition, previous admin of pressor agent; see CI (contraindications) above. Ergometrine-induced vasospasm. Vasoconstriction, acute pulmonary oedema. Postpartum haemorrhage, if bleeding not arrested by *Syntometrine* injection, consider possibility of retained placental fragment, soft tissue injury or clotting defect.
Pregnancy, Lactation: See CI (contraindications) above. Potential for serious adverse events in breastfed newborns/infants; avoid breastfeeding for minimum 12 hours after admin.
ADR: Anaphylactoid reactions (dyspnoea, hypotension, collapse or shock), CVA, headache, dizziness, MI, coronary arteriospasm, bradycardia, arrhythmias, chest pain, hypertension, vomiting, nausea, abdominal pain, rash.
Notes: See 8.1.1 Prostaglandins, Oxytocics.

Syntometrine Parenteral *(Alliance)* A. GMS.
Price, 1mL (5) €8.83.
Injection, ergometrine maleate 500mcg, oxytocin 5 IU (equiv. to 8.5mcg). Clear colourless soln. *Sodium 2.76mg/mL.*

8.1.2　Myometrial Relaxants

Oxytocin

ATC Code: H01BB02. **Sport:** Permitted.
Driving: Not applicable.
Indications: Induction of labour. Stimulation of labour in hypotonic uterine inertia. Caesarean section, following delivery of baby. Prevention and treatment, postpartum uterine atony and haemorrhage. Early stages of pregnancy, adjunctive management of abortion.

Dose: Adult: *Induction, enhancement of labour*, initially 1-4 milliUnits (mU)/min by IV drip infusion or variable-speed infusion pump; titrate at 20-minute intervals until contractions similar to normal labour established; near term usually less than 10mU/min required; max. 20mU/min. Term or near term, if regular contractions not established after 5 IU infusion, recommend cease attempt to induce; repeat following day with 1-4 mU/min.
C-section, 5 IU by slow IV injection immediately after delivery.
Postpartum haemorrhage, prevention, 5 IU by slow IV injection after placenta delivery; *treatment*, 5 IU by slow IV injection; if severe follow with IV infusion of 5-20 IU oxytocin in 500mL diluent at rate to control uterine atony.
Abortion, 5 IU by slow IV injection; if required follow by IV infusion at rate 20-40 mU/min or higher.
CI: Prolonged use with oxytocin-resistant uterine inertia, severe pre-eclamptic toxaemia, severe cardiac disorders.
SP: Induction or enhancement of labour, borderline cephalopelvic disproportion, secondary uterine inertia, mild or moderate pregnancy induced hypertension or cardiac disease, mothers over 35 years, history of lower-uterine-segment C-section, caution. Short-lasting BP drop (rapid IV injection).
ADR: *Common*, headache, tachycardia, bradycardia, nausea, vomiting.
Notes: See Ergometrine, Oxytocin above. See 8.1.1 Prostaglandins, Oxytocics.

Syntocinon Parenteral *(CD Pharma)* A.
Price, (5) 5 IU/mL, €1.40. 10 IU/mL, €1.61.
Infusion or injection, oxytocin 5 IU, 10 IU. Clear colourless soln. *Sodium acetate trihydrate 1.063mg/1mL amp, ethanol.*

8.1.2 - Myometrial Relaxants

In This Chapter: *Atosiban.*

Class Effects
Terbutaline and salbutamol are also used to manage uncomplicated premature labour. See Notes below.
Notes: See 5.1.1 Adrenoreceptor Agonist Bronchodilators (salbutamol, terbutaline).

Atosiban

ATC Code: G02CX01. **Sport:** Permitted.
Driving: Not applicable.
Indications: To delay pre-term birth in pregnant women age 18 years, gestational age 24-33 completed weeks, normal foetal heart rate (FHR) with regular uterine contractions of 30 second duration, rate 4 per 30 minutes. Cervical dilation of 1-3cm (0-3 for nulliparous) and effacement of 50%.
Dose: Adult: Initially 6.75mg over 1-minute bolus then follow with continuous IV infusion of 18mg/hour (3 hours), then 6mg/hour (up to 45 hours). Max. 48 hours; max. 330mg.
Renal Impairment: Not likely to need dose adjustment.
Hepatic Impairment: Caution.
CI: Gestational age below 24 or over 33 completed weeks, premature rupture of membranes at over 30 weeks gestation, intrauterine growth retardation and abnormal FHR, conditions requiring delivery (antepartum uterine haemorrhage, eclampsia, severe pre-eclampsia), intrauterine foetal death, suspected intrauterine infection, placenta praevia, abruptio placenta, where continuation of pregnancy is detrimental to mother or foetus.
SP: Premature rupture of membranes, weigh benefit of delaying delivery against chorioamnionitis risk. Multiple pregnancies, gestational age 24-27 weeks, limited data.

Intrauterine growth retardation, assess foetal maturity. Postpartum bleeding, monitor.
Pregnancy, Lactation: Only for use in pre-term labour (between 24 and 33 completed weeks gestation). Use with caution in case of multiple gestations and/or concomitant admin of other tocolytics. If breastfeeding an earlier child, discontinue during treatment as oxytocin release may augment uterine contractility and counteract effect of tocolytic therapy.
ADR: Nausea, vomiting, hyperglycaemia, headache, dizziness, tachycardia, hot flushes, hypotension, local injection-site reactions, insomnia, pruritus, rash, pyrexia, allergic reactions, haemorrhage/uterine atony.
Notes: See 8.1.1 Prostaglandins, Oxytocics.

Tractocile Parenteral *(Ferring)* A.
Price, injection 0.9mL, €36.44. Conc 5mL, €104.72.
Injection, atosiban acetate (6.75mg/0.9mL), infusion (conc 37.5mg/5mL). Clear colourless conc for soln; particle free.

8.2 - Contraception

8.2.1 - Combined Hormonal Contraceptives

In This Chapter: *Ethinylestradiol (EE) in combination with cyproterone, desogestrel, dienogest, drospirenone, gestodene, levonorgestrel, nomegestrol, norgestimate.*

Class Effects
Combined hormonal contraceptives (CHCs) in oral from are also described as combined oral contraceptives (COCs).
Indications: Indicated for hormonal contraception in adult women of reproductive age; not for use postmenopause. Generally, safety and efficacy under 18 years not established.
The decision to prescribe should consider the individual woman's current risk factors, especially venous thromboembolism (VTE) and VTE risk comparison of any one product compared with other CHCs.
NOTE: There is evidence for differences between CHCs in VTE risk, depending on the type of progestogen. Current data indicate that CHCs with progestogens (levonorgestrel, norethisterone, norgestimate) have lowest VTE risk.
ORAL: **Dose:** Oral preparations may be monophasic, biphasic or triphasic. They may be taken either 1 tab daily for 21 consecutive days (then 7 tablet-free days during which withdrawal bleeding occurs) OR 1 tab daily for 21 days (then 7 placebo tabs during which withdrawal bleed occurs). *Admin*, at approx. same time each day; must be taken regularly to achieve contraceptive protection; usually commenced on day 1 of menstrual cycle i.e. first day of menstrual bleed or day after last active tab of previous CHC. *Changing* to different oral brand, vaginal ring or transdermal patch or instructions regarding missed doses, see manufacturers Full Prescribing Information.
CI: Hypersensitivity to any member of the class. Use in children, post-menopausal women.
Risk of arterial thromboembolism (ATE), thromboembolism (MI), prodromal conditions (angina pectoris), hereditary or acquired ATE predisposition (hyperhomocysteinemia, antiphospholipid-antibodies), migraine with focal neurological symptoms, high ATE risk (diabetes mellitus with vascular symptoms, severe hypertension, severe dyslipoproteinaemia).
Risk of venous thromboembolism (VTE), current VTE (on anticoagulants), history (DVT, pulmonary embolism), hereditary or acquired VTE predisposition (APC-resistance including Factor V Leiden, antithrombin-III-deficiency, protein-C deficiency, protein S deficiency), major surgery with prolonged immobilisation, high VTE risk due to risk factors (obesity, prolonged immobilisation with surgery, temporary immobilisation including air travel, positive family history, medical conditions associated with VTE, increasing age especially over 35 years).
Pancreatitis associated with severe hypertriglyceridaemia, severe hepatic disease, liver tumours (benign or malignant), sex steroid-influenced malignancies (breast, genital organs), undiagnosed vaginal bleeding. See SP below.
Interactions: Effect of Other Drugs on CHCs: *Plasma*

levels decreased (contraceptive efficacy impaired, see SP below): Enzyme inducers* (phenobarbital, bosentan, carbamazepine, eslicarbazepine, felbamate, aprepitant, fosaprepitant, griseofulvin, modafinil, oxcarbazepine, primidone, phenytoin, fosphenytoin, primidone, rifampicin, rifabutin, rufinamide, St John's Wort, topiramate; drugs altering intestinal flora or decrease enterohepatic oestrogen circulation (ampicillin, penicillin, tetracyclines)**; some HIV PIs (nelfinavir, ritonavir, ritonavir-boosted PIs), HCV PIs (boceprevir, telaprevir), NNRTIs (efavirenz, nevirapine); colesevelam. *Plasma levels increased*: Ascorbic acid, paracetamol, CYP3A4 inhibitors (azole antifungals), grapefruit juice, statins, etoricoxib. *Increased intrahepatic cholestasis risk*: Troleandomycin. *(may increase clearance of sex hormones; enzyme induction may be observed within a few days; max. within few weeks; may continue for about 4 weeks after drug cessation; temporarily use a barrier method). **(does not apply to all members of class).

Effect of CHCs on Other Drugs: Oral antidiabetics, insulin: *Dose adjustment, hypoglycaemic effect antagonised.* Antihypertensives, TCADs, coumarins: *Effect antagonised.* Ciclosporin, theophylline, omeprazole, prednisolone, voriconazole: *Plasma levels increased.* Lamotrigine, paracetamol, clofibric acid, morphine, salicylic acid, temazepam: *Plasma levels decreased.* Flunarizine: *Increased galactorrhoea risk.*

SP: *Before starting hormonal contraception, conduct general medical, gynaecological examination (breasts, cervical smear), family history (exclude history of thromboembolic disease e.g. DVT, stroke, MI at young age).*

Reasons for immediate discontinuation, symptoms of thrombosis (venous, arterial), unusual unilateral leg pain and/or swelling. Sudden severe chest pain, breathlessness, coughing, partial or complete loss of vision, severe or prolonged headache, visual disturbances, diplopia, slurred speech or aphasia, vertigo, collapse with or without focal seizure, weakness or marked numbness affecting one side or one part of body, motor disturbances, 'acute' abdomen.

Risk of venous thromboembolic complications increases with, age, thromboembolism family history (early age), prolonged immobilisation, major (surgery, trauma), leg surgery. Discontinue 4 weeks before elective surgery. BMI over 30, varicose veins, superficial thrombophlebitis. CHCs (increased VTE risk).

Risk of arterial thromboembolic complications (life-threatening) increases with, increasing age, smoking (women over 35 years), dyslipoproteinaemia, lipid metabolism disorders, hypertension, valvular heart disease, atrial fibrillation.

Other risk indicators, hypertriglyceridaemia (increased pancreatitis risk), jaundice and/or pruritus related to cholestasis, gallstones, porphyria, SLE, haemolytic uraemic syndrome, Sydenham's chorea, herpes gestationis, otosclerosis-related hearing loss, disturbed liver function, altered peripheral insulin resistance and glucose tolerance. Worsening of endogenous depression, epilepsy, Crohn's disease (new onset, deterioration), ulcerative colitis. Chloasma, avoid exposure to sun, UV radiation. Benign hepatic adenomas, ocular lesions. Hereditary angioedema. Altered laboratory tests. Cervical cancer risk with HPV infection and long-term use.

Enzyme-inducer co-admin, use alternative reliable or barrier contraception during and for up to 28 days after treatment; long term enzyme-inducers, use another reliable non-hormonal form of contraception. NOTE: Efficacy may be reduced if tablets are missed, GI disturbances (vomiting, diarrhoea) or co-admin of medications reducing plasma levels; use additional contraceptive measures.

Long-acting contraceptives, recommend healthcare professionals to participate in training (use of implants and/or insertion of intrauterine devices). Women using progestogen-only products, there may be a slightly increased VTE risk; history of thrombo-embolic disorders advise of possibility of recurrence.

Pregnancy, Lactation: Not indicated for use during pregnancy; exclude before initiation; if occurs, withdraw immediately. Lactation, not recommended.

ADR: *Serious events,* thromboembolic disorders (venous, arterial), hypertension, liver tumours; occurrence or deterioration of conditions where association with CHC use is not conclusive (Crohn's disease, ulcerative colitis, epilepsy, uterine myoma, porphyria, systemic lupus erythematosus, herpes gestationis, Sydenham's chorea, haemolytic uraemic syndrome, cholestatic jaundice); chloasma; acute or chronic liver function disturbances (consider discontinuing until LFTs return to normal); angioedema symptom exacerbation. Application site reactions (transdermal).

Cyproterone, Ethinylestradiol

ATC Code: G03HB01. **Sport:** Permitted.
Driving: Unlikely to impair.

Indications: Oral hormonal contraception; moderate to severe acne related to androgen-sensitivity (with or without seborrhoea) and/or hirsutism in women of reproductive age.

Dose: Adult: See Notes below.

SP: Use only after failure of topical therapy or systemic antibiotics. Not for use with other hormonal contraceptives.

Notes: See 8.2.1 Combined Hormonal Contraceptives. See also 10.1.5 Oral Acne Treatments.

▼ **Dianette 2mg/35mcg** *(Bayer)* B. GMS.
Price, (21) €4.89.
Tablet, cyproterone acetate 2mg, ethinylestradiol 35mcg. Beige s/c. *Lactose, sucrose.*

Desogestrel, Ethinylestradiol

ATC Code: G03AA09. **Sport:** Permitted.
Driving: Unlikely to impair.

Indications: Oral hormonal contraception (adult women).

Dose: Adult: See Notes below.

CI: Known or suspected pregnancy.

Notes: See 8.2.1 Combined Hormonal Contraceptives.

Marvlol 150/30 *(MSD)* B. GMS.
Price, (63) €8.93.
Tablet, desogestrel 150mcg, ethinylestradiol 30mcg. White round. Marked Organon, asterisk (*); TR 4 on reverse. *Lactose.* **Store:** Below 25 deg C; original pack to protect (light).

Mercilon 150/20 *(MSD)* B. GMS.
Price, (63) €10.71.
Tablet, desogestrel 150mcg, ethinylestradiol 20mcg. White round. Marked Organon, asterisk (*); TR 4 on reverse. *Lactose.* **Store:** Below 25 deg C; original pack to protect (light).

Dienogest, Estradiol

ATC Code: G03AB. **Sport:** Permitted.
Driving: Unlikely to impair.

Indications: Oral hormonal contraception; treatment of heavy menstrual bleeding.

Dose: Adult: Phased, estradiol valerate 3mg (2 days), then estradiol valerate 2mg + dienogest 2mg (5 days), then estradiol valerate 2mg + dienogest 3mg (17 days), then estradiol valerate 1mg (2 days), then placebo (2 days).

Notes: See 8.2.1 Combined Hormonal Contraceptives.

Qlaira Tablets *(Bayer)* B. GMS.
Price, (28) €9.17.
Tablet, dienogest (D) 0/2/3/0, estradiol valerate (E) 3/2/2/1. Round f/c. Marked with hexagon. 2x 3mg E: Dark-yellow. Marked DD. 5x (2mg E + 2mg D): Medium-red. Marked DJ. 17x (2mg E + 3mg D): Light-yellow. Marked DH. 2x1mg E: Dark-red. Marked DN. 2x Placebo: White. Marked DT. *Lactose.*

Ethinylestradiol, Drospirenone

ATC Code: G03AA12. **Sport:** Permitted.
Driving: No or negligible effect.

Indications: Oral hormonal contraception (adult women).

Dose: Adult: See Notes below.

Child: Only recommended after menarche; adolescents, safety data no different from women over 18 years.

Renal Impairment: Severe, not recommended.

CI: Pancreatitis (history) if associated with severe hypertriglyceridaemia.

Notes: See 8.2.1 Combined Hormonal Contraceptives.

Elvina 0.03mg/3mg *(Consilient)* B.
Price, (21 x 3) €11.26 (PTW).
Tablet, ethinylestradiol 0.03mg, drospirenone 3mg. White (almost) round. Marked G63. *Lactose, soya lecithin.*

8.2.2 Transdermal

Elvinette 0.02mg/3mg *(Consilient)* B.
Price, (3 x 21) €13.00 (PTW).
Tablet, ethinylestradiol 0.02mg, drospirenone 3mg. White (almost) round f/c. Marked G73. *Lactose, soya lecithin.*
Freedo 0.03mg/3mg *(Rowex)* B. GMS.
Price, (63) €7.29.
Tablet, ethinylestradiol 0.03mg, drospirenone 3mg. Yellow round f/c. *Lactose.*
Freedonel 0.02mg/3mg *(Rowex)* B.
Price, (63) €8.42.
Tablet, ethinylestradiol 0.02mg, drospirenone 3mg. Pink round f/c. *Lactose.*
Yasmin 0.03mg/3mg *(Bayer)* B. GMS.
Price, (21) €3.04.
Tablet, ethinylestradiol 0.03mg, drospirenone 3mg. Light-yellow round. Marked DO in hexagon. *Lactose.* **Store:** Below 25 deg C; original pack.
Yasminelle 0.02mg/3mg *(Bayer)* B. GMS.
Price, (21) €3.51.
Tablet, ethinylestradiol (as betadex clathrate) 0.02mg, drospirenone 3mg. Light-pink round. Marked DS in hexagon. *Lactose.*
Yaz 0.02mg/3mg *(Bayer)* B. GMS.
Price, (28) €8.56.
Tablet, ethinylestradiol (as betadex clathrate) 0.02mg, drospirenone 3mg. Round f/c. Active: Pink. Marked DS*. Placebo: White. Marked DP*. *(in hexagon). *Lactose.*

Gestodene, Ethinylestradiol

ATC Code: G03AA10. **Sport:** Permitted.
Driving: Unlikely to impair.
Indications: Oral hormonal contraception (adult women).
Dose: Adult: See Notes below.
Notes: See 8.2.1 Combined Hormonal Contraceptives.

Estelle 75/30 *(Clonmel)* B. GMS.
Price, (21) €2.31.
Tablet, gestodene 75mcg, ethinylestradiol 30mcg. White round s/c. *Lactose.*
Minulet 75/30 *(Pfizer)* B. GMS.
Price, (21) €2.35.
Tablet, gestodene 75mcg, ethinylestradiol 30mcg. White round s/c. *Lactose, sucrose.* **Store:** Below 25 deg C; outer carton to protect (light).

Levonorgestrel, Ethinylestradiol

ATC Code: G03AB03. **Sport:** Permitted.
Driving: Unlikely to impair.
Indications: Oral hormonal contraception (adult women).
Dose: Adult: See Notes below.
Notes: See 8.2.1 Combined Hormonal Contraceptives.

Logynon Tablets *(Bayer)* B. GMS.
Price, (21) €3.05.
Tablet, levonorgestrel (L) 50/75/125, ethinylestradiol (EE) 30/40/30. EE 30mcg, L 50mcg (light-brown), EE 40mcg, L 75mcg (white), E 30mcg, L 125mcg (ochre-coloured). s/c. Calendar pack. *Lactose, sucrose.*
Leonore 100/20 *(Rowex)* B. GMS.
Price, (63) €9.47.
Tablet, levonorgestrel 100mcg, ethinylestradiol 20mcg. White round coated. *Lactose.*
Microlite 100/20 *(Bayer)* B. GMS.
Price, (21) €4.05.
Tablet, levonorgestrel 100mcg, ethinylestradiol 20mcg. Pink coated. *Lactose, sucrose.*
Mylite 100/20 *(Gerard)* B. GMS.
Price, (63) €9.47.
Tablet, levonorgestrel 100mcg, ethinylestradiol 20mcg. Pink coated. *Lactose, sucrose.*
Ovranette 150/30 *(Pfizer)* B.
Price, (21) €3.75 (PTW).
Tablet, levonorgestrel 150mcg, ethinylestradiol 30mcg. Round white. *Lactose, sucrose.* **Store:** Below 25 deg C.
Ovreena 30/150 *(Consilient)* B. GMS.
Price, (63) €2.30
Tablet, ethinylestradiol 30mcg, levonorgestrel 150mcg. Round white coated. *Sucrose.* **Store:** Below 25 deg C.
Violite 100/20 *(Consilient)* GMS
Price, (63) €6.07.
Tablet, levonorgestrel 100mcg, ethinylestradiol 20mcg. Pink cylindrical f/c. *Lactose.* **Store:** Below 25 deg C.

Nomegestrol, Ethinylestradiol

ATC Code: G03AA14. **Sport:** Permitted.
Driving: No or negligible effect.
Indications: Oral hormonal contraception (adult women).
Dose: Adult: See Notes below.
ADR: *Very common*, acne, abnormal withdrawal bleeding.
Notes: See 8.2.1 Combined Hormonal Contraceptives.

▼ **Zoely 2.5/1.5mg** *(MSD)* B. GMS.
Price, (28) €8.35.
Tablet, nomegestrol acetate 2.5mg, ethinylestradiol hemihydrate 1.5mg. Round f/c. Active (24): White. Marked ne. Placebo (4): Yellow. Marked p. *Lactose.*

Norgestimate, Ethinylestradiol

ATC Code: G03AA11. **Sport:** Permitted.
Driving: Unlikely to impair.
Indications: Oral hormonal contraception (adult women).
Dose: Adult: See Notes below.
Notes: See 8.2.1 Combined Hormonal Contraceptives.

Cilest 250/35 *(Janssen-Cilag)* B. GMS.
Price, (21) €0.94.
Tablet, norgestimate 250mcg, ethinylestradiol 35mcg. Blue round f/c. Marked 0 250; 35 on reverse. *Lactose.*

8.2.2 - Transdermal

In This Chapter: *Ethinylestradiol, norelgestromin combination.*

Ethinylestradiol, Norelgestromin

ATC Code: G03AA13. **Sport:** Permitted.
Driving: Unlikely to impair.
Indications: Transdermal hormonal contraception.
Dose: Adult: 1 patch applied and worn for 7 days. Patch to be changed same day every week, fourth week patch-free starting on cycle day 22.
SP: Strongly advise women over 35 years not to smoke.
Notes: See 8.2.1 Combined Hormonal Contraceptives.

Evra Transdermal *(Janssen-Cilag)* A. GMS.
Price, (3) €8.72. (9) €23.80.
Transdermal patch, ethinylestradiol 600mcg, norelgestromin (NGMN) 6mg; releasing average ethinylestradiol 33.9mcg, NGMN 203mcg/24 hours. Thin matrix 3-layer. Marked Evra.

8.2.3 - Progestogen Only

In This Chapter: *Desogestrel, norethisterone.*

Desogestrel

ATC Code: G03AC09. **Sport:** Permitted.
Driving: No or negligible effect.
Indications: Hormonal contraception.
Dose: Adult: 1 tab daily at about same time each day; start on day 1 of menstrual cycle; take continuously with no break in medication.
Hepatic Impairment: Severe, contraindicated as long as LFTs have not returned to normal.
ADR: *Most common*, bleeding irregularity, acne, mood changes, breast pain, nausea, weight increase.
Notes: See 8.2.1 Combined Hormonal Contraceptives.

Cerazette 75mcg *(MSD)* B. GMS.
Price, (28) €2.89.
Tablet, desogestrel. White round f/c. Marked KV above 2; ORGANON on reverse. *Lactose.* **Store:** Original pack to protect (light, moisture).
Azalia 75mcg *(Consilient)* B. GMS.
Price, (28 x 3), €7.47.
Tablet, desogestrel. White (almost) round. Marked D; 75 on reverse. *Lactose.*
Desogestrel Rowex 75mcg *(Rowex)* B. GMS.
Price, (84) €7.47.
Tablet, desogestrel. White f/c round. *Lactose, soya-bean oil.*

Norethisterone (contraception)

ATC Code: G03AC01. **Sport:** Permitted.
Driving: None known.
Indications: Hormonal contraception.

Dose: Adult: 1 tab daily commencing on day 1 of menstrual cycle and taken continuously with no break in medication.
Notes: See 8.2.1 Combined Hormonal Contraceptives.
Noriday 350mcg *(Pfizer)* B. GMS.
Price, (28) €2.86.
Tablet, norethisterone. White round. Marked Searle; NY on reverse. Lactose.

8.2.4 - Long-Acting Contraceptives

In This Chapter: *Ethinylestradiol, etonogestrel combination, etonogestrel, levonorgestrel.*

Ethinylestradiol, Etonogestrel

ATC Code: G02BB01. **Sport:** Permitted.
Driving: Unlikely to impair.
Indications: Contraception.
Dose: Adult: Age 18-40 years, starting on day 1 of menstrual cycle, insert *NuvaRing* into vagina and leave in continuously for 3 weeks; remove on same day of week as inserted. After a ring-free interval of 1 week, insert a new ring. Starting on days 2-5 is allowed but during first cycle an additional barrier method is recommended (first 7 days). *Changing* from hormonal contraceptive, insert at latest on day following the usual tablet-free, patch-free or placebo tablet interval of previous CHC; from progestogen-only, switch on any day but should use additional barrier as above.
Interactions: Effect of Other Drugs on Etonogestrel, Ethinylestradiol: *Co-admin contraindicated:* Ombitasvir/paritaprevir/ritonavir and dasabuvir, with/without ribavirin (ALT elevation risk); *NuvaRing* can be restarted 2 weeks after drug treatment. See Notes below.
SP: Advise women to regularly check for presence of ring in vagina. If *NuvaRing* is out of the vagina for an unknown amount of time, consider possibility of pregnancy; perform pregnancy test before inserting new ring.
ADR: *Most frequent reported,* headache, vaginal (infection, discharge).
Notes: See 8.2.1 Combined Hormonal Contraceptives.
NuvaRing VDS *(MSD)* A. GMS.
Price, (1-pack) €8.96.
Vaginal delivery system (VDS), ethinylestradiol, etonogestrel 2.7mg/11.7mg releasing 0.015mg/0.120mg per 24 hours over 3 weeks. Flexible transparent colourless ring. **Store:** Refrigerate (before dispensing); below 30 deg C (max. 4 months) (after dispensing).

Etonogestrel

ATC Code: G03AC08. **Sport:** Permitted.
Driving: Unlikely to impair.
Indications: Contraception.
Dose: Adult: Age 18-40 years, insert 1 implant subdermally at inner side of non-dominant upper arm. No preceding hormonal contraception, insert between days 1-5 of menstrual cycle; changing from combined hormonal contraceptive, insert on day after last active tab OR on day of removal of vaginal ring or transdermal patch. Insertion to be performed under aseptic conditions by qualified personnel familiar with the procedure using preloaded applicator.
Postpartum, not breastfeeding, insert between 21-28 days postpartum; breastfeeding, insert after fourth week postpartum.
ADR: Summary, *most common reasons for stopping treatment,* changes in menstrual bleeding pattern (irregular pattern, intensity, duration).
Notes: See 8.2.1 Combined Hormonal Contraceptives.
Implanon NXT Implant 68mg *(MSD)* A. GMS.
Price, (1) 68mg, €120.55.
Subdermal implant, etonogestrel; released at approx. 60-70mcg/day (week 5-6), decreasing to 35-45mcg/day (end year 1), 30-40mcg/day (end year 2), 25-30mcg/day (end year 3). Radio-opaque white (off-white) flexible implant preloaded in applicator.

Levonorgestrel (intrauterine)

ATC Code: G02BA03. **Sport:** Permitted.
Driving: No influence.
Indications: Contraception for up to 3 years *(Jaydess),* up

Long-Acting Contraceptives 8.2.4

to 5 years *(Kyleena).* Contraception, idiopathic menorrhagia, protection from endometrial hyperplasia during oestrogen replacement therapy *(Mirena).*
Dose: Adult: *Jaydess, Kyleena,* insert into uterine cavity within 7 days of onset of menstruation. Can be replaced by a new system at any time in the cycle; can also be inserted immediately after first-trimester abortion; postpartum, not earlier than 6 weeks after delivery. Difficult insertion and/or exceptional pain or bleeding during or after insertion, exclude perforation (physical examination, ultrasound).
Mirena, insert as for brands above. Can be used in women on hormone replacement therapy in combination with oral or transdermal oestrogen preparations without progestogens.
To be inserted by healthcare professional using aseptic technique.
Elderly: No indication post-menopause.
Child: No indication before menarche.
Hepatic Impairment: Acute disease, tumour, severe disease, contraindicated.
CI: Pregnancy, acute/recurrent PID, acute cervicitis or vaginitis, lower genital tract infection, postpartum endometriosis, infected miscarriage/abortion in past 3 months, cervical dysplasia, uterine or cervical malignancy, undiagnosed or abnormal uterine or vaginal bleeding, uterine fibroids, increased infection susceptibility, progestogen-dependent tumours (breast cancer).
SP: Not first choice for young nulligravid women, postmenopausal women with advanced uterine atrophy. Does not protect against HIV infection, other STDs. Before insertion inform woman of efficacy and risk. Consider possibility of pregnancy if menstruation does not occur within 6 weeks of onset of previous menstruation. Risk of pelvic inflammatory diseases. The system can be expelled from the uterine cavity with being noticed (loss of contraceptive protection). Perforation or penetration of uterine corpus or cervix may occur. If the retrieval threads are not visible at the cervix on follow-up examinations, exclude pregnancy. Postpone postpartum insertions until uterus is fully involuted; not earlier than six weeks after delivery.
Pregnancy, Lactation: Insertion during pregnancy, contraindicated. Lactation, appears no deleterious effect on infant growth or development.
ADR: *Very common/common* (all brands), headache, abdominal/pelvic pain, acne/seborrhoea, bleeding changes (increased/decreased menstrual bleeding, spotting, amenorrhoea), ovarian cyst, vulvovaginitis).
Notes: See 8.2.1 Combined Hormonal Contraceptives.
▼ **Jaydess 13.5mg IDS** *(Bayer)* A. GMS.
Price, (1) €104.87.
Intrauterine delivery system (IDS), levonorgestrel 13.5mg delivering 6mcg/24 hours average over 3 years. White (pale-yellow) drug core covered with semi-opaque membrane on vertical stem of T-body (white) with removal threads (brown). Silver ring visibility on ultrasound.
Kyleena 19.5mg IDS *(Bayer)* A. GMS.
Price, (1) €116.51.
Intrauterine delivery system (IDS), levonorgestrel 19.5mg. Whitish (pale-yellow) drug core covered with semi-opaque membrane mounted on vertical stem of T-body with a silver ring; with removal threads (blue) attached.
Mirena 52mg IDS *(Bayer)* A. GMS.
Price, (1) €116.50.
Intrauterine delivery system (IDS), levonorgestrel 52mg delivering 20mcg/24 hours initially reducing to 11mcg/24 hours after 5 years; mean 14mcg/24 hours up to 5 years. White (almost) drug core covered with opaque membrane on vertical stem of T-body with removal threads.

Medroxyprogesterone (contraception)

ATC Code: G03AC06. **Sport:** Permitted.
Driving: Unlikely to impair.
Indications: Contraception including short-term (partners of men undergoing vasectomy until effective; immunisation against rubella; women awaiting sterilisation).
Dose: Adult: 150mg every 3 months; initial injection between day 1-5 of cycle. Deep IM injection into gluteal muscle.
SP: Decreased bone mineral density (BMD); increases with

219

8.2.5 Emergency Contraception

duration of use; during adolescence/early adulthood is critical period of bone accretion. Ensure adequate calcium and Vitamin D intake. Increased fracture risk. Delay in return to normal menstrual cycle and transient infertility (for up to 18 months, occasionally longer) following continuous treatment.

ADR: *Very common*, nervousness, headache, abdominal pain or discomfort, increased or decreased weight.

Notes: See 8.2.1 Combined Hormonal Contraceptives.

Depo-Provera Parenteral 150mg/mL *(Pfizer)* A. GMS.
Price, injection or vial 150mg/mL (1mL) €6.18.
Injection, medroxyprogesterone acetate. White aqueous soln.

8.2.5 - Emergency Contraception

In This Chapter: *Levonorgestrel, ulipristal.*

Class Effects

SP: Emergency contraception is not for regular use; use only as emergency measure; should not replace regular contraception.

Notes: See 8.2.1 Combined Hormonal Contraceptives.

Levonorgestrel (oral)

ATC Code: G03AD01 **Sport:** Permitted.
Driving: Dizziness, fatigue.

Indications: Emergency contraception within 72 hours of unprotected sexual intercourse or contraceptive failure.

Dose: Adult: 1 tab (1500mcg) taken as soon as possible (within 12 hours; no later than 72 hours) after unprotected intercourse; regardless of body weight or BMI. If vomiting occurs within 3 hours of admin, admin another tab immediately. *NorLevo*, if enzyme-inducing drugs have been used during the last 4 weeks and emergency contraception is needed, recommended use of a non-hormonal emergency contraception i.e. Cu-IUD or take a double dose* of levonorgestrel (i.e. 2 tablets taken together) *(not studied).

Child: Not recommended. Under 16 years, limited data.

Hepatic Impairment: Severe, not recommended.

Interactions: Effect of Other Drugs on Levonorgestrel: Ulipristal: *Co-admin not recommended; may interact with progestational activity of levonorgestrel.*

SP: If time of unprotected intercourse is uncertain or longer than 72 hours, consider conception. If no period occurs, exclude pregnancy. Ectopic risk if pregnancy occurs after treatment; if already at risk, salpingitis, ectopic pregnancy, not recommended. Malabsorption syndromes may impair efficacy. Repeated admin within menstrual cycle, not advisable. Thrombolic events; caution, pre-existing risk factors.

Pregnancy, Lactation: Pregnancy, not recommended (cannot interrupt). Lactation, avoid nursing for 6 hours following admin; is excreted in breast milk. Levonorgestrel increases possibility of cycle disturbances; can lead to earlier or later ovulation date and modified fertility date.

ADR: *Common*, dizziness, headache, nausea, low abdominal pain, breast tenderness, delayed/heavy menses, bleeding not related to menses, fatigue, weight increase, depressed mood.

Notes: See 8.2.5 Emergency Contraception.

NorLevo 1.5mg *(HRA)* OTC.
Price, (1) €11.82.
Tablet, levonorgestrel. White round. Marked NL 1.5. *Lactose*.
Store: Blister in outer carton to (light).
Prevenelle 1500mcg *(Consilient)* OTC. GMS.
Price, (1) €6.81.
Tablet, levonorgestrel. Round white. Marked G00. *Lactose*.
Levonorgestrel Rowex 1.5mg *(Rowex)* OTC.
Price, (1) €10.64 (trade).
Tablet, levonorgestrel. Round white. Marked C; I on reverse. *Lactose*.

Ulipristal (contraception)

ATC Code: G03AD02. **Sport:** Permitted.
Driving: Dizziness, somnolence, blurred vision, disturbed attention.
Indications: Emergency contraception within 120 hours of unprotected sexual intercourse or contraceptive failure.

Dose: Adult: 1 tab (30mg) as soon as possible; no later

than 120 hours after unprotected intercourse or contraceptive failure; any time in menstrual cycle.

Child: No indication prepuberty; adolescents, suitable for any women of childbearing age.

Renal Impairment: No specific dose recommendation.

Hepatic Impairment: Severe, not recommended.

Interactions: Effect of Other Drugs on Ulipristal: *Co-admin not recommended (plasma levels decreased):* CYP3A4 inducers (rifampicin, phenytoin, fosphenytoin, phenobarbital, carbamazepine, efavirenz, nevirapine, oxcarbazepine, primidone, rifabutin, St John's Wort; long-term ritonavir).

Effect of Ulipristal on Other Drugs: Levonorgestrel emergency contraception: *Co-admin not recommended.* Combined hormonal and progesterone-only contraceptives: *Effect reduced.*

SP: May reduce action of regular hormonal contraception. After using emergency contraception (including if initiating), use reliable barrier method until next menstrual period. Severe asthma not controlled on oral glucocorticoids, not recommended.

Pregnancy, Lactation: Not intended for use during pregnancy; do not take if pregnancy (suspected or known). Report pregnancy in women who have taken *ellaOne* to www.hra-pregnancy-registry.com. Lactation, breastfeeding not recommended for 1 week following admin.

ADR: *Common*, mood disorders, headache, dizziness, nausea, abdominal pain/discomfort, vomiting, myalgia, pain (back, pelvic), dysmenorrhoea, breast tenderness, fatigue.

Notes: See 8.2.5 Emergency Contraception.

ellaOne 30mg *(HRA)* OTC. GMS.
Price, (1) €16.44.
Tablet, ulipristal acetate. White (marble creamy) round curved. Marked 'ella' both sides. *Lactose*. **Store:** Below 25 deg C; original pack to protect (moisture, light).

8.3 - Vaginal, Vulval Infections

8.3.1 - Fungal Infections

In This Chapter: *Clotrimazole, econazole, miconazole.*

Class Effects

CI: Hypersensitivity to any member of the class. Imidazole hypersensitivity (not ketoconazole). Not for oral or ophthalmic use.

SP: *Consult medical advice if*, pregnant, presence of STDs, age under 16 or over 60, recurrent infection; redness, irritation or swelling associated with treatment, abnormal or irregular vaginal bleeding, blood-stained vaginal discharge, vulval or vaginal sores, ulcers or blisters, lower abdominal pain or dysuria, back pain, associated shoulder pain, fever. All infected areas as well as sexual partner should be treated concurrently. Do not use tampons, intravaginal douches, spermicidal contraceptives or other vaginal products while using these products. Avoid contact with latex products e.g. contraceptive diaphragms, condoms (may damage rubber). Avoid vaginal intercourse (partner infection, reduced safety of latex products, spermicidals inactivated).

Pregnancy, Lactation: Pregnancy, avoid during first trimester; use only if considered necessary; if applicators are used, caution to avoid mechanical trauma. Lactation, caution.

Notes: For systemic effects of topically applied antifungals, see 9.2 Antifungals.

Clotrimazole (gynaecological)

ATC Code: G01AF02. **Sport:** Permitted.
Driving: No or negligible effect.

Indications: Treatment, candidal vaginitis, vulvitis; penis of sexual partner to prevent re-infection.

Dose: Adult: Age 12 years and older, *vaginal pessary* 500mg, insert as high as possible, at night; 200mg, use for 3 consecutive nights; *cream*, apply 2-3 times daily to vulva and surrounding area. Sexual partner (to prevent re-infection), apply 2-3 times daily for up to 2 weeks. Use second treatment if required; recurrent, investigate underlying cause.

Elderly: Over 60 years, seek medical advice.

Child: Under 12 years, not recommended as pessaries are used with an applicator.

Interactions: Effect of Clotrimazole (Vaginal) on Other Drugs: Tacrolimus, sirolimus (oral): *Increased plasma levels with co-admin.*

Pregnancy, Lactation: Pregnancy, avoid during first trimester; during pregnancy use vaginal tabs as they can be inserted without using an applicator. Lactation, stop breastfeeding during treatment.

ADR: Allergic reaction, vulvovaginal discomfort, oedema, burning, genital peeling, irritation, pruritus, pelvic pain, rash, vaginal haemorrhage, erythema, abdominal pain.

Notes: See 8.3.1 Fungal Infections.

> **Canesten Pessary 500mg, Combi** *(Bayer)* B.
> *Price,* (1) €8.22. Combi (1 pessary + 10g cream) €9.87.
> *Vaginal pessary,* clotrimazole. White. Marked Bayer; MU on reverse.
> *Cream,* as above 2% w/w (in Combi). White. *Cetostearyl alcohol.*
> **Canesten Pessary 200mg, Duopak** *(Bayer)* B. GMS.
> *Price,* 200mg (3) €3.21. Duopak, €5.45.
> *Vaginal pessary,* clotrimazole 100mg (in Duopak). White. Marked Bayer; P3 on reverse. 200mg: White. Marked Bayer; NR on reverse. *Lactose.*
> *Cream,* as above 1% w/w (in Duopak). White oil-in-water. *Cetostearyl alcohol.*

Econazole (gynaecological)

ATC Code: G01AF05. **Sport:** Permitted.
Driving: Unlikely to impair.

Indications: Fungal or yeast infections of vagina and vulva.

Dose: Adult, Elderly: Insert 1 pessary deep into vagina. Pregnant women, recommended to admin *without* use of applicator; wash hands thoroughly before self-admin.

ADR: *Common,* pruritus, burning sensation.

Notes: See 8.3.1 Fungal Infections.

> **Gyno-Pevaryl Once 150mg** *(Janssen-Cilag)* B. GMS.
> *Price,* (1) €1.93.
> *Vaginal pessary,* econazole nitrate. Light-beige torpedo-shape.

Ketoconazole (gynaecological)

ATC Code: G01AF11. **Sport:** Permitted.
Driving: Unlikely to impair.

Indications: Cutaneous candidosis (including external application to vulva).

Dose: Adult, Elderly: Apply 1-2 times daily.

Interactions: Effect of Other Drugs on Ketoconazole: *Local irritation:* Topical corticosteroids.

Pregnancy, Lactation: If benefit outweighs risk.

ADR: Local irritation, rash, peri-orbital oedema.

Notes: See 8.3.1 Fungal Infections.

> **Nizoral Cream 2%** *(Janssen-Cilag)* OTC. GMS.
> *Price,* (30g) €4.76.
> *Topical cream,* ketoconazole 2% w/w (20mg/g). White odourless. *Propylene glycol, cetyl/stearyl alcohol.*

Miconazole (gynaecological)

ATC Code: G01AF04. **Sport:** Permitted.
Driving: Unlikely to impair.

Indications: Vulvo-vaginal candidal infections, including superinfection with susceptible Gram-positive bacteria.

Dose: Adult, Elderly: *Vaginal, capsule 1200mg,* insert 1 at night; *cream,* insert 2 applications at night for 7 days OR 1 application for 14 days.

Child: Under 18 years, not recommended.

Interactions: Effect of Miconazole on Other Drugs: Warfarin: *Caution.* Oral hypoglycaemics, phenytoin: *Effects, side effects increased.*

SP: Local sensitisation or allergic reaction, severe hypersensitivity (anaphylaxis, angioedema), discontinue. Does not stain skin or clothes.

ADR: *Post-marketing,* hypersensitivity (anaphylactic, anaphylactoid), angioedema, pruritus, vaginal irritation, application site reactions.

Notes: See 8.3.1 Fungal Infections.

> **Gyno-Daktarin Vaginal Caps, Cream** *(Janssen-Cilag)* B. GMS.
> *Price,* 1200mg (1) €4.58. Cream, €5.88.
> *Vaginal capsule,* miconazole nitrate 1200mg. White (off-white) egg-shaped soft; contains white (cream-coloured) hydrophobic mass. *Parabens.*
> *Vaginal cream,* as above 20mg/g (2% w/w). White homogenous. *Benzoic acid, butylated hydroxyanisole.*

8.3.2 - Other Infections

In This Chapter: *Clindamycin.*

Class Effects
CI: Hypersensitivity to any member of the class.

Clindamycin (gynaecological)

ATC Code: J01FF01. **Sport:** Permitted.
Driving: No special advice.

Indications: Antibiotic management of bacterial vaginosis.

Dose: Adult, Elderly: Insert 1 applicator full (approx. 5g) intravaginally at bedtime for 7 consecutive nights.

Child: Safety/efficacy not established.

CI: Lincomycin hypersensitivity, history of (inflammatory bowel disease, antibiotic-associated colitis).

Interactions: Effect of Other Drugs on Clindamycin: *Cross resistance:* Lincomycin, erythromycin. *Antagonism:* Erythromycin *in vitro.*

Effect of Clindamycin on Other Drugs: Neuromuscular blockers: *Action enhanced, caution with systemic clindamycin.* Vitamin K antagonists (warfarin, acenocoumarol, fluindione): *Increased coagulation tests (PT/INR) and/or bleeding reported, monitor.*

SP: Superinfection. Antibiotic-associated diarrhoea or colitis, discontinue. Co-use of other vaginal products, not recommended.

Pregnancy, Lactation: Pregnancy, first trimester only if clearly needed; second and third trimesters, possibility of foetal harm appears remote. Lactation, if benefit outweighs risk.

ADR: *Very common,* vulvovaginal candidiasis.

Notes: See 8.3.2 Other Infections.

> **Dalacin 2% Vaginal Cream** *(Pfizer)* A. GMS.
> *Price,* (40g) €12.12.
> *Vaginal cream,* clindamycin phosphate 20mg/g. White semi-solid. *Propylene glycol, cetostearyl alcohol.*

8.4 - Urological Disorders

8.4.1 - Benign Prostatic Hyperplasia (BPH)

In This Chapter: *Alfuzosin, dutasteride, finasteride, silodosin, tamsulosin, indoramin and combinations.*

Class Effects
Indications: Doxazosin, prazosin and terazosin have a dual BPH and hypertension indication. See Notes below.

CI: Hypersensitivity to any member of the class. *Alpha-blockers* (alfuzosin, silodosin, tamsulosin, indoramin), orthostatic hypotension, hepatic impairment. *Testosterone-5-alpha-reductase inhibitors* (dutasteride, finasteride), not for use in women, adolescents or children; contraindicated in women who are or may become pregnant.

SP: Exclude other conditions which may cause symptoms same as BPH (prostate cancer) by digital rectal examination.

Alpha-blockers, see Contraindications (CI) above. Intraoperative Floppy Iris Syndrome (IFIS) (increased procedural complications in cataract, glaucoma surgery). Caution, acute cardiac failure, QTc prolongation, drugs increasing QTc interval, orthostatic hypotension, pre-existing cerebral circulatory disturbances (risk of cerebral ischaemic disorders).

Testosterone-5-alpha-reductase inhibitors, large residual urine volume and/or severely diminished urinary flow, monitor (obstructive uropathy). Absorbed through skin; women, adolescents, children to avoid contact (leaking capsules, broken or crushed tabs). Sustained increased PSA levels, evaluate. Causes serum PSA to decrease by

8.4.1 Benign Prostatic Hyperplasia (BPH)

approx. 50% in BPH even in presence of prostate cancer; consider when evaluating PSA data.

Pregnancy, Lactation: *Testosterone-5-alpha-reductase inhibitors,* pregnancy, contraindicated; may inhibit conversion of testosterone to dihydrotestosterone, and may cause abnormalities of external genitalia of a male foetus if admin to pregnant women; avoid exposure to semen of treated males by condom usage. Small amounts of finasteride have been recovered from the semen of subjects receiving finasteride 5mg/day; not known if male foetus adversely affected if mother exposed to this semen. Lactation, not known if excreted in breast milk; not indicated for use in women.

ADR: *Testosterone-5-alpha-reductase inhibitors,* decreased ejaculate volume, impotence, ejaculation disorders, breast enlargement, tenderness, testicular pain, breast secretion/nodules, rash, pruritus, urticaria, localised oedema, angioedema, decreased libido.

Notes: See 2.1.4 Alpha-Blockers.

Alfuzosin

ATC Code: G04CA01. **Sport:** Permitted.
Driving: Dizziness, asthenia, postural hypotension.
Indications: Treatment, lower urinary tract symptoms associated with BPH. Adjunctive, urethral catheterisation for acute urinary retention associated with BPH.
Dose: Adult: STANDARD/R, 2.5mg 3-times daily; max. 10mg/day. Hypertensives, 2.5mg morning and evening. PROLONGED/R, 10mg/day. Acute urinary retention, 10mg/day from first day of catheterisation. Oral after food; swallow tabs whole; do not chew or crush.
Elderly: 2.5mg morning and evening.
Child: Not recommended.
Renal Impairment: Severe, not recommended.
Interactions: Effect of Other Drugs on Alfuzosin: *Co-admin not recommended*: Other alpha-blockers, general anaesthetics (withdraw alpha-blocker 24-hours before surgery). *Co-admin caution (postural hypotension)*: Other antihypertensives, nitrates, CYP3A4 inhibitors (azole antifungals, HIV protease inhibitors).
SP: Another alpha-blocker co-admin, not recommended. Coronary insufficiency, continue specific therapy; if angina pectoris reappears or worsens, discontinue. Pronounced drop in BP reported post-marketing in patients with pre-existing risk factors (cardiac diseases and/or antihypertensive co-admin); hypotension risk may be greater in elderly (caution).
ADR: *Common,* asthenia, nausea, abdominal pain, faintness, dizziness, headache.
Notes: See 8.4.1 BPH.

Xatral 2.5mg, XL 10mg *(SANOFI)* B. GMS.
Price, 2.5mg (60) €17.86. XL 10mg (30) €14.47.
Standard/R tablet, alfuzosin HCl 2.5mg. White round f/c. Marked Xatral/strength. *Lactose.*
Prolonged/R tablet, as above 10mg. 10mg: Round, 3 layered (1 white between 2 yellow). *Mannitol.*
Alfuzosin Rowex 10mg Prolonged/R *(Rowex)* B. GMS.
Price, (30) €11.50.
Prolonged/R tablet, alfuzosin HCl. White round. *Lactose.*
Xatger 10mg Prolonged/R *(Gerard)* B. GMS.
Price, (30) €14.36.
Prolonged/R tablet, alfuzosin HCl. White round u/c. *Lactose.*

Dutasteride

ATC Code: G04CB02. **Sport:** Permitted.
Driving: Unlikely to impair.
Indications: Treatment, lower urinary tract symptoms associated with BPH. Reduction in risk of acute urinary retention (AUR) and surgery (with moderate to severe symptoms of BPH).
Dose: Adult, Elderly: 0.5mg once daily, alone or combination with alpha-blocker tamsulosin 0.4mg. Caps to be swallowed whole with or without food; do not chew or open; contents may result in oropharyngeal mucosa irritation.
Hepatic Impairment: Mild to moderate, caution. Severe, contraindicated.
Interactions: Effect of Other Drugs on Dutasteride: *Increased serum levels*: Moderate CYP3A4 and P-

glycoprotein inhibitors (verapamil, diltiazem), long-term co-admin of potent inhibitors (ritonavir, indinavir, nefazodone, itraconazole, ketoconazole).
SP: Combination therapy, careful benefit/risk assessment; increased adverse event risk including cardiac failure. Breast cancer in men reported. Monitor PSA and evaluate for prostate cancer regularly.
ADR: *Monotherapy, combination,* impotence, decreased libido, ejaculation disorders, breast enlargement and/or tenderness, dizziness, cardiac failure.
Notes: See 8.4.1 BPH.

Avodart 0.5mg *(GSK)* A. GMS.
Price, (30) €23.66.
Capsule, dutasteride. Soft opaque yellow oblong. Marked GXCE2. *Lecithin.*
Dutasteride (TEVA) 0.5mg *(TEVA)* A. GMS.
Price, (30) €9.46.
Capsule, dutasteride. Soft opaque yellow oblong filled with oily yellowish liquid. *Lecithin.* **Store:** Below 30 deg C; original pack to protect (moisture).

Finasteride

ATC Code: G04CB01. **Sport:** Permitted.
Driving: Unlikely to impair.
Indications: Treatment, lower urinary tract symptoms associated with BPH. Reduction in risk of acute urinary retention and surgery (with moderate to severe symptoms of BPH).
Dose: Adult: 5mg daily. Oral, with or without food; tabs to be swallowed whole, not crushed or chewed.
Elderly: Above 70 years, elimination rate slightly decreased.
Hepatic Impairment: Mild to moderate, caution. Severe, contraindicated.
Notes: See 8.4.1 BPH.

Proscar 5mg *(MSD)* A. GMS.
Price, (28) €12.00.
Tablet, finasteride. Blue apple-shaped f/c. Marked Proscar; MSD 72 on reverse. *Lactose.*
Finasteride (Accord) 5mg *(Accord)* A. GMS.
Price, (28) €11.76.
Tablet, finasteride. Round blue. Marked F5. *Lactose.*
Finocar 5mg *(Pinewood)* A. GMS.
Price, (28) €11.76.
Tablet, finasteride. Light-blue spherical f/c. *Lactose.*
Fintrid 5mg *(Rowex)* A. GMS.
Price, (28) €11.76.
Tablet, finasteride. Blue round f/c. *Lactose.*
Profal 5mg *(Accord)* A. GMS.
Price, (28) €11.76.
Tablet, finasteride. Blue round f/c. Marked F5. *Lactose.*

Indoramin

ATC Code: C04CA02. **Sport:** Permitted.
Driving: Caution.
Indications: Treatment, lower urinary tract symptoms associated with BPH.
Dose: Adult: 20mg twice daily; if required increase in 20mg increments at 1-week intervals to max. 100mg/day.
Elderly: 20mg at night.
CI: Cardiac failure.
Interactions: Effect of Other Drugs on Indoramin: *Co-admin not recommended*: MAOIs, antihypertensives, highly protein bound drugs.
SP: Caution, Parkinson's Disease, epilepsy; seizures, depression.
ADR: Drowsiness, sedation.
Notes: See 8.4.1 BPH.

Indoramin 20mg *(Essential Generics)* B. GMS.
Price, (60) €15.12.
Tablet, indoramin HCl. Pale-yellow f/c triangular with small projection on each side. *Lactose.*

Silodosin

ATC Code: G04CA04. **Sport:** Permitted.
Driving: Postural hypotension.
Indications: Treatment, lower urinary tract symptoms associated with BPH.
Dose: Adult, Elderly: 8mg once daily. *Admin,* with food, at

same time of day; swallow whole with water; do not break or chew.

Renal Impairment: CrCl (mL/min) 50-80, initially 4mg once daily; titrate to 8mg/day after 1 week depending on response. Severe, not recommended.

Hepatic Impairment: Severe, not recommended.

Interactions: Effect of Other Drugs on Silodosin: *Co-admin not recommended*: Other alpha-blockers, potent CYP3A4 inhibitors (ketoconazole, itraconazole, ritonavir). *Co-admin, monitor for adverse reactions*: PDE-5 inhibitors, antihypertensives (ACEIs, ARBs, beta-blockers, calcium antagonists, diuretics).

Pregnancy, Lactation: Ejaculation with reduced or no semen observed.

ADR: *Very common*, retrograde ejaculation, anejaculation.

Notes: See 8.4.1 BPH.

Urorec 4mg, 8mg *(Recordati)* B. GMS.
Price, (30) 4mg, €9.60. 8mg, €13.04.
Capsule, silodosin. Hard gelatin opaque. 4mg: Yellow. 8mg: White.

Tamsulosin

ATC Code: G04CA02. **Sport:** Permitted.
Driving: Caution.

Indications: Treatment, lower urinary tract symptoms associated with BPH.

Dose: Adult, Elderly: 0.4mg daily. *Admin*, oral with or without food or after food with glass of water after first meal of day; swallow whole; do not crush or chew (interferes with modified release).

Child: Under 18 years, no data.

Renal Impairment: CrCl (mL/min) below 10, caution.

Hepatic Impairment: Severe, contraindicated.

Interactions: Effect of Other Drugs on Tamsulosin: *Co-admin not recommended*: Strong CYP3A4 inhibitors in patients with poor metaboliser CYP2D6 phenotype. *Co-admin caution*: Strong and moderated CYP3A4 inhibitors. *Potential for increased exposure*: CYP3A4 inhibitors (ketoconazole), CYP2D6 inhibitors (paroxetine). *Elimination rate may be increased*: Warfarin, diclofenac. See Notes below (alfuzosin).

ADR: *Common*, dizziness, ejaculation disorders (retrograde ejaculation, failure).

Notes: See 8.4.1 BPH. See Alfuzosin above.

Interchangeability: Same strengths of all brands of tamsulosin Prolonged/R tablets and capsules and Modified/R capsules listed below are deemed interchangeable.

Reference Price: (30) 400mcg (MR/PR), €4.50.

Omnexel 0.4mg *(Astellas)* B. GMS.
Price, (30) €15.55.
Prolonged/R tablet, tamsulosin HCl. Round yellow f/c.

Tamnexyl XL 400mcg *(Clonmel)* B. GMS.
Price, (30) see reference price above.
Prolonged/R tablet, tamsulosin HCl. White round. Marked T9SL; 0.4 on reverse.

Tamnic 400mcg *(Clonmel)* B. GMS.
Price, (30) see reference price above.
Modified/R capsule, tamsulosin HCl. Orange/olive green with black stripe. Marked TSL 0.4 contains white pellets.

Tamsu 400mcg *(Rowex)* B. GMS.
Price, (30) see reference price above.
Modified/R capsule, tamsulosin HCl. Orange/olive green; contains white (off-white) pellets.

Tamsulosin (Gerard) 400mcg *(Gerard)* B. GMS.
Price, (30) see reference price above.
Modified/R capsule, tamsulosin HCl. Orange/olive-green. Contains white (off-white) spheres.

Tamsulosin, Dutasteride

ATC Code: G04CA52. **Sport:** Permitted.
Driving: Orthostatic hypotension.

Indications: See Notes below (dutasteride).

Dose: Adult, Elderly: 1 cap (0.5mg/0.4mg)/day. *Admin*, approx. 30 minutes before same meal each day; see Notes below (dutasteride).

SP: To minimise postural hypotension risk, patient should be haemodynamically stable on alpha-block before PDE-5 inhibitor initiation.

Notes: See Dutasteride and Tamsulosin above.

Interchangeability: Same strengths of all brands of dutasteride/tamsulosin caps are deemed interchangeable (includes parallel imports).

Combodart *(GSK)* A. GMS.
Price, 0.5/0.4mg (30) €24.74.
Capsule, dutasteride 0.5mg, tamsulosin 0.4mg. Hard oblong brown/orange contains tamsulosin Modified/R pellets + 1 dutasteride soft cap. Marked GS 7CZ. *Sunset Yellow, lecithin.*
Store: Below 30 deg C.

Tamsulosin, Solifenacin

ATC Code: G04CA53. **Sport:** Permitted.
Driving: Dizziness, blurred vision, fatigue, somnolence.

Indications: Treatment, moderate to severe storage symptoms (urgency, increased micturition frequency) and voiding symptoms of BPH in men not adequately responding to monotherapy.

Dose: Adult, Elderly: 1 tablet (6/0.4mg) daily (max. 6/0.4mg). *Admin*, with or without food; swallow whole, intact, without biting or chewing; do not crush tablet.

Child: No relevant use.

Renal Impairment: CrCl(mL/min) below 30, caution (max. 1 tab per day); if also treated with a strong CYP3A4 inhibitor, contraindicated. Haemodialysis, contraindicated.

Hepatic Impairment: Moderate, as for Renal above. Severe, contraindicated.

CI: Severe GI conditions (toxic megacolon), myasthenia gravis, narrow-angle glaucoma, history of orthostatic hypotension.

Interactions: Effect of Other Drugs on Tamsulosin, Solifenacin: *Co-admin caution*: Moderate or strong CYP3A4 inhibitors (verapamil, ketoconazole, ritonavir, nelfinavir, itraconazole), poor CYP2D6 metabolisers with strong CYP2D6 inhibitors. *More pronounced effects and undesirable effects*: Other anticholinergics (allow 1-week dosing interval). *Hypotensive effects*: Other alpha-blockers. *Increased tamsulosin elimination*: Diclofenac, warfarin.

SP: *Caution*, risk of urinary retention, GI obstructive disorders, decreased GI motility, hiatus hernia, GORD, medicinals that may exacerbate oesophagitis, autonomic neuropathy. Pre-existing long QT syndrome and hypokalaemia. Angioedema with airway obstruction (discontinue; do not restart). Anaphylactic reaction. Orthostatic hypotension (dizziness, weakness).

Pregnancy, Lactation: Not for use in women.

ADR: *Summary, most frequent*, dry mouth, constipation, dyspepsia; *common*, dizziness, blurred vision, fatigue, ejaculation disorders; *most serious*, acute urinary retention.

Notes: See 8.4.3 Urinary Incontinence (solifenacin). See Tamsulosin above.

Vesomni 6/0.4mg *(Astellas)* A. GMS.
Price, (30) €39.43.
Modified/R tablet, solifenacin succinate 6mg, tamsulosin HCl 0.4mg. Round red f/c. Marked 6/0.4.

8.4.2 - Erectile Dysfunction, Premature Ejaculation

In This Chapter: *Alprostadil, dapoxetine and PDE-5 inhibitors (avanafil, sildenafil, tadalafil, vardenafil).*

Class Effects

CI: Hypersensitivity to any member of the class. Children. **Women** (except sildenafil in PAH). Men where sexual activity is inadvisable (severe cardiac disorders, unstable angina, severe cardiac failure), see also SP below.

SP: *Erectile dysfunction*: Prior to initiating, complete medical history/physical exam to diagnose ED and underlying cause(s). Consider cardiovascular status (see contraindications); post-MI, stroke, life-threatening arrhythmias, hypotension (BP below 90/50mmHg) or hypertension (BP above 170/100mmHg) (contraindications for avanafil). PDE-5 inhibitors have vasodilator properties; patients with left ventricular outflow obstruction (aortic stenosis, idiopathic hypertrophic sub-aortic stenosis) may be sensitive to vasodilators including PDE-5 inhibitors.

Caution, anatomical deformity of penis (angulation,

8.4.2 Erectile Dysfunction, Premature Ejaculation

cavernosal fibrosis, Peyronie's disease), conditions predisposing to priapism (sickle cell anaemia, multiple myeloma, leukaemia). Priapism reported; if not treated immediately, penile tissue damage and permanent loss of potency could result. Sexual stimulation is required (apomorphine, avanafil, sildenafil, tadalafil, vardenafil).

PDE-5 inhibitors: Visual defects and cases of non-arteritic anterior ischaemic optic neuropathy (NAION); advise patient to report visual changes; sudden visual defect, discontinue and seek medical advice. Decreased or sudden loss of hearing.

Pregnancy, Lactation: Not for use in women except sildenafil (treatment of PAH).

ADR: *PDE-5 Inhibitors,* headache, dizziness, dyspepsia, flushing, nasal congestion, back pain, myalgia. Sudden deafness or hearing loss.

Alprostadil

ATC Code: G04BE01. **Sport:** Permitted.
Driving: Transient hypotension.

Indications: Adult males, treatment, erectile dysfunction (ED) (neurogenic, vasculogenic, psychogenic or mixed aetiology) *(all brands)*; adjunctive, diagnostic evaluation of ED *(Caverject, Muse, Viridal).*

Dose: Adult, Elderly: INTRACAVERNOSAL, *Caverject, treatment,* initially 2.5mcg; if partial response, second dose 5mcg; if no response within 1 hour 7.5mcg; after 1-day interval titrate by 5-10mcg to optimum (erection of duration max. 1 hour); max. once daily, 3-times weekly. Usual range 5-20mcg; above 60mcg not recommended. *Diagnostic,* inject 20mcg into corpus cavernosum and massage through penis. Evidence of neurological dysfunction, initially 5mcg, max. 10mcg.
Viridal Duo, treatment, initially 2.5mcg; ED of neurological origin, initially 1.25mcg. Increase by 2.5-5mcg; usually 10-20mcg per injection is required; over 20mcg, caution with cardiovascular risk factors; max. 40mcg. Max. 2-3 times weekly at 24-hour intervals.
TRANSURETHRAL, *Muse,* patient to urinate before admin; moist urethra aids admin and drug dissolution. *Treatment,* initially 500mcg, then 1000mcg or decrease to 250mcg or 125mcg. Max. 2 doses in 24-hours, 7 doses in 7-days. *Diagnostic,* 500mcg transurethral equiv. to 10mcg intracavernosal.
TOPICAL, *Vitaros,* consider 300mcg starting dose (especially with serious ED, co-morbidity, PDE-5 inhibitor failure); if not tolerated (local side effects), decrease to 200mcg dose (where available). Apply to tip of penis (meatus) within 5-30 minutes prior to attempting intercourse; instruct patient on proper technique. Effect duration 1-2 hours; max. 2-3 times per week; once per 24-hours.

CI: Conditions predisposing to priapism (sickle cell anaemia or trait, multiple myeloma, leukaemia, thrombocytaemia), anatomical deformation of penis, penis implants, if sexual activity is contraindicated. See Notes below. *Vitaros,* underlying disorders (orthostatic hypotension, MI, syncope).

Interactions: Effect of Other Drugs on Alprostadil: *Co-admin not recommended:* Other ED treatments including PDE5 inhibitors, alpha blockers (prolonged erection risk). *Possible increased bleeding risk following injection or topical application:* Warfarin, heparin, other anticoagulants. *Hypotensive crisis risk:* MAOIs. Co-admin *(Muse),* no data: Sildenafil. *Possible reduced alprostadil effect:* Sympathomimetics, decongestants, appetite suppressants.

Effect of Alprostadil on Other Drugs: Antihypertensives, vasodilators, anticoagulants, platelet aggregation inhibitors: *Effect enhanced.*

SP: Use lowest effective dose to minimise priapism risk. Intracavernosal/topical alprostadil does not protect from STDs. Prolonged/painful erection, priapism, penile angulation, cavernosal fibrosis, Peyronie's disease, discontinue. Presence of risk factors for cardiovascular disease and cerebrovascular accident (arterial hypertension), unstable cardiovascular disorders, CHF, TIA, pulmonary disease, (caution); symptomatic hypotension (dizziness), syncope. Abuse potential in patients with psychiatric disorders or addiction. *Vitaros,* intraurethral

exposure may result in penile burning, tingling sensation or pain; apply according to instructions; condom barrier recommended as may cause vaginal irritation (partner).

Pregnancy, Lactation: Use not recommended if female partner is pregnant, unless condom used; women of childbearing potential to ensure adequate contraception. Effect of indirect exposure not known; not recommended in partners who are breastfeeding.

ADR: Summary, *most frequent* (intracavernosal injection, urethral stick, topical), penile/urethral pain.

Notes: See 8.4.2 ED.

Caverject Parenteral *(Pfizer)* A. GMS.
Price, per vial 5mcg, €7.00. 10mcg, €8.91. 20mcg, €11.59.
Intracavernosal injection, alprostadil. White (off-white) lyophilised powder; clear colourless solvent. *Benzyl alcohol, essentially sodium-free.* **Store:** Below 25 deg C.
Muse Urethral Stick *(Meda)* A. GMS.
Price, per stick 125mcg, €11.63. 250mcg, €12.41. 500mcg, €13.43. 1000mcg, €14.49.
Urethral stick, alprostadil. Single-use, contained in applicator tip. **Store:** Unopened; unopened pouches out of refrigerator below 30 deg C (max. 14 days).
Viridal Duo Parenteral *(UCB)* A. GMS.
Price, continuation pack, 10mcg, €21.03. 20mcg, €27.91. 40mcg, €38.10.
Intracavernosal injection, alprostadil (clathrate complex with alfadex 1:1). Lyophilised white odourless powder. Clear solvent (0.9% w/v sodium chloride soln) for injection. **Store:** Below 25 deg; original pack to protect (light).
Vitaros Cream 3mg/g *(Recordati)* A.
Price, not published by company (GMS-pending).
Cream, alprostadil. White (off-white) in single dose container (plunger, barrel, cap in sachet). **Store:** Refrigerate; do not freeze; unopened sachets out of refrigerator below 25 deg C (max. 3 days).

Avanafil

ATC Code: Pending. **Sport:** Permitted.
Driving: Minor influence; dizziness, altered vision.

Indications: Treatment, erectile dysfunction (adult males).

Dose: Adult, Elderly: 100mg as needed approx. 15-30 minutes before sexual activity; based on tolerability increase to max. 200mg/day or decrease to 50mg. Onset may be delayed if taken with food. *Elderly,* over 70 years, limited data.

Renal Impairment: CrCl (mL/min) below 30, contraindicated.

Hepatic Impairment: Mild/moderate, use lowest dose; severe, contraindicated.

CI: Loss of vision in one eye because of non-arteritic anterior ischaemic optic neuropathy, known hereditary retinal disorders. See Notes below.

Interactions: Effect of Other Drugs on Avanafil: *Co-admin contraindicated:* Potent CYP3A4 inhibitors (ketoconazole, ritonavir, atazanavir, clarithromycin, indinavir, itraconazole, nefazodone, nelfinavir, saquinavir, telithromycin), organic nitrates or nitric oxide donors (amyl nitrite) (hypotension). *Co-admin not recommended (reduced avanafil exposure):* CYP3A4 inducers (bosentan, carbamazepine, efavirenz, phenobarbital, rifampicin). *Co-admin avoid:* Grapefruit juice. *Symptomatic hypotension with co-admin:* Alpha-blockers, ALCOHOL, other drugs reducing blood pressure, other treatments for ED. *Avanafil max. 100mg once every 48 hours:* Moderate CYP3A4 inhibitors (erythromycin, amprenavir, aprepitant, diltiazem, fluconazole, fosamprenavir, verapamil).

SP: Bleeding disorders, active peptic ulcer, carefully assess risk/benefit.

ADR: *Common,* headache, flushing, nasal congestion.

Notes: See 8.4.2 ED.

▼ **Spedra 50mg, 100mg, 200mg** *(A.Menarini)* A.
Price, (4), not published by company (GMS-pending).
Tablet, avanafil. Pale-yellow oval. Marked with strength.

Dapoxetine

ATC Code: G04BX14. **Sport:** Permitted.
Driving: Minor or moderate influence; dizziness, disturbed attention, syncope, blurred vision.

Indications: Premature ejaculation (PE) in adult men.

Dose: Adult, Elderly: Age 18-64 years, initially 30mg taken as needed approximately 1-3 hours prior to sexual activity;

may be increased to 60mg. Max. 1 dose in 24 hours. Swallow whole to avoid bitter taste, with full glass of water, with or without food. *Elderly*, over 65 years, no data.

Child: No relevant use.

Renal Impairment: Mild/moderate, caution. Severe, not recommended.

Hepatic Impairment: Moderate/severe, contraindicated.

CI: HF (NYHA Class II-IV), conduction abnormalities, significant (ischaemic heart disease, valvular disease), history of (syncope, mania or severe depression).

Interactions: Effect of Other Drugs on Dapoxetine: *Co-admin contraindicated*: Potent CYP3A4 inhibitors (moderate CYP3A4 inhibitors, restrict dose to 30mg); MAOIs, thioridazine, SSRIs, SNRIs, TCADs, other serotonergics (L-tryptophan, triptans, tramadol, linezolid, lithium, St John's Wort) (or within 14 days of discontinuation; these drugs not to be admin within 7 days of discontinuing dapoxetine), ketoconazole, itraconazole, ritonavir, saquinavir, telithromycin, nefazodone, nelfinavir, atazanavir. *Co-admin caution*: Antiepileptics, antidepressants, antipsychotics, anxiolytics, sedative hypnotics. *Reduced orthostatic tolerance*: Vasodilators, PDE5-inhibitors, alpha-adrenergic receptor antagonists. *Increased exposure*: Potent CYP2D6 inhibitors. *Bleeding abnormalities with co-admin*: Atypical antipsychotics, phenothiazines, acetylsalicylic acid, NSAIDs, anti-platelets, anticoagulants (warfarin).

SP: Indicated only for men with diagnosed premature ejaculation. Not for use in men with ED using PDE5 inhibitors. Perform orthostatic test before initiation; avoid use with orthostatic reaction. Caution, syncope. History of mania, use not recommended. Seizures, discontinue. Use with recreational drugs or alcohol not recommended. Discontinue slowly. **Suicide**, see Notes below (antidepressants).

Pregnancy, Lactation: Not for use in women.

ADR: *Very common*, dizziness, headache, nausea.

Notes: See 8.4.2 ED. See 3.3 Antidepressants and Anxiolytics.

> **Priligy 30mg, 60mg** *(A.Menarini)* A.
> *Price*, not published by company (GMS-pending).
> *Tablet*, dapoxetine HCl. Round f/c. Marked with strength inside a triangle. 30mg: Light-grey. 60mg: Grey. *Lactose.*

Sildenafil (ED)

ATC Code: G04BE03. **Sport:** Permitted.

Driving: Caution. Dizziness, altered vision.

Indications: Treatment of men with erectile dysfunction (ED), which is the inability to achieve or maintain a penile erection sufficient for satisfactory sexual performance. Sexual stimulation is required.

Dose: Adult, Elderly: Age 18 years and over, 50mg as needed 1-hour before sexual activity; titrate up to 100mg or down to 25mg as needed; max. 100mg/day. Max. once daily. If taken with food, onset may be delayed.

Renal Impairment: CrCl (mL/min) below 30, consider 25mg; increase step-wise to 50mg up to 100mg based on efficacy and tolerability.

Hepatic Impairment: Mild to moderate, as for Renal above. Severe, contraindicated.

CI: Severe hypotension (BP below 90/50mmHg), unstable angina, recent history of stroke or MI, known retinal degenerative disorders (retinitis pigmentosa), loss of vision in one eye due to non-arteritic anterior ischaemic optic neuropathy (NAION). See Notes below.

Interactions: Effect of Other Drugs on Sildenafil: *Co-admin contraindicated*: Guanylate cyclase stimulators (riociguat). *Co-admin not recommended*: Other drugs treating pulmonary hypertension (bosentan, epoprostenol, iloprost), other PDE-5 inhibitors, potent CYP3A4 inhibitors (ketoconazole, itraconazole, ritonavir). *Co-admin, consider sildenafil dose adjustment*: Erythromycin, saquinavir, clarithromycin, telithromycin, nefazodone. *Increased sildenafil plasma levels*: CYP3A4 substrates in combination with beta-blockers, grapefruit juice (avoid). *Consider sildenafil 25mg to initiate*: CYP3A4 inhibitors (ketoconazole, erythromycin, cimetidine), ritonavir (co-admin not advised).

Effect of Sildenafil on Other Drugs: Nitrates (nicorandil,

nitric oxide donors, amyl nitrite): *Hypotensive effect potentiated, co-admin contraindicated*. Vitamin K antagonists: *Increased bleeding risk*. Alpha-blockers: *Co-admin caution (hypotension)*.

SP: Consider patient cardiovascular status before initiation; sildenafil has vasodilator properties. Increased susceptibility to vasodilators e.g. left ventricular outflow obstruction (aortic stenosis, hypertrophic obstructive cardiomyopathy) or severely impaired autonomic control of blood pressure; caution hypotension, fluid depletion. Treatment of hypertension, discontinue gradually. Serious cardiovascular events with pre-existing cardiovascular disease (MI, unstable angina, sudden cardiac death, ventricular arrhythmia, cerebrovascular haemorrhage, TIA, hyper- and hypotension), caution. Bleeding disorders, active peptic ulceration (risk assessment). Pulmonary oedema, consider veno-occlusive disease.

ADR: Summary, *most common*, headache, flushing, dyspepsia, nasal congestion, dizziness, nausea, hot flush, visual disturbance, cyanopsia, blurred vision.

Notes: See 8.4.2 ED.

Interchangeability: Same strengths of all brands of sildenafil tabs (chewable, film-coated, orodispersible) listed below are deemed interchangeable.

Reference Price: (4) 25mg €1.33. 50mg (OroDisp, f/c, chew) and 100mg (f/c, chew) €1.41.

> **Viagra 25mg, 50mg, 100mg** *(Pfizer)* A. GMS.
> *Price*, (4) 25mg, €15.81; 50mg, €18.44; 100mg, €22.41.
> *Tablet*, sildenafil citrate. Blue rounded diamond-shaped f/c. Marked Pfizer; VGR/strength on reverse. *Lactose.*
>
> **Blugral 25mg, 50mg, 100mg** *(Niche)* A. GMS.
> *Price*, (4) see reference price. 100mg, €1.51.
> *Tablet*, sildenafil citrate. Blue rounded diamond-shaped f/c. Marked U; strength on reverse. *Lactose.*
>
> **Sidena 25mg, 50mg, 100mg** *(Rowex)* A. GMS.
> *Price*, (4) see reference price. 100mg, €1.50.
> *Tablet*, sildenafil citrate. Light-blue round slightly dotted with breaking notch. Marked with strength. 25mg: Scored (facilitates breaking). 50mg, 100mg: Scored (divisible into equal quarters).
>
> **Sildenafil Accord 25mg, 50mg, 100mg** *(Accord)* A. GMS.
> *Price*, (4) see reference price. 100mg, €1.51.
> *Tablet*, sildenafil citrate. Blue almond-shaped f/c. Marked with strength. *Lactose.*
>
> **Sildenafil Actavis 25mg, 50mg, 100mg** *(Accord)* A. GMS.
> *Price*, (4) see reference price. 100mg, €1.51.
> *Tablet*, sildenafil citrate. Blue elliptical. Marked SL and strength.
>
> **Sildenafil Clonmel 25mg, 50mg, 100mg** *(Clonmel)* A. GMS.
> *Price*, (4) see reference price. 100mg, €1.51.
> *Tablet*, sildenafil citrate. Light-blue pearlscent f/c round. *Lactose, Ponceau 4R, soya lecithin.*
>
> **Sildenafil Mylan 25mg, 50mg, 100mg** *(Gerard)* A. GMS.
> *Price*, (4) see reference price. 100mg, €1.50.
> *Tablet*, sildenafil citrate. Blue round f/c. Marked M; SL over strength on reverse.
>
> **Sildenafil Pfizer 50mg, 100mg** *(Pfizer)* A. GMS.
> *Price*, (4) see reference price. 100mg, €1.51.
> *Tablet*, sildenafil citrate. White (off-white) f/c rounded diamond-shaped. Marked with strength. *Lactose.*
>
> **Vizarsin Tablets, Orodispersible** *(Krka)* A. GMS.
> *Price*, (4) see reference price. 100mg, €1.51.
> *Tablet*, sildenafil citrate 25mg, 50mg, 100mg. White oblong. Marked with strength. *Lactose.*
> *Orodispersible tablet*, sildenafil 25mg, 50mg, 100mg. White (almost) round. *Aspartame, sorbitol.*

Tadalafil (ED)

ATC Code: G04BE08. **Sport:** Permitted.

Driving: Negligible effects; do not drive until effect known (dizziness).

Indications: See Notes below (sildenafil).

Dose: Adult, Elderly: 10mg 30 minutes prior to anticipated sexual activity; titrate to 20mg if needed. Max. once daily. If twice weekly use anticipated, 5mg once daily at approx. same time of day; decrease to 2.5mg once daily based on tolerability; reassess periodically. Oral, with or without food.

Renal Impairment: Severe, max. 10mg for 'on-demand' treatment. Once daily dosing of 2.5mg or 5mg for both ED and BPH not recommended.

Hepatic Impairment: Max. 10mg 'on-demand'. Once daily dosing for both ED and BPH not evaluated; careful benefit/risk evaluation.

8.4.3 Urinary Incontinence

CI: MI within last 90 days, CHF (NYHA II or more), uncontrolled arrhythmias.

Interactions: Effect of Other Drugs on Tadalafil: *Co-admin contraindicated (hypotension)*: Organic nitrates, guanylate cyclase stimulators (riociguat). *Co-admin not recommended (hypotension)*: Alpha-blockers (doxazosin). *Co-admin caution*: 5-alpha reductase inhibitors. *Increased plasma levels (caution)*: Ketoconazole, ritonavir, saquinavir, erythromycin, clarithromycin, itraconazole, grapefruit juice. *Plasma levels decreased*: Rifampicin, phenobarbital, phenytoin, carbamazepine.

Effect of Tadalafil on Other Drugs: Nitrates (nicorandil, nitric oxide donors, amyl nitrite): *Hypotensive effect potentiated (with any dose of tadalafil)*. Vitamin K antagonists: *Increased bleeding risk*. Ethinyloestradiol (oral), terbutaline: *Increased oral bioavailability*.

SP: Visual defects, hearing loss, see Notes below (class effects).

ADR: *Summary, most common*, headache, dyspepsia, back pain, myalgia.

Notes: See Sildenafil above. See 8.4.2 ED.

Cialis 10mg, 20mg *(Lilly)* A.
Price, not published by company.
Tablet, tadalafil. Light-yellow almond-shaped. Marked C/strength.
Lactose. **Store:** Below 30 deg C; original pack to protect (moisture).

Vardenafil

ATC Code: G04BE09. **Sport:** Permitted.
Driving: Abnormal vision, dizziness.
Indications: See Notes below (sildenafil).
Dose: Adult: 10mg as needed 25-60 minutes before sexual activity; titrate up to 20mg or down to 5mg as required; max. 20mg. Max. once daily. Oral, with or without food; onset may be delayed with high fat meal.
Elderly: Age 65 years and older, tolerability at 20mg may be lower. See ADR below.
Renal Impairment: CrCl (mL/min) below 30, initially 5mg; as for Elderly above. ESRD requiring dialysis, contraindicated.
Hepatic Impairment: Mild to moderate, initially 5mg; moderate, max. 10mg. Severe, contraindicated.
CI: Loss of vision in one eye due to non-arteritic anterior ischaemic optic neuropathy. Hypotension (BP below 90/50mmHg), stroke or MI within last 6 months, unstable angina, retinal degenerative disorders (retinitis pigmentosa).
Interactions: Effect of Other Drugs on Vardenafil: *Co-admin contraindicated*: Potent CYP3A4 inhibitors (indinavir, ritonavir); ketoconazole, itraconazole (men over 75 years), nitrates or nitric oxide donors (amyl nitrite), guanylate cyclase stimulators (riociguat). *Co-admin not recommended*: Other ED treatments, other vardenafil formulations. *Co-admin caution (hypotension)*: Alpha-blockers (allow 6-hour dosing interval for terazosin; no interval needed with tamsulosin or alfuzosin; vardenafil max. 5mg). *Co-admin, consider dose adjustment*: Erythromycin or clarithromycin (vardenafil max. 5mg). *Increased plasma levels*: Grapefruit/juice (avoid).
Effect of Vardenafil on Other Drugs: Nitrates (nicorandil, nitric oxide donors, amyl nitrite): *Hypotensive effect potentiated*.
SP: Medicinals prolonging QTc interval where risk factors exist (hyperkalaemia, congenital QT-prolongation, antiarrhythmic co-admin). Visual defects, discontinue. Bleeding disorder or active peptic ulcer, caution.
Pregnancy, Lactation: Contraindicated for use in women.
ADR: *Very common,* headache.
Notes: See 8.4.2 ED. See Sildenafil above.

Levitra 5mg, 10mg, 20mg *(Bayer)* A.
Price, not published by company.
Tablet, vardenafil HCl. Orange round. Marked with Bayer cross; strength on reverse.

8.4.3 - Urinary Incontinence

In This Chapter: *Duloxetine, mirabegron, anticholinergics (fesoterodine, flavoxate, oxybutynin, propiverine, solifenacin, tolterodine, trospium).*

Class Effects

CI: Hypersensitivity to any member of the class.

Anticholinergics, bladder outflow obstruction where urinary retention may be precipitated; GI obstructive disorders (paralytic ileus, intestinal atony, pyloric stenosis); toxic megacolon; severe ulcerative colitis; myasthenia gravis; narrow-angle glaucoma or shallow anterior chamber. High ambient temperature or pyrexia (hyperpyrexia risk due to decreased sweating). Patients with ileostomy, colostomy.

Interactions: Effect of Other Drugs on Anticholinergics: *Co-admin caution*: Azole antifungals (ketoconazole, itraconazole, fluconazole), erythromycin. *Effect enhanced*: Other anticholinergics or products with anticholinergic activity (amantadine), some antihistamines, antiparkinsonian drugs (biperiden, levodopa), antihistamines, antipsychotics (phenothiazine, haloperidol, clozapine), quinidine, digitalis, TCADs, atropine, dipyridamole. *Possible interactions*: Verapamil, diltiazem, rifampicin, phenytoin, carbamazepine. *Drowsiness enhanced*: ALCOHOL.

Effect of Anticholinergics on Other Drugs: GI absorbed drugs: *Enhanced absorption due to reduced GI motility.* Metoclopramide, domperidone: *Effect antagonised.* Sublingual nitrates: *Failure to dissolve due to dry mouth.*

SP: Before initiating, exclude organic causes of frequency, urgency and urge incontinence. *Anticholinergics,* may aggravate symptoms of hyperthyroidism, CHF, cardiac arrhythmia, coronary heart disease, hypertension, tachycardia, prostatic hypertrophy; cognitive disorders (especially elderly); CNS effects (hallucinations, agitation, confusion, somnolence). Porphyria. Dental caries, parodontosis or oral candidiasis due to reduced salivary secretions. UTI. Narrow-angle glaucoma, monitor IOP. Used in high environmental temperatures, can cause heat prostration due to decreased sweating. *Caution*, use in frail, elderly and children (more sensitive to effects), patients with autonomic neuropathy, Parkinson's disease, hepatic or renal impairment, clinically significant bladder outflow obstruction, severe GI motility disorders, GI obstructions (pyloric stenosis), hiatus hernia, reflux oesophagitis. Gastroesophageal reflux and/or taking bisphosphonates, oesophagitis may be exacerbated. Dementia treated with cholinesterase inhibitors, symptoms aggravated.

Pregnancy, Lactation: *Anticholinergics,* pregnancy, only if clearly necessary; lactation, not recommended.

Duloxetine (SUI)

ATC Code: N06AX21. **Sport:** Permitted.
Driving: Caution.
Indications: Moderate to severe stress urinary incontinence (SUI).
Dose: Adult: 40mg twice daily. Oral, with or without food.
Elderly: Caution.
Renal Impairment: CrCl (mL/min) below 30, not recommended.
SP: Suicide, see Notes below (antidepressants). Taper dose for 2 weeks before discontinuing. Consider pelvic floor exercise training.
Pregnancy, Lactation: Pregnancy, only if benefit outweighs risk; discontinuation symptoms may occur in neonates after maternal use near term.
ADR: *Summary, most common*, nausea, dry mouth, fatigue, constipation.
Notes: See 3.3 3 SSRIs, SNRIs (duloxetine). See 8.4.3 Urinary Incontinence.
Interchangeability: Same strengths (20mg, 40mg) of all brands of duloxetine g/r caps listed below are deemed interchangeable.

Yentreve 20mg, 40mg *(Lilly)* A. GMS.
Price, 20mg (28) €10.57. 40mg (56) €21.58.
Capsule, duloxetine HCl. Hard opaque g/r. Marked with strength. 20mg: Blue/blue. Marked 9544. 40mg: Orange/blue. Marked 9545. *Sucrose.*

Loxentia 20mg, 40mg *(Krka)* A. GMS.
Price, (28) €8.40. (56) €16.80.
Capsules, duloxetine HCl. Hard opaque g/r. Marked with strength. Contains white pellets. 20mg: Light-blue. 40mg: Light-orange/light-blue. *Sucrose.*

Fesoterodine

ATC Code: G04BD11. **Sport:** Permitted.
Driving: Blurred vision, dizziness, somnolence.
Indications: Urinary frequency and/or urgency and/or urgency incontinence associated with overactive bladder.
Dose: Adult, Elderly: Initially 4mg/day; titrate to max. 8mg/day if needed. *Co-admin* with potent CYP3A4 inhibitors (atazanavir, clarithromycin, indinavir, itraconazole, ketoconazole, nefazodone, nelfinavir, ritonavir, saquinavir, telithromycin) and normal renal and/or hepatic function, max. 4mg/day. Once daily; swallow whole with water; with or without food.
Child: Under 18 years, not recommended.
Renal Impairment: Not co-administered with *CYP3A4 inhibitors* and mild/moderate impairment, 4-8mg/day; severe 4mg/day. Co-admin with moderate inhibitors and mild/moderate impairment 4mg/day; severe, avoid. Co-admin with potent inhibitors with mild impairment, avoid; moderate/severe impairment, contraindicated.
Hepatic Impairment: Not co-admin with *CYP3A4 inhibitors* and with mild impairment 4-8mg/day; moderate 4mg/day. Co-admin with moderate inhibitors and mild impairment 4mg/day; moderate, avoid. Co-admin with potent inhibitor and mild impairment, avoid; moderate or severe, contraindicated.
CI: See Renal, Hepatic impairment above.
Interactions: Effect of Other Drugs on Fesoterodine: *Co-admin not recommended*: Potent CYP3A4 inducers (carbamazepine, rifampicin, phenobarbital, phenytoin, St John's Wort). *Co-admin caution*: Potent CYP2D6 inhibitors. *Co-admin, adjust dose*: See Dose above. *Increased exposure with co-admin, consider dose adjustment*: CYP2D6 inhibitors.
SP: Clinically significant bladder outflow obstruction, urinary retention risk. Angioedema, discontinue. QT-prolongation risk (hypokalaemia, bradycardia, co-admin with drugs prolonging QT-interval), pre-existing cardiac disease (myocardial ischaemia, arrhythmia, CHF), especially with potent CYP3A4 inhibitors, see Dose and Interactions above.
Pregnancy, Lactation: Not recommended.
ADR: *Very common*, dry mouth. Anticholinergic effects, see Notes below.
Notes: See 8.4.3 Urinary Incontinence.

> Toviaz 4mg, 8mg *(Pfizer)* A. GMS.
> Price, (28) €34.78. 8mg, €39.19.
> *Prolonged/R tablet,* fesoterodine fumarate. Oval f/c. 4mg: Light-blue. Marked FS. 8mg: Blue. Marked FT. *Lactose.*

Flavoxate

ATC Code: G04BD02. **Sport:** Permitted.
Driving: Possible drowsiness, blurred vision, vertigo; caution.
Indications: Dysuria, urgency, nocturia, vesical supra-pubic pain, frequency and incontinence. Vesico-urethral spasm associated with catheterisation, cystoscopy, indwelling catheters; prior to cystoscopy or catheterisation, sequelae of surgical intervention of lower urinary tract.
Dose: Adult, Elderly: 1 tab 3-times daily.
Child: Under 12 years, not recommended.
ADR: *Very rarely,* eosinophilia, leucopenia, hypersensitivity, drowsiness, dizziness, headache, mental confusion, nervousness, vertigo, blurred vision, disturbed eye accommodation, increased ocular tension, palpitations, tachycardia, diarrhoea, dry mouth, dyspepsia, dysphagia, nausea, vomiting, angioedema, urticaria, erythema, rash, pruritus, dysuria, fatigue, hyperpyrexia.
Notes: See 8.4.3 Urinary Incontinence.

> Urispas 200mg *(Recordati)* B. GMS.
> Price, (90) €12.45. (250) €34.61.
> *Tablet,* flavoxate HCl. White f/c. Marked F200. *Lactose.*

Mirabegron

ATC Code: G04BD12. **Sport:** Permitted.
Driving: No or negligible effect.
Indications: Symptomatic treatment, urgency, increased micturition frequency and/or urgency incontinence as with overactive bladder syndrome.

Dose: Adult, Elderly: 50mg once daily. *Admin,* with fluid, with or without food; do not divide, crush or chew.
Child: Under 18 years, not recommended.
Renal Impairment: Mild/moderate, as for Adult above. Admin with strong CYP3A4 inhibitor, 25mg once daily; severe impairment, 25mg once daily. Co-admin with inhibitor or ESRD, not recommended.
Hepatic Impairment: Mild, as for Renal (mild/moderate). Moderate, as for Renal (severe). Severe, not recommended.
CI: Severe uncontrolled hypertension (systolic BP 180mmHg or above and/or diastolic 110mmHg or above).
Interactions: Effect of Mirabegron on Other Drugs: CYP2D6 substrates especially if individually titrated or with narrow therapeutic index (thioridazine, flecainide, propafenone, imipramine, desipramine), P-gp substrates (dabigatran): *Possible inhibitory effect; caution.* Digoxin: *Monitor serum levels.*
SP: Measure BP at baseline and then periodically, especially in hypertensive patients. *Caution,* congenital or acquired QT prolongation. Urinary retention (patients with bladder outlet obstruction or taking antimuscarinic medication).
Pregnancy, Lactation: Not recommended.
ADR: *Summary, most common,* tachycardia, UTI; *serious,* atrial fibrillation.
Notes: See 8.4.3 Urinary Incontinence.

> ▼ *(Betmiga 25mg, 50mg (Astellas)* B. GMS.
> Price, both strengths (30) €35.64.
> *Prolonged/R tablet,* mirabegron. Oval. Marked with company logo.
> 25mg: Brown. Marked 325. 50mg: Yellow. Marked 355.

Oxybutynin

ATC Code: G04BD04. **Sport:** Permitted.
Driving: Drowsiness, somnolence, blurred vision.
Indications: Management, urinary frequency and urgency, incontinence, bladder dysfunction (especially elderly) in unstable bladder due to neurogenic bladder disorders (detrusor hyperreflexia) or in conditions including MS and spina bifida, or idiopathic detrusor instability (motor urge incontinence). Nocturnal enuresis associated with detrusor overactivity. Control of vesical hyperactivity.
Paediatric (over 5 years; not transdermal formulations), urinary incontinence, urgency and frequency in unstable bladder conditions due to idiopathic overactive bladder or neurogenic bladder disorders (detrusor overactivity); nocturnal enuresis associated with detrusor overactivity, with non-drug therapy (other treatment has failed).
Dose: Adult: STANDARD/R, 10-20mg/day in divided doses. *Admin,* with plenty of water.
PROLONGED/R, initially 5mg once daily; titrate by 5mg increments at 1 week intervals; max. 20mg/day. *Admin,* oral with or without food; swallow tabs whole with liquid; do not chew, break or crush.
TRANSDERMAL, apply one 3.9mg transdermal patch twice weekly (every 3-4 days). *Admin,* abdomen, hip or buttock; new site with each new patch; avoid reapplication to same site within 7 days.
Elderly: *Ditropan, Oxybutynin (Accord),* initially 2.5mg twice daily; titrate to 5mg twice daily if needed. All other brands, as for Adult above.
Child: STANDARD/R, PROLONGED/R, age 5 years and over, range 5-15mg/day. *Admin,* with plenty of fluid; Standard/R in divided doses or Prolonged/R once daily. *Oxybutynin Accord,* age 5-9 years, 2.5mg 3-times daily; age 9-12 years, 5mg twice daily; over 12 years, 5mg 3-times daily. All brands, under 5 years, not recommended.
TRANSDERMAL, safety/efficacy not established.
Renal Impairment: Caution.
Hepatic Impairment: Caution.
Interactions: Effect of Oxybutynin on Other Drugs: Prokinetic therapies: *May be antagonised.*
SP: Angioedema of face, lips, tongue and/or larynx.
Pregnancy, Lactation: Not recommended.
ADR: *Very common, oral,* constipation, nausea, dry mouth, dizziness, headache, somnolence, blurred vision, dry skin. *Common, transdermal,* UTI, blurred vision, dizziness, dry mouth, constipation, diarrhoea, nausea, abdominal pain.

227

8.4.3 Urinary Incontinence

Notes: See 8.4.3 Urinary Incontinence.

Cystrin 3mg, 5mg *(SANOFI)* B. GMS.
Price, (56) 3mg, €9.69. (84) 5mg, €14.54.
Standard/R tablet, oxybutynin HCl. Light-blue round. Marked OXB/strength. 5mg: Scored. *Lactose.*
Ditropan 2.5mg, 5mg *(SANOFI)* B. GMS.
Price, (84) 2.5mg, €7.64. 5mg, €15.56.
Standard/R tablet, oxybutynin HCl. Pale-blue. Marked OBX/strength. 2.5mg: Oval. 5mg: Round scored. *Lactose.*
Kentera Transdermal 3.9mg *(Recordati)* B. GMS.
Price, 3.9mg/24 hours (8) €34.60.
Transdermal patch, oxybutynin. 36mg releasing 3.9mg/24 hours. Clear plastic. **Store:** Do not (refrigerate, freeze).
Lyrinel XL 5mg, 10mg *(Janssen-Cilag)* B. GMS.
Price, (30) 5mg, €14.44. 10mg, €28.24.
Prolonged/R tablet, oxybutynin HCl. Round. Marked strength/XL. 5mg: Yellow. 10mg: Pink. *Lactose.* NOTE: Tablet membrane may pass through GI tract unchanged.
Oxybutynin (Accord) 2.5mg, 5mg *(Accord)* B. GMS.
Price, (84) 2.5mg, €4.01. 5mg, €7.79.
Standard/R tablet, oxybutynin HCl. White (off-white) round. 2.5mg: Marked BS. 5mg: Scored (divisible into equal halves). Marked B and R either side of score. *Lactose.*

Propiverine

ATC Code: G04BD06. **Sport:** Permitted.
Driving: Drowsiness, blurred vision; sedatives may enhance drowsiness.

Indications: Urinary incontinence and/or increased urinary frequency and urgency as in overactive bladder (OAB).

Dose: Adult, Elderly: Standard treatment, 1x 30mg (XL) cap once daily. Increase to 1x 45mg cap once daily if needed. *Admin,* before food (high fat meal increases bioavailability); swallow whole, do not crush or chew.

Child: Not recommended.

Renal Impairment: Severe, contraindicated. See Adult above (admin).

Hepatic Impairment: Mild, caution. Moderate/severe, contraindicated. See Adult above (admin).

CI: Tachyarrhythmias.

Interactions: Effect of Other Drugs on Propiverine: *Co-admin caution:* Potent CYP3A4 inhibitors + methimazole. *Increased effects:* Benzodiazepines. *BP reduced:* Patients treated with isoniazid. *Drowsiness enhanced:* Other sedatives.

SP: Autonomic neuropathy. Hiatus hernia with reflux oesophagitis, aggravated.

Pregnancy, Lactation: Pregnancy, not recommended. Lactation, stop breastfeeding or stop drug.

ADR: *Very common,* dry mouth; *common,* headache, abnormal/disturbed eye accommodation, constipation, abdominal pain, dyspepsia, fatigue.

Notes: See 8.4.3 Urinary Incontinence.

Detrunorm XL 30mg, 45mg *(Concordia)* B. GMS.
Price, (28) 30mg, €34.89; 45mg, €52.33.
Modified/R capsule, propiverine HCl. Contain white (off-white) pellets. 30mg: Orange/white. 45mg: Orange. *Lactose.* **Store:** Below 25 deg C; original pack to protect (moisture).

Solifenacin

ATC Code: G04BD08. **Sport:** Permitted.
Driving: Blurred vision, somnolence, fatigue.
Indications: Urge incontinence and/or increased urinary frequency and urgency as in overactive bladder (OAB).

Dose: Adult, Elderly: 5mg/day; titrate to 10mg/day if needed. Oral, with or without food; swallow whole with liquid.

Child: Not recommended.

Renal Impairment: CrCl (mL/min) below 30, caution; max. 5mg once daily. Haemodialysis, not recommended.

Hepatic Impairment: Moderate, max. 5mg once daily. Severe, not recommended.

Interactions: Effect of Other Drugs on Solifenacin: *Co-admin caution (max. dose 5mg/day):* Ketoconazole, other potent CYP3A4 inhibitors (ritonavir, nelfinavir, itraconazole). *Co-admin not recommended (severe renal, moderate hepatic impairment):* Potent CYP3A4 inhibitors.

SP: Hiatus hernia or gastro-oesophageal reflux taking bisphosphonates, oesophagitis exacerbated, autonomic neuropathy. QT-prolongation, Torsade de Pointes (presence of risk factors, existing long QT syndrome, hypokalaemia). Angioedema, anaphylaxis, discontinue.

ADR: *Very common,* dry mouth.

Notes: See 8.4.3 Urinary Incontinence.

Vesitirim 5mg, 10mg *(Astellas)* B. GMS.
Price, (30) 5mg, €33.13. 10mg, €41.63.
Tablet, solifenacin succinate. Round f/c. Marked with logo. 5mg: Light-yellow. Marked 150. 10mg: Light-pink. Marked 151. *Lactose.*

Tolterodine

ATC Code: G04BD07. **Sport:** Permitted.
Driving: Caution.
Indications: Urge incontinence and/or increased urinary frequency and urgency as in overactive bladder (OAB).

Dose: Adult, Elderly: STANDARD/R, 2mg twice daily or PROLONGED/R 4mg once daily. Swallow whole; with or without food.

Child: Not recommended.

Renal Impairment: GFR (mL/min) of 30 or less, Standard/R 1mg twice daily or Prolonged/R (SR) 2mg once daily.

Hepatic Impairment: As for Renal above.

Interactions: Effect of Other Drugs on Tolterodine: *Increased plasma levels (poor CYP2D6 metabolisers):* Macrolides (erythromycin, clarithromycin), azole antifungals (ketoconazole, itraconazole), anti-proteases.

Effect of Tolterodine on Other Drugs: Metoclopramide, cisapride: *Effect decreased.*

SP: QT-prolongation risk factors (existing QT-prolongation, electrolyte disturbances, bradycardia, cardiac disease), caution.

ADR: *Very common,* headache, dry mouth.

Notes: See 8.4.3 Urinary Incontinence.

Interchangeability: Same strengths of all brands of tolterodine Standard/R film-coated tabs and Prolonged/R caps listed below are deemed interchangeable.

Reference Price: Prolonged/R (SR) (28) 2mg, 4mg, €10.08.

Detrusitol 1mg, 2mg, SR 2mg, 4mg *(Pfizer)* B. GMS.
Price, (56) 1mg, €19.42. 2mg, €21.59. SR (28) 2mg, €15.40. 4mg, €16.80.
Standard/R tablet, tolterodine tartrate. White round. 1mg: Marked TO. 2mg: Marked DT.
Prolonged/R capsule, as above. Marked symbol/strength. 2mg: Blue/green. 4mg: Blue. *Sucrose.*
Tendrotil SR 2mg, 4mg *(Accord)* B. GMS.
Price, (28) see reference price above.
Prolonged/R capsule, tolterodine tartrate. Opaque; contains 2 (2mg) or 4 (4mg) white round tabs. 2mg: Green. 4mg: Light-blue. *Lactose.*
Tolterodine (Accord) 1mg, 2mg *(Accord)* B. GMS.
Price, (56) 1mg, €13.62; 2mg, €13.71.
Tablet, tolterodine tartrate. White (off-white) round f/c. 1mg: Marked S16. 2mg: Marked S042.
Toltertan SR 2mg, 4mg *(Clonmel)* B. GMS.
Price, (28) see reference price above.
Prolonged/R capsule, tolterodine tartrate. Hard opaque; contains 2 (2mg) or 4 (4mg) white round coated tablets. 2mg: Green. 4mg: Blue. *Lactose.*
Tolusitol PR 2mg, 4mg *(Rowex)* B. GMS.
Price, (28) see reference price above.
Prolonged/R capsule, tolterodine tartrate. Contains 2 (2mg) or 4 (4mg) white round coated tabs. 2mg: Green. 4mg: Light-blue. *Lactose.*
Trusitev SR 2mg, 4mg *(TEVA)* B. GMS.
Price, (28) see reference price above.
Prolonged/R capsule, tolterodine tartrate. Opaque; contains 2 (2mg) or 4 (4mg) white round coated tabs. 2mg: Green. 4mg: Light-blue. *Lactose.*

Trospium

ATC Code: G04BD09. **Sport:** Permitted.
Driving: Disturbed visual accommodation.
Indications: Urinary frequency, urge incontinence, urgency associated with detrusor instability or hyperreflexia (overactive bladder).

Dose: Adult, Elderly: 20mg twice daily. Swallow tabs whole before food on empty stomach. Assess need for continuing treatment at regular 3-6 month intervals.

Child: Under 12 years, not recommended.

Renal Impairment: CrCl (mL/min) 10-30, 20mg once daily or 20mg every second day. Dialysis, not recommended.

Hepatic Impairment: Slight/moderate, caution; severe, discourage use.

CI: Urinary retention, narrow-angle glaucoma, tachyarrhythmias, myasthenia gravis, ulcerative colitis, toxic megacolon.

Interactions: Effect of Other Drugs on Trospium: *Co-admin, absorption inhibited:* Guar, colestyramine, colestipol.

Effect of Trospium on Other Drugs: Beta-sympathomimetics: *Reinforced tachycardic effects.*

Pregnancy, Lactation: Pregnancy, caution. Lactation, stop drug or stop breastfeeding.

ADR: *Very common,* dry mouth.

Notes: See 8.4.3 Urinary Incontinence.

> **Flotros 20mg** *(Galen)* B. GMS.
> *Price,* (60) €14.45.
> *Tablet,* trospium chloride. Round white f/c. *Lactose.*

8.4.4 - Urinary Alkalinisers, Urolithiasis

In This Chapter: *Potassium citrate.*

Class Effects
CI: Hypersensitivity to any member of the class.

Potassium Citrate
ATC Code: G01. **Sport:** Permitted.
Driving: No effect.
Indications: Symptomatic relief of mild urinary tract infections.

Dose: Adult, Elderly: Dissolve the contents of 1x 3g sachet (granules) in 200mL of cold water; take 3-times daily for 2 days; all 6 sachets to be taken to complete treatment. *Admin,* after food to minimise gastric irritation.

Child: Under 6 years, not recommended.

Renal Impairment: Contraindicated.

Interactions: Effect of Other Drugs on Potassium Citrate: *Hyperkalaemia:* ACEI. *Caution:* Cardiac glycosides.

SP: Short-term treatment only. Cardiac disease, caution.

Pregnancy, Lactation: Pregnancy, can be used if there is no safer alternative; pregnant women should seek medical advice for cystitis.

ADR: Gastric irritation.

Notes: See 8.4.4 Urinary Alkalinisers, Urolithiasis.

> **Cystopurin 3g Granules** *(Bayer)* OTC.
> *Price,* (6) €5.19.
> *Granules* (sachets), potassium citrate. Pink-brown granules for oral soln. *Aspartame.*

8.4.5 - Dialysis

In This Chapter: *Calcium acetate, cinacalcet, lanthanum, sevelamer, sucroferric oxyhydroxide.*

Class Effects
CI: Hypersensitivity to any member of the class. Children under 18 years.

SP: With non-calcium phosphate binders, monitor calcium and consider supplements.

Pregnancy, Lactation: Pregnancy, if benefit outweighs risk. Lactation, stop breastfeeding or stop drug.

Notes: See 15.1 Specific Substance Antagonists (iron). See also 16.3.8 Vitamin D and 16.3.1 Calcium.

Calcium Acetate
ATC Code: V03AE04. **Sport:** Permitted.
Driving: Unlikely to impair.
Indications: Hyperphosphataemia in chronic renal insufficiency with regular haemodialysis or peritoneal dialysis.

Dose: Adult, Elderly: Usually 500-1000mg (up to 2g in special cases) 3-times daily with meals; individualise according to phosphate levels.

SP: Hypercalcaemia (high dose), discontinue; chronic

hypercalcaemia, vascular/soft tissue calcification. Renal dysfunction, monitor blood-calcium.

Pregnancy, Lactation: No data; no problems documented.

ADR: GI disturbances, hypercalcaemia.

Notes: See 8.4.5 Dialysis and 16.3.1 Calcium.

> **Calcium Acetate 500mg** *(Pinewood)* B. GMS.
> *Price,* (100) €16.99.
> *Tablet,* calcium acetate. White round scored. *Lactose.*
> **Phosex 1000mg** *(Pharmacosmos)* B. GMS.
> *Price,* (180) €29.47.
> *Tablet,* calcium acetate. Oval yellow scored. Marked PHOS-EX.

Calcium Acetate, Magnesium Carbonate
ATC Code: V03AE04. **Sport:** Permitted.
Driving: Unlikely to impair.
Indications: Hyperphosphataemia associated with chronic renal insufficiency with haemodialysis or peritoneal dialysis.

Dose: Adult, Elderly: Initially 3 tabs daily; usually 3-10 tabs per day depending on serum phosphate; divided according to meals. Dose may be increased to 12 tabs/day. *Admin,* with meals; do not crush or chew; tabs may be broken to facilitate swallowing.

Child: Under 18 years, not recommended.

Interactions: Effect of Calcium Acetate/Magnesium Carbonate on Other Drugs: Other oral medicinals: *Rate/extent of absorption may vary; allow interval of 2 hours before or 3 hours after admin.* Digitalis: *Admin calcium/magnesium under ECG control and serum calcium monitoring.* Levothyroxine: *Increased absorption due to magnesium.* Digoxin, nitrofurantoin, penicillamine: *Adsorption by magnesium salts in gut may decrease bioavailability.*

SP: Caution, severe hyperphosphataemia with calcium-phosphate-product of more than 5.3mmolL2/L2 if (refractory to therapy, refractory hyperkalaemia, bradycardia or AV-block II with bradycardia), vascular and soft tissue calcifications. Constipation due to precipitation of fatty acids and bile acid as calcium soap. Diarrhoea, reduce dose.

Pregnancy, Lactation: Pregnancy, if benefit outweighs risk. Lactation, not recommended; passes into breast milk.

ADR: *Common,* soft stools, GI irritation, hyper- (calcaemia, magnesaemia).

Notes: See 8.4.5 Dialysis.

> **OsvaRen 435/235** *(Fresenius)* B. GMS.
> *Price,* (180) €27.66.
> *Tablet,* calcium acetate 435mg, magnesium carbonate 235mg. White (yellowish) oblong f/c scored (facilitates breaking). *Sucrose, sodium 5.6mg/tab.*

Cinacalcet
ATC Code: H05BX01. **Sport:** Permitted.
Driving: May impair ability.
Indications: Secondary hyperparathyroidism in ESRD on dialysis adjunctive to phosphate binders and/or Vitamin D sterols. Hypercalcaemia in parathyroid carcinoma or primary hyperparathyroidism.

Dose: Adult, Elderly: *Hyperparathyroidism,* 30mg once daily; titrate over 2-4 weeks to 180mg once daily to achieve target PTH levels.

Parathyroid carcinoma, primary hyperparathyroidism, 30mg twice daily; titrate at 2-4 week intervals to 60mg twice daily, 90mg twice daily, then 90mg three or four times daily; max. 90mg 4-times daily. *Admin,* with or shortly after food; tabs to be taken whole, not divided.

Child: Not recommended.

Hepatic Impairment: Moderate to severe, caution; monitor closely during titration.

Interactions: Effect of Other Drugs on Cinacalcet: *Caution (consider dose adjustment):* Strong CYP3A4 inhibitors (ketoconazole, itraconazole, telithromycin, voriconazole, ritonavir) or CYP3A4 inducers (rifampicin) and/or CYP1A2 inducers or inhibitors, CYP2D6 substrates with narrow therapeutic window, CYP1A2 inducers (smoking) or CYP1A2 inhibitors (fluvoxamine, ciprofloxacin).

Effect of Cinacalcet on Other Drugs: CYP2D6 substrates (flecainide, propafenone, metoprolol in HF, desipramine, nortriptyline, clomipramine): *Consider dose adjustment.*

8.4.5 Dialysis

SP: Seizure threshold lowered by significant serum calcium reductions; do not initiate if serum calcium below the lower limit of normal. Life-threatening events/fatal outcome associated with hypocalcaemia; manifestations (paraesthesias, myalgias, cramping, tetany, convulsions); decreased serum calcium may prolong QT-interval (ventricular arrhythmia). If parathyroid hormone levels fall below recommended target, reduce dose or discontinue.

ADR: Summary, *most common*, nausea, vomiting.

Notes: See 8.4.5 Dialysis.

Mimpara 30mg, 60mg, 90mg *(Amgen)* A. HT.
Price, (28) 30mg, €184.55. 60mg, €344.53. 90mg, €506.05.
Tablet, cinacalcet HCl. Light-green oval f/c. Marked AMG; strength on reverse. *Lactose.*

Lanthanum

ATC Code: V03AE03. **Sport:** Permitted.
Driving: Dizziness, vertigo.

Indications: Hyperphosphataemia in chronic renal failure on haemodialysis or CAPD. Chronic kidney disease with serum phosphate levels of 1.78mmoL/L or more uncontrolled by diet.

Dose: Adult, Elderly: Initially 750mg/day; range 1500-3000mg/day; max. 3750mg/day. Chew tabs completely; do not swallow whole; may be crushed to aid chewing; take with or immediately after food; divided doses with meals.

Child: Under 18 years, safety/efficacy not established.

Hepatic Impairment: Monitor LFTs. Probably excreted in bile; reduced bile flow may result in slower elimination, higher plasma levels and increased tissue deposits.

CI: Hypophosphataemia.

Interactions: Effect of Other Drugs on Lanthanum: *Co-admin not recommended*: Compounds interacting with antacids (chloroquine, ketoconazole), tetracycline, doxycycline, fluoroquinolones (allow 2-hour dosing interval).

Effect of Lanthanum on Other Drugs: Levothyroxine: *Absorption reduced; allow 2-hour dosing interval.*

SP: Long-term admin consider risk/benefit. Acute peptic ulcer, ulcerative colitis, Crohn's disease, bowel obstruction. Abdominal X-rays may have radio-opaque appearance typical of imaging agent.

Pregnancy, Lactation: Pregnancy, not recommended.

ADR: Summary, *most common*, headache, allergic skin reactions, GI disorders (minimised by taking with food).

Notes: See 8.4.5 Dialysis.

Foznol 250mg, 500mg, 750mg, 1000mg *(Shire)* B. GMS.
Price, (90) 250mg, €97.78. 500mg, €162.85. 750mg, €216.97. 1000mg, €245.73.
Chewable tablet, lanthanum carbonate. White round flat. Marked S405/strength. *Glucose.*

Sevelamer (hydrochloride, carbonate)

ATC Code: V03AE02. **Sport:** Permitted.
Driving: No data.

Indications: Hyperphosphataemia (chronic renal failure on peritoneal or haemodialysis) (sevelamer HCl, carbonate); chronic kidney disease (not on dialysis), serum phosphorus 1.78mmoL/L or above (sevelamer carbonate).

Dose: Adult, Elderly: *Renagel* (sevelamer HCl), (not on phosphate binders), serum phosphate (mmoL/L) 1.76-2.42, initially 800mg 3-times daily; above 2.42, 1600mg 3-times daily*. *Admin,* swallow tabs whole; do not chew.

Renvela, Sevelamer (Gerard, Rowex) (sevelamer carbonate), serum phosphate (mmoL/L) 1.78-2.42, initially 2.4g/day; above 2.42 admin 4.8g/day in 3 divided doses with meals*. *Admin,* Renvela, disperse powder in 60mL water; ingest within 30 minutes. Tabs, as for *Renagel* above.
*Titrate by 0.8g 3-times daily (2.4g/day) until acceptable serum phosphorus level reached.

CI: Hypophosphataemia, bowel obstruction.

Interactions: Effect of Other Drugs on Sevelamer: *Co-admin caution:* Antiarrhythmics, anti-seizure drugs. *TSH monitoring:* Levothyroxine (hypothyroidism). *Increased phosphate levels (rare):* PPIs.

Effect of Sevelamer on Other Drugs: Ciprofloxacin (not for co-admin), ciclosporin, mycophenolate mofetil: *Bioavailability decreased (allow dosing interval of 1 hour before or 3 hours after sevelamer).*

SP: Hypo- or hypercalcaemia; may develop low vitamin A, D, E, K levels on dialysis. Chronic failure, metabolic acidosis. *Caution,* swallowing disorders, severe gastroparesis, gastric retention, active inflammatory bowel disease, GI motility disorders, abnormal or irregular bowel motion, major GI surgery. Serious inflammatory disorders of GI tract associated with sevelamer crystal reported; causality not demonstrated; re-evaluate patients with GI symptoms. Folate deficiency. Increased serum chloride. Hypothyroidism.

ADR: Summary, *most frequent*, GI disorders.

Notes: See 8.4.5 Dialysis.

Renagel 800mg *(SANOFI)* B. GMS.
Price, (180) €146.81.
Tablet, sevelamer HCl. Off-white oval f/c. Marked Renagel 800.
Store: Below 25 deg C; protect (moisture).
Renvela 800mg, Sachets 2.4g *(SANOFI)* B. GMS.
Price, tabs (180) €99.65. Sachets (60) €169.13.
Tablet, sevelamer carbonate. White (off-white) f/c. Marked name/800. **Store:** Protect (moisture).
Sachets, as above. Pale-yellow powder for oral susp. *Sucralose.*
Sevelamer (Gerard) 800mg *(Gerard)* B. GMS.
Price, (180) €77.37.
Tablet, sevelamer carbonate. White (off-white) oval f/c. Marked SVL. *Lactose.*
Sevelamer Rowex 800mg *(Rowex)* B. GMS.
Price, (180) €77.37.
Tablet, sevelamer carbonate. White (off-white) oval f/c. Marked SVL. *Lactose.*

Sucroferric Oxyhydroxide

ATC Code: V03AE05. **Sport:** Pending.
Driving: No or negligible effect.

Indications: Control of serum phosphorus in adults with chronic kidney disease (CKD) on haemodialysis or peritoneal dialysis (with calcium supplement, Vitamin D3 or analogues or calcimimetics to control development of renal bone disease).

Dose: Adult, Elderly: Initially 1500mg iron (3 tabs) per day divided across meals; titrate up or down by 500mg iron (1 tab) per day every 2-4 weeks until acceptable serum phosphorus obtained; optimum usually 3-4 tabs per day, max. 3000mg iron (6 tabs) per day. Chew tabs; do not swallow whole; tabs may be crushed; take with food to maximise adsorption of dietary phosphate.

Renal Impairment: Early impairment, no data.

Hepatic Impairment: Severe, no data (excluded from evaluation).

CI: Haemochromatosis, other iron accumulation disorders.

Interactions: Effect of Sucroferric Oxyhydroxide on Other Drugs: Medicinals with narrow therapeutic window: *Monitor levels.* Medicinals with potential to interact with iron (alendronate, doxycycline, levothyroxine): *Admin 1 hour before or 2 hours after sucroferric oxyhydroxide.*

SP: Peritonitis (in last 3 months), significant gastric or hepatic disorders, major GI surgery (careful benefit/risk assessment). Contains sucrose, starches. May cause black stools (may mask GI bleeding).

ADR: Summary, *mostly*, GI disorders (diarrhoea, discoloured faeces).

Notes: See 8.4.5 Dialysis.

▼ **Velphoro 500mg Chewable** *(Vifor)* B. GMS.
Price, (90), €194.16.
Chewable tablet, sucroferric oxyhydroxide. Brown round. Marked PA500. *Sucrose, starches.*

230

9

Infectious Diseases

9.1 - Antibacterials

Class Effects
Indications: All antibacterials are indicated for the treatment of infections caused by susceptible organisms.

CI: Hypersensitivity to any member of the class.

Interactions: Effect of Antibacterials on Other Drugs: Oral contraceptives: *Reduced efficacy.*

SP: Therapy duration and dose depends on infection type, susceptibility to antibiotic, severity, site, clinical response, renal function; children/adolescents, body weight.

Clostridium difficile-associated diarrhoea (CDAD) (mild to fatal); prolonged antibacterial use has possibility of emergence of resistant organisms (Enterococci, *Clostridium difficile*) and superinfection (Candida). Patients presenting with severe or persistent diarrhoea, consider possibility of antibiotic-induced pseudomembranous colitis.

9.1.1 - Penicillins

In This Chapter: *Benzylpenicillin (penicillin G), phenoxymethylpenicillin (penicillin V). Semi-synthetic penicillins including narrow spectrum (flucloxacillin), medium (amoxicillin), broad (amoxicillin/clavulanate), extended spectrum (piperacillin as piperacillin/tazobactam combination).*

Class Effects
Driving: Oral formulations unlikely to impair. Parenteral, caution.

CI: History of severe immediate hypersensitivity reaction (anaphylaxis) to other beta-lactams (penicillins, cephalosporins, carbepenems, monobactams).

Interactions: Effect of Other Drugs on Penicillins: *Co-admin not recommended*: Disulfiram, other bacteriostatics (chloramphenicol, erythromycins, sulphonamides, tetracyclines; may interfere with bactericidal action of flucloxacillin). *Increased, prolonged blood levels (renal excretion inhibited)*: Probenecid. *Increased allergic skin reaction risk*: Allopurinol.

Effect of Penicillins on Other Drugs: Methotrexate:

Excretion may be reduced (monitor). Digoxin: *Possible increased absorption.* Oral anticoagulants: *Monitor prothrombin time or INR.* Mycophenolate mofetil: *Monitor levels during combination and shortly after antibiotic treatment.*

SP: NOTE: Beta-lactams and aminoglycosides should not be mixed in same syringe prior to admin. Before initiating, check for previous hypersensitivity reactions to other beta-lactams. Serious or fatal hypersensitivity reactions (anaphylactoid), more likely with history of penicillin allergy and atopic individuals; if allergy occurs, discontinue. Infectious mononucleosis (glandular fever), avoid using beta-lactams (morbilliform rash). With high doses, maintain adequate fluid intake and urinary output to reduce crystalluria risk. Neuromuscular excitability or convulsions (higher than recommended doses IV), especially with impaired renal function. All beta-lactams, neutropenia and agranulocytosis may develop (extended treatment); duration longer than 10 days, monitor blood counts. *Clostridium difficile* associated diarrhoea, see Notes below.

Pregnancy, Lactation: Pregnancy, if benefit outweighs risk. Lactation, if benefit outweighs risk; candidiasis risk, CNS toxicity due to pre-maturity of blood brain barrier, later sensitisation (caution).

ADR: Hypersensitivity (skin rash, pruritus, urticaria; erythema multiforme, Stevens-Johnson syndrome, toxic epidermal necrolysis, bullous and exfoliative dermatitis; acute generalised exanthematous pustulosis; anaphylactic reactions including shock); renal (interstitial nephritis, crystalluria), GI/hepatic (nausea, vomiting, diarrhoea; mucocutaneous candidiasis, antibiotic associated colitis, abdominal pain, elevated liver enzymes, hepatitis, cholestatic jaundice); haematological (reversible leucopenia i.e. severe neutropenia and agranulocytosis, thrombocytopenia, haemolytic anaemia, prolonged bleeding and prothrombin time, eosinophilia, thrombocytosis). Headache, hyperkinesia, dizziness, convulsions especially high doses/renal impairment, altered laboratory tests. Injection site reactions (parenteral).

Notes: See 9.1 Antibacterials.

Amoxicillin

ATC Code: J01CA04. **Sport:** Permitted.
Driving: Allergic reactions, dizziness, convulsions may influence (oral); parenteral (caution).

Indications: Treatment, (adults, children), acute (bacterial sinusitis, otitis media, streptococcal tonsillitis and pharyngitis, exacerbations of chronic bronchitis), community acquired pneumonia, asymptomatic bacteriuria in pregnancy, acute (cystitis, pyelonephritis), typhoid and paratyphoid fever, dental abscess (severe*) with spreading cellulitis, prosthetic joint infections, *Helicobacter pylori* eradication, Lyme disease. Prophylaxis, endocarditis. *Parenteral; also bacterial meningitis, bacteraemia associated with any of above.

Dose: Adult, Elderly: ORAL (adult, children 40kg and above):

Treatment, acute (bacterial sinusitis, pyelonephritis, cystitis), asymptomatic bacteriuria in pregnancy, dental abscess with spreading cellulitis, 250-500mg 8-hourly or 750-1000mg 12-hourly; for severe infections 750mg-1000mg 8-hourly. Acute cystitis may be treated with 3g twice daily for 1 day.

Treatment, acute (otitis media, streptococcal tonsillitis and pharyngitis, exacerbations of chronic bronchitis), 500mg 8-hourly or 750mg-1000mg 12-hourly; for severe infections 750-1000mg 8-hourly for 10 days. Community acquired pneumonia, prosthetic joint infections, 500-1000mg 8-hourly. Typhoid and paratyphoid fever, 500-2000mg 8-hourly.

Helicobacter pylori eradication, 750-1000mg twice daily + PPI (omeprazole, lansoprazole) + another antibiotic (clarithromycin, metronidazole) for 7 days.

Lyme Disease, *early stage*, 500-1000mg 8-hourly up to max. 4g/day in divided doses for 14 days (range 10-21 days); *late stage* (systemic involvement), 500-2000mg 8-hourly up to max. 6g/day in divided doses (10-30 days).

9.1.1 Penicillins

Prophylaxis of endocarditis, 2g orally as single dose 30-60 minutes before procedure.

PARENTERAL (IV), *treatment*, severe infections (ear, nose, throat) with severe systemic signs/symptoms, acute (exacerbations of chronic bronchitis, cystitis, pyelonephritis), community acquired pneumonia, severe dental abscess, prosthetic joint infections, 750-2000mg 8-hourly or 2g every 12 hours; max. 12g/day. Lyme disease, *late stage*, 2g every 8 hours.

Endocarditis, *prophylaxis* 2g as single dose 30-60 minutes prior to procedure; *treatment* endocarditis and bacterial meningitis, 1-2g every 4-6 hours; bacteraemia, 1-2g every 4, 6 or 8 hours. Max. 12g/day.

PARENTERAL (IM), max. single dose 1g; max. daily dose, 4g/day.

Admin, oral formulations with/without food; swallow whole without opening capsules. Put contents of sachet in 10-20mL of water, shake to form a susp and admin immediately. Admin IV parenteral by slow IV injection (over 3-4 minutes) directly into a vein or via a drip tube or by infusion over 20-30 minutes. IM, inject max. 1g at one time (adults) or 60mg/kg (child).

Child: ORAL, weight under 40kg, *treatment*, acute (bacterial sinusitis, otitis media, pyelonephritis, cystitis), community acquired pneumonia, dental abscess, 20-90mg/kg/day*. Acute streptococcal tonsillitis and pharyngitis, 40-90mg/kg/day*. Typhoid and paratyphoid fever, 100mg/kg/day in 3 divided doses. Lyme Disease, *early stage*, 25-50mg/kg/day in 3 divided doses; *late stage* (systemic involvement), 100mg/kg/day in 3 divided doses (10-30 days). *(in divided doses; consider twice daily only when in upper dose range).

Prophylaxis of endocarditis, 50mg/kg orally as single dose 30-60 minutes before procedure. Above 40kg and for admin, as for Adult above.

PARENTERAL (IV), infants and toddlers over 3 months and children under 40kg: *Treatment*, severe infections (ear, nose, and throat) with severe systemic signs/symptoms, acute (exacerbations of chronic bronchitis, cystitis, pyelonephritis, community acquired pneumonia), severe dental abscess, 20-200mg/kg/day in 2-4 equally divided doses.

Endocarditis, *prophylaxis*, 50mg/kg as single dose 30-60 minutes before procedure; *treatment*, 200mg/kg/day in 3-4 equally divided doses. Bacterial meningitis, 100-200mg/kg/day in 3-4 equally divided doses. Bacteraemia, 50-150mg/kg/day in 3 equally divided doses. Lyme disease, *early stage*, 25-50mg/kg/day in 3 divided doses for 10 days (range 10-21 days); *late stage*, 50mg/kg/day in 3 divided doses.

PARENTERAL (IV), neonates 4kg and above and infants up to 3 months: *Treatment*, most infections, usually 20-150mg/kg/day in 3 equally divided doses. Endocarditis and bacterial meningitis, 150mg/kg in 3 equally divided doses. Bacteraemia, 50-150mg/kg/day in 3 divided doses. Lyme disease, as for infants and toddlers above.

PARENTERAL (IV), premature neonates under 4kg: *Treatment*, most infections, usually 20-100mg/kg/day in 2 equally divided doses. Endocarditis and bacterial meningitis, 100mg/kg in 2 divided doses. Bacteraemia, 50-100mg/kg/day in 2 equally divided doses. Lyme disease, *early stage*, 25-50mg/kg/day in 2 divided doses for 10 days (range 10-21 days); *late stage*, 50mg/kg/day in 2 divided doses.

NOTE: Divided doses (IV) are up to 25mg/kg or infusions of up to 50mg/kg.

PARENTERAL (IM), max 120mg/kg/day as 2-6 equally divided doses.

Renal Impairment: GFR (mL/min) above 30, no adjustment (all ages).

GFR 10-30, adults and children over 40kg, oral 500mg twice daily (children under 40kg*, 15mg/kg twice daily, max. 500mg twice daily); parenteral (IV), 1000mg immediately, then 500-1000mg twice daily (child*, 25mg/kg twice daily); parenteral (IM), 500mg 12-hourly (child*, 15mg/kg 12-hourly).

GFR 10-30, adults and children over 40kg, oral 500mg twice daily (children under 40kg*, 15mg/kg twice daily, max. 500mg twice daily); parenteral (IV), 1000mg immediately, then 500-1000mg twice daily (child*, 25mg/kg twice daily); parenteral (IM), 500mg 12-hourly (child*, 15mg/kg 12-hourly).

GFR below 10, adults and children over 40kg, oral max. 500mg/day (child*, 15mg/kg as single dose; max. 500mg); parenteral (IV), 1000mg immediately, then 500mg/day (child*, 25mg/kg/day as single dose); parenteral (IM), 500mg/day as single dose (child*, 15mg/kg/day as single dose). *(children under 40kg; parenteral therapy preferred in majority of cases).

Dialysis, adults and children over 40kg: Peritoneal dialysis, oral max. 500mg/day; parenteral (IV), 1000mg immediately, then 500mg/day; parenteral (IM), 500mg/day as single dose. Haemodialysis, oral 15mg/kg/day as single daily dose; prior to dialysis, admin one additional dose of 15mg/kg then 15mg/kg after dialysis to restore circulating drug levels; parenteral (IV), 1000mg at end of dialysis, then 500mg 24-hourly; parenteral (IM), 500mg during dialysis, 500mg at end, then 500mg 24-hourly.

Dialysis, children under 40kg: Peritoneal dialysis, parenteral (IV), 25mg/kg/day as single dose; parenteral (IM), 15mg/kg/day as single dose. Haemodialysis, parenteral (IV), 25mg/kg immediately and 12.5mg/kg at end of dialysis, then 25mg/kg/day; parenteral (IM), 15mg/kg during dialysis, 15mg/kg at end, then 15mg/kg 24-hourly.

Hepatic Impairment: Caution. Monitor function regularly.

SP: Not suitable for some types of infection unless pathogen is known OR is highly likely to be susceptible (especially UTI, severe infections of ear, nose, throat). Convulsions may occur especially with impaired renal function, high dose, predisposing factors (history of seizures, epilepsy, meningeal disorders). Feverish generalised erythema with pustule may indicate acute generalised exanthemas pustulosis (AGEP); discontinue; subsequent admin contraindicated. Jarisch-Herxheimer reaction seen following treatment of Lyme disease.

Pregnancy, Lactation: Use only if benefit outweighs risk. Is excreted into breast milk with possible sensitisation of infant.

ADR: *Most common*, diarrhoea, nausea, skin rash.

Notes: See Class Effects 9.1.1 Penicillins.

Amoxil Paed Susp, Sachet, Parenteral *(GSK)* A. GMS.D*.
Price, Paed susp sachet (20mL) €3.84. Sachets 3g* (2) €3.78. Injection 500mg* (10) €6.96.
Oral susp (Paed), amoxicillin trihydrate 125mg/1.25mL (20mL). White powder with yellowish granules for susp. *Aspartame, parabens, sulphur dioxide, maltodextrin.* **Store:** Below 25 deg C.
Injection, amoxicillin sodium 500mg. White (off-white) sterile powder for soln. *Sodium 38mg/vial; lidocaine and benzyl alcohol may only be used for IM injection (not IV).* **Store:** As above.
Sachet (3g), as above. White (off-white) free-flowing powder; forms white (off-white) susp on reconstitution. *Sorbitol.* **Store:** As above; original pack to protect (moisture).

Geramox 250mg, 500mg *(Gerard)* A. GMS.D.
Price, 250mg (100) €8.49; (500) €40.18. 500mg (100) €16.15; (500) €78.06.
Capsule, amoxicillin trihydrate. Hard gelatin red/yellow contains white (off-white) granular powder. Marked AX/strength and G.

Oramox 250mg, 500mg, Oral Susp *(Fannin)* A. GMS.D*.
Price, 250mg* (100) €8.49. (500) €40.18. 500mg* (100) €16.15. (500) €78.06. Susp (100mL) 125mg/5mL, €2.05; 250mg/5mL*, €3.02.
Capsule, amoxicillin trihydrate. Hard gelatin scarlet/ivory containing off-white granular powder. Marked Amox and strength.
Oral susp, as above 125mg(250mg)/5mL. Pale-yellow crystalline powder for susp; lemon odour/flavour. *Sucrose, sodium 3.79mg (6.47mg)/5mL.*

Pinamox 250mg, 500mg, Oral Susp *(Pinewood)* A. GMS.D*.
Price, 250mg* (100) €8.49. (500) €40.18. (1000) €78.01. 500mg* (100) €16.15. (500) €78.06. Susp (100mL) 125mg/5mL, €2.05; 250mg/5mL*, €3.02.
Capsule, amoxicillin trihydrate. Hard scarlet/ivory; contains off-white granular powder. Marked P, logo, Pinamox and strength.
Oral susp, as above 125mg(250mg)/5mL. Pale-yellow powder for oral susp; lemon odour and flavour.

Amoxicillin, Clavulanate

ATC Code: J01RA01. **Sport:** Permitted.
Driving: Unlikely to impair (oral); parenteral (caution).
Indications: Treatment, see Notes below (amoxicillin). Prophylaxis, wound infection associated with GI, pelvic cavity, head/neck and biliary tract surgery.

Dose: Adult: ORAL, (amoxicillin/clavulanate) 1x (250/125mg) tab OR 1x (500/125mg) tab 3-times daily OR 1x (875/125mg) tab twice daily; higher dose (otitis media, sinusitis, lower RTI), 1x (875/125mg) tab 3-times daily. *Admin,* at start of meal to minimise potential GI intolerance; tabs not to be broken.
PARENTERAL, *treatment,* 1g/0.2g 8-hourly; *surgical prophylaxis,* 1-2g/0.2g at induction of anaesthesia; repeat up to 3 doses in 24 hours for procedures over 1 hour. *Admin,* by slow IV injection over 3-4 minutes directly into vein or via drip tube or by IV infusion over 30-40 minutes; not for IM admin.

Elderly: Prolonged/R, 60 years and older, caution; consider liver function testing.

Child: ORAL, under 40kg, *susp (125mg/31.25mg)/5mL,* 20/5 to 60/15mg/kg/day in 3 divided doses; *susp (400/57mg)/5mL,* 25/3.6mg/kg/day to 45/6.4mg/kg/day in 2 divided doses. Some infections (otitis media, sinusitis, lower RTI), up to 70/10 mg/kg/day as 2 divided doses may be needed. Weight 40kg and over, as for Adult above. Under 25kg and under 6 years, use paediatric formulations.
PARENTERAL, under 40kg, age 3 months and over, 25mg/5mg per kg 8-hourly; under 3 months and under 4kg, 25mg/5mg per kg 12-hourly by IV infusion only. Weight 40kg and over, as for Adult above.

Renal Impairment: *Adult,* CrCl (mL/min) 10-30, oral 250/125mg or oral 500/125mg 12-hourly OR parenteral 1g/0.2g initially, then 500mg/100mg 24-hourly (875/125 not recommended); CrCl (mL/min) below 10, oral 250/125mg or oral 500/125mg 24-hourly OR parenteral 1g/0.2g initially, then 500/100mg 24-hourly.
Child, under 40kg, CrCl (mL/min) 10-30, oral 15/3.75mg/kg 12-hourly or oral 250/125mg twice daily (max. 500/125mg 12-hourly); parenteral 25/5mg/kg 12-hourly. CrCl (mL/min) below 10, oral 15/3.75mg/kg 24-hourly or oral 250/125mg once daily (max. 500/125mg 24-hourly); parenteral 25/5mg 24-hourly. Immature renal function, CrCl below 30, use 4:1 formulations. Haemodialysis, see manufacturers Full Prescribing Information.

Hepatic Impairment: Caution, monitor function regularly especially with underlying disease.

CI: Previous history of amoxicillin/clavulanate associated jaundice.

Interactions: Effect of Amoxicillin/Clavulanic Acid Combination on Other Drugs: Mycophenolate mofetil: *Monitor levels during combination and shortly after antibiotic treatment.* Allopurinol: *Increased likelihood of allergic skin reactions.*

SP: GI disturbance, nausea, vomiting, oral absorption may be impaired; use parenteral.

ADR: Very common, diarrhoea.

Notes: See Amoxicillin above and Class Effects 9.1.1 Penicillins.

Interchangeability: Same strengths of all brands of amoxicillin/clavulanic acid f/c tabs and paediatric formulations (powder for oral susp) listed below are deemed interchangeable.

Reference Price: Tabs (14) 875/125mg, €8.35. Oral Susp (70mL) 400/57mg, €3.56.

Augmentin Tabs *(GSK)* A. GMS.D.
Price, 250/125mg (21) €3.06. 500/125mg (21) €4.02. 875/125mg (14), see reference price above.
Tablet, amoxicillin trihydrate/potassium clavulanate 250(500, 875)/125. White (off-white) oval f/c. 250: Marked Augmentin. 500(875): Scored (facilitates breaking). Marked AC.
Augmentin Susp DUO 400/57, Paed 125/31 *(GSK)* A. GMS.
Price, Duo (35mL) €1.78; (70mL), see reference price above. Paed 100mL, €1.38.
Oral susp (Duo), amoxicillin trihydrate, potassium clavulanate

400/57mg per 5mL. White powder (with yellowish grains) for susp; characteristic odour. *Aspartame, maltodextrin.*
Oral susp (Paediatric), as above 125/31.25mg per 5mL. White (off-white) powder for susp. *Aspartame, maltodextrin.*
Augmentin Parenteral *(GSK)* A.
Price, (10) 600mg, €13.08; 1.2g, €26.16 (PTW).
Injection or infusion (IV), amoxicillin sodium 500mg (1g), potassium clavulanate 100mg (200mg) (600mg, 1.2g). White (off-white) powder for soln. *Potassium 19.6mg (39.3mg),* sodium *31.4mg (62.9mg) per 500/100mg (1000/200mg)* vial.
Amoclav 250mg, 500mg, Susp 125mg *(Rowex)* A. GMS.D*.
Price, tabs 250/125mg* (100) €14.26. Forte 500/125mg (21)* €3.79. Susp 125/31.25mg (100mL) €1.38.
Tablet, amoxicillin trihydrate, potassium clavulanate 250 (500)/125mg. Oblong f/c scored (facilitates breaking). 250/125: Off-white. Marked ACX 375; G on reverse. *Cetyl alcohol.* 500/125: White notched both sides.
Oral susp, as above 125/31.25mg/5mL. Off-white powder. *Aspartame.*
Clavamel, Forte, Paed Susp *(Clonmel)* A. GMS.D*.
Price, tabs 250/125mg (21) €3.79. Forte 500/125mg (21)* €3.79. Paed susp 125/31.25mg (100mL) €1.38.
Tablet, amoxicillin trihydrate, potassium clavulanate 250/125mg, Forte 500/125mg. 250: Yellow oblong. Marked 625. Forte: White oval.
Powder for oral susp, as above 125/31.25mg/5mL. White (off-white) powder for reconstitution with water. *Aspartame, ethanol, sulphites, gum arabic.*
Co-Amoxiclav (Actavis) Tabs *(Accord)* A. GMS.D.
Price, tabs 500/125mg (21) €3.79.
Tablet, amoxicillin trihydrate, potassium clavulanate 500/125. White oval f/. Marked A; 64 on reverse.
Co-Amoxiclav Bluefish 500mg *(Bluefish)* A. GMS.D.
Price, tabs 500/125mg (21) €3.79.
Tablet, amoxicillin trihydrate, potassium clavulanate 500/125. White (off-white) oval.
Co-Amoxiclav (Brown & Burk) Tabs, Susp *(Fannin)* A. GMS.D*.
Price, tabs 250/125mg* (21) €2.99. 500/125mg* (21) €3.78. 875/125mg* (14), see reference price above. Susp 400/57mg/5mL (30mL) €1.52, (70mL) €3.56.
Tablet, amoxicillin trihydrate, potassium clavulanate 25(500) (875)/125mg. White cap-shaped f/c. 250/125: Marked I05. 500/125: Marked I06. 875/125: Marked I07. **Store:** Below 25 deg C.
Powder for oral susp (Sugar-Free), as above 400/57mg/5mL. White (off-white) powder; reconstituted has fruity aromatic odour. *Aspartame.* **Store:** Original pack to protect (moisture).
Germentin 250mg, 500mg, Susp 125mg *(Gerard)* A. GMS.D*.
Price, tabs 250/125mg (21)* €2.99. 500/125mg (16) €3.07; (21)*, €3.79. Susp 125/31.25mg (100mL) €1.38.
Tablet, amoxicillin trihydrate, potassium clavulanate 250 (500)/125mg. Off-white scored (facilitates breaking). 250/125mg: Oblong. Marked AXC 375; twice G on reverse. *Potassium 24.5mg.* 500/125mg: Oval.
Powder for oral susp, as above 125/31.25mg/5mL. Off-white granules. *Aspartame, sorbitol, glucose.*

Flucloxacillin

ATC Code: J01CF05. **Sport:** Permitted.
Driving: Unlikely to impair.
Indications: Infection due to sensitive penicillinase producing staphylococci, other Gram-positive infections including osteomyelitis, endocarditis. Prophylaxis, major surgical procedures (cardiothoracic, orthopaedic).

Dose: Adult: ORAL, 250-500mg 3-times daily or 250mg 4-times daily. *Osteomyelitis, endocarditis,* up to 8g daily in divided doses; 6-8 hourly. Take half to one hour before meals.
PARENTERAL, IM or IV usually 750-1500mg in divided doses. *Intrapleural, intra-articular,* 500mg once daily; *osteomyelitis, endocarditis,* as for oral.
Surgical prophylaxis, 1-2g IV at induction of anaesthesia; then 500mg 6-hourly IV, IM, or oral for up to 72 hours.

Elderly: Caution.

Child: Age 2-10 years, half adult dose; under 2 years, quarter adult dose OR 25-50mg/kg.

Renal Impairment: CrCl (mL/min) below 10, reduce dose or extend dosing interval; max. 1g every 8-12 hours. Dialysis, supplementary doses not needed.

Hepatic Impairment: Caution.

CI: Ocular or subconjunctival admin (parenteral).

SP: Newborn, caution hyperbilirubinaemia risk, high serum levels due to reduced excretion. Prolonged treatment, monitor hepatic/renal function. *Caution,* evidence of

9.1.1   Penicillins

hepatic dysfunction, age 50 years and over, serious underlying disease; hepatic events may be severe; rarely deaths reported. At initiation, occurrence of feverish generalised erythema with pustula may be a symptom of acute generalised exanthematous pustulosis (AGEP); if diagnosed, discontinue flucloxacillin; subsequent use contraindicated.

ADR: *Common*, minor GI disturbances.

Notes: See Class Effects 9.1.1 Penicillins.

Interchangeability: Same strengths of all flucloxacillin capsules and powder for oral suspension listed below are deemed interchangeable.

> **Floxapen Caps, Syrup, Parenteral** *(TEVA)* A. GMS.D*.
> *Price*, (28) caps 250mg*, €4.81. 500mg*, €9.60. Syrup (100mL) 125mg/5mL, €2.76. Forte 250mg/5mL*, €8.51. Parenteral* (10) 250mg, €11.89. 500mg, €23.81. Parenteral 1g, 2g, not published by company (non-GMS/D).
> *Capsule*, flucloxacillin sodium 250mg, 500mg. Hard gelatin caramel/black. Marked with name/strength. *Sodium 51mg/g.*
> *Powder for oral susp*, flucloxacillin magnesium 125(250)mg/5mL. White free-flowing.
> *Injection, infusion*, flucloxacillin sodium 250mg, 500mg, 1g, 2g. Powder for soln.

> **Flucillin 250mg, 500mg** *(Pinewood)* A. GMS.D.
> *Price*, 250mg (100) €16.29; (250) €40.51; (500) €84.13. 500mg (100) €32.58; (250) €81.01; (500) €166.99.
> *Capsule*, flucloxacillin sodium. Grey/brown. Marked FXN/strength; logo on reverse.

> **Fluclon 250mg** *(Clonmel)* A. GMS.D.
> *Price*, (250) 250mg, €40.51.
> *Capsule*, flucloxacillin sodium. Blue. Marked FXN/strength, logo.

> **Flucloxacillin GAP Caps, Oral Soln** *(Fannin)* A. GMS.D*.
> *Price*, 250mg* (100) €16.61. (500) €83.15. 500mg* (100) €33.24. (500) €166.31. Oral soln (100mL) 125mg/5mL, €2.68. 250mg/5mL*, €6.43.
> *Capsule*, flucloxacillin sodium 250mg, 500mg. Hard opaque caramel/grey. Marked FXN and strength. *Sodium 52.3mg/1g flucloxacillin.*
> *Oral soln*, as above 125(250)mg/5mL. Free-flowing pink powder for soln. *Sodium 18mg/5mL, sucrose.*

> **Gerifiox 500mg** *(Gerard)* A. GMS.D.
> *Price*, (100) 500mg, €30.41.
> *Capsule*, flucloxacillin sodium monohydrate. Grey/brown. Marked G and FN/strength. *Sodium 13mg (250mg), 26mg (500mg).*
> **Store:** Below 25 deg C; original pack.

Penicillin G

ATC Code: J01CE01. **Sport:** Permitted.
Driving: Unlikely to impair.

Indications: Bacterial endocarditis, meningitis, RTI, septicaemia in children, syphilis.

Dose: Adult, Elderly: 600-1200mg/day IM or IV in 2-4 divided doses.

Child: 1 month-12 years, 100mg/kg/day in 4 divided doses; max. 4g/day; infants 1-4 weeks, 75mg/kg/day in 3 divided doses; neonates, 50mg/kg/day in 2 divided doses.

Notes: See Class Effects 9.1.1 Penicillins.

> **Crystapen Parenteral 600mg** *(Genus)* A. GMS.D.
> *Price*, (25) €13.50.
> *Injection or infusion*, benzylpenicillin sodium. Powder for soln.

Penicillin V

ATC Code: J01CE02. **Sport:** Permitted.
Driving: Unlikely to affect.

Indications: Treatment, infections due to susceptible staphylococci, pneumococci, gonococci, haemolytic streptococci including tonsillitis, pharyngitis, skin infections. Prophylactic management of rheumatic fever.

Dose: Adult, Elderly: *Treatment*, 1-2g/day in 3-4 divided doses depending on severity. Oral, half an hour before meals or three quarters of an hour after.

Prophylaxis, 250mg twice daily (long-term); treat beta-haemolytic streptococci infections for 10 days to avoid later complications.

Child: Over 6 years, 0.5-1g/day; age 1-6 years, 250-500mg/day; under 1 year, 125mg-250mg/day. Admin in 3-4 divided doses.

Renal Impairment: Lower dose may be required.

Interactions: Effect of Other Drugs on **Phenoxymethylpenicillin:** *Reduced absorption:* Aminoglycosides (neomycin), guar gum.

Effect of Phenoxymethylpenicillin on Other Drugs: Oral contraceptives: *Reduced effectiveness*. Methotrexate: *Reduced excretion, increased toxicity risk.*

SP: Severe GI impairments with vomiting and diarrhoea, sufficient absorption not ensured; use parenteral.

Notes: See Class Effects 9.1.1 Penicillins.

> **Calvepen 333mg, 666mg, Susp** *(Clonmel)* A. GMS.D.
> *Price*, (100) 333mg, €8.42. 666mg, €14.44. Susp (100mL) 250mg/5mL, €3.07.
> *Tablet*, phenoxymethylpenicillin calcium. White f/c. Marked with symbol. 333mg: Oval. Marked 105. 666mg: Marked 104.
> *Powder for oral susp*, as above 250mg/5mL. White.

> **Kopen 250mg, Oral Soln** *(Fannin)* A. GMS.D.
> *Price*, tabs 250mg* (100) €4.37; (1000) €39.63. Elixir (100mL) 125mg/5mL, €1.57; 250mg/5mL*, €2.51.
> *Capsule*, phenoxymethylpenicillin calcium. White. Marked Pen 250.
> *Powder for oral soln*, as above, 125mg(250mg)/5mL (sugar free). Off-white. *Sorbitol, Sunset Yellow, Ponceau 4R.*

Piperacillin, Tazobactam

ATC Code: J01CA12. **Sport:** Permitted.
Driving: No data.

Indications: Severe pneumonia (nosocomial, ventilator-associated), complicated infections e.g. UTI (pyelonephritis), intra-abdominal, skin and soft tissue (diabetic foot) associated with bacteraemia. Neutropenics with fever (suspected bacterial infection). Complicated intra-abdominal infections, neutropenia in children.

Dose: Adult: *Complicated infections, intra-abdominal, skin and soft tissue*, usually piperacillin/tazobactam 4g/0.5g 8-hourly (6-hourly for nosocomial pneumonia, neutropenia) for 5-14 days depending on severity. *Admin*, slow IV infusion over 20-30 minutes.

Elderly: CrCl (mL/min) above 40, no adjustment.

Child: Age 2-12 years, neutropenia, piperacillin/tazobactam 80mg/10mg/kg 6-hourly; complicated intra-abdominal infections, 100mg/12.5mg/kg 8-hourly. Admin, see Adult above.

Renal Impairment: *Adult*, CrCl (mL/min) 20-40, piperacillin/tazobactam 4g/0.5g 8-hourly; below 20, 4g/0.5g 12-hourly. On dialysis, additional 2g/0.25g at end of dialysis. *Age 12 years and under*, CrCl (mL/min) below 50, 70mg/8.75mg/kg 8-hourly. On dialysis, additional 40mg/5mg/kg at end of dialysis.

Interactions: Effect of Other Drugs on Piperacillin, Tazobactam Combination: *Co-admin, admixture not recommended (physical incompatibility):* Aminoglycosides (admin separately; if co-admin essential, use Y-site infusion only). *Co-admin (longer half-life, lower renal clearance):* Probenecid. *Acute kidney injury (increased incidence):* Vancomycin.

Effect of Piperacillin, Tazobactam Combination on Other Drugs: Heparin, oral anticoagulants, other drugs affecting coagulation: *Perform regular coagulation tests*. Vecuronium: *Prolonged neuromuscular blockade*. Methotrexate: *Excretion reduced*.

SP: Altered laboratory tests. Prolonged therapy, monitor (haematopoietic, renal, hepatic function). Severe cutaneous reactions (Stevens-Johnson syndrome, toxic epidermal necrolysis, DRESS, acute generalised exanthematous pustulosis).

ADR: Summary, *most common*, diarrhoea; *most serious*, pseudo-membranous colitis, toxic epidermal necrolysis, pancytopenia, anaphylactic shock, Stevens-Johnson syndrome.

Notes: See Class Effects 9.1.1 Penicillins.

> **Piperacillin/Tazobactam Parenteral** *(Gerard)* A.
> *Price*, (vial x 10) 2/0.25g, €56.00. 4/0.5g, €120.00.
> *Infusion*, piperacillin sodium 2g (4g), tazobactam sodium 0.25g (0.5g). White (off-white) powder for soln. *Sodium 108mg (216mg)/vial.* **Store:** Below 25 deg C.

> **Piperacillin/Tazobactam TEVA Parenteral** *(TEVA)* A.
> *Price*, not published by company.
> *Infusion*, piperacillin sodium 4g, tazobactam sodium 0.5g. *Sodium 216mg/vial.*

> **Pipercin Parenteral** *(Clonmel)* A.
> *Price*, not published by company.
> *Infusion*, piperacillin sodium 2g (4g), tazobactam sodium 0.25g (0.5g). White (off-white) powder for soln. *Sodium 108mg (216mg)/vial.*

9.1.2 - Cephalosporins, Carbepenems, Monobactams, Other Cephalosporins

In This Chapter: *Cephalosporins, first generation (cephalexin), second generation (cefaclor, cefuroxime), third generation (cefixime, cefotaxime, ceftriaxone, ceftazidime); fifth generation ceftolozane (tazobactam combination). Carbepenems (ertapenem, meropenem). Monobactams (aztreonam). Other cephalosporins (ceftaroline).*

Class Effects
Driving: Oral and inhaled formulations unlikely to impair. Parenteral, caution (dizziness).

Cephalosporins have a similar profile to penicillins. For additional information, see Notes below (penicillins).

CI: History of severe immediate hypersensitivity reaction (anaphylaxis) to other beta-lactams (penicillins, cephalosporins, carbepenems, monobactams).

SP: *Cephalosporins*, false positive Direct Coombs' tests (antiglobulin test) possible; reaction for glucose in urine may occur with Benedict's or Fehling's soln. Changes/decline in renal function (especially with nephrotoxic drugs e.g. aminoglycosides, potent diuretics), monitor function. Caution, severe allergy, asthma, rash, urticaria. *Clostridium difficile* associated diarrhoea, see Notes below, (antibacterials). Drug-induced haemolytic anaemia (severe, fatal), cases of convulsions, reported. Resistance to penems of Enterobacteriaceae, *Pseudomonas aeruginosa*, Acinetobacter spp. varies across the European Union; consult local resistance patterns.

ADR: Beta-lactam antibiotics have similar adverse events. See Notes below (penicillins).

Notes: See 9.1 Antibacterials. See 9.1.1 Penicillins.

Aztreonam

ATC Code: J01DF01. **Sport:** Permitted.
Driving: No or negligible effect.

Indications: *Parenteral*, aerobic Gram-negative infections (UTI, gonorrhoea, lower RTI, bacteraemia, septicaemia, meningitis, bone and joint, skin and soft tissue, intra-abdominal, gynaecological). Adjunctive to surgery (abscesses, infections complicating hollow viscous perforations, cutaneous, serous surfaces). *Inhaled*, suppressive therapy of chronic pulmonary infections, *Pseudomonas aeruginosa*, in cystic fibrosis patients.

Dose: Adult: PARENTERAL, usually 3-4g daily; max. 8g/day; range 1-8g/day in equally divided doses. *UTI*, 0.5-1g every 8-12 hours IM or IV; *gonorrhoea, cystitis*, 1g as single dose IM; *cystic fibrosis*, 2g every 6-8 hours IV.
Moderate to severe infections, 1-2g every 8-12 hours IM or IV; *severe, life-threatening* infections, 2g every 6-8 hours IM or IV. Other infections, 1g 8-hourly IM or IV OR 2g 12-hourly IV. Admin IM, IV injection or infusion; doses above 1g, IV recommended.
NEBULISER (INHALATION) SOLN, 75mg 3-times per 24 hours by inhalation (min. 4 hours apart) for 28 days; use bronchodilator before each dose, 15 minutes for short-acting; 30 minutes to 12 hours for long-acting. With several respiratory therapies, dose order: Bronchodilator, mucolytics, lastly *Cayston*.
Child: PARENTERAL, older than 1 week, 30mg/kg/dose every 6-8 hours; *severe infections*, 2 years and older, 50mg/kg/dose every 6-8 hours, max. 8g/day.
NEBULISER (INHALATION) SOLN, age 6 years and older, as for Adult; under 6 years, safety/efficacy not established.

Renal Impairment: *Parenteral*, CrCl (mL/min/1.73m2) 10-30, half initial dose; below 10 or on haemodialysis, one fourth of initial dose at intervals of 6, 8 or 12 hours. Serious, life-threatening infections, additional one-eighth of initial dose after each dialysis session. See Hepatic Impairment below. *Inhalation*, serum creatinine above 2xULN, caution.

Hepatic Impairment: *Parenteral*, dose reduction of 20-25% recommended for long-term treatment with chronic liver disease with cirrhosis especially alcoholic cirrhosis

and with renal impairment. *Inhalation*, no dose adjustment; severe, no data.

Interactions: Effect of Aztreonam on Other Drugs: Oral anticoagulants: *Prolonged prothrombin time*. Aminoglycoside co-admin: *Monitor for potential nephro/ototoxicity*.

SP: *Parenteral*, serious blood and skin disorders. Medication inhibiting intestinal peristalsis not recommended. Parenteral formulation not for inhalation; contains arginine known to cause pulmonary inflammation. *Inhalation*, bronchospasm. Efficacy/safety not tested where FEV1 % predicted below 25% or above 75%. Rash may indicate allergic reaction. Haemoptysis, use only if benefit outweighs risk of further haemorrhage.

Pregnancy, Lactation: *Parenteral*, pregnancy, contraindicated; crosses placenta, enters foetal circulation. Lactation, not recommended. *Inhalation*, pregnancy, only if required by clinical condition. Lactation, can be used.

ADR: Parenteral, *very common*, common, none reported. Inhalation, *most frequent*, cough, nasal congestion, wheezing, pharyngolaryngeal pain, pyrexia, dyspnoea.

Notes: See 9.1.2 Cephalosporins.

Azactam Parenteral 1g, 2g *(BMS)* A.
Price, (1) 1g, €12.27. 2g, €24.51.
Injection or infusion, aztreonam. White (off-white), sodium-free powder for soln.
Cayston Nebuliser Soln 75mg *(Gilead)* A. HT.
Price, (84) €2763.78.
Nebuliser soln, aztreonam lysine 75mg/vial. White (off-white) powder; solvent for soln. **Store:** Refrigerate; outside of refrigerator below 25 deg C (max. 28 days).

Cefaclor

ATC Code: J01DC04. **Sport:** Permitted.
Driving: No known effects.

Indications: RTI, otitis media, skin and soft tissue, UTI. Eradication of nasopharyngeal streptococci.

Dose: Adult, Elderly: STANDARD/R, 250mg 8-hourly; severe infection, 500mg 8-hourly; max. 4g/day.
PROLONGED/R, *pharyngitis*, tonsillitis, skin/soft tissue infection, usually 375mg twice daily; *pneumonia*, 750mg twice daily; max. 1.5g/day; *bronchitis*, *UTI*, 375mg twice daily OR 500mg once daily. Tabs should not be crushed or chewed; for oral admin with or without food.
Child: STANDARD/R, age 1 month and over, usually 20mg/kg/day in divided doses 8-hourly (bronchitis, pneumonia) or 12-hourly (otitis media, pharyngitis); severe infection, up to 40mg/kg/day; max. 1g.
Renal Impairment: Severe, caution. Haemodialysis, admin loading dose 250mg-1g prior to dialysis and 250-500mg 6-8 hourly between dialysis.

Interactions: Effect of Cefaclor on Other Drugs: Warfarin: *Monitor prothrombin time*.

SP: Severe allergy, asthma, caution.

Notes: See 9.1.2 Cephalosporins.

Distaclor LA, Susp *(Flynn)* A. GMS.
Price, tabs (14) LA 375mg, €8.08. LA Forte 500mg, €11.71.
Susp (100mL) 125mg/5mL, €4.01. 250mg/5mL, €7.11.
Prolonged/R tablet, cefaclor monohydrate. Blue cap-shaped f/c. 375mg: Marked GP5. *Mannitol*.
Oral susp, as above 125(250)mg/5mL. Dry pink free-flowing granular powder for susp (strawberry flavour). *Sucrose*.
Keftid 250mg *(Co-pharma)* A. GMS.
Price, (21) €7.27.
Capsule, cefaclor. Purple/white. Marked CEF250.
Pinaclor 250mg *(Pinewood)* A. GMS.
Price, caps 250mg (100) €33.38. Susp (100mL) 125mg/5mL, €3.86. 250mg/5mL, €6.90.
Capsule, cefaclor. Purple/white. Marked Cefaclor 250.
Powder for oral susp, as above 125(250)mg/5mL. Strawberry flavour.

Cefixime

ATC Code: J01DD08. **Sport:** Permitted.
Driving: Unlikely to impair.

Indications: Infections due to sensitive organisms including Streptococci (pneumoniae, pyogenes), E. coli, H. influenza, B. catarrhalis, Klebsiella, Enterobacter. Most

235

9.1.2 Cephalosporins, Carbepenems, Monobactams, Other Cephalosporins

Enterococci, Staphylococci, Pseudomonas, Clostridia, *Bacteroides fragilis*, *Listeria monocytogenese* are resistant.

Dose: Adult, Elderly: Usually 200-400mg in 1-2 divided doses; uncomplicated upper RTI or UTI, 200mg/day.
Child: Over 12 years or above 50kg body weight, 200-400mg daily*. Uncomplicated upper respiratory tract infections or UTI, 200mg/day may be sufficient. Under 12 years, oral susp is required. Age 9-12 years, 300mg/day*; age 5-8 years, 200mg/day*; age 2-4 years, 100mg/day*; age 6 months to 2 years, usually 8mg/kg/day*. Under 6 months, safety and efficacy not established. *(in single or twice daily dose regimen).
Renal Impairment: CrCl (mL/min) below 20, CAPD or haemodialysis, max. 200mg/day.
SP: *Discontinue*, severe cutaneous reactions (toxic epidermal necrolysis, Stevens-Johnson syndrome, DRESS), severe GI disturbances (vomiting, diarrhoea), acute renal failure. *Caution*, poor oral nutrition, on parenteral nutrition, elderly, debilitated. Bleeding tendency due to Vitamin K deficiency in elderly.
Pregnancy, Lactation: Safety not established. Not known if excreted in human milk.
Notes: See 9.1.2 Cephalosporins.

Suprax 200mg *(SANOFI)* A. GMS.
Price, tabs 200mg (7) €11.39.
Tablet, cefixime trihydrate. Off-white (cream) round. Marked ORO.

Cefotaxime

ATC Code: J01DD01. **Sport:** Permitted.
Driving: Dizziness, impaired concentration or reaction, refrain from driving.

Indications: Septicaemia, RTI, UTI, skin and soft tissue, bone and joint, obstetric and gynaecological, gonorrhoea, meningitis. Prophylaxis, post-op sepsis. Active *in vitro* against Gram-negative organisms sensitive or resistant to first or second generation cephalosporins; similar to other cephalosporins against Gram-positive organisms.
Dose: Adult, Elderly: Mild to moderate infection, 1g 12-hourly; severe, up to 12g/day in 3-4 divided doses. Pseudomonal spp. sensitive infection, usually above 6g/day required. Gonorrhoea, 1g as single dose. Admin IM or slow IV injection or infusion.
Child: 100-150mg/kg/day; severe infection up to 200mg/kg/day. Neonates, 50mg/kg/day; severe infection 150-200mg/kg/day. Daily dose in 2-4 divided doses. See Contraindications.
Renal Impairment: GFR (mL/min) below 5, 1g loading then half of daily dose at same frequency.
CI: Reconstituted with lidocaine, caution, hypersensitivity to amide type anaesthetics, non-paced heart block, severe HF, IV admin, infants under age 30 months.
Interactions: Effect of Other Drugs on Cefotaxime: *Delayed excretion, plasma levels increased:* Probenecid.
Effect of Cefotaxime on Other Drugs: Nephrotoxic drugs: *May potentiate nephrotoxicity.*
SP: Treatment longer than 7-10 days, monitor white cell counts; neutropenia, discontinue.
Pregnancy, Lactation: Pregnancy, if benefit outweighs risk; crosses placental barrier. Lactation, passes into human milk; stop breastfeeding or stop drug.
ADR: *Very common*, injection site pain with IM admin.
Notes: See 9.1.2 Cephalosporins.

Claforan Parenteral 500mg, 1g *(SANOFI)* A. HOS.
Price, (10) 500mg, €21.36; 1g, €51.95 (PTW).
Injection or infusion, cefotaxime sodium. White (pale-yellow-white) crystalline powder for soln. *Sodium 48mg/1g cefotaxime sodium*.
Store: Unopened, below 25 deg C; reconstituted infusion soln can be refrigerated (max. 24 hours).

Ceftaroline

ATC Code: J01DI02. **Sport:** Permitted.
Driving: Dizziness may occur.
Indications: Complicated skin and soft tissue infections (cSSTI), community-acquired pneumonia (CAP).
Dose: Adult: Age 12 years and over (33kg and above), 600mg 12-hourly by IV infusion over 60 minutes (for all

infusion volumes); duration 5-14 days (cSSTI), 5-7 days (CAP). cSSTI due to S. *aureus*, 600mg every 8-hours using 2-hour infusions. *Admin*, IV infusion over 60 or 120 minutes for all infusion volumes (50mL, 100mL or 250mL). Infusion soln conc during preparation and admin, max. 12mg/mL ceftaroline fosamil.
Elderly: CrCl (mL/min) above 50, no adjustment.
Child: Age 12 years to under 18 years (under 33kg) and age 2 years to under 12 years, 12mg/kg admin every 8-hours; max. 400mg 8-hourly. Age 2 months to under 2 years, 8mg/kg every 8-hours. Under 2 months, safety/efficacy not established. *Admin*, as for Adult above.
Renal Impairment: Age 12 to under 18 years (33kg and above), CrCl (mL/min) above 30 to 50, 400mg 12-hourly; 15-30, 300mg 12-hourly. ESRD including haemodialysis*, 200mg 12-hourly. Age 2 to under 12 years and age 12 to under 18 years (under 33kg), CrCl (mL/min) above 30 to 50, 8mg/kg every 8 hours; max. 300mg 8-hourly; 15-30, 6mg/kg every 8 hourly; max. 200mg 8-hourly. *Admin*, as for Adult above. *(admin after haemodialysis on haemodialysis days).
Hepatic Impairment: No adjustment.
SP: Serious, fatal hypersensitivity reactions. Caution, pre-existing seizure disorder.
Pregnancy, Lactation: Pregnancy, avoid unless necessary. Lactation, stop breastfeeding or drug.
ADR: *Summary*, *most common*, diarrhoea, headache, nausea, pruritus. Greater rash incidence in Asian patients.
Notes: See 9.1.2 Cephalosporins.

Zinforo Parenteral *(AstraZeneca)* A. HOS.
Price, 600mg (10) €555.00 (PTW).
Infusion, ceftaroline fosamil 600mg. Pale yellowish-white (light-yellow) powder for conc for soln. **Store:** Below 30 deg C; original pack to protect (light).

Ceftazidime

ATC Code: J01DD02. **Sport:** Permitted.
Driving: Dizziness.
Indications: Spectrum mainly Gram-negative aerobic. Indications, see Dose below.
Dose: Adult: *Intermittent admin*, broncho-pulmonary infections in cystic fibrosis (CF), 100-150mg/kg/day, admin 8-hourly; max. 9g/day. Febrile neutropenia, nosocomial pneumonia, bacterial meningitis, bacteraemia*, 2g every 8 hours. Bone and joint infections, complicated (skin and soft tissue, intra-abdominal) infections, peritonitis**, otitis media (chronic suppurative), malignant otitis externa, 1-2g every 8 hours. Peri-operative prophylaxis, transurethral resection of prostate, 1g at anaesthetic induction; second dose at catheter removal.
Continuous infusion, febrile neutropenia, nosocomial pneumonia, broncho-pulmonary infections (CF), bacterial meningitis, bacteraemia*, bone and joint infections, complicated (skin and soft tissue, intra-abdominal) infections, peritonitis**, 2g loading dose, then by continuous infusion 4-6g every 24-hours.
*(associated with any of infections listed). **(associated with dialysis in patients on CAPD). Admin by IV injection or infusion or deep IM injection; IM should only be considered when IV not possible or less appropriate.
Elderly: Max. 3g/day, especially over 80 years.
Child: Weight 40kg and over, as for Adult above. Over 2 months and under 40kg, *intermittent admin*, complicated UTI, chronic suppurative otitis media, malignant otitis externa, infections (bone and joint, complicated skin and soft tissue, complicated intra-abdominal), peritonitis**, 100-150mg/kg/day in 3 divided doses; max. 6g/day. Neutropenics, broncho-pulmonary infections (CF), bacterial meningitis, bacteraemia*, 150mg/kg/day in 3 divided doses; max. 6g/day.
Continuous infusion, febrile neutropenia, nosocomial pneumonia, broncho-pulmonary infections (CF), bacterial meningitis, bacteraemia*, infections (bone and joint, complicated skin and soft tissue, complicated intra-abdominal), peritonitis**, 60-100mg/kg loading dose, then continuous infusion 100-200mg/kg/day; max. 6g/day.

236

Neonates, infants under 2 months, most infections, 25-60mg/kg/day in 2 divided doses by intermittent admin.

Admin, bacteraemia* and peritonitis** see Adult above.

Renal Impairment: *Adults and children 40kg and over,* 1g loading dose; maintenance CrCl (mL/min), 50-31, 1g 12-hourly (intermittent) or 2g loading then 1-3g/24-hours (continuous infusion); 30-16, 1g 24-hourly (intermittent) or 2g loading then 1g/24-hours (continuous infusion); 15-6, 0.5g 24-hourly (intermittent); below 5, 0.5g 48-hourly (intermittent). Severe infection, increase unit dose by 50% or increase dosing frequency. *Children under 40kg,* intermittent admin, maintenance CrCl (mL/min) 50-31, 25mg/kg 12-hourly; 30-16, 25mg/kg 24-hourly; 15-6, 12.5mg/kg 24-hourly; below 5, 12.5mg/kg 48-hourly. *Dialysis,* see manufacturers Full Prescribing Information.

Hepatic Impairment: Severe, close clinical monitoring.

ADR: *Most common,* eosinophilia, thrombocytosis, phlebitis, thrombophlebitis (IV admin); diarrhoea, increased hepatic enzymes, rash (maculopapular, urticarial), pain and/or inflammation (IM admin), positive Coomb's test.

Notes: See 9.1.2 Cephalosporins.

Fortum Parenteral *(GSK)* A. GMS.
Price, vials 500mg, €4.55. 1g, €9.02. 2g, €19.02.
Injection or infusion, ceftazidime pentahydrate. White (cream) powder for soln. *Sodium 26(52)(104)mg/500mg(1g)(2g) vial.*

Ceftolozane, Tazobactam

ATC Code: J01DI54. **Sport:** Permitted.
Driving: Minor influence; dizziness.
Indications: Complicated (intra-abdominal infections, UTI), acute pyelonephritis.

Dose: Adult, Elderly: 1g ceftolozane/0.5g tazobactam every 8 hours infused over 1 hour; complicated intra-abdominal infections* (4-14 days), complicated UTI, acute pyelonephritis (7 days). *(use with metronidazole if anaerobes suspected).

Child: Under 18 ears, safety/efficacy not established.

Renal Impairment: CrCl (mL/min), 30-50, 500mg ceftolozane/250mg tazobactam 8-hourly; 15-29, 250mg ceftolozane/125mg tazobactam 8-hourly; ESRD on haemodialysis, single loading of 500mg ceftolozane/250mg tazobactam, then 100mg ceftolozane/50mg tazobactam 8-hourly; admin as early as possible after haemodialysis on dialysis days.

Hepatic Impairment: No adjustment.

Interactions: Effect of Other Drugs on Ceftolozane, Tazobactam: *Tazobactam levels increased:* Active substrates inhibiting OAT1 or OAT3 (probenecid).

SP: Patients (immunocompromised, severe neutropenia) excluded from clinical trials.

Pregnancy, Lactation: Pregnancy, if benefit outweighs risk. Lactation, stop drug or stop breastfeeding.

ADR: Summary, *most common,* nausea, headache, constipation, diarrhoea, pyrexia.

Notes: See 9.1.2 Cephalosporins.

▼ **Zerbaxa Parenteral** *1g/0.5g (MSD)* A. HOS.
Price, (10) €891.75 (PTW).
Infusion, ceftolozane sulfate 1g, tazobactam sodium 0.5g. White (yellowish) powder for conc for soln. *Sodium 230mg/vial.*

Ceftriaxone

ATC Code: J01DD04. **Sport:** Permitted.
Driving: Caution. Dizziness.
Indications: See Dose below.

Dose: Adult, Elderly: Age 12 years and over, (50kg and above), 1-2g* (community-acquired pneumonia, acute exacerbations of COPD, intra-abdominal infections, complicated UTI); 2g* (hospital-acquired pneumonia, complicated skin and soft tissue infections, bone and joint infections); 2-4g*(neutropenics with fever, bacterial endocarditis/meningitis). *dosed once daily; consider twice daily (12-hourly) admin with doses above 2g/day.

Acute otitis media, 1-2g as single IM dose or 1-2g for 3 days if severely ill. Pre-operative prophylaxis, single 2g dose. Gonorrhoea, single 500mg IM dose. Syphilis, 500mg-1g once daily increased to 2g once daily for neurosyphilis for

10-14 days. Disseminated Lyme borreliosis, 2g once daily for 14-21 days.

For IM admin the solvent used is lidocaine; NOT for IV admin; deep IM injection, max. 1g per injection site. Diluents containing calcium should not be used for reconstitution or dilution as precipitate can form. IV admin can be by IV infusion (over minimum 30 minutes; preferred route) or by slow IV injection over 5 minutes.

Child: Age 15 days to 12 years (under 50kg), 50-80mg/kg* (intra-abdominal infections, complicated UT, community-acquired and nosocomial pneumonia); 50-100mg/kg* (skin and soft tissue, bones and joint infections, neutropenics with fever); 80-100mg/kg* (bacterial meningitis); 100mg/kg* (bacterial endocarditis). *Dosed once daily; twice daily (12-hourly) admin may be considered with doses above 2g/day; max. 4g.

Acute otitis media, 50mg/kg as single IM dose or 50mg/kg for 3 days if severely ill. Pre-operative prophylaxis, single 50-80mg/kg dose pre-operatively. Syphilis, 75-100mg/kg (max. 4g) once daily for 10-14 days. Disseminated Lyme borreliosis, 50-80mg/kg once daily for 14-21 days.

Neonates (0-14 days), 20-50mg/kg once daily (all infections except bacterial meningitis/endocarditis); 50mg/kg once daily (bacterial meningitis/endocarditis). Acute otitis media, single 50mg/kg IM dose; pre-operative prophylaxis, single 20-50mg/kg pre-operatively. Syphilis, 50mg/kg once daily for 10-14 days.

Renal Impairment: CrCl (mL/min) 10, max. 2g/day. Severe, with hepatic impairment, monitor plasma levels.

Hepatic Impairment: Severe, as for Renal above.

CI: Premature neonates (up to postmenstrual age 41 weeks) or full-term neonates (up to 28 days) with jaundice or are hypoalbuminaemic or acidotic (bilirubin encephalopathy risk), OR if IV calcium treatment is needed or calcium-containing infusion is needed (risk of ceftriaxone-calcium precipitation). Exclude lidocaine contraindications before IM if using lidocaine as solvent; solns containing lidocaine are not for IV admin.

Interactions: Effect of Other Drugs on Ceftriaxone: *Possible calcium-ceftriaxone precipitates (lungs, kidneys in premature/newborn) with ceftriaxone IV:* Calcium-containing IV solns (see Contraindications). No reports of interaction between ceftriaxone and oral calcium-containing products or between ceftriaxone IM and calcium-containing products (IV or oral).

Effect of Ceftriaxone on Other Drugs: Oral anticoagulants: *Monitor INR.*

SP: Severe (cutaneous reactions, haemolytic anaemia; including fatal). Long-term treatment, perform complete blood counts regularly. Shadows mistaken for gallstones detected by gallbladder sonograms, usually at 1g/day and above; disappear on discontinuation. Pancreatitis, biliary obstruction. Presence of ceftriaxone may falsely lower estimated blood glucose values (some monitoring systems). Ceftriaxone precipitation in urinary tract; mostly children, treated with high doses, with other risk factors (dehydration, confined to bed). Caution, hyperbilirubinaemic neonates, see Contraindications (CI) above. IM admin without lidocaine is painful.

ADR: Summary, *most frequent,* eosinophilia, leucopenia, thrombocytopenia, diarrhoea, rash, increased liver enzymes.

Notes: See 9.1.2 Cephalosporins.

Rocephin Parenteral IM 1g, IM/IV 1g *(Roche)* A. GMS.
Price, (1) IM 1g, €14.42. IM/IV 1g, €14.41. HOS: IM 1g, €8.28 (PTW).
IM injection (not for IV admin), ceftriaxone sodium 1g. White (yellowish-orange) crystalline powder; clear colourless solvent (contains lidocaine HCl) for IM injection. *Sodium 3.6mmol/1g.*
Injection or infusion, as above. White (yellowish-orange powder).

Cefuroxime

ATC Code: J01DC02. **Sport:** Permitted.
Driving: Unlikely to affect.
Indications: Mild to moderately severe, upper RTI (acute otitis media, sinusitis, tonsillitis, pharyngitis); acute bronchitis including acute exacerbations, pneumonia), UTI (lower uncomplicated, cystitis), skin and soft tissue

237

9.1.2 Cephalosporins, Carbepenems, Monobactams, Other Cephalosporins

(furunculosis, pyoderma, impetigo), early Lyme disease and prevention of late complications. Sequential therapy, gonorrhoea. Surgical prophylaxis (abdominal, orthopaedic), meningitis, septicaemia.

Dose: Adult, Elderly: ORAL, *RTI, skin soft tissue,* 250-500mg twice daily; *UTI,* 125-250mg twice daily; *Lyme disease,* 500mg twice daily for 20 days. *Uncomplicated gonorrhoea,* 1g as single dose.

Sequential therapy, pneumonia, 1.5g IV or IM 2-3 times daily for 48-72 hours; then 500mg orally twice daily for 7-10 days. *Acute exacerbations of chronic bronchitis,* 750mg IV or IM for 48-72 hours; then 500mg orally twice daily for 5-10 days. Admin after food.

PARENTERAL (IV injection over 3-5 minutes OR IV infusion over 30-60 minutes OR deep IM injection; doses above 1.5g, use IV route), usually 750mg IM or IV, 3-times daily; range 1.5-6g/day in divided doses. *Gonorrhoea,* 1.5g IM as single dose at 2 different sites; *meningitis,* 3g IV 8-hourly.

Surgical prophylaxis, 1.5g IV with induction of anaesthesia; 750mg IM 8-16 hours later if required in abdominal, pelvic, orthopaedic surgery OR 3-times daily for 24-48 hours in cardiac, pulmonary, oesophageal, vascular. *Joint replacement,* 1.5g powder mixed dry with cement before adding liquid monomer.

Child: ORAL, (3 months and over), usually 125mg OR 10mg/kg twice daily; max. 250mg/day; (age 2 years and older), otitis media, severe infections, 250mg OR 15mg/kg twice daily; max. 500mg/day. Under 5 years, use oral susp.

PARENTERAL, range 30-100mg/kg in divided doses; usually 60mg/kg. *Meningitis,* infants and children, 200-240mg/kg/day IV in 3-4 divided doses; reduce to 100mg/kg/day after 3 days or when clinical improvement; neonates, initially 100mg/kg/day reduced to 50mg/kg/day as above.

Renal Impairment: GFR (mL/min) 10-20, 500mg twice daily; below 10, 750mg once daily. Haemodialysis, additional 750mg IV or IM at end of each dialysis; peritoneal dialysis, 250mg/2L dialysis fluid; continuous peritoneal dialysis, 750mg twice daily; high flux haemofiltration, 750mg twice daily; low flux as for renal impairment above.

Hepatic Impairment: Not recommended.

Interactions: Effect of Other Drugs on Cefuroxime: *Lower bioavailability*: Drugs reducing gastric acidity.

SP: Reserve parenteral use for serious or severe infection. Jarisch-Herxheimer reaction reported following treatment of Lyme disease. Meningitis, mild to moderate hearing loss. Avoid admixture with other IV medications.

ADR: Summary, *most common,* eosinophilia, increased LFTs*; neutropenia, increased bilirubin* (parenteral); Candida overgrowth, headache, dizziness, GI disturbances. *(with pre-existing liver disease).

Notes: See 9.1.2 Cephalosporins.

Zinacef Parenteral *(GSK)* A. GMS.
Price, injection (5) 250mg, €5.53. 750mg, €16.56. Non-GMS, (IV) injection or infusion 1.5g, €7.22.
Injection, cefuroxime sodium 250(750)mg. White (cream) powder.
Injection or infusion, as above 1.5g. White (cream) powder.

Zinnat 125mg, 250mg 500mg, Oral Susp *(GSK)* A. GMS.
Price, tabs (14) 125mg, €1.90. 250mg, €4.73. 500mg, €8.99.
Susp (70mL) 125mg/5mL, €5.30. 250mg/5mL, €5.11.
Tablet, cefuroxime axetil. White (off-white) f/c cap-shaped. Marked GXE. 125mg: Marked S5. 250mg: Marked S7. 500mg: Marked G2. *Parabens.*
Oral susp, as above 125 (250)mg/5mL. Contains white (off-white) free-flowing granules. *Sucrose, aspartame.*

Ceftal 250mg, 500mg *(Rowex)* A. GMS.
Price, (14) 250mg, €4.63. 500mg, €8.80.
Tablet, cefuroxime axetil. White round f/c. *Mannitol, aspartame.*

Cefuroxime Parenteral *(Flynn)* A.
Price, (vial x 10) 500mg, €23.20. 1.5g, €28.00.
Injection, cefuroxime sodium 750mg (1.5g). White powder for susp/soln. *Sodium 40.6mg(81.3mg)/vial.*

Cefuroxime TEVA 250mg, 500mg *(TEVA)* A. GMS.
Price, (14) 250mg, €4.63. 500mg, €8.48.
Tablet, cefuroxime axetil. Light-blue f/c. Marked with strength. 250mg: Marked P125. 500mg: Marked P126.

Cephalexin

ATC Code: J01DB01. **Sport:** Permitted.
Driving: None known.

Indications: RTI, otitis media, skin and soft tissue, bone and joint, GU including acute prostatitis, dental infections.

Dose: Adult, Elderly: Oral, range 1-4g/day in divided doses; usually 500mg 8-hourly. *Skin and soft tissue,* streptococcal pharyngitis, uncomplicated UTI, usually 250mg 6-hourly OR 500mg 12-hourly. *Severe* infection, max. 4g/day; consider parenteral treatment.

Child: Usually 25-50mg/kg in divided doses; under 5 years, 125mg 8-hourly; age 5 years and over, 250mg 8-hourly. Severe infection, double dosage. Otitis media, 75-100mg/kg/day in 4 divided doses. Treat beta-haemolytic streptococcal infections for 10 days.

Renal Impairment: Severe, caution. Dialysis, max. 500mg/day.

Notes: See 9.1.2 Cephalosporins.

Keflex 250mg, 500mg, Susp *(Flynn)* A. GMS.D*.
Price, caps 250mg* (28) €2.03; (100) €15.12. Tabs 500mg* (21) €2.89; (100) €29.58. Susp (100mL) 125mg/5mL, €0.99. 250mg/5mL*, €1.94.
Capsule, cephalexin monohydrate 250mg. Hard green/white. Marked GP1.
Tablet, as above 500mg. Peach f/c scored (facilitates breaking) pillow-shaped. Marked GP4.
Powder for oral suspension, as above 125 (250)mg/5mL. White free flowing. *Sucrose.*

Ertapenem

ATC Code: J01DH03. **Sport:** Permitted.
Driving: Dizziness, somnolence.

Indications: Treatment, community-acquired pneumonia, intra-abdominal, acute gynaecological, skin and soft tissue and diabetic foot infections. Infection prophylaxis following elective colorectal surgery.

Dose: Adult, Elderly: Treatment, 1g once daily. Prophylaxis, 1g as single IV dose 1 hour prior to surgical incision. IV infusion over 30 minutes; usually 3-14 days. *Elderly,* as for Renal below.

Child: Treatment, age 3 months to 12 years, 15mg/kg twice daily; max. 1g/day; age 13-17 years, as for Adult above.

Renal Impairment: Severe or haemodialysis, not recommended.

Interactions: Effect of Ertapenem on Other Drugs: Valproic acid/sodium valproate: *Co-admin not recommended; valproic acid levels decreased; inadequate seizure control.*

SP: Serious anaphylactic reactions require immediate emergency treatment. Seizures, caution elderly, pre-existing CNS disorders (brain lesions, seizure history).

Pregnancy, Lactation: Pregnancy, if benefit outweighs risk. Lactation, not recommended.

ADR: *Common,* headache, infused vein complication, phlebitis, thrombophlebitis, diarrhoea, nausea, vomiting, rash, pruritus; diaper dermatitis, infusion site pain, elevated ALT/AST/ALP, increased platelets, decreased neutrophils.

Notes: See 9.1.2 Cephalosporins.

Invanz Parenteral *(MSD)* A.
Price, (1) €52.94.
Infusion, ertapenem sodium 1g. White (off-white) powder for conc for soln. *Sodium 137mg/1g.*

Meropenem

ATC Code: J01DH02. **Sport:** Permitted.
Driving: Headache, paraesthesiae, convulsions reported.

Indications: See Dose below.

Dose: Adult, Elderly: Severe pneumonia (including hospital and ventilator-associated), complicated (UTI, intra-abdominal, skin and soft tissue), intra/post-partum infections, 500mg or 1g 8-hourly. Broncho-pulmonary infections associated with cystic fibrosis, acute bacterial meningitis, 2g 8-hourly. Febrile neutropenics, 1g 8-hourly. Up to 2g 3-times daily (adults, adolescents) and up to 40mg/kg 3-times daily (children) may be needed with infections due to less susceptible bacterial species

(Enterobacteriaceae, *Pseudomonas aeruginosa,* Acinetobacter spp.) or very severe infections. Admin usually by IV infusion over 15-30 minutes OR doses of 1g (20mg/kg in children) may be given by IV bolus over approx. 5 minutes; limited data to support 2g dose (40mg/kg in children) by IV bolus. *Elderly,* as for Renal below.

Child: Age 3 months to 11 years (up to 50kg), severe pneumonia, complicated (UTI, intra-abdominal, skin and soft tissue) infections, 10 or 20mg/kg 8-hourly. Bronchopulmonary infections (CF), acute bacterial meningitis, 40mg/kg 8-hourly. Management, febrile neutropenics, 20mg/kg 8-hourly. Over 50kg, as for Adult above. *Under 3 months,* limited data suggest 20mg/kg 8-hourly may be appropriate. Admin by IV bolus over 5 minutes (doses up to 20mg/kg) or IV infusion over 15-30 minutes, see Adult.

Renal Impairment: CrCl (mL/min) 26-50, one unit dose (as for Adult) 12-hourly; 10-25, half unit dose 12-hourly; below 10, half unit dose 24-hourly. Haemodialysis, admin unit dose on completion. Children, no data.

Hepatic Impairment: Monitor function, hepatic toxicity risk (cholestasis, cytolysis). Children, no data.

Interactions: Effect of Meropenem on Other Drugs: Valproic acid, sodium valproate, valpromide: *Co-admin not recommended; valproic acid levels rapidly/extensively decreased.*

SP: Caution, monotherapy in *Pseudomonas aeruginosa* lower RTI infection. Not recommended for use for MRSA.

ADR: Summary, *most frequent,* diarrhoea, rash, nausea/vomiting, injection-site inflammation; *laboratory,* thrombocytosis, increased hepatic enzymes.

Notes: See 9.1.2 Cephalosporins.

Meronem Parenteral 500mg, 1g *(AstraZeneca)* A. HOS. *Price,* (10) 500mg, €136.11. 1g, €241.14 (PTW). *Injection or infusion,* meropenem trihydrate. White (light-yellow) powder for soln.

Meroponia Parenteral 500mg, 1g *(Clonmel)* A. *Price,* not published by company. *Injection or infusion,* meropenem trihydrate. White (light-yellow) powder for soln. *Sodium 45mg(90mg)/500mg(1g) vial.*

9.1.3 - Aminoglycosides

In This Chapter: *Amikacin, gentamicin, tobramycin.*

Class Effects
CI: Hypersensitivity to any member of the class. Use with other nephrotoxic or ototoxic drugs.

Interactions: Effect of Other Drugs on Aminoglycosides: *Increased toxicity risk, co-admin caution:* Other nephro- or ototoxic drugs (bacitracin, cisplatin, amphotericin B, ciclosporin, tacrolimus, paromomycin, viomycin, colistin, vancomycin, other aminoglycosides), diuretics (rapidly acting, especially IV; frusemide, etacrynic acid), cephalosporins (especially cephaloridine), fludarabine; polymyxins (nephrotoxicity), platinum compounds (oto- and nephrotoxicity). *Co-admin caution (neuromuscular blockade, paralysis):* Anaesthetics or muscle relaxants (halothane, d-tubocurarine, succinylcholine, decamethonium), botulinum toxin. *Increased plasma levels (neonates):* Indomethacin. *Reduced activity, co-admin (with renal impairment):* Penicillin-type drugs. *Synergism:* Penicillin. *Possible cross-sensitivity:* Kanamycin. *Should not be physically mixed:* Penicillin.

Effect of Aminoglycosides on Other Drugs: Oral anticoagulants: *Increased hypoprothrombinaemic effect.* Botulinum toxin: *Increased toxicity risk (enhanced neuromuscular block).* Bisphosphonates: *Increased hypocalcaemia risk.* Neostigmine, pyridostigmine: *Antagonism.* Thiamine (vitamin B1): *May be destroyed by sodium bisulfate (in amikacin sulfate formulations).*

SP: NOTE: Aminoglycosides should not be mixed with any other drug in same syringe prior to admin. Ensure adequate hydration. Ototoxicity, especially with renal impairment, infants, possibly elderly; vestibular, auditory function, monitor (during, after) treatment. Subclinical renal or 8th nerve damage induced by prior nephro or ototoxic drugs (streptomycin, dihydrostreptomycin, gentamicin,

tobramycin, kanamycin, neomycin, polymyxin B, colistin, cephaloridine), caution (additive toxicity); use only if benefit outweighs risk. Neuromuscular disorders (Parkinson's disease), conditions characterised by myasthenia (myasthenia gravis), muscle weakness may be aggravated due to potential curare-like effect on neuromuscular function. *Clostridium difficile* associated diarrhoea, see Notes below. Caution, premature and neonatal infants because of renal immaturity (prolonged of serum half-life).

Pregnancy, Lactation: Pregnancy, if benefit outweighs risk/considered essential by physician; can cause foetal harm. Crosses placenta with reports of total irreversible bilateral congenital deafness in children where mothers received streptomycin during pregnancy. Lactation, if benefit outweighs risk unless specified.

ADR: Blood dyscrasias, anaemia, pancytopenia, electrolyte disturbances including hypomagnesaemia, allergic reactions, anaphylaxis, ototoxicity, vestibular damage, tinnitus, headache; neuromuscular blockade; central neurotoxicity (encephalopathy, convulsions, confusion, hallucinations, mental depression), nausea, vomiting, stomatitis, pseudomembranous colitis, liver dysfunction, nephrotoxicity, renal failure, tubular necrosis, interstitial nephritis, rash, pruritus, urticaria. Retinal toxicity with intravitreal injection.

Notes: See Class Effects 9.1 Antibacterials.

Amikacin
ATC Code: J01GB06. **Sport:** Permitted.
Driving: Some adverse events may impair.

Indications: Infections due to sensitive Gram-negative organisms.

Dose: Adult: 15mg/kg/day in 1-2 equally divided doses; max. 1.5g by IM or IV route; endocarditis, febrile neutropenia, dose twice daily. *Life-threatening* infection, pseudomonal, 500mg 8-hourly; max. 10 days; max. 1.5g/day (total 15g). *UTI,* 7.5mg/kg in 2 equally divided doses (equiv. to 250mg twice daily); activity enhanced by increased urinary pH (urinary alkaliniser may be co-admin). *Other routes,* 0.25% irrigation soln for abscess cavities, pleural space, peritoneum.

Elderly: As for Renal below.

Child: Age 4 weeks to 12 years, IM or slow IV infusion, 15-20mg/kg/day as single daily dose or as 7.5mg/kg 12-hourly; endocarditis, febrile neutropenia, as for Adult above. Age 12 years and over, as for Adult above. *Neonates,* initially 10mg/kg followed by 7.5mg/kg 12-hourly; premature infants, 7.5mg/kg 12-hourly. Infuse over 30-60 minutes; infants, infuse over 1-2 hours.

Renal Impairment: CrCl below 50mL/min, use either normal doses at prolonged intervals or reduced doses at fixed intervals.

SP: Not recommended for intraperitoneal use in young children, patients under anaesthesia or with muscle relaxing drugs.

Notes: See Class Effects 9.1.3 Aminoglycosides.

Amikin Parenteral *(BMS)* A. GMS. *Price,* 50mg/mL 2mL (5) €13.13. *Injection,* amikacin sulfate 50mg/mL. Clear colourless soln. *Sodium 3mg/vial, sodium metabisulphite.*

Gentamicin (systemic)
ATC Code: J01GB03. **Sport:** Permitted.
Driving: Unlikely to impair.

Indications: Treatment, systemic infections due to susceptible bacteria (bacteraemia, septicaemia, UTI, severe chest infections). Severe neonatal infections *(Cidomycin).*

Dose: Adult: Systemic infections, 3-6mg/kg/day as 1 single dose (preferred) up to 2 single doses. Usually IM admin; can be given IV (over 3 minutes or short infusion); divided doses 6-8 hourly; max. 6mg/kg/24-hours. Caution, significant obesity; gentamicin is poorly distributed in fatty tissue; monitor serum levels, consider dose reduction; calculate on lean body weight.

Elderly: As for Renal below.

Child: Infants after first month of life, 4.5-7.5mg/kg/day

9.1.4 Macrolides

as 1 (preferred) up to 2 single doses; newborns, 4-7mg/kg/day as single dose; children, as for Adult above.
Renal Impairment: CrCl (mL/min) above 70, 80mg 8-hourly; 30-70, 80mg 12-hourly; 10-30, 80mg 24-hourly; 5-10, 80mg 48-hourly. Twice weekly intermittent haemodialysis, GFR (mL/min) below 5, 80mg after dialysis. Body weight under 60kg, admin 60mg instead of 80mg. Gentamicin is dialysable.
Hepatic Impairment: Caution, liver disease can be a risk factor for nephrotoxicity.
CI: Myasthenia gravis.
Pregnancy, Lactation: Pregnancy, use only in life-threatening circumstances. Lactation, in absence of GI inflammation, amount ingested in breast milk unlikely to produce significant blood levels in infant.
Notes: See Class Effects 9.1.3 Aminoglycosides.

Cidomycin Paed Parenteral *(SANOFI)* A. GMS.
Price, 10mg/mL, 2mL (5) €4.31.
Injection, gentamicin sulfate equiv. to gentamicin base 10mg/mL. Clear colourless soln. *Sodium below 23mg/2mL vial*. **Store:** Below 25 deg C; do not (refrigerate, freeze).

Genticin Parenteral 80mg/2mL *(Concordia)* A. GMS.
Price, 40mg/mL 2mL (10) €16.52.
Injection, gentamicin sulfate equiv. to 4% gentamicin base. Clear colourless (pale-yellow) soln. *Preservative free.*

Tobramycin

ATC Code: J01GB01. **Sport:** Permitted.
Driving: No or negligible effect.
Indications: Cystic fibrosis (CF) (6 years and older), long-term management of chronic pulmonary infection due to *Pseudomonas aeruginosa* (nebuliser), or suppressive therapy of (Podhaler).
Dose: Adult: 300mg *(nebuliser)* OR 112mg *(Podhaler)* admin twice daily (12-hourly intervals) for 28 days + standard care; then stop for 28 days with standard care only (cycle 1). Admin for 3 cycles. *Admin*, nebuliser for inhalation only over 15 minutes; NOT for parenteral use. Podhaler for oral inhalation using Podhaler device; caps NOT to be swallowed. Where several different inhaled medicinals and chest physiotherapy used, use Podhaler last.
Elderly: As for Renal below.
Child: Over 6 years, as for Adult above. Under 6 years, no data.
Renal Impairment: Caution, nephrotoxicity; discontinue until trough serum below 2mcg/mL.
Interactions: Effect of Other Drugs on Tobramycin: *Inhaled*: *Co-admin contraindicated*: Diuretics (etacrynic acid, furosemide), urea, mannitol IV.
SP: Auditory, vestibular dysfunction, caution; patients with hearing loss frequently reported tinnitus; modest hypoacusis, vertigo. Bronchospasm following inhalation. Cough induced by nebulised solns; active severe haemoptysis, use only if benefit outweighs risk.
ADR: Summary, *most common* cough, dysphonia *(Tobi, Bramitob)*; productive cough, pyrexia, dyspnoea, oropharyngeal pain, haemoptysis *(Tobi Podhaler, Nebuliser Soln)*; pharyngitis, asthenia, rhinitis, lung disorder, headache, chest pain, discoloured sputum, anorexia, decreased pulmonary function test, asthma, vomiting, abdominal pain, nausea, weight loss *(Tobi Nebuliser Soln)*.
Notes: See Class Effects 9.1.3 Aminoglycosides.

Tobi Nebuliser, Podhaler *(Novartis)* A. HT.
Price, amps 300mg/5mL (56) €1964.16. Podhaler (5) + 224 caps (28mg) €2357.24.
Nebuliser soln, tobramycin 300mg/5mL. Clear slightly yellow. *Inhalation powder*, as above (28mg cap). Clear colourless hard; contains white powder. Marked NVR AVCI and logo.

Bramitob Nebuliser *(Chiesi)* A. HT.
Price, 56 amps, €1799.53.
Nebuliser soln, tobramycin 300mg/4mL. Clear yellowish. **Store:** Refrigerate.

9.1.4 - Macrolides

In This Chapter: *Azithromycin, clarithromycin, erythromycin.*

240

Class Effects

CI: Hypersensitivity to any member of the class including ketolides. QT-prolongation (congenital or family history) or hypokalaemia.
Interactions: Effect of Other Drugs on Macrolides: *Co-admin contraindicated*: Ergot derivatives (ergotamine or dihydroergotamine); acute ergot toxicity; vasospasm, ischaemia of extremities and other tissues including CNS).
Effect of Macrolides on Other Drugs: Lovastatin, simvastatin, atorvastatin: *Co-admin contraindicated; increased rhabdomyolysis risk (consider using fluvastatin; not CYP3A dependent)*. Drugs metabolised by CYP450 (cilostazol, carbamazepine, methylprednisolone, sildenafil, alprazolam, triazolam, midazolam, phenytoin, ciclosporin, tacrolimus, vinblastine, valproate, cisapride, omeprazole, pimozide, terfenadine, astemizole, hexobarbital, alfentanil, bromocriptine, zopiclone): *Co-admin caution, increased plasma levels.* Theophylline, carbamazepine: *Increased circulating levels.* Oral anticoagulants (warfarin): *Monitor prothrombin time.* Rifabutin: *Plasma levels increased, neutropenia risk.* Digoxin: *Monitor serum levels.* Zidovudine: *Plasma levels decreased due to absorption interference (stagger dosing with clarithromycin).* Quinidine, disopyramide: *Torsade de Pointes risk.* Colchicine: *Increased exposure, toxicity risk, monitor.* Insulin, other oral hypoglycaemic agents (sulphonylureas): *Caution, hypoglycaemia.* Sildenafil, tadalafil, vardenafil, tolterodine (in CYP2D6 poor metabolisers): *Consider dose reduction.*
SP: Caution, possible cross-resistance (other macrolides, lincomycin, clindamycin). Rare serious allergic reactions, angioedema, anaphylaxis. Presence/history of prolonged cardiac repolarisation and QT-interval (congenital or documented) or ventricular cardiac arrhythmia (Torsades de Pointes), caution. Caution, impaired renal or hepatic function, co-admin with hepatotoxic drugs (excreted primarily by liver). *Myasthenia gravis*, weakness may be exacerbated (erythromycin, clarithromycin); acute respiratory failure with rapid onset, caution (telithromycin). *Clostridium difficile* associated diarrhoea, see Notes below.
Pregnancy, Lactation: Pregnancy, lactation, use only if benefit outweighs risk.
Notes: See 9.1 Antibacterials.

Azithromycin (systemic)

ATC Code: J01FA10. **Sport:** Permitted.
Driving: No evidence to suggest an effect.
Indications: Treatment of bacterial infections including bronchitis, community-acquired pneumonia, sinusitis, pharyngitis/tonsillitis, otitis media, skin and soft tissue infections, uncomplicated genital infections (*Chlamydia trachomatis, Neisseria gonorrhoeae*).
Dose: Adult: Adult, elderly, children over 45kg, 500mg once daily for 3 days. *Genital infections*, single 1g oral dose (*Chlamydia trachomatis*) or 2g as single oral dose (with ceftriaxone 500mg IM as single dose) (*Neisseria gonorrhoeae*). *Elderly*, caution, presence of proarrhythmic conditions; cardiac arrhythmia, Torsades de Pointes risk. *Admin*, oral as single daily dose 1 hour before or 2 hours after food *(Zithromax)* OR with/without food *(all other brands)*; susp can be taken with food.
Child: Under 45kg (caps not suitable; use susp), 10mg/kg/day as a single dose for 3 days (under 6 months, no data). Up to 15kg, measure dose using 10mL oral dosing syringe (graduated in 0.25mL divisions providing 10mg in every graduation). Weight 15-25kg (3-7 years), 200mg/day (3 days); 26-35kg (8-11 years), 300mg/day; 36-45kg (12-14 years), 400mg/day; over 45kg, as for Adult above. *Admin*, as single daily dose; susp can be taken with food.
Renal Impairment: GFR (mL/min) below 10, caution (33% increase in systemic exposure).
Hepatic Impairment: Severe, not recommended.
CI: Hypersensitivity to other macrolides or ketolides.
Interactions: Effect of Other Drugs on Azithromycin: *Co-admin not recommended*: Antacids (admin 1 hour before or 2 hours after antacid).
SP: Dermatological reactions (Stevens Johnson Syndrome,

toxic epidermal necrolysis, DRESS). Caution with significant hepatic disease; fulminant hepatitis with potential life-threatening liver failure. Infantile hypertrophic pyloric stenosis reported with use in neonates (up to 42 days of life). Prevention or treatment of Mycobacterium Avium Complex in children (safety/efficacy not established). Azithromycin is generally effective against oropharyngeal streptococci; efficacy in preventing acute rheumatic fever (no data).

Pregnancy, Lactation: Pregnancy, if benefit outweighs risk. Lactation, reported to be secreted in human breast milk.

ADR: Very common, diarrhoea.

Notes: See Class Effects 9.1.4 Macrolides.

Zithromax 250mg, Susp (Pfizer) A. GMS.
Price, caps 250mg (4) €5.09; (6) €8.72. Susp 200mg/5mL (15mL) €4.59; (22.5mL) €7.00.
Capsule, azithromycin dihydrate. Hard gelatin white. Marked Pfizer ZTM 250. Lactose.
Oral susp, as above 200mg/5mL. Dry white powder. Sucrose.
Store: Below 30 deg C (dry powder); below 25 deg C (reconstituted); do not (refrigerate, freeze).
Azithromycin Actavis 250mg (Accord) A. GMS.
Price, (6) €6.97.
Tablet, azithromycin dihydrate. White (off-white) f/c oval. Marked with strength. Lactose.
Azithromycin Clonmel 250mg (Clonmel) A. GMS.
Price, (6) €6.97.
Tablet, azithromycin monohydrate. White (off-white) oblong f/c. Soya lecithin.
Azithromycin Krka 250mg (Krka) A. GMS.
Price, (6) €6.97.
Tablet, azithromycin dihydrate. White (almost) cap-shaped f/c. Marked S19.
Azithromycin TEVA 250mg (TEVA) A. GMS.
Price, (6) €6.97.
Tablet, azithromycin dihydrate. White oblong. Marked AI250.
Azromax 250mg (Gerard) A. GMS.
Price, (6) €6.97.
Tablet, azithromycin monohydrate. White (off-white) elongated f/c. Soya lecithin.

Clarithromycin

ATC Code: J01FA09. **Sport:** Permitted.
Driving: Dizziness, vertigo, confusion, disorientation.
Indications: Bronchitis, pneumonia, pharyngitis/tonsillitis, sinusitis; skin and soft tissue infections. H. pylori eradication (with acid suppression). Treatment, localised or disseminated Mycobacterium infection; prophylaxis, disseminated in HIV patients.

Dose: Adult, Elderly: ORAL, STANDARD/R, most infections, 250mg twice daily; severe 500mg twice daily for 6-14 days. Mycobacterial infection, 500mg twice daily; disseminated infections (AIDS patients), continue as long as there is microbiological benefit.
H. pylori eradication, dual therapy* (14 days), 500mg 3-times daily + PPI; triple therapy (7 days), 500mg twice daily + PPI + amoxicillin 1g twice daily OR (7 days) 500mg twice daily + PPI + metronidazole 400mg twice daily OR (7-10 days), 500mg twice daily + amoxicillin 1g twice daily + omeprazole 20mg twice daily. *Not all brands have this dosing regimen (e.g. Klacid).
MODIFIED/R, PROLONGED/R, 500mg once daily; severe infection, 2x 500mg tabs as single dose once daily at same time. Usually 6-14 days. Swallow tabs whole, do not crush or chew; with food.
PARENTERAL, usually 1g/day in 2 divided doses. IV infusion over 60 minutes; not for IV bolus or IM injection.
Child: ORAL, STANDARD/R, under 12 years, use paed susp (dose based on 7.5mg/kg twice daily; severe infection, up to 500mg twice daily); age 1-2 years (8-11kg), 62.5mg*; age 3-6 years (12-19kg), 125mg*; age 7-9 years (20-29kg), 187.5mg*; age 10-12 years (30-40kg), 250mg*; over 12 years, as for Adult above. Under 12 years or body weight under 30kg, solid Standard/R, Prolonged/R and Parenteral formulations, not recommended. *(twice daily)
Renal Impairment: CrCl (mL/min) 30-60, no adjustment; below 30, 250mg once daily; severe infection, max. 250mg Standard/R twice daily OR 500mg Prolonged/R once daily; usually 6 to max. 14 days. Paediatric below 30, reduce dose by one-half. Co-admin with ritonavir or atazanavir or

saquinavir and clarithromycin 500mg 12-hourly, CrCl (mL/min) 30-60, reduce clarithromycin dose by 50%; under 30, reduce by 75%.
Hepatic Impairment: Mild/moderate or co-admin with hepatotoxic drugs, caution. Severe (with renal impairment), contraindicated. Paediatric, as for Renal above.
CI: QT-prolongation (congenital, documented acquired) ventricular cardiac arrhythmia including Torsades de Pointes, hypokalaemia.
Interactions: Effect of Other Drugs on Clarithromycin: Co-admin contraindicated: Cisapride, pimozide, terfenadine, astemizole (QT-prolongation); ergotamine, dihydroergotamine (ergot toxicity), statins* (simvastatin, lovastatin); colchicine (elderly and/or with renal impairment), ticagrelor, ranolazine. Co-admin caution: IV or oromucosal midazolam, triazolam, verapamil, amlodipine, diltiazem. Plasma levels decreased (adjust dose or consider alternative): Efavirenz, nevirapine, rifampicin, rifabutin, rifapentine; known or suspected to be metabolised by CYP3A (alprazolam, astemizole, carbamazepine, cilostazol, cisapride, ciclosporin, disopyramide, ergot alkaloids, lovastatin, methylprednisolone, midazolam, omeprazole, oral anticoagulants (warfarin), quetiapine, pimozide, quinidine, rifabutin, sildenafil, simvastatin, sirolimus, tacrolimus, terfenadine, triazolam, vinblastine); CYP3A inducers (rifampicin, phenytoin, carbamazepine, phenobarbital, St John's Wort). Co-admin (monitor for increased or prolonged effect): Itraconazole. Co-admin, see Renal Impairment above: Ritonavir, atazanavir (bi-directional drug interaction), saquinavir. Use alternative for treating Mycobacterium avium complex (MAC) with co-admin: Etravirine. *If required use fluvastatin.
Effect of Clarithromycin on Other Drugs: Digoxin, phenytoin, valproate, quinidine, disopyramide: Monitor levels. Rifabutin: Increased plasma levels, increased uveitis risk. Nateglinide, repaglinide: Careful glucose monitoring. Sildenafil, tadalafil, vardenafil, theophylline, carbamazepine, tolterodine: Increased exposure; consider dose reduction. Zidovudine (tablets): Allow 4-hour dosing interval.
SP: Signs/symptoms of hepatitis, (anorexia, jaundice, dark urine, pruritus, tender abdomen), discontinue. Signs, acute hypersensitivity. QT-prolongation or hypokalaemia, use not recommended (see Notes below). Sensitivity testing, to be performed for community-acquired pneumonia (emerging Streptococcus pneumoniae resistance), nosocomial pneumonia (use in combination), skin and soft tissue infections (mild/moderate) (Staphylococcus aureus, Streptococcus pyogenes both resistant to macrolides).
Pregnancy, Lactation: Pregnancy, careful risk/benefit (especially first trimester). Lactation, is excreted in human milk; safety not established.
ADR: Summary, most frequent and common (adult, paediatric), abdominal pain, diarrhoea, nausea, vomiting, taste perversion. Parenteral, very common, injection site phlebitis.
Notes: See Class Effects 9.1.4 Macrolides.
Interchangeability: Same strengths of all brands of clarithromycin Standard/R film-coated (f/c) tabs and Prolonged/Modified Release tabs listed below are deemed interchangeable.
Reference Price: (14) 250mg, €2.97; 500mg, €5.94. Prolonged/R (7) 500mg, €6.11.
Klacid 250mg, Forte/LA, Susp/Paed (BGP) A. GMS.D*.
Price, tabs (14) 250mg*, see reference price above; Forte 500mg* €10.82. LA 500mg* (7) €6.11. Susp 125mg/5mL (70mL) €2.84; (100mL) €7.17. 250mg/5mL (70mL) €5.69.
Standard/R tablet, clarithromycin 250mg, 500mg (Forte). Yellow oval f/c. Store: Below 25 deg C.
Modified/R tablet, as above (LA) 500mg. Yellow oval f/c. Lactose, sodium 15.3mg/tab. Store: Below 30 deg C.
Oral susp, as above 125(250)mg per 5mL sachet. 250mg: White (off-white) free-flowing granules for susp; fruit odour. Sucrose 2.276g/5mL. Paed 125mg: White (off-white) granules. Sucrose 2.75g/5mL. Store: Below 25 deg C; do not refrigerate.

9.1.5 Quinolones

Klacid Parenteral 500mg *(BGP)* A.
Price, (1) €13.95 (PTW).
Infusion, clarithromycin. White (off-white) caked lyophilised powder for soln. *Sodium 0.273mg/vial.* *Store:* Below 30 deg C; outer carton to protect (light).

Clarithromycin (Ranbaxy) Tablets *(Pinewood)* A. GMS.D.
Price, see reference price above.
Tablet, clarithromycin 250mg, 500mg. Light-yellow oval f/c. 250mg: Marked C1. 500mg: Marked C2.

Clarithromycin Parenteral *(Concordia)* A.
Price, (1) €10.30 (PTW).
Infusion, clarithromycin lactobionate 2mg/mL (500mg). White crystalline powder for conc for soln.

Clarithromycin Actavis 250mg, 500mg *(Accord)* A. GMS.D.
Price, see reference price above.
Tablet, clarithromycin. Yellow oval f/c. Marked CL and strength. Glucose.

Clarithromycin TEVA 250mg, 500mg *(TEVA)* A. GMS.D.
Price, see reference price above.
Tablet, clarithromycin. Oval f/c. Marked 93. 250mg: Yellow. Marked 7157. 500mg: Light-yellow. Marked 7158. *Tartrazine, Allura Red.*

Clonocid 250mg, 500mg *(Clonmel)* A. GMS.D.
Price, see reference price above.
Tablet, clarithromycin. Light-yellow oval f/c. 250mg: Marked C1. 500mg: Scored. Marked C2.

Clorom 250mg, 500mg, XL 500mg *(Rowex)* A. GMS.D.
Price, see reference price above.
Tablet, clarithromycin. White oblong f/c scored (divisible into equal halves). *Lactose.*
Prolonged/R (XL) tablet, as above. Yellow f/c oblong. *Lactose.*

Klaram LA 500mg *(Accord)* A. GMS.D.
Price, see reference price above.
Prolonged/R tablet, clarithromycin citrate. Yellow oblong f/c. *Lactose.*

Klariger 500mg *(Gerard)* A. GMS.D.
Price, see reference price above.
Tablet, clarithromycin. Yellow oval f/c. Marked C/strength; G on reverse.

Minatev LA 500mg *(TEVA)* A. GMS.D.
Price, see reference price above.
Prolonged/R tablet, clarithromycin. Light-yellow (yellow) f/c oval. Marked C; 500 on reverse. *Lactose.*

Erythromycin (systemic)

ATC Code: J01FA01. **Sport:** Permitted.
Driving: Dizziness, blurred vision.

Indications: Prophylaxis and treatment of infections caused by erythromycin-sensitive organisms.

Dose: Adult, Elderly: ORAL, 1-2g/day; *severe*, up to 4g/day in divided doses with or without food.

PARENTERAL, *severe and immunocompromised* patients, 50mg/kg/day (adult 4g) by continuous infusion; *mild/moderate*, oral route not suitable, 25mg/kg/day. Rapid admin by direct IV injection (IV push), contraindicated; admin by continuous or intermittent IV infusion only.

Child: ORAL, (age up to 2 years), 30mg/kg/day; *severe* infections, up to 50mg/kg/day; normal dose, 125mg 4-times daily or 50mg twice daily; (age 2-8 years), as for up to 2 years; normal dose 250mg 4-times daily or 500mg twice daily; (over 8 years), as for Adult above. Daily dose given in divided doses with or without food.

PARENTERAL, as for Adult above.

Hepatic Impairment: Severe, not recommended (excreted principally by liver).

Interactions: Effect of Other Drugs on Erythromycin: *Co-admin contraindicated:* Astemizole, terfenadine, cisapride, pimozide; lovastatin, simvastatin (increased myopathy risk including rhabdomyolysis; consider fluvastatin; use lowest dose). *Co-admin not recommended:* Penicillin, cephalosporins (except where specifically warranted) *Avoid co-admin (QT-prolongation):* Antiarrhythmics Class Ia (quinidine, procainamide), Class III (dofetilide, amiodarone, sotalol). *Plasma levels decreased:* Theophylline. *Metabolism altered (cardiovascular events):* Terfenadine, astemizole, pimozide.

SP: Interferes with fluorometric urinary catecholamine detection. Does not reach foetus in adequate conc. to prevent congenital syphilis. Risk of developing visual impairment after erythromycin exposure; mitochondrial

dysfunction may play role. Elderly more susceptible to drug-associated effects on QT-prolongation.

Pregnancy, Lactation: Use only if clearly necessary. Lactation, use of macrolides increased the risk of infantile hypertrophic pyloric stenosis.

ADR: *Most frequent*, nausea, vomiting, diarrhoea, abdominal discomfort, anorexia, pancreatitis, infantile hypertrophic pyloric stenosis.

Notes: See Class Effects 9.1.4 Macrolides.

Erythroped 500mg, Susp *(Concordia)* A. GMS.D*.
Price, tabs 500mg* (100) €29.42. Susp (140mL) per 5mL, PI SF 125mg, €4.06. SF* 250mg, €7.91. Forte SF* 500mg, €14.01.
Tablet, erythromycin ethylsuccinate. Oval yellow f/c. Marked with Abbott logo. *Sodium starch glycolate, quinoline yellow.*
Granules for oral susp, as above (per 5mL), 125mg (PI SF), 250mg (SF), 500mg (SF Forte). White free-flowing granules with banana flavour. *Parabens, sorbitol, saccharin; sodium 60mg/5mL (PI SF).*

Erythrocin Tablets, Parenteral *(Concordia)* A. GMS.D.
Price, tabs 250mg (100) €15.12; (500) €73.65. 500mg (100) €30.36. Injection 1g, €10.64.
Tablet, erythromycin stearate 250mg, 500mg. White elongated f/c. Marked with logo.
Infusion, erythromycin lactobionate 1g. White (off-white) powder for soln.

Primacine Susp 125mg, 250mg *(Pinewood)* A. GMS.D*.
Price, (100mL) 125mg/5mL, €2.06. 250mg/5mL*, €3.19.
Oral susp, erythromycin ethylsuccinate 125mg(250mg)/5mL. Pale-yellow free-flowing granules; banana odour. *Sucrose.*

9.1.5 - Quinolones

In This Chapter: *Ciprofloxacin, levofloxacin, moxifloxacin, ofloxacin.*

Class Effects

CI: Hypersensitivity to any member of the class, other quinolones; quinolone-induced tendon disorder. Children and growing adolescents unless epiphyseal closure of long bones is complete or benefit outweighs risk. Epilepsy, see SP below.

Interactions: Effect of Other Drugs on Quinolones: *Absorption interference*: Multivalent cations and mineral supplements (calcium, magnesium, aluminium, iron) (allow 4-hour dosing interval; moxifloxacin, 6 hours; ofloxacin, 2 hours), polymeric phosphate binders (sevelamer, lanthanum carbonate), sucralfate, antacids, highly buffered drugs (anti-retrovirals), dairy products, fortified drinks. *Plasma levels increased (reduced renal clearance)*: Probenecid, cimetidine (levofloxacin). *Accelerated absorption*: Metoclopramide. *Caution*: Drugs prolonging QT-interval (Class IA, III antiarrhythmics, TCADs, macrolides). **Effect of Quinolones on Other Drugs:** Vitamin K antagonists (warfarin): *Prolonged clotting time.* Ciclosporin: *Increased serum creatinine (monitor).*

SP: Tendon inflammation, rupture (may occur several months after discontinuing), especially in elderly or corticosteroid co-admin; signs of pain or inflammation, discontinue. Photosensitivity, avoid sun or UV exposure. Hypersensitivity, discontinue. Severe bullous reactions. Epilepsy, existing CNS disorders, convulsive disorders (history), use only if benefit outweighs risk; quinolones known to trigger seizures. Depression or psychoses (suicidal thought and self-endangering behaviour), discontinue. Caution, psychotic patients or psychiatric illness (history).

Caution, presence of QT-prolongation risk factors including medicines prolonging QTc-interval (elderly and women more susceptible). Diabetics (especially elderly) on oral hypoglycaemics or insulin, monitor (dysglycaemia). Ensure adequate hydration, avoid excessive urinary alkalinity (crystalluria risk). G-6-PD defects, caution haemolytic reactions. Sensory or sensorimotor peripheral neuropathy (paraesthesias, hypoaesthesias, dysaesthesias, weakness). Caution, myasthenia gravis (symptoms exacerbated). Signs/symptoms of hepatic disease (anorexia, jaundice, dark urine, pruritus, tender abdomen) or neuropathy (pain, burning, tingling, numbness, weakness), seek medical advice. *Clostridium difficile* associated diarrhoea, see Notes below. Resistance to fluoroquinolones of *E. coli* (urinary infections) varies across the European Union; consult local prevalence.

Pregnancy, Lactation: Pregnancy, women at risk of pregnancy, lactation, contraindicated.

ADR: Increased ALP, LFTs; nausea, diarrhoea; vomiting, dyspepsia, anorexia, flatulence, bilirubinaemia; moniliasis, jaundice, pseudomembranous colitis, dysphagia, abdominal pain, asthenia; pain (extremities, back, chest), tachycardia, migraine, syncope, vasodilation, hypo/hypertension; QT-prolongation (patients with hypokalaemia), eosinophilia, leucopenia; anaemia, leucocytosis, altered prothrombin time, thrombocytopenia, increased creatinine, BUN; oedema, hyperglycaemia, arthralgia, myalgia, joint disorder; myasthenia, tendonitis, tendon rupture, headache, dizziness, insomnia, agitation, confusion; hallucination, sweating, aesthesia, anxiety, abnormal dreams, depression, tremor, convulsion, somnolence, sensorimotor peripheral neuropathy, dyspnoea, skin rash, pruritus, urticaria; photosensitivity, taste perversion; tinnitus, diplopia, allergic reactions, drug fever, anaphylactic reactions, serum sickness like reaction, angioedema, acute renal failure, haematuria, crystalluria, interstitial nephritis. See SP above.

Notes: See 9.1 Antibacterials.

Ciprofloxacin (systemic)

ATC Code: J01MA02. **Sport:** Permitted.
Driving: Caution, may affect reaction time; may be enhanced with ALCOHOL.

Indications: See Dose below.

Dose: Adult: ORAL and IV: Infections of, *lower respiratory tract, upper respiratory tract* (acute exacerbation of chronic sinusitis, chronic suppurative otitis media), 500-750mg twice daily (oral) OR 400mg 2-3 times daily (IV) (7-14 days); malignant external otitis, 750mg twice daily (oral) OR 400mg 3-times daily (IV) (28 days up to 3 months).

UTI, uncomplicated cystitis, 250-500mg (oral) (3 days); pre-menopausal women, 500mg as single dose may be used (oral); complicated cystitis, uncomplicated pyelonephritis, 500mg twice daily (7 days), complicated pyelonephritis, 500-750mg twice daily (oral) (at least 10 days; up to 21 days or more) OR complicated and uncomplicated pyelonephritis, 400mg 2-3 times daily (IV) (7-21 days or longer); prostatitis, 500-750mg twice daily (oral) (acute, 2-4 weeks; chronic, 4-6 weeks) OR 400mg 2-3 times daily (IV) (acute, 2-4 weeks).

Genital tract infections (gonococcal urethritis, cervicitis), prophylaxis of invasive *Neisseria meningitidis*, 500mg (oral) (single dose); epididymo-orchitis, pelvic inflammatory disease, 500-750mg (oral) OR 400mg 2-3 times daily (IV) (at least 14 days).

GI infections, diarrhoea, 500mg twice daily (oral) OR 400mg twice daily (IV) (pathogens other than *Shigella dysenteriae*, severe travellers' diarrhoea) (duration 1 day); caused by *Shigella dysenteriae* type 1 (5 days); caused by *Vibrio cholerae* (3 days); typhoid fever (7 days). Intra-abdominal (Gram negative), 500-750mg twice daily (oral) OR 400mg 2-3 times daily (IV) (5-14 days).

Skin, soft tissue, 500-750mg twice daily (oral) OR 400mg 2-3 times daily (7-14 days); *bone and joint* (max. 3 months); *neutropenics* with fever (continue over entire neutropenic period). Inhalation anthrax post-exposure prophylaxis and treatment, 500mg twice daily (oral) OR 400mg twice daily (IV) (60 days from confirmation of exposure).

Admin, (oral), swallow tabs whole with adequate liquid, do not chew; absorption more rapid without food; not to be taken with dairy products or mineral fortified drinks (calcium fortified); (parenteral), IV infusion over 60 minutes (400mg) OR over 30 minutes (200mg) (adult); over 60 minutes (child). Slow infusion into large vein will minimise discomfort and reduce venous irritation risk.

Elderly: Dose for infection severity and creatinine clearance.

Child: Use in children and adolescents should follow official guidance.

ORAL and IV, *cystic fibrosis*, 20mg/kg twice daily; max. 750mg/dose (oral) OR 10mg/kg 3-times daily; max.

400mg/dose (IV) (10-14 days); other severe infections, duration according to infection type. *Complicated UTI, pyelonephritis*, 10-20mg/kg twice daily; max. 750mg/dose (oral) OR 6mg/kg 3-times daily; max. 400mg/dose (IV) (10-21 days). *Inhalation anthrax* post-exposure prophylaxis and treatment, 10-15mg/kg twice daily; max. 500mg/dose (oral) or max. 400mg/dose (IV) (60 days from confirmation of exposure). *Admin*, see Adult above.

Renal Impairment: *Adult*, CrCl (mL/min), above 60, usual dose; 30-60, 250-500mg 12-hourly (oral) OR 200-400mg 12-hourly (IV); below 30, 250-500mg 24-hourly (oral) OR 200-400mg 24-hourly IV. Haemodialysis, 250-500mg 24-hourly (oral) OR 200-400mg IV 24-hourly (after dialysis); CAPD, 250-500mg 12-hourly OR 200-400mg 24-hourly IV. *Child*, no data.

Hepatic Impairment: No adjustment.

Interactions: Effect of Other Drugs on Ciprofloxacin: *Co-admin contraindicated*: Tizanidine (hypotension, somnolence). *Plasma levels reduced*: Omeprazole.

Effect of Ciprofloxacin on Other Drugs: Theophylline (reduce dose, monitor), clozapine, olanzapine, ropinirole, duloxetine, agomelatine, tizanidine, sildenafil, zolpidem: *Plasma levels increased; co-admin not recommended/caution*. Phenytoin: *Levels altered*. Methotrexate: *Renal tubular transport inhibited; increased plasma levels*. Lidocaine: *Clearance reduced*.

SP: *Elderly and women*, may be more sensitive to QTc-prolonging medications, caution. Not recommended for streptococcal infections. Epididymo-orchitis, pelvic inflammatory disease, gonococcal urethritis use only if ciprofloxacin-resistant *Neisseria gonorrhoea* can be excluded. When treating UTI, consider local prevalence of *E. coli* resistance to fluoroquinolones. Single dose in uncomplicated cystitis in pre-menopausal women expected to have lower efficacy than longer duration treatment. Intra-abdominal infection post-operative, limited data. Travellers' diarrhoea, consult local information on resistant pathogens. Bone/joint infections, use in combination. Inhalation anthrax, refer to consensus documents regarding anthrax treatment. Impaired vision or any eye effects, consult specialist advice.

ADR: *Summary*, (oral) *most common*, nausea, diarrhoea; (parenteral), injection or infusion site reactions. See Notes below.

Notes: See Class Effects 9.1.5 Quinolones.

Ciproxin 250mg, 500mg, 750mg *(Bayer)* A. GMS.
Price, 250mg (10) €3.66; (20) €7.33; (100) €36.63. 500mg (10) €6.81; (20) €13.63; (100) €68.19. 750mg (10) €9.67.
Tablet, ciprofloxacin HCl. Nearly white (slightly yellowish) f/c. 250mg: Round scored*. Marked with Bayer cross; CIP/strength on reverse. 500mg: Oblong scored*. Marked Bayer; CIP strength. 750mg: Oblong. Marked Bayer; CIP/strength on reverse. *(divisible into equal doses).

Ciproxin Parenteral 2mg/mL *(Bayer)* A.
Price, (5) 200mg/100mL, €70.30; 400mg/200mL, €120.13.
Infusion, ciprofloxacin lactate. Clear nearly colourless (slightly yellowish) soln. pH 3.9-4.5. Sodium 900mg (1800mg)/100mL (200mL) soln. **Store:** Do not (refrigerate, freeze).

Cifloxager 250mg, 500mg *(Gerard)* A. GMS.
Price, 250mg (10) €3.59; (20) €7.18. 500mg (10) €6.67; (20) €13.36.
Tablet, ciprofloxacin HCl. White f/c scored (facilitates breaking). Marked CF/strength; G on reverse. 250mg: Round. 500mg: Cap-shaped. *Polydextrose (glucose, sorbitol)*.

Cifox 250mg, 500mg, 750mg *(Rowex)* A. GMS.
Price, 250mg (10) €3.59; (20) €7.18. 500mg (10) €6.67; (20) €13.36. 750mg (10) €9.46.
Tablet, ciprofloxacin HCl. White round scored f/c. Marked cip/strength.

Ciplox 250mg, 500mg, 750mg *(Accord)* A. GMS.
Price, 250mg (10) €3.59; (20) €7.18. 500mg (10) €6.67; (20) €13.36. 750mg (10) €9.46.
Tablet, ciprofloxacin HCl. White (yellowish) f/c scored (divisible into equal halves). Marked C/strength.

Ciprofloxacin (Hospira) Parenteral 2mg/mL *(Hospira)* A.
Price, not published by company.
Infusion, ciprofloxacin lactate. Clear colourless (slightly yellow) soln. *Glucose 45mg/1mL*. **Store:** Below 25 deg C; do not (refrigerate, freeze).

9.1.5 Quinolones

Ciprofloxacin Krka 250mg, 500mg, 750mg *(Krka)* A. GMS.
Price, 250mg (10) €3.59; (20) €7.18. 500mg (10) €6.67; (20) €13.36. 750mg (10) €9.46.
Tablet, ciprofloxacin. White f/c scored (divisible into equal halves). 250mg: Round. 500mg, 750mg: Oval.
Ciprofloxacin Mylan Parenteral 2mg/mL *(Gerard)* A.
Price, (bag) 200mg (30) €520.00. 400mg (15) €348.00.
Infusion, ciprofloxacin. Clear colourless (slightly yellow) soln. *Glucose.* **Store:** Below 25 deg C; do not (refrigerate, freeze).
Ciprofloxacin TEVA 250mg, 500mg, 750mg *(TEVA)* A. GMS.
Price, 250mg (10) €3.53. (20) €7.07. 500mg (10) €6.58. (20) €13.15.
Tablet, ciprofloxacin HCl. White f/c scored (divisible into equal halves). Marked CIP strength. 250mg: Round. 500mg: Cap-shaped.
Ciprofloxacin (TEVA) Parenteral *(TEVA)* A.
Price, not published by company.
Infusion, ciprofloxacin lactate 2mg/mL. Clear yellowish (slightly yellow) soln. *Sodium 354mg/100mL.* **Store:** Do not (refrigerate, freeze).
Profloxin 250mg, 500mg *(Clonmel)* A. GMS.
Price, 250mg (10) €3.59; (20) €7.18. 500mg (10) €6.67; (20) €13.36.
Tablet, ciprofloxacin HCl. White (yellowish) f/c scored. 250mg: Round. 500mg: Oblong.
Truoxin 250mg, 500mg *(Fannin)* A. GMS.
Price, 250mg (10) €3.57; (20) €7.17. 500mg (10) €6.66; (20) €13.35.
Tablet, ciprofloxacin HCl. White (yellowish) f/c scored (divisible into equal halves). Marked C/strength. 250mg: Round. 500mg: Oval.
Truoxin Parenteral *(Fannin)* A.
Price, not published by company.
Infusion, ciprofloxacin lactate 2mg/mL. Clear colourless (slightly yellow) soln. *354mg sodium/100mL soln.* **Store:** Do not (refrigerate, freeze).

Levofloxacin

ATC Code: J01MA12. **Sport:** Permitted.
Driving: Caution.
Indications: Acute sinusitis, acute exacerbations of chronic bronchitis, community-acquired pneumonia, UTI uncomplicated and complicated including pyelonephritis, chronic bacterial prostatitis, skin and soft tissue infections.
Dose: Adult, Elderly: 500mg once daily for acute sinusitis (10-14 days), chronic bacterial prostatitis (28 days). 250mg once daily for uncomplicated UTI (oral, 3 days), complicated UTI (7-10 days).
Chronic bronchitis, acute exacerbations, 250-500mg once daily (oral, 7-10 days). *Community acquired pneumonia,* 500mg once or twice daily (7-14 days).
Skin, soft tissue, 250mg once daily to 500mg once or twice daily (7-14 days). Oral, once or twice daily; tabs to be swallowed whole with liquid; do not crush or chew; with or without food. Parenteral, slow IV infusion (250mg over 30 minutes; 500mg over 60 minutes) once or twice daily.
Renal Impairment: CrCl (mL/min) 50-20, initially 250mg, then 125mg 24-hourly OR initially 500mg, then 250mg (24-hourly OR 12-hourly); 19-10, initially 250mg, then 125mg 48-hourly OR initially 500mg, then 125mg (24-hourly OR 12-hourly); below 10 or on dialysis, initially 250mg, then 125mg 48-hourly OR initially 500mg, then 125mg 24-hourly. No additional dose required after dialysis.
Interactions: Effect of Levofloxacin on Other Drugs: Theophylline, NSAIDs, other drugs lowering seizure threshold: *Cerebral seizure threshold lowered.*
SP: During parenteral infusion, tachycardia, BP drop; if profound, discontinue; circulatory collapse risk.
ADR: See Notes below.
Notes: See Class Effects 9.1.5 Quinolones.

Tavanic 250mg, 500mg *(SANOFI)* A. GMS.
Price, (10) 250mg, €11.82. 500mg, €17.12.
Tablet, levofloxacin hemihydrate. Pale-yellowish-white (reddish-white) f/c scored (facilitates breaking).
Tavanic Parenteral *(SANOFI)* A. HOS.
Price, 500mg (1) €30.18 (PTW).
Infusion, levofloxacin 5mg/mL. Clear greenish-yellow soln.
Levofloxacin Bluefish 250mg, 500mg *(Bluefish)* A. GMS.
Price, (10) 250mg, €9.45. 500mg, €13.69.
Tablet, levofloxacin hemihydrate. Pink cap-shaped f/c scored (divisible into equal halves). 250mg: Marked L and F. 500mg: Marked L and V.

Levofloxacin KrKa 250mg, 500mg *(Krka)* A. GMS.
Price, (10) 250mg, €9.45. 500mg, €13.69.
Tablet, levofloxacin hemihydrate. Oblong f/c scored (divisible into equal doses). 25mg: Pink. 500mg: Orange. *Sunset Yellow.*
Levofloxacin TEVA Parenteral *(TEVA)* A.
Price, not published by company.
Infusion, levofloxacin hemihydrate 5mg/mL. Clear greenish-yellow soln. pH 4.3-5.3. *Sodium chloride 3.5mg/mL.*
Tavager 500mg *(Gerard)* A. GMS.
Price, (10), €13.69.
Tablet, levofloxacin hemihydrate. White (off-white) cap-shaped f/c scored (divisible into equal halves). Marked LVO and strength; G score G on reverse.

Moxifloxacin (systemic)

ATC Code: J01MA14. **Sport:** Permitted.
Driving: Dizziness; acute, transient loss of vision or acute and short lasting loss of consciousness or syncope.
Indications: Acute, bacterial sinusitis, exacerbations of chronic bronchitis, community-acquired pneumonia. Pelvic inflammatory disease (PID) without tubo-ovarian or pelvic abscess in combination (usually cephalosporin), complicated skin and skin structure infections.
Dose: Adult, Elderly: 400mg once daily (oral or IV); sinusitis (7 days), bronchitis (5-10 days), community-acquired pneumonia (10 days), PID (14 days). Swallow tabs whole with liquid; with or without food. Constant IV infusion over 60 minutes.
Child: Under 18 years, contraindicated.
Hepatic Impairment: Child-Pugh C, transaminases above 5xULN, not recommended.
CI: Congenital or QT-prolongation, electrolyte disturbances (hypokalaemia), bradycardia, HF with reduced LVEF, symptomatic arrhythmias.
Interactions: Effect of Other Drugs on Moxifloxacin: *Co-admin caution:* Medications reducing potassium (loop and thiazide diuretics, laxatives, enemas, corticosteroids, amphotericin B), medications causing bradycardia. *Absorption prevented (reduced systemic availability):* Charcoal.
Effect of Moxifloxacin on Other Drugs: Antiarrhythmics Class Ia (quinidine, hydroquinidine, disopyramide), Class III (amiodarone, sotalol, dofetilide, ibutilide), antipsychotics (phenothiazines, pimozide, sertindole, haloperidol, sultopride), TCADs, antimicrobials (sparfloxacin, erythromycin IV, pentamidine, antimalarials particularly halofantrine), antihistamines (terfenadine, astemizole, mizolastine), others (cisapride, vincamine IV, bepridil, diphemanil): *Additive effect on QT-prolongation.* Anticoagulants: *Monitor INR; precautionary.*
SP: Visual impairment. Ongoing proarrhythmic conditions, especially women, elderly (acute myocardial ischaemia), QT-prolongation, ventricular arrhythmias (Torsades de Pointes). Cardiac arrhythmia, discontinue. Liver function, monitor; fulminant hepatitis (asthenia with jaundice, dark urine, bleeding tendency or hepatic encephalopathy) leading to liver failure, including fatal; monitor; early signs/symptoms of liver or skin reactions (serious bullous). Suicidal ideation/thoughts, or suicide attempt. Myasthenia gravis. Not recommended for treatment of MRSA. Caution hypokalaemia associated with bradycardia.
ADR: See Notes below.
Notes: See Class Effects 9.1.5 Quinolones.

Avelox 400mg *(Bayer)* A. GMS.
Price, (5) €12.68.
Tablet, moxifloxacin HCl. Dull-red f/c oblong. Marked M400; BAYER on reverse. *Lactose.*
Avelox Parenteral *(Bayer)* A.
Price, (1) 400mg/250mL, €36.32.
Infusion, moxifloxacin 400mg/250mL. Clear yellow soln. *Sodium 34mmoL/250mL.*

Ofloxacin (systemic)

ATC Code: J01MA01. **Sport:** Permitted.
Driving: Caution.
Indications: RTI, UTI. Prophylaxis in neutropenia, skin and soft tissue infection.
Dose: Adult, Elderly: ORAL, range 200-800mg/day; up to

400mg as single dose preferably in morning; above 400mg/day admin in 2 divided doses.

RTI, 400mg/day. Lower, 400mg/day increasing to 400mg twice daily if needed; pneumococcal pneumonia (second-line), 800mg/day.

UTI, lower, 200-400mg/day; upper, 200-400mg/day increasing to 400mg twice daily if needed. *Gonorrhoea* (uncomplicated), non-gonococcal urethritis, cervicitis, 400mg as single dose.

Prophylaxis in neutropenia, 400-800mg/day for up to 2 months.

Skin, soft tissue, 400mg twice daily. Tabs to be swallowed with liquid, with or without food.

PARENTERAL, slow IV infusion over 30 minutes. *RTI*, 200mg twice daily; *UTI*, 100mg once or twice daily; *skin*, soft tissue, 400mg twice daily.

Renal Impairment: CrCl (mL/min) 50-20, 100-200mg 24-hourly; below 20 or on dialysis, 100mg 24-hourly OR 200mg 48-hourly.

Hepatic Impairment: Severe, max. 400mg/day.

Interactions: Effect of Other Drugs on Ofloxacin: *Absorption reduced (tabs)*: Antacids containing aluminium (including sucralfate), magnesium hydroxides, aluminium phosphate, zinc, iron (allow 2-hour dose interval). *Caution:* Drugs prolonging QT interval.

Effect of Ofloxacin on Other Drugs: Theophylline, NSAIDs, other drugs lowering seizure threshold: *Cerebral seizure threshold lowered.* Glibenclamide: *Increased serum conc (monitor).* Detection of opiates or porphyrins in urine: *False-positive results.* Bacteriological TB diagnosis: *False-negative result.* Phenylpropionic acid derived NSAIDs: *Increased toxicity.*

ADR: *Common, oral,* none; *parenteral,* phlebitis, infusion-site reaction (pain, reddening). See Notes below.

Notes: See Class Effects 9.1.5 Quinolones.

Tarivid 200mg, Parenteral 2mg/mL *(SANOFI)* A. GMS.
Price, (20) 200mg, €7.23. Parenteral HOS: 100mg, €11.73.
200mg, €18.87 (PTW)
Tablet, ofloxacin. Yellowish (white) oblong f/c scored. Marked MXI and logo. *Lactose.*
Infusion, ofloxacin HCl. Clear greenish yellow soln.

Biravid 200mg *(Sinclair)* A. GMS.
Price, (20) €7.07.
Tablet, ofloxacin. White round f/c scored (divisible into equal halves). Marked FXN and 200. *Lactose*

9.1.6 - Tetracyclines

In This Chapter: *Doxycycline, lymecycline, minocycline, tigecycline.*

Class Effects
Tigecycline is structurally similar to tetracyclines and may have similar adverse events.

CI: Hypersensitivity to any member of the class. Obstructive oesophageal disorders (stricture, achalasia, surgery that bypasses or excludes duodenum) *(oral). Children,* under 12 years use during tooth development including pregnancy, infancy, to age 12 years may cause yellow-grey tooth discolouration, enamel hypoplasia. *Tigecycline,* not recommended under 18 years. *Tigecycline, lymecycline,* contraindicated in children under 8 years due to tooth discolouration.

Interactions: Effect of Other Drugs on Tetracyclines: *Nephrotoxicity risk increased (volume depletion)*: Diuretics. *Co-admin not recommended*: Penicillin, other beta-lactam antibiotics. *Absorption impaired*: Antacids, drugs containing aluminium, calcium, magnesium; oral zinc, iron salts, bismuth chelates, cholestyramine, sucralfate, quinapril (high magnesium content), drugs inhibiting gastric acid secretion. *Increased ergotism risk*: Ergot alkaloids. *Plasma levels decreased*: Carbamazepine, barbiturates, phenytoin.

Effect of Tetracyclines on Other Drugs: Warfarin, coumarins: *Prolonged prothrombin time; consider downward dose adjustment.* Oral contraceptives: *Efficacy may be reduced (few cases reported; usually with diarrhoea).*

SP: Tetracyclines are absorbed in developing bones and teeth; may produce tooth staining and enamel hypoplasia; admin only if essential and for shortest duration; avoid repeated course; effect related to total dose *and* duration. *Solid dosage forms,* may cause oesophageal injury; admin with plenty of water in upright position.

Allergic reactions less than half as common as with penicillins; consider use with allergic reactions to other antibiotics. Hepatic impairment or co-admin of hepatotoxic drugs, caution; rare auto-immune hepatotoxicity including acute failure. Photosensitivity, avoid sun or UV exposure including sunbeds. Bulging fontanelles (infants), benign intracranial hypertension (headache, visual disturbance including blurred vision, scotoma, diplopia; permanent vision loss), discontinue. Anti-anabolic action may cause increased blood urea nitrogen (BUN). Caution, myasthenia gravis (can cause weak neuromuscular blockade). All have potential for diarrhoea; colitis, see Notes below.

Pregnancy, Lactation: Pregnancy, lactation, not recommended; second and third trimesters, contraindicated.

ADR: Flushing, abdominal pain, anorexia, nausea, vomiting, diarrhoea, glossitis, dysphagia, dyspepsia, enterocolitis, pseudomembranous colitis, *Clostridium difficile* diarrhoea (mild diarrhoea to fatal colitis), anogenital inflammatory lesions with candidal overgrowth, oesophagitis, oesophageal ulceration, tinnitus, abnormal function, hepatitis, jaundice, arthralgia, myalgia, maculopapular and erythematous rash, exfoliative dermatitis, erythema multiforme, Stevens-Johnson syndrome, toxic epidermal necrolysis, photosensitivity, increased BUN, hypersensitivity e.g. anaphylactic shock, anaphylaxis, anaphylactoid reaction, anaphylactoid purpura, hypotension, pericarditis, angioedema, SLE exacerbation, dyspnoea, serum sickness, peripheral oedema, tachycardia, urticaria; haemolytic anaemia, thrombocytopenia, neutropenia, eosinophilia, dizziness, light-headedness, headache, bulging fontanelles, benign intracranial hypertension.

Notes: See 9.1 Antibacterials.

Doxycycline

ATC Code: J01AA02. **Sport:** Permitted.
Driving: No or negligible effect.

Indications: *Strength 50mg, 100mg,* treatment, pneumonia, other lower RTI, chronic bronchitis, sinusitis, UTI, *Chlamydia trachomatis* infection, non-gonococcal urethritis, alternative in gonorrhoea, syphilis, acne, ophthalmic infections, Rickettsial infections (Rocky Mountain spotted fever, typhus, Q-fever, Coxiella endocarditis), other infections including psittacosis, brucellosis, cholera, bubonic plague, louse and tick-borne relapsing fever including stage 1 and 2 Lyme disease, leptospirosis, tularaemia glanders, chloroquine-resistant falciparum malaria, acute intestinal amoebiasis (adjunctive), gas gangrene, tetanus. Prophylaxis, scrub typhus, travellers' diarrhoea, leptospirosis, malaria, cholera. *Strength 40mg,* facial rosacea.

Dose: Adult, Elderly: *Strength 100mg,* TREATMENT, *acute infections,* usually 200mg on day 1 (as a single dose or 2 divided doses, with a 12-hour interval) then 100mg/day maintenance; severe infection (especially chronic UTI), 200mg/day for treatment duration.

STDs, uncomplicated, 100mg twice daily (gonococcal, with IM ceftriaxone for 7 days); *epididymo-orchitis,* acute, 100mg twice daily with IM ceftriaxone for 10 days; *syphilis,* primary and secondary, 100mg twice daily for 2 weeks as penicillin alternative.

Louse, tick-borne relapsing fevers, typhus, 100-200mg as single dose; *Lyme disease,* early (stage 1 and 2), 100mg twice daily for 10-30 days; *chloroquine-resistant* falciparum malaria, 200mg/day for 7 days; *leptospirosis,* 100mg twice daily for 7 days; *Bacillus anthracis,* 100mg twice daily for 60 days.

Strength 50mg, TREATMENT, *acne vulgaris,* 50mg/day.

Strength 40mg, TREATMENT, *facial rosacea,* 40mg/day in morning.

PROPHYLAXIS, *malaria,* 100mg/day starting 1-2 days

9.1.6 Tetracyclines

before travel to malaria area, during stay and for 4 weeks after leaving area. *Scrub typhus*, 200mg as single dose once weekly. *Travellers' diarrhoea*, 200mg in 1-2 divided doses on day 1 then 100mg/day for duration of stay; max. 21 days. *Leptospirosis*, 200mg once weekly for duration of stay, then 200mg on completion of trip; max. 21 days.

Admin, oral caps to be taken with fluid in upright position; well before bedtime to avoid oesophageal irritation which may be reduced by taking with milk or food.

Child: Under 12 years, not recommended.

Interactions: Effect of Other Drugs on Vibramycin: *Co-admin contraindicated:* Oral retinoids (intracranial hypertension). *Serum half-life shortened:* ALCOHOL, barbiturates, carbamazepine, phenytoin.

SP: Suspected syphilis, ensure full diagnostic procedure. Beta-haemolytic streptococcal infection, treat for minimum 10 days. *Efracea* yields anti-inflammatory plasma levels below antimicrobial threshold.

ADR: *Very common*, photosensitivity.

Notes: See Class Effects 9.1.6 Tetracyclines.

Vibramycin 100mg *(Pfizer)* A. GMS.D.
Price, (12) €3.16.
Capsule, doxycycline hyclate. Hard dark green opaque. Marked Pfizer and Vibracina. *Lactose*. **Store:** Below 25 deg C.

By-Mycin 50mg, 100mg *(Fannin)* A. GMS.D.
Price, (28) 50mg, €6.26. (8) 100mg, €2.05.
Capsule, doxycycline. Hard gelatin opaque; contains spherical yellowish micro granules. 50mg: Pale-green/white. 100mg: Dark-blue/white. *Sucrose*.

Doxycycline TEVA 100mg *(TEVA)* A. GMS.D.
Price, (8) €1.99.
Capsule, doxycycline. Hard green; contains yellow granules. Marked with logo and DOX 100. *Lactose*.

Efracea 40mg *(Galderma)* A. GMS.
Price, (56) €33.35.
Modified/R capsule, doxycycline monohydrate. Beige. Marked CGPI 40. *Sucrose*.

Lymecycline

ATC Code: J01AA04. **Sport:** Permitted.
Driving: No studies. See ADR below.

Indications: Acne vulgaris. Other infections caused by tetracycline-sensitive organisms.

Dose: Adult, Elderly: Age over 12 years or bodyweight 50kg: *Acne*, 300mg daily for 8 weeks. *Other tetracycline-sensitive infections* infections, 300mg twice daily; increase to 1200mg/day if needed. *Admin*, with a glass of water to reduce risk of oesophageal irritation and ulceration.

Child: Under 12 years, not recommended; under 8 years, contraindicated (dental dyschromia and/or enamel hypoplasia risk). Over 12 years, see Adult above.

Renal Impairment: Caution, accumulation (increased toxicity); consider dose reduction. Nephrotoxic (high doses). Use of expired tetracyclines can lead to renal tubular acidosis.

Hepatic Impairment: Caution, accumulation.

Interactions: Effect of Other Drugs on Lymecycline: *Co-admin contraindication (increased benign intracranial hypertension risk):* Oral retinoids. *Increased kidney failure risk:* Methoxyflurane.

ADR: See Notes below. Visual disturbance (unknown frequency).

Notes: See Class Effects 9.1.6 Tetracyclines.

Tetralysal 300mg *(Galderma)* A. GMS.
Price, (28) €7.81.
Capsule, lymecycline. Hard gelatin red/yellow. **Store:** Below 25 deg C; original pack to protect (light, moisture).

Lycimor 300mg *(TEVA)* A. GMS.
Price, (28) €4.26.
Capsule, lymecycline. Hard blue/white. **Store:** Below 25 deg C; original pack to protect (light).

Minocycline

ATC Code: J01AA08. **Sport:** Permitted.
Driving: Light-headedness, dizziness, vertigo.

Indications: Acne, ear, nose and throat infections, acute and chronic bronchitis, bronchiectasis, lung abscess, pneumonia, prostatitis, PID, venereal diseases, UTI, skin and soft tissue infections, ophthalmological infections,

nocardiosis. Prophylaxis, asymptomatic meningococcal carriers, before and after surgery. Actinomycosis, anthrax (presence of penicillin allergy).

Dose: Adult, Elderly: *Acne*, Standard/R 50mg twice daily; routine antibiotic use, 200mg/day in divided doses. Modified/R 100mg every 24 hours; duration minimum 6 weeks, max. 6 months.

Gonorrhoea, males, initially 200mg, then 100mg 12-hourly (minimum 4 days); females, as for male (10-14 days).

Prophylaxis, asymptomatic meningococcal carriers, 100mg twice daily for 5 days followed by rifampicin. Swallow with plenty of water.

Child: Over 12 years, as for Adult above. Under 12 years, not recommended.

Renal Impairment: Failure, not recommended. Complete failure, contraindicated.

Hepatic Impairment: Severe, not recommended.

Interactions: Effect of Other Drugs on Minocycline: *Co-admin avoid (just before, during, just after minocycline):* Isotretinoin (other systemic retinoids).

SP: Hyperpigmentation at various body sites.

ADR: See Notes below.

Notes: See Class Effects 9.1.6 Tetracyclines.

Minocin SA 100mg *(Meda)* A. GMS.
Price, (56) €35.65.
Modified/R capsule, minocycline HCl dihydrate. Opaque orange/brown; contains yellow and off-white spherical pellets.

Minosil 100mg *(Dexcel)* A. GMS.
Price, (56) €32.59.
Modified/R capsule, minocycline. Hard gelatin opaque buff/brown: contains 1 pink f/c tab and 1 peach e/c tab.

Minox 50mg *(Rowex)* A. GMS.
Price, (100) €32.36.
Tablet, minocycline. Round yellow-brown f/c.

Tigecycline

ATC Code: J01AA12. **Sport:** Permitted.
Driving: Dizziness.

Indications: Complicated skin and soft tissue excluding diabetic foot, intra-abdominal infections. Only for use where other alternatives are not suitable.

Dose: Adult, Elderly: Age 18 years and over, initially 100mg, then 50mg 12-hourly (5-14 days). Admin by IV infusion over 30-60 minutes.

Child: Age 8 to under 12 years, 1.2mg/kg every 12-hours IV; max. 50mg 12-hourly (5-14 days); age 12 to under 18 years, 50mg 12-hourly (5-14 days); under 8 years, should not be used (lack of safety/efficacy data, tooth discolouration). IV infusion over 60 minutes.

Hepatic Impairment: Severe, initially 100mg loading dose, then 25mg 12-hourly; caution.

CI: Tetracycline hypersensitivity.

Interactions: Effect of Other Drugs on Tigecycline: *Pharmacokinetics could be affected:* P-gp inhibitors (ketoconazole, ciclosporin), P-gp inducers (rifampicin).

Effect of Tigecycline on Other Drugs: Anticoagulants (warfarin): *Effect potentiated (monitor prothrombin time).* Oral contraceptives: *Reduced efficacy.*

SP: Impaired surgical wound healing, monitor for superinfection (associated with poorer outcomes, especially with nosocomial pneumonia). Use in non-approved indications not recommended. Anaphylactic or anaphylactoid reactions, potentially life-threatening. Liver injury including hepatic failure (fatal). Acute pancreatitis, consider discontinuation. Use with other severe underlying disease, limited data. May be associated with tooth discolouration if used during tooth development. *Paediatrics*, use only if there is no alternative. Nausea, vomiting; caution dehydration. Monitor, LFTs, coagulation and haematology parameters, amylase, lipase (before initiation, regularly during treatment).

Pregnancy, Lactation: Pregnancy, only if clinical condition requires tigecycline treatment. Lactation, stop drug or stop breastfeeding.

ADR: Summary (adults, paediatrics), *most common*, reversible nausea and vomiting. *Glycylcycline class* antibiotics (adverse reactions similar to tetracyclines):

Photosensitivity, pseudotumour cerebri, pancreatitis, anti-anabolic action (increased BUN, azotaemia, acidosis, hyperphosphataemia).
Notes: See Class Effects 9.1.6 Tetracyclines.

Tygacil Parenteral 50mg *(Pfizer)* A.
Price, not published by company.
Infusion, tigecycline 10mg/mL. Lyophilised orange cake or powder for soln.

9.1.7 - Anaerobic Infections

In This Chapter: *Clindamycin, metronidazole.*

Class Effects
CI: Hypersensitivity to any member of the class.
SP: *Clostridium difficile* associated diarrhoea, see Notes below.
Notes: See 9.1 Antibacterials.

Clindamycin (systemic)
ATC Code: J01FF01. **Sport:** Permitted.
Driving: No or negligible influence.
Indications: Serious infection due to clindamycin sensitive organisms; does not penetrate blood/brain barrier in therapeutically effective quantities.
Dose: Adult, Elderly: ORAL, 150-450mg 6-hourly.
PARENTERAL (IM or IV), complicated or serious infection (intra-abdominal, female pelvis), 1800-2700mg/day in 2-4 equal doses; less complicated, 1200-1800mg/day in 3-4 equal doses; up to 4800mg/day been used. Max. single IV of 1.2g in a single 1-hour infusion; max. single IM 600mg.
NOTE: Parenteral **must** be diluted prior to admin and infused slowly over 10-60 minutes. Max. clindamycin conc in diluent 18mg/mL; max. infusion rate 30mg/min.
Child: ORAL, over 1 month, 12-24mg/kg in 4 divided doses; under 1 year (10kg or less), 37.5mg 8-hourly.
PARENTERAL (over 1 month), serious infections, 15-25mg/kg/day*; more severe infections, 25-40mg/kg/day* but no less than 300mg/day regardless of bodyweight. Neonates under 1 month, IM or IV admin 15-20mg/kg/day*. *Admin daily dose in 3 or 4 equally divided doses; IM or IV, see Adult above.
CI: Lincomycin hypersensitivity, diarrhoea, intestinal inflammatory disease. Benzyl alcohol, see SP below.
Interactions: Effect of Other Drugs on Clindamycin: *Co-admin contraindicated:* Erythromycin; lincomycin (if previously hypersensitive). *Physically incompatible:* Ampicillin, phenytoin sodium, barbiturates, aminophylline, calcium gluconate, magnesium sulfate, ceftriaxone sodium, diphenylhydantoin, idarubicin hydrochloride, ranitidine hydrochloride; alkaline preparations or drugs unstable at low pH.
Effect of Clindamycin on Other Drugs: Neuromuscular blockers: *Caution, action may be enhanced by clindamycin.* Oral contraceptives: *Efficacy can be reduced.* Vitamin K antagonists (warfarin, acenocoumarol, fluindione): *Increased coagulation tests (PT/INR) and/or bleeding.*
SP: Parenteral formulation contains benzyl alcohol; associated with fatal 'gasping syndrome' (premature infants); toxic reactions, anaphylactoid reactions (infants, children up to 3 years). Serious infections, caution diarrhoea, colitis (discontinue). Monitor renal/hepatic function, haematology (prolonged use, infants). Superinfection (prolonged use). Atopic syndrome (asthma, allergy), caution. Not for treatment of meningitis (does not diffuse into CSF). Severe hypersensitivity reactions including severe skin reactions; discontinue.
Pregnancy, Lactation: Pregnancy, if considered essential; both clindamycin and benzyl alcohol cross placenta. Lactation, not recommended (parenteral), reported to appear in human breast milk; potential for serious adverse reactions in nursing infant; caution (oral), unlikely infant can absorb significant amount from GI tract.
ADR: *Common,* pseudomembranous colitis, abnormal LFTs; *oral,* abdominal pain, diarrhoea; *parenteral,* thrombophlebitis, maculopapular rash.
Notes: See Class Effects 9.1.7 Anaerobic Infections.

Dalacin C 150mg, Parenteral *(Pfizer)* A. GMS.D.
Price, caps 150mg (24) €7.65; (100) €32.54. Injection 150mg/mL (5) 2mL, €31.97; 4mL, €63.68. HOS: Injection 150mg/mL (5) 2mL, €25.65; 4mL, €33.57 (PTW).
Capsule, clindamycin HCl. Opaque white/white; contains white powder. Marked CLIN 150 and Pfizer. Lactose. **Store:** Below 25 deg C.
Injection or infusion, clindamycin phosphate 150mg/mL. Clear colourless sterile conc for soln; pH 5.5-7. Benzyl alcohol. **Store:** Below 25 deg C; do not (refrigerate, freeze).

Metronidazole (systemic)
ATC Code: J01XD01. **Sport:** Permitted.
Driving: Confusion, dizziness, hallucinations, convulsions, eye disorders (parenteral).
Indications: Infections due to *E. histolytica, G. lamblia,* including carrier states; acute dental infections, non-specific vaginitis, other anaerobic infections (Bacteroides spp., anaerobic streptococci, fusobacteria, clostridia) including severe (parenteral), chronic pressure sores and ulcers.
Dose: Adult: ORAL, *ulcerative gingivitis,* 600mg/day in 3 divided doses (3 days); *dental* infections, 600-800mg in divided doses (3-7 days).
Amoebiasis, 400-800mg 3-times daily (5-10 days); *giardiasis,* 2g once daily (3 days) OR 400mg 3-times daily (5 days). *Urogenital trichomoniasis,* 2g as single dose OR 200mg 3-times daily (7 days) OR 400mg twice daily (5-7 days); *bacterial vaginitis,* 2g as single dose OR 400mg twice daily (7 days).
Anaerobic infections, treatment initially 800mg then 400mg 8-hourly (7 days); prophylaxis, 400mg 8-hourly for 24 hours before surgery; then IV or rectal post-operative until oral can be resumed. Chronic *pressure sores, ulcers,* 1.2g/day in 3 divided doses.
PARENTERAL, treatment, 500mg 8-hourly; prophylaxis, 500mg immediately before, during or after surgery and then 8-hourly until oral resumed. Admin by IV infusion, rate 5mL/min.
Elderly: Caution at high doses.
Child: ORAL, *ulcerative gingivitis,* age 7-10 years, 300mg/day in 3 divided doses; 3-7 years, 200mg/day in 2 divided doses; 1-3 years, 150mg/day in 3 divided doses (all for 3 days).
Amoebiasis, age 7-10 years, 200-400mg 3-times daily; 3-7 years, 100-200mg 4-times daily; 1-3 years, 100-200mg 3-times daily (all for 5-10 days) OR 35-50mg/kg/day in 3 divided doses; max. 2.4g/day; *giardiasis,* age 7-10 years, 1g/day; 3-7 years, 600-800mg/day; 1-3 years, 500mg/day (all once daily for 3 days) OR 15-40mg/kg/day in 2-3 divided doses; *urogenital trichomoniasis,* under 10 years, 40mg/kg as single dose OR 15-30mg/kg/day in 2-3 divided doses (7 days); max. 2g/dose.
Bacterial vaginitis, dental infections, children over 10 years, as for Adult above.
PARENTERAL, *anaerobic infections,* treatment, age 8 weeks to 12 years, 20-30mg/kg/day as single dose OR 7.5mg/kg 8-hourly increasing to 40mg/kg/day if needed (7 days); under 8 weeks, 15mg/kg as single dose OR 7.5mg/kg 12-hourly. Newborn (gestational age under 40 weeks), monitor (accumulation during first week of life).
Prophylaxis, as single dose before surgery, age under 12 years, 20-30mg; newborns, 10mg/kg. *H. pylori eradication,* 20mg/kg; max. 500mg twice daily; adjunctive.
Renal Impairment: Removed by haemodialysis, admin at end of procedure.
Hepatic Impairment: Hepatic encephalopathy, caution; reduce dose to one third; may dose once daily. Trichomoniasis treatment, consider risk/benefit. Substantial impairment of clearance may occur with advanced hepatic insufficiency.
CI: Active or chronic severe peripheral and CNS disease, caution neurological aggravation.
Interactions: Effect of Other Drugs on Metronidazole: *Co-admin not recommended (or for 48 hours after treatment):* Alcohol, drugs containing alcohol. *Plasma levels decreased:* Phenytoin, phenobarbital. *Admixture (inj) not*

247

9.1.8   Drugs Used In Urinary Tract Infections

recommended: Cefamandole, cefoxitin, dextrose, sodium lactate, penicillin G.

Effect of Metronidazole on Other Drugs: Anticoagulants: *Effect potentiated (monitor prothrombin time).* Lithium, ciclosporin, busulphan: *Plasma levels increased.* Disulfiram: *Psychotic reactions.* 5-fluorouracil: *Reduced clearance; increased toxicity.*

SP: Peripheral neuropathy, leucopenia risk (prolonged use); transient epileptiform seizures at high dose. Regular blood tests recommended. Active CNS disease, except brain abscess, caution. Intensive or prolonged therapy only under specialist care. Darkened urine. *Caution,* warn patients not to take alcohol during treatment or for 48 hours afterwards (disulfiram reaction; flushing, vomiting, tachycardia).

Pregnancy, Lactation: If benefit outweighs risk; avoid high doses.

ADR: Epigastric pain, nausea, vomiting, diarrhoea; oral mucositis, taste disorder, dry mouth, anorexia; pancreatitis (reversible); tongue (discolouration, furry); angioedema, anaphylactic shock; peripheral sensory neuropathy, headache, convulsions, dizziness, encephalopathy (confusion) and subacute cerebellar syndrome, aseptic meningitis; confusion, hallucinations, depressed mood; diplopia, myopia, blurred vision, decreased visual acuity, changed colour vision, optic neuropathy/neuritis; hearing (impaired, loss), tinnitus; agranulocytosis, neutropenia, thrombocytopenia; abnormal LFTs, cholestatic or mixed hepatitis, hepatocellular liver injury, jaundice, liver failure; rash, pruritus, flushing, urticaria, eruptions (pustular, fixed drug), Stevens-Johnson syndrome, toxic epidermal necrolysis; fever.

Notes: See Class Effects 9.1.7 Anaerobic Infections.

Flagyl 200mg, 400mg, Oral Susp *(SANOFI)* A. GMS.D.
Price, tabs 200mg (21) €1.08. 400mg (14) €1.52; (100) €10.84. Susp (100mL) 200mg/5mL, €5.66.
Tablet, metronidazole. White (off-white) f/c. Marked Flagyl and strength. 200mg: Round. 400mg: Cap-shaped.
Oral susp, metronidazole benzoate 200mg/5mL. White (creamy-yellow) redispersible (shake gently). *Sucrose, parabens, ethanol.*

Flagyl Parenteral *(SANOFI)* A. HOS.
Price, 100mL (20) 5mg/mL, €61.57 (PTW).
Infusion, metronidazole 5mg/mL. Clear pale-yellow soln. *Sodium 0.31g/100mL.*

9.1.8 - Drugs Used In Urinary Tract Infections

In This Chapter: *Fosfomycin, nitrofurantoin, trimethoprim and combination (sulphamethoxazole).*

Class Effects

CI: Hypersensitivity to any member of the class.
Notes: See 9.1 Antibacterials.

Fosfomycin

ATC Code: J01XX01. **Sport:** Permitted.
Driving: Unlikely to impair.

Indications: Acute uncomplicated UTI.

Dose: Adult: Single 3g dissolved in water and taken on empty stomach before bedtime.

Elderly: Not recommended.

Child: Not recommended.

Renal Impairment: CrCl (mL/min) below 80, not recommended.

Interactions: Effect of Other Drugs on Fosfomycin: *Serum/urine levels lowered:* Metoclopramide.

SP: Use only one single dose to treat a single acute cystitis episode.

Pregnancy, Lactation: Pregnancy, caution. Lactation, not recommended.

ADR: *Common,* headache, dizziness, diarrhoea, nausea, dyspepsia, vulvo-vaginitis, asthenia.

Notes: See Class Effects 9.1.8 Drugs Used in UTI.

Monuril 3g Sachets *(Fannin)* A. GMS.
Price, (1) €5.22.
Granules for oral soln, fosfomycin. White powder; mandarin odour, flavour. *Sucrose.*

Nitrofurantoin

ATC Code: J01XE01. **Sport:** Permitted.
Driving: Major influence; dizziness, drowsiness.

Indications: UTI, pyelitis. Prophylaxis, GU surgery. Long-term suppression.

Dose: Adult, Elderly: *UTI,* age 10 years and older including elderly (Standard/R) or 12 years and older (Prolonged/R), *acute uncomplicated,* 50mg 4-times daily (Standard/R) OR 100mg twice daily (Prolonged/R) (7 days); *severe chronic recurrent,* 100mg 4-times daily (Standard/R) (7 days); *long-term suppression,* 50mg or 100mg once daily at bedtime. *Surgical prophylaxis,* 50mg 4-times daily (Standard/R) or 100mg twice daily (Prolonged/R) on day of procedure and then for 3 days. Admin with food or milk.

Child: Age 3 months and over, *acute UTI,* 3mg/kg/day in 4 divided doses (7 days); *suppressive therapy,* 1mg/kg once daily. Infants under 3 months and pregnant patients at term (during labour and delivery), contraindicated (haemolytic anaemia possibility in foetus or newborn due to immature erythrocyte enzyme systems). Ages 10-12 years and older, see Adult. Prolonged/R not for use under 12 years.

Renal Impairment: Monitor renal function during treatment. Mild/moderate impairment, dose adjustment may be needed. eGFR (mL/min) between 30-44, short-course therapy only; if benefit outweighs risk otherwise under 45, contraindicated.

Hepatic Impairment: Long-term treatment, monitor (especially elderly).

CI: G-6-PD deficiency, acute porphyria.

Interactions: Effect of Other Drugs on Nitrofurantoin: Co-admin not recommended: Magnesium trisilicate (reduced nitrofurantoin absorption); probenecid, sulphinpyrazone (renal tubular secretion inhibited), quinolones. *Decreased antibacterial activity:* Carbonic anhydrase inhibitors, urinary alkalinisers.

SP: Acute pulmonary reactions (may be associated with ECG changes), peripheral neuropathy. Caution, anaemia, diabetes, electrolyte imbalance, Vitamin B deficiency, debilitation. Haematological effects, GI reactions (minimised by taking with food), hepatotoxicity, false positive reaction for glucose in urine.

Pregnancy, Lactation: Pregnancy, contraindicated at term, see Child above. Lactation, caution.

ADR: Superinfection, allergic reactions including anaphylaxis, psychiatric disorders, cardiac collapse, acute pulmonary reactions, skin reactions, asthenia, acute porphyria. Yellow or brown urine discolouration. See SP above.

Notes: See Class Effects 9.1.8 Drugs Used in UTI.

MacroBID 100mg *(Concordia)* A. GMS.
Price, (14) €4.89.
Prolonged/R Capsule, nitrofurantoin (anhydrous, monohydrate). Opaque blue/yellow. Marked GS100. *Lactose, sucrose.*
Macrodantin 50mg, 100mg *(Concordia)* A. GMS.
Price, (30) 50mg, €3.92. 100mg, €6.73.
Capsule, nitrofurantoin. Opaque; contains yellow odourless powder. Marked Eaton. 50mg: Yellow/white. Marked 008. 100mg: Yellow/yellow. Marked 009. *Lactose.*

Trimethoprim

ATC Code: J01EA01. **Sport:** Permitted.
Driving: None known.

Indications: Treatment, infections caused by trimethoprim-susceptible organisms including UTI, RTI. Prophylaxis, recurrent UTI.

Dose: Adult: TREATMENT, respiratory and urinary tract infections, 200mg twice daily for 7-10 days. PROPHYLAXIS, 100mg at night.

Elderly: As for Renal below.

Child: *Monotrim* (under 12 years), TREATMENT, 6mg/kg/day (divided doses); age 6 weeks to 5 months, 25mg twice daily; 6 months to 3 years (8-15kg), 25-50mg twice daily; 4-7 years (15-25 kg), 50-75mg twice daily; 8-12 years (25-40kg), 75-125mg twice daily (7-10 days; dose on day 1 can be doubled).
PROPHYLAXIS, 2.5mg/kg/day in evening. Premature

infants, neonates under 6 weeks, contraindicated. Tablets 100mg, 200mg, over 12 years, as for Adult above. *Trimoptin*, over 12 years, as for Adult; under 12 years, not recommended.

Renal Impairment: CrCl (mL/sec) 0.25-0.45, normal dose for 3 days, then half normal dose; under 0.25, half normal dose. Removed by dialysis. Severe, where blood levels cannot be monitored, contraindicated.

Hepatic Impairment: Severe, contraindicated.

CI: Blood dyscrasias.

Interactions: Effect of Other Drugs on Trimethoprim: *Increased nephrotoxicity:* Ciclosporin.

Effect of Trimethoprim on Other Drugs: Folate antagonists, anticonvulsants: *Folate deficiency induced.* Diuretics (primarily thiazides): *Increased incidence of thrombocytopenia (with purpura), particularly elderly.* Warfarin, other coumarins: *Anti-coagulatory effect increased.* Repaglinide: *Effect enhanced; monitor blood glucose.* Bone marrow depressants: *Increased bone marrow aplasia risk.* Cytotoxics (azathioprine, mercaptopurine, methotrexate): *Increased haematological toxicity risk.* Phenytoin, digoxin: *Increased plasma level by increasing elimination half-life.* ACEI, other drugs causing hyperkalaemia, spironolactone: *Increased hyperkalaemia risk.* Procainamide: *Increased plasma levels.* Oestrogens: *Possible reduced efficacy.* Dapsone: *Mutually increased plasma levels.*

SP: Depressed haemapoeisis (long-term therapy, monitor for pancytopenia). Folate deficiency aggravated; if deficient, admin calcium folinate; consider discontinuing trimethoprim. Hyperkalaemia; increased risk (impaired renal function, elderly, drugs causing hyperkalaemia), monitor electrolytes. Haemapoeisis affected.

Pregnancy, Lactation: Pregnancy, contraindicated. Lactation, consider that is excreted in breast milk *(Monotrim)*, contraindicated *(Trimoptin)*.

ADR: *Very common*, hyperkalaemia. See SP above.

Notes: See 9.1.8 Drugs Used in UTI.

> **Monotrim 100mg, 200mg, Oral Susp** *(Chemidex)* A. GMS.
> *Price,* (100) 100mg, €4.96. 200mg, €10.67. Susp 10mg/mL (100mL) €27.33.
> *Tablet,* trimethoprim. White round scored (facilitates breaking). 100mg: Marked AE/2. 200mg: Marked DE/5. *Lactose.*
> *Oral susp,* as above 10mg/mL. White homogenous; aniseed odour. Sorbitol, parabens. **Store:** Below 25 deg C.
> **Trimoptin 100mg, 200mg** *(Fannin)* A. GMS.
> *Price,* (100) 100mg, €6.83. 200mg, €13.48.
> *Tablet,* trimethoprim. White flat. Marked TR and strength. *Lactose.*

Trimethoprim, Sulphamethoxazole (Co-Trimoxazole)

ATC Code: J01EE01. **Sport:** Permitted.
Driving: Caution.

Indications: UTI, RTI (second-line in COPD, other RTI including acute otitis media). Management of *Pneumocystis carinii (jirovecii)* pneumonia, nocardiosis, toxoplasmosis, brucellosis.

Dose: Adult: Usually sulphamethoxazole 800mg + trimethoprim 160mg (2x 400/80 tabs or 1x 800/160 tab) 12-hourly. *Severe infection and septicaemia,* 3x 400/80 tabs twice daily.

Pneumocystis carinii (jirovecii) pneumonitis, sulphamethoxazole 100mg + trimethoprim 20mg per kg per day in divided doses 6-hourly for 14 days (with facilities for monitoring sulphamethoxazole plasma levels).

Elderly: Caution, shortest possible duration.

Child: Sulphamethoxazole 30mg + trimethoprim 6mg per kg per 24 hours at 12-hourly intervals. Age 6-12 years, sulphamethoxazole 400mg + trimethoprim 80mg; age 6 months to 5 years, sulphamethoxazole 200mg + trimethoprim 40mg; age 6 weeks to 5 months, sulphamethoxazole 100mg + trimethoprim 20mg.

Renal Impairment: CrCl (mL/min) 15-30, half standard dose; below 15, not recommended.

Hepatic Impairment: Severe, not recommended.

CI: Sulfonamide, trimethoprim or co-trimoxazole

hypersensitivity. Serious haematological disorders. Blood dyscrasias, glucose-phosphate dehydrogenase deficiency.

Interactions: Effect of Other Drugs on Co-Trimoxazole: *Co-admin caution:* Strongly protein bound drugs (oral hypoglycaemics, anti-coagulants), drugs causing hyperkalaemia. *Increased thrombocytopenia risk:* Diuretics (thiazides in elderly). *Megaloblastic anaemia risk:* Pyrimethamine (dose above 25mg/week). *Increased haematological adverse event risk:* Zidovudine (monitor haematology). *Plasma levels mutually increased:* Procainamide, amantadine.

Effect of Co-Trimoxazole on Other Drugs: Methotrexate, phenytoin: *Increased toxicity (methotrexate plasma levels increased; phenytoin half-life prolonged).* Sulphonylureas: *Effect potentiated.* Folate antagonists, anticonvulsants, pyrimethamine (which may cause folate deficiency): *Folate deficiency precipitated.* Ciclosporin: *Reversible renal deterioration.* Lamivudine: *Increased exposure (due to trimethoprim).* Warfarin: *Anticoagulant effect potentiated.* Digoxin: *Plasma levels increased (elderly).*

SP: Skin hypersensitivity, rash, life-threatening cutaneous reactions (caution, discontinue). Elderly, folate-deficiency (adverse events severe, fatal), prolonged use, monitor blood counts. Ensure adequate urinary output to prevent crystalluria and calculus formation; increased risk in malnutrition. G-6-PD, haemolytic anaemia, methaemoglobinaemia risk. Serious haematological disorders, careful supervision. Severe allergy, bronchial asthma, caution. At risk for hyperkalaemia, hyponatraemia, monitor (sodium, potassium). Laboratory tests altered.

Pregnancy, Lactation: Not recommended.

ADR: Nausea (with/without vomiting), skin rash, hypersensitivity (exfoliative dermatitis, erythema multiforme bullosa, toxic epidermal necrolysis; photosensitivity); leucopenia, neutropenia, thrombocytopenia, agranulocytosis, anaemia (megaloblastic, aplastic, haemolytic), methaemoglobinaemia; haemolysis (G-6-PD patients); elevated (serum transaminases, bilirubin); cholestatic jaundice, hepatic necrosis; aseptic meningitis. Interstitial nephritis; allergic reactions e.g. serum sickness, anaphylaxis, allergic myocarditis, angioedema, drug fever; periarteritis nodosa, SLE; cough, shortness of breath, pulmonary infiltrates, diarrhoea, glossitis, stomatitis, anorexia; pseudomembranous colitis, pancreatitis; monilial overgrowth, convulsions, peripheral neuritis, ataxia, vertigo, tinnitus; headache, depression, dizziness, hallucinations, hyperkalaemia, hyponatraemia, arthralgia, myalgia. At high doses used for *Pneumocystis carinii (jirovecii)* pneumonitis in AIDs patients, rash, fever, neutropenia, thrombocytopenia, raised liver enzymes, hyperkalaemia, hyponatraemia (discontinue; admin calcium folinate), rhabdomyolysis.

Notes: See Class Effects 9.1.8 Drugs Used in UTI.

> **Septrin, Forte, Susp Adult, Paed** *(Aspen)* A. GMS.D*.
> *Price,* (100) tabs 80/400mg*, €13.91. Forte 160/800mg*, €23.21. Susp Adult* (100mL), €5.48; Paed (50mL), €1.70. 100mL, €2.47.
> *Tablet,* trimethoprim/sulphamethoxazole. White scored. 80/400: Round. Marked S2. Forte 160/800: Elongated. Marked S3.
> *Oral susp (Adult 80/400/5mL, Paed 40/200/5mL),* as above. Off-white (adult), pink (paed) aniseed flavoured. *Sucrose (adult), sorbitol (paed), parabens, ethanol.*
> **Septrin Parenteral** *(Aspen)* A.
> *Price,* (10) €22.00.
> *Infusion,* trimethoprim/sulphamethoxazole 80/400mg/5mL. Clear faintly yellow (brown) soln. *Sodium 38.87mg/5mL, ethanol, propylene glycol.*

9.1.9 - Other Antibacterials, Enzymes

In This Chapter: *Colistin, colistimethate, daptomycin, fidaxomicin, fusidic acid, linezolid, rifaximin, tedizolid, teicoplanin, vancomycin.*

Class Effects

CI: Hypersensitivity to any member of the class.

Notes: See 9.1 Antibacterials.

9.1.9 Other Antibacterials, Enzymes

Colistimethate

ATC Code: J01XB01. **Sport:** Permitted.
Driving: Neurotoxicity (dizziness, confusion, visual disturbances).
Indications: *Pseudomonas aeruginosa* pulmonary infection in cystic fibrosis (CF) *(both brands)*. Serious infections (selected Gram-negative pathogens), patients with limited treatment options *(Colomycin)*.

Dose: Adult, Elderly: *Colomycin* PARENTERAL, up to 60kg, 50-75 (max.) thousand units/kg/day in 3 divided doses 8-hourly; over 60kg, 1-2 million units (MU) 3-times daily; max. 6 MU in 24 hours. *Admin*, by IV infusion (50mL) over 30 minutes; totally implantable venous access device (TIVAD) may tolerate bolus up to 2 MU (in 10mL) over not less than 5 minutes.

Colomycin INHALATION, dissolve powder in 2-4mL of water for injection or 0.9% sodium chloride IV infusion; use in a nebuliser; usually 1-2 MU twice daily. Cystic fibrosis, 500 thousand to 2 MU 3-times daily nebulised.

Colobreathe, INHALATION POWDER, 1 cap inhaled twice daily (12-hourly). Caps must not be swallowed. Treatment order: Inhaled bronchodilators, chest physiotherapy, other inhaled medicinals, *Colobreathe*.

Child: *Colomycin*, PARENTERAL as for Adult above. Caution, infants under 1 year (renal function not fully matured). INHALATION, over 2 years, as for Adult; under 2 years, 500 thousand to 1 MU twice daily nebulised.

Colobreathe, INHALATION, age 6 years and older, as for Adult above; under 6 years, no data.

Renal Impairment: *Colomycin*, parenteral (60kg and over), CrCl (mL/min) 20-50, 1-2 MU 8-hourly; 10-20, 1 MU every 12-18 hours; below 10, 1 MU every 18-24 hours.

Cl: Polymyxin B hypersensitivity.

Interactions: Effect of Other Drugs on Colistimethate Sodium: *Co-admin caution*: Other neurotoxic and/or nephrotoxic drugs e.g. aminoglycosides (gentamicin, amikacin, netilmicin, tobramycin), other colistimethate formulations. *Increased nephrotoxicity risk*: Cephalosporins. *Co-admin, extreme caution*: Neuromuscular blockers, ether. *Co-admin caution (with myasthenia gravis)*: Azithromycin, clarithromycin, norfloxacin, ciprofloxacin.

SP: Consider IV colistimethate co-admin with other antibacterials (resistance reported with monotherapy). For use only when other more commonly prescribed antibiotics are not effective or appropriate. All patients, monitor renal function (initiation, then regularly during treatment); increased nephropathy risk (hypovolaemia, receiving other nephrotoxics). Decreased urinary output (shock), toxicity risk (caution). Porphyria, caution; myasthenia gravis, extreme caution. Neurotoxicity (overdose, failure to reduce dose in renal impairment, use of curariform agents or other drugs with similar neurological effects). Allergic reactions, discontinue. IV colistimethate does not cross the blood brain barrier to a clinically relevant extent. *Colobreathe*, haemoptysis, weigh benefit/risk of inducing haemorrhage. Acute respiratory exacerbation, consider IV or oral antibiotics. Rinse mouth after use to reduce risk of fungal super-infection. Caution, porphyria. Bronchospasm or coughing on inhalation.

Pregnancy, Lactation: Pregnancy and women of childbearing potential not using contraception, not recommended. Lactation, stop breastfeeding or stop drug.

ADR: *Colomycin, systemic*, neurotoxicity, see SP above. Hypersensitivity, skin rash, drug fever, injection-site reaction; *Inhalation*, cough, bronchospasm, sore throat/mouth, *Candida albicans* infection. *Colobreathe*, very common, dyspnoea, cough, dysphonia, throat irritation, dysgeusia.

Notes: See Class Effects 9.1.9 Other Antibacterials, Enzymes.

Colomycin Parenteral (Forest) A. GMS.
Price, (10) 1 MU, €22.98. 2 MU, €45.96.
Injection, infusion or inhalation, colistimethate sodium 1 MU, 2 MU. White powder for soln.

Colobreathe Inhalation 125mg (Forest) A. HT.
Price, (56 caps) €1300.00.
Inhalation powder in hard capsule, colistimethate sodium 1662500 IU (125mg). Transparent hard gelatin; contains fine white powder.

Daptomycin

ATC Code: J01XX09. **Sport:** Permitted.
Driving: Unlikely to impair.
Indications: Treatment, complicated skin and soft-tissue infections (cSSTI) (adults, children). Right-sided infective endocarditis (RIE) due to *Staphylococcus aureus*; *Staphylococcus aureus* bacteraemia (SAB) associated with RIE or cSSTI (adults). Only for use against Gram-positive organisms.

Dose: Adult, Elderly: *cSSTI* without Staph, 4mg/kg every 24 hours (7-14 days or until infection resolved); with Staph, 6mg/kg once every 24 hours (14 days). *RIE* due to Staph, 6mg/kg every 24 hours. IV infusion over 30 minutes. *Elderly*, adjust dose only with severe renal impairment.

Child: *cSSTI*, age 12-17 years, 5mg/kg/24-hours; 7-11 years, 7mg/kg/24-hours; 2-6 years, 9mg/kg/24-hours; 1 year to under 2 years, 10mg/kg/24-hours. Duration, up to 14 days. Admin by IV infusion over 30 minutes (age 7-17 years) OR over 60 minutes (age 1-6 years). Not for use under 1 year (risk of potential effects on muscular, neuromuscular and/or nervous systems). Other indications, under 18 years, safety/efficacy not established.

Renal Impairment: CrCl (mL/min) below 80, use only if benefit outweighs risk. cSSTI without Staph, CrCl 30 and above, 4mg/kg once daily; below 30, 4mg/kg every 48 hours. RIE or cSSTI with Staph, CrCl 50 and above, 6mg/kg once daily; below 30, 6mg/kg every 48 hours.

Hepatic Impairment: Severe, caution.

Interactions: Effect of Other Drugs on Daptomycin: *Co-admin not recommended*: Other drugs which may cause myopathy (temporarily discontinue unless benefit of co-admin outweighs risk). *Plasma levels increased, caution*: Drugs reducing renal filtration (NSAIDs, COX-2 inhibitors).

SP: Concurrent bacteraemia, not recommended. Pneumonia, not effective. Increased plasma CPK levels (muscular pains, weakness, myositis, myoglobinaemia, rhabdomyolysis); monitor baseline, then regularly once weekly; CPK above 5xULN or at higher myopathy risk, monitor more frequently; signs/symptoms (muscle pain, tenderness, weakness, cramp), monitor every second day. Peripheral neuropathy signs, investigate, discontinuation. Eosinophilic pneumonia; discontinue, treat with systemic steroids. Obese (BMI over 40kg/m2), limited data. Possible interference with lab test (prothrombin time/INR).

Pregnancy, Lactation: Pregnancy, if benefit outweighs risk. Lactation, not recommended.

ADR: *Common*, fungal infections, UTI, candida infection, anaemia, anxiety, insomnia, dizziness, headache, hyper/hypotension, pain (GI, abdominal), nausea, vomiting, constipation, diarrhoea, flatulence, bloating, distention, abnormal laboratory values (LFTs, CPK), rash, pruritus, limb pain, infusion-site reactions, pyrexia, asthenia; *less frequent, more serious*, hypersensitivity reactions, eosinophilic pneumonia, drug rash with eosinophilia (DRESS), angioedema, rhabdomyolysis.

Notes: See Class Effects 9.1.9 Other Antibacterials, Enzymes.

Cubicin Parenteral (MSD) A. HOS.
Price, (1) 350mg, €73.98; 500mg, €103.11 (PTW).
Infusion, daptomycin 350mg, 500mg. Pale yellow (light brown) lyophilised cake or powder/conc for soln: Injection or infusion (350mg) or infusion (500mg). 7mL (350mg) or 10mL (500mg) of 9mg/mL NaCl per mL. NOTE: Not physically or chemically compatible with glucose-containing solns. **Store:** Refrigerate.

Fidaxomicin

ATC Code: A07AA12. **Sport:** Permitted.
Driving: No or negligible effect.
Indications: Treatment, *Clostridium difficile* infections (CDI) (*C. difficile*-associated diarrhoea).

Dose: Adult, Elderly: 200mg twice daily (12-hourly) for 10 days. *Admin,* oral with or without food.

Child: Under 18 years, safety/efficacy not established.

Renal Impairment: Severe, caution.

Hepatic Impairment: Moderate/severe, caution.

Interactions: Effect of Other Drugs on Fidaxomicin: *Co-admin not recommended*: Potent P-gp inhibitors (ciclosporin, ketoconazole, erythromycin, clarithromycin, verapamil, dronedarone, amiodarone).

Effect of Fidaxomicin on Other Drugs: Digoxin, dabigatran: *Effect on exposure cannot be excluded.*

SP: Caution, patients with inflammatory bowel disease (enhanced absorption), pseudomembranous colitis, fulminant or life-threatening CDI. Severe allergic reactions, discontinue; known macrolide allergy, caution.

Pregnancy, Lactation: Pregnancy, avoid. Lactation, stop breastfeeding or stop drug.

ADR: Summary, *most common*, vomiting, nausea, constipation.

Notes: See Class Effects 9.1.9 Other Antibacterials, Enzymes.

> **Dificlir 200mg** *(Astellas)* A. HT.
> *Price,* (20) €1620.00.
> *Tablet,* fidaxomicin. White (off-white) cap-shaped. Marked FCX; 200 on reverse.

Fusidic Acid (systemic)

ATC Code: J01XC01. **Sport:** Permitted.
Driving: No or negligible effect.

Indications: Systemic infections due to sensitive organisms including Staphylococci.

Dose: Adult, Elderly: Oral tablets 1500mg/day; severe infection, double dose or use in combination. Oral suspension 1500-2000mg/day. Admin daily dose in 3 equally divided doses.

Child: Tablets and oral susp, 20-50mg/kg/day in 3 equally divided doses.

Hepatic Impairment: Caution, see SP below.

Interactions: Effect of Other Drugs on Fusidic Acid: *Co-admin contraindicated*: HMG-CoA reductase inhibitors (statins), possible fatal rhabdomyolysis. *Co-admin caution:* Hepatotoxic drugs, drugs with biliary excretion (lincomycin, rifampicin), CYP3A4 transformed drugs.

Effect of Fusidic Acid on Other Drugs: Oral anticoagulants (coumarins), ciclosporin: *Plasma levels increased.* Statins (rhabdomyolysis, muscle weakness, pain), HIV protease inhibitors including ritonavir, saquinavir (hepatotoxicity): *Plasma levels mutually increased.*

SP: Metabolised in liver, excreted in bile; high dose, monitor function with liver impairment, other hepato-toxic drugs, biliary obstruction, other drugs with similar excretion pathway. Theoretical kernicterus risk in neonates.

Pregnancy, Lactation: Pregnancy, avoid. Lactation, stop breastfeeding or stop drug weighing benefit/risk.

ADR: Summary *most frequent*, GI (abdominal discomfort/pain, diarrhoea, dyspepsia, nausea, vomiting). Anaphylactic shock reported.

Notes: See Class Effects 9.1.9 Other Antibacterials, Enzymes.

> **Fucidin 250mg, Oral Susp** *(LEO)* A. GMS.
> *Price,* tabs (100) €82.44. Susp (50mL) €8.79.
> *Tablet,* sodium fusidate. White (off-white greyish) marbled oval f/c. Unmarked. *Lactose, sodium 11mg/tab.*
> *Oral susp,* fusidic acid hemihydrate 250mg/5mL. Cream-coloured; banana odour. *Glucose, sorbitol, orange flavour (sucrose), sodium 2mg/1mL.*

Linezolid

ATC Code: J01XX08. **Sport:** Permitted.
Driving: Dizziness.

Indications: Gram-positive infections, nosocomial or community-acquired pneumonia, complicated skin and soft tissue infections. Not active against Gram-negative pathogens.

Dose: Adult, Elderly: Initiate in hospital, usually 600mg twice daily for 10-14 days; duration max. 28 days depending on response. IV admin over 30-120 minutes; oral to be taken with or without food.

Child: Under 18 years, not recommended.

Renal Impairment: Severe, caution, use if benefit outweighs risk. Haemodialysis, approx. 30% removed over 3 hours; admin after dialysis.

Hepatic Impairment: Use if benefit outweighs risk.

CI: Uncontrolled hypertension, phaeochromocytoma, carcinoid, thyrotoxicosis, bipolar depression, schizoaffective disorder, acute confusional states. See Interactions below.

Interactions: Effect of Other Drugs on Linezolid: *Co-admin contraindicated*: MAOIs (phenelzine, isocarboxazide, selegiline, moclobemide) or within 2 weeks of admin; SSRIs, TCADs, serotonin 5-HT1 receptor agonists (triptans), directly and indirectly acting sympathomimetics (including adrenergic bronchodilators, pseudoephedrine and phenylpropanolamine), vasopressives (epinephrine, norepinephrine), dopaminergics (dopamine, dobutamine), pethidine, buspirone.

SP: Caution tyramine-rich diet. Myelosuppression (anaemia, leucopenia, pancytopenia, thrombocytopenia), monitor blood counts weekly; discontinue unless benefit outweighs risk. Pseudomembranous colitis. Metabolic acidosis needs immediate medical attention. Mitochondrial protein synthesis inhibited (lactic acidosis, anaemia, peripheral and optic neuropathy); more common used longer than 28 days. Serotonin syndrome, co-admin with serotonergic agents (SSRIs), see Interactions above. Diabetic foot lesions, decubitus, ischaemic lesions, severe burns, gangrene, limited data. Advise patients to report history of seizures, visual impairment; optic/peripheral neuropathy, weigh benefit against risk.

Pregnancy, Lactation: Pregnancy, if benefit outweighs risk; potential risk for humans exists. Lactation, contraindicated; stop breastfeeding throughout admin.

ADR: Summary, *most common, leading to discontinuation*, diarrhoea, headache, nausea, vomiting.

Notes: See Class Effects 9.1.9 Other Antibacterials, Enzymes.

> **Zyvox 600mg, Oral Susp, Parenteral** *(Pfizer)* A. HT.
> *Price,* tabs 600mg (10) €283.49. Susp (150mL) €246.36.
> *Tablet,* linezolid. White ovaloid f/c. Marked ZYV; 600 on reverse.
> *Oral susp,* as above 100mg/5mL. White (light-yellow) granules; orange flavour. *Aspartame, sucrose, sorbitol, mannitol, sodium 8.5mg/5mL.* **Store:** Keep bottle tightly closed.
> *Infusion,* as above 2mg/mL (600mg). Isotonic, clear colourless (yellow) soln. *Glucose; sodium 114mg/300mL.* **Store:** Original pack to protect (light).
> **Linezolid (Accord) 600mg** *(Accord)* A. HT.
> *Price,* (10) €226.79.
> *Tablet,* linezolid. White (off-white) f/c oval. Marked EQ1. *Soya lecithin.*
> **Linezolid (Actavis) 600mg** *(Accord)* A. HT.
> *Price,* (10) €226.79.
> *Tablet,* linezolid. White f/c oval. Marked L; 600 on reverse.
> **Linezolid (Rowex) 600mg** *(Rowex)* A. HT.
> *Price,* (10) €226.78.
> *Tablet,* linezolid. White (off-white) f/c oval. Marked LZ600.
> **Linezolid Clonmel 600mg** *(Clonmel)* A. HT.
> *Price,* (10) €226.78.
> *Tablet,* linezolid. White (off-white) f/c oblong.
> **Linezolid Krka 600mg** *(Krka)* A. HT.
> *Price,* (10) €226.78.
> *Tablet,* linezolid. White (almost white) f/c oval.
> **Linezolid Rowex Parenteral** *(Rowex)* A.
> *Price,* (1) €24.70.
> *Infusion,* linezolid 2mg/mL (300mL bag). Clear colourless (yellow) soln. *Glucose; sodium 114mg/bag.*
> **Linezolid TEVA 600mg** *(TEVA)* A. HT.
> *Price,* (10) €226.78.
> *Tablet,* linezolid. White cap-shaped f/c scored (facilitates breaking). Marked 600. *Lactose.*

Rifaximin

ATC Code: A07AA11. **Sport:** Permitted.
Driving: No or negligible effect; dizziness reported.

Indications: Reduction in recurrence of episodes of overt hepatic encephalopathy.

Dose: Adult, Elderly: Age 18 years and over, 550mg twice daily. *Admin,* with or without food with water.

9.1.9   Other Antibacterials, Enzymes

Renal Impairment: Caution.

Hepatic Impairment: Severe, ESRD, caution.

CI: Intestinal obstruction.

Interactions: Effect of Other Drugs on Rifaximin: Co-admin not recommended: Other rifamycins. Co-admin caution: Ciclosporin.

Effect of Rifaximin on Other Drugs: Oral oestrogen contraceptives: Effectiveness decreased. CYP3A4 substrates (warfarin*, antiepileptics, antiarrhythmics): Possible decreased exposure (with hepatic impairment). *(monitor INR).

SP: Reddish discolouration of urine.

Pregnancy, Lactation: Pregnancy, not recommended. Stop breastfeeding or drug.

ADR: Common, depression, dizziness, headache, dyspnoea, abdominal pain/distention, diarrhoea, nausea, vomiting, ascites, rash, pruritus, muscle spasm, arthralgia, peripheral oedema.

Notes: See Class Effects 9.1.9 Other Antibacterials, Enzymes.

> **Targaxan 550mg** (Norgine) A. GMS.
> Price, (56) €283.40.
> Tablet, rifaximin. Pink oval f/c. Marked RX.

Tedizolid

ATC Code: J01XX11. **Sport:** Permitted.

Driving: Minor influence; dizziness, fatigue, somnolence.

Indications: Treatment (adults), acute bacterial skin and skin structure infections (ABSSSI).

Dose: Adult: 200mg/day (6 days; no safety/efficacy data after 6 days). Admin, oral once daily with or without food (use IV if rapid effect needed). Admin parenteral by IV infusion over 60 minutes.

Elderly: Age 75 years and older, limited clinical experience.

Child: Under 18 years, safety/efficacy not established.

Interactions: Effect of Tedizolid on Other Drugs: Narrow therapeutic window substrates of CYP3A4 (oral midazolam, triazolam, alfentanil, ciclosporin, fentanyl, pimozide, quinidine, sirolimus, tacrolimus), CYP2B6 (efavirenz), CYP2C9 (warfarin), P-gp (digoxin); oral hormonal contraceptives: Reduced efficacy. BCRP substrates (imatinib, lapatinib, methotrexate, pitavastatin, rosuvastatin, sulfasalazine, topotecan), OATP1B1 (atorvastatin, fluvastatin, pitavastatin, lovastatin, repaglinide, bosentan, valsartan, olmesartan, glyburide): Increased exposure (consider break during 6-day tedizolid treatment).

SP: Neutropenia with ABSSSI (consider alternative). Mitochondrial protein synthesis inhibited (lactic acidosis, anaemia, optic and peripheral neuropathy). Myelosuppression (decreased platelets, haemoglobin, neutrophils). Advise patients to report visual changes (changed visual acuity, colour vision; blurred vision; visual field defect). Lactic acidosis, optic and peripheral neuropathy not reported with 6-day treatment duration. Clostridium difficile associated diarrhoea (mild to fatal colitis). Serotonin syndrome reported with other members of oxazolidinone class. Generally not active against Gram negative bacteria.

Pregnancy, Lactation: Pregnancy, avoid. Lactation, stop breastfeeding or stop drug.

ADR: Summary, most frequent, nausea, headache, diarrhoea, vomiting.

Notes: See Class Effects 9.1.9 Other Antibacterials, Enzymes.

> ▼ **Sivextro 200mg** (MSD) A. HT.
> Price, (6) €1134.00.
> Tablet, tedizolid phosphate. Oval f/c yellow. Marked TZD; 200 on reverse.
> ▼ **Sivextro Parenteral 200mg** (MSD) A.
> Price, not published by company.
> Infusion, tedizolid phosphate. White (off-white) powder for conc for soln.

Teicoplanin

ATC Code: J01XA02. **Sport:** Permitted.

Driving: Minor influence.

Indications: Treatment, infections and associated bacteraemia e.g. complicated (skin and soft tissue, UTI), bone and joint, hospital and community-acquired pneumonia, infective endocarditis, peritonitis associated with ambulatory peritoneal dialysis. Alternative oral treatment, Clostridium difficile-associated diarrhoea and colitis.

Dose: Adult, Elderly: Complicated (skin and soft tissue, UTI) infections, pneumonia, 400mg 12-hourly (3 loading doses), then maintenance 6mg/kg once daily IV or IM. Bone and joint, infective endocarditis, 800mg IV 12-hourly (3-5 loading doses), then maintenance 12mg/kg IV or IM once daily. Admin, IV bolus over 3-5 minutes or as 30-minute infusion. Monitor trough serum concentrations after loading regimen. Target trough levels, Gram-positive infections, 10mg/L, endocarditis, other severe infections, 15-30mg/L (measured by HPLC). Endocarditis, duration minimum 21 days.

Clostridium difficile diarrhoea and colitis, 100-200mg orally twice daily (7-14 days).

Child: Up to 2 months, 16mg/kg single loading dose by IV infusion (day 1) then maintenance, 8mg/kg by IV infusion once daily (use only infusion admin for neonates); age 2 months to 12 years, loading dose of 10mg/kg as single dose 12-hourly repeated 3 times then maintenance 6-10mg/kg as single IV dose once daily.

Renal Impairment: From day 4 of treatment, CrCl (mL/min) 30-80, admin dose once every two days or half dose once daily; below 30, on haemodialysis, admin dose every third day or one-third dose daily. CAPD, after 6mg/kg single IV loading dose, then 20mg/L in the bag of dialysis soln (week 1), 20mg/L in alternate bags (week 2), then 20mg/L in overnight bag (week 3).

Interactions: Effect of Other Drugs on Teicoplanin: Co-admin or sequential admin (caution): Nephrotoxic or ototoxic drugs (aminoglycosides, colistin, amphotericin B, ciclosporin, cisplatin, frusemide, etacrynic acid).

SP: Serious, life-threatening hypersensitivity reactions (fatal). Infusion-related reactions, rarely, even at first dose (red man syndrome); stopping or slowing infusion may stop reactions. Life-threatening (fatal) cutaneous reactions; discontinue immediately. Has limited spectrum of activity (Gram-positive). Not for intraventricular use. Monitor haematology (thrombocytopenia reported; include full blood counts), hepatic, renal, auditory function (with prolonged treatment, renal insufficiency and/or concomitant ototoxic and/or nephrotoxic drugs). NOTE: Teicoplanin and aminoglycoside solns are not compatible; must not be mixed for injection; they are compatible in dialysis fluid; can be freely used in CAPD-related peritonitis.

Pregnancy, Lactation: Pregnancy, use only if clearly necessary; cannot exclude risk of inner ear and renal damage to foetus. Lactation, stop drug or stop breastfeeding.

ADR: Common, rash, erythema, pruritus, pain, pyrexia.

Notes: See Class Effects 9.1.9 Other Antibacterials, Enzymes.

> ▼ **Targocid Parenteral or Oral Soln** (SANOFI) A. GMS.
> Price, (1) 200mg, €33.46. 400mg, €66.06. HOS: 400mg (1) €61.57.
> Injection, infusion or oral soln, teicoplanin 200mg(400mg)/3mL. Spongy ivory-coloured powder; clear colourless solvent for soln.
> ▼ **Teicoplanin Parenteral or Oral Soln** (Rowex) A. GMS.
> Price, (1) 200mg, €13.38. 400mg, €26.76.
> Injection, infusion or oral soln, teicoplanin 200mg(400mg)/3mL. White (light-yellow) powder; clear colourless solvent for soln. Sodium 24mg/vial.

Vancomycin

ATC Code: A07AA09 (oral); J01XA01 (parenteral). **Sport:** Permitted.

Driving: No or negligible effect.

Indications: ORAL, treatment of pseudomembranous colitis and Staphylococcal enterocolitis due to C. difficile (poorly absorbed from GI tract; not suitable for other infections). PARENTERAL, treatment of severe potentially life-threatening infections due to susceptible Gram-positive organisms (cannot be treated with or failed to respond or are resistant to other antibiotics e.g. penicillins, cephalosporins) (endocarditis, osteomyelitis, pneumonia, soft tissue infection); where appropriate, co-admin with other antibacterials, especially treatment of endocarditis. Endocarditis prophylaxis in patients at risk from dental or surgical procedures.

Dose: Adult: ORAL, usually 500mg in divided doses (7-10 days); severe, up to max. 2g/day in 3-4 divided doses. Use caps or contents of 500mg vial.

PARENTERAL, recommended, 500mg 6-hourly OR 1g 12-hourly OR 30-40mg/kg/day in 2-4 divided doses. *bacterial endocarditis*, generally 1g IV 12-hourly for 4 weeks alone or in combination; enterococcal endocarditis is treated for 6 weeks in combination. Therapeutic vancomycin levels should be 30-40mg/L (max. 50mg/L) 1-hour after end of infusion; minimum level, prior to next admin, 5-10mg/L. Obese patients may need modification of daily dose. *Prophylaxis* of endocarditis, 1g prior to induction of anaesthesia for surgery and depending of surgery type and/or duration, another 1g after 12 hours. *Admin*, by slow IV infusion (max. 10mg/min over at least 60 minutes) diluted to at least 100mL/500mg or 200mL/1g; if fluid restriction is needed, 500mg/50mL or 1g/100mL.

Elderly: Dosage reduction may be needed because of decreasing renal function.

Child: ORAL, 40mg/kg body weight in 3-4 divided doses (7-10 days); max. 2g. See Adult above.

PARENTERAL, age 1 month to 12 years, usually 10mg/kg 6-hourly; total 40mg/kg/day. Neonates, young infants, initially 15mg/kg, then 10mg/kg 12-hourly (age 0-7 days) or 8-hourly (age 7-30 days). *Admin*, IV over 60 minutes, see Adult above. Monitor serum levels closely.

Renal Impairment: CrCl (mL/min/kg) 2, admin 30.9mg/kg/24-hours; 1.5mg, admin 23.2mg/kg/24-hours; 1, admin 15.4mg/kg/24-hours; 0.5, admin 7.7mg/kg/24-hours; 0.2, admin 3.1mg/kg/24-hours. *Functionally anephric patients*, loading dose 15mg/kg and then 1.9mg/kg/24-hours. As maintenance doses of 250mg to 1g are convenient, in marked impairment a dose may be given every several days rather than daily; in anuria, recommended 1g every 7-10 days.

Interactions: Effect of Other Drugs on Vancomycin: *Increased nephro and/or ototoxicity*: Co-admin with other neurotoxic or nephrotoxics e.g. aminoglycosides, amphotericin B, ciclosporin, cisplatin, colistin, loop diuretics, polymyxins. *Ototoxicity aggravated*: Diuretics (etacrynic acid, frusemide). *Effect antagonised (oral vancomycin)*: Colestyramine (admin several hours apart).

Effect of Vancomycin on Other Drugs: Anaesthetics: *Hypersensitivity (histamine-like flushing, anaphylactoid reactions, erythema)*. Suxamethonium: *Effect enhanced*.

SP: Infuse as per Dose above to avoid rapid infusion related reactions (severe hypotension e.g. shock/cardiac arrest, histamine-like responses, maculopapular or erythematous rash). Nephrotoxic, ototoxic, use with care in renal insufficiency; ototoxic risk increased by high blood conc or prolonged treatment. Avoid with previous hearing loss; elderly more susceptible to auditory damage. Irritating to tissue, injection-site pain, thrombophlebitis may occur; necrosis if injected IM. Periodic blood monitoring, urine analysis, liver, renal function. May enhance anaesthetic-induced myocardial depression. Oral, offensive taste; significant systemic absorption with inflammatory disorders of intestinal mucosa.

Pregnancy, Lactation: Pregnancy, only if clearly needed after care risk/benefit evaluation. Lactation, vancomycin is excreted in human milk; use only during lactation if other antibiotics have failed; caution, potential adverse reactions in infants (disturbed intestinal flora with diarrhoea, colonisation with yeast-like fungi).

ADR: *Common*: decreased blood pressure, dyspnoea, stridor, exanthema and mucosal inflammation, pruritus, urticaria, renal insufficiency (increased serum creatinine), phlebitis, redness of upper body and face (Red Man Syndrome). See SP above.

Notes: See Class Effects 9.1.9 Other Antibacterials, Enzymes.

Vancocin Matrigel 125mg *(Flynn)* A. HT.
Price, (28) €112.19.
Capsule, vancomycin HCl. Hard dark-blue/brown. Marked 3125 (red ink). **Store:** Below 25 deg; original pack.
Vancocin Parenteral and Oral Soln *(Flynn)* A.
Price, (1 vial) 500mg, €9.84. 1g, €15.20.
Infusion or oral soln, vancomycin HCl 50mg/mL (500mg, 1g). Off-white powder for conc (clear soln). **Store:** Below 25 deg C.
Vancomycin Parenteral *(TEVA)* A.
Price, not published by company.
Infusion, vancomycin HCl 500mg, 1g. White (off-white) powder for soln.
Vancomycin (Hospira) Parenteral *(Hospira)* A. GMS.
Price, 500mg (1) €11.40. 1g, not published by company (non-GMS).
Infusion, vancomycin HCl 500mg, 1g. White (almost) solid powder for soln.
Vancomycin (Pfizer) Parenteral *(Pfizer)* A.
Price, not published by company.
Infusion, vancomycin HCl 500mg, 1g. White (cream) porous cake for reconstitution for conc for soln.

9.2 - Antifungals

In This Chapter: *Amphotericin B, anidulafungin, caspofungin, fluconazole, flucytosine, itraconazole, micafungin, posaconazole, terbinafine, voriconazole.*

Class Effects
CI: Hypersensitivity to any member of the class.
SP: Dose and duration of therapy depends on infection type, severity, clinical response.
Pregnancy, Lactation: Pregnancy, not recommended unless benefit outweighs risk unless otherwise specified. Women of childbearing potential to ensure adequate contraception. Lactation, not recommended; stop drug or stop breastfeeding.
Notes: See 9.1 Antibacterials. See also 6.3 Oropharyngeal Preparations (nystatin).

Amphotericin B
ATC Code: J02AA01. **Sport:** Permitted.
Driving: Some undesirable effects may impact.
Indications: Cryptococcus, North American blastomycosis, disseminated candidosis, coccidioidomycosis, aspergillosis, histoplasmosis, mucormycosis *(AmBisome, Fungizone)*. Febrile neutropenics unresponsive to broad-spectrum antibacterials, visceral leishmaniasis *(AmBisome)*.
Dose: Adult, Elderly: *AmBisome*, test dose of 1mg over 10 minutes. *Mycoses*, 1mg/kg increasing stepwise to 3mg/kg; *empiric*, febrile neutropenia, 3mg/kg/day until temperature normalises for 3 consecutive days; max. 42 days; *visceral leishmaniasis*, 21-30mg/kg given over 10-21 days. Infuse over 30-60 minutes; above 5mg/kg/day, infuse over 2-hours.
Fungizone, IV infusion, admin 1mg test dose over 20-30 minutes and observe patient for 30 minutes. Initially 0.25mg/kg/day; titrate to 1mg/kg/day if needed; severe infection, max. 1.5mg/kg/day. Infuse over 2-6 hours. *Bladder* irrigation/instillation, continuous irrigation 50mg/1L sterile water daily. *Lung inhalation*, 8-40mg/day nebulised in sterile water or 5% glucose in divided doses. *Intrathecal*, range 0.1-1.5mg per dose ranging from daily to weekly beginning at low dose and increasing until appearance of intolerance.
Child: As for Adult above, on bodyweight basis.
Renal Impairment: Dose range 1-3mg/kg/day and no frequency adjustment *(AmBisome)*.
Hepatic Impairment: *AmBisome*, no dose recommendation.
CI: Hypersensitivity unless the condition is life-threatening and amenable only to such treatment.
Interactions: Effect of Other Drugs on Amphotericin B: *Co-admin caution*: Nephrotoxic drugs (ciclosporin, aminoglycosides, polymyxins, tacrolimus, pentamidine), hypokalaemia potential (corticosteroids unless needed to

9.2   Antifungals

control drug reactions otherwise avoid; corticotrophin, diuretics), leukocyte transfusions (acute pulmonary reactions; separate infusion), antineoplastics (enhanced renal toxicity, bronchospasm, hypotension). *Co-admin (monitor renal and haematological function)*: Zidovudine. *Potassium loss increased*: Corticosteroids.

Effects of Amphotericin B on Other Drugs: Digitalis, antiarrhythmics, skeletal muscle relaxants: *Effect/toxicity potentiated (by hypokalaemia)*. Flucytosine: *Toxicity enhanced*.

SP: Hospital use; facilities for resuscitation available; admin test dose to detect idiosyncratic anaphylactic reactions. Premedication (aspirin, paracetamol, diphenhydramine, pethidine and/or hydrocortisone, other antihistamine, anti-emetics) and/or slower infusion rate may reduce infusion-related reactions (hyperkalaemia, arrhythmias with rapid infusion). Nephrotoxic (serum creatinine over 260micromoL/L, discontinue or decrease dose); liposomal less nephrotoxic than conventional amphotericin; monitor renal function. Increased serum creatinine, hypo- kalaemia, magnesaemia at higher dose 5-10mg/kg. Abnormal LFTs, discontinue. Acute pulmonary toxicity if given during/shortly after leucocyte transfusion. Leucoencephalopathy in patients who have received total body irradiation. *Fungizone*: verify product name and dose before admin especially if dose exceeds 1.5mg/kg to prevent overdose (potentially fatal cardiac or cardiorespiratory arrest). Neurological events (arachnoiditis, myelopathy, paresis, paralysis) associated with intrathecal route.

Pregnancy, Lactation: If benefit outweighs risk in life-threatening disease. See Notes below.

ADR: *AmBisome, very common*, hypokalaemia, nausea, vomiting, rigors, pyrexia. *Fungizone, very common*, hypokalaemia, hypotension, dyspnoea, nausea, vomiting, abnormal renal function, chills (within 15-20 minutes after initiation), pyrexia, increased blood creatinine. Adverse reactions may be made less severe by admin (aspirin, other antipyretics, antihistamine or anti-emetic). Pethidine (25-50mg IV) has been used to decrease duration or intensity of shaking chills and fever following therapy. Febrile reactions may be decreased by small doses of adrenal corticosteroids (25mg hydrocortisone) IV just prior to or during infusion. Amphotericin B admin on alternate days may decrease anorexia and phlebitis. Addition of heparin (1000 U per infusion), injection site rotation, the use of paediatric scalp-vein needle and alternate-day therapy, may lessen thrombophlebitis incidence. Extravasation may cause chemical irritation.

Notes: See 9.2 Antifungals.

AmBisome (Liposomal) Parenteral *(Gilead)* A.
Price, (10) 50mg, €1563.18 (PTW).
Infusion, amphotericin B in liposome 4mg/mL (50mg). Yellow lyophilised cake or powder for dispersion. *Hydrogenated soy phosphatidylcholine, essentially sodium-free.*

Fungizone Parenteral *(BMS)* A.
Price, (1) 50mg, €5.07.
Infusion, amphotericin 50mg. Yellow (orange) fine fluffy powder for conc for soln.

Anidulafungin

ATC Code: J02AX06. **Sport:** Permitted.
Driving: Caution.

Indications: Treatment, invasive candidiasis (adults).

Dose: Adult, Elderly: Loading, 200mg (day 1), then 100mg/day; duration based on response and to continue for at least 14 days after last culture; longer than 35 days, no data. Reconstitute with solvent to conc 3.33mg/mL and dilute to conc 0.77mg/mL before use. IV infusion rate max. 1.1mg/min   equiv.   to   1.4mL/min.   when reconstituted/diluted; not for bolus injection.

Child: Under 18 years, no dose recommendation.

CI: Hypersensitivity to echinocandin class of drugs.

Interactions: Effect of Other Drugs on Anidulafungin: *Co-admin caution (infusion-related reactions)*: Anaesthetics.

Effect of Anidulafungin on Other Products: Effect of other medicine may be altered: *High ALCOHOL content in formulation*.

254

SP: Increased hepatic enzymes, monitor; evidence of worsening hepatic function, evaluate risk/benefit. Anaphylactic reactions. Infusion-related reactions; caution when co-admin with anaesthetic agents.

Pregnancy, Lactation: Caution high alcohol content. See Notes below.

ADR: *Very common*, hypokalaemia, diarrhoea, nausea. See SP above.

Notes: See 9.2 Antifungals.

ECALTA Parenteral *(Pfizer)* A. HOS.
Price, (1) 100mg, €393.33 (PTW).
Infusion, anidulafungin 100mg. White (off-white) lyophilised solid powder; clear colourless solvent for soln. Reconstituted soln (pH 4-6). *Fructose.* **Store:** Refrigerate.

Caspofungin

ATC Code: J02AX04. **Sport:** Permitted.
Driving: No studies performed.

Indications: Treatment, invasive candidiasis, invasive aspergillosis refractory to or intolerant of amphotericin B conventional or lipid and/or itraconazole; empiric, presumed fungal infections in febrile neutropenics.

Dose: Adult: Loading, 70mg (day 1), then 50mg/day (over 80kg, 70mg/day); continue until up to 72 hours after neutropenia resolution. Slow IV infusion over 60 minutes as single daily infusion.

Elderly: Over 65 years, limited data.

Child: Age 12 months to 17 years, loading dose 70mg/m2 BSA (day 1), then 50mg/m2/day; well tolerated, no adequate clinical response, increase to 70mg/m2. Co-admin dose adjustment, see Interactions below. Max. 70mg/day.
Under 12 months, caution; 25mg/m2/day in neonates and infants under 3 months and 50mg/m2/day in children 3-11 months.

Hepatic Impairment: Moderate, 35mg/day after 70mg loading dose; severe and paediatrics, no data.

Interactions: Effect of Other Drugs on Caspofungin: *Co-admin if benefit outweighs risk*: Ciclosporin (monitor liver enzymes). *Plasma levels decreased (consider dose increase to 70mg/day after loading)*: Efavirenz, nevirapine, rifampicin, dexamethasone, phenytoin, carbamazepine. *Not for admixture/co-infusion*: Other IV products (no data), diluents containing glucose (not stable).

Effect of Caspofungin on Other Drugs: Tacrolimus: *Trough conc reduced (monitor blood conc)*.

SP: Hypersensitivity reactions (anaphylaxis and possibly histamine-mediated adverse reactions); if occur, discontinue. If abnormal LFTs develop during treatment, monitor for worsening hepatic failure; consider risk/benefit.

ADR: *Common*, decreased Hb, haematocrit, WBC count; hypokalaemia, headache, phlebitis, dyspnoea, nausea, diarrhoea, vomiting, elevated liver enzymes, rash, pruritus, erythema, hyperhidrosis, arthralgia, pyrexia, chills, infusion-site pruritus, decreased blood potassium/blood albumin. Paediatrics, see manufacturers Full Prescribing Information.

Notes: See 9.2 Antifungals.

Cancidas Parenteral *(MSD)* A. HOS.
Price, (1) 50mg, €445.98; 70mg, €567.80 (PTW).
Infusion, caspofungin acetate 50mg, 100mg. White (off-white) compact lyophilised powder for conc for soln. *Sucrose.* **Store:** Refrigerate.

Fluconazole

ATC Code: J02AC01. **Sport:** Permitted.
Driving: Dizziness, seizures.

Indications: *Treatment*, cryptococcal meningitis, coccidioidomycosis, candidiasis (invasive, mucosal, oral atrophic, vaginal, balanitis). Dermatomycosis (tinea and dermal candida), onychomycosis (tinea). *Prophylaxis, relapse* (cryptococcal meningitis), oropharyngeal candidiasis, vaginal candidiasis (to reduce incidence of recurrence), prophylaxis of candidal infections in neutropenics. *Children (0-17 years)*, treatment of candidiasis (mucosal, invasive), cryptococcal meningitis.

Prophylaxis, candidal infections in immunocompromised, to prevent cryptococcal meningitis relapse.

Dose: Adult: *Cryptococcosis,* treatment, 400mg (day 1), then 200-400mg/day (6-8 weeks); life-threatening infections, 800mg/day can be used; maintenance, to prevent relapse, 200mg/day (indefinitely). *Coccidioidomycosis,* 200-400mg/day (11-24 months or longer); 800mg/day can be used (meningeal disease).

Invasive candidiasis, 800mg loading dose (day 1), then 400mg/day (usually 2 weeks after first negative blood culture).

Mucosal candidiasis: Oropharyngeal (7-21 days), oesophageal (14-30 days), 200-400mg loading dose (day 1), then 100-200mg daily; candiduria, 200-400mg/day (7-21 days); chronic atrophic candidiasis, 50mg/day (14 days); chronic mucocutaneous candidiasis, 50-100mg/day (up to 28 days).

Prevention of mucosal candidiasis relapse (HIV or at high risk), oropharyngeal and oesophageal, 100-200mg/day or 20mg 3-times weekly (indefinitely).

Genital candidiasis: Acute vaginal, balanitis, 150mg as single dose; treatment and prophylaxis, recurrent vaginal candidiasis, 150mg (days 1, 4, 7), then maintenance 150mg once weekly (6 months).

Dermatomycosis (parenteral not indicated): Tinea (pedis, corporis, cruris), candida infections, 150mg once weekly or 50mg/day (2-4 weeks; pedis may need 6 weeks); tinea versicolor, 300-400mg once weekly (1-3 weeks) OR 50mg/day (2-4 weeks); tinea unguium (onychomycosis), 150mg once weekly until infected nail replaced.

Prophylaxis in prolonged neutropenia, 200-400mg/day starting several days before neutropenia onset; continue until 7 days after recovery. *Admin,* with or without food. Transferring from IV to oral or vice versa, no need to change daily dose.

Elderly: As for Renal below.

Child: Age 28 days to 11 years: *Mucosal candidiasis,* 6mg/kg (day 1), then 3mg/kg/day; invasive candidiasis, cryptococcal meningitis, 6-12mg/kg/day*. Maintenance to prevent cryptococcal relapse, 6mg/kg/day*. Candida prophylaxis in immunocompromised, 3-12mg/kg/day depending on extent/duration of neutropenia. Max. 400mg/day.

Term infants (0-14 days), max. 12mg/kg, every 72 hours; (15-27 days), every 48 hours. *(depending on severity of disease).

Age 12-17 years generally as for Adult above. *Admin,* as for Adult above.

Renal Impairment: CrCl (mL/min) 50 and below, 50% recommended dose; regular dialysis, 100% dose after each dialysis. No adjustment for single dose treatment.

Hepatic Impairment: Caution.

CI: Hypersensitivity to related azoles.

Interactions: Effect of Other Drugs on Fluconazole: *Co-admin contraindicated:* Terfenadine (multiple doses of 400mg/day or higher), cisapride, astemizole, pimozide, quinidine. *Co-admin avoid/caution:* Halofantrine, amiodarone (QTc interval prolongation), erythromycin. *Plasma levels increased:* Hydrochlorothiazide, other diuretics; ivacaftor (reduce dose to 150mg once daily). *Plasma levels decreased (consider dose increase):* Rifampicin.

Effect of Fluconazole on Other Drugs: Warfarin, coumarins: *Increased prothrombin time (monitor).* Sulphonylureas (chlorpropamide, glibenclamide, glipizide, tolbutamide): *Serum half-life prolonged; possible hypoglycaemic episode.* Phenytoin, theophylline, zidovudine, tacrolimus, rifabutin, midazolam, other benzodiazepines (short-acting), fentanyl, alfentanil, amitriptyline, carbamazepine, celecoxib (consider halving dose), methadone, vinca alkaloids: *Plasma levels increased; consider dose adjustment.* Ciclosporin, NSAIDs, saquinavir, sirolimus, tacrolimus, zidovudine: *Monitor plasma levels, consider dose adjustment.* HMG-CoA reductase inhibitors (atorvastatin, simvastatin, fluvastatin): *Plasma levels increased, elimination half-life increased; caution (monitor creatinine kinase,*

myopathy/rhabdomyolysis. Calcium channel blockers: *Increased systemic exposure (monitor for adverse effects).* Cyclophosphamide: *Increased serum bilirubin/creatinine risk.* Losartan: *Metabolism to active metabolite inhibited; monitor BP.* Long-term prednisone + fluconazole: *Monitor for adrenal cortex insufficiency when fluconazole discontinued.* Vitamin A: *Caution.* Compounds metabolised by CYP3A4, 2C9, 2C19: *Caution, monitor patient.*

SP: Abnormal hepatic, renal, haematological, other biochemical markers (especially with serious underlying disease). Rarely, serious hepatotoxicity (including fatal), anaphylaxis; hepatotoxicity signs, rash (discontinue). QT-prolongation (caution, proarrhythmic conditions); may be amplified with e.g. amiodarone. Exfoliative cutaneous reactions (Stevens-Johnson syndrome, toxic epidermal necrolysis).

DOSE CONVERSION of powder for oral susp from mg/mL to mL/kg body weight (BW) for paediatric dosing: Dose in mL/day = [child weight (kg) x prescribed dose (mg/kg)] divided by [product strength (mg/mL)].

Pregnancy, Lactation: Pregnancy, if benefit outweighs risk in life-threatening infection; otherwise avoid. Observational study suggests increased spontaneous abortion risk in women treated with fluconazole in first trimester. See Notes below.

ADR: *Common,* headache, rash, abdominal pain, diarrhoea, nausea, vomiting, elevated ALP, ALT, AST, rash.

Diflucan 50mg, 150mg, 200mg, Susp *(Pfizer)* B. GMS.D*.
Price, caps (7) 50mg*, €8.37. 200mg, €33.45. 150mg (1) €3.59. Susp (35mL) 50mg/5mL*, €17.06. 200mg/5mL, €67.55.
Capsule, fluconazole. Marked Pfizer FLU/strength. 50mg: Turquoise/white. 150mg: Turquoise. 200mg: Purple/white. *Lactose.* **Store:** Below 30 deg C.
Oral susp, as above 10mg(40mg)/mL. White (off-white) powder providing white (off-white) susp; orange flavour. *Sucrose.* **Store:** Below 25 deg C.

Diflucan Parenteral 2mg/mL *(Pfizer)* A. GMS.
Price, (1) €18.15
IV infusion, fluconazole (100mL). Clear colourless. *Sodium 0.154mmoL/mL.* **Store:** Do not freeze.

Diflazole 50mg, 150mg, 200mg *(TEVA)* B. GMS.D*.
Price, (7) 50mg*, €8.20. 200mg, €32.78. 150mg (1) €3.51.
Capsule, fluconazole. Hard caps. 50mg: Green/white. 150mg: Yellow. 200mg: White.

Flucol 50mg, 150mg, 200mg *(Rowex)* B. GMS.D*.
Price, (7) 50mg*, €8.20. 200mg, €32.78. 150mg (1) €3.51.
Capsule, fluconazole. Hard. 50mg: Turquoise blue/white. 150mg: White. 200mg: Purple/white. *Lactose*

Flucol Parenteral 2mg/mL *(Rowex)* A.
Price, not published by company.
Infusion, fluconazole. Transparent colourless without visible particles. *Sodium 9mg/mL.*

Fluconazole (Accord) Capsules *(Accord)* A. GMS.D*.
Price, (7) 50mg*, €7.94. 200mg, €31.68. 150mg (1) €3.39.
Capsule, fluconazole. 50mg, 150mg, 200mg, 50mg: White/green. 150mg: Blue/blue. 200mg: White/white. *Lactose.*

Fluconazole (Niche) Capsules *(Niche)* B. GMS.D*.
Price, (7) 50mg*, €8.20. 200mg, €32.78. 150mg (1) €3.51.
Capsule, fluconazole 50mg, 150mg, 200mg. 50mg: Light blue/white. 150mg: Medium blue/white. 200mg: Dark blue/white. *Lactose.*

Fluconazole Actavis Capsules *(Accord)* A. GMS.D*.
Price, (7) 50mg*, €7.91. 200mg, €31.58. 150mg (1) €3.38.
Capsule, fluconazole 50mg, 150mg, 200mg. Hard. Pale-blue/white. Contains white powder. *Lactose.*

Fluconazole TEVA Parenteral 2mg/mL *(TEVA)* A.
Price, not published by company.
Infusion, fluconazole. Clear colourless soln. *Sodium 354mg/100mL; 709mg/200mL.*

Flucytosine

ATC Code: J02AX01. **Sport:** Permitted.
Driving: Not applicable.

Indications: Systemic fungal infections. Cryptococcal meningitis and severe systemic candidiasis, recommend combination, see SP below.

Dose: Adult: 200mg/kg/day divided into 4 divided doses over 24 hours; extremely sensitive organisms, 100-150mg/kg/day may be sufficient. Admin by IV infusion over 20-40 minutes balanced with fluid requirements of patient. May be admin directly in vein, through central venous

9.2 Antifungals

catheter or by intra-peritoneal infusion. Duration dependent on patient response.
Elderly: Caution, renal function.
Child: As for Adult above. Neonates, as for Elderly above. Monitor serum flucytosine levels. With renal impairment extend dose interval; if no impairment but serum levels above recommended, reduce dose.
Renal Impairment: CrCl (mL/min) above 40, 25-50mg/kg 6-hourly; 20-40, 25-50mg/kg 12-hourly; CrCl 10-20, 25-50mg/kg 24-hourly; below 10, initial single dose 25-50mg/kg; then according to serum conc; max. 80mcg/mL; blood levels 25-50mcg/mL normally effective. 65-70% of flucytosine is excreted by haemodialysis.
Hepatic Impairment: Careful monitoring.
Interactions: Effect of Other Drugs on Flucytosine: *Co-admin contraindicated*: Antiviral nucleosides (ganciclovir, valganciclovir, brivudine, sorivudine and analogues; potent DPD inhibitors, see SP below). *Increased toxicity, decreased excretion*: Amphotericin. *Plasma levels decreased*: Cytarabine (strict blood level monitoring).
Effect of Flucytosine on Other Drugs: Phenytoin: *Increased phenytoin levels reported (monitor)*. Nephrotoxics: *Monitor renal function*.
SP: Cryptococcal meningitis, severe systemic candidiasis, use with amphotericin B (where toxicity of combination is dose limiting, use with fluconazole; lower cure rate than with amphotericin B). Bone marrow depression or blood dyscrasias. Monitor renal/hepatic function. Dihydropyrimidine dehydrogenase (DPD) deficiency, severe drug toxicity risk.
Pregnancy, Lactation: Pregnancy, do not use in women* not using contraception unless strictly necessary in case of life-threatening infections and lack of effective alternative treatment. Women* and male patients or their female partners* to use effective contraception during and for 1 month (women) or 3 months (men) after treatment. Lactation, contraindicated. *(of childbearing potential).
ADR: Primarily, GI tract, liver, bone marrow; *serious*, may occur with elevated flucytosine serum concentrations (e.g. renal insufficiency, dose is not adjusted to reduced renal excretion capacity). See SP above.
Notes: See 9.2 Antifungals.

> **Ancotil Parenteral** *(Meda)* A.
> Price, (5) 2.5g/250mL, £272.70.
> *Infusion*, flucytosine 2.5g/250mL. Clear colourless (slightly yellow) soln. *Sodium 316mg per 100mL*.

Itraconazole

ATC Code: J02AC02. **Sport:** Permitted.
Driving: Dizziness, visual disturbances, hearing loss.
Indications: Candidosis (vulvovaginal, oral), pityriasis versicolor, fungal keratitis, systemic mycosis, onychomycosis *(capsules)*. Candidosis (oral, oesophageal) in HIV-positive or other immunocompromised patients; prophylaxis of deep fungal infections (anticipated susceptible to itraconazole, standard therapy inappropriate) in patients with haematological malignancy, bone marrow transplant, expected to become neutropenic *(oral soln)*. Treatment, histoplasmosis, systemic fungal infections when first-line ineffective or inappropriate, aspergillosis, candidosis, cryptococcosis (including cryptococcal meningitis) in immunocompromised patients with cryptococcosis and all patients with cryptococcosis of CNS *(parenteral)*.
Dose: Adult: ORAL *(capsules), short-term use* (max. 4 weeks): Vulvovaginal candidosis, 200mg twice daily (day 1) OR 200mg once daily (3 days). Oral candidosis, 100mg once daily (2 weeks). Tinea (pedis, manuum), 100mg once daily (4 weeks). Pityriasis versicolor 200mg once daily (7 days), fungal keratitis (3 weeks). Tinea (corporis, cruris), 100mg once daily (2 weeks) OR 200mg once daily (7 days). *Long-term treatment*, 200mg once daily, onychomycosis (3 months), aspergillosis (2-5 months), non-meningeal cryptococcus (1-6 months); candidosis, 100-200mg once daily (3 weeks-7 months), chromomycosis (6 months). Cryptococcal meningitis, 200mg twice daily (2 months-1 year). Histoplasmosis, 200mg 1-2 times daily (8 months); 100mg once daily, sporotrichosis (3 months),

paracoccidioidomycosis (6 months); blastomycosis, 100mg once daily to 200mg twice daily (6 months). Caps to be swallowed whole; admin immediately after food.
ORAL *(oral soln)*, candidosis (oral, oesophageal), 200mg/day in either 1 or 2 intakes (1 week); no response, continue for another week; fluconazole resistant, 100-200mg twice daily for 2 weeks; no response continue for max. another 2 weeks. Prophylaxis, 5mg/kg/day in 2 intakes. Admin without food; take no food for 1 hour after intake.
PARENTERAL, loading dose 200mg as 1-hour infusion twice daily for 2 days; then 200mg as 1-hour infusion once daily; max. 14 days. Dedicated extension and in-line filter must be used to ensure correct admin.
NOTE: Not recommended that oral capsules and oral soln are used interchangeably; drug exposure greater with oral soln than with caps with the same dose.
Elderly: If benefit outweighs risk (consider renal, hepatic, cardiac function; concomitant disease or other drugs).
Child: Neutropenia prophylaxis, 5mg/kg/day in 2 intakes of oral soln; ADR incidence higher than in adults. Use caps/IV only if benefit outweighs risk.
Renal Impairment: Oral itraconazole, caution (exposure may be lower, consider dose adjustment). CrCl (mL/min) below 30, IV contraindicated due to excipient hydroxypropyl-B-cyclodextrin eliminated by glomerular filtration.
Hepatic Impairment: As for Renal above.
CI: Evidence of ventricular dysfunction (CHF) unless treatment of life-threatening infection. Not for use when Sodium Chloride Injection, contraindicated (IV).
Interactions: Effect of Other Drugs on Itraconazole: *Exposure decreased, co-admin not recommended*: Potent CYP3A4 inducers (rifampicin, rifabutin, isoniazid, carbamazepine, phenobarbital, phenytoin, efavirenz, nevirapine, St John's Wort). *Exposure increased, co-admin caution*: Potent CYP3A4 inhibitors (ciprofloxacin, clarithromycin, erythromycin, ritonavir-boosted darunavir and fosamprenavir, indinavir, ritonavir). *Absorption impaired*: Decreased gastric acidity (antacids; admin 2 hours apart), achlorhydria (H2-antagonists, PPIs; admin with acid beverage e.g. non-diet cola).
Effect of Itraconazole on Other Drugs: Disopyramide, dofetilide, dronedarone, quinidine, dabigatran, halofantrine, mizolastine, terfenadine, ergot alkaloids, irinotecan, oral midazolam, pimozide, quetiapine, sertindole, triazolam, bepridil, lercanidipine, nisoldipine, aliskiren, ivabradine, ranolazine, eplerenone, cisapride, domperidone, lovastatin, simvastatin; fesoterodine, solifenacin, colchicine (with renal or hepatic impairment); sildenafil (in PAH): *Co-admin contraindicated**. Fentanyl, rifabutin, rivaroxaban, carbamazepine, ebastine, eletriptan, dasatinib, lapatinib, nilotinib, trabectedin, felodipine, ciclesonide, everolimus, temsirolimus, atorvastatin, salmeterol, tolterodine, vardenafil (men 75 years and older): *Co-admin not recommended**. Alfentanil, buprenorphine (IV, sublingual), oxycodone, methadone, digoxin, coumarins, cilostazol, repaglinide, saxagliptin, praziquantel, bortezomib, busulphan, docetaxel, erlotinib, gefitinib, imatinib, ixabepilone, trimetrexate, vinca alkaloids, alprazolam, aripiprazole, brotizolam, buspirone, haloperidol, midazolam IV, perospirone, risperidone, maraviroc, indinavir, ritonavir, saquinavir, nadolol, dihydropyridines (not contraindicated) e.g. verapamil, aprepitant, budesonide, ciclosporin, dexamethasone, fluticasone, methylprednisolone, sirolimus (rapamycin), tacrolimus, reboxetine, fesoterodine, sildenafil (for ED), solifenacin, tadalafil, alitretinoin (oral), cinacalcet, tolvaptan: *Co-admin caution**. *(plasma levels increased). Meloxicam: *Caution, plasma levels decreased*.
SP: Caution, cross-hypersensitivity (other azoles). Transient LVEF decrease (IV). CHF, use only if benefit outweighs risk; consider CHF risk factors (ischaemic and valvular cardiac disease, pulmonary disease including COPD, renal failure, oedematous disorders). Rare serious hepatotoxicity (monitor); advise patient to report signs of hepatitis (anorexia, nausea, vomiting, fatigue, abdominal pain, dark urine). Oral bioavailability may be decreased in immunocompromised (neutropenic, AIDS, organ

256

transplant) or at risk of systemic candidosis; do not initiate with oral. Neuropathy, discontinue. CF patients, variability in itraconazole therapeutic levels; no response, consider alternative. Transient or permanent hearing loss; reports included quinidine co-admin. If fluconazole-resistant strains suspected, test sensitivity before initiation.

Pregnancy, Lactation: See Notes below.

ADR: *Most frequent,* (oral soln) dizziness, headache, dysgeusia, dyspnoea, cough, abdominal pain, diarrhoea, vomiting, nausea, dyspepsia, rash, pyrexia; (caps), headache, abdominal pain, nausea; (IV) cough, diarrhoea, vomiting, nausea, rash, oedema. All formulations, *most serious,* serious (allergic, skin) reactions, cardiac failure, CHF, pulmonary oedema, pancreatitis, serious hepatotoxicity (fatal acute liver failure).

Notes: See 9.2 Antifungals.

Sporanox 100mg, Oral Soln *(Janssen-Cilag)* B. GMS.
Price, 100mg (15) €10.69. Soln 10mg/mL (150mL) €60.10.
Capsule, itraconazole. Opaque blue/pink containing coated beads. *Sucrose.*
Oral soln, as above 10mg/mL. Clear yellow (slightly amber); cherry odour. *Sorbitol.*

Sporanox Parenteral 250mg/25mL *(Janssen-Cilag)* A. HOS.
Price, (1) 250mg, €55.65 (PTW).
Infusion, itraconazole trihydrochloride. Conc and solvent (0.9% NaCl) for soln. *Propylene glycol, hydroxypropyl-beta-cyclodextrin.*

Micafungin

ATC Code: J02AX05. **Sport:** Permitted.
Driving: Caution.

Indications: Treatment, oesophageal candidiasis, invasive candidiasis. Prophylaxis, Candida infection in allogeneic haematopoietic stem cell transplantation OR where neutropenia expected for 10 days or more. Decision to use should consider potential risk for liver tumour development; use only where other antifungals are not appropriate.

Dose: Adult, Elderly: *Invasive* candidiasis, over 40kg, 100mg/day; increase to 200mg/day if response inadequate; 40kg and under, 2mg/kg/day; increase to 4mg/kg/day if response inadequate.
Oesophageal candidiasis, over 40kg, 150mg/day; 40kg and under, 3mg/kg/day.
Prophylaxis of candida infection, over 40kg, 50mg/day; 40kg and under, 1mg/kg/day. IV infusion over approx. 1 hour; more rapid infusion, more frequent histamine-mediated reactions. Duration, see manufacturers Full Prescribing Information.

Child: Under 16 years (including neonates), *invasive* candidiasis, as for Adult; *prophylaxis* of candida infection, over 40kg, 50mg/day; 40kg and under, 1mg/kg/day. Age 16 years and older, as for Adult above.

Hepatic Impairment: Severe, not recommended.

CI: Hypersensitivity to other echinocandins.

Interactions: Effect of Micafungin on Other Drugs: Sirolimus, nifedipine, itraconazole: *Increased exposure, monitor for toxicity; consider dose reduction.* Amphotericin B desoxycholate: *30% increased exposure; co-admin only if benefit outweighs risk; monitor for amphotericin toxicity.*

SP: Monitor hepatic function during treatment; to minimise risk of adaptive regeneration, potential liver tumour formation, discontinue early if significant and persistent ALT/AST elevation; careful risk/benefit with severe impairment or chronic liver diseases representing preneoplastic conditions; significant impairment (increased ALT, AST or total bilirubin; above 3xULN); severe dysfunction, hepatitis, hepatic failure (fatal) reported; under age 1 year, greater liver injury risk. Anaphylactoid reactions (shock), discontinue. Exfoliative cutaneous reactions, monitor (discontinue if lesions progress). Haemolysis (acute intravascular haemolysis, haemolytic anaemia); monitor for worsening, evaluate risk/benefit. Monitor renal function. See Interactions above.

Pregnancy, Lactation: See Notes below.

ADR: *Common,* leucopenia, neutropenia, anaemia, headache, phlebitis, nausea, vomiting, diarrhoea, abdominal pain, abnormal LFTs, rash, pyrexia, rigors, hypo-(kalaemia, magnesaemia, calcaemia). See SP above.

Notes: See 9.2 Antifungals.

Antifungals 9.2

Mycamine Parenteral 50mg, 100mg *(Astellas)* A. HOS.
Price, (1) 50mg, €255.32. 100mg, €426.19 (PTW).
Infusion, micafungin sodium. White compact powder for soln.

Posaconazole

ATC Code: J02AC04. **Sport:** Permitted.
Driving: Dizziness, somnolence.

Indications: Invasive aspergillosis, fusariosis, chromoblastomycosis and mycetoma, coccidioidomycosis (refractory or intolerant to first-line treatment). Prophylaxis, invasive fungal infections with remission-induction chemotherapy for acute myelogenous leukaemia (AML) or myelodysplastic syndromes (MDS), haematopoietic stem cell transplant (HSCT) recipients on high-dose immunosuppressants *(tabs, oral susp, parenteral).* Oropharyngeal candidiasis, first-line (severe disease or immunocompromised) *(oral susp).*

Dose: Adult, Elderly: Treatment, *refractory invasive fungal infection,* ORAL TABS, PARENTERAL, loading dose of 300mg twice daily (day 1), then 300mg once daily. *Admin,* tabs with or without food; swallow whole with water; do not crush, chew or break. Parenteral by slow IV infusion over 90 minutes after dilution, through a central venous line; not for bolus admin. ORAL SUSP, 200mg 4-times daily OR if meal or nutritional supplement can be tolerated then 400mg twice daily after food/supplement.
Prophylaxis, *invasive fungal infections,* ORAL TABS, as for treatment above; with AML or MDS, commence several days before neutropenia onset and continue for 7 days after neutrophil count above 500 cells/mm3. ORAL SUSP, 200mg 3-times daily with meal/supplement to enhance oral absorption and ensure adequate exposure.
Oropharyngeal candidiasis, ORAL SUSP, 200mg once daily (day 1), then 100mg once daily for 13 days.
NOTE: Oral tabs and oral suspension are not interchangeable; follow specific dosing for each formulation.

Child: Under 18 years, no dose recommendation.

Renal Impairment: CrCl (mL/min) below 50, accumulation of IV vehicle expected; use oral formulations. Monitor serum creatinine.

Hepatic Impairment: Caution, potentially higher plasma exposure.

Interactions: Effect of Other Drugs on Posaconazole: *Co-admin contraindicated:* CYP3A4 substrates (terfenadine, astemizole, cisapride, pimozide, halofantrine, quinidine; plasma levels increased; QTc prolongation risk); simvastatin, lovastatin, atorvastatin, ergot alkaloids (plasma levels increased). *Co-admin avoid:* Rifabutin, efavirenz, cimetidine, vincristine*, vinblastine. *Possible reduced bioavailability (avoid co-admin):* H2-antagonists, PPIs. *Plasma levels increased:* CYP3A4 inhibitors (verapamil, ciclosporin, quinidine, clarithromycin, erythromycin), vinca alkaloids (vincristine, vinblastine; *neurotoxicity risk, consider dose reduction),* benzodiazepines (midazolam, triazolam, alprazolam). *Plasma levels decreased (may be significant):* Rifamycin, rifampicin, rifabutin, certain anticonvulsants (phenytoin, carbamazepine, phenobarbital, primidone), fosamprenavir, efavirenz. *Absorption of oral susp increased significantly:* Food. *(co-admin associated with neurotoxicity and other serious adverse events e.g. seizures, peripheral neuropathy, SIADH, paralytic ileus; use only if no alternative).*
Effect of Posaconazole on Other Drugs: Tacrolimus, sirolimus, atazanavir; midazolam (IV), triazolam, alprazolam (prolonged sedation): *Increased exposure; consider benzodiazepine dose adjustment.* Calcium channel blockers (diltiazem, verapamil, nifedipine, nisoldipine): *Consider dose adjustment; monitor (adverse events, toxicity).* Digoxin: *Monitor levels (initiation, discontinuation).* Sulphonylureas (glipizide): *Monitor glucose.*

SP: Severe GI dysfunction (e.g. severe diarrhoea), limited data; monitor for breakthrough fungal infection. Azole hypersensitivity, caution. Altered LFTs (reversible on discontinuation); more severe reactions (rare); evaluate LFTs (initially, during therapy). QTc prolongation, caution

257

9.2 Antifungals

(congenital or acquired QTc prolongation, cardiomyopathy, especially with cardiac failure, sinus bradycardia, symptomatic arrhythmias), see Interactions above. Correct electrolyte disturbances (potassium, magnesium, calcium).

Pregnancy, Lactation: See Notes below.

ADR: Summary, *most frequent serious*, nausea, vomiting, diarrhoea, pyrexia, increased bilirubin.

Notes: See 9.2 Antifungals.

> **Noxafil 100mg, Oral Susp** *(MSD)* A. HT.
> Price, tab (24) €788.49; susp (105mL) €666.54.
> Tablet, posaconazole. Yellow cap-shaped g/r. Marked with strength.
> Oral susp, as above 40mg/mL. White. *Glucose*. **Store:** Do not freeze.
> **Noxafil Parenteral 300mg** *(MSD)* A. HOS.
> Price, (1) €415.78 (PTW).
> Infusion, posaconazole. Clear colourless (yellow) conc for soln. *Sodium 462mg (20mmoL)/vial*. **Store:** Refrigerate.

Terbinafine (systemic)

ATC Code: D01BA02. **Sport:** Permitted.
Driving: Dizziness.

Indications: Treatment, Tinea infections (corporis, cruris, pedis), onychomycosis (dermatophytes). Fungal skin infections caused by Trichophyton (rubrum, mentagrophytes, verrucosum, violaceum), *Microsporum canis, Epidermophyton floccosum.*

Dose: Adult, Elderly: 250mg once daily. Tinea cruris (2-4 weeks), Tinea corporis (4 weeks), Tinea pedis (2-6 weeks), onychomycosis (6-12 weeks). *Elderly*, consider renal/hepatic function. *Admin*, oral with water at same time each day; on empty stomach or after food.

Child: *Lamisil*, age 2 years and over, 20-40kg, 125mg/day; over 40kg, 250mg/day. *Admin*, once daily; see Adult above. *All other brands*, not recommended.

Renal Impairment: Not recommended.

Hepatic Impairment: Severe or chronic or active disease, contraindicated.

Interactions: Effect of Other Drugs on Terbinafine *Plasma levels increased*: Cimetidine. *Plasma levels decreased*: Rifampicin.

Effect of Terbinafine on Other Drugs: Caffeine, CYP2D6 substrates (TCADs, beta-blockers, SSRIs, antiarrhythmics Class Ia, Ib and Ic, MAOIs type B), desipramine: *Plasma levels/effect increased*. Ciclosporin: *Plasma levels/effect decreased*. Desipramine: *Decreased clearance*

SP: Hepatotoxicity (nausea, anorexia, fatigue, vomiting, right upper abdominal pain, jaundice, dark urine, pale stools), discontinue. Haematological effects (fever, sore throat); blood dyscrasias (neutropenia, agranulocytosis, thrombocytopenia, pancytopenia). Serious skin reactions (Stevens-Johnson syndrome, toxic epidermal necrolysis, DRESS), if progressive, discontinue. Pre-existing psoriasis/SLE, caution (exacerbation).

Pregnancy, Lactation: Passes into breast milk. See Notes below.

ADR: *Very common*, headache, abdominal distention, decreased appetite, dyspepsia, nausea, mild abdominal pain, diarrhoea, rash, urticaria, arthralgia, myalgia.

Notes: See 9.2 Antifungals.

> **Lamisil 250mg** *(Novartis)* B. GMS.
> Price, (14) €11.01. (28) €21.23.
> Tablet, terbinafine HCl. Round white (off-white) scored. Marked Lamisil 250. **Store:** Below 30 deg; protect from light.
> **Fungasil 250mg** *(Clonmel)* B. GMS.
> Price, (28) €20.81.
> Tablet, terbinafine HCl. White round scored. Marked with strength. **Store:** Original pack.
> **Lamater 250mg** *(Pinewood)* B. GMS.
> Price, (28) €20.04.
> Tablet, terbinafine HCl. White (off-white) scored (divisible into equal halves). Marked T. **Store:** Original pack.
> **Nailderm 250mg** *(Gerard)* B. GMS.
> Price, (28) €20.81.
> Tablet, terbinafine HCl. White (off-white) round scored (facilitates breaking). Marked TF/strength; G on reverse.

> **Terbasil 250mg** *(Accord)* B. GMS.
> Price, (28) €20.81.
> Tablet, terbinafine HCl. White round flat scored (divisible into equal halves). Marked T above and 1 below score.
> **Ternaf 250mg** *(Rowex)* B. GMS.
> Price, (28) €20.81.
> Tablet, terbinafine HCl. White (almost) round scored. Marked TER/strength. **Store:** Original pack.

Voriconazole

ATC Code: J02AC03. **Sport:** Permitted.
Driving: Caution.

Indications: Treatment, invasive aspergillosis, candidaemia (non-neutropenics), fluconazole-resistant serious invasive Candida infections (including *C. krusei*), serious fungal infections (Scedosporium spp., Fusarium spp.). Use primarily with progressive, possibly life-threatening infections. Prophylaxis, invasive fungal infections in high risk allogeneic haematopoietic stem cell transplant (HSCT) recipients.

Dose: Adult, Elderly: ORAL (40kg and over*), loading dose 400mg 12-hourly (first 24 hours), then 200mg twice daily; increase to 300mg twice daily if needed; (under 40kg*), loading dose 200mg 12-hourly (for 24 hours), then 100mg twice daily; increase to 150mg twice daily if needed. If higher doses not tolerated, decrease by 50mg steps to usual maintenance. *Admin*, take tabs 1 hour before or 1 hour after food; susp 1 hour before or 2 hours after food (reconstitute to total volume 46mL). Oral bioavailability is high (96%); switch between oral and parenteral is appropriate. *(this also applies to patients aged 15 years and older).

PARENTERAL, loading dose 6mg/kg 12-hourly (first 24 hours), then maintenance 4mg/kg twice daily; if 4mg/kg not tolerated reduce to 3mg/kg twice daily. *Admin*, max. rate 3mg/kg/hour over 1-3 hours.

Co-admin (parenteral or oral), with phenytoin, rifabutin, efavirenz, see manufacturers Full Prescribing Information.

Initiate prophylaxis on day of transplant; admin for up to 100 days; up to 180 days after transplant with continuing immunosuppression or graft versus host disease. Dose as for treatment above.

Child: Age 2-14 years, under 50kg, loading dose 9mg/kg 12-hourly IV for 24-hours (oral not recommended), then maintenance 8mg/kg twice daily IV OR oral susp 9mg/kg twice daily (max. 350mg twice daily). Age 12-14 years (50kg and over), age 15-17 years, as for Adult above.

Renal Impairment: *Adult*, parenteral, CrCl (mL/min) below 50, IV not recommended; use oral. Haemodialysis, cleared at 121mL/min; 4-hour dialysis does not warrant dose adjustment. IV vehicle (SBECD) haemodialysed at clearance 55mL/min. *Child*, age 2-12 years, no data.

Hepatic Impairment: Severe, if benefit outweighs risk. Mild to moderate cirrhosis, use standard loading dose, reduce maintenance to half standard dose. Monitor for toxicity. *Children*, as for Renal above.

CI: Hypersensitivity to other azoles.

Interactions: Effect of Other Drugs on Voriconazole: *Co-admin contraindicated*: Drugs prolonging QT-interval (terfenadine, astemizole, quinidine, cisapride, pimozide), rifampicin, carbamazepine, barbiturates (phenobarbital, mephobarbital), sirolimus (sirolimus plasma levels significantly increased), ergot alkaloids, ritonavir (oral high dose, 800mg/day), St John's Wort, efavirenz (dose 400mg and above once daily), ritonavir (400mg and above twice daily). *Co-admin avoid (unless benefit outweighs risk)*: Ritonavir (oral low dose, 100mg twice daily), phenytoin, rifabutin. *Co-admin caution*: Protease inhibitors (saquinavir, amprenavir, nelfinavir); NNRTIs. *Plasma levels increased (no dose adjustment)*: Cimetidine.

Effect of Voriconazole on Other Drugs: Everolimus, ciclosporin (halve dose), methadone*, short-acting opiates (alfentanil, fentanyl)*, long-acting opiates (oxycodone)*, tacrolimus (reduce dose to one-third); warfarin, other oral anticoagulants (monitor prothrombin time); sulphonylureas (tolbutamide, glipizide, glyburide; caution hypoglycaemia), statins* (rhabdomyolysis), benzodiazepines (midazolam, triazolam) (prolonged sedative effect); vinca alkaloids (vincristine, vinblastine; neurotoxicity), prednisolone, omeprazole (halve dose with voriconazole initiation), NSAIDs*: *Plasma levels increased.* *Consider dose reduction.

SP: Correct electrolytes (hypo- kalaemia, magnesaemia, calcaemia) before initiating, during therapy. QT-prolongation risk; caution with proarrhythmic conditions (QT-prolongation, cardiomyopathy especially with HF, sinus bradycardia, symptomatic arrhythmias, medication prolonging QT-interval). Infusion-related reactions, flushing, nausea (severe, discontinue). Blurred vision, optic neuritis, papilloedema. Monitor, renal, pancreatic function, hepatic, LFTs (initiation, weekly for first month of treatment); hepatic toxicity, discontinue. Exfoliative cutaneous reactions, discontinue if lesions progress; photosensitivity. *Long-term use*, skin squamous cell carcinoma reported. Non-infectious periostitis, consider discontinuation.

Pregnancy, Lactation: See Notes below.

ADR: Summary, *most common*, visual impairment, pyrexia, rash, vomiting, nausea, diarrhoea, headache, peripheral oedema, abnormal LFTs, respiratory distress, abdominal pain.

Notes: See 9.2 Antifungals.

VFEND 50mg, 200mg, Susp *(Pfizer)* A. HT.
Price, tabs (28) 50mg, €222.34. 200mg, €886.79. Oral susp 40mg/mL (75mL) €624.69.
Tablet, voriconazole. White (off-white) f/c. Marked Pfizer; VOR/strength on reverse. 50mg: Round. 200mg: Cap-shaped. *Lactose.*
Oral susp, as above 40mg/mL. White (off-white) powder. *Sucrose.*
Store: Refrigerate; keep tightly closed.
VFEND Parenteral 200mg *(Pfizer)* A. HOS.
Price, (1) €128.56 (PTW).
Infusion, voriconazole 200mg/vial. White lyophilised powder for soln. *Sodium 217.6mg/vial.* **Store:** In-use stability (chemical, physical) 24 hours refrigerated.
Voriconazole Accord 50mg, 200mg *(Accord)* A. HT.
Price, (28) 50mg, €130.93; 200mg, €515.17.
Tablet, voriconazole. White (off-white) f/c. Marked V and strength. 50mg: Round. 200mg: Oval. *Lactose.*
Voriconazole Rowex 200mg *(Rowex)* A. HT.
Price, (28) €515.17.
Tablet, voriconazole. White (off-white) cap-shaped f/c. Marked 200. *Lactose.*
Voriconazole TEVA 200mg *(TEVA)* A. HT.
Price, (28) €515.17.
Tablet, voriconazole. White oblong f/c. Marked V; strength on reverse. *Lactose.*

9.3 - Antivirals Used In HIV Infection

Class Effects

Driving: If no specific data available, consider clinical status and adverse reaction (ADR) profile.

Dose: To be prescribed by physicians experienced in HIV infection management. When used in combination always consult the manufacturers Full Prescribing Information for each individual drug (duration, dose adjustments based on tolerability and/or toxicity, guidance for missed doses).

Indications: Antiretroviral combination therapy for the treatment of Human Immunodeficiency Virus-1 (HIV-1) in adults, children (where specified). Additional indications, see individual drugs.

CI: Hypersensitivity to any member of the class.

SP: Effective viral suppression with antiretroviral therapy does not preclude (opportunistic infection, other HIV infection complications); may reduce but does not prevent risk of HIV or hepatitis B transmission through blood contact; may reduce risk of sexual transmission (cannot exclude residual risk). Ensure precautions to prevent transmission in accordance with national guidelines. *Metabolic*, increased weight, metabolic parameters (blood lipids, glucose) may occur; monitor (may be linked to disease control, lifestyle). Manage lipid disorders. Monitor pre-existing liver dysfunction (chronic active hepatitis); evidence of worsening, interrupt or discontinue. Increased risk for severe, potentially fatal hepatic adverse events when HIV (with hepatitis B or C co-infection) is treated with antiretrovirals. *Mitochondrial dysfunction* reported in HIV-negative infants exposed in-utero and/or postnatal

(haematological, metabolic, late-onset neurological disorders). *Immune reactivation syndrome* (immune reconstitution inflammatory syndrome), with initiation of combination antiretroviral therapy (CART) (inflammatory reaction, asymptomatic or residual pathogens causing serious CMV retinitis, mycobacterial infection, *Pneumocystis jirovecii* pneumonia). Autoimmune disorders (Grave's disease) reported with immune reactivation. *Osteonecrosis*, especially advanced HIV-disease and/or long-term CART exposure. Motor weakness with CART, associated with hyperlactataemia or lactic acidosis syndrome; may mimic Guillain-Barre syndrome.

Pregnancy, Lactation: Recommended that HIV infected women do not breast-feed their infants under any circumstances to avoid HIV transmission.

ADR: See Manufacturers Full Prescribing Information.

9.3.1 - Nucleoside Reverse Transcriptase Inhibitors (NRTIs) (HIV)

In This Chapter: *Abacavir and combinations, didanosine, emtricitabine and combinations, lamivudine and combinations, stavudine, zidovudine and combinations.*

Class Effects

Driving, Dose Adjustments: See Notes below.

Dosing Instructions: To ensure admin of entire dose, tab(s) to be swallowed whole without crushing. If unable to swallow tab(s), crush, add to small amount of semi-solid food or liquid and consume immediately *(Ziagen, Epivir, Combivir).*

SP: Lactic acidosis associated with hepatomegaly hepatic steatosis reported with *some* nucleoside analogues; hyperlactataemia symptoms include benign (nausea, vomiting, abdominal pain), non-specific malaise, appetite/weight loss, rapid and/or deep breathing, neurological symptoms. Lactic acidosis has high mortality (pancreatitis, liver or renal failure). Symptomatic hyperlactataemia and metabolic and/or lactic acidosis, progressive hepatomegaly, or rapidly elevating transaminases, discontinue. *Caution*, hepatomegaly, hepatitis, other risk factors for liver disease, hepatic steatosis (medicinals, alcohol), particularly obese women. Monitor, pre-existing liver dysfunction (chronic hepatitis); special risk for severe, potentially fatal hepatic adverse reactions with hepatitis B or C co-infection if treated with alpha interferon + ribavirin + CART. Fixed combinations, titrate dose with separate components. Mitochondrial toxicity (subcutaneous fat loss), see Pregnancy; immune reactivation syndrome, osteonecrosis, Graves' disease, see Notes below.

Pregnancy, Lactation: Pregnancy, use if benefit outweighs risk unless otherwise stated. Nucleoside analogues may affect mitochondrial function; most pronounced with (stavudine, didanosine, zidovudine). Mitochondrial dysfunction in infants exposed to nucleoside analogues (in utero, post-natal) reported. Adverse reactions: Haematological (anaemia, neutropenia), metabolic (hyperlactataemia, hyperlipasaemia), late onset neurological disorders (hypertonia, convulsion, abnormal behaviour). Lactation, see Notes below.

ADR: See Notes below.

Notes: See 9.3 Antivirals Used In HIV Infection.

Abacavir

ATC Code: J05AF06. **Sport:** Permitted.
Driving: Consider patient clinical status; ADR profile below.
Dose: Adult, Elderly: Weight at least 25kg, 600mg/day (1 or 2 divided doses). *Admin*, oral with or without food. HLA-B*5701 allele, see SP below. *Elderly*, over 65 years, no data. Admin instructions, see Notes below.

Child: Weight under 25kg, from age 1 year, 8mg/kg twice daily or 16mg/kg once daily; max. 600mg/day. Age 3 months to 1 year, 8mg/kg twice daily; once daily, as above, can be considered. Under 3 months, limited data.

Renal Impairment: ESRD, not recommended.

Hepatic Impairment: Primarily metabolised by liver. Mild,

9.3.1 Nucleoside Reverse Transcriptase Inhibitors (NRTIs) (HIV)

close monitoring including abacavir plasma levels. Moderate or severe, not recommended unless necessary. **Interactions: Effect of Other Drugs on Abacavir:** *Plasma levels increased*: Ethanol. *Plasma levels slightly decreased*: Rifampicin, phenobarbital, phenytoin.

Effect of Abacavir on Other Drugs: Methadone: *Plasma levels decreased*. Retinoids: *Possible interaction*.

SP: Before initiation, screen for HLA-B*5701 allele irrespective of racial origin. NOT for use in patients carrying HLA-B*5701 allele (increased hypersensitivity risk). *Caution*, hypersensitivity reactions (life threatening/fatal; skin rash, fever, GI, respiratory symptoms, lethargy, malaise, musculoskeletal symptoms); usually within first 6 weeks, but can occur at any time; if diagnosed, MUST discontinue immediately; NEVER restart (risk lower in blacks than other racial groups). Caution drugs causing skin toxicity (NNRTIs); difficult to differentiate between rash and hypersensitivity. After interruption, restart with caution. Ensure patients fully informed of risk. Pancreatitis. MI, minimise risk factors (smoking, hypertension, hyperlipidaemia). Autoimmune disorders (Graves' disease) with immune reactivation.

Pregnancy, Lactation: Pregnancy, malformative risk unlikely; reports of mitochondrial dysfunction in HIV-negative infants exposed in utero and/or postnatally, see Notes below. Lactation, see Notes below.

ADR: See Notes below.

Notes: See 9.3.1 NRTIs.

Ziagen 300mg, Oral Soln *(ViiV)* A. HOS.
Price, 300mg (60) €254.99. Oral soln (240mL) €66.68 (PTW).
Tablet, abacavir sulfate. Yellow cap-shaped scored (divisible into equal halves). Marked GX623.
Oral soln, as above 20mg/mL. Clear (slightly opalescent) yellowish aqueous; strawberry, banana flavour. *Sorbitol, parabens*.

Abacavir, Lamivudine

ATC Code: J05AR02. **Sport:** Permitted.
Driving: Consider clinical status, ADR profile below.

Dose: Adult, Elderly: Weight 25kg and above, 1 tab once daily; *Elderly*, over 65 years, no data; consider renal profile. *Admin*, oral with or without food.

Child: 25kg and over, as for Adult; under 25kg, use individual components.

Renal Impairment: CrCl (mL/min) below 50, not recommended; use individual components.

Hepatic Impairment: Monitor function. Moderate, not recommended unless necessary; severe, contraindicated. See Notes below (abacavir).

Interactions: Effect of Other Drugs on Abacavir, Lamivudine: *Co-admin not recommended*: Emtricitabine, cladribine, other lamivudine-containing products. *Co-admin caution*: Ribavirin + abacavir. *Clinical monitoring with co-admin*: Co-trimoxazole (avoid high doses).

Effect of Abacavir, Lamivudine on Other Drugs: Phenytoin, methadone: *Monitor plasma levels; consider dose adjustment*.

SP: HLA-B*5701 allele, see Notes below (abacavir).

ADR: See Notes below (NRTIs).

Notes: See Abacavir above, Lamivudine below. See 9.3.1 NRTIs.

Kivexa 600/300 Tablets *(ViiV)* A. HOS.
Price, (30) €406.83 (PTW).
Tablet, abacavir sulfate 600mg, lamivudine 300mg. Orange cap-shaped f/c. Marked GSFC2. *Sunset Yellow*.

Abacavir/Lamivudine Mylan 600/300 *(Gerard)* A.
Price, (30) €193.47 (trade).
Tablet, abacavir sulfate 600mg, lamivudine 300mg. Orange cap-shaped f/c. Marked 300; 600 on reverse. *Sunset Yellow*. **Store:** Below 25 deg C.

Abacavir, Lamivudine, Zidovudine

ATC Code: J05AR04. **Sport:** Permitted.
Driving: Consider patient clinical status; ADR profile below.

Indications: Consider fixed combination under special circumstances (TB co-infection); replaces 3 components.

Dose: Adult, Elderly: Age 18 years and over, 1 tab twice daily. *Admin*, oral with or without food.

Renal Impairment: ESRD, not recommended.

Hepatic Impairment: See Notes below (abacavir).

SP: HLA-B*5701 allele, see Notes below (abacavir).

ADR: See individual components below.

Notes: See 9.3.1 NRTIs. See Abacavir above, Lamivudine and Zidovudine below.

Trizivir 300/150/300 Tablets *(ViiV)* A. HOS.
Price, (60) €593.62 (PTW).
Tablet, abacavir sulfate 300mg, lamivudine 150mg, zidovudine 300mg. Blue-green cap-shaped f/c. Marked GXLL1.

Didanosine

ATC Code: J05AF02. **Sport:** Permitted.
Driving: Unlikely to impair.

Indications: HIV-1 infection (combination) when other antiretrovirals cannot be used.

Dose: Adult, Elderly: 60kg and over, 400mg/day; under 60kg, 250mg/day. *Admin*, as single daily dose or 2 divided doses; oral on empty stomach, 2 hours before or 1 hour after food; swallow whole with water. *Elderly*, as for Renal below.

Child: Age 6 years and over 240mg/m2 BSA.

Renal Impairment: CrCl (mL/min) 30-59 (60kg and over) 200mg/day; (under 60kg) 150mg/day; 10-29 (60kg and over) 150mg/day; (under 60kg) 100mg/day; below 10 (60kg and over) 100mg/day; (under 60kg) 75mg/day. Admin after dialysis; no supplemental dose required.

Hepatic Impairment: Monitor for toxicity.

Interactions: Effect of Other Drugs on Didanosine: *Co-admin contraindicated*: Stavudine. *Co-admin not recommended*: Tenofovir (if benefit outweighs risk), allopurinol, hydroxyurea. *Co-admin avoid (pancreatitis)*: Drugs causing peripheral neuropathy or pancreatic toxicity (pentamidine). *Co-admin caution*: Ribavirin. *Decreased exposure*: Methadone.

SP: Extreme caution, pancreatitis. Toxic peripheral neuropathy, discontinue. Retinal or optic nerve changes/lesions (at above recommended dose). Monitor liver function. Non-cirrhotic portal hypertension, leading to liver transplantation or death; monitor (thrombocytopenia, splenomegaly).

ADR: See Notes below.

Notes: See 9.3.1 NRTIs.

Videx EC Capsules *(BMS)* A. HOS.
Price, (30) 125mg, €82.94. 200mg, €102.60. 250mg, €130.92. 400mg, €172.04 (PTW).
Capsule, didanosine, 125mg, 200mg, 250mg, 400mg. Opaque white g/r. Marked BMS, strength. 125mg: Marked 6671. 200mg: Marked 6672. 250mg: Marked 6673. 400mg: Marked 6674. *Sodium*.

Emtricitabine

ATC Code: J05AF09. **Sport:** Permitted.
Driving: Caution.

Dose: Adult, Elderly: 200mg/day (caps) or 240mg/day (oral soln). *Over 65 years*, as for Renal below. *Admin*, once daily, with or without food. NOTE: Caps and oral soln NOT bioequivalent.

Child: Age 4 months and over, weight 33kg and over, 200mg/day (caps if able to swallow) OR 6mg/kg/day (oral soln; max. 240mg). *Admin*, once daily.

Renal Impairment: Adults, CrCl (mL/min) 50 or more, 200mg cap* or 240mg oral soln*; 30-49, 200mg cap 48-hourly or 120mg oral soln*; 15-29, 200mg cap 72-hourly or 80mg oral soln*; below 15 (functionally anephric; intermittent haemodialysis), 200mg cap every 96 hours or 60mg oral soln*. *(24-hourly).

Hepatic Impairment: See SP below.

Interactions: Effect of Other Drugs on Emtricitabine: *Co-admin not recommended*: Zalcitabine, lamivudine, combinations containing emtricitabine or lamivudine. *Plasma levels mutually increased*: Drugs eliminated by active tubular secretion.

SP: Co-infection (HIV and HBV) with advanced liver disease or cirrhosis, do not discontinue.

ADR: See Notes below.

Notes: See 9.3.1 NRTIs.

Nucleoside Reverse Transcriptase Inhibitors (NRTIs) (HIV) 9.3.1

Emtriva 200mg, Oral Soln *(Gilead)* A.
Price, not published by company.
Capsule, emtricitabine. Hard opaque white/light blue. Marked 200mg, GILEAD and logo.
Oral soln, as above 10mg/mL (70mL). Clear orange (dark-orange). Parabens, Sunset Yellow. **Store:** Unopened, refrigerate; below 25 deg C after opening.

Emtricitabine, Tenofovir (alafenamide, disoproxil)

ATC Code: J05AR03. **Sport:** Permitted.
Driving: Dizziness.
Indications: HIV-1 infection. Pre-exposure prophylaxis (PrEP).

Dose: Adult, Elderly: *Descovy* (12 years and over; at least 35kg), dose based on THIRD agent in regimen: Dose 200/10/day* with atazanavir or darunavir + (ritonavir or cobicistat) or lopinavir + (ritonavir). Dose 200/25/day* with dolutegravir, efavirenz, maraviroc, nevirapine, rilpivirine, raltegravir. *Admin*, with or without food; swallow whole; do not chew, crush or split. *(once daily).

Truvada (12 years and over, weighing at least 35kg), treatment and prophylaxis, 1 tab once daily. *Admin*, with food; swallowing difficulty, disintegrate tab in 100mL water or juice (orange, grape), admin immediately. *Over 65 years*, as for Renal below.

Child: *Descovy*, under (12 years, 35kg), no data. *Truvada*, under 12 years, not recommended; see Adult above.

Renal Impairment: *Descovy*, CrCl (mL/min) 30 and above, no adjustment; below 30, do not initiate; if CrCl declines to below 30 during treatment, discontinue. *Truvada*, treatment, CrCl (mL/min) 50-80, dose once daily; 30-49, every 48 hours; below 30, not recommended; prophylaxis, CrCl (mL/min) 60-80, dose once daily; under 60, not recommended.

Hepatic Impairment: No adjustment.
CI: PrEP with unknown or positive HIV-1 status.

Interactions: Effect of Other Drugs on Emtricitabine, Tenofovir Combination: *Descovy*: Co-admin not recommended: Boceprevir, telaprevir, tipranavir + ritonavir, oxcarbazepine, carbamazepine, phenobarbital, phenytoin, rifampicin, rifabutin, St John's Wort. *Decreased tenofovir (TAF)*: Efavirenz. *Increased tenofovir (TAF)*: ritonavir, ciclosporin, ketoconazole, itraconazole, fluconazole, isavuconazole (may increase), atazanavir + (cobicistat or ritonavir), darunavir + (cobicistat or ritonavir), lopinavir + ritonavir.

Truvada: Co-admin not recommended: Other nephrotoxics, medicinals containing individual components including TAF, adefovir dipivoxil, cytidine analogues (lamivudine), didanosine. *Co-admin caution (monitor renal function):* Darunavir + ritonavir + (efavirenz or tenofovir or emtricitabine).

SP: NOTE: Tenofovir may be tenofovir disoproxil fumarate or tenofovir alafenamide fumarate (TAF). *Descovy*, worsening liver disease, interrupt or discontinue. *Truvada*, hypophosphataemia, monitor. Cirrhosis, advanced liver disease, recommend not to discontinue; post-treatment hepatitis exacerbation may lead to hepatic decompensation. Renal precautions, see Notes below (tenofovir).

Pregnancy, Lactation: Pregnancy, if benefit outweighs risk *(Descovy)*. Consider use *(Truvada)*. Lactation, not recommended; passes into human milk *(both)*.

ADR: See Notes below.

Notes: See 9.3.1 NRTIs. See Emtricitabine above, 9.4.2 Viral Hepatitis (tenofovir, brand *Viread*).

▼ **Descovy 200/10(25)** *(Gilead)* A.
Price, not published by company (30).
Tablet, emtricitabine, tenofovir alafenamide fumarate (TAF). Rectangular. Marked GSI. 200/10: Grey. Marked 210. 200/25: Blue. Marked 225. **Store:** Original pack to protect (moisture).

Truvada 200/245 *(Gilead)* A.
Price, not published by company.
Tablet, emtricitabine, tenofovir disoproxil 200/245mg. Blue cap-shaped f/c. Marked Gilead; 701 on reverse. *Lactose*. **Store:** Original pack to protect (moisture).

Emtricitabine, Tenofovir, Cobicistat, Elvitegravir

ATC Code: J05AR09. **Sport:** Permitted.
Driving: Dizziness.
Indications: HIV-1 infection (antiretroviral treatment-naive or without known mutations with any of components).

Dose: Adult, Elderly: Age 18 years and over, 1 tab once daily. *Admin*, with food; do not crush or chew. Elderly, caution; no dose recommendation over 65 years.

Child: Age 6-18 years, safety/efficacy not established; 0-6 years, not recommended (safety concerns).

Renal Impairment: CrCl (mL/min) below 70, do not initiate; below 90 initiate only if considered preferred treatment. During treatment, if CrCl falls below 70, consider risk/benefit; below 50mL/min, discontinue.

Hepatic Impairment: Severe, not recommended.
CI: Previous discontinuation of tenofovir due to renal toxicity with/without reversal of effects post-discontinuation.

Interactions: Effect of Other Drugs on Emtricitabine, Tenofovir, Cobistat, Elvitegravir Combination: *Co-admin contraindicated*: Alfuzosin, amiodarone, quinidine, carbamazepine*, phenobarbital*, phenytoin*, rifampicin*, ergot alkaloids, cisapride, St John's Wort*, lovastatin, simvastatin, pimozide, sildenafil (in PAH), oral midazolam, triazolam. *Co-admin not recommended*: Boceprevir, salmeterol, atorvastatin; corticosteroids (cobicistat + corticosteroid interaction). *Co-admin avoid*: Progestogens (not norgestimate); other nephrotoxics (aminoglycosides, amphotericin B, foscarnet, ganciclovir, pentamidine, vancomycin, cidofovir, aldesleukin), if unavoidable, monitor renal function weekly; medicinals reducing renal function or compete for active tubular secretion (cidofovir). *Co-admin caution*: Fluticasone, disopyramide, flecainide, systemic lidocaine, mexiletine, propafenone, amlodipine, diltiazem, felodipine, nicardipine, nifedipine, verapamil, pitavastatin. *Separate dosing by at least 4 hours*: Antacids, multivitamin supplements. *(significantly decreased cobicistat and elvitegravir plasma levels; loss of therapeutic effect, resistance development).

Effect of Emtricitabine, Tenofovir, Cobistat, Elvitegravir Combination on Other Drugs: Azole antifungals, rifabutin (reduce dose to 150mg 3-times weekly), certain macrolides, H2-antagonists, PPIs, metformin, digoxin, metoprolol, timolol, tadalafil (PAH), sildenafil (ED), colchicine, sedatives/hypnotics, immunosuppressants, antidepressants: *Consider dose adjustment*. Bosentan: *Consider alternative*. Warfarin: *Monitor INR*. Dabigatran: *Monitor*.

SP: Not for co-admin with other antivirals (complete regimen). Determine creatinine clearance (CrCl), urine (glucose, protein) in all patients, monitor (also serum phosphate), every 4 weeks (year 1), then 3-monthly; more frequently with renal impairment risk. Cobicistat inhibits tubular creatinine secretion; serum creatinine increased above 0.3mg/dL from baseline, monitor for renal safety. Serum phosphate below 0.48 mmoL/L (1.5mg/dL) or CrCl below 70 mL/min, evaluate renal function within 1 week including blood (glucose, potassium), urine glucose; serum phosphate below 0.32mmoL/L (1mg/dL), discontinue. Poor CYP2B6 metabolisers switching from efavirenz-regimen, monitor viral load. Bone abnormalities (fractures) associated with proximal renal tubulopathy. Renal precautions, see Notes below (tenofovir, brand *Viread*).

Pregnancy, Lactation: Pregnancy, use only if benefit outweighs risk. Use with effective contraception; females of childbearing potential to use hormonal contraceptive with at least 30mcg ethinylestradiol + norgestimate as the progestogen OR alternative reliable contraceptive method. Lactation, not recommended.

ADR: See Notes below.

Notes: See 9.3.1 NRTIs. See Emtricitabine, Tenofovir above. See 9.4.2 Viral Hepatitis (tenofovir brand *Viread*). See 9.3.2 Protease Inhibitors (HIV) (cobicistat).

261

9.3.1 Nucleoside Reverse Transcriptase Inhibitors (NRTIs) (HIV)

▼ **Stribild 150/150/200/245mg** (Gilead) A.
Price, not published by company.
Tablet, elvitegravir 150mg, cobicistat 150mg, emtricitabine 200mg, tenofovir disoproxil 245mg. Green cap-shaped f/c. Marked GSI; 1 on reverse. Lactose. **Store:** Original pack to protect (moisture).

Emtricitabine, Tenofovir, Efavirenz

ATC Code: J05AR06. **Sport:** Permitted.
Driving: Caution.
Dose: Adult, Elderly: Age 18 years and over, 1 tab daily. Admin, swallow whole with water on empty stomach at bedtime; admin with food may increase. Co-admin with rifampicin, efavirenz, rifabutin (dose adjustment); see Interactions below. Elderly, caution.

Renal Impairment: CrCl (mL/min) below 50, not recommended.

Hepatic Impairment: Mild/moderate, monitor CNS symptoms (efavirenz). Severe, not recommended.

Interactions: Effect of Other Drugs on Emtricitabine, Tenofovir, Efavirenz: Co-admin contraindicated: Terfenadine, astemizole, cisapride, midazolam, triazolam, pimozide, bepridil, ergot alkaloids and derivatives, (inhibited metabolism; serious and/or life threatening adverse events), voriconazole (efavirenz plasma levels increased). Co-admin not recommended: Any components of combination, tenofovir alafenamide fumarate (TAF), lamivudine, atazanavir + ritonavir, didanosine, ritonavir (dose 600mg), saquinavir (as sole PI), adefovir, other NNRTIs, Ginkgo biloba extracts, simeprevir (interacts with efavirenz). Co-admin avoid*: Other nephrotoxics (aminoglycosides, amphotericin B, foscarnet, ganciclovir, pentamidine, vancomycin, cidofovir, interleukin-2). Co-admin caution*: Darunavir + ritonavir + (efavirenz or tenofovir or emtricitabine), efavirenz, emtricitabine, tenofovir. Reduced plasma levels: St John's Wort. No dose recommendation with co-admin: Indinavir, lopinavir + ritonavir combination, saquinavir + ritonavir combination. Adjust dose: Rifampicin (adjust efavirenz dose); rifabutin (increase rifabutin daily dose by 50%). *(monitor renal function)

Effect of Emtricitabine, Tenofovir, Efavirenz on Other Drugs: Didanosine: Co-admin not recommended. Voriconazole: artemether, dihydroartemisinin, lumefantrine: Plasma levels decreased. Clarithromycin: Plasma levels changed; significance unknown. Itraconazole, carbamazepine: No dose recommendation; use alternative. Anticonvulsant (CYP450 substrate): Monitor anticonvulsant levels. Sertraline, diltiazem, calcium channel blockers: Adjust dose according to response. Statins: Consider dose adjustment; monitor cholesterol. Methadone: Consider dose increase (withdrawal). Tacrolimus: Consider dose adjustments; decreased tacrolimus exposure. Telaprevir: Use telaprevir 1125mg 8-hourly if co-admin with Atripla.

SP: HIV-1 with K65R, M184V/I or K103N mutation, avoid. Discontinuation, note long half-life (efavirenz); long intracellular half-life (tenofovir, emtricitabine). Severe depression; suicide, delusions, psychosis-like behaviour, impaired concentration, seizures. Renal failure or impairment, elevated creatinine, hypophosphataemia, proximal tubulopathy (including Fanconi syndrome); monitor renal function every 4 weeks (year 1), then 3-monthly. Decreased bone mineral density. See Notes below (tenofovir).

Pregnancy, Lactation: Pregnancy, avoid. Lactation, not recommended. See Notes below (NRTIs) (HIV).

ADR: See Notes below.

Notes: See 9.3.1 NRTIs (HIV). See Emtricitabine, Emtricitabine, Tenofovir above, 9.4.2 Viral Hepatitis (tenofovir brand Viread).

Atripla 600/200/245 (Gilead) A.
Price, not published by company.
Tablet, efavirenz 600mg, emtricitabine 200mg, tenofovir disoproxil (as fumarate) 245mg. Pink cap-shaped f/c. Marked 123. Sodium 23.6mg/dose.

262

Emtricitabine, Tenofovir, Rilpivirine

ATC Code: J05AR08. **Sport:** Permitted.
Driving: Fatigue, dizziness, somnolence.
Indications: HIV-1 infection (no known mutations associated with NNRTI resistance).

Dose: Adult, Elderly: Age 18 years and over, 1 tab once daily. Co-admin with rifabutin, additional rilpivirine 25mg/day recommended. Admin, oral; MUST be taken with food. Elderly, over 65 years, caution.

Renal Impairment: Mild, if benefit outweighs risk. Moderate/severe, not recommended.

Hepatic Impairment: Moderate, caution. Severe, not recommended.

Interactions: Effect of Other Drugs on Emtricitabine, Tenofovir, Rilpivirine: Co-admin contraindicated: Carbamazepine, oxcarbazepine, phenobarbital, phenytoin, rifampicin, rifapentine, PPIs (omeprazole, esomeprazole, lansoprazole, pantoprazole, rabeprazole), dexamethasone (except as single dose), St John's Wort. Co-admin not recommended: Adefovir dipivoxil, lamivudine, other NNRTIs. Co-admin avoid: Nephrotoxics (aminoglycosides, amphotericin B, foscarnet, ganciclovir, pentamidine, vancomycin, aldesleukin, cidofovir). Co-admin caution, reduced absorption (rilpivirine): H2-antagonists, antacids. Increased serum levels: Cidofovir.

Effect of Emtricitabine, Tenofovir, Rilpivirine on Other Drugs: Didanosine: Increased exposure; co-admin not recommended. Digoxin (no dose adjustment needed), dabigatran: Potential increased exposure. Metformin: No dose adjustment required.

SP: Caution, co-admin with medicinals with Torsade de Pointes risk (rilpivirine). Severe skin reactions. Renal precautions, see Notes below.

Pregnancy, Lactation: Pregnancy, use if clearly needed. Women of childbearing potential to ensure adequate contraception. Lactation, not recommended.

ADR: See Notes below.

Notes: See 9.3.1 NRTIs. See Emtricitabine, Tenofovir above. See 9.4.2 Viral Hepatitis (tenofovir brand Viread).

Eviplera 200/25/245 (Gilead) A.
Price, not published by company.
Tablet, emtricitabine 200mg, tenofovir disoproxil 245mg, rilpivirine HCl 25mg. Purplish-pink f/c cap-shaped. Marked GSI. Lactose, Sunset Yellow.

Lamivudine (HIV)

ATC Code: J05AF05. **Sport:** Permitted.
Driving: No specific studies performed.
Dose: Adult: Weight at least 25kg, 300mg once daily or 150mg twice daily. Admin, oral with or without food.
Elderly: Special care (altered renal function or haematological parameters).
Child: TABS, weight 20-25kg, 225mg/day (75mg morning and 150mg evening) OR 225mg once daily); weight 14-20kg, 150mg/day (75mg twice daily or 150mg once daily); under 3 months, no dose recommendation. ORAL SOLN, weight under 25kg, from age 1 year, 4mg/kg twice daily or 8mg/kg once daily; max. 300mg/day; age 3 months to 1 year, 4mg/kg twice daily; 8mg once daily can be considered (limited data); under 3 months, no dose recommendation.

Renal Impairment: Adults, children over 12 years, initially 150mg (dose 1) then CrCl (mL/min) 50 or above, 150mg twice daily; all once daily, 30-49, 150mg/day; 15-29, 100mg/day; 5-14, 50mg/day. CrCl (mL/min) below 5, 50mg (first dose) then once daily. Children 3 months to 12 years, initially 4mg/kg (dose 1), then CrCl (mL/min) 50 or over, 4mg/kg twice daily; all once daily, 30-49, 4mg/kg/day; 15-29, 2.6mg/kg/day; 5-14, 1.3mg/kg/day; CrCl (mL/min) below 5, 1.3mg (first dose) then 0.7mg/kg once daily. Doses under 150mg, use oral soln. Admin, see Adult above.

Hepatic Impairment: Decompensated liver disease, use in combination with second agent without lamivudine cross-resistance.

Interactions: Effect of Other Drugs on Lamivudine: Co-admin not recommended: IV (ganciclovir, foscarnet), cytidine analogues (emtricitabine), cladribine, other lamivudine-containing products. Co-admin caution: Drugs eliminated by active renal secretion (trimethoprim).

SP: Not for monotherapy in HIV. Pancreatitis, discontinue. HBV DNA in HBeAg, monitor. Spontaneous chronic hepatitis B exacerbations (transient ALT increases); acute exacerbations when hepatitis B therapy discontinued. Autoimmune disorders (Graves' disease, polymyositis, Guillain-Barre syndrome), see Notes below.

Pregnancy, Lactation: Pregnancy, can be used if clinically needed. Hepatitis co-infection (treated with lamivudine) and subsequently become pregnant; possibility of hepatitis recurrence with lamivudine discontinuation. Lactation, passes into breast milk; total amount ingested by breastfed infant very low; breastfeeding may be considered.

ADR: See Notes below.

Notes: See 9.3.1 NRTIs. See also 9.4.2 Viral Hepatitis (lamivudine).

> **Epivir 150mg, 300mg, Oral Soln** (ViiV) A. HOS.
> Price, 150mg (60) €133.16; 300mg (30) €128.63. Soln (240mL) €39.48 (PTW).
> Tablet, lamivudine. Diamond-shaped f/c. 150mg: White. Marked GXCJ7. 300mg: Grey. Marked GXEJ7.
> Oral soln, as above 10mg/mL. Clear colourless (pale-yellow). Sucrose, parabens.

Lamivudine, Zidovudine

ATC Code: J05AR01. **Sport:** Permitted.
Driving: Unlikely to impair.

Dose: Adult, Elderly: Weight 30kg and over (including adolescents), 1 tab twice daily. Admin, see Notes below (NRTIs). Haematological adverse events, adjust dose using individual components. Elderly, special care (altered renal function or haematological parameters).

Child: Weight 21-30kg, half tab in morning, 1 full tab at night; 14-21kg, half tab twice daily; under 14kg, use separate components.

Renal Impairment: CrCl (mL/min) 50 or less, use individual components.

Hepatic Impairment: Severe, as for Renal above.

Cl: Neutrophils below 0.75microL/L or Hb below 7.5g/dL or 4.65mmoL/L.

SP: Haematological reactions, monitor. Pancreatitis, discontinue. Autoimmune disorders (Graves' disease), see Notes below. Loss of subcutaneous fat (linked to mitochondrial toxicity).

Pregnancy, Lactation: Not recommended.

ADR: See individual components below.

Notes: See 9.3.1 NRTIs. See Lamivudine above, Zidovudine below.

> **Combivir 150/300** (ViiV) A. HOS.
> Price, (60) €320.23 (PTW).
> Tablet, lamivudine 150mg, zidovudine 300mg. White (off-white) cap-shaped f/c scored. Marked GXFC3.

Stavudine

ATC Code: J05AF04. **Sport:** Permitted.
Driving: Dizziness, somnolence.

Indications: Indicated when other antiretrovirals cannot be used.

Dose: Adult, Elderly: Under 60kg, 30mg 12-hourly; 60kg and over, 40mg 12-hourly. Admin, oral on empty stomach; optimal absorption 1 hour before food; cap may be opened and contents mixed with food. Over 65 years, no data.

Child: 30 kg and over, as for Adult above. Caps, over 3 months and under 30kg, 1mg/kg 12-hourly. Oral soln, birth to 13 days, 0.5mg/kg 12-hourly; 14 days and under 30kg, 1mg/kg 12-hourly.

Renal Impairment: Under 60kg, CrCl (mL/min) 26-50, 15mg twice daily; 25 or less, 15mg 24-hourly. Weight 60kg and over, CrCl (mL/min) 26-50, 20mg twice daily; 25 and under, 20mg 24-hourly. Haemodialysis, as for CrCl (mL/min) 25 and under, admin on completion.

Interactions: Effect of Other Drugs on Stavudine: Co-admin contraindicated: Didanosine (serious and/or life-threatening events; lactic acidosis, liver function abnormalities, pancreatitis, peripheral neuropathy;

mitochondrial toxicity). Co-admin not recommended: Zidovudine. Co-admin caution: Drugs eliminated by active renal secretion (trimethoprim). Activation inhibited: Doxorubicin, ribavirin.

SP: Severe side effects (lactic acidosis, lipoatrophy*, polyneuropathy), assess risk/benefit (probably mitochondrial toxicity). Peripheral neuropathy, change treatment. High pancreatitis risk, monitor. *Loss of subcutaneous fate (face, limbs, buttocks).

ADR: See Notes below.

Notes: See 9.3.1 NRTIs.

> **Zerit 20mg, 30mg, 40mg** (BMS) A. HOS.
> Price, (56) 20mg €226.29. 30mg, €170.69. 40mg, €152.05. Soln 1mg/mL (200mL) €37.13 (PTW).
> Capsule, stavudine. Hard opaque. Marked BMS/strength. 20mg: Brown. Marked 1965. 30mg: Light-orange/dark-orange. Marked 1966. 40mg: Dark-orange. Marked 1967. Lactose.

Zidovudine

ATC Code: J05AF01. **Sport:** Permitted.
Driving: Consider patient clinical status; ADR profile below.

Indications: Treatment, HIV infection. Prophylaxis, HIV (maternal-foetal transmission, infection in new-born infants) (oral, parenteral). Short-term management, serious manifestations of HIV infection in AIDS patients.

Dose: Adult, Elderly: ORAL, weight 30kg or more, 250-300mg twice daily. Prevention of maternal-foetal transmission, 500mg/day in 5 divided doses until beginning of labour; during labour, 2mg/kg IV over 1-hour, then continuous IV infusion at 1mg/kg/hour until umbilical cord clamped.
PARENTERAL, 1-2mg/kg 4-hourly; similar exposure as oral 1.5-3mg/kg 4-hourly OR 600-1200mg/day (70kg patient) by slow IV infusion over 1-hour; NOT for IM admin; MUST be diluted prior to admin. Over 65 years, no data.

Child: Weight 22-30kg, 200mg twice daily; 14-21kg, 100mg morning and 200mg evening; 8-13kg, 100mg cap twice daily; under 4kg, no data.
Prevention of maternal-foetal transmission, newborn infant, 2mg/kg orally 6-hourly starting within 12 hours after birth OR 1.5mg/kg IV by 30-minute infusion 6-hourly. See also Adult above. Newborn infants, see Contraindications (CI) below.

Renal Impairment: CrCl (mL/min) below 10 or ESRD on dialysis, 100mg 6-8 hourly.

Hepatic Impairment: Consider dose reduction.

Cl: Neutrophils below 0.75microL/L or Hb below 7.5g/dL or 4.65mmoL/L. Newborns with hyperbilirubinaemia needing treatment or transaminases above 5xULN.

Interactions: Effect of Other Drugs on Zidovudine: Co-admin avoid: Rifampicin, ribavirin, stavudine. Co-admin caution (monitor renal function; haematology): Systemic pentamidine, dapsone, pyrimethamine, co-trimoxazole, amphotericin, flucytosine, ganciclovir, interferon, vincristine, vinblastine, doxorubicin. Plasma levels increased: Probenecid, atovaquone, valproic acid, fluconazole, methadone. Absorption reduced: Clarithromycin oral (allow 2-hour dosing interval).

Effect of Zidovudine on Other Drugs: Phenytoin: Monitor levels.

SP: Haematological adverse events, at higher dose (1200-1500mg/day), monitor; Hb 7.5-9g/dL or neutrophils 0.75-1 G (Giga)/L, reduce dose or interrupt. HCV co-infection, ribavirin + zidovudine co-admin not recommended (increased anaemia risk).

Pregnancy, Lactation: Pregnancy, can be used if clinically needed; mitochondrial dysfunction in HIV-negative infants exposed in utero and/or postnatally, reported. Lactation, not recommended.

ADR: See Notes below.

Notes: See 9.3.1 NRTIs.

> **Retrovir 100mg, Oral Soln** (ViiV) A. HOS.
> Price, caps (100) €119.13. Oral soln (200mL) €20.45 (PTW).
> Capsule, zidovudine. Hard gelatin opaque white with blue band. Marked Wellcome, strength, Y9C. Store: Below 30 deg C; original pack.
> Oral soln, as above 50mg/5mL. Clear pale-yellow strawberry-flavoured sugar-free Maltitol, parabens. Store: As above.

9.3.2 Protease Inhibitors (HIV)

Retrovir Parenteral (ViiV) A. HOS.
Price, (5) €61.71 (PTW).
Infusion, zidovudine 200mg/20mL. Clear nearly colourless aqueous conc (soln); pH 5.5. **Store:** Below 30 deg C; outer carton.

9.3.2 - Protease Inhibitors (HIV)

In This Chapter: *Atazanavir, cobicistat (and combinations), fosamprenavir, indinavir, ritonavir (and combinations), simeprevir, tipranavir.*

Class Effects
Protease inhibitors (PI) may be used in combination with ritonavir or cobicistat (pharmacokinetic enhancer).

Driving, Dose Adjustments: See Notes below.

CI: See Interactions below. Severe hepatic impairment, use in children under 18 years, unless otherwise specified.

Interactions: Effect of Other Drugs on Protease Inhibitors: *Co-admin contraindicated (plasma levels decreased):* Rifampicin, St John's Wort, other potent CYP3A4 inducers (phenobarbital, carbamazepine, phenytoin, dexamethasone). *PI absorption reduced:* Didanosine (not e/c formulations), buffered preparations, drugs reducing gastric acid and/or increasing gastric pH (antacids, H2-antagonists, PPIs) (allow 1-hour dosing interval).

Effect of Protease Inhibitors on Other Drugs: CYP3A4 substrates with narrow therapeutic window e.g. benzodiazepines (alprazolam, triazolam oral, clorazepate, diazepam, estazolam, flurazepam, midazolam *oral*; midazolam *parenteral*, extreme caution, prolonged sedation and/or respiratory depression); calcium channel blockers (diltiazem, nicardipine, nifedipine, nimodipine; increased toxicity); antiarrhythmics (amiodarone, bepridil, quinidine, systemic lidocaine, flecainide, propafenone, metoprolol), neuroleptics (pimozide, sertindole), GI motility agents (cisapride), antihistamines (astemizole, terfenadine), alfuzosin, ergot alkaloids, PDE-5 inhibitors (sildenafil, vardenafil, tadalafil; increased adverse events), TCADs (amitriptyline, imipramine), immunosuppressants (ciclosporin, tacrolimus, rapamycin), beta-2 agonists (salmeterol): *Co-admin not recommended, plasma levels increased (contraindication for some members of class).* Lovastatin, simvastatin, atorvastatin: *Increased myopathy risk (rhabdomyolysis).* Phenytoin, methadone (usually no dose adjustment): *Plasma levels decreased.* Oral contraceptives: *Efficacy may be reduced; ensure other contraceptive methods.* Rifabutin: *Plasma levels increased (usually halve dose).* Warfarin: *Monitor INR.*

SP: Pre-existing liver dysfunction (chronic hepatitis), monitor; hepatitis B or C co-infection (treated with alpha interferon + ribavirin + CART) at special risk. Increased spontaneous skin haematomas, haemarthrosis (type A and B haemophiliacs). Diabetes (new onset, exacerbation), hyperglycaemia.

Pregnancy, Lactation: Pregnancy, only if benefit outweighs risk. Recommended that HIV infected women do not breast-feed under any circumstances to avoid HIV transmission.

ADR: Laboratory values altered with HIV-protease inhibitors. See Manufacturers Full Prescribing Information.

Notes: See 9.3 Antivirals Used In HIV Infection.

Atazanavir

ATC Code: J05AE08. **Sport:** Permitted.
Driving: Dizziness.
Indications: HIV-1 infection, in combination (from age 6 years).
Dose: Adult, Elderly: 300mg/day + ritonavir* 100mg/day; didanosine co-admin, allow 2-hour dosing interval. *Admin,* once daily with food; swallow caps whole. *See Notes below.
Child: Age 6-18 years, weight minimum 15 kg: 15-35kg, 200mg + ritonavir 100mg; at least 35kg, 300mg + ritonavir 100mg. See Adult above.
Renal Impairment: Haemodialysis, not recommended.
Hepatic Impairment: Mild, caution; maintain unboosted*,

400mg/day. Moderate, maintain unboosted*, 300mg/day. Severe, contraindicated; unboosted not to be used.

Interactions: Effect of Other Drugs on Atazanavir: Atazanavir + Ritonavir: *Co-admin contraindicated:* Rifampicin, quetiapine, alfuzosin, astemizole, terfenadine, cisapride, pimozide, quinidine, bepridil, triazolam, midazolam (oral), ergot alkaloids, St John's Wort, sildenafil (in PAH), simvastatin, lovastatin. *Co-admin not recommended*: Pls (indinavir, efavirenz, nevirapine, voriconazole); PPIs; tenofovir, H2-antagonist (atazanavir exposure decreased); glucocorticoids, oral contraceptives, atorvastatin, salmeterol, boceprevir. *Co-admin avoid:* Tenofovir + H2 antagonist. *Co-admin caution:* Clarithromycin, ketoconazole, itraconazole (not recommended above 200mg/day), carbamazepine, phenytoin, phenobarbital, verapamil, pravastatin, fluvastatin, midazolam (parenteral; only in ICU). *Allow dosing interval*: Didanosine, H2-antagonists, antacids/buffered medicinals. *Dose reduction*: Rifabutin, diltiazem. *Monitor*: Warfarin (INR); ciclosporin, tacrolimus, sirolimus (plasma levels); amiodarone, systemic lidocaine (therapeutic conc); tenofovir, irinotecan; PDE5-inhibitors (sildenafil, tadalafil, vardenafil) (ED treatment, increased adverse events); buprenorphine (sedation).

Atazanavir Unboosted: *Co-admin not recommended:* Nevirapine, indinavir; efavirenz (if combination required, increase to atazanavir 400mg + ritonavir 200mg*). *Co-admin caution:* Drugs inducing PR prolongations, drugs increasing QT-interval. *Plasma levels decreased:* PPIs, tenofovir (without ritonavir). *(see manufacturers Full Prescribing Information).

Effect of Atazanavir on Other Drugs: Atazanavir + Ritonavir: Oral contraceptives: *Caution under ethinyloestradiol 30mcg and progestogens other than norgestimate (use alternative methods).* **Atazanavir Unboosted:** Glucocorticoids, voriconazole: *Co-admin not recommended.* Ketoconazole, itraconazole: *Co-admin caution.* Opioids (buprenorphine, norbuprenorphine): *Monitor; consider dose reduction.* Ironectin: *Increased toxicity.*

SP: Caution, bradycardia, long congenital QT, electrolyte imbalance. Hyperbilirubinaemia. Cholelithiasis, nephrolithiasis, interrupt or discontinue. Atazanavir + ritonavir + efavirenz, consider increasing ritonavir to 200mg once daily.

Pregnancy, Lactation: Only if benefit outweighs risk. Consider Therapeutic Drug Monitoring to ensure adequate exposure (second, third trimester).

ADR: See Notes below.

Notes: See 9.3.2 Protease Inhibitors Used in HIV. *Ritonavir may be withdrawn under restrictive conditions.

Reyataz 150mg, 200mg, 300mg (BMS) A. HOS.
Price, (60) 150mg, €428.90. 200mg €436.18. (30) 300mg, €419.82 (PTW).
Capsule, atazanavir sulfate. Hard opaque. Marked BMS/strength. 150mg: Blue/light-blue. Marked 3624. 200mg: Blue. Marked 3631. 300mg: Red/blue. Marked 3622. *Lactose.* **Store:** Below 25 deg C.

Cobicistat

ATC Code: V03AX03 **Sport:** Permitted.
Driving: No specific studies performed.
Indications: Pharmacokinetic enhancer of once daily (atazanavir 300mg OR darunavir 800mg) as part of antiretroviral combination therapy.
Dose: Adult: Cobicistat 150mg once daily + HIV-1 protease inhibitor (atazanavir 300mg OR darunavir 800mg) once daily. *Admin,* once daily with food; do not chew or crush.
Elderly: Over 65 years, no dose recommendation.
Child: Under 18 years, safety/efficacy not established.
Renal Impairment: No adjustment; do not initiate below CrCl 70mL/min if any co-admin agent (emtricitabine, lamivudine, tenofovir disoproxil fumarate, adefovir) required dose adjustment based on CrCl. Dialysis, no dose recommendation. Cobicistat decreases estimated creatinine clearance due to inhibition of tubular secretion of creatinine.
Hepatic Impairment: Severe, not recommended.

Interactions: Effect of Other Drugs on Cobicistat:

Co-admin contraindicated: Elevated plasma levels with serious and/or life-threatening events (dihydroergotamine, ergotamine, ergometrine, oral midazolam, triazolam, amiodarone, quinidine, cisapride, pimozide, alfuzosin, simvastatin, lovastatin, sildenafil); decreased plasma levels, loss of therapeutic effect, possible resistance development (strong CYP3A inducers e.g. carbamazepine, phenobarbital, phenytoin, rifampicin, St John's Wort). *Co-admin not recommended:* Decreased plasma levels (weak CYP3A inducers e.g. etravirine, efavirenz, nevirapine, boceprevir, bosentan); plasma levels increased (CYP3A inducers e.g. itraconazole, ketoconazole both max. 200mg/day, voriconazole, consider risk/benefit); another antiviral requiring pharmacokinetic enhancement (another protease inhibitor, elvitegravir); clarithromycin (consider alternative); dasatinib, nilotinib, vinblastine, vincristine (increased plasma levels, increased adverse events); corticosteroids (increased systemic side effect risk; consider risk/benefit); norgestimate/ethinyloestradiol (use alternative); rivaroxaban, salmeterol; warfarin (monitor INR); dabigatran (clinical monitoring). *Co-admin caution:* Disopyramide, flecainide, systemic lidocaine, mexiletine, propafenone.

Effect of Cobicistat on Other Drugs: Maraviroc 150mg twice daily; rifabutin 150mg 3-times weekly; metformin (consider adjustment); digoxin (initiate with lowest dose); metoprolol, timolol, statins, perphenazine, risperidone, thioridazine, buspirone, clorazepate, diazepam, estazolam, flurazepam, zolpidem, colchicine (consider reduction; not recommended with renal or hepatic impairment); amlodipine, diltiazem, felodipine, nicardipine, nifedipine, verapamil (clinical monitoring); sildenafil, tadalafil, vardenafil (consider dose reduction), trazodone (dose titration); ciclosporin, sirolimus, tacrolimus (therapeutic monitoring): *Dose adjustment considerations.*

SP: See Interactions above.

Pregnancy, Lactation: Pregnancy, use only if required by clinical condition.

ADR: See Notes below.

Notes: See 9.3.2 Protease Inhibitors Used in HIV.

▼ **Tybost 150mg** *(Gilead)* A.
Price, not published by company.
Tablet, cobicistat. Orange round f/c. Marked GSI. *Sunset Yellow.*

Darunavir

ATC Code: J05AE10. **Sport:** Permitted.
Driving: Dizziness.

Indications: Treatment, HIV-1 infection (with ritonavir or cobicistat) in adults, children from 3 years and at least 15kg (100mg/mL, 75mg, 150mg tabs) and at least 40kg (400mg, 800mg tabs).

Dose: Adult, Elderly: *ART-naive,* 800mg/day* + cobicistat 150mg/day* OR ritonavir 100mg/day*. *ART-experienced,* genotype testing not available, 600mg twice daily + ritonavir 100mg twice daily; no resistant mutations, as for ART-naive. *Admin,* *(once daily) with food; always in combination with low dose ritonavir or cobicistat. *Elderly,* 65 years and over, caution.

Child: Age 3-17 years, *ART-naive* (with ritonavir 100mg) all dosed once daily, (15-30kg) 600mg (6mL oral susp); (30-40kg) 675mg (6.8mL); (40kg and above) 800mg (8mL). *ART-experienced* (with ritonavir) all dosed twice daily, (weight 15-30kg), 380mg (3.8mL oral susp) + ritonavir 50mg; (weight 30-40kg), 460mg (4.6mL) + 60mg ritonavir; (weight 40kg and over), 600mg (6mL) + ritonavir 100mg; the once daily regimen as per ART-naive may also be used. Not for use in children under 3 years (safety concerns).

Hepatic Impairment: Mild/moderate, caution. Severe, contraindicated.

CI: See Interactions below.

Interactions: Effect of Other Drugs on Darunavir, Ritonavir: *Co-admin contraindicated:* Cobicistat boosted: CYP3A inducers (carbamazepine, phenobarbital, phenytoin; reduced exposure); Cobicistat or ritonavir boosted: Lopinavir + ritonavir, CYP3AV inducers (rifampicin, St John's Wort; reduced plasma levels); alfuzosin, antiarrhythmics/antianginals (amiodarone, bepridil,

Protease Inhibitors (HIV)   9.3.2

dronedarone, quinidine, ranolazine, systemic lidocaine), antihistamines (astemizole, terfenadine), colchicine (with renal impairment), ergot derivatives, elbasvir + grazoprevir, cisapride, lurasidone, pimozide, quetiapine, sertindole, oral (triazolam, midazolam*), sildenafil (in PAH), avanafil, simvastatin, lovastatin, ticagrelor. *Co-admin not recommended:* Anticonvulsants (phenobarbital, phenytoin), PIs (amprenavir, fosamprenavir, nelfinavir, tipranavir, saquinavir) telaprevir, boceprevir + ritonavir, St John's Wort. *Co-admin caution:* Clarithromycin. *Co-admin (increased plasma levels):* Indinavir, systemic azoles, clotrimazole. *Allow dosing interval (1 hour before, 2 hours after darunavir):* Didanosine. *Monitor for toxicity:* Efavirenz (CNS), tenofovir (renal). *IV midazolam only for ICU/close clinical monitoring.

Effect of Darunavir, Ritonavir on Other Drugs: Maraviroc: *Max. 150mg twice daily.* Warfarin, methadone, paclitaxel, rosiglitazone, repaglinide, oestrogen-based contraceptives: *Decreased systemic exposure.* Flecainide, propafenone, metoprolol, buprenorphine/naloxone, rifabutin, calcium channel blockers (felodipine, nicardipine, nifedipine), statins: *Increased plasma levels with co-admin.* Digoxin: *Use lowest dose.* Voriconazole: *Co-admin (if benefit outweighs risk).* Ketoconazole, itraconazole: *Max. 200mg/day, monitor.* Clotrimazole, SSRIs (paroxetine, sertraline), warfarin, ciclosporin, sirolimus, tacrolimus: *Clinical monitoring required.* Carbamazepine: *May need dose reduction.* Etravirine: *Can be used only at 200mg twice daily.* Colchicine: *Reduce dose or interrupt treatment.* Artemether/lumefantrine, dexamethasone: *Caution.* Corticosteroids (betamethasone, budesonide, fluticasone, mometasone, prednisone, triamcinolone): *Co-admin not recommended; may need dose adjustment.* Bosentan: *Monitor patient tolerability.*

SP: Sulfonamide allergics, caution. Severe skin rash with fever and/or elevated transaminases; DRESS, Stevens-Johnson Syndrome, toxic epidermal necrolysis, acute generalised exanthematous pustulosis; higher rash incidence (raltegravir combination). Drug-induced hepatitis, elevated transaminases; new or worsening liver dysfunction, interrupt or discontinue. Hyperglycaemia, diabetes.

ADR: See Notes below.

Notes: See 9.3.2 Protease Inhibitors Used in HIV.

PREZISTA Tablets, Oral Susp 100mg/mL *(Janssen-Cilag)* A. HOS.
Price, (60) 600mg, €619.20; 800mg once daily, €415.93 (PTW).
Tablet, darunavir ethanolate 600mg, 800mg. Oval f/c. Marked with strength; TMC on reverse (except 800mg marked T). 600mg: Orange. 800mg: Dark-red. *Sunset Yellow E110.*
Oral susp, as above. White (off-white) opaque. *Parabens.* **Store:** Below 30 deg C; do not (refrigerate, freeze, expose to excessive heat).

Darunavir, Cobicistat

ATC Code: J05AR14. **Sport:** Permitted.
Driving: Dizziness.

Indications: Treatment, HIV-1 infection (adults).

Dose: Adult, Elderly: *ART-naive,* 1x tab daily. *ART-experienced or HIV-1 genotyping not available, use not recommended. Elderly,* over age 65 years, caution. *Admin,* swallow whole within 30 minutes after completion of meal. NOTE: Unlike ritonavir, cobicistat is not an inducer of CYP1A2, CYP2B6, CYP2C8, CYP2C9, CYP2C19, UGT1A1; switch from ritonavir (pharmacokinetic enhancer) to cobicistat, caution during first 2 weeks especially if doses of other co-admin medicinals have been titrated or adjusted during ritonavir use.

Child: Age 3-17 years, safety/efficacy not established; under 3 years, not recommended (safety concerns).

Renal Impairment: CrCl (mL/min) below 70, do not initiate if any co-admin agents require dose adjustment based on CrCl.

Hepatic Impairment: Mild/moderate, no dose adjustment, caution. Severe, contraindicated.

Interactions: Effect of Other Drugs on Darunavir, Cobicistat: *Co-admin not recommended:* Efavirenz, etravirine, nevirapine, rifabutin, rifapentine (recommendations different from Darunavir, Ritonavir).

265

9.3.2 Protease Inhibitors (HIV)

Effect of Darunavir, Cobicistat on Other Drugs: Apixaban, dabigatran, rivaroxaban: *Anticoagulant plasma levels increased* (recommendations different from Darunavir, Ritonavir). Corticosteroids (betamethasone, budesonide, fluticasone, mometasone, prednisone, triamcinolone): *Co-admin not recommended; monitor for systemic corticosteroid effects.*

SP: See Notes below.

ADR: See Notes below.

Notes: See Darunavir above. See Cobicistat above. For more information, see Ritonavir below. See 9.3.2 Protease Inhibitors Used in HIV.

▼ REZOLSTA 800/150 *(Janssen-Cilag)* A. HOS.
Price, (30), €443.41 (PTW).
Tablet, darunavir ethanolate, cobicistat 800/150mg. Pink oval f/c. Marked 800; TG on reverse.

Fosamprenavir

ATC Code: J05AE07. **Sport:** Permitted.
Driving: Consider adverse reaction profile.

Dose: Adult, Elderly: Antiretroviral naive and experienced, 700mg* + 100mg* ritonavir. *Admin,* *twice daily, with or without food* (oral susp, see Child below). *Over 65 years,* no dose recommendation.

Child: Age 6-17 years, (weight 39kg or more, able to swallow tabs), as for Adult above; (33-38kg), 18mg/kg* oral susp + 100mg ritonavir*; max. as for Adult; (25-32kg), 18mg/kg* oral susp + 3mg/kg ritonavir*; under 25kg, no dose recommendation. *Admin,* oral susp to be taken WITH food in paediatrics (aid palatability, assist compliance); adults to take without food on empty stomach. *(twice daily).

Hepatic Impairment: Mild, once daily (700mg + 100mg ritonavir); moderate, twice daily (450mg + ritonavir 100mg).

CI: Hypersensitivity to amprenavir, ritonavir.

Interactions: Effect of Other Drugs on Fosamprenavir: *Co-admin contraindicated:* Flecainide, propafenone, rifampicin, alfuzosin, sildenafil. *Co-admin not recommended:* Halofantrine, lidocaine, PIs (lopinavir + ritonavir; significantly reduced amprenavir conc), integrase inhibitors (raltegravir; reduced amprenavir and raltegravir exposure), PDE-5 inhibitors (sildenafil*, tadalafil, vardenafil), maraviroc (reduced amprenavir exposure), fluticasone, other glucocorticoids (unless benefit outweighs risk); ketoconazole, itraconazole (at high doses). *Co-admin caution:* Carbamazepine, phenobarbital, clarithromycin, erythromycin. *Telzir dose adjustment may be needed:* Etravirine. *Contraindicated (sildenafil used for PAH).* See Notes below (ritonavir).

NOTE: Fosamprenavir + ritonavir, the ritonavir metabolic drug interaction profile may dominate.

Effect of Fosamprenavir on Other Drugs: CYP3A4 substrates with narrow therapeutic window (see Notes below, Class Effects); paritaprevir, simvastatin, lovastatin; ergotamine, ergonovine and derivatives; cisapride, astemizole, terfenadine, pimozide, quetiapine: *Contraindicated.* Paroxetine: *Decreased exposure; titrate according to response.* Rifabutin: *Reduce dose by at least 75%.* Oral contraceptives: *Recommend alternative non-hormonal methods.* Ciclosporin, tacrolimus, rapamycin, TCADs (desipramine, nortriptyline): *Therapeutic monitoring required.* Warfarin: *Monitor INR.*

SP: Fosamprenavir and amprenavir, not for co-admin. Liver disease, increased risk for severe/potentially fatal hepatic adverse events. Sulfonamide allergics, increased rash risk. Mild/moderate rash, continue; severe/life-threatening, permanently discontinue. Autoimmune disorders (Graves' disease) reported with immune reactivation.

ADR: See Notes below.

Notes: See 9.3.2 Protease Inhibitors Used in HIV.

Telzir 700mg, Oral Susp 50mg/5mL *(ViiV)* A. HOS.
Price, (60) €356.41. Susp 50mg/5mL (225mL) €82.71 (PTW).
Tablet, fosamprenavir calcium. Pink cap-shaped f/c. Marked GXLL7.
Oral susp, as above. White (off-white). *Parabens.* **Store:** Do not freeze.

Indinavir

ATC Code: J05AE02. **Sport:** Permitted.
Driving: Caution.

Dose: Adult, Elderly: 800mg 8-hourly OR 800mg + ritonavir 100mg (both admin twice daily). Co-admin (itraconazole, ketoconazole) consider dose reduction to 600mg 8-hourly. *Admin,* oral caps to be swallowed whole without food, with water; 1 hour before or 2 hours after food; can be admin with light low-fat meal; ensure adequate hydration; with ritonavir, admin with or without food.

Child: Age 4-17 years, 300mg (BSA 0.5m2), 400mg (BSA 0.75m2), 500mg (BSA 1m2), 600mg (BSA 1.25m2), 800mg (BSA 1.5m2) 8-hourly; max. 800mg 8-hourly. Children, adolescents, consider benefit versus increased nephrolithiasis risk.

Hepatic Impairment: Mild or moderate due to cirrhosis, reduce dose to 600mg 8-hourly.

CI: See Interactions and Notes below. Ritonavir not for admin in decompensated liver disease, see Notes below.

Interactions: Effect of Other Drugs on Indinavir: Indinavir Unboosted: *Co-admin contraindicated:* Rifampicin, St John's Wort, lovastatin, simvastatin. *Co-admin not recommended:* Rifabutin, rosuvastatin. *Co-admin caution:* Quinidine, atorvastatin (use lowest dose*); pravastatin, fluvastatin*. *Plasma levels increased:* Itraconazole, ketoconazole (see Dose above), delavirdine (reduce indinavir to 400-600mg 8-hourly), saquinavir (no dose recommendation). *Plasma levels decreased:* Nevirapine (increase indinavir to 1000mg 8-hourly), efavirenz. *Caution, nephrolithiasis risk:* Ritonavir.

Indinavir + Ritonavir: *Co-admin contraindicated:* Alfuzosin, meperidine, piroxicam, propoxyphene, bepridil, encainide, flecainide, propafenone, quinidine, fusidic acid, clozapine, clorazepate, diazepam, estazolam, flurazepam, rifampicin. *Co-admin not recommended in children (toxicity risk of oral soln excipients):* Ritonavir oral soln + amprenavir oral soln. *Co-admin not recommended:* Rifabutin. *Co-admin caution*:* Atovaquone, erythromycin, itraconazole, ketoconazole, fentanyl, morphine, warfarin, carbamazepine, divalproex, lamotrigine, phenytoin, trazodone, fexofenadine, itraconazole, diltiazem (consider dose adjustment), HMG-CoA reductase inhibitors (as for Indinavir unboosted), ciclosporin A (consider dose adjustment), tacrolimus, sildenafil, tadalafil (as for Indinavir unboosted), vardenafil (max. 2.5mg in 72-hour period), buspirone, midazolam, dexamethasone. *(monitor).

Effect of Indinavir on Other Drugs: Sildenafil (max. 25mg in 48-hour period), vardenafil (max. 2.5mg in 24-hour period), tadalafil (max. 10mg in 72-hour period): *Dosing for indinavir co-admin.*

SP: Nephrolithiasis, tubulo-interstitial nephritis, ensure adequate hydration (adults to drink minimum 1.5L in 24 hours; children under 20kg, 75mL/kg/day; 20-40kg, 50mL/kg/day); higher incidence in paediatrics. Acute haemolytic anaemia, consider discontinuation.

ADR: See Notes below.

Notes: See 9.3.2 Protease Inhibitors Used in HIV. See Ritonavir below.

Crixivan 200mg, 400mg *(MSD)* A.
Price, 200mg (60) €322.96. 400mg (90) €161.49; (180) €322.96.
Capsule, indinavir sulfate. Hard semi-translucent white. Marked Crixivan/strength. *Lactose.*

Ritonavir

ATC Code: J05AE03. **Sport:** Permitted.
Driving: Caution.

Dose: Adult, Elderly: *Pharmacokinetic enhancer* (in combination), ritonavir 100mg* with (amprenavir, fosamprenavir, saquinavir, darunavir)* OR ritonavir 100mg once daily with once daily (atazanavir, darunavir) OR ritonavir 200mg* with (tipranavir)*. Lopinavir co-formulated with ritonavir (lopinavir/ritonavir) 400mg/100mg or 800mg/200mg.
Antiretroviral agent, initially 300mg* for max. 3 days;

Protease Inhibitors (HIV) 9.3.2

increase by 100mg* over max. 14 days to 600mg*. *Admin,* oral with food. *(twice daily).*

Child: *Pharmacokinetic enhancer,* age 2 years and older, see Notes below for PIs approved for co-admin with ritonavir.

Antiretroviral, age 2 years and over, initially 250mg/m2 twice daily increased at 2-3 day intervals by 50mg/m2 twice daily to 350mg/m2 BSA twice daily; max. 600mg twice daily.

Renal Impairment: Caution; dosing with other protease inhibitors, see Notes below.

Hepatic Impairment: Decompensated liver disease, not recommended. As for Adult above.

Interactions: Effect of Other Drugs on Ritonavir: *Co-admin contraindicated (ritonavir plasma levels decreased):* St John's Wort. *Co-admin not recommended:* Saquinavir + ritonavir + rifampicin (hepatotoxicity); amprenavir + ritonavir oral solns (toxicity from excipients of both solutions in children), simeprevir, riociguat, vorapaxar (avoid). *Co-admin caution:* Afatinib, ceritinib. *Plasma levels decreased:* Phenytoin.

Effect of Ritonavir on Other Drugs: Alfuzosin (severe hypotension), pethidine, piroxicam, propoxyphene (respiratory depression, haematological abnormalities), amiodarone, dronedarone, bepridil, encainide, flecainide, propafenone, quinidine, astemizole, terfenadine, cisapride (arrhythmias), rifabutin (uveitis with ritonavir 600mg twice daily), clozapine, pimozide (serious haematological abnormalities), quetiapine (coma), ergot alkaloids (ergot toxicity, vasospasm, ischaemia), lovastatin, simvastatin (myopathy, rhabdomyolysis), avanafil, sildenafil (in PAH), vardenafil, clorazepate, diazepam, estazolam, flurazepam, oral midazolam and triazolam (extreme sedation, respiratory depression): *Co-admin contraindicated (plasma levels increased).* Fusidic acid: *Co-admin contraindicated (plasma levels mutually increased).* Voriconazole: *Co-admin contraindicated (plasma levels decreased).* Trazodone, tadalafil: *Co-admin caution.* Rivaroxaban, salmeterol, fluticasone (risk/benefit): *Co-admin not recommended.* Amprenavir, atazanavir, darunavir, fosamprenavir, indinavir, nelfinavir, saquinavir, tipranavir, maraviroc, digoxin, dasatinib, nilotinib, vincristine, vinblastine, carbamazepine, amitriptyline, fluoxetine, imipramine, nortriptyline, paroxetine, sertraline, desipramine, colchicine (contraindicated with renal impairment; potential serious or life-threating reactions), fexofenadine, loratadine, clarithromycin (caution, renal failure), erythromycin, itraconazole, ketoconazole, haloperidol, risperidone, thioridazine, amlodipine, diltiazem, nifedipine, bosentan, atorvastatin, rosuvastatin, ciclosporin, tacrolimus, everolimus, alprazolam, buspirone, zolpidem (monitor, excessive sedation), dexamethasone, prednisone: *Plasma levels increased.* Raltegravir, zidovudine (minimally), theophylline, warfarin (monitor), divalproex, lamotrigine, atovaquone, ethinyl oestradiol, buprion: *Plasma levels decreased.* Amphetamine, bedaquiline: *Increased plasma levels; prolonged effect/increased adverse events.* Methadone, morphine: *Increased biotransformation, decreased/shortened therapeutic effect.* Delamanid: *Increased exposure; QT-prolongation risk; VERY frequent ECG monitoring.*

SP: Diarrhoea, malabsorption, monitor. Pancreatitis. PR-interval prolongation; second or third degree AV block (structural heart disease, conduction system abnormalities, drugs prolonging PR-interval). Immune Reconstitution Inflammatory Syndrome.

ADR: See Notes below.

Notes: See 9.3.2 Protease Inhibitors Used in HIV.

Norvir 100mg *(AbbVie)* A. HOS.
Price, 100mg (30), €27.22 (PTW).
Tablet, ritonavir. White oval f/c. Marked with logo and NK. **Store:** Original pack to protect (moisture).

Ritonavir, Lopinavir

ATC Code: J05AR10. **Sport:** Permitted.
Driving: Caution.
Dose: Adult, Elderly: 2 tabs twice daily; swallowing difficulties, use oral soln 5mL twice daily. 4 tabs once daily

can be used (increased diarrhoea risk). *Admin,* swallow whole with or without food. Increase *Kaletra* dose to 500/125mg TWICE daily, combination with efavirenz (600mg 4-times daily) or nevirapine (200mg twice daily). Decrease maraviroc to 150mg twice daily with *Kaletra* 400/100mg twice daily.

Child: Oral soln, age 2 years and over, *dose by body surface area (BSA),* 230/57.5mg/m2 twice daily; max. 400/100mg twice daily. Consider 300/75mg/m2 when co-admin with nevirapine or efavirenz; *dose by weight,* 15-40kg, 10/2.5mg/kg twice daily if not co-admin with nevirapine or efavirenz. Over 40kg or BSA above 1.4m2, as for Adult above. Should NOT be dosed once daily in children.

Renal Impairment: Significant removal by dialysis unlikely.

Hepatic Impairment: Mild to moderate, 30% increase in lopinavir exposure. Severe, contraindicated. Chronic hepatitis B or C (CART treated), increased hepatic adverse event risk.

Interactions: Effect of Other Drugs on Ritonavir, Lopinavir Combination: *Co-admin contraindicated:* Alfuzosin, amiodarone, fusidic acid, astemizole, terfenadine, pimozide, quetiapine, ergot alkaloids, cisapride, simvastatin, lovastatin, avanafil, sildenafil, vardenafil, oral midazolam, triazolam, St John's Wort. *Co-admin not recommended:* Tipranavir, fosamprenavir, amprenavir, simeprevir; ketoconazole, itraconazole (high dose); colchicine, efavirenz, nevirapine, phenytoin, carbamazepine, phenobarbital, riociguat, vorapaxar. *Co-admin avoid:* Voriconazole. *Co-admin caution:* Atorvastatin, rosuvastatin, trazodone; drugs prolonging PR interval (verapamil, atazanavir) (cardiac adverse events); afatinib, ceritinib (adjust dose). *No combination dose established:* Indinavir, nelfinavir.

Effect of Ritonavir, Lopinavir Combination on Other Drugs: Vincristine, vinblastine; digoxin, bepridil, lidocaine systemic, quinidine (possible); clarithromycin (renal impairment, consider dose reduction): *Plasma levels increased.* Phenytoin, amprenavir (significant): *Plasma levels decreased.* Bupropion (monitor efficacy): *Caution, exposure reduced.* Fentanyl: *Increased respiratory depression, sedation.* Dasatinib, nilotinib, vincristine, vinblastine: *Careful monitoring for tolerance.* Rifabutin (monitor, neutropenia, uveitis), rivaroxaban (bleeding risk): *Increased exposure.* Lamotrigine, valproate: *Monitor levels.* Trazodone: *Caution, consider lower dose.* Delamanid: *Increased exposure, QT-prolongation risk; VERY frequent ECG monitoring.*

SP: If statin is needed, use pravastatin or fluvastatin. Elevated transaminases with/without elevated bilirubin (early as 7 days after initiation); serious hepatic dysfunction. Caution, bedaquiline combination, more frequent monitoring (ECG, transaminases).

ADR: See Notes below.

Notes: See 9.3.2 Protease Inhibitors Used in HIV. See Ritonavir above.

Kaletra Tablets, Oral Soln *(AbbVie)* A. HOS.
Price, 100/25mg (60), €111.27. 200/50 (120), €413.40. Oral soln 80/20mg (300mL), €409.51. (PTW).
Tablet, lopinavir 100(200)mg, ritonavir 25(50)mg. f/c. Marked with logo. 100/25: Pale-yellow. Marked KC. 200/50mg: Yellow. Marked KA.
Oral soln, lopinavir 80mg, ritonavir 20mg/mL. Light-yellow. *Alcohol, fructose, polyethylene glycol, castor oil, acesulfame.*
Store: Refrigerate; or store below 25 degrees C (max. 42 days).

Tipranavir

ATC Code: J05AE09. **Sport:** Permitted.
Driving: Dizziness, somnolence, fatigue; Aptivus caps contain alcohol.
Indications: Treatment, highly pre-treated patients with resistance to multiple protease inhibitors with ritonavir.
Dose: Adult, Elderly: Age 12 years and older, 500mg tipranavir + ritonavir 200mg both twice daily. Over 65 years, insufficient data. Oral, with food. See SP.
Child: Using oral soln, age 2-12 years, 375mg/m2 admin with 150mg/m2 ritonavir twice daily; max. 500mg/200mg dose. See SP.

267

9.3.3 Non-Nucleoside Reverse Transcriptase Inhibitors (NNRTIs) (HIV)

Hepatic Impairment: Mild, caution. Moderate or severe, contraindicated.

Interactions: Effect of Other Drugs on Tipranavir: Tipranavir + Ritonavir: *Co-admin contraindicated:* Antiarrhythmics (amiodarone, bepridil, quinidine), antihistamines (astemizole, terfenadine), ergot derivatives (dihydroergotamine, ergonovine, ergotamine, methylergonovine), GI motility agents (cisapride), antipsychotics (pimozide, sertindole, quetiapine), sedatives/hypnotics (oral midazolam and triazolam), HMG-CoA reductase inhibitors (simvastatin, lovastatin), rifampicin, St John's Wort, alpha-1 adrenoceptor antagonist (alfuzosin), sildenafil (used for PAH), low dose ritonavir, substrates highly dependent on CYP2D6 for clearance (flecainide, propafenone; metoprolol in CHF). *Co-admin not recommended:* Zidovudine, abacavir (unless no alternative), other protease inhibitors (amprenavir, atazanavir, lopinavir, saquinavir); halofantrine, lumefantrine (Torsades de Pointes risk); disulfiram, metronidazole (disulfiram-like reaction); fluticasone, other glucocorticoids (if benefit outweighs risk); buprenorphine/naloxone (decreased buprenorphine efficacy; monitor for withdrawal), colchicine, bosentan. *Allow 2-hour dosing interval:* Didanosine.

Effect of Tipranavir on Other Drugs: Amprenavir, lopinavir, saquinavir: *Co-admin not recommended.* Fluconazole, itraconazole, ketoconazole: *Max. 200mg/day.* Theophylline: *Plasma levels decreased (monitor plasma conc).* Desipramine, trazodone (caution): *Plasma levels increased (reduce dose).* Digoxin: *Monitor until steady state.* Omeprazole, esomeprazole: *Plasma levels decreased (tipranavir-ritonavir).* Bupropion: *Metabolism induced, monitor efficacy.* Clarithromycin: *Reduce dose in renal impairment.* Fusion inhibitors (enfuvirtide), see manufacturers Full Prescribing Information.

SP: Always admin with low dose ritonavir (pharmacokinetic enhancer). Not for use in treatment-naive patients. Hepatic monitoring every 2 weeks (first 3 months). Rash (urticarial, maculopapular), photosensitivity. Increased bleeding risk with antiplatelets, anticoagulants or supplemental Vitamin E (max. 1200 IU/day). NOTE: Caps and oral soln are not interchangeable (higher tipranavir exposure with oral soln); oral soln has high vitamin E content; do not switch from caps to oral soln; switching from oral soln to caps at age 12, monitor closely for virological response.

Pregnancy, Lactation: Women of childbearing potential to ensure adequate contraception; tipranavir adversely interacts with oral contraceptives.

ADR: See Notes below.

Notes: See 9.3.2 Protease Inhibitors Used in HIV.

Aptivus Caps, Soln 100mg/mL *(Boehringer)* A.
Price, 250mg (120) €725.00. Oral soln (95mL) €229.59.
Capsule, tipranavir 250mg. Soft pink oblong. Marked TPV 250.
Ethanol, macrogolglycerol ricinoleate, sorbitol. **Store:** Refrigerate.
Oral soln, as above 100mg/mL. Clear yellow viscous liquid. **Store:** Do not (store below 15 deg C, refrigerate, freeze).

9.3.3 - Non-Nucleoside Reverse Transcriptase Inhibitors (NNRTIs) (HIV)

In This Chapter: *Efavirenz, etravirine, nevirapine.*

Class Effects
Driving, Dose Adjustments: See Notes below.

CI: Hypersensitivity to any member of the class.

Notes: See 9.3 Antivirals Used In HIV Infection.

Efavirenz

ATC Code: J05AG03. **Sport:** Permitted.
Driving: Dizziness, impaired concentration, somnolence.
Dose: Adult, Elderly: Adults, adolescents over 40kg, 600mg once daily (in combination). *Admin,* caps and tabs without food on an empty stomach; admin with food may lead to increased adverse events; preferably at bedtime to improve tolerability/CNS. Dose adjustments (in combination), see Notes below.
Child: *Sustiva* CAPSULES (dose in mg), body weight 3.5kg to under 5kg, efavirenz 100mg; 5kg to under 7.5kg, 150mg;

7.5kg to under 15kg, 200mg; 15kg to under 20kg, 250mg; 20kg to under 25kg, 300mg; 25 to under 32.5kg, 350mg; 32.5kg to under 40kg, 400mg; 40kg and over, 600mg (as for Adult). Under 3 months old and weight at least 3.5kg who cannot swallow caps, cap contents can be admin with a small amount of food using the capsule sprinkle method; consume no additional food for 2 hours after admin.
TABS, are not suitable for children under 40kg. Under 3 months or under 3.5kg, no data.

Renal Impairment: Minimal impact on elimination.

Hepatic Impairment: Mild to moderate, monitor. Severe, contraindicated.

Interactions: Effect of Other Drugs on Efavirenz: *Co-admin not recommended:* Voriconazole, atazanavir + ritonavir, lopinavir + ritonavir (adjust dose); ritonavir (high dose); saquinavir (as sole protease inhibitor); amprenavir + saquinavir, efavirenz + emtricitabine + tenofovir fixed combination. *Co-admin avoid:* Posaconazole, atovaquone + proguanil. *Co-admin caution:* Darunavir + ritonavir (adjust dose). *Plasma levels decreased:* Rifampicin (50kg and above, adjust efavirenz dose), St John's Wort (co-admin contraindicated). *Possible increased adverse effects:* Low-dose ritonavir. Dose adjustments, see Notes below.

Effect of Efavirenz on Other Drugs: Terfenadine, astemizole, cisapride, midazolam, triazolam, pimozide, bepridil, ergot alkaloids and derivatives: *Co-admin contraindicated (metabolism inhibited, plasma levels increased).* Indinavir, lopinavir + ritonavir, rifabutin (increase dose by 50%; consider doubling when given in a 2 or 3 times weekly regimen), statins (pravastatin, atorvastatin, simvastatin; consider dose adjustment), methadone; calcium channel blockers, diltiazem, sertraline (increase dose based on clinical response): *Plasma levels decreased.* Clarithromycin, carbamazepine: *Increased adverse events, seek alternative.* Oral contraceptives: *Ensure other adequate contraception.* Voriconazole, simeprevir: *Co-admin not recommended unless dose adjusted.* Immunosuppressants, warfarin, acenocoumarol, bupropion: *Dose adjustment may be required.* Telaprevir: *Use 1125mg 8-hourly if co-admin with efavirenz.*

SP: Not for monotherapy. Not recommended with severe/life-threatening cutaneous reaction with other NNRTIs. Psychiatric events; possible CNS effects, caution (seizure history). Osteonecrosis. Consider monitoring liver enzymes.

Pregnancy, Lactation: Pregnancy, not for use unless needed for clinical condition; caution first trimester (potential neural tube defect risk). Use barrier contraception in combination with other methods by males and females during and up to 12 weeks after treatment. Lactation, not recommended.

ADR: See Notes below.

Notes: See 9.3.3 NNRTIs.

Sustiva Capsules, Tablets *(BMS)* A. HOS.
Price, caps (30) 50mg, €14.75. 100mg, €34.02. (90) 200mg, €177.05. Tabs (30) 600mg, €178.02 (PTW).
Capsule, efavirenz 50mg, 100mg, 200mg. Hard. Marked Sustiva/strength. 50mg: Dark-yellow/white. 100mg: White. 200mg: Dark-yellow. *Lactose.*
Tablet, as above 600mg. Dark yellow cap-shaped f/c. Marked Sustiva on both sides. *Lactose.*

Efavirenz Rowex 600mg *(Rowex)* A. HOS.
Price, (30) €83.78 (trade).
Tablet, efavirenz. Yellow f/c cap-shaped scored both sides (divisible into equal doses). *Lactose.*

Etravirine

ATC Code: J05AG04. **Sport:** Permitted.
Driving: Caution.
Indications: Combination treatment, ART-experienced adults and children from age 6 years.
Dose: Adult, Elderly: 200mg twice daily after food; tabs may be dispersed in water. *Elderly,* over 65 years, caution.
Child: Age 6-18 years, weight 16-20kg, 100mg twice daily; 20-25kg, 125mg twice daily; 25-30kg, 150mg twice daily; over 30kg, as for Adult above.

Hepatic Impairment: Moderate, caution. Severe, not recommended.

Interactions: Effect of Other Drugs on Etravirine: Co-admin not recommended *(reduced exposure)*: Tipranavir + ritonavir; carbamazepine, phenobarbital, phenytoin, rifampicin, rifapentine, St John's Wort, other NNRTIs. *Co-admin, discourage*: Clopidogrel. *Co-admin caution*: Rifabutin (mutually decreased exposure; adjust rifabutin dose). *Etravirine plasma levels decreased, co-admin not recommended*: CYP (3A4, 2C9, 2C19) inducers; efavirenz, nevirapine, dexamethasone (systemic); can be dosed in combination with atazanavir or darunavir with ritonavir without dose adjustment. *Plasma levels increased*: CYP (3A4, 2C9, 2C19) inhibitors. *Increased monitoring for HIV/HCV suppression*: Boceprevir.

Effect of Etravirine on Other Drugs: CYP3A4 substrates; indinavir, ciclosporin, sirolimus, tacrolimus, rilpivirine, artemether/lumefantrine: *Plasma levels decreased.* CYP (2C9, 2C19) substrates; nelfinavir, diazepam (use alternative): *Plasma levels increased.* Amprenavir + ritonavir, fosamprenavir + ritonavir: *Consider dose reduction.* Maraviroc (recommended 150mg twice daily): *Co-admin with etravirine + potent CYP3A4 inhibitor (PIs).* Maraviroc (recommended 300mg twice daily): *Co-admin with fosamprenavir + ritonavir.* Digoxin: *Monitor levels.* Antiarrhythmics (amiodarone, bepridil, disopyramide, flecainide, lidocaine (systemic), mexiletine, propafenone, quinidine): *Caution, monitor therapeutic concentrations.* Clarithromycin: *Consider alternatives in treatment of Mycobacterium avium complex.* Warfarin: *Monitor INR.* Atorvastatin, PDE-5 inhibitors: *Adjust dose based on clinical response.*

SP: Decreased virological response (with various mutations). Caution, HBV or HCV co-infection (increased liver enzymes). Cutaneous reactions; severe (Stevens-Johnson Syndrome, erythema multiforme); discontinue (incidence higher in women). Severe hypersensitivity (DRESS, toxic epidermal necrolysis); discontinue, treat with corticosteroids.

Pregnancy, Lactation: Pregnancy, only if benefit outweighs risk; no dose adjustment required during pregnancy and postpartum (caution medications increasing etravirine exposure). Lactation, not recommended.

ADR: See Notes below.

Notes: See 9.3.3 NNRTIs.

INTELENCE 100mg, 200mg *(Janssen-Cilag)* A. HOS.
Price, 100mg (120) €390.69. 200mg (60) €395.64 (PTW).
Tablet, etravirine. White (off-white). 100mg: Oval. Marked T125; 100 on reverse. 200mg: Oblong. Marked T200. *Lactose.*

Nevirapine

ATC Code: J05AG01. **Sport:** Permitted.
Driving: Fatigue.
Dose: Adult, Elderly: Age 16 years and older, STANDARD/R, 200mg once daily for 14 days (lead-in to lessen rash frequency), then 200mg twice daily; max. 400mg/day; rash in first 14-days, do not increase dose until resolved; 200mg/day for max. duration 28 days.

PROLONGED/R, use only after 14-day lead-in, 400mg once daily. With or without food; Prolonged/R not to be broken or chewed. See SP below. *Over 65 years*, no data.

Child: STANDARD/R (under 16 years) 150mg/m2 BSA once daily (14 days), then 150mg/m2 twice daily OR (up to 8 years) 4mg/kg body weight once daily (14 days), then 7mg/kg twice daily; (8 years and over) 4mg/kg once daily (14 days) then 4mg/kg twice daily.

PROLONGED/R, initiate with Standard/R 200mg or oral susp 50mg/5mL as above, then Prolonged/R.

Dose by BSA, 0.58-0.83 BSA, 200mg/day; 0.84-1.16 BSA, 300mg/day; 1.17 BSA and above, 400mg/day. *Dose by Weight* (up to 8 years) weight 12.5-17.8kg OR (8 years and over) weight 17.9-31.2kg, 200mg/day. Age (up to 8 years) weight 17.9-24.9kg OR (8 years and over) weight 31.3-43.7kg, 300mg/day. Age (up to 8 years) weight 25kg and above OR (8 years and over) 43.8kg and above, 400mg/day. Under 3 years, not recommended.

Renal Impairment: Dialysis, additional 200mg (Standard/R) following each dialysis (children, additional 50% of daily dose).

Hepatic Impairment: Severe, contraindicated. Pretreatment ASAT or ALAT above 5xULN, do not initiate until stabilised below 5xULN. Recurrence of liver function abnormalities, do not re-admin. Hepatotoxicity more frequent in women.

CI: Severe rash, hypersensitivity, hepatitis due to nevirapine.

Interactions: Effect of Other Drugs on Nevirapine: Co-admin contraindicated: St John's Wort. Co-admin not recommended: Ketoconazole, fluconazole (caution); fosamprenavir (if not co-admin with ritonavir); rifampicin; NNRTIs (efavirenz, delavirdine, etravirine, rilpivirine, elvitegravir + cobicistat); atazanavir + ritonavir, boceprevir. *Co-admin caution*: Tipranavir + ritonavir (low dose), rifabutin, telaprevir. *Plasma levels mutually altered*: Protease inhibitors. *Co-admin (granulocytopenia risk)*: Zidovudine.

Effect of Nevirapine on Other Drugs: Clarithromycin: *Co-admin caution.* Oral contraceptives: *No dose recommendation (except depot-medroxyprogesterone acetate).* Efavirenz: *Plasma levels decreased, increase to 800mg once daily.* Lopinavir + ritonavir: *Increase dose.* Methadone: *Plasma levels decreased.* Warfarin: *Monitor coagulation time.*

SP: During first 18 weeks closely monitor for severe hepatitis/hepatic failure (higher risk females, higher CD4 counts), severe life-threatening skin reactions (toxic epidermal necrosis, Stevens-Johnson syndrome), hypersensitivity (rash, constitutional findings, visceral involvement); permanently discontinue. Suspected rash, monitor. Caution, prodromal signs of hepatitis (anorexia, nausea, jaundice, bilirubinuria, acholic stools, hepatomegaly, liver tenderness), rhabdomyolysis. Not for monotherapy. Autoimmune disorders (Graves' disease) with immune reactivation. Remnants in faeces resembling intact tablets; does not affect therapeutic response.

Pregnancy, Lactation: Pregnancy, caution. Women of childbearing potential *not* to use oral contraceptives as sole birth control method. Lactation, not recommended; crosses placenta, found in breast milk.

ADR: See Notes below.

Notes: See 9.3.3 NNRTIs.

Viramune Tablets, Oral Susp *(Boehringer)* A. HOS.
Price, 200mg (60) €143.27. Prolonged/R, 100mg (90), €139.60; 400mg (30), €171.33. Susp 50mg/5mL (240mL) €41.82 (PTW).
Tablet (Standard/R), nevirapine anhydrate 200mg. White oval scored (not to be broken). Marked 54 and 193; logo on reverse. *Tablet (Prolonged/R)*, as above 100mg, 400mg. Yellow. 100mg: Round. Marked V01. 400mg: Oval. Marked V04. *Lactose.*
Oral susp, nevirapine hemihydrate 50mg/mL. White (off-white) homogenous. *Parabens, sorbitol, sucrose.*
Nevirapine TEVA 200mg *(TEVA)* A.
Price, €201.91.
Tablet, nevirapine (as anhydrate). White oval scored (facilitates breaking). Marked N/strength. *Lactose.*

9.3.4 - Other Antiretrovirals (HIV)

In This Chapter: Dolutegravir, maraviroc, raltegravir.

Class Effects
Driving, Dose Adjustments: See Notes below.
CI: Hypersensitivity to any member of the class.

SP: Before initiation of abacavir-containing products, screen for carriage of HLA-B*5701 allele irrespective of racial origin; not to be used in if carrying HLA-B*5701 allele. Opportunistic infections, lipodystrophy, mitochondrial dysfunction, immune reactivation syndrome, osteonecrosis, see Notes below.

Pregnancy, Lactation: Pregnancy, if benefit outweighs risk unless otherwise specified. Recommended that HIV infected women do not breast-feed their infants under any circumstances to avoid HIV transmission.

Notes: See 9.3 Antivirals Used In HIV Infection.

9.3.4 Other Antiretrovirals (HIV)

Dolutegravir

ATC Code: J05AX12. **Sport:** Permitted.
Driving: Dizziness.

Indications: Treatment in combination, HIV infection.

Dose: Adult, Elderly: No resistance* and including adolescents (age 12-17 years, 40kg or more), 50mg once daily. Admin twice daily when co-admin with efavirenz, nevirapine, tipranavir/ritonavir, rifampicin. With resistance*, 50mg twice daily. *Admin, with/without food; with integrase class resistance, preferably with food to enhance exposure. *(documented or clinically suspected resistance to integrase class).

Child: No resistance: Age 12 years and older (at least 40kg), 50mg once daily; age 6 years to under 12 years (at least 15kg), 15kg to under 20kg, 20mg once daily; 20kg to under 30kg, 25mg once daily; 30kg to under 40kg, 35mg once daily; 40kg and above, 50mg once daily. Under 6 years or under 15kg, no data. *Admin, see Adult above.*
With resistance: No data, no dose recommendation.

Renal Impairment: No adjustment; Dialysis, differences in pharmacokinetics not expected.

Hepatic Impairment: Severe, caution.

Interactions: Effect of Other Drugs on Dolutegravir: Co-admin contraindicated: Dofetilide (increased plasma levels; potential life-threatening toxicity). Co-admin avoid (with integrase class resistance): Efavirenz, nevirapine, tipranavir + ritonavir, fosamprenavir + ritonavir; reduced exposure (magnesium, aluminium antacids*, iron and calcium supplements*, multivitamins*), inducing agents, rifampicin, certain anti-epileptics). Co-admin strongly discouraged: St John's Wort. Decreased dolutegravir exposure: UGT1A (1, 3, 9), CYP3A4, P-gp, BCRP substrates. Decreased plasma levels: Etravirine, oxcarbamazepine, phenytoin, phenobarbital, carbamazepine. *(admin 6 hours before or 2 hours after dolutegravir).

Effect of Dolutegravir on Other Drugs: Excretion dependent on OCT2 or MATE (dofetilide, metformin) or OAT3: Plasma levels increased.

SP: Hypersensitivity (severe rash, rash with raised liver enzymes, fever, malaise, fatigue, muscle/joint aches, blisters, oral lesions, conjunctivitis, facial oedema, eosinophilia, angioedema), discontinue; monitor liver aminotransferases, bilirubin. Increased risk in combination with abacavir (HLA-B*5701 allele).

Pregnancy, Lactation: Pregnancy, if benefit outweighs risk. Lactation, not recommended.

ADR: See Notes below.

Notes: See 9.3.4 Other Antiretrovirals.

▼ **Tivicay 50mg** (ViiV) A. HOS.
Price, (30) €562.42 (PTW).
Tablet, dolutegravir sodium. Yellow f/c round. Marked SV572; 50 on reverse.

Dolutegravir, Abacavir, Lamivudine

ATC Code: J05AR13. **Sport:** Permitted.
Driving: Dizziness.

Indications: Treatment, HIV infection.

Dose: Adult, Elderly: 1 tablet daily (above age 12 years, weight 40kg or more; under 40kg, not recommended). Admin, oral with or without food. Elderly, caution (decreased renal function, altered haematology).

Child: Under 12 years, under 40kg, not recommended.

Renal Impairment: CrCl (mL/min), below 50, not recommended.

Hepatic Impairment: Mild, consider abacavir dose reduction (using separate components). Moderate/severe, not recommended.

Interactions: Effect of Other Drugs on Dolutegravir, Abacavir, Lamivudine: Co-admin not recommended: Etravirine without co-admin (atazanavir, darunavir, lopinavir, tipranavir) + ritonavir; efavirenz, nevirapine, emtricitabine-containing products (lamivudine, emtricitabine are cytidine analogues), rifampicin, carbamazepine, phenobarbital, phenytoin, oxcarbazepine, cladribine. Co-admin caution: Ribavirin. See Notes below (dolutegravir).

Effect of Dolutegravir, Abacavir, Lamivudine on Other Drugs: See Notes below (dolutegravir).

SP: Hypersensitivity reactions (HSR) (may occur at any time during therapy), discontinue immediately; do not re-initiate with medicinals containing (abacavir, dolutegravir). Respiratory, GI hypersensitivity may lead to misdiagnosis of HSR as respiratory disease (pneumonia, bronchitis, pharyngitis) or gastroenteritis. See Notes below. Not for use with integrase inhibitor resistance.

ADR: See Notes below.

Notes: See Dolutegravir above. See Class Effects 9.3.1 Nucleoside Reverse Transcriptase Inhibitors (NRTIs) (abacavir and abacavir, lamivudine). See 9.3.4 Other Antiretrovirals.

▼ **Triumeq 50/600/300** (ViiV) A. HOS.
Price, (30) €917.06 (PTW).
Tablet, abacavir sodium, abacavir sulfate, lamivudine. Purple f/c oval. Marked 572 Tri. **Store:** Original pack; do not remove desiccant.

Maraviroc

ATC Code: J05AX09. **Sport:** Permitted.
Driving: Dizziness.

Indications: Treatment-experienced, infected with only CCR5-tropic HIV-1 detectable in combination.

Dose: Adult, Elderly: 150mg, 300mg or 600mg twice daily; with or without food. Over 65 years, caution. Co-admin with other antivirals, see Notes below.

Child: Not recommended.

Renal Impairment: Adjust dose when co-admin with protease inhibitors (except tipranavir + ritonavir), ketoconazole, itraconazole, clarithromycin, telithromycin; CrCl (mL/min) below 80, dose interval 24-hourly (caution); co-admin saquinavir + ritonavir, CrCl (mL/min) 50-80, dose interval 24-hourly; 30-50, dose interval 48-hourly; below 30, dose interval 72-hourly.

Hepatic Impairment: Caution, limited data.

CI: Peanut or soya hypersensitivity.

Interactions: Effect of Other Drugs on Maraviroc: Co-admin not recommended: Combinations (rifampicin + efavirenz, amprenavir/fosamprenavir + ritonavir), St John's Wort. Postural hypotension risk: Drugs causing hypotension. Plasma levels reduced (reduced therapeutic effect): CYP3A4 inducers. Plasma levels increased (consider dose reduction): CYP3A4 inhibitors.

SP: Use when only CCR5-tropic HIV-1 detectable. Not for monotherapy or in treatment-naive patients. Postural hypotension, severe cardiac disease, caution. Impaired immunity, caution active TB, invasive fungal infections. Pre-existing liver dysfunction (chronic active hepatitis, increased frequency of liver function abnormalities, acute hepatitis), discontinue. Hypersensitivity reactions (severe, potentially life-threatening). Hepatitis B and/or C co-infection, limited data.

ADR: See Notes below.

Notes: See 9.3.4 Other Antiretrovirals.

Celsentri 150mg, 300mg (ViiV) A. HOS.
Price, (60) 150mg, €738.33; 300mg, €737.62 (PTW).
Tablet, maraviroc. Oval f/c. Marked Pfizer; MVC/strength on reverse. Soya lecithin.

Raltegravir

ATC Code: J05AX08. **Sport:** Permitted.
Driving: Dizziness.

Indications: Combination treatment of HIV-1 infection.

Dose: Adult, Elderly: Tab (f/c), including adolescents and children weighing at least 25kg and able to swallow a tablet, 400mg twice daily with or without food; do not chew, crush or split tab; chewable tab, not studied in age 12-18 years or adults. Elderly, caution, limited data.

NOTE: Formulations are NOT bioequivalent; chewable tabs should not be substituted for 400mg f/c tab.

Child: At least 11kg, weight based dose of chewable tab to max. 300mg twice daily (approx. 6mg/kg/dose twice daily), see Adult above.

Hepatic Impairment: Severe, caution.

Interactions: Effect of Other Drugs on Raltegravir: Co-admin not recommended (plasma levels decreased): Antacids (aluminium or magnesium). Co-admin caution (plasma levels decreased): Rifampicin (if co-admin required, consider doubling raltegravir dose). Plasma levels increased: UGT1A1 inhibitors (atazanavir, tipranavir, efavirenz, etravirine, indinavir, saquinavir, tenofovir, maraviroc), midazolam, ethinyl estradiol, norelgestromin, methadone (no dose adjustment); medicinals increasing gastric pH (PPIs, H2-antagonists).

SP: Depression, including suicidal ideation and behaviour reported (especially with pre-existing history, caution). Always admin in combination to minimise resistance. HBV, HCV co-infection, increased hepatic adverse event risk. Phenotypic Sensitivity Score (PSS)=0 (higher risk, resistance development). May be associated with cancer risk. Autoimmune disorders (Graves' disease) in setting of immune reactivation.

Pregnancy, Lactation: Not recommended.

ADR: See Notes below.

Notes: See 9.3.4 Other Antiretrovirals.

> **Isentress 400mg, Chewable** (MSD) A. HOS.
> Price, (60) 400mg, €582.99. Chewable 100mg, €146.69. 25mg, €36.62 (PTW).
> Tablet, raltegravir potassium. Pink oval f/c. Marked 227. Lactose. Chewable tablet, as above 25mg, 100mg. Marked with logo. 25mg: Pale-yellow round. Marked 473. 100mg: Pale-orange oval scored (divisible into equal halves). Marked 477. Fructose, phenylalanine, sorbitol.

9.4 - Antivirals Used In Other Viral Infections

Class Effects

Dose: For dose adjustments (required for toxicity or renal or hepatic impairment), or for combination therapy, see manufacturers Full Prescribing Information.

9.4.1 - Herpes, CMV Infection

In This Chapter: Aciclovir, famciclovir, ganciclovir, inosine acedoben dimepranol, valaciclovir, valganciclovir.

Class Effects

Herpes virus family has 8 members i.e. Herpes simplex (HHV-1 and 2), Varicella zoster (HHV-3), Epstein-Barr (HHV-4) and cytomegalovirus (CMV) (HHV-5).

CI: Hypersensitivity to any member of the class.

SP: Initiate earliest after start of infection. Genital herpes is a sexually transmitted disease (STD). Transmission risk increased during acute episodes. Advise patients to avoid intercourse when symptomatic even with antiviral treatment (frequency of viral shedding is reduced, risk of transmission still theoretically possible).

Notes: See 9.4 Antivirals Used In Other Viral Infections.

Aciclovir (systemic)

ATC Code: J05AB01. **Sport:** Permitted.

Driving: Unlikely to impair (oral). Not applicable (parenteral).

Indications: Oral, treatment, Herpes simplex infection of skin, mucous membrane including initial and recurrent genital Herpes. Herpes simplex infections, suppression (prevention of recurrences), recurrent Herpes simplex (immunocompetent); prophylaxis in immunocompromised. Treatment, Varicella (chickenpox) and Herpes zoster (shingles) infections. Parenteral, severe initial genital herpes, recurrent Varicella zoster, Herpes simplex encephalitis in immunocompromised; Herpes simplex infection treatment and prophylaxis, primary and recurrent Varicella zoster, Herpes simplex encephalitis.

Dose: Adult: ORAL, treatment, Herpes simplex 200mg 5-times daily at 4-hourly intervals omitting night-time dose; severely immunocompromised or impaired absorption, increase to 400mg or use IV; Varicella, Herpes zoster, 800mg 5-times daily 4-hourly; early treatment of shingles can reduce incidence of post-herpetic neuralgia. Suppression, immunocompetent, 200mg 4-times daily 6-hourly OR 400mg 12-hourly. Immunocompromised

prophylaxis, 200mg 4-times daily 6-hourly; severely immunocompromised, increase to 400mg or use IV.

PARENTERAL, treatment, Herpes simplex infection (except encephalitis) or Varicella zoster, 5mg/kg 8-hourly. Immunocompromised with Varicella zoster infection or patients with herpes encephalitis, 10mg/kg 8-hourly provided renal function not impaired (usually 10 days). Admin by slow IV infusion over 1-hour.

Elderly: As for Renal below. Parenteral (IV), caution.

Child: ORAL, treatment, Herpes simplex, prophylaxis in immunocompromised, age 2 years and over, as for Adult; under 2 years, half adult dose. Treatment, varicella, age 6 years and over, 800mg 4-times daily; 2 to under 6 years, 400mg 4-times daily; under 2 years, 200mg 4-times daily OR 20mg/kg (max. 800mg) 4-times daily.

PARENTERAL, neonates and infants up to 3 months (dose calculated by body weight), 20mg/kg IV 8-hourly for 21 days (disseminated or CNS disease) or 14 days (skin, mucous membrane)*. Children age 3 months-12 years (dose calculated by body surface area), Herpes simplex (excluding encephalitis), Varicella zoster, 250mg/m2 BSA 8-hourly*. Immunocompromised infants, children with Varicella zoster infections or herpes encephalitis, 500mg/m2 8-hourly*. *(if renal function is normal).

Renal Impairment: Oral, treatment, Varicella and Herpes zoster, CrCl (mL/min) below 10, 800mg twice daily 12-hourly; CrCl 10-25, 800mg 3-times daily 8-hourly.

Parenteral, CrCl 25-50, 5-10mg/kg 12-hourly (child, 250-500mg/m2 BSA or 20mg/kg body weight); CrCl 10-25, 5-10mg/kg (child, 250-500mg/m2 BSA or 20mg/kg body weight) every 24 hours; CrCl 10 and less, peritoneal dialysis (CAPD) and haemodialysis, half dose, admin every 24 hours after haemodialysis.

Hepatic Impairment: IV, caution.

CI: Valaciclovir hypersensitivity.

SP: Elderly, renal impairment, increased neurological side effect risk; high oral doses, ensure adequate hydration (especially elderly). IV not for bolus admin. Prolonged or repeated course in severely immunocompromised may result in selection of virus strains, reduced sensitivity.

Pregnancy, Lactation: Pregnancy, if benefit outweighs risk. Lactation, caution.

ADR: Common, headache, dizziness, nausea, vomiting, diarrhoea, abdominal pains, pruritus, rash including photosensitivity, fatigue, fever, phlebitis, increased liver enzymes, increased blood urea and creatinine (parenteral).

Notes: See 9.4.1 Herpes, CMV Infection.

> **Zovirax OroDisp, Susp, Double Strength** (GSK) A. GMS.D*.
> Price, OroDisp 200mg (25)* €10.88. 800mg (35) €42.24. Susp (per 5mL) 200mg (125mL)* €29.42. Double Strength 400mg (100mL) €23.16.
> OroDisp tablet, aciclovir 200mg, 800mg. White f/c. 200mg: Round. Marked GXCF3. 800mg: Elongated. Marked GXCG1.
> Oral susp, as above 200mg/5mL, Double Strength 400mg/5mL. Off-white. 200mg/5mL: Banana-flavour. 400mg/5mL: Orange flavour. Sorbitol, parabens
> **Zovirax Parenteral** (GSK) A. HOS.
> Price, Zovirax (5) €42.65 (PTW).
> Infusion (IV), aciclovir sodium 250mg. White (off-white) freeze-dried powder for soln. Sodium 26mg/vial.

Famciclovir

ATC Code: J05AB09. **Sport:** Permitted.

Driving: CNS disturbances, dizziness, somnolence, confusion.

Indications: Adults, treatment, herpes zoster, ophthalmic zoster (immunocompetent), herpes zoster (immunocompromised); treatment, first and recurrent episodes of genital herpes (immunocompetent), recurrent episodes of genital herpes (immunocompromised); suppression, recurrent genital herpes (immunocompetent and immunocompromised).

Dose: Adult, Elderly: Age 18 years and over, treatment Herpes zoster and ophthalmic zoster, 500mg 3-times daily for 7 days (immunocompromised 10 days). Genital herpes, first episode, 250mg 3-times daily for 5 days; recurrent, 125mg twice daily for 5 days (immunocompromised 500mg twice daily for 7 days).

9.4.1 Herpes, CMV Infection

Suppression, 250mg twice daily (immunocompromised 500mg twice daily). Admin with or without food.
Renal Impairment: Dose reduction required. Admin after haemodialysis.
Hepatic Impairment: No dose adjustment; severe, no data.
CI: Penciclovir hypersensitivity.
Interactions: Effect of Other Drugs on Famciclovir: *Monitor for toxicity (increased metabolite plasma levels):* Probenecid. *Monitor clinical efficacy:* Raloxifene.
Pregnancy, Lactation: Pregnancy, if benefit outweighs risk. Lactation, not recommended; not known if excreted into human breast milk.
ADR: *Very common*, headache.
Notes: See 9.4.1 Herpes, CMV Infection.

Famvir 125mg, 250mg, 500mg *(Novartis)* A. GMS.
Price, 125mg (10) €7.17. 250mg (15) €33.35. 500mg (21) €86.10.
Tablet, famciclovir. White f/c. 125mg, 250mg: Round. Marked FV; strength on reverse. 500mg: Oval. Marked FV500. *Lactose*.

Famciclovir 125mg, 250mg *(TEVA)* A. GMS.
Price, 125mg (10) €7.17. 250mg (15) €32.31.
Tablet, famciclovir. White (off-white) round f/c. Marked 93. 125mg: Marked 8117. 250mg: Marked 8118.

Ganciclovir

ATC Code: J05AB06. **Sport:** Permitted.
Driving: May have a major influence.
Indications: Treatment, cytomegalovirus (CMV) infections in immunocompromised patients. Prevention of CMV in patients with drug-induced immunosuppression (cancer chemotherapy, organ transplantation).
Dose: Adult: *CMV treatment* (age 12 years and older), induction, 5mg/kg as IV infusion every 12 hours for 14-21 days; maintenance 5mg/kg as IV infusion once daily for 7 days per week OR 6mg/kg once daily for 5 days per week. If CMV disease progresses either on maintenance or discontinuation, re-treat using induction regimen.
CMV prophylaxis, 5mg/kg as IV infusion once daily for 7 days per week OR 6mg/kg once daily for 5 days per week. *CMV pre-emptive therapy*, as for prophylaxis; duration based on risk of CMV disease.
Admin, by IV infusion over 1 hour at infusion conc max. 10mg/mL, not recommended. Not for rapid or bolus IV injection as resulting excessive plasma levels may increase ganciclovir toxicity. Not for IM or SC injection; may result in severe tissue irritation due to high pH.
Elderly: Consider renal status.
Child: Under 12 years, limited safety and efficacy data.
Renal Impairment: CrCl (mL/min) 70 or above, induction 5mg/kg 12-hourly, maintenance 5mg/kg/day; 50-69, induction 2.5mg/kg 12-hourly, maintenance 2.5mg/kg/day; 25-49, induction 2.5mg/kg/day, maintenance 1.25mg/kg/day; 10-24, induction 1.25mg/kg/day, maintenance 0.625mg/kg/day. Below 10, induction 1.25mg/kg, maintenance 0.625mg/kg (both dosed 3-times per week after haemodialysis).
Interactions: Effect of Other Drugs on Ganciclovir: *Co-admin not recommended (only if benefit outweighs risk):* Imipenem-cilastatin (convulsions), trimethoprim. *Caution, monitor for toxicity:* Didanosine, myelosuppressives (zidovudine), drugs affecting renal function or nephrotoxic drugs (cidofovir, foscarnet), mycophenolate mofetil, zalcitabine, drugs inhibiting rapidly dividing cells (dapsone, pentamidine, flucytosine, vincristine, vinblastine, adriamycin, amphotericin B, trimethoprim/sulpha combinations, nucleoside analogues, hydroxyurea). *Decreased renal clearance:* Probenecid.
SP: Cross-hypersensitivity (aciclovir, penciclovir), caution. Congenital or neonatal CMV infection, not recommended. Potentially carcinogenic. Severe myelosuppression (severe leucopenia, neutropenia, anaemia, thrombocytopenia, pancytopenia, bone marrow depression, aplastic anaemia); do not initiate if neutrophils below 500 cells/microL, platelets below 25000/microL, Hb below 8g/dL; caution, pre-existing or drug-related haematological cytopenia, patients on radiotherapy. Monitor complete blood counts including platelets during therapy (every

second day for first 14 days; low baseline neutrophils or have developed leucopenia or with renal impairment, monitor daily).
Pregnancy, Lactation: Pregnancy, potentially teratogenic; potential to cause birth defects; not for use unless clinical need outweighs reproductive toxicity. Women of childbearing potential to ensure adequate contraception. May cause temporary or permanent inhibition of human spermatogenesis. Lactation, contraindicated.
ADR: Summary, *most serious and common*, haematological (neutropenia, anaemia, thrombocytopenia). NOTE: Valganciclovir is a pro-drug of ganciclovir; adverse reactions associated with valganciclovir can be expected with ganciclovir.
Notes: See 9.4.1 Herpes, CMV Infection. See Valganciclovir below.

Cymevene Parenteral 500mg *(Roche)* A. HOS.
Price, (5) €171.61 (PTW).
Infusion, ganciclovir sodium. White (off-white) powder for soln for conc for soln. *Sodium 43mg/500mg.*

Inosine Acedoben Dimepranol

ATC Code: J05AX05. **Sport:** Permitted.
Driving: Unlikely to impair.
Indications: SSPE, varicella, *Herpes simplex* including recurrent, genital warts (adjunctive).
Dose: Adult, Elderly: 50mg/kg/day in 3-4 divided doses; max. 4g. *SSPE*, 100mg/kg/day; max. 3-4g. *Genital warts*, 3g/day adjunctive (low risk patients, 14-28 days; high risk, 5 days per week for 1-2 consecutive weeks per month for 3 months). Oral, tabs may be crushed and dissolved to facilitate ingestion.
Child: Older than 1 year, 50mg/kg/day (1 tab/10kg up to 20kg); over 20kg, as for Adult above.
Renal Impairment: Caution.
CI: Active gout or elevated uric acid.
Interactions: Effect of Other Drugs on Inosine Acedoben Dimepranol: *Co-admin caution:* Xanthine oxidase inhibitors, uricosurics agents, diuretics. *Co-admin not recommended (but may be admin after):* Immunosuppressive agents.
Effect of Inosine Acedoben Dimepranol on other Drugs: Zidovudine: *Effect increased.*
SP: Gout, hyperuricaemia, urolithiasis, caution. Ureteric biliary calculi may occur. Hypersensitivity (urticaria, angioedema, anaphylaxis), discontinue.
Pregnancy, Lactation: Pregnancy, lactation, if benefit outweighs risk.
ADR: Summary, *consistently observed*, elevated urine and serum uric acid.
Notes: See 9.4.1 Herpes, CMV Infection.

Imunovir 500mg *(KoRa)* A. GMS.
Price, (100) €46.08.
Tablet, inosine acedoben dimepranol. White (off-white) oblong scored (facilitates breaking). Marked DN. *Wheat starch.*

Valaciclovir

ATC Code: J05AB11. **Sport:** Permitted.
Driving: Caution.
Indications: *Herpes zoster* (VZV) treatment (adults), shingles (immunocompetent); mild/moderate immunosuppression); ophthalmic zoster (immunocompetent). *Herpes simplex* (HSV), treatment and suppression (immunocompetent adults, adolescents); immunocompromised adults), skin and mucous membrane infection (first episode genital herpes, recurrences, suppression or recurrences); recurrent ocular HSV infections. *Cytomegalovirus* (CMV), prophylaxis following solid organ transplant (adults, adolescents).
Dose: Adult: Treatment, *Herpes zoster*, 1g 3-times daily for 7 days; continue for 2 days after lesion crusting (immunocompromised). *Herpes simplex*, 500mg twice daily; initial episode (10 days); recurrent (3-5 days). *Herpes labialis (cold sores)*, 2g 12-hourly for 1 day. *HSV, immunocompromised*, 1g twice daily (5 days); initial episode (10 days).
Suppression of HSV recurrences, 500mg once daily OR

250mg twice daily (immunocompetent), 500mg twice daily (immunocompromised HIV patients).

Prophylaxis CMV Infection, 2g 4-times daily usually for 90 days; may need to be extended in high risk.

Elderly: Consider dose reduction, see Renal below.

Child: Under 12 years, no data.

Renal Impairment: *Herpes zoster*, CrCl (mL/min) 50 and above, 1g 3-times daily; 30-49, 1g twice daily; 10-29, 1g/day*; below 10, 500mg/day*. *Herpes simplex*, treatment (immunocompetent), CrCl (mL/min) 30 and above, 500mg twice daily; below 30, 500mg/day*; (immunocompromised) CrCl (mL/min) 30 and above, 1g twice daily; below 30, 1g/day*. *Herpes labialis (cold sores)*, CrCl (mL/min) 50 and above, 2g twice in one day; 30-49, 1g twice in one day; 10-29, 500mg twice in one day; below 10, 500mg as single dose. *Suppression*, immunocompetent, CrCl (mL/min) 30 and above, 500mg once daily; below 30, 250mg once daily; immunocompromised, CrCl (mL/min) 30 and above, 500mg twice daily; below 30, 500mg once daily.

CMV, solid organ transplantation, CrCl (mL/min) 75 and above, 2g 4-times daily; 50-75, 1.5g 4-times daily; 25-50, 1.5g 3-times daily; 10-25, 1.5g twice daily; below 10 on dialysis, 1.5g once daily after dialysis. *(once daily)*.

Hepatic Impairment: 4g/day in liver disease, caution. Liver transplantation, no data.

CI: Aciclovir hypersensitivity.

Interactions: Effect of Other Drugs on Valaciclovir: *Plasma levels mutually increased:* Mycophenolate mofetil. *Caution, monitor:* Drugs affecting renal function (aminoglycosides, organo/iodinated contrast media, methotrexate, pentamidine, ciclosporin, tacrolimus), drugs affecting tubular secretion.

SP: Ensure adequate hydration (especially elderly). Suppressive therapy reduces genital herpes transmission risk; does not cure or completely eliminate risk.

Pregnancy, Lactation: Pregnancy, if benefit outweighs risk. Lactation, passes into breast milk, caution; at therapeutic doses, no effects on the breastfed newborn/infant anticipated.

ADR: *Most common*, headache, nausea; *more serious*, thrombotic thrombocytopenic purpura/haemolytic uraemic syndrome, acute renal failure, neurological disorders. See SP above.

Notes: See 9.4.1 Herpes, CMV Infection. See Aciclovir and Ganciclovir above.

Valtrex 250mg, 500mg *(GSK)* A. GMS.D*.
Price, tabs (60) €66.12. 500mg* (10) €9.50; (30) €28.51; (42) €39.92.
Tablet, valaciclovir HCl. Elongated white (off-white) f/c. 250mg: Marked GXCE7. 500mg: Marked GXCF1.

Valaciclovir Actavis 500mg *(Accord)* A. GMS.D.
Price, (10) €9.50. (30) €28.51. (42) €39.92.
Tablet, valaciclovir hydrochloride monohydrate. Oval white f/c. Marked VC2.

Valaciclovir Bluefish 500mg *(Bluefish)* A. GMS.
Price, €23.40.
Tablet, valaciclovir hydrochloride monohydrate. White cap-shaped f/c. Marked V; 500 on reverse.

Valaciclovir TEVA 500mg *(TEVA)* A. GMS.D.
Price, (30) €28.51.
Tablet, valaciclovir hydrochloride dihydrate. White f/c oblong scored (divisible into equal halves). Marked VL and D.

Valotix 500mg *(Rowex)* A. GMS.D.
Price, (10) €9.50.
Tablet, valaciclovir HCl. White (off-white) cap-shaped f/c. Marked 500.

Valganciclovir

ATC Code: J05AB14. **Sport:** Permitted.
Driving: Convulsions, sedation, dizziness, ataxia and/or confusion reported; may affect ability.
Indications: Treatment, CMV retinitis (AIDS patients). Prevention, CMV disease in CMV-negative adults and children (birth to 18 years) following solid organ transplantation from CMV-positive donor.
Dose: Adult, Elderly: *CMV retinitis*, induction 900mg *twice* daily (21 days); maintenance 900mg *once* daily.
Prevention, CMV disease in solid organ transplant, 900mg once daily starting within 10 days of transplant; continue to 100 days post-transplant. Kidney transplant, may continue to 200 days post-transplant (leucopenia risk). *Elderly*, safety/efficacy not established. *Admin*, oral, with food wherever possible; do not break or crush tabs; reconstitute powder for oral soln.
NOTE: Caution, strict adherence to dosage recommendations essential. Oral valganciclovir 900mg twice daily is equiv. to IV ganciclovir 5mg/kg twice daily.
Child: *CMV prevention, solid organ transplant* (age from birth): Paed dose (mg) = 7 x BSA x CrCl. Kidney transplant, start within 10 days post-transplant, continue for 200 days post-transplant; other transplants, 100 days post-transplant. *CMV retinitis*, safety and efficacy not established.
Renal Impairment: CrCl (mL/min) 40-59, induction 450mg twice daily; maintenance, 450mg once daily; 25-39, induction 450mg once daily; maintenance, 450mg every 2 days; 10-24, induction 450mg every 2 days; maintenance, 450mg twice weekly; below 10, not recommended.
Hepatic Impairment: No data.
CI: Ganciclovir, aciclovir, valaciclovir hypersensitivity.
Interactions: Effect of Other Drugs on Valganciclovir: See Notes below (ganciclovir).
SP: Potential to cause carcinogenicity and reproductive toxicity long-term; caution handling product. Monitor regularly, complete blood counts, platelets; paediatrics or with renal impairment, monitor at each attendance at transplant clinic.
Pregnancy, Lactation: Pregnancy, use only if benefit outweighs risk. Women of childbearing potential to ensure adequate contraception; males to practise barrier contraception during and for 90 days after treatment if female partner at risk for pregnancy. Lactation, not recommended.
ADR: *Very common*, severe neutropenia, anaemia, diarrhoea; *adults*, dyspnoea; *children*, hypertension, upper RTI, nausea, vomiting, constipation, pyrexia, transplant rejection.
Notes: See 9.4.1 Herpes, CMV Infection. See Ganciclovir above.

Valcyte 450mg, Oral Soln *(Roche)* A. HT.
Price, tabs 450mg (60) €896.86. Oral soln (100mL) €288.63.
Tablet, valganciclovir HCl. Pink oval f/c. Marked VGC; 450 on reverse.
Oral soln, as above 50mg/mL. White (slightly yellow) granular powder; forms clear colourless (brown) soln. Sodium 0.188mg/mL.

Valganciclovir Accord 450mg *(Accord)* A. HT.
Price, (60) €635.05.
Tablet, valganciclovir HCl. Pink oval f/c. Marked J; 156 on reverse.

Valganciclovir Rowex 450mg *(Rowex)* A. HT.
Price, (60) €616.00
Tablet, valganciclovir HCl. Pink oval f/c. Marked J; 156 on reverse.

9.4.2 - Viral Hepatitis

In This Chapter: *Adefovir, daclatasvir, dasabuvir, elbasvir/grazoprevir, entecavir, lamivudine, ledipasvir/sofosbuvir, ombitasvir/paritaprevir/ritonavir, peginterferon alfa-2a, ribavirin, simeprevir, tenofovir.*

Class Effects
Dose: For treatment duration, combination drugs, dose adjustments for combination use and/or missed doses, see manufacturers Full Prescribing Information.
CI: Hypersensitivity to any member of the class.
Interactions: Effect of Other Drugs on Nucleoside Analogues: *Possible mutually increased plasma levels:* Drugs eliminated by tubular excretion or altering tubular function.
SP: *Some nucleoside analogues*, lactic acidosis with severe hepatomegaly and hepatic steatosis, discontinue; increased risk (HIV co-infection receiving HAART). Benign symptoms (nausea, vomiting abdominal pain) may indicate lactic acidosis; severe (pancreatitis, liver failure/hepatic steatosis, renal failure, higher levels of serum lactate).

9.4.2　Viral Hepatitis

Caution, particularly obese women, underlying hepatomegaly, hepatitis, other liver disease risk factors. Spontaneous exacerbations (during and/or after treatment), may be severe. Treatment does not reduce hepatitis B transmission risk. *Alpha interferons* including in combination (ribavirin), severe CNS/psychiatric effects (depression, suicidal ideation, attempted suicide; aggressive behaviour, homicidal ideation, bipolar disorders, mania, confusion, altered mental status), monitor. Severe psychiatric conditions (or history), manage before initiating; increased risk of developing or exacerbation with substance use disorder (alcohol, cannabis). Severe (ocular, dental, periodontal) disorders, growth inhibition in children and adolescents (may be irreversible). *Direct-acting antivirals* (daclatasvir, dasabuvir, elbasvir/grazoprevir, ledipasvir, ombitasvir, paritaprevir, simeprevir, sofosbuvir), used to treat viral hepatitis (hepatitis B re-activation risk); screen for HBV before initiation; HBV/HCV co-infection, monitor/manage.

Pregnancy, Lactation: Pregnancy, if benefit outweighs risk. Women of child-bearing age and male partners to ensure adequate contraception. Lactation, not recommended (adefovir, entecavir, peginterferon alfa-2a and 2b). Ribavirin, contraindicated. Nucleoside analogues may impact mitochondrial function; most pronounced with stavudine, didanosine, zidovudine. Reports of mitochondrial dysfunction in infants exposed in utero and/or post-natal to nucleoside analogues. Main adverse reactions are haematological (anaemia, neutropenia), metabolic (hyperlactataemia, hyperlipasaemia), late onset neurological disorders (hypertonia, convulsion, abnormal behaviour).

ADR: See manufacturers Full Prescribing Information.

Notes: See 9.4 Antivirals Used In Other Viral Infections. See 13.2.3 Interferons used in Oncology.

Adefovir

ATC Code: J05AF08. **Sport:** Permitted.
Driving: No or negligible effect.

Indications: Treatment, chronic Hepatitis B with (compensated liver disease with active viral replication, persistently elevated ALT levels, histological evidence of active liver inflammation/fibrosis) OR decompensated liver disease (combination with second agent without cross-resistance to *Hepsera*).

Dose: Adult, Elderly: Age 18 years and over, 10mg once daily. *Over 65 years*, no dose recommendation. Oral, with or without food.

Renal Impairment: CrCl (mL/min) 30-49, 10mg every 48 hours; below 30 and on dialysis, not recommended. Only if benefit outweighs risk, CrCl (mL/min) 10-29, 10mg every 72 hours; haemodialysis, 10mg every 7 days following 12-hour continuous dialysis (or 3 dialysis sessions of 4-hours); below 10, not dialysed, no dose interval recommendation.

Interactions: Effect of Other Drugs on Adefovir: *Co-admin, monitor renal function*: Tenofovir *(Viread)*, tacrolimus, ciclosporin, any medicinal affecting renal function. *Caution*: Pegylated interferon.

SP: Renal impairment risk (long-term use), monitor frequently; calculate CrCl prior to initiation; monitor function every 4 weeks (year 1), then every 3 months. Renal insufficiency and advanced liver disease or cirrhosis, adjust dose interval or change treatment. HIV co-infection, monitor virological response.

ADR: See Notes below.

Notes: See 9.4.2 Viral Hepatitis.

Hepsera 10mg *(Gilead)* A. HT.
Price, (30) €461.47.
Tablet, adefovir dipivoxil. White (off-white) round flat. Marked Gilead/strength; shape of a liver on reverse. *Lactose*.

Daclatasvir

ATC Code: J05AX14. **Sport:** Pending.
Driving: Dizziness, disturbed attention, blurred vision, reduced visual acuity (in combination).

Indications: Treatment, chronic hepatitis C (HCV).

Dose: Adult, Elderly: 60mg once daily; duration depends on genotype. *Combination*, strong CYP3A4 inhibitors

(boceprevir, telaprevir, atazanavir/ritonavir, cobicistat, clarithromycin, telithromycin, ketoconazole), reduce to 30mg once daily; moderate CYP3A4 inducers (efavirenz), increase to 90mg once daily. Admin with or without food; always in combination (consult prescribing information of combination drugs before initiation) and never as monotherapy; swallow whole, do not crush or chew (unpleasant taste of active substance).

Child: Under 18 years, no data.

Renal Impairment: No adjustment.

Hepatic Impairment: As for Renal; decompensated cirrhosis, no data.

Interactions: Effect of Other Drugs on Daclatasvir: *Co-admin contraindicated*: Strong CYP3A4 and P-gp inducers (phenytoin, carbamazepine, oxcarbazepine, phenobarbital, rifampicin, rifabutin, rifapentine, systemic dexamethasone, St John's Wort). *Co-admin not recommended*: Darunavir, lopinavir, etravirine, nevirapine. *Co-admin caution*: Erythromycin, calcium channel blockers, rosuvastatin. *Severe bradycardia and heart block*: Sofosbuvir + amiodarone. *Daclatasvir dose adjustment recommended*: Moderate CYP3A4 and P-gp inducers (plasma levels decreased), strong CYP3A4 inhibitors (plasma levels increased). *Combination not evaluated*: Sofosbuvir.

Effect of Daclatasvir on Other Drugs: Substrates of P-gp, OATP1B1, OCT1 or BCRP: *Systemic exposure may be increased*. Dabigatran, other intestinal P-gp substrates with narrow therapeutic window: *Safety monitoring advised*. Digoxin: *Caution, monitor; use lowest dose*. Buprenorphine/naloxone: *Monitor for opiate toxicity*. See Dose above.

SP: HCV genotypes 5 and 6, retreatment with prior NS5A inhibitor exposure, post organ transplant, (no data). Hepatitis B virus (HBV) reactivation reported (including fatal); screen for HBV before initiation.

Pregnancy, Lactation: Pregnancy, not recommended. Women of childbearing potential to ensure highly effective contraception during and up to 5 weeks after treatment.

ADR: See Notes below.

Notes: See 9.4.2 Viral Hepatitis.

▼ **Daklinza 30mg, 60mg** *(BMS)* A. HOS.
Price, both strengths (28) €8717.09 (PTW).
Tablet, daclatasvir dihydrochloride. Pentagonal. Marked BMS. 30mg: Green. Marked 213. 60mg: Light-green. Marked 215. *Lactose*.

Dasabuvir

ATC Code: Pending. **Sport:** Permitted.
Driving: Fatigue reported (in combination).

Indications: Treatment, adults with chronic hepatitis C, in combination.

Dose: Adult, Elderly: 250mg twice daily (morning, evening) always in combination, see SP below. Genotype 1b* (GT1b) (without cirrhosis or with compensated cirrhosis), GT1a (without cirrhosis), duration 12 weeks; GT1a (with compensated cirrhosis) and liver transplant recipients, duration 24 weeks. *(8 weeks may be considered; previously untreated GT1b; minimal to moderate fibrosis). *Admin*, swallow tabs whole; do not break, chew or dissolve; to maximise absorption, admin with food without regard to fat and calorie content.

Child: Under 18 years, no safety/efficacy data.

Renal Impairment: No adjustment. Ribavirin co-admin, see Notes below (ribavirin).

Hepatic Impairment: Moderate, not recommended. Severe, should not be used.

Interactions: Effect of Other Drugs on Dasabuvir (in combination): *Co-admin contraindicated*: Ethinyloestradiol (combined oral contraceptives, contraceptive vaginal rings), enzyme inducers (carbamazepine, phenytoin, phenobarbital, efavirenz, nevirapine, etravirine, enzalutamide, mitotane, rifampicin, St. John's Wort), strong CYP2C8 inhibitors (gemfibrozil), ketoconazole. *Co-admin not recommended*: Fluvastatin, pitavastatin. *Co-admin caution (increased exposure)*: Deferasirox, teriflunomide. For co-admin of HIV antivirals, see manufacturers Full Prescribing Information.

Effect of Dasabuvir (in combination) on Other Drugs: BCRP substrates (sulfasalazine, imatinib; rosuvastatin max. 5mg/day; pravastatin reduce dose by 50%), UGT1A1 substrates (levothyroxine), imatinib, dabigatran; amlodipine, furosemide (reduce dose by 50%), alprazolam: *Increased exposure (consider dose reduction).* CYP2C19 substrates (lansoprazole, esomeprazole, omeprazole; consider higher doses), s-mephenytoin: *Decreased exposure.* Digoxin, warfarin, other Vitamin K antagonists: *Monitor levels.* Ciclosporin (reduce dose to one-fifth of daily dose), tacrolimus (reduce dose to 0.5mg once weekly): *Monitor levels.*

SP: Not for use as monotherapy or HIV co-infection without suppressive antiretrovirals. Efficacy established for HCV genotype 1 with (ombitasvir, paritaprevir, ritonavir with/without ribavirin). No efficacy data (previous dasabuvir exposure or cross-resistant medicinals). Elevated ALT (up to 5xULN), more frequent with ethinyloestradiol co-admin; switch to alternative prior to initiation (progestin only, non-hormonal). Hepatic decompensation, failure (liver transplant or fatal outcomes); most severe with advanced or decompensated cirrhosis prior to initiation. Hepatitis B virus (HBV) reactivation reported (including fatal); screen for HBV before initiation.

Pregnancy, Lactation: Used in combination with ribavirin, extreme caution. See Notes below (ribavirin). Ethinylestradiol contraindicated. Lactation, stop drug or stop breastfeeding.

ADR: See Notes below.

Notes: See 9.4.2 Viral Hepatitis. See Ribavirin below.

▼ **Exviera 250mg** *(AbbVie)* A. HOS.
Price, (56) €1060.60 (PTW).
Tablet, dasabuvir sodium monohydrate. Beige ovaloid f/c. Marked AV2. *Lactose.*

Elbasvir, Grazoprevir

ATC Code: J05AX658. **Sport:** Pending.
Driving: Not likely to affect; fatigue.

Indications: Treatment, chronic HCV.

Dose: Adult, Elderly: 1 tablet once daily; HCV genotype 1a*, 1b, 4* (12 weeks). *(16 weeks + ribavirin with HCV RNA above 800000 IU/mL to minimise treatment failure). *Admin,* swallow tabs whole; with or without food.

Child: Under 18 years, no safety/efficacy data.

Renal Impairment: No adjustment.

Hepatic Impairment: Moderate/severe, contraindicated.

Interactions: Effect of Other Drugs on Elbasvir, Grazoprevir: *Co-admin contraindicated:* OATP1B inhibitors (rifampicin; atazanavir, darunavir, lopinavir, saquinavir, tipranavir *all* + ritonavir; cobicistat, ciclosporin), CYP3A4 or P-gp inducers (efavirenz, phenytoin, carbamazepine, bosentan, etravirine, modafinil, St John's Wort), elvitegravir/cobicistat/emtricitabine/tenofovir fixed combination. *Co-admin not recommended:* Ketoconazole. **Effect Elbasvir, Grazoprevir on Other Drugs:** Dabigatran (bleeding risk), sunitinib (caution, consider dose adjustment): *Increased plasma levels.* Atorvastatin (max. 20mg/day); rosuvastatin (max. 10mg/day); fluvastatin, lovastatin, simvastatin (max. 20mg/day): *Max. doses with co-admin.* Tacrolimus: *Monitor levels, renal function, adverse events.* Vitamin K antagonists: *Monitor INR closely.*

SP: ALT elevations (above 5xULN); monitor LFTs (prior to initiation, week 8, then as needed); on 16-week therapy, monitor at week 12. Fatigue, weakness, lack of appetite, nausea, vomiting, jaundice, discoloured faeces, advise to seek medical advice. ALT above 10xULN or with signs of liver inflammation or increasing (conjugated bilirubin, ALP, INR), discontinue. Not for use in genotypes 2, 3, 5, 6. Efficacy with retreatment (or medicinals of same class) or HCV/HBV co-infection, no data.

Pregnancy, Lactation: Pregnancy, weigh risk/benefit. Lactation, stop breastfeeding or stop drug. With ribavirin, see Notes below (ribavirin).

ADR: See Notes below.

Notes: See 9.4.2 Viral Hepatitis. See Ribavirin below.

▼ **Zepatier 50/100mg** *(MSD)* A. HOS.
Price, (28) €11934.37 (PTW).
Tablet, elbasvir 50mg, grazoprevir 100mg. Beige oval f/c. Marked 770. *Lactose; sodium 69.85mg/tab.*

Entecavir

ATC Code: J05AF10. **Sport:** Permitted.
Driving: Caution.

Indications: Treatment (adults), chronic HBV infection (compensated* or decompensated liver disease); nucleoside naive children (2-18 years) (compensated liver disease*). *(active viral replication, persistently elevated serum ALT levels, active inflammation and/or fibrosis).

Dose: Adult, Elderly: Compensated liver disease, nucleoside naive, 0.5mg/day with or without food; lamivudine-refractory or decompensated liver disease, 1mg once daily which must be taken on empty stomach; 2 or more hours before or after food. Presence of lamivudine resistance mutations, consider combination use in preference to monotherapy. *Elderly,* as for Renal below.

Child: Age 2-18 years, body weight at least 32.6kg, 1x 0.5mg tab or 10mL oral soln with or without food; under 32.6kg, see manufacturers Full Prescribing Information.

Renal Impairment: CrCl (mL/min) 30-49, 0.25mg once daily or 0.5mg 48-hourly (nucleoside naive) OR 0.5mg once daily (lamivudine-refractory); 10-29, 0.15mg once daily or 0.5mg 72-hourly (nucleoside naive) OR 0.3 once daily or 0.5mg 78-hourly (lamivudine-refractory); below 10 on dialysis, 0.05 once daily or 0.5mg every 5-7 days (nucleoside naive) OR 0.1mg once daily or 0.5mg 72-hourly (lamivudine-refractory). Doses under 0.5mg, use soln.

SP: Renal impairment, monitor virological response. Hepatitis exacerbations; cirrhosis, higher hepatic decompensation risk; decompensated liver disease, higher risk of serious hepatic adverse events. Hepatorenal syndrome risk, monitor. Liver transplant, monitor renal function (with ciclosporin or tacrolimus). Entecavir not recommended with hepatitis C or D, HIV co-infection not receiving HAART. Lamivudine-refractory, see manufacturers Full Prescribing Information. Some children may need long-term (lifetime) treatment of chronic HBV infection; consider impact of entecavir on future treatment options.

ADR: See Notes below.

Notes: See 9.4.2 Viral Hepatitis.

Baraclude 0.5mg, 1mg, Oral Soln *(BMS)* A. HT.
Price, tabs (30) 0.5mg, €450.92. 1mg, €473.73. Oral susp (210mL) €585.37.
Tablet, entecavir monohydrate. Triangular f/c. Marked BMS. 0.5mg: White (off-white). Marked 1611. 1mg: Pink. Marked 1612. *Lactose.*
Oral soln, as above 0.05mg/mL. Clear colourless (pale-yellow). *Maltitol, parabens.*

Lamivudine (HBV)

ATC Code: J05AF05. **Sport:** Permitted.
Driving: Caution.

Indications: Chronic Hepatitis B, decompensated (with second agent); compensated with other factors, use only if alternative antiviral agent with a higher genetic barrier is not available or appropriate.

Dose: Adult, Elderly: 100mg once daily. *Admin,* with or without food.

Child: Under 18 years, not recommended.

Renal Impairment: Using oral soln 5mg/mL (where available), CrCl (mL/min) 30-49, 100mg (dose 1) then 50mg; 15-29, 100mg (dose 1) then 25mg; 5-14, 35mg (dose 1) then 15mg; below 5, 35mg (dose 1) then 10mg. *Admin,* once daily.

Interactions: Effect of Other Drugs on Lamivudine: See Notes below (lamivudine).

SP: Discontinuation, recurrent hepatitis may occur; marginal liver function, caution severe/fatal decompensation. Can be used if clinically needed.

Pregnancy, Lactation: Data on more than 1000 exposed outcomes indicate no malformative toxicity; can be used if clinically needed. Lactation, weigh risk/benefit (risk of emergence of lamivudine-resistant mutants in infant).

9.4.2   Viral Hepatitis

ADR: See Notes below.

Notes: See 9.4.2 Viral Hepatitis. See also 9.3.1 NRTIs (lamivudine in HIV).

Zeffix 100mg *(GSK)* A. HT.
Price, tabs (28) €54.83.
Tablet, lamivudine. Butterscotch-coloured f/c. Marked GXCG5.
Store: Below 30 deg C.

Ledipasvir, Sofosbuvir

ATC Code: J05AX65. **Sport:** Permitted.
Driving: No or negligible influence; fatigue.

Indications: Treatment, chronic hepatitis C (CHC) (adults).

Dose: Adult, Elderly: Recommended, 1 tab (90/400) once daily in combination. Treatment duration and recommended use of co-admin ribavirin for certain subgroups, see Full Prescribing Information. *Admin,* swallow table whole with or without food; do not crush or chew as f/c tablet is bitter.

Child: Under 18 years, safety/efficacy not established.

Renal Impairment: Severe or ESRD on dialysis, safety not assessed.

Hepatic Impairment: No adjustment. Decompensated cirrhosis, safety/efficacy not established.

Interactions: Effect of Other Drugs on Ledipasvir, Sofosbuvir: *Co-admin contraindicated*: Rosuvastatin, potent P-gp inducers (rifampicin, rifabutin, St John's Wort, carbamazepine, phenobarbital, phenytoin). *Co-admin not recommended*: Telaprevir, boceprevir; *Harvoni* levels decreased (increased gastric pH e.g. antacids, allow 4-hour dose interval; H2-antagonists, dose equiv. to famotidine 40mg; PPI, dose equiv. to omeprazole 20mg), tipranavir (ritonavir boosted); plasma levels mutually increased (simeprevir, oxcarbazepine). *Co-admin only if benefit outweighs risk*: Other direct-acting antivirals. *Severe bradycardia, heart block (monitor)*: Amiodarone (use only if not alternative available), other drugs lowering heart rate.

Effect of Ledipasvir, Sofosbuvir on Other Drugs: Digoxin, dabigatran: *Increased plasma levels, monitor.* Tenofovir + atazanavir (darunavir, lopinavir, elvitegravir) + ritonavir or cobicistat + *Harvoni*: Tenofovir and atazanavir plasma levels increased. Statins: *Plasma level increased, consider dose reduction.* Vitamin K antagonists: *Monitor INR (due to liver function changes).*

SP: Use in patients infected with HCV genotype 2, 3, 6, limited data. Hepatitis B virus (HBV) reactivation reported (including fatal); screen for HBV before initiation.

Pregnancy, Lactation: Used in combination with ribavirin, see Notes below (ribavirin). Pregnancy, avoid. Lactation, not recommended.

ADR: See Notes below.

Notes: See 9.4.2 Viral Hepatitis. See Ribavirin below.

▼ **Harvoni 90/400** *(Gilead)* A.
Price, not published by company.
Tablet, ledipasvir 90mg, sofosbuvir 400mg. Orange diamond-shaped f/c. Marked GSI; 7985 on reverse. *Lactose, Sunset Yellow.*

Ombitasvir, Paritaprevir, Ritonavir

ATC Code: Pending. **Sport:** Permitted.
Driving: Fatigue (in combination).

Indications: Chronic hepatitis C, genotypes 1a, 1b, 4 in adults.

Dose: Adult, Elderly: 2 tabs (12.5/75/50) once daily in combination (dasabuvir, or ribavirin or dasabuvir + ribavirin), depending on genotype. Genotype 1b* (GT1b) and Genotype 4 (without cirrhosis or with compensated cirrhosis), GT1a (without cirrhosis), duration 12 weeks; GT1a (with compensated cirrhosis) and liver transplant recipients, duration 24 weeks. *(8 weeks may be considered; previously untreated GT1b; minimal to moderate fibrosis). Admin,* with food without regard to fat and calorie content; swallow whole, do not chew, break or dissolve.

Child: Under 18 years, no safety/efficacy data.

Renal Impairment: No adjustment. Ribavirin co-admin, see Notes below (ribavirin).

Hepatic Impairment: Mild, no adjustment. Moderate, not

recommended. Severe, contraindicated. Liver transplant recipients, individualise dose.

Interactions: Effect of Other Drugs on Ombitasvir, Paritaprevir, Ritonavir: *Co-admin contraindicated*: Ethinyloestradiol (combined oral contraceptives, contraceptive vaginal rings), CYP3A4 substrates e.g. alfuzosin, amiodarone, astemizole, terfenadine, cisapride, colchicine (with renal or hepatic impairment), dronedarone, ergotamine and derivatives, fusidic acid, lovastatin, simvastatin, atorvastatin, lurasidone oral (midazolam, triazolam), pimozide, quetiapine, quinidine, ranolazine, salmeterol, sildenafil (in PAH), ticagrelor; enzyme inducers (carbamazepine, phenytoin, phenobarbital, efavirenz, nevirapine, etravirine, enzalutamide, mitotane, rifampicin, St John's Wort); CYP3A4 strong inhibitors e.g. cobicistat, indinavir, lopinavir/ritonavir, saquinavir, tipranavir, itraconazole, ketoconazole, posaconazole, voriconazole, clarithromycin, telithromycin, conivaptan. *Co-admin not recommended*: Other antivirals except dasabuvir and/or ribavirin. *Increase hyperbilirubinaemia risk*: Atazanavir. *Caution, with ECG monitoring*: Rilpivirine.

Effect of Ombitasvir, Paritaprevir, Ritonavir on Other Drugs: Glucocorticoids (metabolised by CYP3A4), inhaled glucocorticoids: *Increased exposure; systemic effects.* Colchicine: *Reduce dose or interrupt (normal renal/hepatic function); otherwise contraindicated.* Rosuvastatin: *Max. 5mg/day (with dasabuvir); max. 10mg/day (without dasabuvir).* Pitavastatin, fluvastatin: *Temporary suspend or reduce pravastatin, rosuvastatin dose.* Sulfasalazine, valsartan, erythromycin, imatinib, dabigatran, trazodone, fexofenadine; amlodipine, furosemide (decrease dose by 50%); diltiazem, verapamil, nifedipine; ciclosporin (decrease to one fifth of daily dose), tacrolimus (0.5mg every 7 days), sirolimus, everolimus (co-admin not recommended; weigh risk/benefit), repaglinide, alprazolam, levothyroxine: *Increased plasma levels.* Digoxin, warfarin, other Vitamin K antagonists: *Monitor serum digoxin, INR.* S-mephenytoin: *Plasma levels decreased.* Omeprazole, esomeprazole, lansoprazole: *Consider dose increase.*

SP: Use not recommended (monotherapy, HCV genotypes 2, 3, 5, 6, HIV co-infection not treated with antiretrovirals). Hepatic decompensation and failure (liver transplant or fatal outcomes); associated with advanced or decompensated cirrhosis prior to initiation. Counsel patients to watch for early signs of liver inflammation (fatigue, weakness, lack of appetite, nausea, vomiting, jaundice, discoloured faeces). Hepatitis B virus (HBV) reactivation reported (including fatal); screen for HBV before initiation.

Pregnancy, Lactation: Used in combination with ribavirin, see Notes below (ribavirin). Pregnancy, avoid. Lactation, not recommended. Patients using ethinyloestradiol-containing medicinals must switch to alternative contraception (progestin only or non-hormonal methods) prior to initiation. Counsel patients to watch for early signs of liver inflammation (fatigue, weakness, lack of appetite, nausea, vomiting, jaundice, discoloured faeces).

ADR: See Notes below.

Notes: See 9.4.2 Viral Hepatitis. See Ribavirin below.

▼ **Viekirax 12.5/75/50** *(AbbVie)* A. HOS.
Price, (56), €12100.12 (PTW).
Tablet, ombitasvir, paritaprevir, ritonavir. Pink oblong f/c. Marked AV1.

Peginterferon Alfa-2a

ATC Code: L03AB11. **Sport:** Permitted.
Driving: Caution.

Indications: Treatment, chronic hepatitis B and C.

Dose: Adult, Elderly: HBV, HCV, HIV-HCV co-infection (HBeAg positive and negative), 180mcg once weekly; HCV, HIV-HCV co-infection, monotherapy (only if other medicinals contraindicated) OR combination (ribavirin). *Admin,* SC injection. Combination medicines and duration, see Notes below. Should no compare potency with other pegylated or non-pegylated proteins of same therapeutic class.

children up to 3 years, formulations containing benzyl alcohol are contraindicated.

Renal Impairment: Mild, moderate, no adjustment; severe, ESRD, 135mcg weekly (monitor).

Hepatic Impairment: Decompensated cirrhosis, bleeding oesophageal varices, no data.

CI: Autoimmune hepatitis, pre-existing cardiac disease.

Interactions: Effect of Other Drugs on Peginterferon-2a: *Co-admin contraindicated:* Telbivudine. *Co-admin avoid (peginterferon-2a + ribavirin):* Azathioprine.

Effect of Peginterferon-2a on Other Drugs: Theophylline: *Monitor serum levels, adjust dose.* Methadone: *Monitor for methadone toxicity (high dose), QTc prolongation risk.*

SP: *Before initiation,* liver biochemistry, standard haematology, biochemistry; repeat haematology after 2 and 4 weeks, biochemical after 4 weeks; additional tests periodically; treatment associated with (decreased WBC, absolute neutrophils, platelets, anaemia, pancytopenia, bone marrow depression), altered glycaemic control. Thyroid (abnormalities, worsening of pre-existing disorders). Cardiovascular disease, caution (hypertension, supraventricular arrhythmias, CHF, chest pain, MI). Hepatic decompensation, discontinue. Hypotension (fluid depletion), ensure adequate hydration. Auto-antibody development. Hypertriglyceridaemia. Increased ketoacidosis risk with HAART. Dental, periodontal disorders. Zidovudine induced anaemia (combination). *Use only if benefit outweighs risk,* acute hypersensitivity reactions (urticaria, angioedema, bronchoconstriction, anaphylaxis), persistent fever, retinal (haemorrhage, exudates, serous detachment, retinal artery or vein obstruction), pulmonary infiltrates, pneumonitis, pneumonia, psoriatic disease (exacerbation) and sarcoidosis, retreatment after haematological adverse events. Liver, renal graft rejections reported. *Psychiatric, CNS precautions,* see Notes below.

ADR: See Notes below.

Notes: See 9.4.2 Viral Hepatitis (psychiatric precautions). See Ribavirin below.

Pegasys Parenteral *(Roche)* A. HT.
Price, (0.5mL) injection 135mcg (1) €160.88. 180mcg (4) €795.72. PFP 135mcg (1) €166.76. PFP 180mcg (4) €811.00.
Injection, peginterferon alfa-2a 135mcg, 180mcg. Produced by rDNA technology. Clear colourless (light-yellow) soln in PFS or PFP. *Benzyl alcohol.* **Store:** Refrigerate; do not freeze.

Ribavirin

ATC Code: J05AB04. **Sport:** Permitted.

Driving: Caution, combination (peginterferon/interferon alfa-2a).

Indications: Treatment, chronic Hepatitis C (CHC) in combination.

Dose: Adult, Elderly: *Copegus,* combination with direct acting antivirals (DAA) or peginterferon alfa-2a with DAA or peginterferon alfa-2a/interferon alfa-2a without DAA, (genotype 1/4, 2/3 treatment experienced, 1 with HIV co-infection), (under 75kg), 1000mg/day; (75kg and over), 1200mg/day; combination peginterferon alfa-2a without DAA, (genotype 2/3 treatment naive, 2/3/4 with HIV co-infection), 800mg/day. Peginterferon alfa-2b with or without DAA (under 65kg), 800mg/day, (65-80kg), 1000mg/day, (81-105kg), 1200mg/day, (above 105kg), 1400mg/day. *Admin,* in 2 divided doses. Duration of treatment and dose modifications (treatment emergent anaemia) depend on combination drugs.

Moderiba, in combination with direct-acting antivirals (DAA) OR peginterferon (pegIFN) alfa-2a + DAA, HCV genotype (1,4 or 2,3 treatment experienced or 1 with HIV co-infection), under 75kg, 1000mg/day; 75kg and over, 1200mg/day; pegIFN alfa-2a without DAA, genotype (2,3) treatment naive, genotype (2, 3, 4) with HIV co-infection, 800mg/day. IFN alfa-2a without DAA, under 75kg, 1000mg/day; 75kg and over, 1200mg/day. PegIFN alfa-2b, with or without DAA, under 65kg, 800mg/day; 65-80kg, 1000mg/day; 81-105kg, 1200mg/day; over 105kg, 1400mg/day. Dose modification is required for treatment-emergent anaemia. *Admin,* in 2 divided doses (morning and evening) with food; do not break, crush or handle tabs (teratogenic potential).

Rebetol, dose and duration depend on patient weight and medicinals used in combination*. If there is no specific dose recommendation, under 75kg, 1000mg; over 75kg, 1200mg. *(check licenses for further prescribing information). Admin in 2 divided doses (morning, evening) with food.

Child: *Rebetol,* age 3 years and older (not previously treated; without liver decompensation), in combination with peginterferon alfa-2b or interferon alfa-2b. Above 47kg, able to swallow caps, used with adult alfa 200mg caps in 2 divided doses (47-49kg, 600mg/day; 50-65kg, 800mg/day; above 65kg, as for Adult above). Under 47kg and unable to swallow capsules, use oral soln (40mg/mL) at dose of 15mg/kg. Under 3 years, no data.
Copegus, Moderiba, under 18 years, not recommended.

Renal Impairment: CrCl (mL/min) 30-50, alternate doses of 200mg/day and 400mg/day every other day; under 30 or on haemodialysis, 200mg/day.

Hepatic Impairment: See Notes below.

CI: Severe pre-existing cardiac disease including (unstable, uncontrolled) in previous six months, haemoglobinopathies (thalassemia, sickle-cell anaemia).

Interactions: Effect of Other Drugs on Ribavirin: *Co-admin not recommended:* Didanosine (mitochondrial toxicity/lactic acidosis risk), zidovudine (increased anaemia risk), abacavir (lactic acidosis risk). *Decreased bioavailability:* Antacids (magnesium, aluminium, simeticone).

Effect of Ribavirin on Other Drugs: Azathioprine: *Co-admin if benefit outweighs risk; myelotoxicity, closely monitor haematology.*

SP: *Psychiatric, CNS,* caution, see Notes below. Not for use as monotherapy. Potentially teratogenic and/or carcinogenic, caution handling broken tabs. Acute hypersensitivity (urticaria, angioedema, bronchoconstriction, anaphylaxis), hepatic decompensation), discontinue. HIV co-infection receiving HAART, increased adverse event risk (lactic acidosis, peripheral neuropathy, pancreatitis). Prior to initiation, monitor renal function, full blood chemistry (pancytopenia/bone marrow suppression, decreased Hb). Gout. History of CHF, MI, arrhythmic disorders, monitor. Monitor co-infected patients for hepatic decompensation. *Children,* weight loss, growth inhibition (assess risk/benefit).

Pregnancy, Lactation: Pregnancy, contraindicated; exclude before initiation; ensure extreme care to avoid pregnancy in female patients or female partners of male patients; advise patient of significant teratogenic risk if pregnancy occurs. Females of childbearing potential and males (or their female partners) to ensure adequate and effective contraception during and up to 4 months (males/female partners, 7 months) after treatment. Conduct routine monthly pregnancy tests. Lactation, contraindicated.

ADR: See Notes below.

Notes: See 9.4.2 Viral Hepatitis. See Peginterferon Alpha-2a above.

Copegus 200mg, 400mg *(Roche)* A. HT.
Price, 200mg (42) €113.55; (112) €302.80; (168) €454.20. 400mg (56) €309.24.
Tablet, ribavirin. Oval f/c. Marked RIB/strength; Roche on reverse. 200mg: Light-pink. 400mg: Reddish-brown.

Moderiba 200mg, 400mg, 600mg *(AbbVie)* A. HT.
Price, (168) 200mg €273.28; (56) 400mg, €182.20, 600mg, €273.28.
Tablet, ribavirin. Blue cap-shaped f/c unscored. Marked with 3RP logo; strength on reverse. *Lactose.*

Rebetol 200mg, Oral Soln *(MSD)* A. HT.
Price, caps 200mg (84) €275.21; (140) €420.12; (168) €537.54. Oral soln (118mL) €88.21.
Capsule, ribavirin. Hard white opaque. Blue marking. *Lactose.*
Oral soln, as above 40mg/mL. Clear colourless pale (light-yellow) soln. *Sorbitol, sucrose.*

9.4.3 Influenza

Simeprevir

ATC Code: J05AE14. **Sport:** Permitted.
Driving: No or negligible influence.
Indications: Treatment, chronic hepatitis C (adults, genotype 1, 4).
Dose: Adult, Elderly: 150mg once daily in combination. Based on race, no dose adjustment. Recommended medicinals for co-admin, treatment duration, discontinuation (stopping rules), see Notes below. *Admin*, swallow whole with food. *Elderly*, over 65 years, limited data; over 75 years, no data.
Renal Impairment: CrCl (mL/min) below 30, caution.
Hepatic Impairment: Mild, no adjustment. Moderate to severe, not recommended.
Interactions: Effect of Other Drugs on Simeprevir: *Co-admin not recommended*: Other direct-acting antivirals, telaprevir, boceprevir; CYP3A4 inducers or inhibitors (altered exposure); systemic (erythromycin, azole antifungals, dexamethasone), astemizole, terfenadine, clarithromycin, telithromycin; rifampicin, rifabutin, rifapentine; cisapride, milk thistle, St John's Wort, efavirenz, delavirdine, etravirine, nevirapine, darunavir/ritonavir, ritonavir, HIV protease inhibitors with/without ritonavir, cobicistat, ciclosporin. *Co-admin caution*: Oral (midazolam, triazolam).
Effect of Simeprevir on Other Drugs: Digoxin, antiarrhythmics (amiodarone, disopyramide, flecainide, mexiletine, propafenone, quinidine), sirolimus, tacrolimus: *Therapeutic drug monitoring (see SP below).* Warfarin: *Monitor* INR. Carbamazepine, oxcarbazepine, phenobarbital, phenytoin: *Co-admin not recommended; loss of anticonvulsant effect.* Amlodipine, bepridil, diltiazem, felodipine, nicardipine, nifedipine, nisoldipine, verapamil: *Caution, clinical monitoring.* Statins except fluvastatin: *Use lowest dose, titrate carefully.* PDE-5 inhibitors: *Consider dose adjustment (PAH).*
SP: Not for monotherapy. Efficacy reduced with hepatitis C genotype 1a with NS3 Q80K polymorphism. Photosensitivity reactions, rash. Interferon-free regimens, treatment with HBV co-infection, organ transplant patients (no data). *Monitor*, HCV RNA levels (weeks 4, 12)*; LFTs before initiating* (those at high risk for hepatic decompensation or failure); when initiating in combination with sofosbuvir and concomitant amiodarone. *(then as clinically indicated).
Pregnancy, Lactation: Pregnancy, only if benefit justifies risk. Women of childbearing potential to ensure adequate contraception.
ADR: See Notes below.
Notes: See 9.4.2 Viral Hepatitis.

▼ **OLYSIO 150mg** *(Janssen-Cilag)* B. HOS.
Price, (7) €2076.07.
Capsule, simeprevir sodium. White hard gelatin. Marked TMC435 150. *Lactose.* **Store:** Original pack to protect (light).

Tenofovir

ATC Code: J05AF07. **Sport:** Permitted.
Driving: Caution.
Indications: HIV-1 infection, in combination. Chronic hepatitis B with (compensated liver disease, lamivudine-resistant hepatitis B or decompensated liver disease).
Dose: Adult, Elderly: 245mg/day with food. Swallowing difficulty, disintegrate tab in 100mL fluid. Over 65 years, no data.
Child: Age 12-18 years and 35kg or over, as for Adult; under 12 years, see manufacturers Full Prescribing Information.
Renal Impairment: CrCl (mL/min) 30-49, 245mg 48-hourly; 10-29, 245mg every 72-96 hours; haemodialysis, 245mg every 7 days after dialysis. Monitor clinical response and renal function.
Interactions: Effect of Other Drugs on Tenofovir: *Co-admin avoid*: Nephrotoxic drugs (aminoglycosides, amphotericin B, foscarnet, ganciclovir, pentamidine, vancomycin, cidofovir, interleukin-2), adefovir, cidofovir (monitor renal function). *Plasma levels increased*: Lopinavir, ritonavir. *Renal injury risk (in presence of risk factors)*: NSAIDs. *Co-*

admin caution (monitor renal function): Darunavir + ritonavir + (efavirenz or tenofovir or emtricitabine), efavirenz, emtricitabine, tenofovir (disoproxil fumarate, alafenamide).
Effect of Tenofovir on Other Drugs: Didanosine: *Co-admin not recommended; plasma levels increased.*
SP: Renal impairment risk, monitor renal function more frequently; decline in function, consider treatment interruption. Decreased bone mineral density (fractures). CART-experienced patients with K65R mutation, avoid use. Liver disease, monitor function; spontaneous exacerbations in chronic Hepatitis B common during and after treatment. Autoimmune disorders (Graves' disease) in setting of immune reactivation.
Pregnancy, Lactation: Pregnancy, if benefit outweighs risk. Women of child-bearing potential to ensure adequate contraception.
ADR: See Notes below.
Notes: See 9.4.2 Viral Hepatitis.

Viread 245mg *(Gilead)* A. HT.
Price, (30) €369.75.
Tablet, tenofovir disoproxil fumarate. Light-blue almond-shaped f/c. Marked Gilead, 4331; 300 on reverse. *Lactose.*

9.4.3 - Influenza

In This Chapter: *Oseltamivir, zanamivir.*

Class Effects
CI: Hypersensitivity to any member of the class.
SP: Not a substitute for influenza vaccination. Neuropsychiatric events reported (especially children, adolescents), monitor for behavioural changes and evaluate benefit/risk of continued treatment.

Oseltamivir

ATC Code: J05AH02. **Sport:** Permitted.
Driving: No influence expected.
Indications: Treatment, (adults, children including full term neonates) with symptoms typical of influenza (virus is circulating in the community). Post-exposure prevention (age 1 year and older) following contact with clinically diagnosed influenza case.
Dose: Adult, Elderly: Adults, adolescents 13 years and over, body weight 40kg and above:
TREATMENT, 75mg TWICE daily for 5 days.
PREVENTION, post exposure, 75mg ONCE daily for 10 days; during epidemic, 75mg ONCE daily for up to 6 weeks. Caps and susp are bioequivalent.
Child: TREATMENT (age 1-12 years), 10-15kg body weight, 30mg (TWICE daily); over 15kg-23kg, 45mg (TWICE daily); over 23kg-40kg, 60mg (TWICE daily); above 40kg as for Adult above; (infants age 0-12 months excluding premature infants with a post-conceptual age under 36 weeks), 3mg/kg (TWICE daily) for 5 days.
PREVENTION post exposure, as for treatment, but admin ONCE daily. Prevention during influenzae epidemic, children 0-12 months, no controlled clinical trial data.
Renal Impairment: *Age 13 years and over,* TREATMENT, CrCl (mL/min) above 60, 75mg twice daily; 30-60, 30mg twice daily; 10-30, 30mg once daily; below 10, not recommended. Haemodialysis, 30mg after each dialysis session; peritoneal, 30mg single dose.
PREVENTION, CrCl (mL/min) above 60, 75mg once daily; 30-60, 30mg once daily; 10-30, 30mg every second day; below 10, not recommended. Haemodialysis, 30mg after every dialysis session; peritoneal, 30mg once weekly.
Interactions: Effect of Other Drugs on Oseltamivir: *Co-admin caution*: Co-excreted agents with narrow therapeutic margin (chlorpropamide, methotrexate, phenylbutazone).
SP: Safety/efficacy in treatment/prophylaxis of influenza in immunocompromised not firmly established. Circulating influenza virus strain susceptibility is highly variable; prescribers should consult most recent information available on susceptibility patterns of currently circulating viruses. Neuropsychiatric disorders, especially children,

278

adolescents; monitor for behavioural changes; weigh benefit/risk of continuing treatment.

Pregnancy, Lactation: Pregnancy, may be used after considering (available safety information, pathogenicity of circulating influenza virus strain, underlying condition of the pregnant woman). Lactation, consider use where there are clear potential benefits to mother.

ADR: Summary, *most common*, nausea, vomiting; *serious*, anaphylactic and anaphylactoid reactions, hepatic disorders, angioedema, Stevens-Johnson syndrome, toxic epidermal necrolysis, GI bleeding, neuropsychiatric disorders.

Notes: See 9.4.3 Influenza.

> **Tamiflu 30mg, 45mg, 75mg, Oral Susp** *(Roche)* A. GMS.
> *Price*, caps (10) 30mg, €10.76. 45mg, €18.62. 75mg, €20.70. Susp 6mg/mL (100mL) €11.28.
> *Capsule*, oseltamivir phosphate. Hard opaque. Marked ROCHE and strength (in blue). 30mg: Light-yellow. 45mg: Grey. 75mg: Grey/light-yellow. **Store:** Below 25 deg C.
> *Powder for oral susp*, as above 6mg/mL. White (light-yellow) granulate or clumped granulate. *Sorbitol*. **Store:** Below 30 deg C. NOTE: *Tamiflu* is not a substitute for influenza vaccination. Use only syringe included in package with doses indicated in **mg**; cannot be replaced with syringe with **mL** markings.

Zanamivir

ATC Code: J05AH01. **Sport:** Permitted.
Driving: Unlikely to impair.
Indications: Treatment, prevention post-exposure, influenza A and B. Seasonal prophylaxis, influenza A and B during a community outbreak.

Dose: Adult: TREATMENT, 2x inhalations (10mg) twice daily (5 days).
PREVENTION, 2x inhalations (10mg) once daily for 10 days (post exposure), for up to 28 days (seasonal prophylaxis). Admin within 48 hours (adults) or 36 hours (children) after symptom onset.
Elderly: 65 years and over, no data.
Child: Age 5 years and over, as for Adult above.
SP: Severe asthma, weigh risk/benefit; COPD, bronchospasm risk. NOTE: Zanamivir inhalation powder must not be made into extemporaneous soln for admin by nebulisation or mechanical ventilation; use only device provided.
Pregnancy, Lactation: Pregnancy, if benefit outweighs risk. Lactation, not recommended.
ADR: See Notes below.
Notes: See 9.4.3 Influenza.

> **Relenza 5mg Inhalation** *(GSK)* A.
> *Price*, not published by company.
> *Inhalation powder*, zanamivir 5mg/dose. White (off-white). *Lactose*.

9.5 - Antiprotozoals

9.5.1 - Antimalarials

In This Chapter: *Atovaquone, proguanil combination; piperaquine, dihydroartemisinin combination; quinine sulfate.*

Class Effects
Doxycycline is also used in malaria prophylaxis.
CI: Hypersensitivity to any member of the class or related compounds.
SP: Always seek local professional advice regarding resistant malaria strains, prophylaxis and/or treatment of choice. Ensure routine measures to protect against mosquito bites. All travellers to inform their doctor of exposure to risk of malaria, should they fall ill, either during their stay, or after returning home.
Pregnancy, Lactation: Pregnant women should be made aware of the risks of contracting malaria during pregnancy, and should be advised not to undertake unnecessary journeys to endemic areas.
Notes: See 9.1.6 Tetracyclines (doxycycline).

Atovaquone, Proguanil

ATC Code: P01BB51. **Sport:** Permitted.
Driving: Dizziness.
Indications: Treatment, acute uncomplicated *P. falciparum* malaria. Prophylaxis, *P. falciparum* malaria.
Dose: Adult, Elderly: TREATMENT, 4 tabs as single dose for 3 consecutive days.
PROPHYLAXIS, 1 tab daily starting 24-48 hours before entering malaria area, continue during stay, and for 7 days after leaving area. Persons under 40kg, not recommended. *Admin*, oral, with food or milky drink to ensure max. absorption; take at same time each day.
Child: TREATMENT, single dose once daily for 3 consecutive days, weight 11-20kg, 1 tab/day; 21-30kg, 2 tabs/day; 31-40kg, 3 tabs/day; over 40kg, as for Adult above. PROPHYLAXIS, over 40kg, as for Adult above.
Renal Impairment: CrCl (mL/min) below 30, treatment, seek alternative if possible; prophylaxis, contraindicated.
Hepatic Impairment: No adjustment.
Interactions: Effect of Other Drugs on Atovaquone, Proguanil Combination: *Co-admin not recommended (plasma levels decreased):* Rifampicin, rifabutin, metoclopramide, tetracycline (monitor parasitaemia). *Co-admin avoid:* Efavirenz, boosted protease inhibitors. *Absorption (proguanil) reduced, co-admin not recommended:* Magnesium trisilicate.
Effect of Atovaquone, Proguanil Combination on Other Drugs: Warfarin, other coumarin anticoagulants: *Effect potentiated (proguanil).* Etoposide (and metabolites): *Plasma levels increased.*
SP: Diarrhoea, vomiting (absorption may be reduced). Severe allergic reactions (anaphylaxis), discontinue. Atovaquone/proguanil has no efficacy against hypnozoites; intense exposure to *P. vivax* or *P. ovale* may require additional drug active against hypnozoites. Haematological changes (proguanil). Recrudescence, chemoprophylaxis failure, acute malaria with diarrhoea or vomiting, seek alternative.
Pregnancy, Lactation: Pregnancy, if benefit outweighs risk. Lactation, not recommended.
ADR: *Very common*, headache, abdominal pain, nausea, vomiting, diarrhoea. See SP above.
Notes: See 9.5.1 Antimalarials.

> **Malarone Tablets** *(GSK)* A. GMS.
> *Price*, (12) €15.78.
> *Tablet*, atovaquone 250mg, proguanil HCl 100mg. Pink round f/c. Marked GXCM3.
> **Atovaquone/Proguanil 250mg/100mg** *(Gerard)* A. GMS.
> *Price*, (12) €15.78.
> *Tablet*, atovaquone 250mg, proguanil HCl 100mg. Buff-coloured round f/c. Marked A-P over 2; M on reverse. *Lactose*.

Piperaquine, Artenimol

ATC Code: P01BF05. **Sport:** Permitted.
Driving: Unlikely to affect.
Indications: Treatment, uncomplicated *P. falciparum* malaria.
Dose: Adult: 3 doses over 3 consecutive days, same time each day. Per dose (piperaquine tetraphosphate; PQP/artenimol) based on body weight 5-7kg, 80/10mg; 7-13kg, 160/20mg; 13-24kg, 320/40mg; 24-36kg, 640/80mg; 36-75kg, 960/120mg; 75-100kg, 1280/160mg; above 100kg, no dose recommendation. Max. 2 courses in 12-month period; second course not for admin within 2 months after first (long PQP half-life). *Admin*, oral with water, without food (no food 3 hours before or 3 hours after dose). Tabs may be crushed and mixed with water; admin immediately.
Elderly: Age 65 years and older, no dose recommendation. Caution.
Child: See Adult above. Under (6 months or 5kg), no data.
Renal Impairment: Moderate to severe, caution.
Hepatic Impairment: As for Renal above.

9.5.2   Other Antiprotozoals

CI: Severe malaria, sudden death (family history), congenital Qtc-interval prolongation, cardiac arrhythmia, bradycardia, conditions predisposing to arrhythmia (severe hypertension, LVH, CHF with reduced LVEF), electrolyte disturbances (hypo-, kalaemia, calcaemia, magnesaemia).

Interactions: Effect of Other Drugs on Piperaquine, Artenimol: *Co-admin contraindicated:* Antiarrhythmics (amiodarone, disopyramide, dofetilide, ibutilide, procainamide, quinidine, hydroquinidine, sotalol), neuroleptics (phenothiazines, sertindole, sultopride, chlorpromazine, haloperidol, mesoridazine, pimozide, thioridazine), antidepressants, certain antimicrobials e.g. macrolides (erythromycin, clarithromycin), fluoroquinolones (moxifloxacin, sparfloxacin), imidazole and triazole antifungals, pentamidine, saquinavir, certain non-sedating antihistamines (terfenadine, astemizole, mizolastine), cisapride, droperidol, domperidone, bepridil, diphemanil, probucol, levomethadyl, methadone, vinca alkaloids, arsenic trioxide, medicinals prolonging QTC interval (mefloquine, halofantrine, lumefantrine, chloroquine, quinine, other antimalarials). *Piperaquine plasma levels increased (QTc effects):* Protease inhibitors, nefazodone, verapamil, strong CYP3A4 inhibitors, moderate CYP3A4 inhibitors (oral contraceptives). *Piperaquine plasma levels decreased:* Rifampicin, phenytoin, phenobarbital, St John's Wort. *Increased absorption, increased piperaquine levels:* Fatty food, grapefruit juice. *Co-admin caution:* Mild CYP3A4 inhibitors.

Effect of Piperaquine, Artenimol on Other Drugs: Antiretrovirals, ciclosporin: *Increased plasma levels.* Omeprazole: *Reduced metabolism, increased plasma levels.* Paracetamol, theophylline, enflurane, halothane, isoflurane: *Increased metabolism, decreased plasma levels.*

SP: NOTE: Long piperaquine half-life. ECG monitoring, with risk for arrhythmia or QTc-prolongation; caution, females, elderly as they have longer QTc intervals.

Pregnancy, Lactation: Pregnancy, not recommended. Lactation, not recommended.

ADR: Summary, *P. falciparum* infection; *most frequent,* (adults, children), headache, prolonged ECG QTc, anaemia, eosinophilia, decreased (haemoglobin, haematocrit, red cell count), sinus bradycardia, asthenia, pyrexia; (children 6 months to 5 years), cough, pyrexia, influenza, diarrhoea, vomiting, anorexia.

Notes: See 9.5.1 Antimalarials.

▼ **Eurartesim 320/40mg** *(Sigma-Tau)* A. GMS.
Price, (12) €44.92.
Tablet, piperaquine tetraphosphate, dihydroartemisinin. White oblong f/c scored (divisible into equal halves). Marked with 2 letters. **Store:** Below 30 deg C.

Quinine Sulfate

ATC Code: P01BC01. **Sport:** Permitted.
Driving: Caution.
Indications: Treatment, chloroquine resistant malaria. Nocturnal leg cramps.

Dose: Adult, Elderly: 600mg 8-hourly for 7 days.

Child: Under 12 years, 10mg/kg 8-hourly for 7 days.

CI: Haemoglobinuria, optic neuritis, myasthenia gravis.

Interactions: Effect of Other Drugs on Quinine: *Co-admin avoid (increased ventricular arrhythmia risk):* Amiodarone, moxifloxacin, pimozide. *Increased plasma levels:* Cimetidine.

Effect of Quinine on Other Drugs: Digoxin, flecainide: *Increased plasma levels.* Mefloquine: *Increased convulsion risk.*

SP: Atrial fibrillation, conduction defects, G-6-PD deficiency.

Pregnancy, Lactation: Pregnancy, if benefit outweighs risk; seek medical advice in first trimester.

ADR: Tinnitus, headache, flushing, abdominal pain, rash, visual disturbances, confusion, vomiting, vertigo, fever. Hypersensitivity (angioedema, thrombocytopenia, intravascular coagulation). Acute renal failure.

Notes: See 9.5.1 Antimalarials.

Quinine Sulphate 300mg *(TEVA)* B. GMS.
Price, (28) €9.08.
Tablet, quinine sulfate. White s/c. *Sucrose.* NOTE: Quinine base 100mg=quinine sulfate 122mg. **Store:** Below 25 deg C; original pack.

9.5.2 - Other Antiprotozoals

In This Chapter: *Pentamidine.*

Class Effects
CI: Hypersensitivity to any member of the class.

Pentamidine

ATC Code: P01CX01. **Sport:** Permitted.
Driving: Dizziness.

Indications: *Pneumocystis carinii (jirovecii)* pneumonia, treatment; prophylaxis in HIV patients.

Dose: Adult, Elderly: TREATMENT, 600mg by inhalation once daily for 3 weeks. PROPHYLAXIS, 300mg once monthly OR 150mg every 2 weeks.

Hepatic Impairment: No data.

Interactions: Effect of Other Drugs on Pentamidine: *Caution:* Drugs prolonging QT-interval (TCADs, terfenadine and astemizole, IV erythromycin, halofantrine, quinolones). *Hypocalcaemia risk:* Foscarnet.

SP: Establish baseline BP; monitor (during admin, regular intervals until completion). Patients should receive drug lying down. Severe adverse events with IM and IV (hypotension, hypoglycaemia, acute pancreatitis, cardiac arrhythmias); inhalation, monitor closely. High risk of pneumothorax, weigh risk/benefit. QT-prolongation, caution in coronary heart disease, ventricular arrhythmias, uncorrected hypokalaemia, hypomagnesaemia, bradycardia (below 50 bpm); QTc above 500 msec, consider continuous cardiac monitoring. *Monitor,* blood urea, serum creatinine, complete blood, platelets, urine analysis, electrolytes (daily*); fasting blood glucose (daily*, regular intervals after); LFTs (daily*, weekly after); serum calcium (weekly); ECG (regular intervals). *(during therapy). NOTE: 4mg pentamidine isethionate equiv. to 2.3mg pentamidine base. 1mg pentamidine base equiv. to 1.74mg pentamidine isethionate.

Pregnancy, Lactation: Pregnancy, only if considered essential. Lactation, contraindicated.

ADR: *Common,* local reactions including cough, shortness of breath, wheezing, bronchospasm especially with asthma but controllable with bronchodilators, taste disturbance, nausea.

Pentacarinat Nebuliser *(SANOFI)* A.
Price, 300mg/5mL (1) €24.06.
Nebuliser soln, pentamidine isethionate 60mg/mL equiv. to 172.4mg/mL pentamidine base (300mg/5mL Ready-to-Use). Clear colourless.

9.6 - Tuberculosis, Leprosy

In This Chapter: *Bedaquiline, rifabutin, rifampicin and (isoniazid, pyrazinamide) combinations.*

Class Effects
CI: Hypersensitivity to any member of the class (including other rifamycins).

SP: *Rifamycins,* reddish colour of urine, sweat, sputum, tears (advise patients); permanent staining of soft contact lenses.

Bedaquiline

ATC Code: J04AK05. **Sport:** Permitted.
Driving: Minor influence; dizziness.

Indications: Combination treatment, multidrug-resistant TB.

Dose: Adult, Elderly: Recommended, 400mg once DAILY (weeks 1-2); then 200mg 3-times per WEEK (weeks 3-24) with minimum 48 hours between doses. Duration 24 weeks. *Elderly,* 65 years and older, limited data. Advise patients to take doses exactly as prescribed and to complete full course. Admin with food (food increases oral bioavailability); swallow whole with water. Combination drugs, see SP below.

Child: Under 18 years, safety/efficacy not established.

Renal Impairment: Mild/moderate, no adjustment. CrCl (mL/min) below 30 or ESRD on haemodialysis or peritoneal dialysis, caution.

Hepatic Impairment: Mild/moderate, no adjustment. Moderate, caution. Severe, not recommended.

Interactions: Effect of Other Drugs on Bedaquiline: *Co-admin caution:* Other drugs prolonging QTc interval. *Co-admin not recommended:* Gatifloxacin, moxifloxacin, sparfloxacin (potential for significant QT prolongation). *Co-admin avoid:* Strong/moderate CYP3A4 inducers (efavirenz, etravirine, rifampicin, rifapentine, rifabutin, carbamazepine, phenytoin, St John's Wort), reduced exposure, reduced bedaquiline effect; strong/moderate CYP3A4 inhibitors for more than 14 days (ciprofloxacin, erythromycin, fluconazole, clarithromycin, ketoconazole, ritonavir) lopinavir/ritonavir (if benefit outweighs risk); increased exposure, may increase adverse reaction risk).

SP: Always use in combination with at least 3 medicinals (isolates susceptible *in vitro*) OR 4 medicinals (isolates likely to be susceptible but no *in vitro* testing available). Use in extra-pulmonary TB (CNS, bone), infections other than OR latent infections of *Mycobacterium tuberculosis,* HIV co-infection (no data). Bedaquiline prolongs QTc interval; conduct ECG (before initiation, then monthly). Correct electrolytes before initiation; monitor if QTc prolongation is detected. Use not recommended unless benefit outweighs risk: HF, QTcF above 450ms, history of (or congenital QT prolongation; Torsade de Pointes), ongoing (hypothyroidism, bradyarrhythmia), hypokalaemia. Discontinue if patient develops significant ventricular arrhythmia, QTcF interval above 500ms. Monitor liver enzymes throughout treatment.

Pregnancy, Lactation: Pregnancy, avoid unless benefit outweighs risk. Lactation, stop breastfeeding or stop drug.

ADR: Summary, *most frequent,* nausea, arthralgia, headache, vomiting, dizziness.

Notes: See Class Effects 9.6 Tuberculosis, Leprosy.

▼ **SIRTURO 100mg** *(Janssen-Cilag)* A. HOS.
Price, (188) €22572.77 (PTW).
Tablet, bedaquiline fumarate. White (almost) uncoated round. Marked T over 207; 100 on reverse. *Lactose.*

Rifabutin

ATC Code: J04AB04. **Sport:** Permitted.
Driving: Unlikely to impair.
Indications: Second-line treatment, TB.

Dose: Adult, Elderly: 150-450mg/day in combination. Reduce dose to 300mg/day (combination with clarithromycin, fluconazole, related compounds); by 50% (combination with nelfinavir, amprenavir, indinavir), by 75% (combination with fosamprenavir, lopinavir, ritonavir).

Child: Not recommended.

Renal Impairment: CrCl (mL/min) below 30, reduce dose by 50%.

Hepatic Impairment: Severe, caution, reduce dose.

CI: Porphyria.

Interactions: Effect of Other Drugs on Rifabutin: *Plasma levels increased:* Clarithromycin, fluconazole (others of same classes). *Co-admin at 8-12 hour interval:* Aminosalicylic acid. *Plasma levels increased:* Indinavir, nelfinavir and amprenavir, fosamprenavir, lopinavir, ritonavir (dose adjustment), ritonavir (uveitis risk, avoid co-admin). *Rifabutin monitoring recommended:* Tipranavir/ritonavir combination. See Dose above.

Effect of Rifabutin on Other Drugs: Oral contraceptives: *Efficacy reduced.* Analgesics, anticoagulants, to

corticosteroids, ciclosporin, digitalis (not digoxin), dapsone, oral hypoglycaemics, narcotics, phenytoin, quinidine: *Activity reduced.* Saquinavir, indinavir: *Plasma levels decreased.* Delavirdine (dose 400mg 8-hourly): *Co-admin not recommended.* Tacrolimus: *Trough levels decreased.*

SP: Uveitis.

Pregnancy, Lactation: Not recommended.

ADR: *Very common,* leucopenia.

Notes: See 9.6 Tuberculosis, Leprosy.

Mycobutin 150mg *(Pfizer)* A. GMS.
Price, (30) €102.74.
Capsule, rifabutin. Opaque red/brown hard gelatin.

Rifampicin

ATC Code: J04AB02. **Sport:** Permitted.
Driving: Dizziness, faintness, impaired vision.
Indications: Combination treatment, TB and certain mycobacterial infections, pulmonary TB. All TB forms, where parenteral indicated, for life-threatening severe infections.

Dose: Adult: ORAL, 450-600mg/day (10mg/kg/day); under 50kg, usually 450mg/day; 50kg or more, 600mg/day. Oral, on empty stomach, not less than 30 minutes before food or 2 hours after food.
PARENTERAL, IV only (not IM or SC), 600mg (8-12mg/kg) by IV infusion over 2-3 hours once daily. *Non-TB infection,* 50kg and over, 450mg twice daily OR 300mg 3-times daily.

Elderly: Caution, consider lower dose.

Child: Over 3 months, 15mg (10-20)mg/kg/day; max. 600mg/day *(oral, parenteral).* Non-tuberculous infections up to 20mg/kg/day in divided doses *(parenteral).* Admin, see Adult above.

Hepatic Impairment: Only if necessary; max. 8mg/kg/day.

CI: Jaundice.

Interactions: Effect of Other Drugs on Rifampicin: *Co-admin contraindicated:* Saquinavir + ritonavir (hepatotoxicity). *Co-admin at 8-hour interval:* Aminosalicylic acid. *Plasma levels increased:* Atovaquone. *Plasma levels decreased:* Ketoconazole. *Absorption reduced:* Antacids (admin 1-hour apart). *Hepatotoxicity:* Halothane, isoniazid.

Effect of Rifampicin on Other Drugs: Anticonvulsants (phenytoin), antiarrhythmics (disopyramide, mexiletine, quinidine, propafenone, tocainide), anti-oestrogens (tamoxifen, toremifene), antipsychotics (haloperidol), oral anticoagulants (warfarin), antifungals (fluconazole, itraconazole, ketoconazole), antiretrovirals (zidovudine, saquinavir, indinavir, efavirenz), barbiturates, beta-blockers, benzodiazepines (diazepam) and related drugs (zopiclone, zolpidem), calcium channel blockers (diltiazem, nifedipine, verapamil), chloramphenicol, clarithromycin, corticosteroids, cardiac glycosides, clofibrate, systemic hormonal contraceptives, dapsone, doxycycline, oestrogens, fluoroquinolones, gestrinone, oral hypoglycaemic agents (sulphonylureas), immunosuppressives (ciclosporin, tacrolimus, irinotecan), levothyroxine, losartan, narcotic analgesics, methadone, praziquantel, progestins, quinine, riluzole, selective 5-HT3 receptor antagonists (ondansetron), statins metabolised by CYP3A4, telithromycin, theophylline, thiazolidinediones (rosiglitazone), TCADs (amitriptyline, nortriptyline): *Accelerated metabolism, reduced activity.* Atovaquone, ketoconazole, enalapril (enalaprilat): *Plasma levels decreased.*

SP: Monitor SGPT, SGOT, hyperbilirubinaemia. Caution combination with isoniazid (impaired liver function, elderly, malnourished, children under 2 years). Hypersensitivity (platelets, vascular tissue); caution intermittent therapy. Porphyria exacerbation. *Parenteral,* avoid extravasation (local irritation, inflammation).

Pregnancy, Lactation: If benefit outweighs risk. Last few weeks of pregnancy, caution post-natal haemorrhage potential in mother and infant (treat with Vitamin K). Lactation, is excreted in breast milk; only if benefit outweighs risk.

9.7 Infestations

ADR: *Common*, thrombocytopenia (with or without purpura), nausea, vomiting, increased (blood bilirubin, AST, ALT). Reddish discolouration of urine, sputum, tears. May permanently stain contact lenses. *Serious*, renal failure, thrombocytopenia, haemolytic anaemia.

Notes: See 9.6 Tuberculosis, Leprosy.

Rifadin 150mg, 300mg, Syrup *(SANOFI)* A. GMS.
Price, (100) 150mg, €23.21. 300mg, €44.46. Syrup 100mg/5mL (120mL) €4.33.
Capsule, rifampicin. Opaque hard gelatin. Marked R-strength. 150mg: Scarlet/light-blue. 300mg: Scarlet. **Store:** Below 25 deg C; original pack to protect (moisture).
Oral susp, as above 100mg/5mL. Homogenous dark red; raspberry odour. *Sucrose, parabens, metabisulphite.* **Store:** Below 25 deg C.

Rifadin Parenteral *(SANOFI)* A.
Price, not published by company.
Infusion, rifampicin 600mg. Red lyophilised powder; solvent of soln for conc. *Sodium 16mg/vial.* **Store:** Below 25 deg C.

Rifampicin, Isoniazid

ATC Code: J04AM03. **Sport:** Permitted.
Driving: Unlikely to impair.

Indications: See Notes below.

Dose: Adult: *Continuous therapy,* 450-600mg OR 10mg/kg/day as single dose with isoniazid 5mg/kg/day. *Intermittent therapy,* 450-600mg either 2-3 times weekly. Oral 30 minutes before food or 2 hours after.

Elderly: Caution.

Child: Not recommended.

Renal Impairment: Severe, caution, monitor.

CI: Manic, hypomanic psychoses.

Interactions: Effect of Other Drugs on Rifampicin, Isoniazid Combination: *Co-admin contraindicated:* Saquinavir/ritonavir. *Plasma levels increased (isoniazid), co-admin contraindicated:* Para-aminosalicylic acid. *Avoid:* Tyramine (cheese, red wine), histamine (tuna) containing food. *Caution:* Drugs metabolised by CYP450 (rifampicin; inducer), (isoniazid; inhibitor).

Effect of Rifampicin, Isoniazid Combination on Other Drugs: Carbamazepine, phenytoin: *Metabolism inhibited*.

SP: *Isoniazid,* pyridoxine supplements if elderly, malnourished, predisposition to neuropathy e.g. diabetics, adolescents. Drug-induced peripheral neuropathy. Combination, greater potential to induce liver function abnormalities; chronic liver disease, monitor. Prodromal symptoms of hepatitis (fatigue, weakness, malaise, anorexia, nausea, vomiting), discontinue.

ADR: *Isoniazid,* eosinophilia, agranulocytosis, thrombocytopenia, anaemia, anaphylactic reactions, pellagra, polyneuritis, convulsions, toxic encephalopathy, optic neuritis and atrophy, memory impairment, toxic psychosis, vasculitis, pancreatitis, nausea, vomiting, epigastric distress, severe and sometimes fatal hepatitis, rash, acne, Stevens-Johnson syndrome, exfoliative dermatitis, pemphigus, toxic epidermal necrolysis, DRESS, SLE-like syndrome, fever.

Notes: See Rifampicin above. See 9.6 Tuberculosis, Leprosy.

Rifinah Tablets *(SANOFI)* A. GMS.
Price, 150mg (84) €19.31. 300mg (56) €25.52.
Tablet, rifampicin 150mg, isoniazid 100mg ('150'); rifampicin 300mg, isoniazid 150mg ('300'). Smooth shiny f/c, s/c. '150': Cyclamen round. '300': Orange cap-shaped. *Sucrose, sodium 0.9mg(1.3mg)/tab.* **Store:** Below 25 deg C; original pack to protect (moisture).

Rifampicin, Isoniazid, Pyrazinamide

ATC Code: J04AM05. **Sport:** Permitted.
Driving: Unlikely to impair.

Indications: See Notes below.

Dose: Adult, Elderly: Under 40kg, 3 tabs daily; 40-49kg, 4 tabs daily; 50-64kg, 5 tabs daily; over 65kg, 6 tabs daily. Initial intensive phase, daily, continuous. Oral, as single dose 1-2 hours before food.

Child: No data.

Renal Impairment: Reduce dose.

Hepatic Impairment: Not recommended. See SP below.

SP: Liver function abnormalities (pre-existent liver disease, elderly, very young, malnourished). Caution, diabetes mellitus, alcoholism, convulsive disorders, manic or hypomanic psychosis. Sideroblastic anaemia, peptic ulceration, discontinue. *Pyrazinamide,* gout or history of (caution); hyperuricaemia with acute gouty arthritis, discontinue. Haemoptysis, caution.

ADR: *Pyrazinamide,* gout, anorexia, sideroblastic anaemia, thrombocytopenia with/without purpura, nausea, vomiting, aggravated peptic ulcer, hepatic reaction is most common; varies from symptomless hepatic cell function abnormality, through mild syndrome of fever, malaise and liver tenderness, to more serious reactions e.g. clinical jaundice; rare cases of acute yellow atrophy, death), DRESS, urticaria, pruritus, erythema, rash, arthralgia, dysuria, malaise, fever.

Notes: See Rifampicin and Rifampicin, Isoniazid Combination above. See Class Effects 9.6 Tuberculosis, Leprosy.

Rifater 50/300/120 *(SANOFI)* A. GMS.
Price, (100) €23.54.
Tablet, isoniazid/pyrazinamide/rifampicin 50/300/120mg. Smooth round pink-beige s/c. *Sucrose.* **Store:** Below 25 deg C; original pack.

9.7 - Infestations

In This Chapter: *Mebendazole.*

Class Effects
CI: Hypersensitivity to any member of the class.
Notes: See 9.5.1 Antimalarials (chloroquine) and 9.1.7 Anaerobic Infections (metronidazole).

Mebendazole

ATC Code: P02CA01. **Sport:** Permitted.
Driving: Unlikely to impair.

Indications: GI infestations caused by nematodes and cestodes (enterobiasis, ascariasis, trichuriasis, ankylostomiasis, strongyloidiasis, taeniasis).

Dose: Adult, Elderly: *Ascariasis, trichuriasis, mixed infections, ankylostomiasis,* 100mg twice daily for 3 consecutive days. *Enterobiasis,* 100mg as single dose; repeat after 2-4 weeks. *Taeniasis, strongyloidiasis,* 200mg twice daily for 3 consecutive days. Oral, tabs may be chewed or swallowed whole; young children, crush tab.

Child: Age 2 years and older, as for Adult above, except *taeniasis, strongyloidiasis,* 100mg twice daily for 3 consecutive days.

Interactions: Effect of Other Drugs on Mebendazole: *Co-admin avoid:* Metronidazole. *Increased plasma levels:* Cimetidine.

Pregnancy, Lactation: Not recommended.

ADR: *Common,* abdominal pain.

Notes: See 9.7 Infestations.

Vermox 100mg, Susp 100mg/5mL *(J&J)* OTC. GMS.
Price, 100mg (6) €1.98. Susp (30mL) €2.28.
Tablet, mebendazole. Pale-orange round flat scored (facilitates breaking). Marked ME 100; Janssen on reverse. *Sunset Yellow.* **Store:** Below 25 deg C; original pack to protect (light).
Oral susp, as above. Banana flavour; opaque white. *Sucrose, parabens.* **Store:** As for tabs above.

282

10

Dermatology

10.1 - Acne, Rosacea, Actinic Keratosis

Class Effects

CI: No data for use in children or elderly as acne does not usually present in these patient groups.

SP: Generally for topical external use only applied to affected area. Avoid contact with eyes, other mucous membranes. The affected area should be cleansed prior to application. Generally not be applied to broken or abraded skin. Systemic effects may occur, see Notes below (antibacterials). Prolonged antibacterial use may result in superinfection due to resistant micro-organisms.

Notes: See 9.1 Antibacterials.

10.1.1 - Topical Retinoids and Related Compounds

In This Chapter: *Adapalene, isotretinoin.*

Class Effects

CI: Hypersensitivity to any member of the class. Not for use in children unless otherwise specified (generally no data).

Interactions: Effect of Other Drugs on Topical Retinoids: *Co-admin, not recommended:* Other retinoids or drugs with similar mode of action. *Co-admin avoid:* Peeling agents, astringents, irritants, oxidising agents (benzoyl peroxide) (additive irritant effects).

SP: Avoid angles of nose, lips; not for application to broken or eczematous skin, in severe acne or acne involving large areas of body. Avoid repeated exposure to excessive sunlight or UV irradiation or use of sunlamps. Cosmetics used should be non-comedogenic and non-astringent.

Pregnancy, Lactation: Pregnancy, contraindicated. Tretinoins are TERATOGENIC when absorbed systemically, see Notes below (isotretinoin). Women of childbearing age to ensure adequate contraception. Lactation, avoid; stop drug or stop breast feeding. Not to be used on chest of mother to avoid contact exposure to infant.

ADR: Skin irritation, erythema, dryness, scaling, burning, fragility; stinging on application, eyelid oedema or irritation. Undue irritation, interrupt treatment and resume when reaction subsides.

Notes: See 10.1 Acne. See 10.1.5 Oral Acne Treatments (isotretinoin).

Adapalene

ATC Code: D10AD03. **Sport:** Permitted.
Driving: Unlikely to impair.

Indications: Mild to moderate acne vulgaris where comedones, papules and pustules predominate.

Dose: Adult: Apply once daily at bedtime.

SP: Sensitivity, severe irritation, discontinue; some irritation, reduce use frequency or discontinue temporarily.

ADR: *Common,* dry skin, skin (irritation, burning sensation, erythema).

Notes: See 10.1.1 Topical Retinoids.

  Differin Cream, Gel *(Galderma)* A. GMS.
  Price, (30g) €7.39.
  Topical cream/gel, adapalene 0.1% w/w. White shiny/smooth. *Parabens.*

Isotretinoin (acne)

ATC Code: D10AD04. **Sport:** Permitted.
Driving: No or negligible effect.

Indications: Mild to moderate acne vulgaris.

Dose: Adult: Apply once or twice daily.

Renal Impairment: Not expected to result in sufficient systemic exposure.

Hepatic Impairment: As for Renal above.

SP: May be 6-8 weeks before therapeutic effect observed. Caution, family history (cutaneous epitheliomata, skin cancer, photoallergy). More rapid results will be not be obtained if applied excessively; marked redness, peeling, discomfort may occur. Flammable (avoid smoking or being near open flame while or immediately after applying).

Notes: See 10.1.1 Topical Retinoids.

  Isotrex Gel *(Stiefel)* A.
  Price, (30g) €10.67.
  Topical gel, isotretinoin 0.05% w/w. Soft greenish-yellow; ethanol odour. *Butylated hydroxytoluene.*

Isotretinoin, Erythromycin

ATC Code: D10AD54. **Sport:** Permitted.
Driving: Unlikely to impair.

Indications: Mild to moderate acne vulgaris.

Dose: Adult: Apply in a thin film once or twice daily.

Child: Under 12 years, not recommended.

Renal Impairment: Not expected to result in sufficient systemic exposure.

Hepatic Impairment: As for Renal above.

Notes: See Isotretinoin above. See 10.1.2 Topical Antibacterials (erythromycin).

  Isotrexin Gel *(Stiefel)* A. GMS.
  Price, (30g) €8.07.
  Topical gel, isotretinoin 0.5mg/g, erythromycin 20mg/g. Soft pale-yellow; ethanol odour. *Butylated hydroxytoluene.*

10.1.2 - Topical Antibacterials Used In Acne

In This Chapter: *Clindamycin (and tretinoin combination), erythromycin combinations.*

Class Effects

Systemic antibacterials are also used in the treatment of acne. Adolescents, dose generally as for Adult.

CI: Hypersensitivity to any member of the class. Not for use in children under 12 years unless otherwise specified.

Interactions: Effect of Other Drugs on Topical Antibacterials: *Co-admin caution:* Other topical treatments (cumulative local adverse events).

SP: For systemic effects and/or *Clostridium difficile* associated diarrhoea, see Notes below (antibacterials).

Pregnancy, Lactation: Pregnancy, generally no data. Lactation, caution.

10.1.3   Benzoyl Peroxide, Azelaic Acid

ADR: Local irritation, erythema, dryness especially with alcohol based formulations.

Notes: See 10.1 Acne. See 9.1 Antibacterials.

Clindamycin (acne)

ATC Code: D10AF01. **Sport:** Permitted.
Driving: Unlikely to impair.

Indications: Acne vulgaris, pustular or papular.

Dose: Adult: Apply thinly twice daily *(Dalacin T)*; once daily *(Zindaclin)*.

CI: Lincomycin sensitivity, (history of) inflammatory bowel disease or antibiotic-associated colitis; patients with systemic infections being treated with antimicrobials.

Interactions: Effect of Clindamycin on Other Drugs: Neuromuscular blockers: *Action enhanced, caution (systemic clindamycin).* Vitamin K antagonists (warfarin, acenocoumarol, fluindione): *Increased coagulation tests (PT/INR) and/or bleeding reported, monitor.*

SP: Antibiotic-associated diarrhoea or colitis (infrequent), discontinue. Caution applying around mouth, unpleasant taste.

Pregnancy, Lactation: Pregnancy, avoid oral clindamycin; topical, no data. Lactation, stop drug or stop breastfeeding.

ADR: *Very common,* skin irritation, urticaria, dry skin.

Notes: See 10.1.2 Topical Antibacterials.

> **Dalacin T Topical** *(Pfizer)* A. GMS.
> *Price,* (30mL) lotion, €8.04. Soln, €6.57.
> *Cutaneous lotion,* clindamycin phosphate 10mg/mL. Smooth white (off-white) emulsion. *Cetostearyl alcohol, parabens.*
> *Cutaneous soln,* as above. Clear colourless. *Propylene glycol.*
> **Zindaclin Gel** *(Fannin)* A. GMS.
> *Price,* (30g) €10.26.
> *Topical gel,* clindamycin phosphate 1%.

Clindamycin, Tretinoin

ATC Code: D10AF51. **Sport:** Permitted.
Driving: Unlikely to impair.

Indications: Acne vulgaris (comedones, papules, pustules present).

Dose: Adult, Elderly: Age 12 years and over, apply once daily at bedtime; squeeze pea-sized amount of gel onto finger, dot onto chin, cheeks, nose, forehead; gently rub over entire face (after cleansing). Max. duration 12 weeks. *Elderly,* over 65 years, safety/efficacy not established.

Child: Under 12 years, not recommended.

Renal Impairment: No data; individual decisions advisable if severe.

Hepatic Impairment: As for Renal above.

CI: Regional enteritis, ulcerative colitis, history of antibiotic-associated colitis, history of skin cancer, acute eczema, rosacea, perioral dermatitis, pustular and deep cystic nodular acne (conglobata, fulminans). See Notes below (clindamycin).

Interactions: Effect of Other Drugs on Clindamycin, Tretinoin: *Co-admin caution:* Topicals with strong drying effect or with high alcohol conc, astringents.

Effect of Clindamycin, Tretinoin on other Drugs: Vitamin K antagonists (warfarin, acenocoumarol, fluindione): *Increased coagulation tests (PT/INR) and/or bleeding with clindamycin co-admin.*

SP: Not for oral, ophthalmic, intranasal use. Not recommended for mild acne. Avoid contact with mouth, eyes, mucous membranes, abraded or eczematous skin. More than recommended amount or too frequent application may cause redness, stinging, discomfort. Caution, atopic subjects. Not for application at same time as other topicals; tretinoin enhances permeability for other topicals. Photosensitivity (minimise sun exposure).

Pregnancy, Lactation: Not for use in pregnancy, especially first trimester and in women who may become pregnant. Use in women of childbearing potential only if effect

284

contraception is used during and for one month after treatment. Lactation, not to be used.

ADR: *Uncommon,* skin disorders, application site reactions.

Notes: See Clindamycin above. See 10.1.2 Topical Antibacterials.

> **Treclin Gel** *(Meda)* A. GMS.
> *Price,* (30g) €15.66.
> *Topical gel,* clindamycin phosphate 1%, tretinoin 0.025% (w/w). Translucent yellow. *Parabens, butylhydroxytoluene.*

Erythromycin, Zinc

ATC Code: D10AF52. **Sport:** Permitted.
Driving: Unlikely to impair.

Indications: Acne vulgaris.

Dose: Adult: Apply twice daily.

CI: Macrolide, zinc, di-isopropyl sebacate, ethanol hypersensitivity.

SP: Cross-resistance with other macrolides, lincomycin, clindamycin. Avoid contact with mucous membranes of nose and mouth. Superinfection.

Pregnancy, Lactation: Use if benefit outweighs risk. Pregnancy, systemic absorption low. Lactation, not for use in chest area to avoid accidental infant ingestion.

ADR: *Uncommon,* pruritus, erythema, skin irritation/burning, dry skin, exfoliation.

Notes: See 10.1.2 Topical Antibacterials.

> **Zineryt Cutaneous Soln** *(LEO)* A. GMS.
> *Price,* 30mL, €9.29.
> *Cutaneous soln,* erythromycin 40mg, zinc acetate 12mg per mL. White crystalline powder; clear colourless solvent for soln. *Ethanol.*

10.1.3 - Benzoyl Peroxide, Azelaic Acid

In This Chapter: *Azelaic acid, benzoyl peroxide and combinations.*

Class Effects

Adolescents, dose generally as for Adult.

CI: Hypersensitivity to any member of the class. Not for use in children under 12 years unless otherwise specified.

SP: Amount of irritation, peeling or drying can be reduced by reducing amount or frequency of application.

ADR: Application site burning, stinging. Pruritus, erythema, skin irritation, dry skin, scaling and/or feeling of skin tension, exfoliation. Contact dermatitis, skin discolouration, facial oedema.

Notes: See 10.1 Acne.

Azelaic Acid

ATC Code: D10AX03. **Sport:** Permitted.
Driving: No influence.

Indications: Mild to moderate papular-pustular facial acne, papulopustular rosacea.

Dose: Adult: Apply sparingly twice daily; massage in gently.

CI: Propylene glycol hypersensitivity.

SP: Avoid contact with eyes/mucous membranes. Wash hands after applying. Avoid use of alcoholic cleansers, tinctures/astringents, abrasives, peeling agents, occlusion. Worsening of asthma. Renal/hepatic impairment, elderly, no data.

Pregnancy, Lactation: Pregnancy, caution. Lactation, infants must not come into contact with treated skin/breast.

ADR: *Very common,* application site (burning, pain, pruritus).

Notes: See 10.1.3 Benzoyl Peroxide, Azelaic Acid.

> **Skinoren Gel** *(Bayer)* B. GMS.
> *Price,* (30g) €8.75.
> *Topical gel,* azelaic acid 15%. White (yellowish-white) opaque. *Benzoic acid, propylene glycol.*

Benzoyl Peroxide, Clindamycin

ATC Code: D10AE51. **Sport:** Permitted.
Driving: Not relevant.
Indications: Acne vulgaris (inflammatory lesions).

Dose: Adult: Apply once daily.

Interactions: Effect of Other Drugs on Benzoyl Peroxide, Clindamycin Combination: Co-admin not recommended: Preparations containing Vitamin A derivatives, other drugs with desquamative, irritant or drying effects. Transient skin discolouration: PABA-containing sunscreens (co-admin).

SP: History of antibiotic-associated colitis. Antibiotic cross-resistance. Undue redness or discomfort, discontinue; consult medical advice. May bleach hair and coloured fabrics. Application to neck, other sensitive areas, caution (benzoyl peroxide).

Notes: See 10.1.3 Benzoyl Peroxide, Azelaic Acid. See 10.1.2 Topical Antibacterials Used in Acne (clindamycin).

> **Duac Once Daily Gel** (Stiefel) A. GMS.
> Price, (30g) €15.79.
> Topical gel, anhydrous benzoyl peroxide 50mg, clindamycin phosphate 10mg per g. White (slightly yellow) homogenous. **Store:** Refrigerate; do not freeze; after dispensing, below 25 deg C.

10.1.4 - Other Topicals Used In Acne, Rosacea

In This Chapter: Brimonidine, ivermectin, metronidazole.

Class Effects
CI: Hypersensitivity to any member of the class.
Notes: See 10.1 Acne.

Brimonidine (topical)

ATC Code: D11AX21. **Sport:** Permitted.
Driving: No or negligible effect.
Indications: Symptomatic treatment, facial erythema of rosacea (adults).

Dose: Adult, Elderly: 1 application per 24 hours at any suitable time for as long as facial erythema present; max. 1g/day. Apply smoothly and evenly as thin layer across entire face; avoid eyes, eyelid, lips, mouth, membrane of inner nose. Other products should be applied after Mirvaso has dried. Elderly, over 65 years, limited data.

Child: Under 18 years, not recommended; under 2 years, contraindicated (serious systemic safety risk).

Interactions: Effect of Other Drugs on Brimonidine: Co-admin contraindicated: MAOI (selegiline, moclobemide), TCADs (imipramine), tetracyclic antidepressants (maprotiline, mianserin, mirtazapine). Co-admin caution: Substances affecting metabolism and uptake of circulating amines (chlorpromazine, methylphenidate, reserpine), substances which may interact with alpha-adrenergic receptor agonists (isoprenaline, prazosin), antihypertensives and/or cardiac glycosides. Additive or potentiating effect: CNS depressants (alcohol, barbiturates, opiates, sedatives, anaesthetics).

SP: Not for use on irritated skin or open wounds; severe irritation or contact allergy, discontinue. Initiate on small areas of face (test tolerance). May exacerbate rosacea symptoms. Erythema and flushing. Do not exceed recommended dose or frequency of use. Co-admin with other systemic alpha-receptor agonists may potentiate undesirable effects with (severe or unstable or uncontrolled cardiovascular disease; depression, cerebral or coronary insufficiency, Raynaud's phenomenon, orthostatic hypotension, thromboangiitis obliterans, scleroderma, Sjogren's syndrome).

Pregnancy, Lactation: Pregnancy, avoid. Lactation, not recommended.

ADR: Common, flushing, erythema, pruritus, skin burning sensation.

> **Mirvaso Gel** (Galderma) B. GMS.
> Price, 30g, €38.88.
> Topical gel, brimonidine 3.3mg/1g. White (light-yellow) opaque aqueous. Parabens, propylene glycol. **Store:** Do not freeze.

Ivermectin

ATC Code: D11AX22. **Sport:** Permitted.
Driving: No or negligible effect.
Indications: Topical treatment, inflammatory lesions of rosacea (papulopustular) in adults.

Dose: Adult, Elderly: Apply once daily (up to 4 months); may repeat treatment course. No improvement after 3 months, discontinue. Spread a thin layer over entire face; avoid eyes, lips, mucosa.

Child: Under 18 years, no safety/efficacy data.

Hepatic Impairment: Severe, caution.

Interactions: Effect of Other Drugs on Ivermectin: Co-admin caution (plasma exposure increased): Potent CYP3A4 inhibitors.

SP: Allergic reactions or skin irritation (excipients).

Pregnancy, Lactation: Pregnancy, not recommended. Lactation, stop breastfeeding or stop drug.

ADR: Summary, most common, skin burning sensation, irritation, pruritus, dry skin.

Notes: See 10.1.4 Other Topicals Used In Acne.

> **Soolantra Cream 10mg/g** (Galderma) B. GMS.
> Price, 30g, €23.76.
> Topical cream, White (pale-yellow) hydrophilic. Cetyl/stearyl alcohol, propylene glycol, parabens.

Metronidazole (topical)

ATC Code: D06BX01. **Sport:** Permitted.
Driving: Unlikely to impair.
Indications: Acute inflammatory exacerbations of rosacea.

Dose: Adult: Apply thin film twice daily, morning and evening.

Interactions: Effect of Other Drugs on Metronidazole (topical): Possible disulfiram-like reaction: ALCOHOL.
Effect of Metronidazole (topical) on Other Drugs: Coumarins: INR values modified (rarely)

SP: Local irritation, use less frequently or discontinue temporarily. Blood dyscrasias, caution. Avoid prolonged use, exposure to UV or strong sunlight.

Pregnancy, Lactation: Pregnancy, if considered essential. Lactation, stop drug or stop breastfeeding.

ADR: Common, dry skin, erythema, pruritus, discomfort including burning/stinging, irritation, rosacea worsening.
Notes: See 10.1.4 Other Topicals Used In Acne. See 9.1.7 Anaerobic Infections (metronidazole, systemic).

> **Rozex Cream, Gel** (Galderma) A. GMS.
> Price, (30g) cream, €7.03. Gel, €6.05.
> Topical cream, metronidazole 0.75%. White (slightly beige) shiny. Cetostearyl alcohol.
> Topical gel, as above. Colourless (pale-yellow); may turn slightly brown over time. Propylene glycol, parabens.

10.1.5 - Oral Acne Treatments

In This Chapter: Isotretinoin.

Class Effects
Indications: The combined oral contraceptive (cyproterone, ethinylestradiol) is indicated for the treatment of severe acne vulgaris in women (Dianette).
CI: Hypersensivity to any member of the class.
Notes: See 8.2.1 Combined Hormonal Contraceptives (Dianette).

10.1.6 Photodamage, Actinic Keratosis

Isotretinoin (systemic)

ATC Code: D10BA01. **Sport:** Permitted.
Driving: Caution. Decreased night vision; may be of sudden onset; may persist after therapy. Drowsiness, dizziness, visual disturbances. See ADR below.

Indications: Severe forms of acne (nodular or conglobate with risk of permanent scarring) resistant to standard therapy with systemic antibacterials and topical therapy.

Dose: Adult: Initially 0.5mg/kg/day; range, 0.5-1mg/kg/day. Take caps with food once or twice daily.

Child: Adolescents, as for Adult above. Under 12 years, not recommended.

Renal Impairment: Severe, commence at 10mg/day; if needed titrate up to 1mg/kg/day or max. tolerated dose.

Hepatic Impairment: Not recommended.

CI: Excessively elevated blood lipids, hypervitaminosis A, peanut or soya hypersensitivity.

Interactions: Effect of Other Drugs on Isotretinoin: Co-admin not recommended: Tetracyclines (benign intracranial hypertension), other topical keratolytics or exfoliative agents (local reactions), vitamin A (hypervitaminosis A risk).

SP: This medicinal is TERATOGENIC. Counsel both male and female patients not to share medication and to return unused caps to pharmacist at end of treatment. Blood may NOT be donated during or for 1 month after treatment. *Depression*, anxiety, aggressive tendencies through to suicidal ideation, attempts and suicide; caution. *Acute acne exacerbation*, avoid exposure to UV or sunlight, use SPF 15 and moisturisers; severe skin reactions (erythema multiforme, Stevens-Johnson Syndrome, toxic epidermal necrolysis), discontinue. *Eye dryness*, corneal opacities, decreased night vision, keratitis; contact lens intolerance; myalgia, arthralgia, increased serum CPK with vigorous activity; bone changes; benign intracranial hypertension (caution, tetracycline co-admin). Liver enzymes, serum lipids, monitor. Inflammatory bowel disease. *Allergic reactions* (severe, interrupt treatment, monitor); serious cases of allergic vasculitis, often with purpura (bruises, red patches) of extremities and extracutaneous involvement. High risk patients (diabetes, obesity, alcoholism, lipid metabolism disorders), monitor.

Pregnancy, Lactation: This medicinal is TERATOGENIC. Pregnancy is an absolute contraindication and women should understand the teratogenic risk and understand and accept the need for effective contraception without interruption 1 month before, during, and 1 month after treatment. Perform regular pregnancy testing. Not for use in women of childbearing potential, unless all conditions of the Pregnancy Prevention Programme are met. Lactation, contraindicated; likely to pass into human milk.

ADR: *Very common*, anaemia, increased ESR, thrombocytopenia, thrombocytosis, blepharitis, conjunctivitis, dry eye, eye irritation, transaminase increased, cheilitis, dermatitis, dry skin, localised exfoliation, pruritus, erythematous rash, skin fragility, arthralgia, myalgia, back pain particularly children/adolescents, increased blood triglycerides. See SP above.

Notes: See 10.1.5 Oral Acne Treatments.

> **Roaccutane 10mg, 20mg** *(Roche)* A. GMS.
> *Price*, (30) 10mg, €11.07. 20mg, €20.37.
> *Soft capsules*, isotretinoin. Oval opaque. Marked ROA/strength.
> 10mg: Brown-red. 20mg: Brown-red/white. *Soya bean oil, sorbitol*.
> NOTE: See manufacturers Full Prescribing Information for Pregnancy Prevention Programme.

10.1.6 - Photodamage, Actinic Keratosis

In This Chapter: *Diclofenac sodium, ingenol mebutate*

Class Effects
Imiquimod is also indicated for the treatment of actinic keratoses. See Notes below.

CI: Hypersensivity to any member of the class.

Notes: See 10.6 Warts (imiquimod).

Diclofenac Sodium (keratosis)

ATC Code: D11AX18. **Sport:** Permitted.
Driving: Unlikely to impair.

Indications: Treatment, actinic keratoses.

Dose: Adult, Elderly: Apply thinly twice daily for 60-90 days; max. 8g/day.

Child: Not recommended.

CI: Benzyl alcohol, macrogol monomethyl ether 350, sodium hyaluronate hypersensitivity; previous reactions with aspirin or other NSAIDs (asthma, allergic rhinitis, urticaria).

SP: Systemic side effects (larger areas, prolonged period); caution, GI ulceration or bleeding, reduced heart, liver, renal function, intracranial haemorrhage, bleeding diathesis. Avoid direct sunlight, solarium; hypersensitivity, discontinue. Systemic effects, see Notes below (NSAIDs).

Pregnancy, Lactation: Pregnancy, first and second trimesters, use only if clearly necessary. Third trimester, contraindicated. Lactation, no effect on suckling child anticipated at prescribed dose; not for application to breast area while nursing.

ADR: *Common*, conjunctivitis, application site reactions including inflammation, irritation, pain, tingling, blistering, hyperesthesia, hypertonia, localised paraesthesia, contact dermatitis, eczema, dry skin, erythema, oedema, pruritus, rash, scaly skin, hypertrophy, ulcer, vesiculobullous rash.

Notes: See 10.1.6 Photodamage, Actinic Keratosis. For systemic effects, see 4.4.2 NSAIDS (Non-Selective).

> **Solaraze Gel** *(Almirall)* B. GMS.
> *Price*, 25g, €21.95. 50g, €51.68.
> *Topical gel*, diclofenac sodium 3% w/w. Clear transparent colourless (pale-yellow). **Store:** Below 25 deg C.

Ingenol Mebutate

ATC Code: D06BX02. **Sport:** Pending.
Driving: No or negligible effect.

Indications: Non-(hyperkeratotic, hypertrophic) actinic keratosis.

Dose: Adult, Elderly: Apply 1 tube (either 150mcg/g or 500mcg/g*) once daily to area (3 consecutive days); using fingertips, spread evenly over entire treatment area; allow to dry for 15 minutes. Do not apply immediately after showering or less than 2 hours before bedtime; do not wash area for 6 hours after application; do not occlude. Single use, discard tube after use. *Not for use on face or scalp.

SP: Avoid contact with eyes; can cause chemical conjunctivitis and corneal burns. Do not ingest. Do not apply to open wounds or damaged skin, near eyes, inside of (nostrils, ears) or on lips. Avoid or minimise sun exposure. Localised erythema, flaking, scaling, crusting.

Pregnancy, Lactation: Pregnancy, avoid. Lactation, newborn/infant to avoid physical contact with treated area for minimum 6 hours after application.

ADR: Summary, *most frequent*, erythema, flaking, scaling, crusting, swelling, vesiculation, pustulation, erosion, ulceration. Infection when treating face, scalp.

Notes: See 10.1.6 Photodamage, Actinic Keratosis.

> ▼ **Picato Gel** *(LEO)* A. GMS.
> *Price*, (47g) 150mcg/g (3), €85.16; 500mcg/g (2), €86.53.
> *Topical gel*, ingenol mebutate 150mcg(500mcg)/g. Clear colourless gel. **Store:** Refrigerate.

10.2 - Topical Anti-Infectives

10.2.1 - Topical Antibacterials

In This Chapter: *Bacitracin, neomycin, amino acid combination, fusidic acid, gramicidin, mupirocin, silver sulphadiazine.*

Class Effects

Indications: In severe infections, concomitant systemic therapy may be indicated.

CI: Hypersensivity to any member of the class.

SP: Cleanse application area prior to application; remove debris (pus, crusts). Avoid contact with eyes; wash hands after use. Prolonged use may result in overgrowth by non-susceptible organisms and/or development of antibiotic resistance.

ADR: Prolonged and extensive use may lead to systemic absorption and systemic adverse events.

Notes: For systemic effects, see 9.1 Antibacterials.

Fusidic Acid (topical)

ATC Code: D06AX01. **Sport:** Permitted.
Driving: Unlikely to impair.

Indications: Topical infections especially *Staphylococcus aureus.*

Dose: Adult, Elderly: Apply 3-4 times daily; less frequent may be adequate with covered lesions.

Pregnancy, Lactation: Can be used (negligible systemic exposure); avoid applying on breast if breastfeeding.

ADR: *Uncommon*, dermatitis including contact dermatitis, eczema, rash, pruritus, erythema, application site pain/irritation.

Notes: See 10.2.1 Topical Antibacterials, 9.1.9 Other Antibacterials, Enzymes (fusidic acid).

Fucidin Cream, Ointment 2% *(LEO)* A. GMS.D.
Price, cream (15g) €3.70; (30g) €6.26; ointment (15g) €3.02; (30g) €5.13.
Topical cream, fusidic acid 20mg/g. White. *Cetyl alcohol, butylhydroxyanisole, potassium sorbate.* **Store:** Below 30 deg C.
Topical ointment, as above. Off-white viscous. *Cetyl alcohol, wool fat, butylhydroxytoluene.*

Mupirocin (topical)

ATC Code: D06AX09. **Sport:** Permitted.
Driving: No or negligible effect.

Indications: Acute primary bacterial skin infection e.g. impetigo, folliculitis due to sensitive organisms.

Dose: Adult, Elderly: Apply up to 3 times daily; cover with dressing or occlude if needed. *Elderly*, no restrictions unless moderate or severe renal impairment.

Renal Impairment: Moderate to severe, caution.

CI: Topical not suitable for ophthalmic or intranasal use.

Interactions: Effect of Other Drugs on Mupirocin: *Admixture with other preparations not recommended*: Reduction in antibacterial activity, potential loss of stability of mupirocin.

SP: Sensitisation or severe local irritation, discontinue. Not suitable for ophthalmic or intranasal use, use with cannulae, at site of central venous cannulation or where absorption of large quantities of polyethylene glycol is possible (especially with moderate or severe renal impairment). Avoid contact with eyes.

Pregnancy, Lactation: Pregnancy, insufficient data; animal studies do not indicate reproductive toxicity. Lactation, inadequate data.

ADR: *Common*, burning (localised to application area).

Notes: See 10.2.1 Topical Antibacterials.

Bactroban 2% Ointment *(GSK)* A. GMS.
Price, (15g) €4.83.
Topical ointment, mupirocin 20mg/g. White translucent water-soluble.

Silver Sulphadiazine

ATC Code: D06BA01. **Sport:** Permitted.
Driving: Unlikely to impair.

Indications: Burns, wound infection, leg ulcers, pressure sores.

Dose: Adult, Elderly: Apply in 3-5mm layer; change dressing 3-times weekly (ulcers), daily (burns).

Child: Under 3 months, not recommended.

Renal Impairment: Caution.

Hepatic Impairment: As for Renal above.

Pregnancy, Lactation: Not recommended.

Notes: See 10.2.1 Topical Antibacterials.

Flamazine Cream *(Smith&Nephew)* A. GMS.
Price, 50g, €5.59. 250g, €15.00. 500g, €22.26.
Topical cream, silver sulphadiazine 1%.

10.2.2 - Topical Antifungals

In This Chapter: *Amorolfine, ketoconazole, miconazole, terbinafine, tioconazole, calcium undecylenate, zinc undecenoate.*

Class Effects

Fungal infections with inflammation, consider antifungal + corticosteroid combination.

CI: Hypersensitivity to any member of the class.

Notes: For systemic antifungals, see 9.2 Antifungals. For corticosteroid combinations, see 10.4 Topical Corticosteroids.

Amorolfine

ATC Code: D01AE16. **Sport:** Permitted.
Driving: Unlikely to impair.

Indications: Onychomycoses caused by dermatophytes, yeasts, moulds.

Dose: Adult, Elderly: Apply to nails once weekly.

Child: Not for use.

CI: Hypersensitivity.

SP: Avoid contact (eyes, ears, mucous membranes); avoid use (nail varnish, artificial nails). Do not apply to nail bed.

Pregnancy, Lactation: Use only if clearly necessary.

ADR: *Rare*, nail disorder/discoloration, brittle/broken nails.

Notes: See 10.2.2 Topical Antifungals.

Loceryl Nail Lacquer *(Galderma)* B. GMS.
Price, (5mL) €26.07.
Nail lacquer, amorolfine HCl 5%. Clear colourless (almost colourless) medicated.

Ketoconazole (topical)

ATC Code: D01AC08. **Sport:** Permitted.
Driving: Not applicable.

Indications: Dermatophyte infections of skin (Tinea corporis, cruris, manuus, pedis) due to Trichophyton, Microsporum, Epidermophyton spp. Treatment and prophylaxis, seborrhoea capitis, seborrhoeic dermatitis of the body, pityriasis versicolor.

Dose: Adult, Elderly: Cream, *Tinea pedis*, apply twice daily (1 week); more severe, 4-6 weeks; pityriasis versicolor, yeast infection (2-3 weeks), *Tinea cruris*, seborrhoeic dermatitis (2-4 weeks), *Tinea corporis* (3-4 weeks).

Shampoo, seborrhoea capitis, apply to scalp, leave for 3-5 minutes, rinse *(Nizoral, Ketozol)*; seborrhoeic dermatitis, wash area with shampoo, leave for 3-5 minutes, rinse; twice weekly for 2-4 weeks; prophylaxis, use once every 1-2 weeks *(Nizoral)*.

Pityriasis versicolor, use once daily (up to 5 days); prophylaxis, once daily (up to 3 days) before prolonged sun exposure.

10.2.3 Topical Antivirals

Interactions: Effect of Other Drugs on Ketoconazole: *Local irritation:* Topical corticosteroids.

SP: Not for ophthalmic use; if shampoo gets into eyes, bathe with water.

Pregnancy, Lactation: Pregnancy, lactation, no known risk.

ADR: *Uncommon,* dysgeusia, folliculitis, irritation, increased lacrimation, acne, alopecia, rash, urticaria, skin irritation, dry skin, changed hair texture, contact dermatitis, exfoliation, application site reaction, hypersensitivity.

Notes: See 10.2.2 Topical Antifungals.

Nizoral Cream 2%, Shampoo 2% *(McNeil)* OTC. GMS.
Price, cream (30g) €4.76. Shampoo (120mL) €4.28.
Topical cream, ketoconazole 20mg/g. White odourless. *Propylene glycol, cetyl/stearyl alcohol.*
Shampoo, as above 20mg/g. Pink viscous.

Ketozol 2% Shampoo *(Rowex)* OTC. GMS.
Price, (120mL) €4.19.
Shampoo, ketoconazole 20mg/g. Clear reddish. *Potassium sorbate.*

Miconazole (topical)

ATC Code: D01AC02. **Sport:** Permitted.
Driving: Not applicable.

Indications: Fungal skin infections, secondary infection due to Gram-positive organisms.

Dose: Adult, Elderly: Apply twice daily; rub in cream until fully penetrated; duration 2-6 weeks depending of localisation and severity of lesion.

SP: Sensitivity, irritation, discontinue. Avoid contact with eyes. Powder contains talc, avoid inhalation; caution with infants or children.

Pregnancy, Lactation: Pregnancy, if benefit outweighs risk. Lactation, caution.

ADR: *Uncommon,* local skin reactions, application site reactions.

Notes: See 10.2.2 Topical Antifungals.

Daktarin 2% Cream, Powder 2% *(McNeil)* OTC. GMS.
Price, cream (30g) €2.60. Powder (20g) €1.85.
Topical cream, miconazole 20mg/g. White homogenous. *Benzoic acid, butylated hydroxyanisole.*
Cutaneous powder, as above. White.

Terbinafine (topical)

ATC Code: D01AE15. **Sport:** Permitted.
Driving: No influence.

Indications: Fungal skin infections caused by Trichophyton spp., *Microsporum canis, Epidermophyton floccosum.* Yeast skin infections caused by Candida. Pityriasis (tinea) versicolor.

Dose: Adult, Elderly: Apply once daily, tinea (pedis, corporis, cruris) (1 week). Apply 1-2 times daily, cutaneous candidiasis (1-2 weeks); pityriasis versicolor (2 weeks).

Child: Not recommended.

SP: Intertriginous infections, application may be covered with gauze strip, especially at night. External use only. Avoid contact with eyes.

Pregnancy, Lactation: Pregnancy, if benefit outweighs risk and if clearly necessary. Lactation, not recommended.

ADR: *Common,* skin exfoliation, pruritus.

Notes: See 10.2.2 Topical Antifungals.

Lamisil 1% Cream *(GSK Consumer)* B. GMS.
Price, (15g) €5.71. (30g) €10.92.
Topical cream, terbinafine HCl. White smooth (almost) glossy. *Benzyl, cetyl-, -stearyl alcohol.*
Fungasil 1% Cream *(Clonmel)* B. GMS.
Price, (7.5g) €2.22.
Topical cream, terbinafine HCl 10mg/g. White (almost). *Cetostearyl alcohol.*

Tioconazole

ATC Code: D01AC07. **Sport:** Permitted.
Driving: Unlikely to impair.

Indications: Topical treatment, nail infections due to susceptible fungi (dermatophytes, yeasts) and bacteria.

Dose: Adult, Elderly: Apply soln to nail and immediate surrounding skin every 12 hours. Allow to dry for 10-15 minutes after application. Duration, 6 months; 12 months may be needed.

Child: As for Adult above.

SP: Not for ophthalmic use.

Pregnancy, Lactation: Pregnancy, contraindicated. Lactation, stop nursing.

ADR: Local irritation. Sensitivity reactions, discontinue.

Notes: See 10.2.2 Topical Antifungals.

Trosyl Nail Soln *(Pfizer)* B. GMS.
Price, (12mL) €27.67.
Topical soln, tioconazole 283mg/mL. Clear pale-yellow.

10.2.3 - Topical Antivirals

In This Chapter: Aciclovir.

Class Effects
CI: Hypersensitivity to any member of the class.

Aciclovir (topical)

ATC Code: D06BB03. **Sport:** Permitted.
Driving: Unlikely to impair.

Indications: Treatment, *Herpes simplex* infections of skin e.g. genital herpes, herpes labialis.

Dose: Adult, Elderly: Apply 5-times daily at 4-hourly intervals, omitting night-time dose. See SP below.

Child: As for Adult above.

SP: Start treatment as early as possible (prodromal/erythema stage); can be started later (papule/blister) stages. Avoid contact with eyes; not for application to mucous membranes (mouth, eye, vagina). Severely immunocompromised, consider oral treatment.

Pregnancy, Lactation: Pregnancy, if benefit outweighs risk. Lactation, dosage received by nursing infant insignificant.

ADR: Transient burning, stinging, drying or flaking, itch; erythema, contact dermatitis, immediate hypersensivity (angioedema).

Notes: See 10.2.3 Topical Antivirals.

Zovirax 5% Cream *(GSK)* A. GMS.D*.
Price, (10g) €19.27. (2g)* €3.84.
Topical cream, aciclovir 5% w/w. Smooth white (off-white). *Cetostearyl alcohol, propylene glycol.*

10.3 - Emollients, Barriers, Topical Antipruritics

Class Effects
SP: Caution, slipping in bath or shower with bath additives or shower gels.

Pregnancy, Lactation: No special precautions for use.

Notes: See 10.7 Scabies, Head Lice (crotamiton).

Paraffins

ATC Code: D02AC. **Sport:** Permitted.
Driving: Unlikely to impair.

Indications: Emollient, moisturiser *(all brands).* Ointment base, soap substitute, (chronic dermatitis, lichenification, eczema, other dry skin conditions) *(Silcock's, Aqueous Cream).* Protective ointment (follow-up or spacing treatment or diluent for topical steroids); symptomatic treatment (red inflamed, damaged/dry chapped skin, protection of raw skin area, pre-bathing emollient for dry/eczematous skin) *(Diprobase).* Treatment, dermatitis (contact, atopic), senile pruritus, ichthyosis *(Oilatum),* dry skin (eczema, psoriasis, ichthyosis) *(Doublebase).*

Dose: Adult, Elderly: *Cream, ointment,* apply as often as required to prevent itching and flaking dry skin *(all brands). Gel,* smooth across skin in same direction as hair growth;

do not rub vigorously; allow time for excess to soak in. Diprobase, rub cream in well; ointment, apply thinly. Bath additive, 1-3 capfuls in 20cm bath of water; soak for 10-20 minutes, pat dry. Skin cleansing, rub small amount onto wet skin, rinse, pat dry.

Child: *Cream, ointment, gel,* as for Adult above. *Bath additive,* infants, add 0.5-1 capfuls (Junior, 0.5-2 capfuls) to small bath/basin of water; sponge on gently over entire body and pat dry.

SP: Do not use *(Silcock's)* to dilute steroid creams, ointments.

Pregnancy, Lactation: Can be used.

ADR: Allergic reaction to excipients. Local skin reactions.

Notes: See 10.3 Emollients.

Aqueous Cream *(Ovelle)* OTC. GMS.
Price, 500g, €2.11.
Cream, white soft paraffin 15%, emulsifying wax 9%, liquid paraffin 6% (w/w). Smooth white homogenous. *Cetostearyl alcohol.*
Diprobase Cream, Ointment *(Bayer)* OTC.
Price, not published by company.
Cream, paraffins. Smooth white uniform. *Chlorocresol, cetostearyl alcohol.*
Ointment, as above. Smooth white uniform.
Doublebase Emollient Gel *(Dermal)* OTC.
Price, (1) 100g, €3.42; 250g, €6.21 (trade).
Topical gel, liquid paraffin 15%, isopropyl myristate 15% (w/w). White opaque. **Store:** Below 25 deg C; do not freeze.
Oilatum Emollient Bath, Cream *(GSK Consumer)* OTC.
Price, not published by company (150mL, 250mL, 500mL). Junior (150mL, 300mL). Cream 40g.
Bath additive including Junior, light liquid paraffin 63.4% (w/w). Pale-yellow oily liquid with faint perfume.
Cream, light liquid paraffin 6%, white soft paraffin 15% (w/w). White (off-white). *Cetostearyl alcohol, potassium sorbate.*
Silcock's Base Cream *(Ovelle)* OTC. GMS.
Price, 500g, €2.03.
Cream, white soft paraffin 20%, emulsifying wax 15% (w/w). Smooth white homogenous. *Parabens, cetostearyl alcohol.*

10.4 - Topical Corticosteroids And Combinations

In This Chapter: *Alclometasone, betamethasone, clobetasone, diflucortolone, hydrocortisone, mometasone, triamcinolone and combinations.*

Class Effects
Corticosteroids are classed as mild (hydrocortisone 0.5%, 1%, hydrocortisone acetate 1%), moderately potent (alclometasone dipropionate 0.05%, betamethasone valerate 0.025%, clobetasone butyrate 0.05%, hydrocortisone butyrate 0.1%), potent (betamethasone dipropionate 0.05%, betamethasone valerate 0.1%, diflucortolone valerate 0.1%, mometasone furoate 0.1%, triamcinolone acetonide 0.1%), very potent (clobetasol propionate 0.05%, diflucortolone valerate 0.3%).

Driving: Systemic glucocorticoids may cause mood changes (euphoria, depression) or visual disturbances; caution in driving or operating machinery. Topical, unlikely to impair.

Indications: Corticosteroid responsive dermatoses. Topical corticosteroids generally not indicated in wide-spread plaque psoriasis.

CI: Primary skin infections: Bacterial (impetigo, pyoderma), fungal (candida, dermatophyte), viral (herpes simplex/zoster, varicella, verrucae vulgares, condylomata acuminata, molluscum contagiosum), tuberculosis or parasites (untreated or uncontrolled). Acne, rosacea, perioral dermatitis, atrophic skin, striae atrophicae, fragility of skin veins, ichthyosis, ulcers, wounds, pruritus without inflammation. Children under 12 years only with medical supervision. Not for use on broken skin.

SP: *Prolonged use:* Avoid (especially face); use for shortest duration; acne vulgaris management, avoid; thinning of skin (especially elderly); caution, children under 12 years.

If applied topically (to large areas, broken skin, with occlusive dressing), may be absorbed and cause systemic effects, see Notes below.

Keep away from eyes, glaucoma risk; avoid mucous membranes. Secondary infection, withdraw (start antimicrobial treatment); persistent infection (consider systemic treatment).

Cream formulations usually used for moist, weeping surfaces; ointments for dry, lichenified or scaly lesions. Thickened plaques of psoriasis on elbows and knees, effect can be enhanced with occlusion with polythene film overnight. Psoriasis, possibility of rebound relapses, development of tolerance, risk of generalised pustular psoriasis, local or systemic toxicity (impaired skin barrier function); careful supervision. Phaeochromocytoma crisis (fatal) reported.

Pregnancy, Lactation: Only if considered essential; benefit outweighs risk. If unavoidable, use minimum quantity for shortest duration. Corticosteroids cross placenta. Lactation, caution; stop drug or stop breastfeeding; do not apply to breast to avoid accidental infant ingestion.

ADR: Children (especially infants), more susceptible to side-effects, especially with occlusion. Application site reactions (local irritation, pruritus, burning). Severe hypersensitivity, discontinue. Local skin atrophy, striae, superficial vascular dilatation (especially face) (continuous application without interruption). Superinfection (anti-infective combinations).

Notes: Systemic effects, see 11.1.1 Glucocorticoids. Combinations, see 10.2.1 Topical Antibacterials, 10.2.2 Topical Antifungals.

Alclometasone
ATC Code: D07AB10. **Sport:** Permitted.
Driving: Unlikely to impair.

Indications: Inflammatory and pruritic corticosteroid responsive dermatoses.

Dose: Adult, Elderly: Apply 2-3 times daily.

Notes: See 10.4 Topical Corticosteroids.

Modrasone Cream *(TEVA)* B. GMS.
Price, (15g) €2.13. (50g) €6.04
Topical cream, alclometasone dipropionate 0.05%. Smooth white (off-white). *Propylene glycol, cetostearyl alcohol.*

Betamethasone Dipropionate, Calcipotriol
ATC Code: D07XC01. **Sport:** Permitted.
Driving: No or negligible influence.

Indications: Treatment, stable plaque psoriasis vulgaris; scalp psoriasis (gel).

Dose: Adult, Elderly: Apply directly to affected area once daily; rub in gently. Scalp (4 weeks, using gel) OR non-scalp areas (8 weeks, using ointment/gel or 4 weeks using foam); max. calcipotriol 15g/day; recommend not to bath, shower or wash hair immediately after applying; to remain on skin/scalp during day or during night. Max. 30% BSA treated with calcipotriol.

Child: Under 18, not recommended; age 12-17 years, no dose recommendation.

CI: Disorders of calcium metabolism. Erythrodermic, exfoliative and pustular psoriasis.

SP: Do not apply to skin of face, mouth, eyes, genitals; wash hands after use. Excessive usage, hypercalcaemia risk (calcipotriol). Co-admin with other anti-psoriatics, phototherapy, no data.

ADR: *Most frequent,* pruritus (gel, ointment); skin exfoliation (ointment); application site reactions (foam).

Notes: See 10.4 Topical Corticosteroids.

Dovobet Ointment, Gel *(LEO)* A. GMS.
Price, ointment 30g, €20.37. Gel 60g, applicator pack 60g, €41.01; 2x(60g) €79.38.
Topical ointment, betamethasone dipropionate 0.5mg/g, calcipotriol monohydrate 50mcg/g. Off-white (yellow).

10.4 Topical Corticosteroids And Combinations

Butylhydroxytoluene. **Store:** Below 25 deg C.
Topical gel, as above. Almost clear colourless (slightly off-white) gel. *Butylhydroxytoluene.* **Store:** Do not refrigerate.
Enstilar Foam *(LEO)* A. GMS.
Price, (60g) €43.20.
Cutaneous foam, betamethasone dipropionate 0.5mg/g, calcipotriol monohydrate 50mcg/g. White (off-white) foam. *Butylhydroxytoluene.*

Betamethasone Dipropionate, Clotrimazole

ATC Code: D07CC01. **Sport:** Permitted.
Driving: Unlikely to impair.
Indications: Corticosteroid responsive dermatoses with actual or potential secondary fungal infection.

Dose: Adult, Elderly: Candidiasis, apply morning and evening. Tinea (cruris, corporis), 2 weeks, (pedis), 4 weeks.

Child: Under 12 years, not recommended.

ADR: Local irritation, burning, sensitivity.

Notes: See 10.4 Topical Corticosteroids.

Lotriderm Cream *(MSD)* A. GMS.
Price, (30g) €4.90.
Topical cream, clotrimazole 1%, betamethasone dipropionate 0.064%. Smooth uniform white (off-white). *Propylene glycol, cetostearyl alcohol.*

Betamethasone Dipropionate, Salicylic Acid

ATC Code: D07XC01. **Sport:** Permitted.
Driving: None stated.
Indications: Chronic lichenified eczema, lichen planus, lichen simplex, non-bullous ichthyosiform erythroderma. Psoriasis (scalp, chronic plaque of hands and feet).

Dose: Adult, Elderly: Apply a few drops 1-2 times daily; maintenance, reduce frequency. Review after 2 weeks.

Child: Limit to 5 days.

CI: Rosacea, acne, perioral dermatitis, perianal and genital pruritus, tuberculous and viral skin lesions, napkin eruptions, fungal or bacterial skin infections (unless with antimicrobial therapy).

SP: Occlusive dressings must NOT be used. Irritation, sensitisation, discontinue.

ADR: Prolonged salicylic acid use, dermatitis risk.

Notes: See 10.4 Topical Corticosteroids.

Diprosalic Scalp Application *(MSD)* A. GMS.
Price, (100mL) €12.99.
Scalp application, betamethasone dipropionate, salicylic acid (%) 0.05/2 w/w. Colourless translucent viscous soln.

Betamethasone Valerate

ATC Code: D07AC01. **Sport:** Permitted.
Driving: Unlikely to impair.
Indications: Eczema, including (atopic, infantile, discoid), prurigo nodularis, psoriasis, neurodermatoses, including lichen (simplex, planus); seborrhoeic dermatitis; contact sensitivity reactions; discoid lupus erythematosus, adjunct to systemic therapy in generalised erythroderma, insect bite reactions, prickly heat. *Scalp applications,* scalp psoriasis, seborrhoea capitis, inflammation associated with severe dandruff.

Dose: Adult, Elderly: Apply sparingly 1-3 times daily; maintenance, once daily. Scalp, apply sparingly to scalp night and morning; maintenance once daily.

Child: As for Adult above. Under 1 year, not recommended; under 3 years, avoid use for longer than 3 weeks. *Betamousse* not recommended under 6 years. *Betacap,* seborrhoeic dermatitis, max. 7 days.

CI: Perianal, genital pruritus, widespread plaque psoriasis (topical cream, ointment).

SP: Scalp application is highly flammable; do not use near fire or naked flame. Allow treated scalp to dry naturally.

ADR: Hypersensitivity, discontinue. Prolonged use,

hypercortisolism, dilatation of superficial blood vessels, thinning, striae, pigmentation changes, hypertrichosis, allergic contact dermatitis, pustular psoriasis.

Notes: See 10.4 Topical Corticosteroids.

Betnovate, RD Cream, Ointment, Scalp App *(GSK)* B. GMS.
Price, cream, ointment (30g) €1.77. (100g) €4.94. RD cream, ointment (100g) €3.97. Scalp App (100mL) €6.47.
Topical cream, betamethasone valerate 0.1% w/w. (RD* 0.025% w/w). White homogenous aqueous-based. *Chlorocresol, cetostearyl alcohol.* *Ready Diluted.
Topical ointment, as above. Off-white homogenous.
Scalp application, as above. Colourless hazy slightly viscous soln.
Betacap Scalp Application *(Dermal)* B. GMS.
Price, (100mL) €5.17.
Scalp application, betamethasone valerate 0.1%. Transparent slightly gelled.
Bettamousse Cutaneous Foam *(Recipharm)* A. GMS.
Price, (100g) €10.11.
Topical foam, betamethasone 0.1%. White foam.

Betamethasone Valerate, Clioquinol

ATC Code: D07BC01. **Sport:** Permitted.
Driving: Unlikely to impair.
Indications: Corticosteroid responsive dermatoses complicated by infection including, dermatitis (atopic, nummular, seborrhoeic, irritant or allergic contact), prurigo nodularis, psoriasis, lichen simplex chronicus and lichen planus, insect bite reactions, miliaria (prickly heat), anal and genital intertrigo, otitis externa.

Dose: Adult, Elderly: Apply 2-3 times daily; maintenance, once daily or less often.

Child: Under 2 years, contraindicated.

CI: Rosacea, acne vulgaris, peri-oral dermatitis, perianal and genital pruritus, pruritus without inflammation, primary cutaneous viral infections (herpes simplex, chicken pox), primary infected skin lesions caused by infection (fungi, bacteria), primary or secondary infections (yeasts).

Interactions: Effect of Other Drugs on Betamethasone Valerate, Clioquinol: *Co-admin not recommended (clioquinol):* Vigabatrin

SP: Not to be diluted. May stain hair, skin, fabric; cover application with a dressing to protect clothing. Neurotoxicity risk (clioquinol; prolonged use or under occlusion).

ADR: Clioquinol may be toxic if absorbed from open surfaces. *Common,* pruritus, local skin burning or pain.

Notes: See 10.4 Topical Corticosteroids.

Betnovate-C Cream *(GSK)* B. GMS.
Price, (30g) €2.16.
Topical cream, betamethasone valerate 0.1%, clioquinol 3% w/w. Pale-yellow homogenous aqueous. *Chlorocresol, cetostearyl alcohol.*

Betamethasone Valerate, Fusidic Acid

ATC Code: D07CC01. **Sport:** Permitted.
Driving: No or negligible effect.
Indications: Inflammatory dermatoses *(Fucibet),* eczematous dermatosis (atopic, infantile, discoid, stasis, contact and seborrhoeic eczema) *(Eczibet)* (secondary bacterial infection confirmed or suspected).

Dose: Adult, Elderly: Apply a small quantity twice daily; max. 2 weeks *(both brands).* More resistant lesions, enhance effect with polyethylene film occlusion; overnight usually adequate *(Eczibet).*

Child: Use with care. *Eczibet* contraindicated under 1 year.

CI: Use in presence of non-sensitive organisms. See Notes below.

SP: Systemic absorption (prolonged use with occlusive dressing). Bacterial resistance (fusidic acid). Avoid use near eyes.

ADR: *Most frequent,* pruritus, application site irritation.

Notes: See 10.4 Topical Corticosteroids.

Topical Corticosteroids And Combinations 10.4

Fucibet Cream, Lipid Cream *(LEO)* A. GMS.
Price, cream (15g) €4.87; (30g) €8.16. Lipid Cream (15g) €7.40; (30g) €12.87.
Topical cream, betamethasone 1mg/g, fusidic acid 20mg/g. White. *Cetostearyl alcohol, chlorocresol.* **Store:** Below 30 deg C. Lipid Cream: White highly viscous oil-in-water emulsion. *Cetostearyl alcohol, parabens.* **Store:** Below 25 deg C.
Eczibet Cream *(Gerard)* A. GMS.
Price, (15g) €1.94; (30g) €3.26.
Topical cream, betamethasone 1mg/g, fusidic acid 20mg/g. White (off-white) smooth homogenous. *Cetostearyl alcohol, chlorocresol.* **Store:** Below 30 deg C.

Clobetasol Propionate

ATC Code: D07AD01. **Sport:** Permitted.
Driving: No or negligible effect.
Indications: Corticosteroid responsive dermatoses (psoriasis excluding widespread plaque, recalcitrant dermatoses, lichen planus, discoid lupus erythematosus, other conditions not responding to less potent steroids).

Dose: Adult, Elderly: *Dermovate,* apply once or twice daily (up to 4 weeks) then reduce frequency or change to less potent preparation. Max. 50g/week.
Etrivex, apply once daily to dry scalp, leave for 15 minutes without covering, rinse; max. 4 weeks.
Clarelux, apply twice daily directly onto lesion; massage until foam is absorbed; max. 50g/week, max 2 weeks.
Child: Under 18 years, not recommended *(Etrivex, Clarelux).* Contraindicated under 1 year *(Dermovate);* under 2 years *(Etrivex).*
Hepatic Impairment: Caution.
CI: Ulcerated burns, perianal and genital pruritus, primary infected skin lesions, ulcerous wounds. Not for use on face.
SP: Increased systemic absorption with occlusion. For more resistant lesions (hyperkeratosis), *Dermovate* effect can be enhanced with occlusion. *Clarelux* is NOT for use with occlusion unless with medical supervision. Scalp application is flammable.
ADR: Systemic effects (prolonged use, large amounts, large areas). Application site reactions, local skin burning, skin pain, pruritus.
Notes: See 10.4 Topical Corticosteroids.

Dermovate Cream, Ointment, Scalp App *(GSK)* B. GMS.
Price, cream, ointment (30g) €3.21; (100g) €9.41. Scalp (100mL) €9.60.
Topical cream, clobetasol propionate 0.05% w/w. White (off-white) homogenous. *Cetostearyl alcohol, propylene glycol, chlorocresol.*
Topical ointment, as above. White (off-white) translucent homogenous. *Propylene glycol.*
Scalp application, as above 0.05% w/v. Colourless clear (slightly hazy) slightly viscous cutaneous soln.
CLARELUX Foam *(Pierre Fabre)* B. GMS.
Price, (100g) €14.83.
Cutaneous foam (pressurised container), clobetasol propionate 500mg/g. White; breaks down on skin contact. In pressurised container. *Cetyl and stearyl alcohol, propylene glycol.* **Store:** Below 25 deg C; do not (refrigerate, expose to temp. above 50 deg C).
Etrivex Shampoo *(Galderma)* B. GMS.
Price, (125mL) €14.34.
Shampoo, clobetasol propionate 500mcg/g. Viscous translucent colourless (pale yellow) with alcoholic odour. *Ethanol.*

Clobetasone Butyrate

ATC Code: D07AD01. **Sport:** Permitted.
Driving: Unlikely to impair.
Indications: Relief of steroid responsive dermatoses (inflammatory, pruritic).
Dose: Adult, Elderly: Apply once or twice daily until improvement, then reduce frequency or change to less potent preparation; max. 4 weeks.
Child: Under 12 years, caution; max. 7 days (with medical advice). Under 1 years, use with occlusion (e.g. nappy) contraindicated.
SP: May be used as maintenance between courses of more potent steroids.
ADR: *Common,* burning (localised to application area).

Notes: See 10.4 Topical Corticosteroids.

Eumovate Cream, Ointment *(GSK)* B. GMS.
Price, cream, ointment (30g) €2.19.
Topical cream, clobetasone butyrate 0.05% w/w.
Topical ointment, as above. Smooth white (off-white) translucent.

Diflucortolone Valerate, Isoconazole

ATC Code: D07BC04. **Sport:** Permitted.
Driving: Unlikely to impair.
Indications: Superficial skin fungal infections accompanied by highly inflammatory or eczematous skin conditions (hand, interdigital spaces of feet, inguinal and genital regions).
Dose: Adult, Elderly: Apply twice daily; max. 2 weeks; after regression, follow with emollient.
SP: Use without occlusion. Interdigital spaces, place a strip of gauze smeared with cream between fingers or toes.
ADR: Itching, burning, erythema or vesiculation, skin discolouration.
Notes: See 10.4 Topical Corticosteroids.

Travocort Cream *(Bayer)* B. GMS.
Price, (15g) €2.71.
Topical cream, diflucortolone valerate 0.1%, isoconazole nitrate 1% w/w. White (faintly yellow). *Cetostearyl alcohol.*

Hydrocortisone (topical)

ATC Code: D07AA02. **Sport:** Permitted.
Driving: Unlikely to impair.
Indications: *Prescription,* management of corticosteroid sensitive superficial dermatoses. *Non-prescription,* dermatitis (contact, irritant), insect bite reactions.
Dose: Adult, Elderly: Apply twice daily *(Dioderm);* up to 4-times daily *(Hydrocortisyl).*
Child: As for Adult above. Infants, max. 7 days; under 12 years *(Hydrocortisyl),* use only with medical supervision.
CI: Not for use on eye, face, anogenital region, broken or infected skin.
SP: Skin irritation due to propylene glycol, discontinue.
ADR: Hypersensitivity, discontinue.
Notes: See 10.4 Topical Corticosteroids.

Hydrocortisyl 1% Cream *(SANOFI)* B. GMS.D.
Price, (15g) €1.89.
Topical cream, hydrocortisone 1% w/w. Smooth white uniform.
Dioderm 0.1% Cream *(Dermal)* B. GMS.
Price, (30g) €3.41.
Topical cream, hydrocortisone 0.1% w/w. Smooth white aqueous.

Hydrocortisone Acetate, Fusidic Acid

ATC Code: D07CA01. **Sport:** Permitted.
Driving: No or negligible effect.
Indications: Inflammatory dermatoses where bacterial infection present or likely.
Dose: Adult, Elderly: Apply twice daily; max. 2 weeks.
CI: Infections due to non-sensitive organisms. See Notes below.
ADR: *Common,* application site reactions.
Notes: See 10.4 Topical Corticosteroids.

Fucidin H Cream *(LEO)* A. GMS.
Price, (15g) €4.16. (30g) €7.18.
Topical cream, hydrocortisone acetate 10mg/g, sodium fusidate 20mg/g. White homogenous. *Butylhydroxyanisole, cetyl alcohol, potassium sorbate.*

Hydrocortisone Butyrate

ATC Code: D07AB02. **Sport:** Permitted.
Driving: None known.
Indications: Corticosteroid sensitive dermatoses (eczema, dermatitis, psoriasis) not caused by micro-organisms.
Dose: Adult, Elderly: Apply 2-3 times daily.
Child: Max. 7 days; avoid occlusion.
SP: Use occlusion only for limited areas.
Notes: See 10.4 Topical Corticosteroids.

10.5 Eczema, Psoriasis, Scalp Disorders

Locoid Cream, Lipo, Ointment, Scalp *(LEO)* B. GMS.
Price, cream, ointment (30g) €2.73. (100g) €8.52. Lipo (30g) €2.81. (100g) €9.16. Scalp App (100mL) €9.21.
Topical cream, hydrocortisone butyrate 0.1% w/w. White aqueous. Practically white *(Lipocream)*. *Cetostearyl alcohol, parabens.*
Topical ointment, as above. Translucent light-grey (white) soft fatty.
Scalp lotion, as above. Clear colourless (faintly yellow). *Isopropyl alcohol.*

Hydrocortisone, Clotrimazole

ATC Code: D01AC20. **Sport:** Permitted.
Driving: No or negligible effect.
Indications: Topical treatment of superficial dermatophytes, yeasts, moulds, other clotrimazole-sensitive fungi accompanied by inflammation (itching requiring rapid relief).
Dose: Adult, Elderly: Apply thinly twice daily; rub in gently (max. 7 days).
SP: May cause damage to latex contraceptives.
Notes: See 10.4 Topical Corticosteroids.
  Canesten HC Cream *(Bayer)* B. GMS.
  Price, (30g) €3.97.
  Topical cream, clotrimazole 1%, hydrocortisone 1% w/w. White (pale-yellow) cream. *Benzyl-, cetostearyl alcohol.*

Hydrocortisone, Miconazole

ATC Code: D01AC52. **Sport:** Permitted.
Driving: Unlikely to impair.
Indications: Skin conditions where inflammation and infection of susceptible organisms co-exist.
Dose: Adult, Elderly: Apply 1-3 times daily; rub in gently until completely penetrated skin.
Child: Caution, use on extensive areas or under occlusion. Infants, occlusion contraindicated.
CI: Use on eyes, face. See Notes below.
SP: Miconazole may decrease hydrocortisone metabolism (increased serum hydrocortisone). Vaginal anti-infectives may decrease effectiveness of latex contraceptives; do not use with latex condoms, diaphragms. Severe hypersensitivity (anaphylaxis, angioedema) reported with miconazole topical formulations.
ADR: *Uncommon*, skin irritation, burning sensation, urticaria, pruritus.
Notes: See 10.4 Topical Corticosteroids.
  Daktacort Cream *(Janssen-Cilag)* B. GMS.D.
  Price, (30g) €1.02.
  Topical cream, hydrocortisone 1%, miconazole nitrate 2%. White homogenous odourless. *Benzoic acid, butylated hydroxyanisole.*
  Store: Refrigerate.

Hydrocortisone, Urea

ATC Code: D07XA01. **Sport:** Permitted.
Driving: Unlikely to impair.
Indications: Treatment, dry ichthyotic, eczematous skin conditions including eczema (atopic, infantile, chronic allergic, irritant; asteatotic, hyperkeratotic and lichenified), neurodermatoses, prurigo.
Dose: Adult, Elderly: Apply twice daily.
CI: Not for use on weeping surfaces.
SP: Moist or fissured skin, caution temporary irritation.
Notes: See 10.4 Topical Corticosteroids.
  Alphaderm Cream *(Alliance)* B. GMS.
  Price, (30g) €2.87. (100g) €8.51.
  Topical cream, hydrocortisone 1%, urea 10%. Translucent white.

Hydrocortisone, Urea, Lactic Acid

ATC Code: D07XA01. **Sport:** Permitted.
Driving: Unlikely to impair.
Indications: Dermatoses characterised by hyperkeratosis and inflammation.
Dose: Adult, Elderly: Apply twice daily.
CI: Plaque psoriasis.
SP: Open wounds, mucous membranes, smarting; dilute with equal quantities of aqueous cream.

292

Notes: See 10.4 Topical Corticosteroids.
  Calmurid HC Cream *(Galderma)* B. GMS.
  Price, (30g) €2.91. (100g) €8.47.
  Topical cream, hydrocortisone 1%, lactic acid 5%, urea 10% w/w. Smooth white oil-in-water.

Mometasone (topical)

ATC Code: D07AC13. **Sport:** Permitted.
Driving: Unlikely to impair.
Indications: Management, corticosteroid responsive dermatoses.
Dose: Adult, Elderly: Apply once daily.
Child: Age 2 years and older, caution; under 2 years, not recommended.
CI: Use on wounds or ulcerated skin.
SP: Irritation, sensitisation, discontinue; avoid sudden discontinuation (rebound phenomenon). Use in children or on face, max. 5 days. Not for ophthalmic use (eyelids) or on ulcerated skin. Psoriasis, supervise.
Notes: See 10.4 Topical Corticosteroids.
  Elocon Cream, Ointment, Scalp App *(MSD)* A. GMS.
  Price, cream (30g) €3.53; (100g) €16.20. Ointment (30g) €3.76. Scalp App (30mL) €3.84.
  Topical cream, mometasone furoate 0.1% w/w (equiv. 1mg/g). White (off-white) smooth homogenous. *Hydrogenated soya phosphatidylcholine.*
  Topical ointment, as above. White (off-white) opaque. *Propylene glycol stearate.*
  Scalp application, as above. Colourless (light-yellow) smooth viscous soln. *Propylene glycol.*

10.5 - Eczema, Psoriasis, Scalp Disorders

In This Chapter: *Acitretin, calcipotriol, calcitriol, ciclopirox olamine, coal tar and combinations, dithranol, selenium sulphide, mTOR inhibitor (tacrolimus), tazarotene.*

Class Effects

Topical corticosteroids are used to treat psoriasis. Severe, where conventional treatment (not getting response, not tolerated, contraindicated), drugs used to suppress the rheumatic disease process and immunosuppressants are used. See Notes below.
CI: Hypersensitivity to any member of the class.
SP: Avoid contact with eyes, if contact occurs rinse thoroughly with water; for external use only (all shampoos). Do not use undiluted (bath additives).
Notes: See 10.4 Topical Corticosteroids. See also 4.4.1 Drugs Suppressing Rheumatic Disease Process.

Acitretin

ATC Code: D05BB02. **Sport:** Permitted.
Driving: Caution. Decreased night vision.
Indications: Psoriasis, severe extensive, palmo-plantar pustular. Severe, congenital ichthyosis, Darier's disease (keratosis follicularis), lichen planus.
Dose: Adult, Elderly: Initially 25-30mg/day (2-4 weeks); then range 25-50mg/day (6-8 weeks); max. 75mg/day. *Darier's disease*, initially 10mg; increase cautiously; *severe congenital ichthyosis*, Darier's disease, lichen planus may require treatment longer than 3 months; use lowest effective dose (max. 50mg/day). Oral, once daily with meals or with milk.
Child: If benefit outweighs risk. Usually 0.5mg/kg/day; up to 1mg/kg/day may be needed; max. 35mg/day.
Renal Impairment: Not recommended.
Hepatic Impairment: As for Renal above.
CI: Chronic elevated blood lipids, retinoid hypersensitivity.
Interactions: Effect of Other Drugs on Acitretin: *Co-admin not recommended:-* Tetracyclines (intracranial hypertension); methotrexate (hepatitis), other retinoids or preparations containing high doses of Vitamin A (hypervitaminosis A).

SP: Highly TERATOGENIC. Blood donation not recommended during treatment or for 1 year after. Stop keratolytics before initiation; topical corticosteroids or emollients may be used. *Regular examination* (skeletal hyperostosis, extraosseous calcification) with long-term treatment. Monitor, hepatic function, fasting serum cholesterol, triglycerides, blood sugar. *Warn patients of signs/symptoms of benign intracranial hypertension* (severe headache, nausea, vomiting, visual disturbance). Conjunctivitis or xeophthalmia (due to conjunctival dryness), intolerance to contact lenses. Decreased night vision. Alopecia. Avoid excessive sun exposure.

Pregnancy, Lactation: Highly TERATOGENIC. Not recommended in pregnancy, or women who may become pregnant during or within 2 years of finishing treatment. Lactation, not recommended. For oral contraception, combined oestrogen-progesterone formulation recommended.

ADR: *Very common*, paronychia, dry eyes, nasal dryness, epistaxis, rhinitis, dry mouth, thirst, dysgeusia, dry lips, cheilitis, dry skin, erythema, pruritus, alopecia, skin exfoliation, skin atrophy, increased (blood cholesterol, triglycerides), abnormal LFTs.

Notes: See 10.5 Eczema, Psoriasis, Scalp Disorders. See 10.1.5 Oral Acne Treatments (isotretinoin).

Neotigason 10mg, 25mg *(TEVA)* A. GMS.
Price, (60) 10mg, €33.86. 25mg, €78.62.
Capsule, acitretin. Hard. Marked Roche on both cap and body. 10mg: Brown/white. 25mg: Brown/yellow. *Glucose*. NOTE: Supply Neotigason Patient Information Leaflets to patients. **Store:** Below 25 deg C; original pack to protect (moisture).

Calcipotriol

ATC Code: D05AX02. **Sport:** Permitted.
Driving: Unlikely to impair.
Indications: Severe plaque psoriasis vulgaris.

Dose: Adult, Elderly: Apply once or twice daily; max. 100g/week (4-8 weeks). *Combination*, calcipotriol once daily (morning) with topical steroid (evening).

Child: Apply twice daily. Over 12 years, max. 75g/week; 6-12 years, max. 50g/week.

Renal Impairment: Severe, not recommended.

Hepatic Impairment: As for Renal above.

CI: Calcium metabolism disorders.

Interactions: Effect of Other Drugs on Calcipotriol: *Co-admin may cause inactivation*: Salicylic acid.

SP: Not for use on face. Hypercalcaemia if max. weekly dose exceeded (calcipotriol 5mg/week). Limit or avoid excessive exposure to sunlight; use with UV radiation (risk/benefit). Avoid use in guttate, erythrodermic, exfoliative, pustular psoriasis.

Pregnancy, Lactation: Pregnancy, only if clearly necessary. Lactation, not recommended.

ADR: *Most frequent*, skin irritation, pruritus, erythema. See SP above.

Notes: See 10.5 Eczema, Psoriasis, Scalp Disorders and 10.4 Topical Corticosteroids (used in combination).

Dovonex Cream, Ointment *(LEO)* A. GMS.
Price, cream (30g) €9.87; ointment (60g) €15.16.
Topical cream, calcipotriol hydrate 50mcg/g. Soft white. Cetostearyl alcohol.
Topical ointment, as above. Off-white (yellowish-white) translucent. Propylene glycol.

Calcitriol (topical)

ATC Code: D05AX03. **Sport:** Permitted.
Driving: Unlikely to impair.
Indications: Treatment, mild to moderately severe plaque psoriasis (psoriasis vulgaris).

Dose: Adult, Elderly: Apply twice daily; max. 30g/day; treated area max. 35% of body surface to be treated.

Child: No experience.

Renal Impairment: Not recommended.

Hepatic Impairment: Not recommended.

CI: Systemic treatment of calcium homeostasis, hypercalcaemia, abnormal calcium metabolism.

Interactions: Effect of Other Drugs on Calcitriol: *Co-admin caution*: Thiazides (increased calcium levels), calcium supplements, Vitamin D (high dose). *Additive irritant effect*: Peeling agents, astringents, irritants.

SP: Apply to face with caution (increased irritation risk); avoid contact with eyes. Do not add substances stimulating absorption to ointment; occlusive dressing not recommended; increased absorption may lead to systemic side effects (increased urinary and serum calcium). Severe irritation or contact allergy, discontinue.

Pregnancy, Lactation: Pregnancy, use in restricted amount only if clearly necessary; monitor calcium levels. Lactation, not recommended.

ADR: *Common*, pruritus, skin discomfort/irritation, erythema.

Notes: See 10.5 Eczema, Psoriasis, Scalp Disorders.

Silkis Ointment *(Galderma)* A. GMS.
Price, (100g) €24.67.
Topical ointment, calcitriol 3mcg/g. White translucent.

Ciclopirox Olamine

ATC Code: D01AE14. **Sport:** Permitted.
Driving: Unlikely to impair.
Indications: Scalp disorders including dandruff, seborrhoeic dermatitis.

Dose: Adult, Elderly: Use 2-3 times weekly or as required; apply to wet hair, massage vigorously into scalp, rinse and repeat. Shampoo to remain in contact with scalp for 3-5 minutes over 2 applications. Recommended treatment duration 4 weeks.

Child: Under 12 years, no data.

Pregnancy, Lactation: Pregnancy, no effects anticipated. Lactation, ensure residual product washed off breast before breastfeeding.

ADR: *Common*, application site irritation (pruritus, burning sensation, erythema, rash).

Notes: See 10.5 Eczema, Psoriasis, Scalp Disorders.

Stieprox 15mg/g Shampoo *(Stiefel)* B. GMS.
Price, (100mL) €6.54.
Shampoo, ciclopirox olamine. Clear straw (light-orange) viscous. Dipropylene glycol.

Coal Tar

ATC Code: D05AA. **Sport:** Permitted.
Driving: Unlikely to impair.
Indications: Psoriasis of skin, scalp *(Exorex Lotion)*. Sub-acute, chronic psoriasis *(Psoriderm Bath, Cream)*, of scalp *(Scalp Lotion)*.

Dose: Adult: Apply a thin layer 2-3 times daily, massage gently, let dry. Add 30mL to bath, soak for 5 minutes, pat dry *(Psoriderm Bath)*. Apply to affected area once or twice daily *(Psoriderm Cream)*. Shampoo, wet hair, apply to scalp and massage to rich lather; retain on scalp for few minutes. Rinse and repeat.

Elderly: Dilute emulsion before applying *(Exorex Lotion)*.

Child: As for Adult; *Exorex Lotion*, as for Elderly above.

CI: Presence of folliculitis, acne vulgaris, disease characterised by photosensitivity (lupus erythematosus, sunlight allergy) *(Exorex Lotion)*. Not for application to inflamed or broken skin, open exuding wounds, infection of skin. Acute, sore or pustular psoriasis.

SP: May cause skin irritation, discontinue; photosensitivity enhanced, avoid sun exposure after application; avoid eyes and mucous membranes; not for application to rectal or genital areas; application to face, caution.

Pregnancy, Lactation: No specific safety data; been used

10.5   Eczema, Psoriasis, Scalp Disorders

topically without adverse effects; use intermittently, at low concentration, on small body area; first trimester, avoid.

ADR: Skin irritation, photosensitivity, acne-like eruptions, increased skin cancer risk (psoriatics treated with coal tar and UVB radiation). Excipient hypersensitivity.

Notes: See 10.5 Eczema, Psoriasis, Scalp Disorders.

Exorex 5% Lotion *(Forest)* OTC. GMS.
Price, (100mL) €12.53. (250mL) €25.06.
Cutaneous emulsion, coal tar 5% v/w. Smooth mustard-coloured. *Parabens, castor oil.*

Psoriderm Bath, Cream *(Dermal)* OTC. GMS.
Price, (200mL) bath €3.77. (225mL) cream €4.28.
Bath additive, coal tar 40% (w/v). Buff-coloured liquid.
Cream, coal tar 6%, lecithin 0.4% (w/w). Buff-coloured smooth.

Psoriderm Scalp *(Dermal)* OTC.
Price, not published by company (250mL).
Shampoo, coal tar 2.5%, lecithin 0.3% (w/v). Golden-brown foaming.

Coal Tar, Salicylic Acid

ATC Code: D05AA. **Sport:** Permitted.
Driving: Unlikely to impair.

Indications: Scaly skin disorders of scalp (psoriasis, eczema, seborrhoeic dermatitis, dandruff, cradle cap in children). May also be used to remove previous scalp applications.

Dose: Adult, Elderly: Wet hair thoroughly, massage a small amount of shampoo into scalp, leave for few minutes, wash out. Repeat. Rinse hair well and dry.

Child: As for Adult above.

Pregnancy, Lactation: See Notes below.

Notes: See Coal Tar above. See 10.5 Eczema, Psoriasis, Scalp Disorders.

Capasal Therapeutic Shampoo *(Dermal)* OTC.
Price, not published by company (100mL, 250mL).
Shampoo, coal tar 1%, salicylic acid 0.5%, coconut oil 1% (w/v). Golden-brown foaming.

Coal Tar, Salicylic Acid, Sulphur

ATC Code: D05AA. **Sport:** Permitted.
Driving: Unlikely to impair.

Indications: Scaly skin disorders of scalp (psoriasis, eczema, seborrhoeic dermatitis, dandruff).

Dose: Adult, Elderly: Mild dandruff, apply once weekly. Psoriasis, eczema, seborrhoeic dermatitis, severe dandruff, use daily for 3-7 days until improvement; then use intermittently.

Child: Age 6-12 years, only with medical supervision.

CI: Sulphur, salicylate hypersensitivity. Acute local infection, pustular psoriasis.

SP: Not for use on broken or inflamed skin. If irritation develops, discontinue. May stain fabric and jewellery.

Pregnancy, Lactation: Not recommended.

ADR: Bronchospasm.

Notes: See Coal Tar above. See 10.5 Eczema, Psoriasis, Scalp Disorders.

Cocois Ointment *(Recipharm)* OTC. GMS.
Price, (40g) €5.32. (100g) €10.20.
Topical ointment, coal tar 12%, salicylic acid 2%, sulphur 4% w/w. *Cetostearyl alcohol.*

Dithranol

ATC Code: D05AC01. **Sport:** Permitted.
Driving: Unlikely to impair.

Indications: Subacute and chronic psoriasis including scalp (0.1%, 0.25%); patients failing to respond (0.5%-2%).

Dose: Adult, Elderly: Initially 0.1% (1 week); if needed, increase gradually over 4 weeks to highest tolerated strength; apply once every 24 hours. Either apply and then wash off up to 1 hour after application OR apply at night and wash off in morning. Scalp, comb hair to remove scalar debris and apply; shampoo may be used to remove *Dithrocream* residue; ensure it does not get into eyes.

294

Child: Use cautiously with supervision.

CI: Acute pustular psoriasis, application to face.

SP: Burning on application, if lesions spread, discontinue, re-evaluate dose. Not for use on skin folds. Avoid eyes, mucous membranes. Allow 1-week interval between steroid discontinuation and dithranol initiation. May stain fabrics, plastics, skin, hair.

Pregnancy, Lactation: No adverse effects reported.

ADR: Some skin irritation and/or feeling of warmth when applied; may induce burning sensation if strength too high or left in contact with skin too long.

Notes: See 10.5 Eczema, Psoriasis, Scalp Disorders.

Dithrocream *(Dermal)* B. GMS.
Price, (50g) 0.1%, €5.09. 0.25%, €5.45. 2%, €9.15.
Topical cream, dithranol. Pale-yellow. *Cetostearyl alcohol, chlorocresol.*

Selenium Sulphide

ATC Code: D11AC03. **Sport:** Permitted.
Driving: Unlikely to impair.

Indications: Simple dandruff, seborrhoeic dermatitis of scalp.

Dose: Adult, Elderly: Wet hair thoroughly, massage shampoo to form lather; leave for 2-3 minutes, rinse. Use twice weekly (2 weeks), then once weekly (2 weeks) to control condition, then as needed.

Child: Age 5-14 years, as for Adult; under 5 years, not recommended.

CI: Use on broken or severely inflamed skin.

SP: Remove gold, silver, metallic jewellery before using (discolouration). Keep out of eyes. Do not leave in contact with hair/scalp for longer than recommended (burning, blistering). Rinse thoroughly from hair before dying, tinting or permanent waving; do not apply for 2 days before or after any of these procedures.

Pregnancy, Lactation: Avoid.

ADR: Irritation, sensitisation, burning. Increased hair loss, hair discolouration. Oiliness or hair dryness may occur. Allergic reactions.

Notes: See 10.5 Eczema, Psoriasis, Scalp Disorders.

Selsun Shampoo *(SANOFI)* OTC.
Price, not published by company (50mL, 100mL).
Shampoo, selenium disulphide 2.5% (w/v). Beige (pale-yellow to orange) uniform susp.

Tacrolimus (topical)

ATC Code: D11AH01. **Sport:** Permitted.
Driving: Unlikely to impair.

Indications: Treatment, moderate to severe atopic dermatitis (not adequately responsive or intolerant of conventional treatment). Prevention of flares and prolongation of flare-free intervals where there was initial response to max. 6 weeks treatment.

Dose: Adult, Elderly: *Flares,* initially apply twice daily (0.1%) until cleared, then switch to maintenance; *recurrence,* restart with twice daily (0.1%) then reduce frequency or strength. *Maintenance,* apply once a day twice weekly (2-3 days between applications). Use short- or intermittent long-term treatment; not for continuous use.

Child: Age 16 years and above, as for Adult above. *Flares,* age 2 years and above, initiate twice daily with 0.03% for up to 3 weeks; then once daily until lesions clear. *Recurrence, maintenance,* as for Adult above using 0.03%.

Interactions: Effect of Other Drugs on Tacrolimus: *Co-admin not recommended:* Emollients (allow 2-hour interval); other topicals, systemic steroids, immunosuppressives (no data), live or live-attenuated vaccines (vaccine failure, risk). *Co-admin caution:* CYP3A4 inhibitors (erythromycin, itraconazole, ketoconazole, diltiazem).

SP: Minimise exposure to sunlight; avoid combination use (solarium UV light, UVA or UVB therapy); use sunscreen, protective clothing. Not for application to potentially malignant or pre-malignant lesions. Skin barrier defects (Netherton's syndrome, lamellar ichthyosis, generalised erythroderma, cutaneous Graft vs. Host disease), not recommended (increased systemic absorption). Lymphadenopathy (usually infection-related), lymphoma, cutaneous malignancies. Avoid contact with eyes, mucous membranes; can be applied on any other part of body including face, neck, flexure areas. Caution, use on extensive area over extended time (especially children). Any new change in treated area (different from previous eczema), review.

Pregnancy, Lactation: Not recommended unless clearly necessary.

ADR: *Very common*, application site burning/pruritus.

Notes: See 10.5 Eczema, Psoriasis, Scalp Disorders.

> **Protopic Ointment** *(LEO)* A. GMS.
> *Price*, 0.03% (30g) €24.88; (60g) €48.13. 0.1% (30g) €27.62; (60g) €53.12.
> *Topical ointment*, tacrolimus monohydrate 0.03%, 0.1%. White (slightly) yellowish.

Tazarotene

ATC Code: D05AX05. **Sport:** Permitted.
Driving: Unlikely to impair.

Indications: Mild to moderate plaque psoriasis up to 10% body surface area (BSA).

Dose: Adult, Elderly: Age 18 years and over, initially, use 0.05% to evaluate skin response/tolerance before using 0.1%. Apply thin film of gel once daily (evening); avoid surrounding healthy skin or skin folds (may be covered with zinc paste). Use an emollient adjunctive for improved tolerability. Duration usually 12 weeks.

CI: Treatment, psoriasis pustulosa and psoriasis exfoliativa; application to intertriginous areas, face or hair-covered scalp.

Interactions: Effect of Other Drugs on Tazarotene: *Co-admin (no data)*: Other antipsoriatic agents (including tar shampoos). *Avoid (altered absorption)*: Allow 1-hour interval before emollient/cosmetic application.

SP: Avoid facial skin, eyes. Irritation, interrupt treatment. Avoid excessive UV exposure. Use with occlusion, no data.

Pregnancy, Lactation: Pregnancy, contraindicated; exclude prior to initiation. Women of child-bearing potential should be warned of potential risk and should use adequate contraception; if patient becomes pregnant during treatment, discontinue and warn of potential risk to foetus. Lactation, not recommended.

ADR: Pruritus, burning, erythema, dermatitis, skin pain, worsening psoriasis, skin discolouration.

Notes: See 10.5 Eczema, Psoriasis, Scalp Disorders.

> **Zorac 0.05%, 0.1% Gel** *(Allergan)* B. GMS.
> *Price*, 0.05% (30g) €16.79; (60g) €23.02. 0.1% (30g) €17.74; (60g) €24.21.
> *Topical gel*, tazarotene. Colourless (light-yellow) translucent (cloudy) homogenous. *Butylhydroxyanisole, butylhydroxytoluene.*

10.6 - Warts, Corns, Calluses

In This Chapter: *Green tea extract, imiquimod, salicylic acid, lactic acid and combinations, podophyllotoxin, podophyllum resin.*

Class Effects

Imiquimod is also indicated for the treatment of actinic keratosis. For other drugs used for actinic keratosis, see Notes below.

CI: Hypersensitivity to any member of the class.

SP: Avoid application to healthy skin. Avoid eyes, mucous membranes. Not for application to broken or inflamed skin.

Pregnancy, Lactation: Generally no special precautions unless otherwise specified.

ADR: Excessive irritation, discontinue.

Notes: See 10.1.6 Photodamage, Actinic Keratosis.

Green Tea Extract

ATC Code: D06BB12. **Sport:** Permitted.
Driving: Unlikely to affect.

Indications: Cutaneous treatment, external genital and perianal warts in immunocompetent patients.

Dose: Adult, Elderly: Apply up to 250mg ointment (total single dose) 3-times daily to all external genital and perianal warts; total 750mg/day. Max. 16 weeks. Avoid application into vagina, urethra or anus.

Child: Under 18 years, no data.

Hepatic Impairment: Severe, not recommended (insufficient data).

Interactions: Effect of Other Drugs on Green Tea Extract: *Co-admin avoid*: Other local treatments, high-dose oral green tea extracts.

SP: Do not apply to mucous membranes (eyes, nostrils, lips, mouth), open wounds, broken or inflamed skin. Wash ointment off treated area before sexual activity; may weaken condoms, vaginal diaphragms. Insert tampons prior to application. Avoid occlusive dressings. Ointment stains clothing and bedding. Intense local skin reactions, interrupt treatment.

Pregnancy, Lactation: Pregnancy, avoid. Lactation, no effect on newborn/infant expected.

ADR: Summary, *most frequency*, local skin and application site reactions.

Notes: See 10.6 Warts, Corns, Calluses.

> **Catephen 10% Ointment** *(KoRa)* A. GMS.
> *Price*, (15g) €46.00.
> *Ointment*, green tea extract 100mg/g equiv. to 55-72mg epigallocatechingallate. *Propylene glycol, isopropyl myristate.*

Imiquimod

ATC Code: D06BB10. **Sport:** Permitted.
Driving: No or negligible effect.

Indications: Topical treatment, external genital, perianal warts (condylomata acuminata), small superficial basal cell carcinomas (sBCCs) *(Aldara)*. Non- (hyperkeratotic, hypertrophic) actinic keratosis (AK) on face or balding scalp *(Zyclara)*.

Dose: Adult, Elderly: *Aldara*, external genital warts, AK, apply 3-times weekly*; genital warts max. 16 weeks per episode; actinic keratosis, 4 weeks, max. 8 weeks. sBCCs, apply 5-times weekly for 6 weeks.

Zyclara, AK, apply once daily* before bedtime for 2 treatment cycles of 2-weeks separated by 2-weeks of no-treatment. Do not occlude. *Leave on for 8 hours then remove with soap and water.

Child: Under 18 years, not recommended.

Renal Impairment: Monitor under close supervision.

Hepatic Impairment: As for Renal above.

Interactions: Effect of Other Drugs on Imiquimod: *Caution*: Use with immunosuppressives.

SP: Avoid contact with eyes, lips, nostrils. Potential to exacerbate inflammatory conditions. Autoimmune conditions (worsening), organ transplantation (rejection, GVHD), reduced haematological reserve, caution (weigh risk/benefit). Do not use on broken skin (or not healed after previous treatment) or with occlusive dressing. Uncircumcised males treating warts under foreskin, retract foreskin, wash area daily; local skin reaction, rest period of several days. Actinic keratosis, protect skin from solar exposure.

Pregnancy, Lactation: Pregnancy, caution, weigh risk benefit. Lactation, stop breastfeeding or stop drug.

10.7   Scabies, Head Lice

ADR: *Most frequent* application site pruritus/pain *(Aldara)*; erythema, scab, skin (exfoliation, oedema, ulcer, hypopigmentation), application site reactions *(Zyclara)*.

Notes: See 10.6 Warts, Corns, Calluses.

> **Aldara 5% Cream** *(Meda)* B. GMS.
> *Price,* sachets 5% (12) €76.66.
> *Topical cream,* imiquimod. White (slightly yellow). *Parabens, cetostearyl/cetyl alcohol.* **Store:** Below 25 deg C; do not re-use sachets once opened.
>
> **Zyclara 3.75% Cream** *(Meda)* B. GMS.
> *Price,* sachets 3.75% (28) €130.39.
> *Topical cream,* imiquimod. White (slightly yellow). *Parabens, cetyl/stearyl alcohol.*

Podophyllotoxin

ATC Code: D06BB04. **Sport:** Permitted.
Driving: No effect.

Indications: Condylomata acuminata (warts), affecting penis or female external genitalia.

Dose: Adult, Elderly: Apply twice daily (3 consecutive days); repeat weekly, max. 5 weeks *(Condyline),* max. 4 weeks *(Warticon).* Admin, avoid normal adjacent tissue; treat only a small area/number of warts at any one time.

Child: Not recommended, under 18 years *(Warticon),* under 12 years *(Condyline).*

CI: Co-admin with other podophyllotoxin containing preparations, inflamed/bleeding lesions, open wounds.

SP: Avoid contact with healthy skin, face, eyes (severe irritation). Systemic toxicity risk (treatment of large areas, excessive use, prolonged periods; friable, bleeding, recently removed warts; use on normal skin/mucous membranes). Do not use occlusive dressings.

Pregnancy, Lactation: Pregnancy, not recommended *(Warticon);* contraindicated *(Condyline).* Lactation, stop treatment or stop breastfeeding.

ADR: Skin erosion, local irritation (itching burning, pain, erythema, epithelial ulceration), balanoposthitis.

Notes: See 10.6 Warts, Corns, Calluses.

> **Condyline Cutaneous Soln** *(Takeda)* B. GMS.
> *Price,* (3.5mL) €16.52.
> *Cutaneous soln,* podophyllotoxin 0.5% w/v. Clear colourless alcoholic; with applicators.
>
> **Warticon 0.15% Cream** *(Stiefel)* B. GMS.
> *Price,* (5g) €20.62.
> *Topical cream,* podophyllotoxin 0.15% w/w. Homogenous white. *Parabens, cetyl/stearyl alcohol, butylhydroxyanisole, sorbic acid.*

10.7 - Scabies, Head Lice

In This Chapter: *Crotamiton, malathion, permethrin, phenothrin.*

Class Effects
Phenothrin is also used to treat head lice and pubic lice.

CI: Hypersensitivity to any member of the class.

SP: Scabies treatment should be accompanied by change of clothes and bedding; all contacts should be treated. With both scabies and lice all members of the household should be treated preferably simultaneously.

Crotamiton

ATC Code: D04AX, P03AX. **Sport:** Permitted.
Driving: No influence.

Indications: Treatment, scabies, pediculosis. Management of pruritus of any aetiology.

Dose: Adult, Elderly: *Pruritus,* apply 2-3 times daily.

Scabies, bath thoroughly, apply to all areas below chin, particular attention to interdigital areas; repeat after 24 hours; bath a day after.

Child: Can be used in children; infants, consult medical advice.

CI: Acute exudative dermatoses.

SP: For external use only. Do not use on buccal mucosa, in or around eyes, exudative wounds, acute eczema, broken or very inflamed skin. Genital itching, consult doctor or pharmacist before use.

Pregnancy, Lactation: No evidence of risk during pregnancy. Lactation, do not apply to nipple area.

ADR: Inflammation of conjunctiva (if used near eyes), local skin irritation.

Notes: See 10.7 Scabies, Head Lice.

> **Eurax Cream** *(GSK Consumer)* OTC.
> *Price,* (30g) €3.25. (100g) €5.63.
> *Topical cream,* crotamiton. White (cream-coloured); characteristic perfume. *Parabens, stearyl alcohol.*

Malathion

ATC Code: P03AX03. **Sport:** Permitted.
Driving: Unlikely to impair.

Indications: Head lice, pubic lice, scabies.

Dose: Adult, Elderly: *Lice, head,* apply liberally and leave to dry naturally; shampoo out after 12 hours; *pubic,* apply to whole body, allow to dry; wash off after 12 hours.

Scabies, apply over whole body and leave for 24 hours; wash off.

Child: Under 6 months, only with medical supervision.

SP: Avoid contact with eyes. Not for use on broken skin, local infection. Alcoholic lotions not recommended for head lice in severe eczema, asthma or young children or for scabies or crab lice. Not for prolonged use; max. once per week for 3 consecutive weeks.

Pregnancy, Lactation: Not recommended.

ADR: Local irritation.

Notes: See 10.7 Scabies, Head Lice.

> **Derbac-M Lotion** *(SSL)* OTC. GMS.
> *Price,* 200mL, €5.45. 50mL, €2.17.
> *Topical lotion,* malathion 0.5%.

Permethrin

ATC Code: P03AC04. **Sport:** Permitted.
Driving: Unlikely to impair.

Indications: Pubic lice, scabies *(Dermal),* head lice *(Creme Rinse).*

Dose: Adult, Elderly: *Lyclear Dermal Cream, scabies,* apply to whole body excluding head; up to one 30g tube as a single application; wash thoroughly after 8-12 hours. If needed a second application may be made after not less than 14 days. *Elderly,* as for Adult; face, ears and scalp should also be treated; avoid skin around eyes.

Pubic lice, up to one third (10g) sufficient to treat pubic region, peri-anal region, thighs and trunk. Wash after 8 hours but before 24 hours after application. Re-treat after 7 days if needed. *Elderly,* over 70 years, use with medical supervision.

Lyclear Cream Rinse, head lice, shampoo and towel dry hair, apply enough cream rinse to saturate hair and scalp, leave for 10 minutes, rinse thoroughly; dry in usual way. Not necessary to remove nits except for cosmetic purposes using a fine-toothed comb. *Elderly,* suitable for use.

Child: *Lyclear Dermal,* scabies, age 2 months to 5 years, up to 7.5g (1/4 of 30g tube); age 6-12 years, 15g (half 30g tube); age 12 years and over, as for Adult above; under 2 years, safety/efficacy not established. Pubic lice, under 18 years, seek medical advice before using product. *Lyclear Creme Rinse,* head lice, over 6 months, as for Adult above.

CI: Hypersensitivity to permethrin, pyrethrin group of substances and excipients (chrysanthemums).

SP: Avoid eyes, mucous membranes (nasopharyngeal space, genital area), open wounds. *(Dermal Cream),* children age 2-23 months, limited experience; use with close medical supervision. Direct contacts should be treated. *(Creme Rinse)*, under 6 months, use with medical advice.

Pregnancy, Lactation: Pregnancy and when breastfeeding, use permethrin only after consultation with healthcare professional.

ADR: *Common*, paraesthesia, skin burning sensation, pruritus, erythematous rash, dry skin.

Notes: See 10.7 Scabies, Head Lice.

Lyclear Dermal Cream *(Chefaro)* OTC. GMS.
Price, (30g) €6.39.
Topical cream, permethrin 5% w/w. White (off-white). *Formaldehyde, butylhydroxytoluene.* **Store:** Below 25 deg C; outer carton.
Lyclear Creme Rinse *(Chefaro)* OTC.
Price, not published by company.
Cutaneous soln, permethrin. Orange-coloured. *Parabens, cetyl alcohol, propylene glycol.*

10.8 - Miscellaneous Dermatologicals

In This Chapter: *Aluminium salts, eflomithine, minoxidil.*

Class Effects
CI: Hypersensitivity to any member of the class.

Aluminium (dermatology)
ATC Code: D11AA. **Sport:** Permitted.
Driving: None known.

Indications: Topical treatment of hyperhidrosis (axillae, hands, feet).

Dose: Adult, Elderly: Apply to affected sites at night as required and allow to dry. Wash off in morning.

SP: Do not use in axillae within 12 hours of using depilatories or shaving or immediately after bathing. Avoid direct contact with clothing, polished surfaces, jewellery, metal.

Pregnancy, Lactation: No special precautions.

ADR: Irritation is applied too frequent.

Notes: See 10.8 Miscellaneous Dermatologicals.

Anhydrol Forte *(Dermal)* OTC.
Price, not published by company (60mL).
Cutaneous soln, aluminium chloride hexahydrate 20% (w/v). Clear colourless evaporative soln.

Eflornithine
ATC Code: D11AX16. **Sport:** Permitted.
Driving: No or negligible effect.
Indications: Facial hirsutism in women.

Dose: Adult, Elderly: Apply thin layer of cream twice daily; rub in thoroughly; do not wash off within 4 hours of application. Max. 30g per month.

Child: Under 18 years, no safety/efficacy data.

Renal Impairment: Severe, caution.

SP: Cosmetics may be applied over area after 5 minutes; following hair removal, wait 5 minutes before applying. Consider underlying cause of excessive hair growth before initiation. Avoid contact with eyes, mucous membranes. If applied to broken or abraded skin, transient stinging, burning. Irritation or intolerance, reduce application frequency.

Pregnancy, Lactation: Pregnancy, use alternative method to manage facial hair. Lactation, not recommended.

ADR: *Very common*, acne. *Common*, pseudofolliculitis barbae, alopecia, stinging, burning, tingling or dry skin, pruritus, erythema, irritated skin, folliculitis.

Notes: See 10.8 Miscellaneous Dermatologicals.

Vaniqa Cream *(Almirall)* A. GMS.
Price, (30g) €32.16. (60g) €66.79.
Topical cream, eflornithine HCl 115mg/g. White (off-white). *Cetostearyl/stearyl alcohol, parabens.*

Minoxidil (topical)
ATC Code: D11AX01. **Sport:** Permitted.
Driving: Unlikely to impair.

Indications: Slowing of hair loss and/or regrowth in alopecia androgenetica (adults over 18 years).

Dose: Adult, Elderly: Age 18-65 years, hair and scalp to be thoroughly dry; apply 1mL to total affected scalp area twice daily; max. 2mL/day; continuous use required to maintain results. Application method depends on applicator. *Elderly* over 65 years, children under 18 years, no data.

CI: Hypertension, scalp abnormality (psoriasis, sunburn, shaved scalp), occlusive dressing, application of other topical medication.

Interactions: Effect of Other Drugs on Minoxidil (topical): *Increased systemic absorption*: Dithranol, tretinoin, drugs altering stratum corneum barrier.

SP: Systemic effects (prolonged or excessive use); increased if applied to shaved or abraded skin, or dermatoses. Hair colour or texture change. Avoid contact with eyes, mucous membranes, abraded or broken skin. Avoid inhalation. Hypotension, chest pain, rapid heartbeat, faintness/dizziness, sudden unexplained weight gain, swollen hands/feet, persistent redness or irritation of scalp, discontinue.

Pregnancy, Lactation: Not recommended.

ADR: *Very common*, headache.

Notes: See 10.8 Miscellaneous Dermatologicals.

Regaine Extra Strength 5% *(McNeil)* OTC.
Price, not published by company (soln 60mL, foam 60mg).
Cutaneous soln, minoxidil 50mg/mL. Clear colourless (light-yellow) odourless. *Propylene glycol.* **Store:** Below 25 deg C; flammable.

10.9 - Wound Care

In This Chapter: *Collagenase (clostridiopeptidase A).*

Class Effects
CI: Hypersensitivity to any member of the class.

Clostridiopeptidase A
ATC Code: D03BA02 **Sport:** Permitted.
Driving: Unlikely to affect.

Indications: Enzymatic debridement of necrotising wounds, including leg and decubital ulcers.

Dose: Adult, Elderly: Apply approx. 2mm of ointment to dressing or directly to slightly moistened area, once daily (twice daily may be needed). Ensure close contact with wound surface; sufficient moisture must be present. Protect wound edges and healthy skin to avoid irritation.

Interactions: Effect of Other Drugs on Collagenase: *Not for co-admin*: Tyrothricin, gramicidin, tetracycline. *Collagenase activity inhibited*: Antiseptics, heavy metals, detergents, soap.

SP: Avoid contact with eyes/mucosa. In diabetics, dry gangrene should be moistened with caution to avoid conversion to moist gangrene. If reduction in necrotic tissue not observed within 14 days, discontinue. Can be used with silver and silver sulfadiazine.

Pregnancy, Lactation: Pregnancy, use in first trimester only when strictly indicated. Lactation, excretion into breast milk unlikely.

ADR: Local pain, pruritus, burning, erythema.

Notes: See 10.9 Wound Care.

Iruxol Mono Ointment *(Smith&Nephew)* B. GMS.
Price, (20g) €9.04.
Ointment, clostridiopeptidase A 1.2 units/g. Brown lipophilic with faint odour.

297

11

Endocrinology

11.1 - Systemic Corticosteroids

Class Effects

Steroids synthesised by the adrenal cortex can be divided into two groups i.e. corticosteroids (glucocorticoids, mineralocorticoids) and sex corticoids.

11.1.1 - Glucocorticoids

In This Chapter: *Dexamethasone, hydrocortisone, methylprednisolone and combinations, prednisolone, triamcinolone.*

Class Effects

Driving: Glucocorticoids may cause mood changes (euphoria, depression) or visual disturbances; if affected, exercise caution when driving or operating machinery. Convulsions possible after corticosteroid treatment.

Sport: Glucocorticoids are prohibited and require a TUE when used orally, rectally, or by IV or IM injection; admin by all other routes do not require a TUE. When described as Restricted, these products contain substance(s) which may be either 'Prohibited (in-competition) and require TUE or are 'Permitted' for use depending on route of admin.

CI: Untreated systemic infection (acute, viral, fungal, parasitic). Hypersensitivity to any member of the class.

Interactions: Effect of Other Drugs on Corticosteroids: *Co-admin contraindicated:* Live vaccines. *Enhanced metabolism (reduced effect):* CYP3A4 inducers (rifampicin, rifabutin, carbamazepine, phenobarbitone, phenytoin, primidone, aminoglutethimide, ephedrine, mifepristone). *Co-admin caution:* Fluoroquinolones (increased tendon rupture risk). *Increased plasma levels :* CYP3A4 inhibitors including ketoconazole, itraconazole, clotrimazole, erythromycin, clarithromycin, telithromycin, ethinyloestradiol, other oral contraceptives, ritonavir (metabolism reduced, caution), atazanavir, indinavir, nelfinavir, saquinavir; cobicistat (increased systemic side-effect risk). *Metabolism mutually inhibited:* Ciclosporin (caution, convulsion risk). *Increased GI ulceration risk:* NSAIDs, other ulcerogenic drugs. *Clearance increased or decreased:* Hypo- or hyperthyroid patients (assess thyroid status). *Levels decreased:* Quetiapine.

Effect of Corticosteroids on Other Drugs: Anticholinesterases (use in myasthenia gravis), cholecystographic X-ray media, NSAIDs: *Effect reduced by corticosteroids.* Hypoglycaemic agents (including insulin), anti-hypertensives, diuretics: *Effect antagonised.* Potassium-depleting diuretics (acetazolamide, loop diuretics, thiazides, carbenoxolone): *Hypokalaemic effects enhanced, may result in severe hypokalaemia.* Coumarin anticoagulants: *Effect enhanced, monitor INR.* Salicylates: *Renal clearance increased (caution, salicylate intoxication with steroid withdrawal).* Non-depolarising muscle relaxants: *Prolonged relaxation, acute myopathy.* Digoxin: *Caution, steroid-induced electrolyte disturbances, increased toxicity.* Methotrexate: *Increased haematological toxicity.* Somatropin: *Growth promoting effect inhibited.* Sympathomimetics, high dose (bambuterol, fenoterol, formoterol, ritodrine, salbutamol, salmeterol, terbutaline): *Increased hypokalaemia risk (with high dose corticosteroids).* Tretinoin: *Metabolism enhanced, levels decreased.*

SP: *Dosing/withdrawal,* individualise dose according to (response, disease, severity); use lowest effective dose for shortest duration; withdraw gradually. Rapid withdrawal, can lead to acute adrenal insufficiency, hypotension, death; 'withdrawal syndrome' may occur (fever, myalgia, arthralgia, rhinitis, conjunctivitis, painful itchy skin nodules, weight loss).

Infection, due to reduced (inflammatory response, immune function), increased susceptibility, increased severity (septicaemia, TB may be masked); chickenpox may be fatal (avoid contact with chickenpox, herpes zoster). Avoid exposure to measles; seek medical advice if exposure occurs.

Adrenal suppression, with prolonged use, caution adrenal cortical atrophy (may persist for years after discontinuation); may cause acute adrenocortical insufficiency with circulatory collapse during stress; less when corticosteroid is given as a single dose in morning, or on alternate days or less frequently; re-evaluate dose.

Caution, osteoporosis (post-menopausal females), hypertension, CHF, post MI (myocardial rupture risk), TB (active, restrict to fulminating or disseminated where used adjunctive to TB regimen), myopathy (corticosteroid-induced), liver failure, renal insufficiency, epilepsy, peptic ulcer; diabetes mellitus; glaucoma, ocular herpes simplex (corneal ulceration, perforation). Salt and water retention, increased potassium and calcium excretion; may need dietary salt restriction and potassium supplements. Hypercortisonism (caution, fat embolism). Cerebral malaria, corticosteroids associated with prolongation of coma and higher incidence of pneumonia, GI bleeding. Caution, hypothyroidism, myasthenia gravis; patients predisposed to thromboembolic disorders as thrombosis (including VTE) associated with corticosteroids. Cirrhosis or liver failure (increased blood levels, enhanced effect). Visual disturbances reported (systemic, topical corticosteroid use); blurred vision or other visual disturbances, consider ophthalmologist evaluation for possible causes e.g. cataract, glaucoma or rare diseases such as central serous chorioretinopathy (CSCR) leading to retinal detachment. Reports of epidural lipomatosis (long-term, high doses). May change motility and spermatozoa number. Activation of latent amoebiasis or strongyloidiasis, or exacerbate active disease.

Psychiatric, severe psychiatric reactions may occur with systemic steroids e.g. affective disorders (irritable, euphoric, depressed and labile mood, suicidal thoughts), psychotic reactions (mania, delusions, hallucinations, aggravation of schizophrenia), behavioural disturbances, irritability, anxiety, sleep disturbances, cognitive dysfunction (confusion, amnesia). Dose levels do not allow prediction of reaction (onset, type, severity, duration). Advise patients/carers to seek medical advice if symptoms develop; especially if depressed mood or suicidal ideation suspected.

Special populations, children, dose-related growth retardation (may be irreversible); to minimise HPA-axis suppression and growth retardation, admin single doses on alternate days. More susceptible to systemic toxicity. *Elderly,* adverse events more serious (osteoporosis, hypertension, hypokalaemia, diabetes, infection susceptibility, thinning skin); supervise closely. Patient should carry 'steroid treatment' cards; supply Patient Information Leaflets (PIL).

Pregnancy, Lactation: Pregnancy, if benefit outweighs risk; mothers taking high doses of systemic corticosteroids for prolonged periods, monitor infants for adrenal suppression; cataracts reported in infants. Pre-eclampsia or fluid retention, caution. Corticosteroids cross the placenta; may be a very small risk of cleft palate and intra-uterine growth retardation of foetus. Lactation, advise not to breastfeed; weigh benefit/risk; excreted into breast milk.

ADR: Hypothalamic-pituitary-adrenal (HPA) suppression; depends on drug potency, dose, timing of admin, treatment duration. Endocrine effects include growth suppression, menstrual irregularity, amenorrhoea, Cushingoid face, hirsutism, weight gain, impaired carbohydrate tolerance, negative protein and calcium balance, increased appetite. Increased susceptibility to and severity of infections, suppression of clinical signs and symptoms, dormant TB recurrence.

Osteoporosis, vertebral and long bone fractures, avascular osteonecrosis, tendon rupture, proximal myopathy. Sodium and water retention, hypertension, potassium loss, hypokalaemic alkalosis.

Euphoria, psychological dependence, depression, psychosis, insomnia, aggravation of schizophrenia; increased intra-cranial pressure with papilloedema in children, epilepsy aggravation.

Increased IOP, glaucoma, papilloedema, posterior subcapsular cataracts, corneal or scleral thinning, exacerbation of ophthalmic infection.

Dyspepsia, peptic ulceration with perforation and haemorrhage, acute pancreatitis, candidiasis. Impaired healing, skin atrophy, bruising, telangiectasia, striae, acne. Hypersensitivity including anaphylaxis, leucocytosis, thromboembolism. See SP above.

Notes: See 11.1 Systemic Corticosteroids.

Dexamethasone (systemic)

ATC Code: H02AB02. **Sport:** Prohibited.
Driving: Mood changes, visual disturbances.
Indications: Various inflammatory and autoimmune diseases e.g. rheumatism, collagen disease, allergies, primary and secondary adrenocortical insufficiency, adrenogenital syndromes. Adjunctive, cerebral oedema (not head injury associated), lymphocytic leukaemia, anti-emetic in antineoplastic regimens, palliative in terminal neoplastic disease. Various endocrine and non-endocrine disorders. Diagnostic testing for adrenocortical hyperfunction.

Dose: Adult, Elderly: Usually 0.5-10mg/day *(Dexamethasone 2mg tabs)* OR 0.5-9mg/day *(Dexsol Oral Soln)* depending on severity of condition and patient response. *Admin,* tabs with fluid. Withdrawal after prolonged or repeated use, Tests for Cushing's syndrome, see manufacturers Full Prescribing Information.

Child: Caution, growth retardation; dose to be individually determined. See SP below.

CI: Gastric and duodenal ulcer.

Interactions: Effect of Dexamethasone on Other Drugs: Drugs metabolised by CYP3A4 (indinavir, erythromycin): *Increased clearance, decreased plasma concentrations.*

SP: Evidence suggests long-term neurodevelopmental adverse events after early treatment (under 96 hours) of premature infants with chronic lung disease at starting dose 25mg/kg twice daily. Tumour lysis syndrome (TLS) reported with haematological malignancies; high TLS risk (high proliferative rate, high tumour burden, high sensitivity to cytotoxic agents), monitor.

Glucocorticoids   11.1.1

ADR: The incidence of predictable undesirable effects of glucocorticoids correlates with dosage, timing of admin, treatment duration.

Notes: See 11.1.1 Glucocorticoids.

Dexamethasone 2mg *(Aspen)* A. GMS.
Price, (100) €13.73.
Tablet, dexamethasone. Round flat white. Marked XC/8. *Lactose.*
Store: Below 25 deg C; original pack.
Dexsol Oral Soln *(Fannin)* A. GMS.
Price, 150mL, €46.72.
Oral soln, dexamethasone sodium phosphate. Colourless (faint yellow); mint odour. **Store:** Below 25 deg C; do not refrigerate.

Hydrocortisone (systemic)

ATC Code: H02AB09. **Sport:** Prohibited.
Driving: Side effects may affect ability.
Indications: Replacement therapy (primary, secondary, acute adrenocortical insufficiency), known adrenal insufficiency or doubtful adrenocortical reserve (pre-op, during serious trauma or illness). Conditions requiring rapid and intense corticosteroid effect. Shock secondary to adrenocortical insufficiency.

Dose: Adult, Elderly: *Hydrocortone,* adrenocortical insufficiency, 20-30mg/day OR in combination with 4-6g sodium chloride or 50-300mcg fludrocortisone daily.
Solu-Cortef, rapid corticosteroid effect, IV injection (preferred emergency route) or IV infusion or IM; range 100-500mg by IV injection over 1-10 minutes; repeat at 2, 4 or 6 hour intervals based on response; usually not beyond 48-72 hours (replace with methylprednisolone to minimise sodium retention if needed to be continued).

Child: *Hydrocortone,* adrenocortical insufficiency, 0.4-0.8mg/kg/day in 2-3 divided doses.
Solu-Cortef, not less than 25mg/day based on severity of condition and patient response.

SP: Presence of fungal infection, use only to control life-threatening reactions to amphotericin. Inactivated viral or bacterial vaccines, expected serum antibody response may not be achieved. Rarely, anaphylactic reactions with parenteral corticosteroids.

Notes: See 11.1.1 Glucocorticoids.

Hydrocortone 10mg *(Auden McKenzie)* A. GMS.
Price, (30) €21.60.
Tablet, hydrocortisone. White oval quartersected (facilitates breaking). Marked MSD 619. *Lactose.*
Solu-Cortef Parenteral 100mg *(Pfizer)* A. GMS.
Price, (10) €11.66.
Injection or infusion, hydrocortisone sodium succinate 133.7mg equiv. to hydrocortisone 100mg. White (off-white) powder for soln. *Sodium 10.14mg/vial.*

Methylprednisolone

ATC Code: H02AB04. **Sport:** Restricted.
Driving: Dizziness, vertigo, visual disturbances, fatigue.
Indications: Management, corticosteroid disorders; conditions requiring rapid and intense corticosteroid effect.
Dose: Adult, Elderly: *Depo-Medrone,* usually 20-120mg daily or weekly. Route IM, intra-articular, intralesional, intrarectal, intrabursal, periarticular, into tendon sheath; NOT for intrathecal or IV route.
Solu-Medrone, rapid corticosteroid effect according to severity of condition, initially 10-500mg; graft versus host rejection reaction, up to 1g/day. *Admin,* IM, IV injection over minimum 30 minutes (high doses), up to 250mg (over 5 minutes) or IV infusion.

Child: *Depo-Medrone,* including infants, dose depends on condition, body weight, patient age.
Solu-Medrone, high dose indications, 30mg/kg/day; max. 1g/day. Graft versus host rejection, 10-20mg/kg/day for up to 3 days; max. 1g/day. *Status asthmaticus,* 1-4mg/kg/day for 1-3 days. NOTE: Products containing benzyl alcohol should not be used in pre-term or full-term neonates. *Admin,* IV associated with serious adverse events. See Adult above.

CI: Not for use in Achilles tendon due to absence of true tendon sheath. *Depo-Medrone,* not for intrathecal use. *Solu-Medrone,* not for epidural use.

SP: Hepatobiliary disorders; monitor (oral formulations).

299

11.1.2   Replacement Therapy

Drug-induced liver injury can result from cyclical pulsed IV admin; hepatotoxicity (parenteral formulations). *Depo-Medrone*, not for use by unapproved routes (epidural, intranasal, intra-ocular). Dermal, subdermal, subcutaneous atrophy, depigmentation. Intra-articular route, increased risk of inflammatory response in joint, increased pain with local swelling (septic arthritis risk); avoid injection into previously infected joint or unstable joints. Systemic absorption. Frequent ophthalmic monitoring.

ADR: Hypo- or hyperpigmentation, atrophy (subcutaneous, cutaneous), sterile abscess, post-injection flare (intra-articular), Charcot-like arthropathy; blindness (intralesional therapy around face and head).

Notes: See 11.1.1 Glucocorticoids.

> **Depo-Medrone Parenteral 40mg/mL** *(Pfizer)* A. GMS.
> *Price,* (1) 1mL, €2.44. 2mL, €4.75. 3mL, €8.35.
> *Depot injection,* methylprednisolone acetate. Sterile white aqueous susp. **Store:** Below 25 deg C; outer carton; do not freeze.
> **Solu-Medrone Parenteral** *(Pfizer)* A. GMS.
> *Price,* (1) vial 40mg, €1.63. 125mg, €4.89. Non-GMS 500mg, €10.83. 1g, €19.52.
> *Injection or concentrate for soln for infusion,* methylprednisolone sodium succinate. White (off-white) lyophilised powder for soln. *Sodium.* 40mg, 125mg: Clear colourless soln. *Benzyl alcohol.* 500mg, 1g: Sterile water for soln. **Store:** Below 25 deg C.

Methylprednisolone, Lidocaine

ATC Code: H02BX01. **Sport:** Permitted.
Driving: None known.

Indications: Conditions requiring a glucocorticoid effect; local use where added anaesthetic effect required.

Dose: Adult, Elderly: *Intra-articular,* large joint 20-80mg; medium joint 10-40mg, small joint 4-10mg; *periarticular,* epicondylitis, infiltrate 4-30mg; *intrabursal,* directly into bursae or into tendon sheath 4-30mg.

Notes: See Methylprednisolone above (*Depo-Medrone*).

> **Depo-Medrone With Lidocaine Parenteral** *(Pfizer)* A. GMS.
> *Price,* 1mL (10) €31.71. 2mL (1) €5.76.
> *Depot injection,* methylprednisolone acetate, lidocaine HCl 40/10mg. White aqueous susp. *Benzyl alcohol.* **Store:** Below 25 deg C; outer carton; do not freeze.

Prednisolone (systemic)

ATC Code: H02AB06. **Sport:** Prohibited.
Driving: Unlikely to impair.

Indications: Conditions requiring systemic corticosteroid treatment (allergic, rheumatic, inflammatory).

Dose: Adult, Elderly: *Deltacortril,* initially 5-60mg/day in divided doses depending on disorder type and severity. Allergic, skin disorders, 5-15mg/day; collagenosis, 20-30mg/day; rheumatoid arthritis, 10-15mg/day; blood disorders, lymphoma, 15-60mg/day.
Prednesol, range 10-100mg/day.
Prednisolone (Clonmel), range 5-60mg/day.
Child: *Deltacortril,* dose determined by clinical response; alternate day dosing preferable.
Prednesol, age 1-7 years, 25-50% of adult dose; 7-12 years, 50-75% of adult dose.

Notes: See 11.1.1 Glucocorticoids.

> **Deltacortril Enteric 2.5mg, 5mg** *(Phoenix)* A. GMS.
> *Price,* 2.5mg (30) €2.17; (100) €5.83. 5mg (30) €3.82; (100) €10.69.
> *Tablet,* prednisolone. e/c. 2.5mg: Brown.
> **Prednesol 5mg** *(Phoenix)* A. GMS.
> *Price,* (20) €7.20.
> *Dispersible tablet,* prednisolone sodium phosphate. Pink round scored (divisible into equal halves). Marked Pred 5. *Sodium* (benzoate, acid citrate, bicarbonate), saccharin.
> **Prednisolone 1mg, 5mg** *(Clonmel)* A. GMS.
> *Price,* 1mg (250) €7.95. 5mg (98) €3.06. (1000) €19.09.
> *Tablet,* prednisolone. Round white. 1mg, 5mg: Scored (facilitates breaking). *Lactose.*

Triamcinolone (musculoskeletal)

ATC Code: H02AB08. **Sport:** Permitted.
Driving: None known.

Indications: Inflammation (joints, bursae, tendon sheaths) in rheumatoid arthritis, osteoarthritis, bursitis, synovitis,

tendonitis, epicondylitis, trauma *(intra-articular).* Inflammatory dermal lesions (lichen simplex, lichen planus, psoriasis, granuloma annulare, keloids, alopecia) *(intra-dermal).*

Dose: Adult, Elderly: *Intra-articular,* smaller joints, 2.5-5mg; larger joints, 5-15mg. *Intradermal,* usually 2-3mg depending on lesion size; if several sites are injected, max. 30mg. *NOT* for IV, intrathecal or intraocular use.
Child: Over 6 years, in suitably adjusted dose.

CI: Not for use in Achilles tendon.

SP: Caution history of allergy to any drug; admin in setting with access to emergency care. Not for alleviation of joint pain arising from infectious states (gonococcal, TB arthritis). Warn patients to avoid over-use of joints if symptomatic benefit obtained. Repeated intra-articular injection over prolonged period, caution severe joint destruction (bone necrosis). Vaginal bleeding (post-menopausal women).

ADR: *Common,* increased susceptibility and severity of infections (sepsis, necrotising fasciitis), headache, injection-site reaction.

Notes: See 11.1.1 Glucocorticoids.

> **Adcortyl Parenteral 10mg/mL** *(BMS)* A. GMS.
> *Price,* 1mL (5) €5.05. 5mL (1) €5.19.
> *Intra-articular or intradermal injection,* triamcinolone acetonide. White sterile aqueous susp; slight odour. *Benzyl alcohol.* **Store:** Below 25 deg C; do not (refrigerate, freeze); protect (light).

11.1.2 - Replacement Therapy

In This Chapter: Fludrocortisone.

Class Effects

CI: Hypersensitivity to any member of the class.

Fludrocortisone

ATC Code: H02AA02. **Sport:** Prohibited (in-competition).
Driving: Unlikely to impair.

Indications: Partial replacement therapy, primary adrenocortical insufficiency in Addison's disease; salt-losing adrenogenital syndrome.

Dose: Adult, Elderly: *Addison's disease,* range 0.05-0.3mg/day. For enhanced glucocorticoid effect, co-admin daily cortisone (6.25-25mg) OR hydrocortisone (5-20mg). *Adrenogenital syndrome* (salt-losing), usually 0.1-0.2mg/day; restrict sodium intake; supplementary potassium may be required.
Child: 0.05-0.1mg/day; adjust to age, weight, severity of condition.

CI: Peptic ulcer, active TB, acute psychosis, acute/systemic infection (bacterial, viral).

SP: Dietary salt restriction, potassium supplementation may be needed; corticosteroids increase calcium excretion (osteoporosis). Advise adequate protein intake. See Notes below.

ADR: See Notes below.

Notes: See 11.1.1 Glucocorticoids.

> **Fludrocortisone 0.1mg** *(Aspen)* A. GMS.
> *Price,* (100) €12.10.
> *Tablet,* fludrocortisone acetate. Round white scored (divisible into equal doses). Marked SQUIBB and 429. *Lactose.*

11.2 - Drugs Used In Diabetes

Class Effects

Driving: Anti-diabetic agents themselves may not affect the ability to drive, but there is a potential for hypoglycaemia which may impair ability to concentrate and react. Hypoglycaemia risk is increased with combination use.

Type I Diabetes (insulin-dependent diabetes mellitus; IDDM) and Type 2 Diabetes (non-insulin dependent diabetes; NIDDM), are characterised by hyperglycaemia. Dietary modification and control is important in both types.

Indications: Oral antidiabetic drugs are indicated as adjunctive to diet and exercise to improve glycaemic control. They are used to treat Type 2 diabetes mellitus.

CI: Use in children. Hypersensitivity to any member of the class.

SP: Elderly, debilitated or patients with adrenal or pituitary insufficiency are particularly susceptible to hypoglycaemic action of glucose lowering drugs. Exceptional stress situations (trauma, surgery, febrile infections, shock, anaesthesia), blood glucose regulation may deteriorate; consider temporary dose changes to maintain metabolic control. With any blood-glucose-lowering drug, hypoglycaemia risk exists.

Risk factors for hypoglycaemia, lack of patient co-operation (unwillingness, incapacity); under-nourishment, irregular mealtimes or missed meals; imbalance between physical exertion and carbohydrate intake; alterations of diet; impaired renal and/or liver function; overdosage; uncompensated endocrine disorders affecting carbohydrate metabolism or counter-regulation of hypoglycaemia; co-admin of other drugs. Control hypoglycaemia by immediate carbohydrate intake (glucose or sucrose); if severe, glucose infusion.

Oral antidiabetic drugs, use lowest effective dose, monitor glucose levels; individualise dose. Major surgery, substitute insulin for oral hypoglycaemics.

Pregnancy, Lactation: Pregnancy, oral antidiabetics are not suitable (either recommended or contraindicated); insulin is the drug of first choice for treatment of diabetes during pregnancy. Lactation, contraindicated (risk of neonatal hypoglycaemia).

ADR: *Hypoglycaemia*, symptoms include, headache, ravenous hunger, nausea, vomiting, lassitude, sleepiness, disordered sleep, restlessness, aggressiveness, impaired concentration, alertness, and reactions, depression, confusion, speech disorders, aphasia, visual disorders, tremor, pareses, sensory disturbances, dizziness, helplessness, loss of self-control, delirium, cerebral convulsions, somnolence and loss of consciousness (including coma), shallow respiration, bradycardia.

Lactic acidosis, symptoms include, acidotic dyspnoea, abdominal pain, hypothermia, coma.

Diagnostic laboratory findings, decreased blood pH, plasma lactate levels above 5mmoL/L, increased anion gap and lactate/pyruvate ratio.

11.2.1 - Sulphonylureas

In This Chapter: *Gliclazide, glimepiride.*

Class Effects
Driving: See Notes below.

Indications: Type 2 diabetes, inadequate response to dietary measures alone and not requiring insulin.

CI: Type 1 diabetes, diabetic (ketoacidosis, coma/precoma), severe renal or hepatic impairment (switch to insulin), sulphonylurea or sulfonamide intolerance. Circumstances of unusual stress (infection, surgery, pregnancy, when dietary measures and insulin are essential).

Interactions: Effect of Other Drugs on Sulphonylureas: *Blood-glucose-lowering effect, potentiated (hypoglycaemia risk):* ALCOHOL, NSAIDs (phenylbutazone, azapropazone, oxyfenbutazone), uricosurics (sulfinpyrazone, allopurinol), insulin, other antidiabetic agents (acarbose, metformin, thiazolidinediones, dipeptidyl peptidase-4 inhibitors, GLP-1 receptor agonists); sulfonamides, tetracyclines, quinolones, azole antifungals (miconazole, contraindicated for some brands; fluconazole, voriconazole), chloramphenicol, clarithromycin, p-aminosalicylic acid; salicylates, MAOIs, anabolic steroids, male sex hormones, probenecid, coumarins, fenfluramine, pentoxifylline (high dose parenteral), fibrates, tritoqualine, ACEIs, fluoxetine, cyclo-, tro- and iphosphamides, disopyramide, fenyramidol, H2-antagonists, sympatholytics (beta-blockers, guanethidine). *Effect reduced (hyperglycaemia risk):* Acetazolamide, barbiturates, corticosteroids, diazoxide, diuretics, oestrogens, progestogens, thiazides, thyroid stimulating agents, phenothiazine derivatives, chlorpromazine, adrenaline and sympathomimetics, nicotinic acid (high dosages) and derivatives, laxatives

(long-term use), phenytoin, glucagon, rifampicin; ritodrine, salbutamol, terbutaline (due to beta-2 agonist effect), St John's Wort. *Effect unpredictably potentiated OR reduced:* Clonidine, reserpine, barbiturates, H2-antagonists, alcohol (acute and chronic intake); fluoroquinolones (especially elderly). *Warning hypoglycaemia symptoms masked:* Sympatholytics (beta-blockers, clonidine, guanethidine, reserpine).

Effect of Sulphonylureas on Other Drugs: Coumarins, warfarin: *Effect potentiated or reduced.*

SP: Use limited to maturity onset diabetes mellitus, not ketogenic, unable to be controlled by diet, insulin therapy not appropriate. Dose not taken at prescribed time, meal skipped, extra dose taken (consult medical advice); important not to skip meals after admin. Adjust dose according to weight, life-style changes. Elderly usually require lower dose. Haemolytic anaemia risk in G-6-PD deficient patients.

ADR: Prolonged, life-threatening hypoglycaemia, temporary visual impairment, nausea, vomiting, sensations of pressure or fullness, abdominal pain, diarrhoea, elevated liver enzymes, liver impairment, cholestasis, jaundice, hepatitis, thrombopenia presenting as purpura, haemolytic anaemia, erythrocytopenia, leucopenia, granulocytopenia, agranulocytosis due to myelosuppression, pancytopenia, allergic or pseudoallergic reactions, itching, rash, urticaria, allergic vasculitis, photosensitivity, elevated serum sodium.

Notes: See 11.2 Drugs Used In Diabetes.

Gliclazide

ATC Code: A10BB09. **Sport:** Permitted.
Driving: Hypoglycaemia may influence.
Dose: Adult: STANDARD/R, usually 40-80mg/day; if needed titrate by 40-80mg every 7-14 days until satisfactory control; max. 320mg/day. Maintenance, 80-160mg/day; over 160mg, consider twice daily dosing. Admin with or immediately before breakfast.

MODIFIED/R, initially 30mg/day; if needed titrate by 30mg increments at 1-month intervals; range, 30mg to max. 120mg/day. Admin as single dose at breakfast; swallow tabs whole.

Switch, usually, 80mg Standard/R comparable to 30mg Modified/R.

Elderly: STANDARD/R, initially 40mg/day before breakfast, then as for Adult above; 160mg/day, caution. Modified/R, as for Adult above.

Renal Impairment: Severe, contraindicated.

Hepatic Impairment: Severe, contraindicated.

CI: Secondary failure to sulphonylurea-therapy, adrenal or thyroid dysfunction.

Interactions: Effect of Other Drugs on Gliclazide: *Co-admin not recommended:* Danazol.

Notes: See 11.2 Drugs Used In Diabetes.

Interchangeability: Same strengths (30mg, 60mg) of all brands of gliclazide Prolonged/R and/or Modified/R tablets listed below are deemed interchangeable.

Diamicron MR 30mg, 60mg *(Servier)* B. GMS.
Price, 30mg (60) €3.73. 60mg (30) €3.73.
Modified/R tablet, gliclazide. White oblong. Marked DIA and strength. 30mg: Logo on reverse. 60mg: Scored (divisible into equal halves). *Lactose.*

Diabrezide 80mg *(Fannin)* B. GMS.
Price, (60) €5.26.
Standard/R tablet, gliclazide. White round scored (divisible into equal halves). *Lactose.*

Diaclide MR 30mg *(Gerard)* B. GMS.
Price, (60) €3.52.
Modified/R tablet, gliclazide. White (almost) oval. *Lactose.*

Diacronal MR 30mg, 60mg *(Krka)* B. GMS.
Price, (60) 30mg, 60mg, €3.52.
Modified/R tablet, gliclazide. White oval. *Lactose.*

Diaglyc Modified Release 30mg *(TEVA)* B. GMS.
Price, (60) €3.52.
Modified/R tablet, gliclazide. White oval. *Lactose.*

Vitile MR 30mg *(Accord)* B. GMS.
Price, (60) €3.52.
Modified/R tablet, gliclazide. White oval. Marked G.

11.2.2 Biguanides

Glimepiride

ATC Code: A10BB12. **Sport:** Permitted.
Driving: Concentration, reaction may be impaired.
Dose: Adult, Elderly: Initially 1mg/day. If needed increase by 1mg at 1-2 week intervals until control; max. 6mg/day.
Interactions: Effect of Other Drugs on Glimepiride: *Caution:* CYP2C9 inhibitors (fluconazole) or inducers (rifampicin). See Notes below. *Absorption reduced (allow 4-hour dose interval):* Colesevelam.
Notes: See 11.2 Drugs Used In Diabetes.

> **Amaryl 1mg, 3mg** *(SANOFI)* B. GMS.
> *Price,* (30) 1mg, €1.77. 3mg, €6.89.
> *Tablet,* Oblong scored (divisible into equal halves). 1mg: Pink. 3mg: Pale-yellow. *Lactose.*
> **Glimepiride 1mg, 2mg, 3mg, 4mg** *(Accord)* B. GMS.
> *Price,* (30) 1mg, €1.71; 2mg, €2.98; 3mg, €5.12; 4mg, €4.84.
> *Tablet,* glimepiride. Oval (except 1mg) scored (facilitates breaking) uncoated. 1mg: Pink round. 2mg: Light-pink. 3mg: Pale-yellow. 4mg: White. *Lactose.*

11.2.2 - Biguanides

In This Chapter: *Metformin.*

Class Effects
Driving: See Notes below; caution, combination (sulfonylureas, insulin, meglitinides).
Indications: Management of Type 2 diabetes, when response to diet and exercise inadequate for glycaemic control; particularly if overweight. Monotherapy or combination with oral antidiabetics or insulin (adults) or with insulin (children).
Notes: See 11.2 Drugs Used In Diabetes.

Metformin

ATC Code: A10BA02. **Sport:** Permitted.
Driving: Caution, hypoglycaemia risk especially in combination.
Dose: Adult, Elderly: Normal renal function (GFR 90mL/min and above), initially 500-850mg 2-3 times daily; adjust after 10-15 days; max. 3g/day (3 divided doses). Insulin combination, usually 500-850mg 2-3 times daily, while insulin dose is adjusted. *Elderly,* base dose on renal function. *Admin,* during or after food. Base dose adjustments on blood glucose measurements.
Child: Over 10 years, initially usually 500mg once daily. Titrate as for Adult above; max. 2g/day in 2-3 divided doses during or after food. Caution, age 10-12 years.
Renal Impairment: CrCl (mL/min) 60-89, max. 3g/day* (consider dose reduction in relation to declining renal function); 45-59, max 2g/day* (review factors that may increase lactic acidosis risk before initiating; starting dose at most half of max. dose); 30-44, max. 1g/day (as for 45-59); under 30, contraindicated. Assess function before initiation of metformin-containing products, then annually; every 3-6 months in patients at risk for further renal impairment and elderly. *(2-3 divided doses).
Hepatic Impairment: Contraindicated.
CI: Diabetic (ketoacidosis, pre-coma), any metabolic acidosis (lactic acidosis). Acute conditions with potential to alter renal function (dehydration, severe infection, shock). Disease (acute or worsening chronic) which may cause tissue hypoxia (decompensated heart failure, respiratory failure, recent MI, shock). Hepatic insufficiency, acute alcohol intoxication, alcoholism.
Interactions: Effect of Other Drugs on Metformin: *Co-admin caution:* Glucocorticoids, beta-2-agonists, diuretics, ACEIs, NSAIDs. *Increased lactic acidosis risk:* Alcohol, including alcohol-containing medications (avoid), iodinated contrast media. *Reduced metformin efficacy:* OCT1 inhibitors (verapamil). *Decreased renal elimination, increased plasma levels:* OCT2 inhibitors (cimetidine, dolutegravir, ranolazine, trimethoprim, vandetanib, isavuconazole). *Increased GI absorption and efficacy:* OCT1 inducers (rifampicin). *Altered efficacy and renal elimination:* OCT1 and 2 inhibitors (crizotinib, olaparib).
SP: Lactic acidosis, rare but *serious* metabolic complication; most often with acute worsening of renal function, cardiorespiratory illness or sepsis. Dehydration, temporarily discontinue. Medicinals that may impair renal function e.g. antihypertensives, diuretics or NSAIDs (caution). Other lactic acidosis risk factors e.g. excessive alcohol intake, hepatic insufficiency, poorly controlled diabetes, ketosis, prolonged fasting, conditions associated with hypoxia. Lactic acidosis is characterised by acidotic dyspnoea, abdominal pain, hypothermia followed by coma. *Monitor,* creatinine clearance before initiating, annually (normal function) or 2-4 times yearly if CrCl at lower limit of normal, elderly. Intravascular iodinated contrast media can lead to renal failure, metformin accumulation and lactic acidosis (discontinue metformin prior to or at time of test with normal function or 48 hours before with moderate impairment; resume after 48 hours *and* if renal function normal). *Elective surgery* (general, spinal, peridural anaesthesia), discontinue 48 hours before; restart 48 hours after surgery or resumption of oral nutrition *and* renal function normal.
Metformin alone does not cause hypoglycaemia; caution in combination with e.g. sulfonylureas or meglitinides.
Pregnancy, Lactation: Use insulin. Lactation, if benefit outweighs risk.
ADR: Summary, *most common*, nausea, vomiting, diarrhoea, abdominal pain, loss of appetite (to prevent GI disturbances, admin metformin in 2 or 3 daily doses).
Notes: See 11.2 Drugs Used In Diabetes.
Interchangeability: Same strengths of all brands of metformin f/c tabs and oral soln listed below are deemed interchangeable.
Reference Price: 500mg (84) €2.00. 850mg (56) €2.11. 1g (60) €3.00.

> **Glucophage Tablets** *(Merck Serono)* B. GMS.
> *Price,* see reference price above.
> *Tablet,* metformin HCl 500mg, 850mg, 1g. White f/c. 500mg, 850mg: Round. Marked GL and strength. 1g: Marked with strength, scored (divisible into equal halves).
> **Metformin (Rosemont) Oral Soln** *(Rosemont)* B. GMS.
> *Price,* 500mg/5mL (150mL) €69.43.
> *Oral soln,* metformin HCl 500mg/5mL. Clear brown liquid. *Parabens, maltitol; sodium 5.3mg, potassium 14.5mg per 5mL.* *Store:* Below 25 deg C.
> **Metformin Aurobindo Tablets** *(Rowex)* B. GMS.
> *Price,* (90) 500mg, (60) 850mg, see reference price above.
> *Tablet,* metformin HCl 1000mg. White oval f/c scored (not intended for breaking). Marked 6 and 2; A on reverse.
> **Metformin Bluefish Tablets** *(Bluefish)* B. GMS.
> *Price,* see reference price above. 1g (30) €1.50; (60) €3.00.
> *Tablet,* metformin HCl 500mg, 850mg, 1000mg. White f/c. 500mg A. Round. 850mg: Round. Marked 60. 850mg: Round. Marked 61. 1000mg: Oval with groove (not for breaking). Marked 62.
> **Metformin Mylan Tablets** *(Gerard)* B. GMS.
> *Price,* see reference price above.
> *Tablet,* metformin HCl 500mg, 850mg, 1000mg. White f/c. 500mg, 850mg: Round. 1000mg: Oval scored (divisible into equal halves). Marked MF and 3; G on reverse.
> **Metformin TEVA Tablets** *(TEVA)* B. GMS.
> *Price,* see reference price above. 1g (60) €4.70.
> *Tablet,* metformin HCl 500mg, 850mg, 1g. White oval f/c. 93. 500mg: Marked 48. 850mg: Marked 49. 1g: Oval scored (facilitates breaking). Marked 72/14.
> **Metophage Tablets** *(Rowex)* B. GMS.
> *Price,* (90) 500mg, €2.14. (60) 850mg, €2.26 (reference price pro rata).
> *Tablet,* metformin HCl 500mg, 850mg. Round white f/c. Marked M, strength.

11.2.3 - Alpha-Glucosidase Inhibitors

In This Chapter: *Acarbose.*

Class Effects
Driving: See Notes below.
Indications: Type 2 diabetes, adjunct to diet, alone or combination with insulin or oral hypoglycaemics.
Notes: See 11.2 Drugs Used In Diabetes.

Acarbose

ATC Code: A10BF01. **Sport:** Permitted.
Driving: No specific data available.
Dose: Adult, Elderly: Initially 50mg once or twice daily,

titrate gradually to 50mg 3-times daily; inadequate response after 6-8 weeks, increase to 100mg 3-times daily; max. 200mg 3-times daily (monitor). Oral, tabs to be chewed with first mouthful of food, or swallowed whole with a little liquid before food.

Child: Under 18 years, no data.

Renal Impairment: CrCl (mL/min) below 25, not recommended.

Hepatic Impairment: Not recommended. Severe (cirrhosis), contraindicated.

CI: Inflammatory bowel disease, colonic ulceration, partial intestinal obstruction, chronic intestinal diseases associated with digestion or absorption disorders, conditions which may deteriorate as a result of increased intestinal gas formation (large hernias).

Interactions: Effect of Other Drugs on Acarbose: *Activity altered, avoid co-admin*: Intestinal adsorbents (charcoal), digestive enzymes (amylase, pancreatin), colestyramine. *Increased GI adverse events (frequency, severity)*: Neomycin. *Abdominal discomfort/diarrhoea*: Sucrose, foods containing sucrose (increased colonic carbohydrate fermentation).

Effect of Acarbose on Other Drugs: Digoxin: *Plasma levels increased or decreased (monitor; adjust dose)*. Insulin, metformin, sulphonylureas: *Hypoglycaemic effect potentiated*.

SP: Monitor liver enzymes during first 6-12 months (idiosyncratic response); elevated transaminases, reduce dose or discontinue (fulminant hepatitis reported). Antacids (magnesium, aluminium salts) do not ameliorate acute GI adverse events (not recommended). If hypoglycaemia occurs, treat with glucose (not sucrose). Acarbose delays digestion and absorption of disaccharides, but not monosaccharides; has antihyperglycaemic effect; does not induce hypoglycaemia; co-admin with sulphonylureas, metformin, insulin may lead to hypoglycaemia, adjust co-medication dose.

ADR: *Very common*, flatulence.

Notes: See 11.2 Drugs Used In Diabetes.

Glucobay 50mg *(Bayer)* B. GMS.
Price, (90) €11.34.
Tablet, acarbose. White (yellow-tinged). Round. Marked with Bayer cross; G/strength on reverse.

11.2.4 - PPAR-Gamma Agonists

In This Chapter: *Pioglitazone, and metformin combination(s).*

Class Effects

Driving: See Notes below. PPAR-gamma is primary target of the thiazolidinedione class of drugs which include pioglitazone.

CI: Cardiac failure (or history of, NYHA stages I to IV), hepatic impairment.

SP: See CI above. Thiazolidinediones can cause fluid retention (dose-dependent; may exacerbate or precipitate HF especially with HF history, elderly, renal failure); increased risk with insulin, and/or sulphonylurea (HF risk, reduced cardiac reserve, monitor for signs and symptoms of fluid retention e.g. weight gain, HF). Monitor Hb, liver enzymes, weight gain (increase due to fat accumulation, water retention; especially with insulin combination). *Elderly*, caution. New-onset/worsening macular oedema with decreased visual acuity, caution. Polycystic ovarian syndrome, premenopausal anovulatory women, enhanced insulin action may result in ovulation (pregnancy risk). Cases of cardiac failure reported with pioglitazone in combination with insulin.

Notes: See 11.2 Drugs Used In Diabetes and 11.2.2 Biguanides (metformin).

Pioglitazone

ATC Code: A10BC03. **Sport:** Permitted.
Driving: Visual disturbance, caution.
Indications: Second or third-line therapy of Type 2 diabetes, where inadequate control achieved with diet and exercise; either as *monotherapy*, *dual therapy* with metformin OR

PPAR-Gamma Agonists   11.2.4

with sulphonylurea or as *triple therapy* with sulphonylurea + metformin (particularly overweight patients). Combination with insulin.

Dose: Adult: Initially 15-30mg/day; titrate in increments up to 45mg/day if needed. *Combination with insulin*, maintain current insulin dose; review after 3-6 months to assess response; no adequate response, discontinue. Initiate at lowest dose (especially combination with insulin). Oral with or without food, once daily; swallow with water.

Elderly: Insulin combination, caution (increased serious HF risk); consider risk/benefit.

Renal Impairment: Dialysis, no data.

Hepatic Impairment: ALT above 2.5xULN or other evidence of liver disease, do not initiate.

CI: Diabetic ketoacidosis.

Interactions: Effect of Other Drugs on Pioglitazone: *Plasma levels increased (consider dose reduction)*: Gemfibrozil. *Plasma levels decreased (consider dose increase)*: Rifampicin.

SP: Increased bone fracture incidence in women (studies suggest both men and women); consider with long-term use. Assess bladder cancer risk before initiation (age, smoking history, exposure to occupational or chemotherapy agents, prior radiation).

ADR: Monotherapy, all combinations, *very common*, oedema. Combinations with, *metformin*, anaemia, headache, visual disturbances, arthralgia, haematuria, ED; *sulphonylurea*, flatulence, dizziness; *metformin + sulphonylurea*, hypoglycaemia, arthralgia, increased blood CPK; *insulin* bronchitis, hypoglycaemia, dyspnoea, arthralgia, back pain, oedema.

Notes: See 11.2.4 PPAR-Gamma Agonists.

Actos 15mg, 30mg, 45mg *(Takeda)* B. GMS.
Price, (28) 15mg, €18.12. 30mg, €26.97. 45mg, €27.79.
Tablet, pioglitazone HCl. White (off-white) round. Marked with strength; ACTOS on reverse. *Lactose*.
Pioglitazone Accord 15mg, 30mg, 45mg *(Accord)* B. GMS.
Price, (28) 15mg, €14.50. 30mg, €21.57. 45mg, €20.52.
Tablet, pioglitazone HCl. White (off-white) round. Marked with strength. 15mg: Marked P. 30mg, 45mg: Marked PIO. *Lactose*.
Pioglitazone Actavis 15mg, 30mg, 45mg *(Accord)* B. GMS.
Price, (28) 15mg, €14.50. 30mg, €21.57. 45mg, €20.52.
Tablet, pioglitazone HCl. White round flat. Marked TZ, strength. *Lactose*.

Pioglitazone, Metformin

ATC Code: A10BD05. **Sport:** Permitted.
Driving: Visual disturbance, caution.
Indications: Second-line therapy of Type 2 diabetes (inadequate control on max. tolerated metformin dose alone).

Dose: Adult, Elderly: Normal renal function, pioglitazone 30mg/day + metformin 1700mg/day dosed as 1 tab (15mg/850mg) twice daily. Swallow tabs whole with or just after food to reduce metformin GI symptoms. *Elderly*, monitor renal function.

Renal Impairment: Pioglitazone dose: No adjustment including CrCl (mL/min) below 30; max. 45mg/day. Metformin dose: See Notes below (metformin).

SP: Lactic acidosis risk with metformin. See Notes below (metformin).

Pregnancy, Lactation: Contraindicated.

ADR: Summary, *very common*, abdominal pain, diarrhoea, appetite loss, nausea, vomiting (at initiation); *serious*, lactic acidosis; *other reactions*, bone fracture, increased weight, oedema.

Notes: See Pioglitazone above. See, 11.2.2 Biguanides (metformin).

Competact 15mg/850mg *(Takeda)* B. GMS.
Price, (56) €38.04.
Tablet, pioglitazone, metformin (hydrochloride) 15/850. White (off-white) oblong. Marked 15/850; 4833M on reverse.

11.2.5 - DPP-4 Inhibitors

In This Chapter: *Linagliptin, saxagliptin, sitagliptin, vildagliptin and metformin combinations.*

303

11.2.5 DPP-4 Inhibitors

Class Effects

Driving: See Notes below. Dipeptidyl peptidase-4 (DPP-4) inhibitors include linagliptin, saxagliptin, sitagliptin, vildagliptin.

Pharmacology: Dipeptidyl peptidase-4 inhibitors act as incretin enhancers; incretins are part of an endogenous system involved in physiologic regulation of glucose homeostasis.

Indications: Type 2 diabetes in adults (in addition to diet/exercise) to improve glycaemic control. See individual molecules below.

CI: Hypersensitivity to any member of the class. *Metformin* combinations, diabetic ketoacidosis. Acute conditions altering renal function (dehydration, severe infection, shock, intravascular admin of iodinated contrast agents), acute/chronic disease causing tissue hypoxia (cardiac or respiratory failure, recent MI, shock), acute ALCOHOL intoxication, alcoholism.

SP: *DPP-4 inhibitors* associated with acute pancreatitis; symptoms (persistent severe abdominal pain); if suspected, discontinue; if confirmed, do not restart; advise patients of symptoms. *Sulphonylureas*, caution hypoglycaemia; lower dose may be required with DPP-4 inhibitor. *Metformin* (fixed combinations) is excreted via kidney; monitor renal function. Not for use in Type 1 diabetes or diabetic ketoacidosis. Not a substitute for insulin. Monitor for rash. Discontinue metformin-containing medicines 48 hours before elective surgery with general, spinal or epidural anaesthesia; do not be resume use earlier than 48 hours and only when renal function is normal. Lactic acidosis risk (metformin accumulation), especially in elderly; usually with renal failure; assess risk factors to reduce incidence (poorly controlled diabetes, ketosis, prolonged fasting or malnutrition, excessive alcohol intake, hepatic insufficiency, conditions associated with hypoxia). Monitor serum creatinine; normal function (once yearly) at upper limit of normal and elderly (2-4 times yearly). Admin metformin combinations, with food to reduce metformin-associated GI adverse reactions.

Special Populations: Children (under 18 years), not recommended; elderly (75 years and over), caution unless stated that there is no dose adjustment.

Pregnancy, Lactation: Not for use unless otherwise stated.

Notes: See 11.2 Drugs Used In Diabetes and 11.2.2 Biguanides (metformin).

Linagliptin

ATC Code: A10BH05. **Sport:** Permitted.

Driving: Hypoglycaemia risk, especially in combination.

Indications: Monotherapy or dual therapy in combination (metformin OR sulphonylurea). Combination with other hypoglycaemics including insulin.

Dose: Adult, Elderly: Age 18 years and over, 5mg once daily. Combination with metformin (maintain metformin dose), with sulphonylurea or insulin (caution, consider sulphonylurea or insulin dose reduction). *Admin*, with or without food; any time of day. *Elderly*, see Notes below.

Interactions: Effect of Other Drugs on Linagliptin: Full efficacy may not be achieved: Strong P-gp inducers (rifampicin).

SP: Post-marketing, bullous pemphigoid reported; discontinue.

ADR: *Very common*, pancreatitis; hypoglycaemia (metformin + sulphonylurea combination).

Notes: See 11.2.5 DPP-4 Inhibitors.

Trajenta 5mg (Boehringer) B. GMS.
Price, (28) €36.90.
Tablet, linagliptin. Light-red f/c. Marked D5; logo on reverse.

Linagliptin, Metformin

ATC Code: A10BD11. **Sport:** Permitted.

Driving: Hypoglycaemia risk, especially in combination.

Indications: Type 2 diabetes not controlled by max. dose metformin alone OR already being treated with linagliptin + metformin individually. *Triple therapy*, combination with other antidiabetic agents including insulin (not adequately controlled with these agents + metformin).

Dose: Adult, Elderly: Age 18 years and over, with normal renal function, individualise; max. daily 5mg linagliptin + 2g metformin. Inadequately controlled on metformin alone, 2.5mg linagliptin daily + metformin dose being taken. based on current metformin dose, initiate at 2.5mg linagliptin (50/850 or 50/1000) twice daily; max. 5mg/day (duel therapy). Combination, with sulphonylurea or insulin, as for duel therapy but consider sulphonylurea or insulin dose reduction. *Elderly*, monitor renal function.

Renal Impairment: Linagliptin dose: No adjustment including CrCl (mL/min) below 30. Metformin dose: See Notes below (metformin).

Hepatic Impairment: Not recommended.

SP: Lactic acidosis risk with metformin. See Notes below (metformin).

ADR: Summary, *most frequent*, diarrhoea; hypoglycaemia (with sulphonylurea).

Notes: See Linagliptin above. See 11.2.2 Biguanides (metformin).

Jentadueto Tablets (Boehringer) B. GMS.
Price, (56) 2.5/850mg, €37.41; 2.5/1000mg, €37.49.
Tablet, linagliptin 2.5mg, metformin HCl 850mg (1000mg). Oval f/c. Marked D2, metformin strength and logo. 2.5/850mg: Light-orange. 2.5/1000mg: Light-pink.

Saxagliptin

ATC Code: A10BH03. **Sport:** Permitted.

Driving: Dizziness; hypoglycaemia risk especially in combination.

Indications: Monotherapy or dual therapy in combination (metformin OR sulphonylurea OR thiazolidinediones). Triple therapy in combination with metformin + sulphonylurea. Combination with insulin with or without metformin.

Dose: Adult, Elderly: Age 18 years and over, 5mg once daily. Combination with metformin, insulin, thiazolidinedione OR sulphonylurea, a lower dose of insulin or sulphonylurea may be required to reduce hypoglycaemia risk. Admin with or without food; any time of day; do not split or cut tabs. *Elderly*, no dose adjustment recommended based solely on age.

Renal Impairment: Moderate/severe, 2.5mg once daily. ESRD requiring dialysis, not recommended.

Hepatic Impairment: Moderate, caution. Severe, not recommended.

Interactions: Effect of Other Drugs on Saxagliptin: *Glycaemic lowering effect reduced*: CYP3A4 inducers (carbamazepine, dexamethasone, phenobarbital, phenytoin, rifampicin).

SP: NYHA Class III-IV, limited data, caution.

ADR: *Very common* (sulphonylurea combination) hypoglycaemia.

Notes: See 11.2.5 DPP-4 Inhibitors.

Onglyza 2.5mg 5mg (AstraZeneca) B. GMS.
Price, (28) 2.5mg, €37.82. 5mg, €37.46.
Tablet, saxagliptin HCl. Round f/c. Marked with strength. 2.5mg: Pale-yellow. Marked 4214. 5mg: Pink. Marked 4215. Lactose.

Saxagliptin, Metformin

ATC Code: A10BD10. **Sport:** Permitted.

Driving: Dizziness; hypoglycaemia risk especially in combination.

Indications: Type 2 diabetes not controlled by metformin alone or already treated with saxagliptin + metformin. Combination with insulin (not adequately controlled by insulin + metformin) or with sulphonylurea (not adequately controlled by metformin + sulphonylurea).

Dose: Adult, Elderly: Adults with normal renal function (GFR 90mL/min or above), initiate at 2.5mg saxagliptin twice daily + dose of metformin already being taken e.g. 2.5/850 or 2.5/1000. In combination with insulin or sulphonylurea a lower dose of insulin or sulphonylurea may be required to reduce hypoglycaemia risk. *Admin*, twice daily with food. *Elderly*, monitor renal function.

Child: Under 18 years, no dose.

Renal Impairment: GFR 60-89mL/min, no adjustment. Saxagliptin dose: GFR (mL/min) 60-89, max. 5mg/day; 30-59, max. 2.5mg/day; under 30, contraindicated. Metformin dose: See Notes below (metformin).

Hepatic Impairment: Not recommended.

304

SP: Lactic acidosis risk with metformin. See Notes below (metformin).
ADR: See Notes below.
Notes: See Saxagliptin above. See 11.2.2 Biguanides (metformin).

Komboglyze Tablets *(AstraZeneca)* B. GMS.
Price, (56) 2.5/850mg, €38.71; 2.5/1000mg, €37.51.
Tablet, saxagliptin HCl 2.5mg, metformin HCl (850mg/1000mg).
f/c. 2.5/850mg: Light-brown (brown) round. Marked 2.5/850 and 4246. 2.5/1000mg: Pale-yellow (yellow) oval. Marked 2.5/1000 and 4247. **Store:** Below 25 deg C.

Sitagliptin

ATC Code: A10BH01. **Sport:** Permitted.
Driving: Dizziness, somnolence; hypoglycaemia risk.
Indications: Monotherapy, dual therapy in combination (metformin OR sulphonylurea OR thiazolidinediones); triple therapy in combination (sulphonylurea + metformin OR thiazolidinedione + metformin). Combination with insulin with or without metformin.
Dose: Adult, Elderly: Age 18 years and over, 100mg once daily. Combination with metformin or PPAR-gamma agonist, maintain metformin or PPAR-gamma agonist dose; with sulphonylurea or insulin consider sulphonylurea or insulin dose reduction. With or without food. *Elderly,* no dose adjustment.
Renal Impairment: CrCl (mL/min) 30-50, 50mg once daily; below 30 or ESRD on dialysis, 25mg once daily. Assess function prior to initiation.
Hepatic Impairment: Severe, no data.
Interactions: Effect of Other Drugs on Sitagliptin: *Possible altered pharmacokinetics (with renal insufficiency):* Potent CYP3A4 inhibitors (ketoconazole, itraconazole, ritonavir, clarithromycin).
Effect of Sitagliptin on Other Drugs: Digoxin: *Monitor patients at risk for digoxin toxicity.*
SP: Increased hypoglycaemia incidence (combination). Serious hypersensitivity reactions (anaphylaxis, angioedema, exfoliative skin conditions including Stevens-Johnson syndrome), discontinue.
ADR: *Very common,* hypoglycaemia. *Serious,* pancreatitis, hypersensitivity, see SP above.
Notes: See 11.2.5 DPP-4 Inhibitors.

Januvia 25mg, 50mg, 100mg *(MSD)* B. GMS.
Price, (28) 25mg, €28.80; 50mg, €28.67; 100mg, €36.30.
Tablet, sitagliptin phosphate monohydrate. Round f/c. 25mg: Pink. Marked 221. 50mg: Light-beige. Marked 112. 100mg: Beige. Marked 277.

Sitagliptin, Metformin

ATC Code: A10BD07. **Sport:** Permitted.
Driving: Dizziness, somnolence; hypoglycaemia risk (combination).
Indications: Type 2 diabetes not controlled by metformin alone or already treated with sitagliptin + metformin OR as TRIPLE therapy in combination (sulphonylurea OR thiazolidinediones). Combination with insulin when not adequately controlled by insulin + metformin.
Dose: Adult, Elderly: Age 18 years and over, based on current metformin dose, initiate at 50mg sitagliptin (50/850 or 50/1000) twice daily. Max. 100mg/day. Combination with sulphonylurea or insulin, consider sulphonylurea or insulin dose reduction. Admin twice daily with food. *Elderly,* monitor renal function; no adjustment.
Renal Impairment: Sitagliptin dose: GFR 50-89mL/min, max. 100mg/day; 30-49, max. 50mg/day; under 30, max. 25mg/day (metformin contraindicated). Metformin dose: See Notes below (metformin).
Hepatic Impairment: Contraindicated.
SP: Serious hypersensitivity reactions (anaphylaxis, angioedema, exfoliative skin reaction including Stevens-Johnson syndrome); discontinue and institute alternative. Lactic acidosis risk with metformin. See Notes below (metformin).
Pregnancy, Lactation: Lactation, contraindicated.
ADR: Summary, *serious,* pancreatitis, hypersensitivity; hypoglycaemia (with sulphonylurea).

Notes: See Sitagliptin above. See 11.2.2 Biguanides (metformin).

Janumet Tablets *(MSD)* B. GMS.
Price, (56) 50/850mg, €39.06. 50/1000mg, €38.76.
Tablet, sitagliptin metformin 50mg, metformin HCl (850mg/1000mg). Cap-shaped f/c. 50/850: Pink. Marked 515. 50/1000: Red. Marked 577. **Store:** Below 30 deg C.

Vildagliptin

ATC Code: A10BH02. **Sport:** Permitted.
Driving: Dizziness.
Indications: Monotherapy, dual therapy in combination (metformin OR sulphonylurea OR thiazolidinediones); triple therapy in combination (sulphonylurea + metformin OR thiazolidinedione + metformin). Combination with insulin with or without metformin.
Dose: Adult, Elderly: Age 18 years and over (monotherapy, combination with metformin or thiazolidinediones) 100mg/day in 2 equally divided doses. Combination with sulphonylurea, 50mg/day in morning; max. 100mg/day. With or without food. *Elderly,* see Notes below.
Renal Impairment: Moderate or severe or with ESRD, 50mg once daily. ESRD on haemodialysis, caution.
Hepatic Impairment: Not recommended including where pre-treatment ALT or AST is above 3xULN.
Interactions: Effect of Other Drugs on Vildagliptin: *Hypoglycaemic effect reduced:* Thiazides, corticosteroids, thyroid products, sympathomimetics. *Increased angioedema risk:* ACE-inhibitors.
SP: Hepatic dysfunction (including hepatitis); monitor liver enzymes prior to initiation, at 3-month intervals (year 1), then periodically. Jaundice, discontinue. CHF NYHA Class III-IV, not recommended; combination with metformin, contraindicated. Skin, monitor (blistering, ulceration).
ADR: *Common* (metformin or sulphonylurea combination), tremor, headache, dizziness, nausea; (thiazolidinedione combination), weight increase, peripheral oedema.
Notes: See 11.2.5 DPP-4 Inhibitors.

Galvus 50mg *(Novartis)* B. GMS.
Price, (56) €36.33.
Tablet, vildagliptin. White (light-yellowish) round flat-faced. Marked NVR; FB on reverse. *Lactose.* **Store:** Original pack to protect (moisture).

Vildagliptin, Metformin

ATC Code: A10BD08. **Sport:** Permitted.
Driving: Dizziness.
Indications: Dual therapy in combination with (metformin OR sulphonylurea); triple therapy in (sulphonylurea + metformin). Combination with insulin with or without metformin.
Dose: Adult, Elderly: Age 18 years and over, based on current metformin dose, initiate at either 50mg/850mg (vildagliptin/metformin) or 50mg/1000mg twice daily (morning, evening). Max. vildagliptin 100mg/day. Combination with sulphonylurea or insulin, consider sulphonylurea or insulin dose reduction. *Admin,* with or just after food. *Elderly,* monitor renal function.
Renal Impairment: GFR 60-89mL/min, no adjustment. Vildagliptin dose: GFR (mL/min) 30-59, max. 50mg/day; under 30, max. 50mg/day (metformin contraindicated). Metformin dose: See Notes below (metformin).
Hepatic Impairment: Contraindicated.
SP: Lactic acidosis risk with metformin. See Notes below (metformin).
Pregnancy, Lactation: Lactation, contraindicated.
ADR: *Common,* hypoglycaemia, tremor, headache, dizziness, fatigue, nausea.
Notes: See Vildagliptin above. See 11.2.2 Biguanides (metformin).

Eucreas Tablets *(Novartis)* B. GMS.
Price, (60) 50/850mg, €43.10. 50/1000mg, €40.81.
Tablet, vildagliptin/metformin HCl 50/850mg, 50/1000mg. Ovaloid f/c. Marked NVR. 50/850: Yellow. Marked SHE. 50/1000: Dark-yellow. Marked FLO. **Store:** Below 30 deg C; original pack to protect (moisture).

11.2.6 - SGLT-Inhibitors

In This Chapter: *Canagliflozin, dapagliflozin, empagliflozin and metformin combinations.*

Class Effects

Driving: See Notes below.

SGLT2 (sodium-glucose co-transporter 2) inhibitors include canagliflozin, dapagliflozin, empagliflozin.

Indications: Type 2 diabetes mellitus (monotherapy or add-on), in combination with other glucose-lowering agents including insulin.

CI: Hypersensitivity to any member of the class. Children under 18 years. Metformin combinations: Acute conditions altering renal function (dehydration, severe infection, shock); acute or chronic disease causing hypoxia (cardiac or respiratory failure, recent MI, shock). Acute alcohol intoxication, alcoholism, hepatic impairment. Diabetic ketoacidosis, diabetic pre-coma.

SP: Not for use in Type 1 diabetes, not for ketoacidosis treatment. Increased hypoglycaemia risk (combination with sulphonylurea). Efficacy renal-function dependent (monitor prior to initiation, then once yearly; also prior to initiation of other medicinals that may reduce renal function, then periodically). Renal impairment, moderate (efficacy reduced), severe (likely absent). Due to mechanism of action, increased urinary glucose induces osmotic diuresis; may reduce intravascular volume, decrease BP (caution if drop poses risk e.g. cardiovascular disease, anti-hypertensive therapy, hypotension history, elderly). Use not recommended with volume depletion due to acute illness (GI illness) (monitor volume status, electrolytes). UTI frequently reported; including complicated (empagliflozin); genital mycotic infections. Urine will test positive for glucose. Diabetic ketoacidosis (including life-threatening); if suspected or diagnosed, discontinue; caution, patients at risk for diabetic ketoacidosis (low beta-cell function reserve, conditions leading to restricted food intake or severe dehydration, patients for whom insulin doses are reduced or with increased insulin requirement e.g. due to acute medical illness, surgery, alcohol abuse).

Patients with type 2 diabetes with cardiovascular disease (or at high risk for CVD), increased cases of lower limb amputation (primarily toe) observed (long-term clinical studies); monitor; counsel patients (routine preventative foot care, adequate hydration).

Metformin combinations, lactic acidosis a serious metabolic complication; metformin is excreted by kidney and accumulation may precipitate lactic acidosis. Determine creatinine clearance before initiation, then regularly. Intravascular admin of iodinated contrast agents can lead to renal failure. Discontinue metformin 48 hours before elective surgery (general, spinal, peridural anaesthesia); restart not earlier than 48 hours afterwards. Admin metformin combinations after food to reduce the GI effects. See Notes below (metformin). *Elderly*, frequently have decreased renal function. Monitor regularly to prevent metformin-associated lactic acidosis. Increased volume depletion risk (over 75 years).

Pregnancy, Lactation: Pregnancy, should not be used (insulin recommended). Lactation, not recommended.

ADR: Summary *most commonly*, hypoglycaemia (combination with insulin or sulphonylurea), vulvovaginal candidiasis, UTI, polyuria or pollakiuria (urinary frequency). Rare cases of diabetic ketoacidosis (DKA) (life-threatening, fatal) reported

Notes: See 11.2 Drugs Used In Diabetes. See 11.2.2 Biguanides (metformin).

Canagliflozin

ATC Code: A10BX11. **Sport:** Permitted.

Driving: Hypoglycaemia, especially in combination. See SP below.

Indications: Type 2 diabetes mellitus (monotherapy or add-on) (combination with other glucose-lowering agents including insulin).

Dose: Adult: Initially 100mg once daily; if tolerated *and*

egFR 60mL/min/1.73m2* or CrCl 60mL/min* *and* need for tighter glycaemic control, increase to 300mg once daily. Combination (insulin or sulphonylurea), consider lower dose of insulin or sulphonylurea to reduce hypoglycaemia risk. *Admin*, swallow tabs whole; preferably before first meal of day. *(or above).

Elderly: Age 75 years and older, known cardiovascular disease or where initial diuresis poses a risk, caution; age 65 years and older, as for Renal below.

Renal Impairment: eGFR (mL/min/1.73m2) below 60 or CrCl (mL/min) below 60, do not initiate. If canagliflozin is tolerated and levels (eGFR, CrCl) fall* below 60, adjust dose to or maintain at, 100mg once daily; levels below* 45, discontinue. ESRD or on dialysis, not recommended (not expected to be effective). *(persistently).

Hepatic Impairment: Severe, not recommended.

Interactions: Effect of Other Drugs on Canagliflozin: Co-admin *not recommended*: Loop diuretics, thiazides (dehydration, hypotension). *Decreased exposure (decreased efficacy)*: Enzyme inducers (St John's Wort, rifampicin, barbiturates, phenytoin, carbamazepine, ritonavir, efavirenz), colestyramine (dose 1 hour before or 4-6 hours after colestyramine).

Effect of Canagliflozin on Other Drugs: Digoxin; dabigatran: *Monitor.*

SP: Renal function, see Notes below (SGLT2-inhibitors). Increased haematocrit. Driving, adverse reactions related to volume depletion (postural dizziness).

Pregnancy, Lactation: Pregnancy, not for use; if detected, discontinue. Lactation, not recommended.

ADR: See Notes below.

Notes: See 11.2.8 Other Antidiabetics, Excluding Insulin.

▼ **Invokana 100mg, 300mg** *(Janssen-Cilag)* B. GMS.
Price, (30) 100mg, €45.04; 300mg, €62.21.
Tablet, canagliflozin hemihydrate. Cap-shaped f/c. Marked CFZ; strength on reverse. 100mg: Yellow. 300mg: White. *Lactose*.

Canagliflozin, Metformin

ATC Code: A10BD16. **Sport:** Permitted.

Driving: Hypoglycaemia risk in combination.

Indications: Type 2 diabetes not controlled by metformin alone or already being treated with canagliflozin + metformin OR in combination (other glucose-lowering agents including insulin) + metformin when not controlled.

Dose: Adult: Not controlled on metformin, initial dose providing canagliflozin 50mg twice daily + metformin dose already being taken (nearest appropriate dose). If tolerated and tighter control needed, increase to canagliflozin 150mg twice daily. *Admin*, with food to reduce GI effects (metformin). Combination, see Notes below (canagliflozin).

Elderly: Caution. See Notes below (other antidiabetics).

Renal Impairment: CrCl (mL/min) below 60, not to be used (due to metformin).

Hepatic Impairment: Contraindicated.

Interactions: Effect of Other Drugs on Canagliflozin + Metformin: Co-admin *not recommended*: ALCOHOL (lactic acidosis due to metformin). *Increased metformin exposure*: Cationic substances eliminated by renal tubular secretion (cimetidine), drugs reducing renal function.

Notes: See Canagliflozin above. See 11.2.2 Biguanides (metformin). See Class Effects 11.2.8 Other Antidiabetics, Excluding Insulin.

▼ **Vokanamet Tablets** *(Janssen-Cilag)* B. GMS.
Price, (60) 50/850(1000)mg, €45.04; 150/850(1000), €62.21
Tablets, canagliflozin hemihydrate, metformin HCl. Cap-shaped f/c immediate-release. Marked CM. 50/850: Pink. Marked 358. 50/1000: Beige. Marked 551. 150/850: Light-yellow. Marked 418. 150/1000: Purple. Marked 611. **Store:** Below 30 deg C.

Dapagliflozin

ATC Code: A10BX09. **Sport:** Permitted.

Driving: Hypoglycaemia risk in combination.

Indications: Type 2 diabetes mellitus (monotherapy or add-on) (combination with other glucose-lowering agents including insulin).

Dose: Adult: Monotherapy and add-on combination, 10mg once daily. Combination with insulin or insulin secretagogue (sulphonylurea), consider lower dose of insulin or secretagogue to reduce hypoglycaemia risk. Swallow tabs whole; with or without food at any time of day.

Elderly: Age 75 years and older, initiation of dapagliflozin not recommended.

Renal Impairment: CrCl (mL/min) below 60, not recommended; below 30 or ESRD, no data.

Hepatic Impairment: Severe (increased exposure), initiate with 5mg; if well tolerated, increase to 10mg.

Interactions: Effect of Other Drugs on Dapagliflozin: *Co-admin not recommended*: Loop diuretics, thiazides (dehydration, hypotension).

SP: Renal function, see Notes below; if function approaching moderate impairment, monitor 2-4 times yearly. Co-admin with pioglitazone, not recommended; small increased bladder cancer risk. Increased haematocrit.

Pregnancy, Lactation: Second and third trimesters, not recommended.

ADR: *Very common*, hypoglycaemia (with sulphonylurea or insulin).

Notes: See 11.2.8 Other Antidiabetics, Excluding Insulin.

▼ **Forxiga 5mg, 10mg** *(AstraZeneca)* B. GMS.
Price, (28) 5mg, €41.52; 10mg, €40.94.
Tablet, dapagliflozin propanediol monohydrate. Yellow f/c. Marked with strength. 5mg: Marked 1427. 10mg: Marked 1428. *Lactose*.

Dapagliflozin, Metformin

ATC Code: A10BD15. **Sport:** Permitted.
Driving: Hypoglycaemia risk.

Indications: Type 2 diabetes not controlled by metformin alone or already being treated with dapagliflozin + metformin OR in combination (other glucose-lowering agents including insulin) + metformin when not controlled.

Dose: Adult: 1 tablet (dapagliflozin 5mg + metformin 850mg) twice daily with food to reduce GI effects (metformin). Combination, see Notes below (dapagliflozin).

Elderly: Monitor function. See Notes below (other antidiabetics).

Renal Impairment: GFR (mL/min) below 30, contraindicated; below 60, not recommended (dapagliflozin efficacy is renal function dependent). See Notes below (metformin).

Hepatic Impairment: Contraindicated.

Interactions: Effect of Other Drugs on Dapagliflozin + Metformin: *Co-admin not recommended*: ALCOHOL (lactic acidosis due to metformin). *Increased metformin exposure*: Cationic substances eliminated by renal tubular secretion (cimetidine), drugs reducing renal function.

SP: Renal function, lactic acidosis, see Notes below (metformin).

Pregnancy, Lactation: Second and third trimesters, use during lactation, not recommended.

ADR: *Very common*, hypoglycaemia (with sulphonylurea or insulin), GI symptoms.

Notes: See Dapagliflozin above. See 11.2.2 Biguanides (metformin). See Class Effects 11.2.8 Other Antidiabetics, Excluding Insulin. **Interchangeability:** Same strengths of all brands of metformin/dapagliflozin f/c tablets listed below are deemed interchangeable.

▼ **Xigduo Tablets** *(AstraZeneca)* B. GMS.
Price, (56), 5/850, €40.84; 5/1000, €40.97.
Tablet, dapagliflozin propanediol monohydrate, metformin HCl 5/850, 5/1000 (mg). Oval f/c. Marked with strength. 5/850: Brown. Marked 1067. 5/1000: Yellow. Marked 1069.

Empagliflozin

ATC Code: A10BX12. **Sport:** Permitted.
Driving: Hypoglycaemia risk especially in combination.

Indications: Type 2 diabetes mellitus (monotherapy or add-on) (combination with other glucose-lowering agents including insulin).

Dose: Adult: 10mg once daily (monotherapy and add-on combination with other glucose-lowering agents including insulin); if tolerated AND eGFR 60mL/min/1.73m2 or above AND need for tighter glycaemic control, increase to 25mg once daily. Combination (insulin or sulphonylurea),

consider lower dose of insulin or sulphonylurea to reduce hypoglycaemia risk. *Admin*, with or without food, swallow whole.

Elderly: Age 75 years and older, increased volume depletion risk; age 85 years and older, not recommended.

Renal Impairment: eGFR (mL/min/1.73m2) below 60 or CrCl (mL/min) below 60, do not initiate. If empagliflozin is tolerated and levels (eGFR, CrCl) persistently fall below 60, adjust dose to or maintain at 10mg once daily; below 45, discontinue. ESRD or on dialysis, not recommended (not expected to be effective).

Hepatic Impairment: Severe, not recommended.

Interactions: Effect of Other Drugs on Empagliflozin: *Potential decreased efficacy*: UGT enzyme inducers.

Effect Empagliflozin on Other Drugs: Loop diuretics, thiazides: *Increased diuretic effect (dehydration, hypotension risk).*

SP: Renal function, see Notes below (other antidiabetics). Hepatic injury reported.

Pregnancy, Lactation: Early pregnancy, avoid; second, third trimesters, not recommended. Lactation, not recommended.

ADR: Summary, *most frequent*, hypoglycaemia (with sulphonylurea or insulin).

Notes: See 11.2.8 Other Antidiabetics, Excluding Insulin.

▼ **Jardiance 10mg, 25mg** *(Boehringer)* B. GMS.
Price, (28) 10mg, €39.17; 25mg, €39.94.
Tablet, empagliflozin. Pale-yellow. Marked with logo, S and strength. 10mg: Round. 25mg: Oval. *Lactose*.

Empagliflozin, Metformin

ATC Code: A10BD20. **Sport:** Permitted.
Driving: Caution, hypoglycaemia risk when used in combination.

Indications: Type 2 diabetes not controlled by metformin alone or already being treated with empagliflozin + metformin OR in combination (other glucose-lowering agents including insulin) + metformin when not controlled.

Dose: Adult: Not adequately controlled on metformin, initial dose providing empagliflozin 5mg twice daily + metformin dose already being taken or nearest appropriate dose. To tolerated and tighter control needed, increase to canagliflozin 12.5mg twice daily (25mg/day). *Admin*, with food to reduce GI effects (metformin). Combination, see Notes below (empagliflozin).

Elderly: Caution. See Notes below (other antidiabetics). Age 85 years and older, not recommended.

Renal Impairment: GFR 60-89mL/min, no adjustment. Empagliflozin dose: GFR (mL/min) 60-89, max. 25mg/day; 45-59, max. 10mg/day (empagliflozin should not be initiated); 30-44, not recommended; below 30, not recommended (metformin contraindicated). Metformin dose: See Notes below (metformin).

Hepatic Impairment: Contraindicated.

Interactions: Effect of Other Drugs on Empagliflozin + Metformin: *Co-admin not recommended*: ALCOHOL (lactic acidosis due to metformin). *Increased metformin exposure*: Cationic substances eliminated by renal tubular secretion (cimetidine), drugs reducing renal function.

SP: Renal function, lactic acidosis risk with metformin, see Notes below (metformin and other antidiabetics).

ADR: Summary, *most common*, hypoglycaemia (with insulin and/or sulphonylurea), infections (urinary tract, genital tract), increased urination.

Notes: See Empagliflozin above. See 11.2.2 Biguanides (metformin). See Class Effects 11.2.8 Other Antidiabetics, Excluding Insulin.

▼ **Synjardy Tablets** *(Boehringer)* B. GMS.
Price, (56) 5/850mg, €40.82; 5/1000mg, €40.95. 12.5/850mg, €41.83; 12.5/1000mg, €41.80.
Tablets, empagliflozin, metformin HCl. Oval f/c. Marked S5 (5mg) or S12 (12.5mg) and Boehringer logo; 850 (850mg) or 1000 (1000mg) on reverse. 5/850: Yellowish-white. 5/1000: Brownish-yellow. 12.5/850: Pinkish-white. 12.5/1000: Dark brownish-purple.

11.2.7   GLP-1 Agonists

In This Chapter: Exenatide, dulaglutide, liraglutide.

Class Effects

~~Driving: See Notes below.~~
GLP-1 (glucagon-like peptide-1) agonists include exenatide, dulaglutide, liraglutide.

Indications: Type 2 diabetes mellitus (monotherapy or add-on), in combination with other glucose-lowering agents including insulin.

CI: Hypersensitivity to any member of the class. Children under 18 years.

SP: SC injection (abdomen, thigh, upper arm); not for IV or IM admin. Not for use in Type 1 diabetes, not for ketoacidosis treatment. Increased hypoglycaemia risk (combination with sulphonylurea). Acute pancreatitis; if suspected, discontinue/do not resume. May be associated with GI adverse reactions.

Pregnancy, Lactation: Pregnancy, should not be used (insulin recommended). Discontinue minimum 3 months before planned pregnancy (Bydureon). Lactation, not recommended.

ADR: Very commonly, commonly, hypoglycaemia (in combination). See individual drugs below.

Notes: See 11.2 Drugs Used In Diabetes.

Dulaglutide

ATC Code: A10BX14. **Sport:** Permitted.
Driving: Hypoglycaemia risk especially in combination.
Indications: Treatment, Type 2 diabetes mellitus (monotherapy or combination) with oral glucose-lowering agents including insulin.

Dose: Adult, Elderly: Monotherapy, 0.75mg once weekly. Add-on therapy, 1.5mg once weekly; vulnerable populations (e.g. 75 years and older), consider starting at 0.75mg once weekly. Admin, SC injection. When added to existing metformin and/or pioglitazone, continue current metformin and/or pioglitazone dose; when added to existing sulphonylurea or insulin, consider sulphonylurea or insulin dose reduction to reduce hypoglycaemia risk.

Renal Impairment: Mild/moderate, no adjustment. Severe or ESRD, not recommended.

Hepatic Impairment: No adjustment.

Interactions: Effect of Other Drugs on Dulaglutide: Increased exposure: Sitagliptin.

Effect of Dulaglutide on Other Drugs: Oral medications requiring rapid GI absorption; some Prolonged/R formulations: Gastric emptying delayed by dulaglutide

ADR: Summary, most frequent, GI (nausea, vomiting, diarrhoea); hypoglycaemia (in combination).

Notes: See 11.2.8 Other Antidiabetics, Excluding Insulin.

▼ **Trulicity Parenteral 0.75mg, 1.5mg** (Lilly) A. GMS.
Price, PFP 0.5mL x 4: 0.75mg, €111.73; 1.5mg, €111.41.
Injection, dulaglutide. Clear colourless soln. **Store:** Refrigerate; do not freeze; unrefrigerated below 30 deg C (max. 14 days).

Exenatide

ATC Code: A10BX04. **Sport:** Permitted.
Driving: Caution, hypoglycaemia risk when used in combination.
Indications: Type 2 diabetes mellitus in combination (metformin, sulphonylurea or thiazolidinedione). Adjunctive to basal insulin with or without metformin and/or pioglitazone (Byetta).

Dose: Adult: Byetta, initially 5mcg twice daily; titrate after minimum 1 month to max. 10mcg to improve control. Add-on, continue current metformin and/or pioglitazone dose; consider reducing sulphonylurea or basal insulin (hypoglycaemia risk). Admin, within 60 minutes before morning and evening meal; not for admin after meal; with basal insulin, use 2 separate injections.
Bydureon, 2mg once weekly. Add-on, as above. Admin, same day each week; any time of day with or without meals; max. 1 injection in a 24-hour period.

Elderly: Over 70 years, caution; titrate conservatively from

5mcg to 10mcg (Byetta). Over 75 years, limited data (both brands).

Renal Impairment: CrCl (mL/min) 30-50, limited data (Byetta), Bydureon not recommended. Below 30 or ESRD, not recommended.

Interactions: Effect of Other Drugs on Exenatide: Co-admin not recommended: Insulin, D-phenylalanine derivatives (meglitinides), alpha-glucosidase inhibitors, dipeptidyl peptidase-4 inhibitors, other GLP-1 receptor agonists. Caution: Oral drugs requiring rapid GI absorption, medicinals with narrow therapeutic ratio. Allow dose interval: Drugs dependent on threshold conc (antibiotics) (take 1 hour before exenatide), (g/r) formulations (PPIs) (1 hour before or 4 hours after exenatide).

Effect of Exenatide on Other Drugs: Warfarin, coumarol derivatives: Monitor INR.

SP: Monitor lipid profiles. Pancreatitis, see Notes below. Renal impairment. Rapid weight loss (above 1.5kg/week), may have harmful consequences (cholelithiasis). Admin, SC injection; not for IV or IM admin. After discontinuation, effect may continue (plasma levels decline over 10 weeks). Increased heart rate observed (Bydureon).

ADR: Summary, most frequent, (both brands), GI (nausea, diarrhoea), hypoglycaemia (with sulphonylurea); Bydureon, injection-site reactions, headache; Byetta, vomiting. Acute (pancreatitis, renal failure).

Notes: See 11.2.8 Other Antidiabetics, Excluding Insulin.

Byetta Parenteral (AstraZeneca) A. GMS.
Price, PFP 60-dose: 5mcg, €94.88. 10mcg, €96.22.
Injection (Standard/R), exenatide (synthetic) 5mcg, 10mcg. Clear colourless soln. Essentially sodium-free. **Store:** Refrigerate; do not freeze; in use, store below 25 deg C.
Bydureon Parenteral (AstraZeneca) A. GMS.
Price, 2mg (4): Inj €100.04, (PFP) €97.24.
Injection (Prolonged/R), exenatide 2mg. White (off-white) powder; clear colourless (pale-yellow to brown) solvent for soln. PFP. **Store:** Refrigerate; do not freeze; store below 30 deg C (max. 4 weeks) prior to use.

Liraglutide

ATC Code: A10BX07. **Sport:** Permitted.
Driving: Hypoglycaemia, especially with (sulphonylurea or insulin).
Indications: Treatment, Type 2 diabetes mellitus (monotherapy) or in combination (oral glucose-lowering agents and/or basal insulin).

Dose: Adult: Initially 0.6mg daily to improve GI tolerability. Increase to 1.2mg/day and then max. 1.8mg/day at minimum 1-week intervals. Can be added to existing metformin or metformin + thiazolidinedione; the current metformin or metformin combination dose can continue unchanged; when added to sulphonylurea or metformin + sulphonylurea or basal insulin, adjust sulphonylurea or basal insulin dose to reduce hypoglycaemia risk. Admin, once daily at any time but same time daily independent of meals; NOT for IV or IM use; inject SC in abdomen, thigh or upper arm.

Elderly: Over 75 years, limited experience.

Renal Impairment: CrCl (mL/min) 30-90, no adjustment; below 30 or ESRD, not recommended.

Hepatic Impairment: Mild/moderate, no adjustment. Severe, not recommended.

Interactions: Effect of Liraglutide on Other Drugs: Warfarin: Monitor INR.

SP: CHF NYHA Class I-II/III-IV, no data. Inflammatory bowel disease, diabetic gastroparesis, not recommended. Transient GI reactions (nausea, vomiting, diarrhoea), potential dehydration risk, avoid fluid depletion. Thyroid adverse events (increased blood calcitonin, goitre, thyroid neoplasm). Not a substitute for insulin. Combination with sulphonylurea or basal insulin, increased hypoglycaemia risk. Pancreatitis, see Notes below.

ADR: Summary, most frequent, GI disorders (nausea, diarrhoea, vomiting, constipation, abdominal pain, dyspepsia), headache, nasopharyngitis; hypoglycaemia (sulfonylurea combination).

Notes: See 11.2.8 Other Antidiabetics, Excluding Insulin.

Victoza Parenteral *(Novo Nordisk)* B. GMS.
Price, 3mL (6mg/mL) (2) €99.57. (3) €148.88.
Injection, liraglutide 6mg/1mL. Clear colourless isotonic soln.
Store: Refrigerate*. After first use, below 30 deg C or refrigerate*.
*(do not freeze).

11.2.8 - Other Antidiabetic Drugs Excluding Insulin

In This Chapter: *Repaglinide and metformin combinations.*

Class Effects
Driving: See Notes below.
Indications: Type 2 diabetes mellitus (monotherapy or add-on), in combination with other glucose-lowering agents including insulin.
CI: Hypersensitivity to any member of the class. Children under 18 years. See Notes below (metformin).
SP: Not for use in Type 1 diabetes, not for ketoacidosis treatment. Increased hypoglycaemia risk (combination with sulphonylurea).
Pregnancy, Lactation: Pregnancy, avoid (insulin recommended). Lactation, not recommended.
Notes: See 11.2 Drugs Used In Diabetes. See 11.2.2 Biguanides (metformin).

Repaglinide

ATC Code: A10BX02. **Sport:** Permitted.
Driving: Hypoglycaemia risk.
Indications: Type 2 diabetes, monotherapy (not responding adequately to diet, exercise alone, not requiring insulin) or combination (with metformin) inadequate control with max. tolerated metformin.
Dose: Adult, Elderly: Initially 0.5mg/day (switch from other oral hypoglycaemics, initially 1mg/day); titrate at 1-2 week intervals. Max. single dose, 4mg; max. 16mg/day. To be taken 15 minutes before main meals. Debilitated or malnourished, titrate carefully.
Renal Impairment: Not affected by renal disorders.
Hepatic Impairment: Severe, contraindicated.
CI: Type 1 diabetes (C-peptide negative), diabetic acidosis with or without coma.
Interactions: Effect of Other Drugs on Repaglinide: *Co-admin contraindicated*: Gemfibrozil. *Co-admin caution (increased plasma levels)*: CYP2C8 inhibitors (rifampicin, St John's Wort, deferasirox), CYP3A4 inhibitors (deferasirox), OATP1B1 inhibitors. *Co-admin avoid*: Clopidogrel (careful glucose monitoring). *Enhanced or prolonged effect*: Gemfibrozil, clarithromycin, itraconazole, ketoconazole, trimethoprim, ciclosporin (avoid), other antidiabetic agents, MAOIs, non-selective beta-blockers, ACEIs, salicylates, NSAIDs, octreotide, ALCOHOL, anabolic steroids. *Effect reduced*: Oral contraceptives, rifampicin, barbiturates, carbamazepine, thiazides, corticosteroids, danazol, thyroid hormones, sympathomimetics. *Co-admin, increased hypoglycaemia risk*: Metformin, thiazolidinediones.
SP: Increased incidence of acute coronary syndrome (MI). Over 75 years, limited data. Can produce hypoglycaemia; metformin combination (increased risk).
ADR: Summary, *most frequent*, hypoglycaemia (with sulphonylurea or insulin). *Common*, abdominal pain, diarrhoea.
Notes: See 11.2.8 Other Antidiabetics, Excluding Insulin.

Novonorm 0.5mg, 1mg, 2mg *(Novo Nordisk)* B. GMS.
Price, (120) 0.5mg, €16.51. 1mg, €17.86. 2mg, €19.19.
Tablet, repaglinide. Round. Marked with Novo Nordisk logo. 0.5mg: White. 1mg: Yellow. 2mg: Peach. **Store:** Original pack to protect (moisture).

Repaglinide (Accord) 0.5mg, 1mg, 2mg *(Accord)* B. GMS.
Price, (30) 0.5mg, €2.89. (90) 0.5mg, €8.67; 1mg, €9.67; 2mg, €11.16.
Tablet, repaglinide. Round u/c. Marked R. 0.5mg: White (off-white). 1mg: Light-yellow. 2mg: Peach-coloured.

11.3 - Insulin

In This Chapter: *Insulin human, aspart, detemir, glargine, glulisine, lispro.*

Class Effects
Driving: With all insulin treatment, ability to concentrate and react may be impaired due to hypoglycaemia; caution, driving a car or operating machinery.
Sport: Insulin, and other substances with similar (chemical structure or biological effect) are prohibited in sport, see WADA Prohibited List 2017.
Store: Insulin should be refrigerated i.e. stored between 2-8 degrees Celsius (C); do not freeze; protect from light. After first use, see individual brands below.
Pharmacology: The potency of insulin analogues is expressed in units (U); human insulin is expressed in international units (IU). Insulin may be fast-acting (ATC A10AB), (Actrapid, Humulin S, Insuman Rapid, NovoMix, NovoRapid, Apidra, Humalog), intermediate-acting (ATC A10AC) (Humulin I, Insuman Basal), biphasic (ATC A10AD) (Humulin M3, Insuman Comb) or long-acting (ATC A10AE) (Insulatard, Levemir, Lantus).
Indications: Treatment, diabetes mellitus requiring insulin. For additional indications, see individual products below.
CI: Hypersensitivity to any member of the class. Hypoglycaemia.
Interactions: Effect of Other Drugs on Insulin: *Co-admin caution*: Pioglitazone (cardiac failure reported, especially with risk factors). *Enhanced hypoglycaemic effect*: Oral hypoglycaemics, certain antidepressants (MAOIs, SSRIs), non-selective beta-blockers, salicylates, ALCOHOL, sulfonamides, ACEIs (captopril, enalapril), AIIAs, anabolic steroids, disopyramide, fibrates, pentoxifylline, propoxyphene. *Reduced hypoglycaemic effect*: Thiazides, glucocorticoids, thyroid hormones, beta-sympathomimetics (ritodrine, salbutamol, terbutaline), somatropin, danazol, oral contraceptives (oestrogen, progesterone), diazoxide, diuretics, glucagon, isoniazid, atypical antipsychotics (clozapine, olanzapine), protease inhibitors. *Hypoglycaemia symptoms masked*: Beta-blockers, guanethidine, reserpine. *Increased or decreased insulin requirement*: Octreotide, lanreotide, beta-blockers, clonidine, lithium, alcohol. *Hypoglycaemic effect intensified, prolonged*: ALCOHOL. *Hypoglycaemia (may be followed by hyperglycaemia)*: Pentamidine.
SP: *Individualise* dose (monitor glucose, adjust dose); optimised glycaemic control delays onset of late diabetic complications; increased monitoring (renal or hepatic impairment, elderly). Insulin requirements may be reduced in renal impairment, hepatic impairment (reduced gluconeogenesis capacity, reduced insulin metabolism). Insulin antibody formation, may need insulin dose adjustment. Rotate injection sites to reduce (lipodystrophy risk, injection-site reactions).
Hyperglycaemia, due to inadequate dose or treatment discontinuation; gradual symptom onset (thirst, increased frequency of urination, nausea, vomiting, drowsiness, flushed dry skin, dry mouth, loss of appetite, acetone odour of breath). Untreated, may lead to diabetic ketoacidosis (potentially lethal).
Hypoglycaemia, results with too high dose in relation to insulin requirement, omission of a meal, unplanned, strenuous physical exercise; susceptibility increased by (change in injection area, improved sensitivity, unusual increased or prolonged physical activity, inadequate food intake, missed meals, alcohol consumption, certain endocrine disorders, other medication, changing insulin preparation, intercurrent illness including infection/fever); concomitant disease (kidney, liver, affecting adrenal, pituitary or thyroid gland); consider dose adjustment. Warning signs may be decreased (improved glycaemic control, if hypoglycaemia develops gradually, elderly, autonomic neuropathy present, history of diabetes, psychiatric illness, other drugs); severe hypoglycaemia may result before patient is aware. In children, match insulin doses (especially basal-bolus regimen) with food intake, physical activity to minimise hypoglycaemia.
Changing insulin brand requires strict medical supervision; changes in strength, brand (manufacturer), type (fast-, dual-, long-acting), origin (animal, human, analogue) and/or method of manufacture (recombinant DNA versus animal source) may require dose change; always consult

11.3   Insulin

manufacturers Full Prescribing Information. Caution, medication errors with different insulin types; always check insulin label. Insulin is for SC admin; rotate injection sites. Insulin susp are not for use in insulin infusion pumps.

Travel, seek medical advice before travelling between different time zones, as insulin and meals may need to be taken at different times.

Pregnancy, Lactation: Pregnancy, no restriction on human insulin use; does not pass placental barrier; recommend increased control of diabetic pregnant women as hypo- and hyperglycaemia increase risk of malformations and death *in utero*. Insulin requirements usually fall during first trimester, increase in second and third trimesters and return to pre-pregnancy levels after delivery. Lactation, insulin use presents no risk to baby.

ADR: Summary, *most frequently*, hypoglycaemia (varies with patient type, dose, level of glycaemic control); *beginning of treatment*, refraction anomalies, oedema, injection-site reactions (pain, redness, hives, inflammation, bruising, swelling, itching); usually transient; *rapid improvement in glycaemic control*, acute painful neuropathy (usually reversible); intensification of therapy with abrupt improvement in control, temporary worsening of diabetic retinopathy; long-term improved control decreases risk of diabetic retinopathy progression; *potentially life-threatening*, generalised hypersensitivity reactions (skin rash, itching, sweating, GI, angioedema, breathing difficulty, palpitation, reduction in BP); rare.

Notes: See 11.2 Drugs Used In Diabetes.

Insulin Human, rDNA E. coli

ATC Code: A10AB01 (S), A10AC01 (I), A10AD01 (M3). **Sport:** Prohibited.
Driving: Hypoglycaemia risk.

Indications: Hyperglycaemic coma and ketoacidosis, pre-, intra- and post-op stabilisation in diabetes mellitus.

Dose: Adult, Elderly: *Humulin*, S (Soluble), for SC or IV admin; I (Isophane) and M3 (Mixture 3; biphasic), for SC admin; NOT for IV admin. All can be admin by IM route, but not recommended.

Insuman, average insulin requirement often 0.5-1 international units/kg/day. For SC injection before meal, Basal (45-60 minutes before), Rapid (15-20 minutes before), Comb 15, 25 (30-45 minutes before), Comb 50 (20-30 minutes before). Basal, Comb NOT for IV admin, NOT for use in infusion pumps, external or implanted insulin pumps. Rapid, NOT for use in external or implanted insulin pumps, peristaltic pumps with silicone tubing.

Child: No data.

CI: Where allergy exists to animal insulin intradermal skin testing recommended, may be immunological cross-reactions.

ADR: *Most frequent*, hypoglycaemia.

Notes: See 11.3 Insulin.

> **Humulin S (Soluble), I (Isophane), M3 (Mix3)** *(Lilly)* B. GMS.
> *Price*, 100 IU: Cartridge x 5: (S), €25.94; (M3) €26.97; (I) €26.35. KwikPen x 5: (I) €31.63; (M3) €32.23. Vial 10mL x1: (S), €14.54; (I) (M3), €13.23.
> *Injection*, insulin human 100 IU/mL (rDNA) sterile. S: Clear colourless aqueous soln; pH 7-7.8. I: Susp of white crystalline precipitate in isotonic phosphate buffer. M3: Susp in the proportion 30% soluble insulin to 70% isophane insulin; pH 6.9-7.5. **Store:** After first use, below 30 deg C; do not refrigerate (cartridge, PFP).
>
> **Insuman Basal, Rapid, Comb Parenteral** *(SANOFI)* B. GMS.
> *Price*, (100 IU/mL): Vial 5mL x 1: Basal and Comb 25, €7.49. Cartridge 3mL x 5: Basal, €26.54; Comb 25, €27.98; Comb 50, €29.75; Rapid 100, €28.88.
> *Injection*, insulin human 100 IU (equiv. 3.5mg). Cartridge 3mL, vial 5mL. *Basal*: Isophane susp. *Rapid*: Neutral soln (regular insulin). *Comb*: Biphasic isophane susp; 15%(25%, 50%) dissolved insulin and 85%(75%, 50%) as crystalline protamine insulin. **Store:** After first use, below 25 deg C (max. 4 weeks); do not refrigerate pen containing a cartridge.

310

Insulin Human, rDNA Saccharomyces cerevisiae

ATC Code: A10AB01. **Sport:** Prohibited.
Driving: Hypoglycaemia risk.

Dose: Adult, Elderly: Individual insulin requirement usually 0.3-1 international units/kg/day.

Actrapid, for SC admin (IV only by healthcare professionals). Fast-acting, may be used in combination with long-acting insulin.

Insulatard, for SC admin. Long-acting, may be used alone or with fast-acting insulin or as basal insulin (evening and/or morning) with fast-acting at meals.

Notes: See 11.3 Insulin.

> **Actrapid Parenteral** *(Novo Nordisk)* B. GMS.
> *Price*, 10mL (1) €11.59.
> *Injection*, insulin human 100 international units/mL equiv. to 3.5mg (rDNA). Clear colourless aqueous soln. *Essentially sodium-free*. NOTE: Not for use in insulin pumps for continuous SC insulin infusion; precipitation risk. **Store:** After first use, below 25 deg C; do not refrigerate.
>
> **Insulatard Parenteral** *(Novo Nordisk)* B. GMS.
> *Price*, 100 units/mL: (5) Penfill cartridge, €26.97. Innolet PFP (5) €34.29. Vial 10mL x 1, €12.05.
> *Injection*, insulin human 100 international units/mL (rDNA). Cloudy white susp. *Essentially sodium-free*. **Store:** After first use, below 25 deg C (vial) or 30 deg C (Penfill, Innolet); do not refrigerate.

Insulin Aspart

ATC Code: A10AB05. **Sport:** Prohibited.
Driving: Hypoglycaemia risk.

Dose: Adult: *NovoMix*, Type 2 diabetes, monotherapy or combination (oral antidiabetics). Initially 6 units (breakfast) and 6 units (evening meal) OR 12 units once daily with evening meal; with once daily dosing, when 30 units is reached, split dose (breakfast, dinner). Type 1 diabetes, 0.5-1 units/kg/day. *Admin*, SC immediately before meal; not for IV admin or use in infusion pumps. See SP below.

NovoRapid, usually 0.5-1 units/kg/day. Faster onset and shorter duration than soluble human insulin. *Admin*, SC immediately before a meal; can be used IV by healthcare staff if needed; can be used for Continuous Subcutaneous Insulin Infusion (CSII) in pump system using abdominal wall and rotating sites. Normally used in combination (intermediate- or long-acting insulin).

Elderly: Over 75 years, limited data (combination with oral antidiabetic agents) *(NovoMix)*.

Child: *NovoMix*, can be used age 10 years and over (premixed insulin preferred); age 6-9 years, limited data; under 6 years, no data. *NovoRapid*, over age 1 year, can be used; under 1 year, safety/efficacy not established.

Renal Impairment: Insulin requirement may be reduced; recommend glucose monitoring, dose adjustment.

Hepatic Impairment: As for Renal above.

SP: Combination of pioglitazone with insulin (especially with risk factors); cardiac failure reported; if combination considered, observe patient for signs/symptoms of HF, weight gain, oedema.

Notes: See 11.3 Insulin. Combination, see 11.2.4 PPAR-Gamma Agonists (pioglitazone).

> **NovoMix 30 Parenteral** *(Novo Nordisk)* B. GMS.
> *Price*, 100 units/mL (3mL): (5) FlexPen PFP, €37.47. Penfill Cartridge, €35.94.
> *Injection*, insulin aspart 100 units/mL (soluble, protamine-crystallised in 30/70 ratio; equiv. to 3.5mg). Cloudy white susp. **Store:** After first use, below 30 deg C; do not refrigerate.
>
> **NovoRapid Parenteral** *(Novo Nordisk)* B. GMS.
> *Price*, 100 units/mL: (5) FlexPen, €38.39; Penfill cartridge, €34.78. Vial (1x10mL) €19.48.
> *Injection*, insulin aspart 100 units/mL (equiv. to 3.5mg) in vial, cartridge and PFP (colour coded FlexPen). *Essentially sodium-free*. **Store:** After first use, below 30 deg C; do not refrigerate.

Insulin Degludec

ATC Code: A10AE06. **Sport:** Prohibited.
Driving: Hypoglycaemia risk.

Dose: Adult: Type 2 diabetes, initiate with 10 units/day, then individualise (when GLP-1 receptor agonist added, reduce dose by 20% to minimise hypoglycaemia risk). Type 1 diabetes, use once-daily with meal-time insulin.

Type 2 diabetes, taking once-daily basal, basal-bolus, premix or self-mixed insulin changing basal insulin to *Tresiba* can be done unit-to-unit based on previous basal insulin dose; consider dose reduction of 20% on previous basal insulin when transferring to *Tresiba* from either twice-daily basal insulin or from insulin glargine (300 units/mL). *Type 1 diabetes*, consider 20% dose reduction based on previous basal insulin or basal component of a continuous SC insulin infusion.

Dose steps are different for different strengths: *100 units/mL*, a dose of 1-80 units per injection in steps of 1 unit; *200 units/mL*, a dose of 2-160 units per injection in steps of 2 units. In Type 2 diabetes, admin alone or in combination with oral hypoglycaemics, GLP-1 receptor agonists and bolus insulin. *Admin*, SC only, at any time of day but same time each day. NOT for IV admin (severe hypoglycaemia); not for IM admin as absorption may be changed. Not for use in insulin infusion pumps. NOTE: 1 unit insulin degludec corresponds to 1 international unit human insulin, 1 unit of insulin glargine or 1 unit insulin detemir.

Elderly: 65 years and above, intensified glucose monitoring.

Child: Age 1 year and over, can be used; when switching, consider reducing basal and bolus insulin to minimise hypoglycaemia. No experience with flexibility in dosing time.

Renal Impairment: As for Elderly above.

Hepatic Impairment: As for Elderly above.

SP: Cases of cardiac failure reported with pioglitazone especially with risk factor for cardiac failure; consider if pioglitazone combination is used. *Medication errors*, instruct patients to always check insulin label before each injection to avoid accidental mix-ups between the two different strengths of *Tresiba* as well as other insulin products.

Pregnancy, Lactation: Pregnancy, no clinical experience. Lactation, no metabolic effects anticipated in breast-fed newborn/infant.

ADR: Summary, *most frequent*, hypoglycaemia.

Notes: See 11.3 Insulin.

▼ **Tresiba Parenteral** *(Novo Nordisk)* B. GMS.
Price, 100 units/mL (5x3mL), €67.65. 200 units/mL (3x3mL), €81.18.
Injection (PFP Flextouch), insulin degludec 100 units/mL, 200 units/mL. Produced by rDNA technology. Clear colourless soln. **Store:** After first use, below 30 deg C (max. 8 weeks); can be refrigerated.

Insulin Detemir

ATC Code: A10AE05. **Sport:** Prohibited.
Driving: Hypoglycaemia risk.

Dose: Adult: Initially 0.1-0.2 units/kg or 10 units (adults) once daily in combination with oral antidiabetics and/or GLP-1 receptor agonists (when GLP-1 receptor agonist added, reduce *Levemir* dose by 20% to minimise hypoglycaemia risk). Can be used alone as basal insulin or in combination with bolus insulin as once or twice daily regimen. *Admin*, SC only, at any time of day but same time each day. NOT for IV admin (severe hypoglycaemia), avoid IM admin. Not for use in insulin infusion pumps. NOTE: 1 unit insulin detemir corresponds to 1 international unit human insulin.

Elderly: 65 years and above, intensified glucose monitoring.

Child: Age 1 year and over, can be used; when switching, consider reducing basal and bolus insulin dose to minimise hypoglycaemia.

Renal Impairment: Insulin requirement may be reduced; as for Elderly above.

Hepatic Impairment: As for Renal above.

SP: Severe hypoalbuminaemia, caution, monitor. Avoid mixing with rapid insulin.

Pregnancy, Lactation: Pregnancy, can consider use; weigh benefit/risk. Lactation, not known if excreted in human milk.

ADR: *Very common*, hypoglycaemia.

Notes: See 11.3 Insulin.

Levemir Parenteral *(Novo Nordisk)* B. GMS.
Price, 100 units/mL (5x3mL): FlexPen, €56.57. Cartridge, €56.24. Innolet, €58.60.
Injection, insulin detemir 100 units/mL. Produced by rDNA technology. Clear colourless aqueous soln. **Store:** During use or carried as spare, below 30 deg C; FlexPen can be refrigerated; do not refrigerate (Penfill, InnoLet); do not freeze.

Insulin Glargine

ATC Code: A10AE04. **Sport:** Prohibited.
Driving: Hyper/hypoglycaemia; visual impairment.

Dose: Adult: *Abasaglar, Lantus* (100 units/mL), individualise dose and timing. Prolonged duration of action. *Admin*, SC once daily (any time but same time each day); not for IV use; could result in severe hypoglycaemia. *Switch*, from other insulin (intermediate or long-acting), may need dose change (basal insulin, concomitant antidiabetics); from twice daily NPH, reduce daily basal insulin dose by 20-30% for first few weeks.

Toujeo (300 units/mL), type 2 diabetes, initially 0.2 units/kg then individualise. Not bioequivalent with insulin glargine *(Abasaglar, Lantus)*; not directly interchangeable. Switch from insulin glargine, a higher *Toujeo* dose (approx. 10-18%) may be needed; switch from *Toujeo* to insulin glargine, reduce dose (approx. 20%).

Elderly: As for Renal.

Child: Safety/efficacy, *Lantus, Abasaglar*, above 2 years, has been established (individualise dose); under 2 years, not established; *Toujeo*, under 18 years, not established.

Renal Impairment: Insulin requirements may decrease due to reduced renal function.

Hepatic Impairment: Insulin requirements may decrease due to reduced (capacity for gluconeogenesis, insulin metabolism).

SP: Not insulin of choice for diabetic ketoacidosis. High insulin doses due to antibodies may have improved insulin response with *Lantus, Abasaglar* or *Toujeo*.

Pregnancy, Lactation: Pregnancy, consider use if needed. Lactation, dose may need adjustment; no metabolic effects of ingested insulin glargine anticipated.

ADR: *Very common*, hypoglycaemia.

Notes: See 11.3 Insulin.

▼ **ABASAGLAR Parenteral** *(Lilly)* B. GMS.
Price, 100 units/mL (5x3mL): Cartridge and KwikPen (1-80 Units), €41.96.
Injection, insulin glargine 100 U/mL (equiv. 3.64mg). 3mL (cartridge, KwikPen). rDNA technology. Clear colourless soln. *Note:* Do not mix with other insulin or dilute (can change time/action profile) or may cause precipitation. **Store:** After first use, below 30 deg C (max. 28 days); do not refrigerate.

Lantus Parenteral *(SANOFI)* B. GMS.
Price, 100 U/mL (5x3mL): Cartridge, €47.36; Solostar, €46.55. Vial (1x10mL) €36.94.
Injection, insulin glargine 100 U/mL (equiv. 3.64mg). 3mL (cartridge, Solostar PFP), 5mL vial. rDNA technology. Clear colourless soln. NOTE: Do not mix with other insulin or dilute (can change time/action profile) or may cause precipitation. Potency stated in units exclusive to *Lantus*. **Store:** After first use, below 30 deg C (max. 4 weeks); do not refrigerate. See Class Effects.

Toujeo Parenteral *(SANOFI)* B. GMS.
Price, 300 units/mL (5x1.5mL), €69.00.
Injection, insulin glargine 300 units/mL (1.5mL PFP Solostar). Clear colourless soln. Potency stated in units exclusive to *Toujeo*.
Store: After first use, below 30 deg C (max. 4 weeks); do not refrigerate.

Insulin Glulisine

ATC Code: A10AB06. **Sport:** Prohibited.
Driving: Hypoglycaemia risk.

Dose: Adult, Elderly: Admin 0-15 minutes before meals; use with intermediate or long-acting insulin. SC injection or continuous SC pump infusion.

Child: 6 years and over, as for Adult above.

Pregnancy, Lactation: Pregnancy, caution. Lactation, dose adjustment may be required.

Notes: See 11.3 Insulin.

11.4 Treatment of Hypoglycaemia

Apidra Parenteral *(SANOFI)* B. GMS.
Price, 100 IU/mL: (5) Cartridge, €33.62; Solostar PFP (5) €35.43. Vial (1x10mL) €19.38.
Injection, insulin glulisine 100 U/mL (equiv. 3.49mg). 3mL (PFP Solostar, cartridge), 10mL vial. Clear colourless soln. NOTE: Potency expressed in units exclusive to *Apidra*. Do not mix with any preparations other than NPH (Neutral Protamine Hagedorn) human insulin. **Store:** After first use, below 25 deg C (max. 4 weeks); do not refrigerate.

Insulin Lispro

ATC Code: A10AB04. **Sport:** Prohibited.
Driving: Hypoglycaemia risk.
Indications: *Humalog* also indicated for initial stabilisation.
Dose: Adult, Elderly: *Humalog,* admin shortly before meals; SC or continuous SC infusion pump; can be given IM but not recommended; can be used IV; *Humalog Mix* admin shortly before meals or soon after; SC injection only; NOT for IV use. Duration of action of insulin lispro protamine suspension (NPL) component is similar to that of a basal insulin (NPH isophane).
Child: Only for use in preference to soluble insulin when fast action of insulin might be beneficial.
Notes: See 11.3 Insulin.

Humalog Parenteral *(Lilly)* B. GMS.
Price, 100 units/mL: KwikPen (5x3mL) €37.76. Cartridge, €35.37. Vial (1x10mL) €20.81. 200 units/mL: KwikPen (5x3mL) €74.09.
Injection, insulin lispro 100 units/mL (equiv. to 3.5mg) and 200 units/mL (equiv. to 6.9mg). Clear colourless soln. **Store:** After first use, below 30 deg C; do not refrigerate (vials may be refrigerated).
Humalog Mix Parenteral *(Lilly)* B. GMS.
Price, 100 units/mL: Mix25 (5x3mL): Cartridge, €35.30; KwikPen, €38.45. Mix50 (5x3mL): Cartridge, €35.29. KwikPen, €37.67.
Injection, insulin lispro/insulin lispro protamine 100 U/mL (25%, 75%) and (50%, 50%). White sterile susp. **Store:** After first use, below 30 deg C; do not refrigerate; vials may be refrigerated.

11.4 - Treatment of Hypoglycaemia

In This Chapter: *Glucagon.*

Class Effects
CI: Hypersensitivity to any member of the class.

Glucagon

ATC Code: H04AA01. **Sport:** Permitted.
Driving: Caution.
Indications: Treatment, severe hypoglycaemic reactions (may occur in management of insulin treated diabetics). *Diagnostic,* motility inhibition in examinations of GI tract.
Dose: Adult, Elderly: TREATMENT, severe hypoglycaemia, 1mg SC or IM; patient normally responds within 10 minutes; follow with oral glucose, see SP below; no response in 10 minutes, admin IV glucose.
DIAGNOSTIC, must be admin by medical personnel. Inhibition of motility, 0.2-0.5mg IV (onset of action within 1 minutes, duration 5-20 minutes depending on organ being examined) OR 1-2mg IM (onset of action 5-15 minutes, duration 10-40 minutes depending on organ). Stomach, duodenal bulb, duodenum, small bowel, 0.2-0.5mg IV OR 1mg IM; colon, 0.5-0.75mg IV or 1-2mg IM. Not for IV infusion. See SP below.
Child: Severe hypoglycaemia, over 25kg or 6-8 years, 1mg for Adult; under 25kg or under 6-8 years, 0.5mg SC or IM.
CI: Phaeochromocytoma.
Interactions: Effect of Other Drugs on Glucagon: *Inability to raise blood glucose, hypoglycaemia:* Indomethacin.
Effect of Glucagon on Other Drugs: Insulin: *Antagonised.* Warfarin: *Increased anticoagulant effect.*
SP: *Therapeutic,* after response to treatment, admin oral carbohydrate to restore liver glycogen and prevent secondary hypoglycaemia. *Diagnostic,* if compatible with procedure admin oral carbohydrates; if fasting required, admin IV glucose. Fasting patients may experience discomfort; nausea, hypoglycaemia and BP changes.
Glucagon antagonises insulin. Insulinoma, glucagonoma, caution (hypoglycaemia relapse). Radiographic procedures in diabetics, elderly with cardiac disease, caution diagnostic use.
Pregnancy, Lactation: Pregnancy, reported use with no harmful effects with respect to course of pregnancy and health of unborn/neonate. Lactation, will not exert metabolic effect in child.
ADR: *Therapeutic, Diagnostic,* anaphylactic, shock, abdominal pain, nausea, vomiting. *Diagnostic,* hypoglycaemia, hypoglycaemic coma, hypo-, hypertension; tachy-, bradycardia.
Notes: See 11.4 Treatment of Hypoglycaemia.

GlucaGen HypoKit 1mg *(Novo Nordisk)* A. GMS.
Price, (1) €18.39.
SC or IM injection, glucagon HCl 1mg (1 IU)/mL. White (nearly white) powder; clear colourless solvent (without particles). **Store:** Can be stored below 25 deg C (18 months) provided within expiry date.

11.5 - Thyroid, Antithyroid Hormones

11.5.1 - Thyroid Hormones

In This Chapter: *Levothyroxine.*

Class Effects
CI: Hypersensitivity to any member of the class, thyrotoxicosis. Adrenal insufficiency without adequate corticosteroid cover. Not for initiation in acute MI, acute myocarditis, acute pancarditis.
Interactions: Effect of Other Drugs on Thyroid Hormones: *Metabolism accelerated, plasma levels decreased:* Rifampicin, phenytoin, primidone, barbiturates, carbamazepine. *Co-admin (severe hypertension, tachycardia):* Ketamine.
Effect of Thyroid Hormones on Other Drugs: Warfarin, phenindione: *Anticoagulant effect enhanced.* Cardiac glycosides: *Digoxin dose reduction may be needed.* Sympathomimetics (adrenaline, noradrenaline): *Effect enhanced.* Beta-blockers (propranolol): *Increased clearance in hyperthyroidism; dose reduction may be needed when patient becomes euthyroid.* Erythromycin: *Reduced clearance.* Prednisolone: *Increased clearance.*
SP: Long-standing hypothyroidism, cardiovascular disorders (angina, CAD, hypertension, insufficiency, MI), elderly with potential for cardiac disease, adrenocortical insufficiency may occur (caution, diabetes mellitus and diabetes insipidus). Thyroid replacement therapy may require increased dosage of insulin or other anti-diabetics.
Pregnancy, Lactation: Combination of levothyroxine and an antithyroid agent for hyperthyroidism is not indicated in pregnancy.
ADR: Anginal pain, arrhythmias, palpitation, tachycardia, skeletal muscle cramp, muscular weakness, diarrhoea, vomiting, tremors, restlessness, excitability, insomnia, headache, flushing, sweating, excessive weight loss, fever, heat intolerance. Hypersensitivity reactions (rash, pruritus, oedema).

Levothyroxine (thyroxine)

ATC Code: H03AA01. **Sport:** Permitted.
Driving: Unlikely to impair.
Indications: Hypothyroidism (congenital, acquired), juvenile myxoedema, goitre (diffuse, non-toxic; Hashimoto's thyroiditis), suppression therapy in thyroid carcinoma.
Dose: Adult: Initially 50-100mcg/day before breakfast; if needed titrate by 50mcg at 3-4 week intervals to maintenance; max. 100-200mcg/day. Diffuse non-toxic goitre, 50-200mcg/day. Suppression therapy in thyroid carcinoma, 150-300mcg/day. Cardiac disease, see Elderly below. *Switch* of dosage form, monitor closely.
Elderly: Initially 12.5mcg/day; increase slowly, at lengthy intervals (12.5mcg fortnightly). Clinical response more acceptable criterion for dosage than serum levels.
Child: *Tabs,* infants (congenital hypothyroidism, juvenile myxoedema), initially 25mcg/day titrating in 25mcg increments according to clinical response; over 1 year, initially 2.5-5mcg/kg/day.

Oral soln, infants with congenital hypothyroidism, 10-15mcg/kg/day for first 3 months then according to response/TSH values; acquired hypothyroidism, initially 12.5-50mcg per day; increased every 2-4 weeks according to response/TSH values. Admin half hour before first meal of day.

Interactions: Effect of Other Drugs on Levothyroxine: *Absorption reduced*: Calcium salts and/or oral iron (allow several hours dosing interval), cimetidine, sucralfate, colestyramine, colestipol, sodium polystyrene sulphonate, soy proteins. *Plasma levels (possibly) reduced*: Imatinib. *Increased dose required*: Oestrogen and oestrogen-containing products. *Decreased levothyroxine binding globulins*: Androgens, corticosteroids.

Effect of Levothyroxine on Other Drugs: Amitriptyline, TCADs: *Effect enhanced.*

SP: Use lowest effective dose to minimise osteoporosis risk. Partial hair loss in children; usually transient.

Pregnancy, Lactation: Pregnancy, if benefit outweighs risk of foetal untreated hypothyroidism. Lactation, excreted in breast milk in low conc; interference with neonatal screening, contentious.

Notes: See 11.5.1 Thyroid Hormones.

Eltroxin Tablets, Oral Soln *(Concordia)* B. GMS.
Price, (28) 25mcg, €1.21. 50mcg, €1.64. 100mcg, €1.80. Oral soln (100mL) 25mcg, €50.14. 50mcg, €23.37. 100mcg, €93.71 (PTW; non-GMS).
Tablet, levothyroxine sodium 25mcg, 50mcg, 100mcg. White scored (facilitates breaking). 25mcg: Marked FW 41. 50mcg, 100mcg: Marked with name/strength. *Lactose.*
Oral soln, as above 25mcg (50mcg, 100mcg)/5mL. Clear colourless liquid. *Glycerol, parabens.*

11.5.2 - Antithyroid Drugs

In This Chapter: *Carbimazole.*

Class Effects
CI: Hypersensitivity to any member of the class.

Carbimazole

ATC Code: H03BB01. **Sport:** Permitted.
Driving: Unlikely to impair.
Indications: Conditions where reduction of thyroid function is required (hyperthyroidism, preparation for thyroidectomy in hyperthyroidism, therapy prior to and post radio-iodine treatment).

Dose: Adult, Elderly: Initially 20-60mg in 2-3 divided doses; titrate dose against thyroid function until patient is euthyroid. Maintenance, range 5-15mg/day as single daily dose for 6-18 months. Blocking-replacement, maintain dose at initial level (20-60mg/day) with supplemental levothyroxine, 50-150mcg/day to prevent hypothyroidism; duration 6-18 months.
Child: Age 3-17 years, initially 0.5mg/kg in 2 or 3 divided doses; max. 40mg/day. Maintenance, dose can be reduced depending on response. Levothyroxine may be required to avoid hypothyroidism. Age 2 years and under, not recommended.

SP: Bone marrow depression (neutropenia, eosinophilia, leucopenia, agranulocytosis), including fatalities. Warn patients of signs or symptoms of early bone marrow depression (sore throat, mouth ulcers, pyrexia), discontinue immediately; monitor. Confused patients, or those with poor memory, conduct regular full blood counts. Liver disorders, caution. At time of radio-iodine admin, temporarily stop carbimazole to avoid thyroid crisis.

Pregnancy, Lactation: Non-pregnant women of child-bearing potential, use if benefit outweighs risk. Pregnancy, use lowest dose; consider discontinuing 3-4 weeks before term to reduce risk of neonatal complications. Blocking-replacement regimen, not recommended (very little thyroxine crosses placenta in last trimester). Lactation, not recommended.

ADR: Summary, *most frequent,* nausea, headache, arthralgia, mild gastric distress, skin rash, pruritus; usually self-limiting. See SP above.

Notes: See 11.5.2 Antithyroid Drugs.

11.6 - Hypothalamic and Pituitary Hormones, Anti-Oestrogens

Class Effects
Hypothalamic hormones include: *Anterior Pituitary Hormones,* corticotrophin (ACTH), gonadotropins, follicle-stimulating hormone (FSH), luteinising hormone (LH), growth hormone, lactogenic hormone and thyroid stimulating hormone (TSH). *Posterior Pituitary Hormones,* antidiuretic hormone (vasopressin), oxytocin. Diagnostics, tetracosactide *(Synacthen)* (investigation of adrenocortical insufficiency); gonadorelin, sermorelin.

Notes: See 8.1.1 Prostaglandins, Oxytocics.

11.6.1 - Anterior Pituitary Hormones, Gonadotrophins Used In Infertility

In This Chapter: *Choriogonadotropin alfa, corifollitropin, human chorionic gonadotropin (hCG), follitropin alpha, follicle stimulating hormone (FSH), lutropin alfa, menotrophin.*

Class Effects
Sport: Gonadotropins (LH, hCG) prohibited for use in sport by males only, see WADA Prohibited List 2017.

CI: Hypersensitivity to any member of the class. When effective response cannot be obtained (primary ovarian failure, primary gonadal failure) or incompatible with pregnancy (malformation of sexual organs, fibroid tumours of uterus), postmenopause.
Tumours (ovary, breast, uterus, testis, hypothalamus, pituitary), ovarian enlargement or cyst (other than PCOD), undiagnosed vaginal bleeding.

SP: These drugs are used only within specialised units. Infertility should be assessed before initiation; evaluate contraindications to pregnancy (hypothyroidism, adrenocortical deficiency, hyperprolactinaemia, pituitary or hypothalamic tumours); caution if pregnancy may lead to worsening of systemic disease.
ART, has risk of Ovarian Hyperstimulation Syndrome (OHSS), due to multiple follicular development characterised by large ovarian cysts, prone to rupture, presence of ascites, circulatory dysfunction; avoid by withholding hCG. Perform ultrasonic assessment of follicular development, determine of oestradiol levels, prior to FSH-treatment, then at regular intervals during treatment. Severe OHSS (haemoperitoneum, acute pulmonary distress, ovarian torsion, thromboembolism). Thromboembolic events associated with OHSS or separate; may be venous or arterial.
Multiple pregnancies, miscarriage, increased risk; miscarriage rate higher than normal population. With tubal disease there is risk of ectopic pregnancy due to spontaneous conception or fertility treatment. Prevalence of congenital malformations after ART slightly higher than spontaneous conceptions; may be due to parental characteristics (maternal age, sperm characteristics). Ovarian, other reproductive system neoplasms (benign, malignant), with multiple drug regimens for infertility treatment. hCG may induce precocious puberty in children, discontinue immediately. May cause growth spurt; care where epiphyseal growth still potentially active. Fluid retention (caution, asthma, migraine, epilepsy, cardiac or renal dysfunction). Allergic diathesis, caution; preliminary skin test.

Pregnancy, Lactation: Not recommended.

Notes: See 11.6 Hypothalamic and Pituitary Hormones, Anti-Oestrogens, 11.9 Other Endocrine Drugs (buserelin) and 13.3.2 Prostate Cancer (buserelin, goserelin).

NeoMercazole 5mg, 20mg *(Concordia)* B. GMS.
Price, (100) 5mg, €6.35. 20mg, €23.60.
Tablet, carbimazole. Pink round. Marked Neo/strength. *Lactose, sucrose.*

Choriogonadotropin Alfa

ATC Code: G03GA08. **Sport:** Prohibited (in men).
Driving: No studies performed.

Indications: Superovulation in women prior to assisted reproductive techniques; anovulatory or oligo-ovulatory women.

Dose: Adult: 250mcg by SC injection 24-48 hours after *superovulation* last FSH or hMG admin or *anovulation or oligo-ovulation* optimal stimulation of follicular growth; coitus recommended on day or day after admin.

CI: Thromboembolic disorders.

Interactions: Effect of Choriogonadotropin Alfa on Other Drugs: Immunological determination of serum/urine hCG: False positive pregnancy test.

SP: Minor thyroid stimulation. Self-admin only with adequate training and access to expert advice.

ADR: Nausea, vomiting, abdominal pain, headache, tiredness, injection site local reaction/pain.

Notes: See 11.6.1 Gonadotrophins Used In Infertility.

Ovitrelle Parenteral *(Merck Serono)* A. HT.
Price, 250mcg/0.5mL (1), (PFP) €33.58 (PFS) €33.73.
Injection, choriogonadotropin alfa 250mcg. r-hCG produced by rDNA technology. Clear colourless (slightly yellow) soln in PFP.

Corifollitropin Alfa

ATC Code: G03GA09. **Sport:** Permitted.
Driving: Dizziness.

Indications: Controlled Ovarian Stimulation (COS), combination with GnRH antagonist.

Dose: Adult: Weight 60kg and less, 100mcg; above 60kg, 150mcg admin SC as single dose. Stimulation (day 1), during early follicular phase of menstrual cycle; (day 5 or 6), start GnRH antagonist depending on ovarian response to prevent premature LH surges; (day 8) continue daily recombinant FSH (usually 150 IU) until oocyte maturation; then single hCG injection (5-10 thousand IU).

Renal Impairment: Elimination rate may be reduced, not recommended.

CI: Primary ovarian failure, (history) ovarian hyperstimulation syndrome (OHSS); previous cycle resulting in more than 30 follicles, basal antral follicle count above 20, polycystic ovarian syndrome (PCOS). See Notes below.

SP: Additional injection should not be given in same treatment cycle. For SC injection only. No additional FSH-containing product should be admin prior to stimulation day 8.

ADR: *Common,* headache, nausea, OHSS, pelvic pain/discomfort, breast complaints, fatigue.

Notes: See 11.6.1 Gonadotrophins Used In Infertility.

Elonva Parenteral *(MSD)* A. HT.
Price, PFS (1) 0.5mL, 100mcg, €544.99. 150mcg, €559.65.
Injection (PFS), corifollitropin alfa 100mcg, 150mcg. Clear colourless aqueous soln. Produced by rDNA technology. *Sodium less than 23mg/injection.* **Store:** Refrigerate; do not freeze; can be stored below 25 deg C (max. 1 month).

Human Chorionic Gonadotrophin

ATC Code: G03GA01. **Sport:** Prohibited (in men).
Driving: None known.

Indications: Ovulation induction in subfertility due to anovulation or impaired follicle ripening in females. Hypogonadotrophic hypogonadism, delayed puberty, pre-operative preparation of ectopic testes in males.

Dose: Adult: *Ovulation induction, hyperstimulation,* usually 5000-10000 IU to complete treatment with FSH. Luteal phase support, 1000-3000 IU admin within 9 days following ovulation or embryo transfer.
Hypogonadotrophic hypogonadism, 1000-2000 IU 2-3 times weekly; subfertility, add FSH 2-3 times weekly.
Child: *Delayed puberty in males,* 1500 IU 2-3 times weekly; for 6 months. *Pre-op preparation for ectopic testes,* 500 IU 2-3 times weekly for 1-2 months before surgery. *Cryptorchidism,* under 2 years, 250 IU twice weekly; under 6 years, 500-1000 IU twice weekly; over 6 years, 1500 IU twice weekly for 6 weeks.

CI: Sex hormone-dependant tumours in males (prostate, breast).

Pregnancy, Lactation: Pregnancy, only for luteal phase support. Lactation, not to be used.

ADR: Rash, injection-site reactions. Water, sodium retention (males, high doses).

Notes: See 11.6.1 Gonadotrophins Used In Infertility.

Pregnyl Parenteral *(MSD)* A.
Price, 5000 IU (1) €3.91.
Injection, hCG 5000 IU. White dry cake or powder. Clear colourless solvent for soln. *Essentially sodium-free.*

Follitropin Alfa

ATC Code: G03GA05. **Sport:** Permitted.
Driving: No or negligible effect.

Indications: Anovulation (including polycystic ovarian syndrome) unresponsive to clomifene; superovulation; stimulation of follicular development in severe LH and FSH deficiency in females. Stimulation of spermatogenesis (congenital or acquired hypogonadotrophic hypogonadism) in males.

Dose: Adult: *Anovulation,* usually 75-150 IU FSH daily; titrate to 37.5 IU or 75 IU at 7-14 day intervals; max. 225 IU FSH/day until optimal response; follow with hCG/r-hCG.
Superovulation, 150-225 IU/day commencing on days 2 or 3 of cycle; max. usually 450 IU/day followed by hCG or r-hCG. *Severe LH/FSH deficiency,* initially 75 IU lutropin alfa daily with 75-100 IU FSH; titrate at 7-14 day intervals by 37.5-75 IU increments until optimal response; follow with hCG/r-hCG.
Hypogonadotrophic hypogonadism, 150 IU 3-times weekly with hCG (minimum 4 months). SC injection. See SP below.

Renal Impairment: Safety, efficacy not established.

Hepatic Impairment: As for Renal above.

Interactions: Effect of Other Drugs on Follitropin Alfa: *Follicular response potentiated:* Other agents used to stimulate ovulation (hCG, clomifene). *Increased dosage requirement:* GnRH agonists.

SP: Porphyria, increased risk of acute attack, caution. Generally lower cumulative dose, shorter duration required than with urinary FSH. Thromboembolism may occur very rarely.

Pregnancy, Lactation: Data on limited number of exposed pregnancies indicate no malformative or feto/neonatal toxicity of follitropin alfa. Lactation, not recommended.

ADR: *Very common, common,* injection-site reactions; *females,* headache, abdominal (pain, distension), discomfort), nausea, vomiting, diarrhoea, ovarian cysts, mild OHSS; *males,* acne, gynaecomastia, varicocele, weight gain.

Notes: See 11.6.1 Gonadotrophins Used In Infertility.

Gonal-f Parenteral *(Merck Serono)* A. HT.
Price, injection (1) 75 IU, €23.65. 1050 IU, €394.93. PFP (1) 300 IU, €98.82. 450 IU, €148.12. 900 IU, €333.77.
Injection, follitropin alpha 75 IU (5.5mcg), 300 IU (22mcg), 450 IU (33mcg), 900 IU (66mcg), 1050 IU (77mcg); r-hFSH. White lyophilised pellet. Clear colourless solvent OR clear colourless soln in PFP. *Sodium 23mg/dose (essentially sodium-free).* **Store:** Refrigerate, do not freeze; unrefrigerated below 25 deg C (max. 3 months) then discard.

▼ **Bemfola Parenteral** *(GedeonRichter)* A. HT.
Price, (1) 75 IU, €24.70; 150 IU, €48.99; 225 IU, €73.95; 300 IU, €98.82; 450 IU, €148.13.
Injection, follitropin alpha (IU) 75, 150, 225, 300, 450. Recombinant human follicle stimulating hormone (r-hFSH). Clear colourless soln in PFP. *Essentially sodium-free.* **Store:** Refrigerate, do not freeze; unrefrigerated below 25 deg C (max. 3 months) then discard.

Follitropin Alfa, Lutropin Alfa

ATC Code: G03GA30. **Sport:** Prohibited (in men).
Driving: No or negligible effect.

Indications: Stimulation of follicular development in severe LH and FSH deficiency in women.

Dose: Adult: Follitropin alfa 150 IU, lutropin alfa 75 IU daily by SC injection; if needed adjust dose after 7-14 days by 37.5-75 IU follitropin alfa then hCG or r-hCG.

Renal Impairment: Safety, efficacy not established.

Interactions: Effect of Other Drugs on Follitropin Alfa, Lutropin Alfa Combination: *Not recommended*: Admixture with other medicinals in same injection (except follitropin alfa).

ADR: *Females*, breast pain, pelvic pain. See Notes below (follitropin alfa).

Notes: See Follitropin Alfa above and Lutropin Alfa below.

Pergoveris Parenteral *(Merck Serono)* A. HT.
Price, (1) €79.03; (10) €728.77.
Injection, follitropin alfa 150 IU (11mcg), lutropin alfa 75 IU (3mcg); r-hFSH, r-hLH. White (off-white) lyophilised powder. Clear colourless solvent for soln. **Store**: Below 25 deg C; original pack to protect (light).

Follitropin Beta

ATC Code: G03GA06. **Sport:** Permitted.
Driving: Unlikely to impair.

Indications: Adults (females), anovulation including polycystic ovarian syndrome (PCOS) unresponsive to clomifene in females; controlled ovarian hyperstimulation for assisted reproduction; (males), deficient spermatogenesis in hypogonadotrophic hypogonadism.

Dose: Adult: *Females*, anovulation, initially 50 IU (7 days); controlled ovarian hyperstimulation, 100-225 IU (minimum 4 days); maintenance 75-375 IU (6-12 days). Follow with hCG.

Males, hypogonadotrophic hypogonadism, 150 IU 3-times weekly with hCG (3-4 months). Admin by slow IM or SC injection alternating injection sites.

Interactions: Effect of Other Drugs on Follicle Stimulating Hormone: See Notes below (follitropin alfa).

SP: Exclude presence of uncontrolled non-gonadal endocrinopathies. Admin lower dose than used for urinary FSH. Transient LFT abnormalities. May contain traces of streptomycin and/or neomycin.

Pregnancy, Lactation: Pregnancy, no indication for use. Lactation, may affect milk production.

ADR: Injection site bruising, pain, redness, swelling, itching; headache, nausea; thromboembolism. Gynaecomastia (males).

Notes: See Follitropin Alfa above. See 11.6.1 Gonadotrophins Used In Infertility.

Puregon Parenteral *(MSD)* A. HT.
Price, injection (5mL x 1) 50 IU, €21.05. 100 IU, €39.98. Cartridge 300 IU, €106.81. 600 IU, €210.90. 900 IU, €319.84. *Injection*, FSH. Recombinant. Clear colourless soln. *Essentially sodium-free.*

Ganirelix

ATC Code: H01CC01. **Sport:** Permitted.
Driving: Unlikely to impair.

Indications: Prevention, premature LH surges in women undergoing controlled ovarian hyperstimulation.

Dose: Adult: Initially, 0.25mg by SC injection once daily (day 5 or day 6) of FSH admin or following corifollitropin alfa admin.

Child: No relevant use.

Renal Impairment: Moderate/severe, contraindicated.

Hepatic Impairment: As for Renal above.

Interactions: Effect of Other Drugs on Ganirelix: *Possible interactions*: Histamine liberators.

SP: Hypersensitivity reactions (early as first dose); not recommended with severe active allergic conditions. Under 50kg or over 90kg, no data.

ADR: *Very common*, local injection-site reactions (redness with or without swelling).

Notes: See 11.6.1 Gonadotrophins Used In Infertility.

Orgalutran Parenteral 0.25mg/0.5mL *(MSD)* A. HT.
Price, (1) €34.85.
Injection, ganirelix. GnRH. Clear colourless aqueous. *Essentially sodium-free; natural rubber needle shield.*

Lutropin Alfa

ATC Code: G03GA07. **Sport:** Prohibited (in men).
Driving: No or negligible effect.

Indications: Stimulation of follicular development in adult women with severe LH and FSH deficiency.

Dose: Adult: 75 IU lutropin alfa SC daily with 75-150 IU FSH; if needed titrate FSH after 7-14 days by 37.5 IU-75 IU increments until optimal response. Follow with hCG or r-hCG. Use self-admin only if (patient is adequately trained; has access to expert advice).

Renal Impairment: Safety, efficacy not established.

Hepatic Impairment: As for Renal above.

ADR: *Common*, headache, abdominal pain/discomfort, nausea, vomiting, diarrhoea, mild or moderate OHSS; ovarian cyst, breast/pelvic pain, injection site reaction.

Notes: See 11.6.1 Gonadotrophins Used In Infertility.

Luveris Parenteral *(Merck Serono)* A. HT.
Price, (1) €40.75.
Injection, lutropin alfa (r-hLH) 75 IU. White lyophilised pellet. Clear colourless solvent.

Menotrophin

ATC Code: G03GA02. **Sport:** Prohibited (in men).
Driving: Unlikely to impair.

Indications: Anovulation (including PCOD) unresponsive to clomifene in females. Controlled ovarian hyperstimulation. Stimulation of spermatogenesis (congenital or acquired hypogonadotrophic hypogonadism) in males.

Dose: Adult: *Anovulation, PCOD*, start day 7 of menstrual cycle, initially 75-150 IU/day (minimum 7 days); if required increase every 7 days by 37.5 IU (max. 75 IU); max. 225 IU/day until optimal response. Follow with hCG.

Controlled ovarian hyperstimulation, using down-regulation with GnRH agonist, commence on day 2 or 3 of menstrual cycle, initially 150-225 IU/day for first 5 days; titrate by max. 150 IU increments to max. 450 IU/day (max. 20 days).

Spermatogenesis stimulation, 75-150 units with hCG. Admin SC or IM.

Interactions: Effect of Other Drugs on Menotrophin: *Follicular response potentiated*: Other agents stimulating ovulation (clomifene). *Increased dose requirement*: GnRH agonists.

Pregnancy, Lactation: Contraindicated.

ADR: *Common*, abdominal pain/distention, nausea, headache, OHSS, pelvic pain, injection site reaction/pain.

Notes: See 11.6.1 Gonadotrophins Used In Infertility.

MENOPUR Parenteral *(Ferring)* A. HT.
Price, (10) 75IU, €213.44. (1) 600IU, €170.75; 1200IU, €341.51.
Injection, menotrophin 75 IU, 600 IU, 1200 IU. White (off-white) powder. Clear colourless solvent for soln.

11.6.2 - Anterior Pituitary Hormones, Growth Hormone

In This Chapter: *Mecasermin, somatropin.*

Class Effects
Sport: Growth hormone (hGH) is prohibited for use in sport, see WADA Prohibited List 2017.

CI: Hypersensitivity to any member of the class.

SP: Treatment to be carried out by physicians qualified and experienced in diagnosis and management of growth disorders. Consult manufacturers Full Prescribing Information. Individualise dose, admin schedule. With endocrine disorders, including growth hormone deficiency, slipped epiphyses of the hip may occur more frequently; children limping during treatment, examine clinically.

Mecasermin

ATC Code: H01AC03. **Sport:** Prohibited.
Driving: Caution.

Indications: Growth failure in children and adolescents with severe primary insulin-like growth factor-1 deficiency.

Dose: Adult: Not applicable.

Child: Initially 0.04mg/kg twice daily; if no significant adverse events in week 1, increase by 0.04mg/kg to max. 0.12mg/kg twice daily. SC shortly before or after a food; if hypoglycaemia occurs despite adequate food intake, decrease dose; if patient unable to eat, withhold. Rotate injection sites. Under 2 years, not recommended;

11.6.2 Anterior Pituitary Hormones, Growth Hormone

contraindicated in neonates, premature babies. IV admin contraindicated.

CI: Active/suspected neoplasia; discontinue if evidence of neoplasia develops.

SP: Correct thyroid and nutritional deficiencies before initiation. Not for use if epiphyses closed.

Hypoglycaemia, at initiation avoid high-risk activities within 2-3 hours of dosing; severe hypoglycaemia, and unconscious or unable to ingest food, use glucagon injection. Insulin/other hypoglycaemic dose may need reduction. *ECG*, recommended before initiation and termination. Lymphoid tissue hypertrophy (tonsillar) (snoring, sleep apnoea, chronic middle ear effusions). Intracranial hypertension, with papilloedema, visual changes, headache, nausea and/or vomiting; recommend funduscopic examination.

Rapid growth, slipped capital femoral epiphysis (with potential to lead to avascular necrosis) and progression of scoliosis can occur; limp or hip/knee pain, evaluate. Allergic reactions, antibody response to injected IGF-1. No response after 1 year, reconsider treatment.

Pregnancy, Lactation: Pregnancy, only if clearly necessary. Women of child-bearing potential to ensure adequate contraception. Lactation, not recommended.

ADR: Summary, *most frequent*, headache, hypoglycaemia, vomiting, injection site hypertrophy, otitis media.

Notes: See 11.6.2 Growth Hormone.

▼ **Increlex Parenteral** *(Ipsen)* A. HT.
Price, (1) €646.98.
Injection, mecasermin 10mg/mL. rDNA-derived human IGF-1. Clear colourless aqueous soln. *Benzyl alcohol 9mg/mL.*

Somatropin

ATC Code: H01AC01. **Sport:** Prohibited.
Driving: No influence.

Indications: Children, growth failure due to growth hormone deficiency (GHD), associated with Turner's syndrome (gonadal dysgenesis) *(all brands)*, chronic renal insufficiency/failure (CRF), children born short for gestational age (SGA) *(all brands except Zomacton)*, Prader-Willi syndrome (PWS) for improvement of body growth and composition *(all brands except Zomacton, NutropinAq, Saizen)*. Adults, replacement therapy, childhood and adult onset GHD *(all brands except Zomacton)*.

Dose: Adult: GHD, initial range 0.15-0.3mg/day. Continuation after childhood GHD, restart at 0.2-0.5mg; adult onset, initially 0.15-0.3mg/day. Maintenance, usually 1mg/day; women may require higher doses than men. Individualise dose. *Admin*, SC varying site to prevent lipoatrophy.

Elderly: Over 60 years, initiate at 0.1-0.2mg/day; maintenance seldom exceeds 0.5mg/day. Over 80 years, limited data.

Child: Growth hormone insufficiency, usually 0.025-0.035mg/kg bodyweight per day *(Zomacton 0.02-0.03mg/kg/day)* OR 0.7-1mg/m2 body surface area per day.
Turner's Syndrome, usually 0.045-0.05mg/kg/day *(Norditropin 0.045-0.067mg/kg/day)* OR 1.4mg/m2/day *(Zomacton 1.4-1.63mg/m2/day)*, *(Norditropin 1.3-2mg/m2/day)*.
Chronic Renal Failure, 0.045-0.05mg/kg/day OR 1.4mg/m2 BSA/day.
Short children born SGA, 0.035mg/kg/day OR 1mg/m2/day until final height reached. *PWS*, generally, 0.035mg/kg/day OR 1mg/m2/day; max. 2.7mg/day.

Renal Impairment: Conservative treatment in renal insufficiency (control of acidosis, hyperparathyroidism, nutritional status); discontinue at renal transplant.

Hepatic Impairment: No data.

CI: Evidence of tumour activity. Growth promotion in children with closed epiphyses. Acute critical illness, complications, of surgery (open heart, abdominal), multiple accident trauma, acute respiratory failure. Chronic renal disease, discontinue at renal transplant. Age under 3 years, if solvent contains benzyl alcohol.

Interactions: Effect of Other Drugs on Somatropin: *Somatropin dose increase may be needed*: Oral oestrogen replacement.

Effect of Somatropin on Other Drugs: Drugs metabolised by CYP3A4 (sex steroids, corticosteroids, anticonvulsants, ciclosporin): *Increased clearance*. Insulin: *Dose adjustment*.

SP: Somatropin influences carbohydrate metabolism, monitor glucose, insulin resistance, hyperglycaemia; Type 2 diabetes may develop with risk factors (obesity, PWS obesity, family history, steroid treatment, impaired glucose tolerance); existing diabetes, consider therapy adjustment. Monitor thyroid function; hypothyroidism may prevent optimal response. Malignancy relapse if treating secondary to malignancy (childhood cancer survivors, increased risk of second neoplasm after somatropin treatment). Severe or recurrent headache, visual problems, nausea and/or vomiting, recommend funduscopy for papilloedema; if confirmed, consider benign intracranial hypertension; discontinue. Myositis. Scoliosis. Pancreatitis. Not for use with proliferative or pre-proliferative diabetic retinopathy. Stable background retinopathy should not lead to discontinuation of somatropin replacement therapy.

PWS, NutropinAq not indicated unless GHD diagnosed. Always with calorie-restricted diet. Sudden death in children with PWS, with risk factors (severe obesity, respiratory impairment, sleep apnoea, respiratory infection); assess before initiating; signs of upper airway obstruction (onset or increased snoring, interrupt (obtain ENT assessment). SGA, measure fasting insulin, blood glucose; increased diabetes risk (familial history, obesity, insulin resistance, acanthosis nigricans); overt diabetes, do not use. Monitor IGF-I levels. Some height gain obtained in children born SGA may be lost if treatment stopped before final height reached. Stimulation of growth only expected until epiphyseal closure; not for longitudinal growth promotion with closed epiphyses. *Turner Syndrome*, monitor growth of hands and feet; otological evaluation recommended annually (increased otitis media risk). CRF, monitor renal function. All patients developing acute critical illness, weigh somatropin risk/benefit.

Pregnancy, Lactation: Pregnancy, women of childbearing potential not using contraception, not recommended (interrupt treatment). Lactation, not known if excreted in breast milk; absorption of intact protein from GI tract of infant unlikely; caution.

ADR: *Very common*, arthralgia, myalgia, oedema, peripheral oedema (adults). See SP above. Injection site reactions especially with SC admin.

Notes: See 11.6.2 Growth Hormone.

Genotropin, Miniquick Parenteral *(Pfizer)* A. HT.
Price, cartridge (1) 5.3mg, €141.80; 12mg, €343.87. Miniquick syringe (7) 0.2mg, €42.81. 0.4mg, €85.62. 0.6mg, €123.37. 0.8mg, €166.06. 1mg, €208.91. 1.2mg, €249.08. 1.4mg, €292.65. 1.6mg, €335.37. 1.8mg, €376.72. 2mg, €421.16. PFP Go Quick (1) 5.3mg, €124.47. 12mg, €339.27.
Injection, somatropin cartridge (5.3mg, 12mg), Miniquick (0.2mg to 2mg in 0.2mg increases). White powder and solvent for soln. *Store:* Refrigerate; do not freeze. Unopened, below 25 deg C (max. 6 months, Miniquick; max. 1 month, cartridge), then discard. Protect (light).
Norditropin SimpleXx Parenteral *(Novo Nordisk)* A. HT.
Price, (1) 5mg, €153.24. 10mg, €307.51. 15mg, €476.97.
Injection (cartridge), somatropin 5(10, 15)mg/1.5mL. Clear colourless soln.
NutropinAq Parenteral *(Ipsen)* A. HT.
Price, (1) €279.55.
Injection, somatropin 10mg/2mL. Clear colourless sterile soln.
Saizen Parenteral *(Merck Serono)* A. HT.
Price, injection (1) 6mg, €169.80. 12mg, €348.17. 20mg, €565.87. Click.Easy (1) 8mg, €242.14.
Injection, somatropin (recombinant human growth hormone) 5.83mg/mL (6mg), 8mg/mL (12mg, 20mg). Click.Easy 8mg. 8mg: White lyophilised powder. Clear colourless solvent. 6mg*, 12mg*, 20mg*: Clear slightly opalescent soln. pH 5.6-6.6. (*multiple dose vials).
Zomacton Parenteral 10mg *(Ferring)* A. HT.
Price, 10mg/mL (1) €235.40.
Injection, somatropin. White (off-white) lyophilised powder. Clear colourless solvent.

11.6.3 - Anterior Pituitary Hormones, Growth Hormone Antagonists

In This Chapter: Pegvisomant.

Class Effects
CI: Hypersensitivity to any member of the class.
SP: Treatment to be initiated under supervision of a physician experienced in treatment of acromegaly.
Notes: See 3.5.1 Dopaminergics Used In Parkinson's Disease (bromocriptine), 13.3 Sex Hormones, Hormone Antagonists In Malignancy and 13.3.3 Somatostatin Analogues (octreotide, lanreotide). Consult manufacturers Full Prescribing Information.

Pegvisomant

ATC Code: H01AX01. **Sport:** Permitted.
Driving: Unlikely to impair.
Indications: Treatment, acromegaly (inadequate response to surgery and/or radiation therapy or somatostatin analogue treatment) in adults.
Dose: Adult: Loading dose, 80mg SC; then 10mg SC once daily rotating injection sites; based on IGF-I levels, titrate at 5mg increments to max. 30mg/day.
Interactions: Effect of Pegvisomant on Other Drugs: Insulin, oral hypoglycaemics: *Consider dose decrease.*
SP: Growth hormone-secreting pituitary tumours may expand; monitor to avoid progression. Growth hormone deficient state may arise from treatment; monitor serum IGF-I. Monitor serum ALT every 4-6 weeks (first 6 months) or symptoms of hepatitis; exclude obstructive biliary tract disease. Hypoglycaemia risk.
Pregnancy, Lactation: Pregnancy, only if clearly necessary. Lactation, stop drug.
ADR: Summary, *most common*, headache, arthralgia, diarrhoea.
Notes: See 11.6.3 Growth Hormone Antagonists.

Somavert Parenteral *(Pfizer)* A. HT.
Price, injection (30) 10mg, €2223.50; 15mg, €3330.90; 20mg, €4444.47. 20mg (1) €144.90.
Injection, pegvisomant. White (off-white) powder. Solvent for soln.
Store: Refrigerate; do not freeze.

11.6.4 - Posterior Pituitary Hormones

In This Chapter: Desmopressin, terlipressin.

Class Effects
CI: Hypersensitivity to any member of the class.
SP: Admin under specialist supervision with appropriate laboratory facilities for monitoring (cardiac, haematology, electrolytes). Consult manufacturers Full Prescribing Information. Prevent fluid overload with conditions characterised by fluid and/or electrolyte imbalance.
Pregnancy, Lactation: Pregnancy, if benefit outweighs risk; caution. Lactation, generally amount transferred to child less than required to influence diuresis or haemostasis.

Desmopressin

ATC Code: H01BA02. **Sport:** Prohibited.
Driving: No or negligible effect.
Indications: Diagnosis and treatment, cranial diabetes insipidus. To establish renal concentration capacity. Control, bleeding in mild to moderate haemophilia and Von Willebrand's disease undergoing surgery or following trauma. Nocturia, associated with MS *(Desmospray)*, associated with nocturnal polyuria *(Desmotabs Melt, Nordurine)*. Nocturnal enuresis *(Desmotabs)*.
Dose: Adult: PARENTERAL, 1-4mcg once daily SC, IM or IV. *Cranial diabetes*, diagnosis, 2mcg SC or IM; restrict fluid intake to max. 500mL from 1 hour before until 8 hours after admin. *Haemophilia, Von Willebrand's Disease*, 0.4mcg/kg by IV infusion over 20 minutes immediately prior to surgery or following trauma; admin further doses 12-hourly as long as cover is required. *Renal concentration capacity test*, SC or IM as single dose 2mcg; limit fluid intake as for cranial diabetes.

ORAL, NASAL (sublingual tabs, oral tabs; nasal drops, spray). *Central diabetes insipidus*, diagnosis, single 20mcg dose intranasal with restricted fluid intake as for Parenteral above. Treatment, 10-20mcg intranasal 1-2 times daily OR sublingual, initially 60mcg 3-times daily; maintenance usually 60-120mcg 3-times daily (range 120-720mcg) OR oral tabs initially 0.1mg 3-times daily; maintenance 0.1-0.2mg 3-times daily (range 0.2-1.2mg).
Renal function testing, 40mcg intranasal as single dose.
Primary nocturnal enuresis 0.2mg oral tabs at bedtime, may be increased to 0.4mg; limit fluid intake only to satisfy thirst for 8 hours following admin. *Nocturia* (nocturnal polyuria), initially 60mcg sublingually; if needed increase to 120mcg and then 240mcg at 1-week intervals OR oral tabs initially 0.2mg at bedtime; may be increased to 0.4mg. Sublingual tabs to be placed under tongue where they dissolve; no need for water. Food may reduce intensity and duration of antidiuretic effect with low dose desmopressin.
Elderly: Over 65 years, primary nocturnal enuresis or nocturia, contraindicated. Central diabetes insipidus, as for Adult above.
Child: PARENTERAL, from 0.4mcg may be used, as for Adult above. Renal concentration capacity testing, under 1 year, caution (perform only in hospital under careful supervision).
ORAL, NASAL, *central diabetes insipidus*, diagnosis, as for Adult; treatment, 5-10mcg once or twice daily; lower dose may be required for infants. *Renal function testing*, age 1-15 years, 20mcg as single dose; infants, 10mcg as single dose. *Nocturnal enuresis*, over 5 years, as for Adult above.
Renal Impairment: Caution. CrCl (mL/min) below 50, contraindicated.
CI: Exclude habitual and psychogenic polydipsia; alcohol abuse, known hyponatraemia before initiating. Renal concentration capacity test, nocturnal enuresis (hypertension, heart disease, cardiac insufficiency, other conditions requiring diuretic treatment). Haemostatic (unstable angina pectoris, decompensated cardiac insufficiency, Von Willebrand's Disease Type IIB), desmopressin admin may result in pseudo-thrombocytopenia due to release of clotting factors which cause platelet aggregation. SIADH.
Interactions: Effect of Other Drugs on Desmopressin: *Response magnitude augmented:* Indomethacin. *Additive antidiuretic effect (increased water retention risk):* Drugs releasing antidiuretic hormone (TCADs, SSRIs, chlorpromazine, carbamazepine, sulfonylureas particularly chlorpropamide). *Fluid retention, hyponatraemia:* NSAIDs, loperamide.
SP: Caution, patients at risk for raised intracranial pressure, reduced renal function and/or cardiovascular disease, cystic fibrosis (expect reduced antidiuretic effect with renal insufficiency); immediately post-hypophysectomy (adjust dose based on urinary osmolality); hypertension. *Repeated dosing to control bleeding**; admin only enough fluid to satisfy thirst; IV infusion should not be left up as routine post-surgery. Conditions requiring diuretic treatment*. Monitor BP during injection. Desmopressin does not reduce prolonged bleeding time, thrombocytopenia. *Diagnostic use*, caution*; admin only enough fluid to satisfy thirst. *Nocturnal enuresis*, exclude severe bladder dysfunction, outlet obstruction. Primary nocturnal enuresis and nocturia, limit fluid intake to minimum from 1 hour before to 8 hours after (next morning) admin; monitor BP/weight*. Avoid ingesting water while swimming. Acute intercurrent illness (fluid and/or electrolyte imbalance), interrupt treatment. Symptoms of water retention and/or hyponatraemia (headache, nausea/vomiting, weight gain, convulsions), interrupt treatment until recovery; restart with strict fluid restriction. Infants, elderly, patients with low sodium levels at increased risk for hyponatraemia. *(caution, fluid overload)
Nasal preparations, to be used only when oral formulations not feasible (start at lowest dose, ensure fluid restriction compliance, increase dose with caution, ensure children are supervised to control dose intake). Benzalkonium chloride may cause bronchospasm.
ADR: Summary, *most serious*, hyponatraemia which may

11.6.5   Anti-Oestrogens

cause headache, dizziness, nausea, vomiting, decreased sodium, weight increase, malaise, abdominal pain, muscle cramps, dizziness, confusion, decreased consciousness, convulsions, coma; *Desmospray*, nasal congestion, rhinitis, epistaxis.

Notes: See 11.6.4 Posterior Pituitary Hormones.

DDAVP Desmopressin Parenteral *(Ferring)* C.
Price, 1mL (10) 4mcg/mL, €134.12.
Injection, desmopressin acetate 4mcg/mL. Clear colourless soln. **Store:** Refrigerate; do not freeze.
DDAVP Desmopressin Nasal Soln *(Ferring)* B. GMS.
Price, 2.5mL (1) €12.14.
Nasal drops, desmopressin acetate 100mcg/mL equiv. to 89mcg desmopressin. Clear colourless aqueous soln. **Store:** Refrigerate; do not freeze.
Desmospray *(Ferring)* B. GMS.
Price, 6mL (1) €34.81.
Nasal spray, desmopressin acetate 10mcg/spray. Clear colourless soln. *Benzalkonium chloride*.
Desmotabs Melt *(Ferring)* B. GMS.
Price, (30) 60mcg, €21.12. 120mcg, €42.25. 240mcg, €84.50.
Sublingual tablet, desmopressin acetate 60mcg, 120mcg, 240mcg. White round lyophilisate. Marked with drop-shapes. *Mannitol*.
Nordurine 0.1mg, 0.2mg *(Ferring)* B. GMS.
Price, 0.1mg (30) €21.11; (90) €63.33. 0.2mg (30) €42.25; (90) €126.77.
Oral tablet, desmopressin acetate. White oval scored (facilitates breaking). Marked with strength. *Lactose*.

Terlipressin

ATC Code: H01BA04. **Sport:** Prohibited.
Driving: Not applicable.

Indications: Short-term management, bleeding oesophageal varices. Emergency treatment, Type 1 hepatorenal syndrome.

Dose: Adult: *Bleeding oesophageal varices*, usually 2mg IV bolus repeated every 4-6 hours until bleeding controlled or 72 hours has elapsed. *Hepatorenal syndrome*, 3-4mg every 24 hours as 3 or 4 administrations.

Elderly: Caution.

Renal Impairment: Caution.

CI: Septic shock.

Interactions: Effect of Other Drugs on Terlipressin: *Bradycardia*: Drugs causing bradycardia (propofol).
Effect of Terlipressin on Other Drugs: Non-selective beta-blockers: *Increased hypotensive effect on portal vein.*

SP: Caution, hypertension, dysrhythmias, cardiac/coronary insufficiency. IV admin only to avoid local necrosis. Hepatorenal syndrome, confirm acute functional renal failure before initiating.

Pregnancy, Lactation: Pregnancy, contraindicated. Lactation, stop breastfeeding or stop drug.

ADR: *Common*, headache, bradycardia, peripheral (vasoconstriction, ischaemia), facial pallor, hypertension, transient (abdominal cramp, diarrhoea).

Notes: See 11.6.4 Posterior Pituitary Hormones.

Glypressin Parenteral *(Ferring)* A.
Price, 1mg/5mL (5) €180.20. 1mg/8.5mL, not published by company.
Injection, terlipressin acetate 1mg/5mL and 1mg/8.5mL soln. White sterile powder. *Sodium 17.7mg/5mL vial*. Clear colourless solvent for soln OR clear colourless soln.

11.6.5 - Anti-Oestrogens

In This Chapter: *Clomifene.*

Class Effects
CI: Hypersensitivity to any member of the class.

Clomifene

ATC Code: G03GB02. **Sport:** Prohibited.
Driving: Visual symptoms may impair.
Indications: Treatment, ovulatory failure.

Dose: Adult: *First course*, 50mg daily (5 days); commencing on day 5 of cycle. *Second course*, if ovulation does not appear to have occurred, 100mg as single dose (5 days); may be started as early as 30 days after first course. Max.

318

100mg/day for 5 days. 3 courses are adequate trial; if ovulation has not occurred re-evaluate.

CI: Active liver disease, history of liver dysfunction, bilirubin metabolism disorders. Ovarian dysgenesis, menopause, where response not expected. Abnormal uterine bleeding, hormone-dependent tumours, ovarian cyst (except PCOD).

SP: OHSS reported; severe (pericardial effusion, anasarca, hydrothorax, acute abdomen, renal failure, pulmonary oedema, ovarian haemorrhage, DVT, torsion of the ovary, acute respiratory distress); advise patient to report abdominal or pelvic pain, weight gain, discomfort, distention. Increased risk of multiple or ectopic pregnancy; pregnancy wastage, birth anomalies within general population range. Long-term cyclic therapy, not recommended. Uterine fibroids, caution (potential further enlargement). Increased risk of ovarian cancer (prolonged use). Visual symptoms, spots, flashes; may be irreversible (increased dose, duration). Hypertriglyceridaemia.

Pregnancy, Lactation: Pregnancy, contraindicated; exclude before initiating and next course. Lactation may be reduced; not known if excreted in human milk.

ADR: *Very common*, flushing, ovarian enlargement. See SP above.

Notes: See 11.6.5 Anti-Oestrogens.

Clomid 50mg *(SANOFI)* A. GMS.
Price, (30) €10.27.
Tablet, clomifene citrate. Beige round flat scored (facilitates breaking). Marked with M in 2 circles. *Lactose.*

11.7 - Sex Hormones

11.7.1 - Male Sex Hormones, Androgens

In This Chapter: *Testosterone.*

Class Effects
CI: Hypersensitivity to any member of the class. Use in women unless specified. Men with known/suspected carcinoma of breast or prostate. Hypercalciuria, hypercalcaemia, nephrotic syndrome, ischaemic heart disease, untreated CHF. See SP below.

Interactions: Effect of Other Drugs on Testosterone: *Metabolism stimulated, dose adjustment*: Barbiturates, phenylbutazone. *Increased oedema risk, caution*: ACTH, corticosteroids.

Effect of Testosterone on Other Drugs: Anticoagulants (including oral): *Effect enhanced, monitor especially at initiation and end of androgen therapy*. Oxyphenbutazone: *Serum levels elevated*. Insulin: *Dose adjustment may be required*. Propranolol: *Increased clearance (with testosterone parenteral)*. ACTH, corticosteroids: *Increased oedema*.

SP: Testosterone treatment to be under specialist care. *Medical examination*: Monitor testosterone levels at baseline and regular intervals during treatment. *Exclude*: BPH or sub-clinical prostate cancer, polycythaemia (monitor haematocrits, haemoglobin). Long-term (monitor haematocrit, Hb, LFTs, lipids). *Supervision Required*: Patients (especially elderly) monitor, for tumours (patients with breast carcinoma, hypernephroma, lung carcinoma, bone metastases can develop hypercalcaemia spontaneously or during anabolic/androgenic steroid therapy; monitor serum calcium), pre-existing conditions (severe cardiac, hepatic or renal insufficiency as treatment may cause oedema with or without CHF; MI, hypertension, epilepsy, migraine), diabetes mellitus, anticoagulant treatment, sleep apnoea. Caution, patients with thrombophilia; thrombotic events reported during testosterone therapy. Avoid undue stimulation (physical or mental); evidence of excessive sexual stimulation, discontinue. NOTE: Androgens are NOT for enhancing muscular development in healthy individuals or increasing physical ability or performance in sport.

Pregnancy, Lactation: Not for use in women including during pregnancy (may cause virilising effects on female foetus), women who may become pregnant, or during lactation.

ADR: Increased (haematocrit, RBC count, Hb). *Associated* with androgen therapy, prostate cancer, polycythaemia, fluid retention, depression, nervousness, mood disturbances, libido (increased, decreased), myalgia, hypertension, nausea, pruritus, acne, gynaecomastia, oligozoospermia, priapism, prostatic disorder, ejaculation disorder, abnormal LFTs/lipids, increased PSA. *Topical, parenteral*, injection site or application site reactions.

Testosterone

ATC Code: G03BA03. **Sport:** Prohibited.

Driving: No studies performed.

Indications: Male hypogonadism (testosterone deficiency or absence of endogenous testosterone) *(all brands)*. Osteoporosis due to androgen deficiency *(Restandol)*. Oestrogens used in HRT, see Notes below.

Dose: Adult: PARENTERAL, DEPOT, *Nebido*, 1000mg injection every 10-14 weeks; first interval may be reduced to 6 weeks. Admin very slowly over 2 minutes; strictly IM, extremely slow deep into gluteal muscle; avoid intravasal injection.

ORAL, *Restandol*, initially 120-160mg/day (2-3 weeks); maintenance, 40-120mg/day depending on response. Must admin with food and some fluid; swallow whole, do not chew; 2 divided doses morning, evening.

TOPICAL, TRANSDERMAL, apply once daily (morning, same time of day) to clean, dry, intact skin (shoulders, upper arms, inner thighs) after bath/shower. Initially 50mg/day (1 tube or 1 sachet) or 60mg (3g gel); daily range 40-80mg (2-4g gel); if needed increase to max. 100mg/day.

Elderly: Limited experience on safety and efficacy over 65 years *(Testim)*.

Child: Under 18 years, not recommended.

Renal Impairment: Caution.

Hepatic Impairment: As for Renal above.

SP: Not for use in women; virilisation symptoms (hirsutism, acne; voice changes e.g. deepening, hoarsening) may be irreversible. *Topical*, not for application to genitals; advise not to wash/shower for at least 6 hours after application. Can be transferred to others by close skin contact; not recommended with safety non-compliance risk (severe alcoholism, psychiatric disorders, drug-abuse). Local application site reactions (erythema, oedema, blistering due to hypersensitivity), discontinue. Long-term use, limited data (effect on breast tissue, cardiovascular, increased insulin resistance, breast cancer). With cardiovascular risk factors (hypertension), monitor BP/weight. Use with natural menopause not evaluated.

Nebido, observe for possible signs/symptoms of pulmonary oily micro-embolism during, immediately after each injection. Caution, hyper- (calciuria, calcaemia), nephrotic syndrome, ischaemic heart disease, untreated CHF.

Pregnancy, Lactation: Pregnant women must avoid contact with topical testosterone application sites.

ADR: Summary, *most frequent*, injection or application site reactions; *Nebido*, acne; *Testim Gel*, increased PSA; *Testogel*, erythema, acne, dry skin; *Tostran Gel*, paraesthesia, xerosis, pruritus, rash, erythema.

Notes: See 11.7.1 Male Sex Hormones, Androgens. See 11.7.4 Oestrogens, HRT.

Nebido Parenteral 1000mg/4mL *(Bayer)* A. GMS.
Price, 250mg/mL (1x4mL) €92.13.
Depot injection, testosterone undecenoate equiv. to 631.5mg testosterone. Clear yellowish oily soln (amp).

Restandol Testocaps 40mg *(MSD)* A. GMS.
Price, (60) €19.60.
Capsule, testosterone undecenoate equiv. to 25.3mg testosterone. Soft oval glossy orange transparent; contains yellow oil. Marked Org DV3. *Sunset Yellow, soya lecithin.* **Store:** Below 30 deg C; do not (refrigerate, freeze).

Testim Transdermal Gel 50mg/5g *(Ferring)* A. GMS.
Price, (30g) €45.73.
Transdermal gel, testosterone. Clear (translucent). *Propylene glycol.* **Store:** Below 25 deg C; flammable.

Testogel 50mg/5g *(Besins)* A. GMS.
Price, (30) €40.06.
Topical gel (sachet), testosterone. Transparent (slightly opalescent) colourless.

Tostran Gel 20mg/g *(KyowaKirin)* A. GMS.
Price, (60g) €38.32.
Topical gel, testosterone 2%. Clear colourless gel in metered dose canister. *Butylhydroxytoluene, propylene glycol.* **Store:** Upright; below 25 deg C; do not (refrigerate, freeze).

11.7.2 - Male Sex Hormones, Anti-Androgens

In This Chapter: *Cyproterone.*

Class Effects

CI: Hypersensitivity to any member of the class.

SP: Anti-androgen initiation and treatment to be under specialist supervision.

Notes: Use in females, see 8.2.1 Combined Hormonal Contraceptives.

Cyproterone

ATC Code: G03HA01. **Sport:** Permitted.

Driving: Tiredness, diminished vitality, impaired concentration.

Indications: Combination with ethinyloestradiol for treatment of severe acne vulgaris, oral contraceptive in woman suffering severe acne. Reduction of drive in sexual deviations, anti-androgen treatment of inoperable prostate carcinoma in males.

Dose: Adult, Elderly: *Reduction of drive* (sexual deviation), initially 50mg twice daily; titrate to 100mg 2-3 times daily; once effect obtained, reduce dose by 25-50mg at intervals of several weeks; 25mg twice daily usually sufficient.

Prostate cancer, 100mg twice daily for 5-7 days, then 100mg twice daily with GnRH agonist. Hot flushes, combination with GnRH analogue, with orchiectomy, initially 50-150mg/day; titrating up to 300mg/day if needed. Oral with liquid after meals.

Child: Male children, adolescents under 18 years, not recommended.

Hepatic Impairment: Liver disease, LFTs not returned to normal, contraindicated.

CI: Meningioma. Liver disease, Dubin-Johnson syndrome, Rotor syndrome, liver tumours (only if not due to metastases from prostate carcinoma in prostate indication), wasting diseases, severe chronic depression, thromboembolic disorders, severe diabetes with vascular changes, sickle-cell anaemia.

Interactions: Effect of Other Drugs on Cyproterone: *Metabolism inhibited:* Strong CYP3A4 inhibitors (ketoconazole, itraconazole, clotrimazole, ritonavir). *Metabolism increased:* CYP3A4 inducers (rifampicin, phenytoin, St John's Wort). *Drive-reducing effect diminished:* ALCOHOL (disinhibitory effect).

Effect of Cyproterone on Other Drugs: Insulin, oral antidiabetics: *Dose adjustment.* HMG-CoA Reductase Inhibitors: *Myopathy or rhabdomyolysis may be increased.*

SP: Meningioma reported (longer term use at doses 25mg/day and above); if diagnosed, discontinue. Not for use before conclusion of puberty. Monitor, liver and adrenocortical function, RBC. Hepatic toxicity (jaundice, hepatitis, hepatic failure) observed at dose 100mg and above; if confirmed, discontinue unless due to another cause (continue only if benefit outweighs risk). Severe upper abdominal complaints, liver enlargement, signs of intra-abdominal haemorrhage, consider liver tumour. Diabetes, strict medical supervision. High dose, sensation of shortness of breath. Previous arterial or venous thrombotic or thromboembolic events (DVT, pulmonary embolism, MI), history of CVA, advanced malignancies, increased risk of thromboembolic events. Inoperable prostate carcinoma with history of thromboembolic processes, sickle-cell anaemia, severe diabetes with vascular changes; careful risk/benefit evaluation. Drive-reducing effect can be diminished under disinhibitory influence of alcohol.

ADR: *Very common,* reversible inhibition of spermatogenesis, decreased libido, ED.

Notes: See 11.7.2 Male Sex Hormones, Anti-Androgens.

11.7.3   Female Sex Hormones, Progestogens

Androcur 100mg *(Bayer)* A. GMS.
Price, (60) €72.75.
Tablet, cyproterone acetate. White (faintly yellowish) cap-shaped scored (divisible into equal halves). Marked LA both sides of score; equilateral hexagon on lower face. *Lactose.*

Duphaston 10mg *(BGP)* A. GMS.
Price, (42) €8.81.
Tablet, dydrogesterone. White round f/c scored (facilitates breaking). Marked 155 either side of score. *Lactose.*

11.7.3 - Female Sex Hormones, Progestogens

In This Chapter: *Dydrogesterone, medroxyprogesterone, norethisterone, progesterone.*

Class Effects

CI: Hypersensitivity to any member of the class. Thromboembolic disorder, severe thrombophlebitis, thromboembolism (arterial or venous); hormone dependent breast (known, past or suspected) or genital cancer or undiagnosed breast pathology; undiagnosed irregular vaginal bleeding; porphyria. Adjunctive with oestrogen, consider contraindications relating to oestrogen.

Interactions: Effect of Other Drugs on Progestogens: *Metabolism increased*: Strong inducers (phenobarbital, phenytoin, carbamazepine, rifampicin, rifabutin, nevirapine, efavirenz, St John's Wort); although strong inhibitors (ritonavir, nelfinavir) exhibit enzyme inducing properties when used with steroid hormones.

Effect of Progestogens on Other Drugs: Insulin, oral antidiabetics: *Dose adjustments*. Ciclosporin: *Interfered metabolism.*

SP: Careful observation, conditions influenced by fluid retention (epilepsy, migraine, asthma, cardiac or renal dysfunction). May alter endocrine and biochemical markers. Caution, renal and liver disease, in presence of liver tumour. Sex steroids may increase risk of retinal vascular lesions. Conditions needing supervision and reasons for immediate withdrawal, see Notes below.

Pregnancy, Lactation: Pregnancy, not recommended; exclude before initiation. If used during pregnancy, or if patient becomes pregnant, patient should be advised of potential hazard to foetus.

Notes: Progesterone combinations (including oestrogen combinations) used in HRT, see 11.7.4 Female Sex Hormones, Oestrogens, HRT.

Dydrogesterone

ATC Code: G03DB01. **Sport:** Permitted.
Driving: No or negligible influence.
Indications: Conditions associated with progesterone deficiency (dysmenorrhoea, endometriosis, infertility, irregular menstrual cycles). Adjunctive, with oestrogen, management of dysfunctional bleeding or secondary amenorrhoea; HRT.

Dose: Adult: *HRT*, 10mg daily (last 14 days of 28-day oestrogen treatment cycle); increase to 10mg twice daily if early withdrawal bleeding occurs.
Dysfunctional bleeding, to arrest bleeding 10mg twice daily with oestrogen once daily for 5-7 days; to prevent bleeding, as above (days 11-25 of cycle). *Dysmenorrhoea*, 10mg twice daily (day 5-25 of cycle). *Amenorrhoea*, oestrogen once daily (day 1-25 of cycle), dydrogesterone 10mg twice daily (day 11-25). *Endometriosis*, 10mg 2-3 times daily (day 5-25 of cycle) or continuously.
Infertility or irregular cycles, 10mg twice daily (day 11-25 of cycle); maintain for at least 6 consecutive cycles; after conception, continue 10mg twice daily until week 20 of pregnancy, then gradually reduce dose.
Premenstrual syndrome (PMS), 10mg twice daily (day 12-26 of cycle); increase dose if needed.

CI: Progestogen dependant neoplasms.

SP: See Notes below.

Pregnancy, Lactation: Not indicated for use during pregnancy; if pregnancy occurs, withdraw immediately. Lactation, not recommended; passes into breast milk.

ADR: *Common*, headache, migraine, nausea, abdominal pain, flatulence.

Notes: See 11.7.3 Progestogens.

Medroxyprogesterone (progesterone deficiency)

ATC Code: G03DB02. **Sport:** Permitted.
Driving: Unlikely to impair.
Indications: Dysfunctional uterine bleeding associated with progesterone deficiency, secondary amenorrhoea, endometriosis; adjunctive, to oppose endometrial effect of oestrogen in oestrogen-treated post-menopausal women. Treatment, hormone-dependent neoplasms (renal cell, endometrial), breast carcinoma post-menopause.

Dose: Adult: *Dysfunctional bleeding, amenorrhoea*, 2.5-10mg/day for 5-10 days (day 16-21 of cycle) for 2 consecutive cycles (3 consecutive cycles for secondary amenorrhoea). Adjunctive with conventional oestrogen, 5-10mg for 10 days. *Endometriosis*, 10mg 3-times daily for 90 consecutive days; commencing day 1 of cycle. *Post-menopausal* women treated with oestrogen, 10mg daily for 10-12 days (from day 16) of 28-day oestrogen therapy. *Carcinoma*, endometrial, renal cell, 200-400mg/day; breast, 400-800mg/day.

Hepatic Impairment: Liver disease, LFTs not returned to normal, contraindicated.

Interactions: Effect of Other Drugs on Medroxyprogesterone: *Reduced bioavailability*: Aminoglutethimide.

SP: See Notes below.

Pregnancy, Lactation: Pregnancy, contraindicated. Lactation, drug and metabolites are excreted in breast milk; no evidence to suggest hazard to nursing child.

ADR: *Summary, most frequent*, dysfunctional uterine bleeding, headache, nausea.

Notes: See 11.7.3 Progestogens, 8.2.4 Long-Acting Contraceptives *(Depo-Provera).*

Provera 2.5mg, 5mg, 10mg, 100mg *(Pfizer)* A. GMS.
Price, (30) 2.5mg, €2.32; 5mg, €4.66; (90) 10mg, €19.32. (100) 100mg, €51.49.
Tablet, medroxyprogesterone acetate. Round scored (facilitates breaking). 2.5mg: Orange. Marked U64. 5mg: Blue. Marked 286; U on reverse. 10mg: Half-oval white. Marked Upjohn 50. 100mg: White flat. Marked U-467. *Lactose, sucrose.* **Store:** Below 25 deg C.

Norethisterone (endometriosis)

ATC Code: G03DC02. **Sport:** Permitted.
Driving: Unlikely to impair.
Indications: Dysfunctional bleeding, endometriosis.

Dose: Adult: *Dysfunctional bleeding*, treatment, 5mg 3-times daily for 10 days; withdrawal bleed will occur 2-4 days after completion. Prophylaxis, recurrence, patients with anovulatory cycles, 5mg 1-2 times daily (days 16-25 of cycle) (day 1 of cycle = day 1 of last bleed).
Endometriosis, initiate between day 1-5, 5mg twice daily; spotting, increase to 10mg twice daily; duration 4-6 months. Oral, to be swallowed whole with some liquid.

CI: Active venous thromboembolic disorder, arterial and cardiovascular disease (MI, CVA, ischaemic heart disease). Diabetes mellitus with vascular involvement.

Interactions: Effect of Other Drugs on Norethisterone: *Increased clearance*: Phenytoin, barbiturates, primidone, carbamazepine, rifampicin, oxcarbazepine, St John's Wort, rifabutin; griseofulvin (suspected).

SP: Contraception, use additional non-hormonal methods. Caution, circulatory disorders, tumours, diabetes, chloasma, depression. See Notes below.

Pregnancy, Lactation: Not recommended.

ADR: Visual disturbances, nausea, migraine, headache, dyspnoea, hypersensitivity, rash, urticaria, oedema.

Notes: See 11.7.3 Progestogens.

Primolut N 5mg *(Bayer)* A. GMS.
Price, (20) €1.78.
Tablet, norethisterone. Round white flat. Marked AN in regular hexagon. *Lactose, sucrose, Sunset Yellow (2.5mg).*

Progesterone (infertility)

ATC Code: G03DB04. **Sport:** Permitted.
Driving: Somnolence, drowsiness, dizziness.

Indications: Infertility, due to inadequate luteal phase *(Crinone)*, luteal support for ART *(Lutinus)*.

Dose: Adult: *Crinone*, 1 application (1.125g) every day starting after ovulation or on day 18-21 of cycle. *Lutinus*, 100mg vaginally 3-times daily starting at oocyte retrieval; continue for 30 days if pregnancy confirmed.

Elderly: Over 65 years, no data.

Hepatic Impairment: Mild/moderate, caution.

CI: Missed abortion, ectopic pregnancy, acute porphyria.

SP: Undiagnosed or irregular bleeds, consider non-functional causes. MI, cerebrovascular disorders, arterial/venous thromboembolism, thrombophlebitis, retinal thrombosis, worsening depression, discontinue.

Pregnancy, Lactation: Pregnancy, can be used during first month *(Crinone)*, first trimester *(Lutinus)*. Lactation, not recommended.

ADR: *Common*, headache, somnolence, breast tenderness, uterine spasm, abdominal pain/distension, nausea.

Notes: See 11.7.3 Progestogens.

> **Crinone 8% Vaginal Gel** *(Merck Serono)* A. GMS.
> *Price*, (15 applicator) €45.38.
> *Vaginal gel*, progesterone 8% w/w (90mg/dose). White (off-white) in applicator. *Sorbic acid.*
> **Lutinus 100mg Vaginal Tabs** *(Ferring)* A. GMS.
> *Price*, (21) €26.25.
> *Vaginal tablet*, progesterone. White (off-white) oblong. Marked FPI; strength on reverse. With applicator. *Lactose.*

11.7.4 - Female Sex Hormones, Oestrogens, HRT

In This Chapter: *Estradiol, estradiol combinations (drospirenone, dydrogesterone, medroxyprogesterone), estriol, oestrogen.*

Class Effects

Indications: Hormone replacement therapy (HRT) for the oestrogen deficiency syndromes postmenopause (relief of menopausal symptoms). Also indicated for prevention of osteoporosis in postmenopausal women at high risk for fractures where other medicinals for osteoporosis prevention are not tolerated or contraindicated. See individual molecules and brands below.

CI: Hypersensitivity to any member of the class. Use in Children under 18 years. Undiagnosed genital bleeding, known or suspected oestrogen-dependent malignant tumours (endometrial cancer) or premalignant tumours, untreated endometrial hyperplasia, breast carcinoma, previous or current venous thromboembolism (DVT, pulmonary embolism), thrombophlebitis, known thrombophilic disorder (protein C, protein S, antithrombin deficiency), active or recent arterial thromboembolic disease (CVA, angina, MI), acute liver disease or history of (LFTs not returned to normal), porphyria.

Interactions: Effect of Other Drugs on Oestrogens: *Increased metabolism*: Strong enzyme inducers e.g. phenylbutazone, meprobamate, anticonvulsants (phenobarbital, barbiturates, phenytoin, primidone, carbamazepine), anti-infectives (rifampicin, rifabutin, nevirapine, efavirenz), St John's Wort, bosentan, felbamate, griseofulvin, oxcarbazepine, topiramate. *Plasma levels increased (oestrogens, progestin or both)*: Strong and moderate CYP3A4 inhibitors e.g. azole antifungals (itraconazole, voriconazole, fluconazole), verapamil, macrolides (clarithromycin, erythromycin), diltiazem, grapefruit juice. *Caution, ALT elevations*: Ombitasvir, paritaprevir, ritonavir with/with dasabuvir.

Effect of Oestrogens on Other Drugs: Metyrapone: *Reduced response*. Lamotrigine: *Significantly decreased plasma levels (may reduce seizure control); consider dose adjustment*. Ciclosporin: *Increased plasma levels*.

SP: Elderly, over 65 years, limited data (use lowest effective dose). Initiate HRT only if symptoms adversely affect quality of life (for as long as benefit outweighs risk, lowest dose possible). Premature menopause, risk/benefit may be better than older women. Before initiating take complete medical history (person, family), physical examination (pelvic, breast).

Conditions needing supervision, leiomyoma (uterine fibroids) or endometriosis, thromboembolic disorders (risk factors), oestrogen-dependent tumours (risk factors) (first degree heredity for breast cancer), hypertension, liver disorders (adenoma), diabetes mellitus (with or without vascular involvement), cholelithiasis, migraine or (severe) headache, SLE, endometrial hyperplasia (history), epilepsy, asthma, otosclerosis, meningioma, hereditary angioedema.

Reasons for immediate withdrawal, jaundice or liver function deterioration, significant BP increase, new onset of migraine-type headache, pregnancy.

Endometrial carcinoma or hyperplasia, increased risk for oestrogen-only users; to avoid hyperplasia in non-hysterectomised women, combine oestrogen with progestogen for 12 days per 28-day cycle; progestogen not recommended hysterectomised women. Breast cancer (increased duration dependant risk), ovarian cancer (slightly increased risk in women taking oestrogen-only or combined oestrogen-progesterone HRT; becomes apparent within 5 years; diminishes over time after stopping).

Venous thromboembolism (higher DVT, pulmonary embolism risk), possible increased risk (CAD, stroke), angioedema. *Other conditions*, fluid retention, caution (cardiac or renal dysfunction/failure especially with potassium-sparing medication). Pre-existing hypertriglyceridaemia, monitor. Oestrogens increase thyroid binding globulin (TBG) and increase circulating total thyroid hormone; monitor thyroid hormone levels if on thyroid hormone replacement and HRT. Possible elevated corticoid binding globulin (CBG), sex- hormone-binding globulin (SHBG) leading to increased circulating corticosteroids and sex steroids; other plasma proteins increased (angiotensinogen/renin substrate, alpha-l-antitrypsin, ceruloplasmin). Chloasma (especially with history of chloasma gravidarum); avoid exposure to sun or ultraviolet. Severe anaphylactic or anaphylactoid reactions. Topical or transdermal, contact sensitisation; severe hypersensitivity with continued exposure. Some laboratory tests changed (glucose tolerance, thyroid function).

Pregnancy, Lactation: Pregnancy, not indicated; exclude before initiation; if occurs, withdraw. Lactation, indicated.

ADR: *Commonly*, hypersensitivity, depression, insomnia, anxiety, nervousness, dizziness, migraine, headache, paraesthesia, palpitations, hypertension, varicose vein, vasodilation, nausea, dyspepsia, diarrhoea, abdominal pain/distension, acne, rash, dry skin, pruritus, back pain, arthralgia, breast tension/pain, dysmenorrhoea, menstrual disorder; breast enlargement/pain, menorrhagia, genital discharge, irregular uterine/vaginal bleeding, uterine spasm, vaginal infection, endometrial hyperplasia, pain, asthenia, peripheral oedema, weight fluctuation/increase. *Transdermal*, application site reactions, erythema. See SP above.

Notes: See also 11.7.3 Female Sex Hormones, Progestogens.

Estradiol (oestradiol)

ATC Code: G03CA03. **Sport:** Permitted.
Driving: No or negligible influence.

Indications: HRT in women more than 1 year postmenopause *(Climara/Forte)*; more than 6 months postmenopause *(Evorel Conti, Femata)*, time postmenopause not specified *(Divigel, Estradot, Estrofem, Evorel)*. Prevention, osteoporosis (except *Estradot* 37.5mcg). Treatment, vaginal atrophy due to oestrogen deficiency postmenopause (brand *Vagifem*).

Dose: Adult: TRANSDERMAL (patch), *Climara, Forte*, post-menopause 100mcg/24-hour patch; osteoporosis 50mcg/24-hour patch. Continuous use, apply once weekly; cyclical use, apply for 3 consecutive weeks, then 7 patch-free days.
Estradot, initiate at lowest dose and titrate; apply twice

11.7.4 Female Sex Hormones, Oestrogens, HRT

weekly to buttock, hip or abdomen; should not be exposed to sunlight; not to be applied to breasts. Osteoporosis, initially 50mcg/day. For continuous therapy.

Evorel, initially 50mcg; max. 100mcg/24 hours. Osteoporosis, use 50mcg/24 hours. Apply below waist, change twice weekly using different application site.

TRANSDERMAL (gel), *Divigel*, initially 1mg (1g gel) daily; if needed adjust after 2-3 cycles to 0.5-1.5mg/day. Can be used continuously, cyclical or sequential. Intact uterus, combine with progestogen for at least 12-14 consecutive days per month/28-day cycle. Apply on skin of lower trunk, left or right thighs on alternate day.

ORAL, *Estrofem*, initially 2mg daily without interruption; increase to 4mg if needed; reduce to 2mg as soon as possible.

Fematab, initially 1mg; increase to 2mg if required; use lowest effective dose for shortest duration. Take continuously with or without food.

INTRAVAGINAL, *Vagifem*, 1 vaginal tab (10mcg) daily for 2 weeks, then maintenance, 1 tab twice weekly for shortest possible time.

Elderly: Over 65 years, limited experience.

CI: Non-hysterectomised women without opposing progestogen *(Fematab)*.

SP: Women with an intact uterus, endometrial hyperplasia and carcinoma risk is increased when oestrogens are admin alone, see Notes below.

Notes: See 11.7.4 Oestrogens And HRT.

Climara, Forte *(Bayer)* A. GMS.
Price, (4) 3.9mg, €6.04. Forte 7.8mg, €7.62.
Transdermal patch, estradiol hemihydrate 50mcg (3.8mg), 100mcg, (7.6mg)/24-hour. Oval matrix.
Divigel 0.1% *(Orion)* A. GMS.
Price, (28) €9.33.
Topical gel, estradiol hemihydrate 0.1% w/w, 1mg/dose. Smooth opalescent. *Propylene glycol.*
Estradot Transdermal *(Novartis)* A. GMS.
Price, (8) 37.5mcg, €6.03. 50mcg, €6.47. 75mcg, €7.60. 100mcg, €7.65.
Transdermal patch, estradiol hemihydrate 37.5mcg, 50mcg, 75mcg, 100mcg/24-hour. Rectangular with rounded corners.
Estrofem *(Novo Nordisk)* A. GMS.
Price, (28) €4.98.
Tablet, estradiol hemihydrate. Round blue f/c. Marked Novo 280. *Lactose.*
Evorel Transdermal *(Janssen-Cilag)* A. GMS.
Price, (8) €5.27.
Transdermal patch, estradiol hemihydrate 50mcg/24 hour. Square with rounded corners. Marked CE50.
Fematab 1mg, 2mg *(BGP)* A. GMS.
Price, (28) 1mg, €2.75. 2mg, €2.80.
Tablet, estradiol hemihydrate. Round f/c. Marked 379. 1mg: White. 2mg: Brick-red. *Lactose.*
Vagifem Vaginal 10mcg *(Novo Nordisk)* A. GMS.
Price, (24) €20.65
Vaginal tablet, estradiol hemihydrate. White f/c. 10mcg: Marked Novo 278. *Lactose.*

Estradiol, Drospirenone

ATC Code: G03FA17. **Sport:** Permitted.
Driving: Unlikely to impair.
Indications: HRT, women more than 1 year postmenopause. Prevention, osteoporosis.
Dose: Adult, Elderly: 1 tab daily. *Admin*, swallow whole with liquid; with or without food. Continuous treatment.
Renal Impairment: Severe, contraindicated.
Hepatic Impairment: As for Renal above.
Interactions: Effect of Other Drugs on Estradiol, Drospirenone: *Plasma levels increased or decreased*: HIV/HCV protease inhibitors, NNRTIs.
Effect of Estradiol, Drospirenone on Other Drugs: Antihypertensives: *Additional BP decrease.* NSAIDs, ACEIs: *Increased serum potassium (more pronounced in diabetics).*
ADR: *Most common*, breast pain, bleeding irregularities.
Notes: See 11.7.4 Oestrogens And HRT.
Angeliq 1mg/2mg *(Bayer)* A. GMS.
Price, (84) €39.57.
Tablet, estradiol hemihydrate, drospirenone. Medium-red round f/c. Marked DL in regular hexagon. *Lactose.*

322

Estradiol, Dydrogesterone

ATC Code: G03FA14. **Sport:** Permitted.
Driving: Unlikely to impair.
Indications: HRT in women more than 6 months postmenopause. Prevention, osteoporosis.
Dose: Adult, Elderly: *Femoston* (continuous, sequential) *1/10* and *2/10*: First 14 days of 28-day cycle, 1 white tab (estradiol 1mg; *1/10*) OR 1 brick-red tab (estradiol 2mg; *2/10*) then for next 14 days 1 grey tab (estradiol 1mg + dydrogesterone 10mg; *1/10*) OR 1 yellow tab (estradiol 2mg + dydrogesterone 10mg; *2/10*) daily. Usually commence with *1/10*; adjust dose based on clinical response. *Femoston-conti* (continuous) 0.5/2.5, 1/5, 1 tab daily for a 28-day cycle with no break between packs.
Elderly: Older than 65 years, limited experience.
Pregnancy, Lactation: *Very commonly*, headache, pain (abdominal, back), breast pain/tenderness.
Notes: See 11.7.4 Oestrogens And HRT.
Femoston 1/10, 2/10, conti 0.5/2.5, 1/5 *(BGP)* A. GMS.
Price, (28) 1/10, 2/10, €5.82. Conti 0.5/2.5 (84) €24.40; 1/5 (28) €8.13.
Tablet, estradiol hemihydrate (DHG). 2/10*: EH 2mg (14 days) (brick red); EH 2mg+DHG 10mg (14 days) (yellow). Conti*: EH 1mg+DHG 5mg (salmon-coloured). *Round. Marked 379. Lactose.*

Estradiol, Medroxyprogesterone

ATC Code: G03FA12. **Sport:** Permitted.
Driving: Unlikely to impair.
Indications: HRT in women with intact uterus more than 3 years postmenopause. Prevention, osteoporosis.
Dose: Adult: Initially 1mg/2.5mg; if breakthrough bleeding occurs, increase to 1mg/5mg; if 1mg estradiol insufficient, increase to 2mg/5mg. Continuous.
Notes: See 11.7.4 Oestrogens And HRT.
Indivina Tablets *(Orion)* A. GMS.
Price, (28) 1/2.5mg, €8.36. (84) 1/2.5mg, €28.50; 1/5mg, 2/5mg, €25.08.
Tablet, estradiol valerate + medroxyprogesterone acetate (1mg/2.5mg, 1mg/5mg, 2mg/5mg). White round. Marked with strengths. *Lactose.* **Store:** Below 25 deg C; original pack to protect (moisture)

Estradiol, Norethisterone

ATC Code: G03FA01. **Sport:** Permitted.
Driving: No known effects.
Indications: HRT in women more than 1 year post-menopause; *Evorel conti, Novofem, Trisequens*, 6 months post-menopause. Prevention, osteoporosis (except *Evorel conti*).
Dose: Adult: ORAL, 1 tab daily without interruption. *Novofem*, biphasic oestrogen 16 days, then oestrogen/progestogen 12 days. *Trisequens*, triphasic oestrogen/progestogen with 10 days progestogen.
TRANSDERMAL, patches to be applied to trunk below the waist. *Evorel Conti*, patches to be worn continuously, changed twice weekly.
Notes: See 11.7.4 Oestrogens And HRT.
Activelle *(Novo Nordisk)* A. GMS.
Price, (28) €7.67.
Tablet, estradiol hemihydrate, norethisterone acetate (1mg/0.5mg). White round f/c. Marked Novo 288; APIS on reverse. *Lactose.* **Store:** Below 25 deg C; do not refrigerate.
Evorel Conti *(Janssen-Cilag)* A. GMS.
Price, (8) €15.47.
Transdermal patch, estradiol hemihydrate, norethisterone acetate (50mcg/170mcg)/24 hours. Square; rounded corners. Marked CEN1. **Store:** Below 25 deg C; original sachet/box.
Kliogest *(Novo Nordisk)* A. GMS.
Price, (28) €6.21.
Tablet, estradiol hemihydrate, norethisterone acetate (2mg/1mg). White round f/c. Marked Novo 281. *Lactose.*
Novofem *(Novo Nordisk)* A. GMS.
Price, (3x28) €17.99.
Tablet, estradiol hemihydrate (EH) 1mg, EH 1mg+norethisterone acetate 1mg (EH+N). EH: Red. Marked Novo 282. EH+N: White. Marked Novo 283. *Lactose.*
Trisequens *(Novo Nordisk)* A. GMS.
Price, (28) €4.96.
Tablet, estradiol hemihydrate (EH) 2mg, EH 2mg+norethisterone

acetate 1mg (EH+N), EH 1mg. f/c. Marked Novo. EH 2mg: Blue. Marked 280. EH+N: White. Marked 281. EH 1mg: Red. Marked 282. *Lactose.*

Estriol

ATC Code: G03CA04. **Sport:** Permitted.
Driving: No effect on alertness, concentration.
Indications: HRT for treatment of atrophy of lower urogenital tract due to oestrogen deficiency. Pre- and post-operative, postmenopausal undergoing vaginal surgery.
Dose: Adult, Elderly: *Atrophy of lower genital tract,* 1 application (0.5mg estriol) per day for 2-3 weeks; reduce gradually to maintenance 1 application twice weekly.
Vaginal surgery, 1 application per day for 2 weeks before surgery; 1 application twice weekly for 2 weeks after surgery. Admin using calibrated applicator before going to bed.
Pregnancy, Lactation: Contraindicated.
ADR: Application-site pruritus, vaginal (burning sensation, discharge), breast (discomfort, pain).
Notes: See 11.7.4 Oestrogens And HRT.

Ovestin Vaginal Cream *(Aspen)* B.
Price, not published by company (GMS-pending).
Vaginal cream, estriol 1mg/gram. Homogenous smooth white (nearly white). With applicator. *Cetyl alcohol, stearyl alcohol.* **Store:** Below 25 deg C; do not freeze.

Oestrogens, Conjugated

ATC Code: G03CA57. **Sport:** Permitted.
Driving: Unlikely to impair.
Indications: HRT for oestrogen deficiency symptoms in menopausal and postmenopausal women. Prevention, osteoporosis.
Dose: Adult: Vasomotor symptoms, atrophic vaginitis/urethritis, kraurosis vulvae, 0.625-1.25mg/day. Osteoporosis, minimum effective 0.625mg/day.
ADR: *Common,* depression, alopecia, arthralgias, leg cramp, breakthrough bleeding/spotting, breast (pain, tenderness, enlargement, discharge), weight changes, increased triglycerides.
Notes: See 11.7.4 Oestrogens And HRT.

Premarin 0.625mg, 1.25mg *(Pfizer)* A. GMS.
Price, (28) 0.625mg, €2.69. 1.25mg, €3.18.
Prolonged/R tablet, conjugated oestrogen. Oval coated. Marked with strength. 0.625mg: Maroon. 1.25mg: Yellow. *Lactose, sucrose; Sunset Yellow (1.25mg).*

Oestrogen, Conjugated, Medroxyprogesterone

ATC Code: G03FA12. **Sport:** Permitted.
Driving: Unlikely to impair.
Indications: HRT, women postmenopause with intact uterus. Prevention, osteoporosis.
Dose: Adult: 1 tab daily without interruption.
ADR: *Very common,* breast pain.
Notes: See 11.7.4 Oestrogens And HRT.

Premique 0.625/5mg *(Pfizer)* A. GMS.
Price, (28) €4.83.
Tablet, conjugated oestrogen, medroxyprogesterone acetate. Oval light-blue s/c. Marked 0.625/5. *Lactose, sucrose.* **Store:** Below 25 deg C; original pack.

Oestrogen, Norgestrel

ATC Code: G03FA10. **Sport:** Permitted.
Driving: No studies performed.
Indications: HRT in women postmenopause. Prevention, osteoporosis.
Dose: Adult: Continuous, 12 days norgestrel 0.15mg, with oestrogen 0.625mg on days 17-28 of cycle. Use only in patients with intact uterus.
Notes: See 11.7.4 Oestrogens And HRT.

Prempak-C 0.625mg *(Pfizer)* A. GMS.
Price, 0.625mg, €2.84. Triple Pack, €15.29.
Tablet, conjugated oestrogens 0.625mg (28 tabs) and norgestrel (N) 0.15mg (12 tabs). Oval s/c. Marked with strength. 0.625mg: Maroon. N: Round light-brown. *Lactose, sucrose, Sunset Yellow.* **Store:** Below 25 deg C.

Tibolone

ATC Code: G03CX01. **Sport:** Prohibited.
Driving: Unlikely to impair.
Indications: HRT, relief of menopausal symptoms in women more than 1 year postmenopause. Second-line for prevention of osteoporosis.
Dose: Adult, Elderly: Usually 2.5mg/day; a separate progestogen should not be added.
CI: Tibolone increased the risk of breast cancer recurrence in a placebo-controlled trial.
Interactions: Effect of Other Drugs on Tibolone: *Efficacy reduced*: Certain antibiotics, anti-epileptics, sedatives.
Effect of Tibolone on Other Drugs: Anticoagulants (warfarin): *Effect enhanced.*
SP: Base decision to prescribe on overall risk (especially over 60) with consideration of stroke risk.
Notes: See 11.7.4 Oestrogens And HRT.

Livial 2.5mg *(MSD)* A. GMS.
Price, (28) €12.82.
Tablet, tibolone. White round flat. Marked MK above 2; Organon and star on reverse. *Lactose.*

11.8 - Drugs Affecting Bone Metabolism

11.8.1 - Bisphosphonates

In This Chapter: *Alendronic, clodronic, ibandronic, risedronic, zoledronic acids/salts and combinations.*

Class Effects

CI: Hypersensitivity to any member of the class. Abnormalities of oesophagus, factors delaying oesophageal emptying (stricture, achalasia). Hypocalcaemia. Oral formulations, inability to stand or sit upright for at least 30 minutes (alendronic acid, risedronic acid) or for 60 minutes (ibandronic acid).
Interactions: Effect of Other Drugs on Bisphosphonates: *Co-admin not recommended*: Other bisphosphonates. *Absorption impaired*: Milk, food, drugs containing calcium/other polyvalent cations. *Co-admin caution*: Aminoglycosides, other calcitonin, loop diuretics (additive effect in lowering serum calcium); other nephrotoxic drugs, other drugs causing hypocalcaemia; NSAIDs, acetylsalicylic acid (GI irritation).
SP: Not for use in children under 18 years unless otherwise specified. Once Weekly formulations, not indicated for glucocorticoid induced osteoporosis.
Osteonecrosis of jaw (ONJ) reported with both IV and oral bisphosphonates; risk factors e.g. bisphosphonate potency (highest for zoledronic acid), admin route, cumulative dose, concomitant risk factors (cancer, chemotherapy, angiogenesis inhibitors, radiotherapy, corticosteroids, smoking, dental disease, poor oral hygiene, periodontal disease, invasive dental procedures, poorly fitting dentures). Cancer patients should maintain good oral hygiene; dental examination with preventive dentistry prior to treatment. Consider temporary interruption of bisphosphonate until condition resolves. *Osteonecrosis of external auditory canal* also reported, usually with long-term therapy; risk factors (steroid use, chemotherapy, infection, trauma).
Dietary supplements, admin calcium and Vitamin D if dietary intake inadequate. Before using, treat hypocalcaemia, other bone/mineral metabolism disturbances, Vitamin D deficiency, hypoparathyroidism. Monitor hypercalcaemia-related metabolic parameters (serum calcium, phosphate, magnesium). Hypocalcaemia (severe, requiring hospitalisation; may be life-threatening) with secondary cardiac arrhythmias, neurological adverse events (seizures, numbness, tetany). Post thyroid surgery, particularly susceptible to hypocalcaemia due to relative hypoparathyroidism. Bone, joint and/or muscle pain; may be severe. Atypical femoral fractures, subtrochanteric and diaphyseal, especially with long-term use. Irritation of upper GI mucosa; caution, dysphagia, oesophagitis, oesophageal or gastric ulcers, upper GI surgery, peptic ulcer, active GI bleeding. Known Barrett's oesophagus, benefit/risk. Seek

11.8.1 Bisphosphonates

medical advice if symptoms occur (oesophageal irritation, dysphagia, pain on swallowing, retrosternal pain, new or worsening heartburn). NOTE: Consult dosing instructions for individual drugs. Missed doses, see manufacturers Full Prescribing Information.

Pregnancy, Lactation: Pregnancy, lactation, contraindicated unless otherwise specified; advise of women of childbearing age to avoid becoming pregnant. Colecalciferol/active metabolites do pass into breast milk.

Alendronic Acid

ATC Code: M05BA04. **Sport:** Permitted.
Driving: No or negligible effect; adverse reactions may affect.
Indications: Post-menopausal osteoporosis (adults). Reduces vertebral and hip fracture risk.
Dose: Adult, Elderly: 70mg once weekly; re-evaluate after 5 years. Do not crush or chew; oral soln unit-dose is 100mL. Dosing instructions, see SP below.
Renal Impairment: GFR (mL/min) below 35, not recommended.
SP: *Dosing*, to facilitate delivery to stomach and reduce potential for local irritation of upper GI mucosa, swallow oral soln or tabs whole with full glass of *plain* water upon rising for day; do not crush, chew or allow tabs to dissolve in mouth; dissolve effervescent tabs in half a glass of *plain* water; drink soln once fizzing has subsided and effervescent tab has completely dissolved to give clear soln; follow with minimum 30mL of plain water; additional water can be taken. For *all* formulations, do not lie down for at least 30 minutes after admin and until after first food of day; not to be taken at bedtime or before rising for day.
ADR: *Very common*, bone, muscle, joint pain including severe pain. See SP above.
Notes: See 11.8.1 Bisphosphonates.
Interchangeability: Same strengths of all brands of alendronic acid (sodium alendronate) 70mg tabs listed below are deemed interchangeable.
Reference Price: 70mg (4) €5.04.

Fosamax Once Weekly 70mg *(MSD)* B. GMS.
Price, (4), see reference price above.
Tablet, alendronate sodium trihydrate. Oval white. Marked with bone image; 31 on reverse. *Lactose*.
Alendronic Acid Accord Once Weekly *(Accord)* B. GMS.
Price, (4), see reference price above.
Tablet, alendronate sodium 70mg. White (off-white) oval. Marked AHI. *Lactose*.
Alendronic Acid Bluefish Once Weekly *(Bluefish)* B. GMS.
Price, (4), see reference price above.
Tablet, sodium alendronate 70mg. White oval. Marked 70.
Binosto Once Weekly *(Clonmel)* B. GMS.
Price, (4) €21.21.
Effervescent tablet, alendronate sodium trihydrate 70mg. White (off-white) round flat. *Sodium 602.54mg*.
Bonasol Once Weekly Oral Soln 70mg *(Fannin)* B. GMS.
Price, (4x100mL) €21.06.
Oral soln, alendronate sodium trihydrate 70mg/100mL. Orange opalescent soln. *Benzoate, Sunset Yellow*.
Fostepor Once Weekly 70mg *(Gerard)* B. GMS.
Price, (4), see reference price above.
Tablet, alendronate sodium. White. Marked AD70; G on reverse. *Lactose*.
Fostolin 70mg *(Accord)* B. GMS.
Price, (4), see reference price above.
Tablet, alendronate sodium trihydrate. Round white. Marked 70. *Lactose*.
Osteomel 70mg *(Clonmel)* B. GMS.
Price, (4), see reference price above.
Tablet, alendronate sodium trihydrate. Oval white (off-white). Marked AN70; logo on reverse. *Lactose*.
Romax Once Weekly 70mg *(Rowex)* B. GMS.
Price, (4), see reference price above.
Tablet, alendronate sodium trihydrate. Oval white (off-white). Marked AN70; logo on reverse. *Lactose*.
Tevanate Once Weekly 70mg *(TEVA)* B. GMS.
Price, (4), see reference price above.
Tablet, alendronate sodium monohydrate. White (off-white) flat-faced round. Marked T.

Alendronic Acid, Colecalciferol

ATC Code: M05BB03. **Sport:** Permitted.
Driving: No or negligible effect; blurred vision, dizziness, severe bone, muscle or joint pain (may influence).
Indications: Postmenopausal osteoporosis in patients at risk for Vitamin D deficiency (not receiving Vitamin D supplement). Reduces vertebral and hip fracture risk.
Dose: Adult, Elderly: 1 tab once weekly. *Admin*, swallow whole; do not crush, chew or allow to dissolve in mouth.
Renal Impairment: CrCl (mL/min) below 35, not recommended.
Interactions: Effect of Other Drugs on Colecalciferol: *Absorption impaired*: Olestra, mineral oils, orlistat, bile acid sequestrants (colestyramine, colestipol). *Catabolism increased*: Anticonvulsants, cimetidine, thiazides.
SP: Vitamin D3 may increase hypercalcaemia and/or hypercalciuria in presence of unregulated overproduction of calcitriol (leukaemia, lymphoma, sarcoidosis); monitor calcium (serum, urinary). Patients with malabsorption syndrome may not adequately absorb Vitamin D3. Decreased serum calcium and phosphate (especially patients taking glucocorticoids). Admin, see Notes below (alendronic acid).
ADR: *Summary, most common*, upper GI (abdominal pain/distention, dyspepsia, oesophageal ulcer, dysphagia, acid regurgitation).
Notes: See Alendronic Acid above.
Interchangeability: Same strengths of all brands of alendronic acid/cholecalciferol tabs listed below are deemed interchangeable.
Reference Price: (4) 70mg/2800 IU, €10.65. 70mg/5600 IU, €8.09.

FOSAVANCE 70MG/2800(5600) IU *(MSD)* B. GMS.
Price, (4) 70mg/2800 IU, €22.27. 70mg/5600 IU, €20.23.
Tablet, 70mg/2800(5600) IU; alendronic acid as sodium trihydrate 70mg, colecalciferol (Vitamin D3) 2800(5600) IU. White (off-white). Marked with bone image. 70/2800: Cap-shaped. Marked 710. 70/5600: Modified rectangle-shape. Marked 270. *Lactose, sucrose*. **Store:** Original blister; protect (light, moisture).
Alendronate/Colecalciferol Rowex *(Rowex)* B. GMS.
Price, (4), see reference price above.
Tablet, 70mg/5600 IU, alendronate sodium trihydrate 70mg, colecalciferol (Vitamin D3) 5600. White (almost) oval. Marked 714.
Alendronate/Colecalciferol TEVA *(TEVA)* B. GMS.
Price, (4), see reference price above.
Tablet, 70mg/2800 (5600) IU, alendronate sodium trihydrate 70mg, colecalciferol (Vitamin D3) 2800 IU/5600. White (off-white) cap-shaped. Marked A70; 2800 or 5600 on reverse. *Sucrose*.

Clodronic Acid

ATC Code: M05BA02. **Sport:** Permitted.
Driving: Unlikely to impair.
Indications: Management, increased bone resorption due to malignancy; hypercalcaemia of malignancy.
Dose: Adult, Elderly: *Increased bone resorption*, usually 1.6g as single dose; above 1.6g, take part of dose above 1.6g as second dose; max. 3.2g/day (divided doses). *Hypercalcaemia*, initially 2.4-3.2g/day (divided doses); reduce to 1.6g/day maintenance. Do not crush or dissolve tabs before intake; for ease of swallowing, may be divided into 2 halves and taken at same time. See SP below.
Child: Not recommended unless life-threatening malignant hypercalcaemia.
Renal Impairment: CrCl (mL/min) 30-50, 1.2g/day; below 30, 600mg/day; below 10, no data, avoid.
Interactions: Effect of Other Drugs on Clodronic Acid: *Increased renal dysfunction risk*: NSAIDs (diclofenac).
Effect of Clodronic Acid on Other Drugs: Estramustine: *Increased plasma levels*.
SP: *Dosing*, single daily dose OR divided dose, first dose in morning on empty stomach with a glass of water; refrain from eating, drinking other than plain water, or taking other oral medications for 1 hour; second dose to be taken between meals (2 hours after; 1 hour before eating, as

above). Ensure adequate hydration (especially with hypercalcaemia or renal failure). Monitor renal function before and during treatment (serum creatinine, calcium and phosphate).

Pregnancy, Lactation: Pregnancy, only if benefit outweighs risk. Lactation, not recommended.

ADR: Hypocalcaemia, asymptomatic; increased (serum parathyroid hormone associated with decreased serum calcium; serum ALP, transaminases), diarrhoea, nausea, vomiting, hypersensitivity reactions.

Notes: See 11.8.1 Bisphosphonates.

Bonefos 800mg *(Bayer)* B. HT.
Price, (60) €157.10.
Tablet, clodronate sodium tetrahydrate. White oval scored f/c. Marked L134. *Sodium 128mg/tab.*

Ibandronic Acid

ATC Code: M05BA06. **Sport:** Permitted.
Driving: No or negligible effect.
Indications: Osteoporosis in postmenopausal women at increased risk of vertebral fracture (efficacy on femoral neck fracture not established).

Dose: Adult, Elderly: *Postmenopausal osteoporosis,* 150mg orally once monthly, taken on same date each month OR parenteral 3mg by IV injection over 15-30 seconds, every 3 months; with supplemental calcium and Vitamin D if dietary intake inadequate. Oral dosing instructions, see SP below.

Renal Impairment: CrCl (mL/min) 30 or above, no adjustment; below 30, not recommended.

Hepatic Impairment: No dose adjustment required.

SP: *Dosing,* oral admin, after overnight fast (minimum 6 hours) and before first food or drink of day or any other medicinals and supplements; continue to fast for 30 minutes after admin; swallow tabs whole; do not suck, crush or chew; with a full glass (180-240mL) of plain water while standing or sitting; do not lie down for 60 minutes after taking. If tap water has high calcium concentration, use bottled water. Monitor renal function, serum magnesium. Oesophageal reaction, discontinue. Cardiac failure risk, avoid over hydration. Anaphylactic reaction/shock, including fatal events reported.

ADR: *Common,* hypocalcaemia, dyspepsia, asthenia, headache, skin disorder, oesophagitis, oesophageal reflux, gastritis, abdominal pain, nausea, infection, parathyroid disorder, dizziness, dysgeusia, cataract, bundle branch block, pharyngitis, diarrhoea, vomiting, GI pain, tooth disorder, ecchymosis, osteoarthritis, myalgia, arthralgia, joint disorder, bone pain, pyrexia, flu-like illness, peripheral oedema, thirst, increased (creatinine, gamma-GT).

Notes: See 11.8.1 Bisphosphonates.

Bonviva 150mg *(Roche)* B. GMS.
Price, (1) €14.97.
Tablet, ibandronic sodium monohydrate. White (off-white) oblong f/c. Marked BNVA; 150 on reverse. *Lactose.*
Bonviva Parenteral *(Roche)* A. HOS.
Price, 3mg (1) €59.59 (PTW).
Injection, ibandronic monosodium, monohydrate 3mg. Clear colourless soln in PFS.
Bonefurbit 150mg *(Rowex)* B. GMS.
Price, (1) €11.98.
Tablet, ibandronate sodium hydrate. White f/c oblong scored. Marked LC. *Lactose.*
Ibandronic Acid Clonmel 150mg *(Clonmel)* B. GMS.
Price, (1) €11.98.
Tablet, ibandronic acid sodium monohydrate. White (off-white) oblong f/c. Marked I9BE; 150 on reverse. *Lactose.*
Ibandronic Acid Mylan 150mg *(Gerard)* B. GMS.
Price, (1) €11.98.
Tablet, ibandronate sodium monohydrate. White f/c cap-shaped. Marked G over I-150. *Lactose.*
Ibandronic Acid TEVA 150mg *(TEVA)* B. GMS.
Price, (1) €11.98.
Tablet, ibandronic acid sodium monohydrate. White cap-shaped f/c. Marked I150.
Osbonelle 150mg *(Accord)* B. GMS.
Price, (1) €11.98.
Tablet, ibandronic sodium monohydrate. White (off-white) oblong f/c. Marked I9BE and 150. *Lactose.*

Risedronic Acid, Combinations

ATC Code: M05BA07, M05BB02, M05BB04. **Sport:** Permitted.
Driving: Unlikely to impair.
Indications: Postmenopausal, treatment of osteoporosis in women to reduce risk of vertebral and hip fractures; where calcium/Vitamin D supplementation needed *(Ca/Vitamin D combinations);* prevention, osteoporosis including corticosteroid-induced. Osteoporosis in men at high risk of fractures.

Dose: Adult, Elderly: *5mg and 35mg once weekly strengths,* treatment and prevention of osteoporosis, 5mg/day (women) OR 1x35mg Once Weekly tab (men, women) taken once weekly on same day.
Ca & D combinations (Actonel Combi, Plus), 1x35mg tab (day 1), followed by 1x500mg calcium tab (or calcium/Vitamin D3 sachet) daily for 6 days; repeat this 7-day sequence each week. Dosing instructions, see SP below.

Renal Impairment: CrCl (mL/min) below 30, contraindicated.

CI: Hypocalcaemia. Hypercalcaemia, hypercalciuria, nephrolithiasis *(Combi, Plus).* Hypervitaminosis D *(Plus).*

Interactions: Effect of Other Drugs on Risedronic Acid, Combinations: *Reduced calcium urinary excretion:* Thiazides. *Calcium absorption inhibited:* Foods rich in oxalic and/or phytic acid (allow 2-hour interval). *Reduced Vitamin D absorption:* Colestyramine, laxatives (paraffin oils).

Effect of Risedronic Acid, Combinations on Other Drugs: Tetracyclines, sodium fluoride, foods high in oxalic or phytic acid: *Impaired calcium absorption* (allow 2-hour before or 4-6 hour after dosing interval). Cardiac glycosides: *Increased toxicity (hypercalcaemia).*

SP: *Dosing,* admin at least 30 minutes before first food of day, drink or other medication with *plain* water; may be taken between meals (2 hours before or 2 hours after) or evening 2 hours after last food, at least 30 minutes before bedtime; must be taken on empty stomach. Swallow tabs whole, do not suck or chew; in upright position; do not lie down for 30 minutes after taking tab. *Combi,* calcium tab to be swallowed whole with food. *Plus,* pour contents of sachet into glass of plain water, stir, drink once fizzing stops. *Calcium/Vitamin D3 combinations,* with long-term treatment, monitor serum and urinary calcium, renal function (calcium, phosphates); severe impairment, colecalciferol not metabolised normally. *Elderly* on treatment with cardiac glycosides or diuretics, monitor, high calculus formation tendency. Additional calcium or Vitamin D, only under close medical supervision. Sarcoidosis, caution.

ADR: *Common,* headache, constipation, dyspepsia, nausea, abdominal pain, diarrhoea, pain. See SP above.

Notes: See 11.8.1 Bisphosphonates.

Interchangeability: Same strengths of all brands of risedronic acid (risedronate) film-coated (f/c) tabs, risedronic acid (risedronate)/calcium carbonate film-coated (f/c) tabs listed below are deemed interchangeable.

Reference Price: Risedronic acid (4) 35mg, €5.04.

Actonel 5mg, Once A Week 35mg *(Accord)* B. GMS.
Price, 5mg (28) €22.19. 35mg (4), €16.65.
Tablet, risedronate sodium. Oval f/c. Marked RSN; strength on reverse. 5mg: Yellow. 35mg: Light-orange. *Lactose.*
Actonel Combi *(TEVA)* B. GMS.
Price, (28) €22.43.
Tablet, risedronate sodium 35mg (1 tab); calcium carbonate equiv. to 500mg elemental calcium (6 tabs). 35mg: See Actonel Once A Week. Calcium: Cap-shaped blue f/c. Marked NE2 both sides. *Lactose.*
Actonel Plus Ca & D *(TEVA)* B. GMS.
Price, (1-pack) €29.88.
Tablet + granules, risedronate sodium 35mg (1 tab); calcium carbonate equiv. to 1000mg elemental calcium + colecalciferol 22mcg (880 IU) (24 sachets). 35mg: See Actonel Once A Week. Sachet: White effervescent granules. *Sorbitol, sucrose, soya-bean oil, potassium 163mg.*
Ridate Once A Week 35mg *(Rowex)* B. GMS.
Price, (4), see reference price above.
Tablet, risedronate sodium. Oval orange f/c. Marked 35. *Lactose.*

11.8.2   Other Drugs Affecting Bone Metabolism

Risedronate Actavis Once Weekly 35mg *(Accord)* B. GMS.
Price, (4), see reference price above.
Tablet, risedronate sodium. Orange round f/c. Marked I. *Lactose.*
Risedronate Adamed Once Weekly 35mg *(Niche)* B. GMS.
Price, (4), see reference price above.
Tablet, risedronate sodium. Pale-orange round f/c. *Lactose.*
Risedronate Bluefish 35mg *(Bluefish)* B. GMS.
Price, (4), see reference price above.
Tablet, risedronate sodium. White round f/c. Marked 35. *Lactose.*
Risedronate Mylan Once A Week 35mg *(Gerard)* B. GMS.
Price, (4), see reference price above.
Tablet, risedronate sodium. White round f/c. Marked 35. *Lactose.*
Risonate (TEVA) Once Weekly 35mg *(TEVA)* B. GMS.
Price, (4), see reference price above.
Tablet, risedronate sodium. Orange round f/c. Marked R35.
Lactose, Sunset Yellow.
Ristonel Once A Week 35mg *(Clonmel)* B. GMS.
Price, (4), see reference price above.
Tablet, risedronate sodium. White round f/c. Marked 35. *Lactose.*

Zoledronic Acid Actavis Parenteral 4mg/5mL *(TEVA)* A.
Price, (1) not published by company.
Infusion, zoledronic acid monohydrate. Clear colourless conc for
soln. *Essentially sodium-free.*
Zoledronic Acid Mylan Parenteral 4mg/5mL *(Gerard)* A.
Price, (1), €232.00.
Infusion, zoledronic acid monohydrate 4mg/5mL. Clear colourless
conc for soln. *Essentially sodium-free.*
Zoledronic Acid Parenteral 4mg/5mL *(Intrapharm)* A.
Price, (1) €20.00.
Infusion, zoledronic acid monohydrate 4mg/5mL. Clear colourless
conc for soln.
Zoledronic Acid Sandoz Parenteral 4mg/5mL *(Rowex)* A.
Price, (1) €80.00
Infusion, zoledronic acid monohydrate 4mg/5mL. Clear colourless
conc for soln. *Sodium 5.63mg per dose.*
Zometa Parenteral 4mg/100mL *(Novartis)* A. HOS.
Price, (1) €157.33 (PTW).
Infusion, zoledronic acid monohydrate. Clear colourless soln.

Zoledronic Acid

ATC Code: M05BA08. **Sport:** Permitted.
Driving: Dizziness.
Indications: Paget's Disease of bone. Treatment,
osteoporosis in post-menopausal women, men at
increased risk of fracture including glucocorticoid induced
osteoporosis. Prevention, skeletal events with advanced
malignancies involving bone. Treatment, tumour-induced
hypercalcaemia (TIH).
Dose: Adult, Elderly: *Aclasta 5mg/100mL, Paget's
Disease*, 5mg then calcium 500mg elemental twice daily
for 10 days; if retreatment required, 5mg after 1-year
interval or longer. *Osteoporosis*, 5mg once a year; low-
trauma hip fracture, admin infusion two or more weeks
after fracture repair with loading dose Vitamin D; admin
paracetamol or ibuprofen to reduce post-dose symptoms.
Brands 4mg/100mL OR 4mg/5mL (all except Aclasta),
prevention of skeletal events with advanced malignancies
involving bone 4mg every 3-4 weeks with oral calcium
500mg and Vitamin D 400 IU daily. *Tumour-induced
hypercalcaemia*, 4mg.
Zoledronic Acid Sandoz, prevention of fracture/bone loss
postmenopause with early breast cancer with aromatase
inhibitors 4mg infusion every 6 months with oral calcium
and Vitamin D as above.
Admin all brands as single slow IV infusion over minimum
15 minutes.
Child: *Aclasta*, under 18 years, safety/efficacy not
established. *Other brands*, age 1-17 years, no dose
recommendation.
Renal Impairment: *Aclasta*, CrCl (mL/min) below 35,
contraindicated.
Zometa, Zoledronic Acid Sandoz, prevention of skeletal
events, CrCl (mL/min) 50-60, 3.5mg; 40-49, 3.3mg; 30-
39, 3mg. TIH, severe impairment, if benefit outweighs risk.
SP: Calculate CrCl (based on actual body weight) before
each dose; at-risk, monitor function. Other medicinals
affecting renal function, caution. Ensure adequate
hydration prior to admin especially with diuretic therapy
and elderly (over 65 years); avoid over-hydration if risk of
cardiac failure. Ensure adequate calcium/Vitamin D intake.
Pregnancy, Lactation: Pregnancy, contraindicated; not
recommended in women of childbearing potential.
Lactation, contraindicated.
ADR: Summary, *Aclasta*, after first infusion (pyrexia,
myalgia, influenzae-like symptoms, arthralgia, headache).
Other brands, identified risks e.g. renal impairment,
osteonecrosis of jaw, acute phase reaction (bone pain,
fever, fatigue, arthralgia, myalgia, rigors, arthritis with joint
swelling), hypocalcaemia, atrial fibrillation, anaphylaxis,
interstitial lung disease.
Notes: See 11.8.1 Bisphosphonates.

Aclasta Parenteral 5mg/100mL *(Novartis)* A. HOS.
Price, (1) €297.29 (PTW).
Infusion, zoledronic acid monohydrate. Clear colourless soln.
Zerlinda Parenteral 4mg/100mL *(TEVA)* A.
Price, (1) not published by company.
Infusion, zoledronic acid monohydrate. Clear colourless soln.

11.8.2 - Other Drugs Affecting Bone Metabolism

In This Chapter: *Bazedoxifene, denosumab, parathyroid
hormone, raloxifene, strontium, teriparatide.*

Class Effects

Indications: Treatment, post-menopausal osteoporosis in
women to reduce risk of vertebral fractures *(calcitonin,
bazedoxifene, raloxifene)*, vertebral and non-vertebral
fractures including glucocorticoid-induced *(teriparatide)*,
vertebral *and* hip fractures *(strontium)*, vertebral, non-
vertebral and hip fractures *(denosumab)*.
Treatment, osteoporosis in men at increased risk of
fractures *(denosumab, strontium)* including glucocorticoid-
induced *(teriparatide)*. Bone loss associated with hormone
ablation in men *(denosumab)*.
Prevention, skeletal related events (fracture, bone
radiation, spinal cord compression, bone surgery; adults
with bone metastases from solid tumours); treatment, giant
cell tumour of bone (denosumab brand *Xgeva*).
CI: Hypersensitivity to any member of the class. Use in
children under 18 years. SERMs *(bazedoxifene, raloxifene)*,
VTE including DVT, pulmonary embolism, retinal vein
thrombosis, unexplained uterine bleeding, signs or
symptoms of endometrial cancer. See Pregnancy, Lactation
below.
SP: Admin supplemental calcium and Vitamin D if dietary
intake inadequate. SERMs, increased VTE risk (illness,
prolonged immobilisation, discontinue immediately;
restart only when full mobility resumed). Investigate uterine
bleeding. Monitor liver function. Increased triglycerides,
especially with history of oral oestrogen-induced
hypertriglyceridaemia. Use for osteoporosis treatment and
prevention *after* breast cancer treatment completed. Not
effective for reducing menopausal symptoms associated
with oestrogen deficiency. Osteonecrosis of jaw (ONJ) and
external auditory canal, calcium and Vitamin D
supplementation, fractures, see Notes below.
Pregnancy, Lactation: Unless otherwise stated,
contraindicated for use in women of childbearing potential;
ensure adequate contraception; if pregnancy occurs,
discontinue. Lactation, generally not recommended.
Notes: See Class Effects 11.8 Drugs Affecting Bone
Metabolism.

Bazedoxifene

ATC Code: G03XC02. **Sport:** Prohibited.
Driving: Minor influence; somnolence, visual disturbance.
Indications: See Notes below.
Dose: Adult, Elderly: 20mg max. daily. Admin at any time
of day with or without food.
Renal Impairment: Severe, caution.
Hepatic Impairment: Not recommended.
SP: Use not recommended in women with increased VTE
risk, premenopause, breast cancer. Hypertriglyceridaemia,
caution. Bazedoxifene increased hormone-binding
globulins including (corticosteroid, sex hormone,
thyroxine)-binding globulin.

ADR: Summary, *most frequent*, hot flushes, muscle spasms (including leg cramp).

Notes: See 11.8.2 Other Drugs Affecting Bone Metabolism.

Conbriza 20mg *(Pfizer)* B. GMS.
Price, (28) €22.53.
Tablet, bazedoxifene. White (off-white) cap-shaped f/c. Marked WY20. *Lactose*.

Denosumab

ATC Code: M05BX04. **Sport:** Permitted.
Driving: No or negligible effect.

Indications: See Notes below.

Dose: Adult, Elderly: *Prolia*, 60mg as single SC injection once every 6 months*.

Xgeva, skeletal events (bone metastases from solid tumour), 120mg as single SC injection once every 4 weeks*; giant cell tumour of bone, as for skeletal events with additional 120mg (day 8, 15) of first treatment month. See SP below. *Admin into thigh, abdomen or upper arm.

Child: Under 18, not recommended other than skeletally mature adolescents with giant cell tumour of bone, as for Adult above.

Renal Impairment: Severe or on dialysis, monitor calcium.

CI: Hypocalcaemia, unhealed lesions from dental or oral surgery.

SP: Monitor calcium prior to initiation, within 2 weeks, and if hypocalcaemia symptoms occur; correct pre-existing hypocalcaemia; supplementation, see Notes below. Skin infections; signs of cellulitis, seek medical advice *(Prolia)*. Osteonecrosis of jaw, see Notes below. Supply patient with reminder card (information on ONJ). Atypical femoral fractures.

Pregnancy, Lactation: Pregnancy, not recommended. Lactation, weigh risk/benefit.

ADR: Summary, *most common (Prolia)*, musculoskeletal pain, extremity pain; *common (Xgeva)*, hypocalcaemia.

Notes: See 11.8.2 Other Drugs Affecting Bone Metabolism.

Prolia Parenteral 60mg/mL *(Amgen)* A. GMS.
Price, (1) €213.24.
Injection, denosumab. Human monoclonal antibody (IgG2). Clear colourless (slightly yellow) soln. *Natural rubber (needle cover); sorbitol*. **Store:** Refrigerate; do not freeze.

▼ **Xgeva Parenteral 120mg/mL** *(Amgen)* A. HT.
Price, 120mg (1) €322.12.
Injection, denosumab. Human monoclonal antibody (IgG2). Clear colourless (slightly yellow) soln. *Sorbitol*. **Store:** Refrigerate; do not freeze.

Raloxifene

ATC Code: G03XC01. **Sport:** Prohibited.
Driving: Unlikely to impair.

Indications: See Notes below.

Dose: Adult, Elderly: 60mg daily with or without food.

Renal Impairment: Mild/moderate, caution. Severe, contraindicated.

Hepatic Impairment: Including cholestasis, contraindicated.

Interactions: Effect of Other Drugs on Raloxifene: *Co-admin not recommended*: Systemic oestrogens. *Reduced absorption*: Colestyramine, other anion exchange resins.

Effect of Raloxifene on Other Drugs: Warfarin, other coumarin derivatives: *Monitor prothrombin time*.

ADR: *Very common*, hot flushes, nausea, vomiting, abdominal pain, dyspepsia, flu syndrome, increased BP.

Notes: See 11.8.2 Other Drugs Affecting Bone Metabolism.

Evista 60mg *(Daiichi Sankyo)* B. GMS.
Price, (28) €21.46.
Tablet, raloxifene HCl. White elliptical f/c. Marked 4165. *Lactose*.

Raloxifene Actavis 60mg *(Accord)* B. GMS.
Price, (28) €9.39.
Tablet, raloxifene HCl. White elliptical f/c. *Lactose*.

Strontium

ATC Code: M05BX03. **Sport:** Permitted.
Driving: No or negligible effect.

Indications: Indicated where treatment with other osteoporosis approved products is either contraindicated or not tolerated. Base decision to prescribe on individual patient overall risk. See Notes below.

Dose: Adult, Elderly: One 2g sachet once daily in-between meals or preferably at bedtime at least 2 hours after food. Granules to be taken as suspension in water.

Renal Impairment: CrCl (mL/min) below 30, not recommended.

CI: Ischaemic heart disease, peripheral arterial disease and/or cerebrovascular disease, uncontrolled hypertension.

Interactions: Effect of Other Drugs on Strontium: *Co-admin not recommended*: Oral tetracyclines, quinolones. *Reduced bioavailability*: Food, milk, medicinals containing calcium, antacids (allow 2-hour dosing interval).

SP: Specialist supervision. Before initiation evaluate cardiovascular risk; caution with risk factors (hypertension, hyperlipidaemia, diabetes mellitus, smoking); monitor every 6-12 months. Development of ischaemic heart disease, peripheral artery disease, cerebrovascular disease, hypertension (uncontrolled), discontinue. Increased VTE incidence, contraindicated (venous thromboembolic history); caution, if at VTE risk. Monitor renal function. Hypersensitivity (DRESS), can be fatal. Rash, advise patients to discontinue immediately; life-threatening cutaneous reactions.

ADR: Summary, *most common*, nausea, diarrhoea (generally, beginning of treatment).

Notes: See 11.8.2 Other Drugs Affecting Bone Metabolism.

▼ **Protelos 2g** *(Servier)* B. GMS.
Price, (28) €32.69.
Granules for oral susp, strontium ranelate. Yellow. *Aspartame*.

Teriparatide

ATC Code: H05AA02. **Sport:** Permitted.
Driving: Transient orthostatic hypotension, dizziness.

Indications: See Notes below.

Dose: Adult, Elderly: Usually 20mcg once daily by SC injection (thigh, abdomen); max. 24-month course (should not be repeated over patient lifetime).

Renal Impairment: Severe, contraindicated. Moderate, caution.

Hepatic Impairment: No data.

CI: Pre-existing hypercalcaemia, metabolic bone disease (hyperparathyroidism, Paget's disease of bone), other than primary or glucocorticoid-induced osteoporosis, unexplained elevated ALP, prior external beam or implant radiation to skeleton, skeletal malignancies, bone metastases.

Interactions:Effect of Teriparatide on Other Drugs: Digitalis: *Caution (due to hypercalcaemia)*.

SP: Small increase in urinary calcium excretion. Caution, potential to exacerbate active urolithiasis. Transient orthostatic hypotension. Younger adults, premenopause, weigh risk/benefit.

ADR: Summary, *most common*, nausea, limb pain, headache, dizziness.

Notes: See 11.8.2 Other Drugs Affecting Bone Metabolism.

Forsteo Parenteral *(Lilly)* A. HT.
Price, PFP (1) €373.93.
Injection, teriparatide (rhPTH) 600mcg/2.4mL (250mcg/mL). Clear colourless soln (PFP).

11.9 - Other Endocrine Drugs

In This Chapter: *Buserelin, cetrorelix, metyrapone, nafarelin, ulipristal.*

Class Effects

Cabergoline is also indicated for Parkinson's disease; buserelin brand *(Suprefact)* and triptorelin have a dual endocrine indication as well as for prostate cancer treatment, see Notes below. Ketoconazole (systemic) is used to treat endogenous Cushing's syndrome.

CI: Hypersensitivity to any member of the class, structural analogues or extrinsic peptide hormones.

SP: These drugs should be used under specialist supervision with appropriate monitoring facilities. Consult

11.9 Other Endocrine Drugs

manufacturers Full Prescribing Information. Increased risk of depression (may be severe) with GnRH agonist treatment (buserelin, nafarelin, triptorelin); history of depression, monitor (recurrence, worsening). Androgen deprivation therapy may prolong QT-interval; history or risk factors for QT-prolongation, weigh risk/benefit.

Pregnancy, Lactation: Exclude pregnancy before initiating. Ensure adequate non-hormonal contraception during treatment.

Notes: See 3.5.1 Dopaminergics Used In Parkinson's Disease (cabergoline), 13.3.2 Prostate Cancer (buserelin, triptorelin).

Buserelin (endocrine)

ATC Code: LO2AE01. **Sport:** Prohibited (in men).
Driving: Caution.

Indications: Treatment, endometriosis. Pituitary desensitisation in preparation for ovulation induction regimens using gonadotropins.

Dose: Adult: *Endometriosis*, 150mcg spray in each nostril 3-times daily for 6 months. *Ovulation induction*, adjunctive, 150mcg as spray in each nostril 4-times daily spread over waking hours.

Child: Not recommended.

CI: Undiagnosed vaginal bleeding.

Interactions: Effect of Other Drugs on Buserelin: *Co-admin (allow at least 30-min dosing interval)*: Nasal decongestants. *Carefully evaluate co-admin (QT-prolongation)*: Drugs prolonging QT-interval (quinidine, disopyramide, amiodarone, sotalol, dofetilide, ibutilide, methadone, moxifloxacin, antipsychotics).

Effect of Buserelin on Other Drugs: Antidiabetic agents: *Effect attenuated*.

SP: Discontinue hormonal contraception before initiation. Effect prolonged with hepatic or renal disturbances. Pain exacerbation and increase in nodular mass and pressure. Start treatment on first or second day of menstruation to exclude pregnancy, or pregnancy test. Repeated courses, risk of additive effects of reduction in bone mass; restrict treatment to 6 months. Ovarian cysts may develop. Risks specific to assisted reproduction procedures (increase in miscarriages, ectopic and multiple pregnancies) unaltered adjunctive buserelin; follicle recruitment may be increased. Combination with gonadotrophins, higher OHSS risk. Acute abdomen. Severe thromboembolic events. Depression, monitor; risk of recurrence or worsening. Hypertension, monitor BP.

ADR: Scalp/body hair changes, BP deterioration in hypertensives, hypersensivity reactions including skin, respiratory, anaphylactic/toid shock, nervousness, emotional instability, anxiety, depression, increased thirst, appetite changes, reduced glucose tolerance, neoplasms benign/malignant, pituitary adenomas, tiredness, lipid changes, increased liver enzymes/bilirubin, weight changes, thrombopenia, leucopenia, palpitations, headache, sleep disturbance, fatigue, drowsiness, disturbed memory and concentration, dizziness, tinnitus, hearing disorder, impaired vision, pressure feeling behind eye, nausea, vomiting, diarrhoea, constipation, discomfort, pain, decreased bone density, nasal mucosal irritation.

Notes: See 11.9 Other Endocrine Drugs and 13.3.2 Prostate Cancer (buserelin, brand *Suprefact Injection*).

Supecur Nasal Spray *(SANOFI)* A. GMS.
Price, 150mcg (1) €49.02; (2) €98.04.
Nasal spray, buserelin acetate 150mcg/metered dose. Clear colourless soln. *Benzalkonium chloride.* **Store:** Below 25 deg C; do not freeze.

Cetrorelix

ATC Code: HO1CC02. **Sport:** Permitted.
Driving: No or negligible influence.

Indications: Prevention, premature ovulation in patients undergoing a controlled ovarian stimulation in assisted reproduction.

Dose: Adult: 0.25mg once daily (morning or evening) at 24-hour intervals. Following first admin, keep patient under medical supervision for 30 minutes to ensure no allergic reaction. *Morning admin*, commence on day 5 or 6 of ovarian stimulation; *evening admin*, commence on day 5. *Admin*, by SC injection into lower abdominal wall.

Elderly: No relevant use.

Child: No relevant use.

Renal Impairment: Caution. Severe, contraindicated.

Hepatic Impairment: Caution.

Interactions: Effect of Other Drugs on Cetrorelix: *Caution*: Drugs inducing histamine release.

SP: Cases of allergic/pseudo-allergic reactions (including life-threatening anaphylaxis) reported with first dose. Give luteal phase support. Use in repeated cycles only after careful risk/benefit evaluation.

ADR: Summary, *most common*, injection-site reactions (erythema, swelling, pruritus), mild/moderate ovarian hyperstimulation syndrome (OHSS).

Notes: See 11.9 Other Endocrine Drugs.

Cetrotide Parenteral *(Merck Serono)* A. HT.
Price, (1) €33.20. (7) €226.00.
Injection, cetrorelix acetate 0.25mg. White lyophilised powder. Clear colourless solvent (reconstituted pH 4-6).

Ketoconazole (systemic)

ATC Code: Pending. **Sport:** Permitted.
Driving: Dizziness, somnolence.

Indications: Treatment, endogenous Cushing's syndrome (12 years and older).

Dose: Adult, Elderly: Age 12 years and over, initially 400-600mg/day*; this can be increased rapidly to 800-1200mg/day*. Individualise based on urinary free cortisol and/or plasma cortisol levels; if above normal range, consider dose increase of 200mg/day every 7-28 days. Maintenance 400mg/day to max. 1200mg/day* may be needed to restore normal cortisol levels; maintenance range 600-800mg/day*. *Admin*, oral. *(in 2 or 3 divided doses).

Child: Under 12 years, no dose recommendation.

Renal Impairment: No adjustment.

Hepatic Impairment: Acute or chronic impairment and/or pre-treatment liver enzymes above 2x ULN contraindicated. QTc prolongation (congenital, acquired).

CI: Imidazole hypersensitivity.

Interactions: Effect of Other Drugs on Ketoconazole (systemic): *Co-admin contraindicated*: Statins (simvastatin, atorvastatin, lovastatin), eplerenone, QT-prolonging drugs (methadone, disopyramide, quinidine, dronedarone, pimozide, sertindole, saquinavir, ranolazine, mizolastine, halofantrine), dabigatran, triazolam, oral midazolam, alprazolam, ergot alkaloids, lurasidone, quetiapine, telithromycin, clarithromycin, felodipine, nisoldipine, colchicine, vardenafil, fesoterodine, solifenacin. NOTE: Contraindicated interactions are listed however, the interaction profile is extensive. See manufacturers Full Prescribing Information.

SP: *Before or at initiation*, control 24-hour urinary free cortisol every few days/weeks. Once effective dose is established, monitor urinary free cortisol and/or plasma cortisol every 3-6 months. Case of adrenal insufficiency (depending on severity), decrease to 200mg/day or temporarily discontinue and/or add corticosteroid therapy. Can stop abruptly without tapering dose. At initiation, measure liver enzymes (ASAT, ALAT, gammaGT, alkaline phosphatase) and bilirubin; inform patient of hepatotoxicity risk; do not initiate if liver enzymes are above 2xULN. Measure QTc interval.

After initiation, measure liver enzymes and bilirubin weekly (month 1), then monthly (6 months); weekly (during 1 month with dose increase). Increased liver enzymes below 3xULN, monitor more frequently, decrease daily dose by minimum 200mg; 3xULN or above, discontinue at once; do not restart (hepatotoxicity risk). Monitor QTc interval after 1 week, then as clinically needed. Signs of hepatitis, discontinue. Inflammatory/autoimmune disorders described after Cushing's syndrome remission. Block and replace regimen, see manufacturers Full Prescribing Information. Supply patients with emergency card and equip with emergency glucocorticoid set.

Pregnancy, Lactation: Contraindicated. Provide women

with comprehensive information on pregnancy prevention; women of childbearing potential must use effective contraception.

ADR: Summary, *most frequent*, adrenal insufficiency, nausea, vomiting, abdominal pain, diarrhoea, pruritus, rash, increased hepatic enzymes; *most serious*, hepatotoxicity.

Notes: See 11.9 Other Endocrine Drugs.

▼ **Ketoconazole HRA 200mg** *(HRA)* A.
Price, (60), €705.88.
Tablet, ketoconazole. Off-white (light cream) round. *Lactose.*

Metyrapone

ATC Code: V04CD01. **Sport:** Permitted.
Driving: Minor influence; dizziness, sedation.

Indications: Diagnostic test for ACTH insufficiency and in differential diagnosis of ACTH-dependent Cushing's syndrome. Management, endogenous Cushing's syndrome.

Dose: Adult, Elderly: DIAGNOSTIC, *short single-dose* (ambulatory), 30mg/kg (max. 3g) at midnight; blood sample taken in morning followed by 50mg cortisone acetate prophylactically. *Multiple test* (hospitalised), 500-700mg every 4 hours for 24 hours; total 3-4.5g; max. effect on urinary steroid values should be reached in next 24 hours. Admin with milk or after food to minimise nausea and vomiting.
THERAPEUTIC, *Cushing's Syndrome*, initially 250mg-1g/day depending on severity; usual maintenance 500mg-6g/day.

Child: DIAGNOSTIC, *short single-dose* (ambulatory), as for Adult; *multiple test* (hospitalised), 15mg/kg for 6 doses 4-hourly; minimum 250mg 4-hourly.
THERAPEUTIC, adjust on individual basis.

CI: Primary adrenocortical insufficiency.

Interactions: Effect of Other Drugs on Metyrapone: *Diagnostic results influenced*: Anticonvulsants (phenytoin, barbiturates), antidepressants, neuroleptics (amitriptyline, chlorpromazine), hormones affecting hypothalamo-pituitary axis, corticosteroids, antithyroid agents.
Effect of Metyrapone on Other Drugs: Paracetamol, acetaminophen: *May potentiate toxicity.*

SP: Before using, demonstrate ability of adrenal cortex to respond to exogenous ACTH. Liver cirrhosis, possible delayed response due to delayed cortisol plasma elimination half-life. Thyroid hypofunction, urinary steroid levels may rise very slowly or not at all. Before diagnostic use, discontinue drugs affecting pituitary or adrenocortical function. Transient adrenocortical insufficiency, correct with corticosteroids. Hypertension. Ectopic Cushing's syndrome, at risk for opportunistic infections.

Pregnancy, Lactation: Pregnancy and women of childbearing potential, not recommended unless clearly necessary. Lactation, stop breastfeeding during treatment.

ADR: *Common*, nausea, vomiting, dizziness, sedation, headache, hypotension.

Notes: See 11.9 Other Endocrine Drugs.

Metopirone 250mg *(HRA)* B.
Price, (50) €14.42.
Capsule, metyrapone. Soft gelatin white (yellowish-white) oblong opaque; faintly yellow viscous contents. Marked HRA. *Parabens.*
Store: Below 30 deg C.

Nafarelin

ATC Code: H01CA02. **Sport:** Prohibited (in men).
Driving: Unlikely to impair.

Indications: Hormonal management of endometriosis. Controlled ovarian stimulation prior to *in vitro* fertilisation.

Dose: Adult: *Endometriosis*, initiate between days 2-4 of cycle, 200mcg twice daily as 1 spray in 1 nostril in morning; 1 spray in other nostril in evening for max. 6 months.
Controlled ovarian stimulation, 400mcg twice daily as 1 spray in each nostril morning and evening.

Child: Under 18 years, not recommended.

CI: Hypersensitivity to other GnRH analogues, undiagnosed vaginal bleeding, hormone-dependant neoplasms.

Interactions: Effect of Other Drugs on Nafarelin: *Co-*

admin not recommended: Nasal decongestants (dose 30 minutes after nafarelin).

SP: Missed dose, breakthrough ovulation risk, conception potential. Pituitary-gonadal suppression; exacerbation of symptoms of pain and increased nodular mass and pressure initially. Ovarian cysts. Sneezing during or immediately after dosing may impair absorption; repeat dose. Depression.

Pregnancy, Lactation: Pregnancy, contraindicated. Lactation, contraindicated. If pregnancy occurs during treatment, discontinue; inform of potential risk to foetal development and/or miscarriage.

ADR: *Very common*, increased weight, affected lability, decreased libido, headache, hot flush, rhinitis, acne, seborrhoea, myalgia, breast atrophy, vulvovaginal dryness, oedema.

Notes: See 11.9 Other Endocrine Drugs.

Synarel Nasal Spray *(Pfizer)* A. HT.
Price, (1) €72.86.
Nasal spray, nafarelin acetate 2mg/mL (200mcg/spray). Clear colourless (slightly yellow) aqueous soln.

Ulipristal (uterine fibroids)

ATC Code: G03XB02. **Sport:** Permitted.
Driving: Minor influence; dizziness.

Indications: Intermittent treatment, moderate to severe symptoms of uterine fibroids in adult women of reproductive age.

Dose: Adult: 5mg once daily for treatment courses of up to 3 months; commence during first week of menstruation; commence re-treatment courses during first week of second menstruation following completion of previous course. Up to 4 intermittent courses. Admin with or without food.

Child: Under 18 years, no safety/efficacy data.

Renal Impairment: Severe, not recommended unless closely monitored.

Hepatic Impairment: As for Renal above.

CI: Genital bleeding of unknown aetiology or not due to fibroids; cancer (uterine, cervical, ovarian, breast).

Interactions: Effect of Other Drugs on Ulipristal: *Co-admin not recommended*: CYP3A4 inhibitors (moderate) (erythromycin, grapefruit juice, verapamil), (potent) (ketoconazole, ritonavir, nefazodone, itraconazole, telithromycin, clarithromycin); CYP3A4 inducers (potent) (rifampicin, rifabutin, carbamazepine, oxcarbazepine, phenytoin, fosphenytoin, phenobarbital, primidone, St John's Wort, efavirenz, nevirapine, long-term ritonavir).
Effect of Ulipristal on Other Drugs: Hormonal contraceptives (progestogen only, progestogen-releasing devices, combined hormonal contraceptives): *Co-admin not recommended or within 12 days of stopping ulipristal.* P-gp substrates (dabigatran, digoxin, fexofenadine): *Separate dosing by minimum 1.5 hours.*

SP: Severe insufficiently controlled asthma, use not recommended. Do not mistake Progesterone Receptor Modulator Associated Endometrial Changes (PAEC) for endometrial hyperplasia. Reversible increase of endometrium thickness; with repeated intermittent treatment, monitor endometrium periodically (ultrasound). If thickening persists beyond 3 months after end of treatment and/or altered bleeding pattern noted, exclude other underlying conditions. Hyperplasia (without atypia), monitor. Advise patients of significant reduction in menstrual blood loss or amenorrhoea within first 10 days of treatment (notify physician if excessive bleeding persists).

Pregnancy, Lactation: Contraindicated. Exclude pregnancy before initiation. Non-hormonal contraceptive method recommended during treatment (see Interactions).

ADR: Summary, *most common*, amenorrhoea; *most frequent*, hot flush.

Notes: See 11.9 Other Endocrine Drugs.

Esmya 5mg *(GedeonRichter)* A. HT.
Price, (28) €139.86.
Tablet, ulipristal acetate. White (off-white) round. Marked ES5.

12

Immunology, Vaccines

12.1 - Active Immunisation

In This Chapter: *Cholera; Diphtheria, Tetanus, Poliomyelitis and combinations (Pertussis, H. influenzae, Hepatitis B); Diphtheria, Tetanus, Pertussis combination (DTPa); Measles, Mumps, Rubella (MMR) combination; H. influenzae type b (Hib), Hepatitis A, Hepatitis B (HBV), Human Papilloma Virus (HPV), Influenzae, Japanese encephalitis, Neisseria meningitidis; Rabies, Rotavirus, Streptococcus pneumoniae, Tuberculosis (TB), Typhoid, Varicella, Yellow Fever Vaccines.*

Class Effects

Store: Refrigerate; do not freeze unless otherwise stated. Usually in outer carton to protect (light). Specified per brand: Storage at room temp after removal from refrigerator (usually below 25 degrees C) if applicable.

Indications: Active immunisation in accordance with the Official Guidance.

CI: Hypersensitivity to (any member of class, vaccine component, trace substances after manufacture, after previous admin of similar vaccine). Use of live viruses with immunosuppression (chemo- or radiotherapy, organ or bone marrow transplantation and/or currently on immunosuppressives including corticosteroids); impaired cell-mediated immunity (HIV infection, Severe Combined Immunodeficiency Syndrome, Di George Syndrome or congenital/hereditary immunodeficiency; severe humoral or cellular, primary or acquired immunodeficiency). NOT for use with acute febrile disease/fever over 38.5 degrees C (postpone admin unless delay causes greater risk); minor infection not a contraindication.

Interactions: Effect of Other Drugs on Vaccines: *Co-admin (general rule):* Do not mix with other vaccines or vaccine components in same syringe.

SP: Admin vaccines only if facilities available for management of acute anaphylactoid or serum sickness type reactions; prior to injection, take all precautions to prevent adverse events (possible hypersensitivity history); observe recipients until no immediate adverse reactions seen. Anxiety-related reactions (vasovagal reactions/syncope, hyperventilation, stress-related reactions e.g. psychogenic response to needle injection); can be accompanied by neurological signs (transient visual disturbance, paraesthesia, tonic-clonic limb movements) during recovery; avoid injury from faints. Vaccines may not protect 100% of recipients; reduced immunogenicity in immuno-compromised (immunosuppressive therapy, genetic causes). HIV infection not a contraindication for use *(Hiberix, Infanrix IPV Hib, Boostrix, Infanrix Hexa)*; M-M-R (only if patient is NOT immunocompromised). Guillain-Barre syndrome or brachial neuritis following vaccine with tetanus toxoid (weigh risk/benefit).

After pertussis-containing vaccines, carefully consider admin of further doses if: Severe reaction within 48 hours of preceding injection; fever of 40 degrees C or above within 48 hours of vaccination; inconsolable, persistent crying (more than 3 hours); convulsions with or without hyperthermia; allergic reactions; collapse, shock-like state. New onset or severe, neurological disorders, consider risk/benefit. All vaccines given to (very) preterm infants, apnoea risk (primary immunisation), monitor 48-72 hours.

Admin, vaccines for IM or SC use are **NOT** for intravascular injection. Thrombocytopenia, any coagulation disorder or on anticoagulants, use IM route (weigh risk/benefit); SC preferred. Multiple vaccine admin, use separate injection sites.

ADR: Injection site reactions e.g. erythema, swelling, pain, induration, bruising, nodule formation; pyrexia/fever, headache. See SP above.

Cholera Vaccine

ATC Code: J07AE01. **Sport:** Permitted.
Driving: No evidence of effect.

Indications: Active immunisation against diseases caused by *Vibrio cholerae* serogroup O1 (adults, children) visiting endemic/epidemic areas.

Dose: Adult, Elderly: Age 6 years and above, *primary schedule*, 2 doses (minimum 1-week intervals); interval of over 6 weeks, re-start primary schedule. Complete immunisation minimum 1 week prior to potential exposure; *booster* as single dose recommended within 2 years; if more than 2 years has elapsed, repeat primary course. *Elderly*, age 65 years and above, limited data. *Admin*, oral; vaccine susp to be mixed with buffer solution (effervescent granules) dissolved in approx. 150mL water; see Interactions below.

Child: Age 2 to below 6 years, *primary schedule*, 3 doses as for Adult; 6 years onwards, as for Adult; *booster* as single dose recommended within 6 months; if more than 6 months has elapsed, repeat primary course. Under 2 years, not recommended. *Admin*, as for Adult; use half of buffer soln.

CI: Acute GI or febrile illness.

Interactions: Effect of Other Drugs on Cholera Vaccine: *Avoid co-admin (allow 1-hour dosing interval before and after cholera vaccine):* Food and/or drink (increases stomach acid production), other vaccines and medicinals.

SP: Does not protect against *V. cholerae* serogroup O139 or other Vibrio species. HIV infected subjects, limited data.

Pregnancy, Lactation: Can be used (careful benefit/risk assessment).

ADR: *Most frequent*, GI symptoms (abdominal pain, diarrhoea, loose stools, nausea, vomiting).

Notes: See 12.1 Active Immunisation.

> **DUKORAL Oral Susp** *(Valneva)* A.
> *Price*, 2-doses, €32.19.
> *Oral susp, Vibrio cholerae* O1 strain with buffer. *Sodium 1.1g/dose; formalin trace.* **Store:** See Class Effects. Room temp. (14 days).

Diphtheria, Tetanus Vaccine

ATC Code: J07AM51. **Sport:** Permitted.
Driving: Unlikely to impair.

Indications: Re-vaccination (children, adults); previously received primary immunisation (3 doses of diphtheria + tetanus vaccine).

Dose: Adult, Elderly: Single 0.5mL dose IM; can be admin deep SC. Repeat usually at 10-year intervals.

Child: Age 5 years and over, as for Adult above.

SP: Not for primary immunisation. Too frequent booster vaccination increases adverse reaction risk.

Pregnancy, Lactation: Pregnancy, weigh risk/benefit. Lactation, no evidence of harm to infant.

ADR: *Most common*, injection-site reactions; fever.

Notes: See 12.1 Active Immunisation.

diTeBooster *(SSI)* A. HSEi(Adult).
Price, not published by company.
Injection, purified toxoid (diphtheria 2 IU, tetanus 20 IU)/0.5mL. Adsorbed (aluminium hydroxide). Susp. *Formaldehyde; sodium below 23mg/dose.* **Store:** See Class Effects.

Diphtheria, Tetanus, Poliomyelitis (DTP) Vaccine

ATC Code: J07AM51. **Sport:** Permitted.
Driving: Vertigo.

Indications: Immunisation against diphtheria, tetanus, poliomyelitis (children); booster following primary vaccination (adults).

Dose: Adult, Elderly: Single 0.5mL dose IM only, deltoid; not for intradermal, intravascular use. Bleeding disorders, deep SC.

Child: Age 6 years and over, as for Adult above.

CI: Hypersensitivity (neomycin, streptomycin, polymyxin B). Neurological complications after earlier immunisation against diphtheria and/or tetanus.

SP: Not for (primary immunisation; a primary vaccination course or booster of a diphtheria/tetanus toxoid vaccine within previous 5 years). May be used with tetanus-prone injuries if co-vaccination (diphtheria, poliomyelitis) is needed *(Revaxis).*

Pregnancy, Lactation: Pregnancy, only if urgent to boost immunity. Lactation, may be used.

ADR: Summary, *most common,* injection-site reactions.

Notes: See 12.1 Active Immunisation.

REVAXIS *(SanofiPasteur)* A. HSEi(Restricted).
Price, not published by company.
Injection, purified toxoid (diphtheria 2 IU*, tetanus 20 IU*), IPV antigen units type 1 (40), type 2 (8), type 3 (32). Adsorbed (aluminium hydroxide). Cloudy white susp in PFS. *(not less than).* **Store:** See Class Effects; discard if been frozen.

DTP, Pertussis Vaccine

ATC Code: J07AJ52. **Sport:** Permitted.
Driving: Unlikely to impair.

Indications: Immunisation against diphtheria, tetanus, pertussis, poliomyelitis, *primary vaccination* in infants *(Tetravac). Booster* vaccination (children previously received a primary vaccination with a diphtheria-tetanus-whole-cell or acellular pertussis-poliomyelitis vaccine) *(Tetravac),* children 3 years and older *(IPV-Boostrix)* or age 16 months to 13 years *(IPV Infanrix).*

Dose: Adult, Elderly: *IPV-Boostrix,* single 0.5mL dose. May be admin to (adolescents, adults) with unknown vaccination status or incomplete vaccination against diphtheria, tetanus, pertussis; 2 additional doses (diphtheria and tetanus containing vaccine) recommended at months (1 and 6) after first dose to maximize vaccine response. *IPV-Boostrix* can be used in management of tetanus prone injuries (persons previously received a primary vaccination of tetanus toxoid and for whom a booster against diphtheria and pertussis is indicated). Co-admin tetanus immunoglobulin. Repeat vaccination against diphtheria, tetanus and pertussis at intervals as per official recommendations. *Admin,* deep IM injection (preferably deltoid).

Child: PRIMARY, *Tetravac,* 3 doses at 1-2 month intervals starting at 2-3 months OR 2 doses at 2-month intervals starting at age 3 months; third dose at 12 months.

BOOSTER, *Tetravac,* admin fourth dose within second year of life (children who received 3-dose primary series between age 2-6 months); can be used in children 5-12 years (previous acellular vaccine, or 4 doses of whole-cell vaccine).

BOOSTER, *IPV-Boostrix,* single 0.5mL dose from age 4 years onwards. *IPV-Infanrix,* single 0.5mL dose from age 16 months to 13 years. Not for primary vaccination. Deep IM, antero-lateral aspect of upper thigh (infants), deltoid muscle (older children); NOT for intradermal or intravascular use.

Active Immunisation 12.1

CI: Evolving encephalopathy. Hypersensitivity to pertussis vaccines. Neurological complications with previous immunisation (any antigens in vaccine). Hypersensitivity to neomycin, polymyxin *(IPV-Boostrix, IPV-Infanrix),* formaldehyde *(IPV Infanrix);* transient thrombocytopenia *(IPV-Boostrix).*

SP: Caution, hypersensitivity (glutaraldehyde, thiomersal, neomycin, streptomycin, polymyxin B) *(Tetravac).*

Pregnancy, Lactation: *IPV-Boostrix,* first and second trimester weigh risk/benefit; can be considered in third trimester. Lactation, if benefit outweighs risk; no risk to infant expected.

ADR: *Very common,* somnolence, injection-site reactions, headache, malaise. *Premature infants,* apnoea. *(Tetravac).*

Notes: See 12.1 Active Immunisation.

IPV-Boostrix *(GSK)* A. HSEi(Restricted).
Price, not published by company.
Injection, toxoid (diphtheria 2 IU, tetanus 20 IU, pertussis 8mcg), filamentous haemagglutinin 8mcg, pertactin 2.5mcg, IPV antigen units type 1 (40), type 2 (8), type 3 (32). Adsorbed (aluminium hydroxide). Turbid white susp, PFS. **Store:** See Class Effects. After refrigeration, 21 deg C (8 hours).

IPV-Infanrix *(GSK)* A. HSEi(Child).
Price, not published by company.
Injection, toxoid (diphtheria 30 IU, tetanus 40 I*, pertussis 25mcg), filamentous haemagglutinin 25mcg, pertactin 8mcg, IPV antigen units type 1 (40), type 2 (8), type 3 (32). Adsorbed (aluminium hydroxide). Turbid white susp, PFS. **Store:** See Class Effects.

TETRAVAC (4 in 1) *(SanofiPasteur)* A. HSEi(Child).
Price, not published by company.
Injection, purified toxoid (diphtheria 30 IU, tetanus 40 IU, pertussis 25mcg), filamentous haemagglutinin 25mcg, IPV antigen units type 1 (40), type 2 (8), type 3 (32). Adsorbed (aluminium hydroxide). Sterile whitish turbid susp. **Store:** See Class Effects.

DTP, Pertussis, H. influenzae, Hepatitis B Vaccine

ATC Code: J07CA09. **Sport:** Permitted.
Driving: Not applicable.

Indications: Primary immunisation and booster (infants), against diphtheria, tetanus, pertussis, hepatitis B, poliomyelitis, *Haemophilus influenzae* type b, children under 36 months.

Dose: Adult, Elderly: Not for Adult use.

Child: PRIMARY, 3x 0.5mL doses at (2, 3, 4 months OR 3, 4, 5 months OR 2, 4, 6 months) OR 2x 0.5mL doses at (3, 5 months) with at least 1-month interval. Age 6, 10, 14 weeks may be used only if a dose of hepatitis B vaccine was given at birth.

BOOSTER, after vaccination with 2 doses as above (booster between age 11-13 months) OR after 3 doses as above (booster preferably before age 18 months). Admin booster at least 6 months after last priming dose. Deep IM; NOT for intravascular injection.

CI: Encephalopathy of unknown aetiology within 7 days after previous vaccination with pertussis containing vaccine. See Notes below.

SP: See Notes below, (Pertussis Vaccine, special precautions). New onset or progression of severe neurological disorder, weigh risk/benefit. Caution, thrombocytopenia, bleeding disorders. Hepatitis B component does not protect against hepatitis A, C or E; Hib component only protects against *Haemophilus influenzae* type b. Co-admin with pneumococcal saccharide conjugated vaccine *(Prevenar),* incidence of convulsions (with or without fever) and hyporesponsive episode were higher; initiate antipyretic treatment.

ADR: *Very common,* abnormal crying, irritability, restlessness, appetite loss, fever, fatigue.

Notes: See 12.1 Active Immunisation.

Infanrix Hexa (6 in 1) *(GSK)* A. HSEi(Child).
Price, not published by company.
Injection (0.5mL), toxoid (diphtheria 30 IU, tetanus 40 IU, pertussis 25mcg), filamentous haemagglutinin 25mcg, pertactin 8mcg, HBV surface antigen 10mcg, IPV antigen units type 1 (40),

331

12.1   Active Immunisation

type 2 (8), type 3 (32), Hib 10mcg, conjugate vaccine (adsorbed). Turbid white susp (DTpa-HBV-IPV); white powder (Hib) for susp. *Traces, formaldehyde, neomycin, polymyxin.* **Store:** See Class Effects; below 25 deg C (max. 72 hours then discard).

Diphtheria, Tetanus, Pertussis Vaccine

ATC Code: J07AJ52. **Sport:** Permitted.
Driving: Unlikely to impair.

Indications: Booster vaccination against diphtheria, tetanus, pertussis (age 4 years and older).

Dose: Adult, Elderly: Single 0.5mL dose, from age 4 years onwards. May be admin to (adolescents, adults) with unknown vaccination status or incomplete vaccination (diphtheria, tetanus, pertussis); 2 additional doses (diphtheria, tetanus containing vaccine) recommended at months (1 and 6) after first dose (maximise vaccine response). *Boostrix* can be used in management of tetanus prone injuries (previous primary vaccination of tetanus toxoid and a booster against diphtheria and pertussis is indicated). Co-admin tetanus immunoglobulin. Repeat vaccination against diphtheria, tetanus and pertussis generally at 10-year intervals. *Admin,* deep IM injection (preferably deltoid).

Child: See Adult above.

CI: Encephalopathy of unknown aetiology within 7 days following previous pertussis-containing vaccine. Transient thrombocytopenia or neurological complications after earlier immunisation against diphtheria and/or tetanus.

SP: Can be used to manage tetanus prone injuries with previous primary vaccination series of tetanus toxoid vaccine and where a diphtheria and pertussis booster is indicated.

Pregnancy, Lactation: Pregnancy, first two trimesters*; may be considered during third trimester. Lactation, only if clearly needed*; no risk to breastfed infant expected. *(weigh risk/benefit).

ADR: *Very common,* irritability, somnolence, injection-site reactions, headache.

Notes: See 12.1 Active Immunisation.

Boostrix *(GSK)* A. HSEi(Restricted).
Price, not published by company.
Injection, toxoid (diphtheria 2 IU, tetanus 20 IU, pertussis 8mcg), filamentous haemagglutinin 8mcg, pertactin 2.5mcg. Adsorbed (aluminium hydroxide/phosphate). Turbid white susp, PFS. **Store:** See Class Effects. Below 21 deg C (max. 8 hours).

Haemophilus influenzae Vaccine

ATC Code: J07AG01. **Sport:** Permitted.
Driving: Not applicable.

Indications: Immunisation against *H. influenzae* type b (infants from age 2 months).

Dose: Adult, Elderly: Not for Adult use.

Child: PRIMARY, infants 2 months and over, 3x 0.5mL doses at 2-month intervals (normally at same time as DTP or combination); children 13 months and over, 1x 0.5mL dose (with MMR).

BOOSTER, additional Hib conjugate dose may be given after completion of 3-dose primary series in infancy. Admin IM; SC with thrombocytopenia or bleeding disorders; NOT for IV injection.

SP: *H. influenzae* type b disease may occur in first week after vaccination. Not a substitute for routine tetanus admin.

Pregnancy, Lactation: Not for use (not intended for use in adults).

ADR: *Very common,* loss of appetite, irritability, crying, restlessness, somnolence, diarrhoea, injection-site reactions.

Notes: See 12.1 Active Immunisation.

Hiberix Parenteral *(GSK)* A. HSEi(Child).
Price, not published by company.
Injection, H. influenzae type b polysaccharide 10mcg conjugated (tetanus protein approx. 25mcg)/0.5mL. White powder. Clear colourless solvent. *Sodium 77micromoL per dose.* **Store:** See Class Effects.

Hepatitis A Vaccine

ATC Code: J07BC02. **Sport:** Permitted.
Driving: No or negligible effect.

Indications: Against infection caused by Hepatitis A virus in susceptible *(Avaxim),* non-immune *(Havrix)* adults and adolescents (16 years and over). Includes travellers to high risk areas, other high risk non-immune groups (see SP), during Hepatitis A infection outbreaks *(Havrix).* Against Hepatitis A infection (age 1-15 years), particularly if at increased risk of infection or transmission.

Dose: Adult, Elderly: PRIMARY, age 16 years and over, initial protection, 1 single dose.

BOOSTER, long-term protection, admin second dose between 6-12 months, up to 36 months after first dose; provides up to 10 years protection *(Avaxim)* or up to 5 years *(Havrix).* For IM injection ONLY, deltoid region and not gluteal; not for intradermal or intravascular use (exceptionally, with thrombocytopenia or bleeding disorders, subcutaneous admin may be used; may have suboptimal response).

Child: *Havrix Junior,* PRIMARY, 1 single dose IM.

BOOSTER, single dose, schedule as per Adult above. Under 16 years, not recommended *(Havrix)*; age 15 years or under not recommended *(Avaxim).*

Hepatic Impairment: Caution.

CI: Neomycin hypersensitivity *(Avaxim, Havrix Junior).* Hypersensitivity after previous Hepatitis A vaccine.

SP: Seropositivity against hepatitis A is not a contraindication for use. Not for injection in buttocks. Symptoms of hypersensitivity, further injection not recommended. High risk, non-immune groups e.g. recent contact with infection, child- and health-care workers; staff, residents (institutions for mentally handicapped); haemophilia and recipient of plasma-derived clotting factors, chronic liver disease, food handlers, sewage workers, prison officers, renal failure (prior to dialysis), military and diplomatic personnel, IV drug abusers, homosexual men.

Havrix Monodose can be co-admin with monovalent and combination vaccines (measles, mumps, rubella, varicella).

Pregnancy, Lactation: Pregnancy, not recommended unless high infection risk and if clearly needed. Lactation, not recommended *(Avaxim),* caution *(Havrix).*

ADR: Appetite loss, irritability, headache, drowsiness, asthenia, myalgia, arthralgia, nausea, vomiting, diarrhoea, abdominal pain, mild fever, elevated serum transaminases, allergic reactions, injection-site reactions.

Notes: See 12.1 Active Immunisation.

AVAXIM Vaccine *(SanofiPasteur)* A. HSEi(Restricted).
Price, not published by company.
Injection, Hepatitis A virus, GBM strain (inactivated) 160 U*. Produced in human diploid MRC-5 cells; adsorbed (aluminium hydroxide). *In-house reference.* **Store:** See Class Effects.
Havrix Monodose, Junior *(GSK)* A. HSEi(Restricted).
Price, not published by company.
Injection, Hepatitis A virus (HM175 strain) (inactivated) (produced on MRC-5 human diploid cell) 1440 ELISA units (Junior, 720 ELISA units). Adsorbed (aluminium hydroxide). Slightly white susp, PFS *(Havrix Monodose). Essentially sodium and potassium-free.* **Store:** See Class Effects.

Hepatitis A, Hepatitis B Vaccine

ATC Code: J07BC20. **Sport:** Permitted.
Driving: Unlikely to impair.

Indications: Immunisation against Hepatitis A and B infection age 16 years and over *(Twinrix Adult)* or 1 year to (including) 15 years *(Twinrix Paediatric).*

Dose: Adult, Elderly: PRIMARY, 3x 1mL doses at 0, 1 and 6 months; exceptionally, when standard schedule not possible, 3x 1mL doses at 0, 7 and 21 days and a fourth dose 12 months after dose 1.

BOOSTER, of hepatitis A and/or B is required, a monovalent or combined vaccine can be used. Safety/immunogenicity when used as booster following 3-dose primary course not evaluated *(Twinrix Paed)*. *Admin*, IM injection, deltoid (thrombocytopenia or bleeding disorders, SC; may result in suboptimal immune response). Not for intradermal use or IM into gluteal muscle use or intravascular admin.

Child: Use 0.5mL dose, as per Adult schedule.

CI: Hypersensitivity to previous admin or monovalent Hepatitis A or B vaccine.

SP: Not recommended, post-exposure prophylaxis (needle stick injury); can be co-admin with HPV vaccine *(Twinrix)*. Reduced immune response to Hepatitis B vaccines, see Hepatitis B below, hepatitis A vaccines, obesity; BMI of 30kg/m2 or more.

Pregnancy, Lactation: Pregnancy, delay vaccination until after delivery unless urgent need. Lactation, not known if excreted in human milk; discontinue therapy or breastfeeding.

ADR: *Very common*, injection-site reaction; (adult) headache, fatigue.

Notes: See 12.1 Active Immunisation.

Twinrix Adult, Paed Vaccine *(GSK)* A. HSEi(Restricted).
Price, not published by company.
Injection, inactivated HAV 720 (Paed, 360) ELISA units, HBV surface antigen recombinant (S protein) 20mcg (Paed, 10mcg). Produced in human diploid cells and *(Saccharomyces cerevisiae)* by rDNA technology. Susp in PFS. *Traces neomycin.* **Store:** See Class Effects.

Hepatitis B Vaccine

ATC Code: J07BC01. **Sport:** Permitted.
Driving: Caution.

Indications: Immunisation against Hepatitis B (HBV) infection, in non-immune subjects; in renal insufficiency including pre-haemodialysis, dialysis.

Dose: Adult, Elderly: *Engerix 20mcg, HBVAXPRO 10mcg*, PRIMARY, age 16 years and over 20mcg *(Engerix)* OR 10mcg *(HBVAXPRO)*, schedule 0, 1 and 6 months; admin fourth dose at month 12. Rapid Protection, *Engerix 20mcg* age 18 years and over, schedule 0, 7 and 21 days; fourth dose at month 12; age 11-15 years, 20mcg can be used as 2-dose schedule, 0 and 6 months. Known or presumed exposure, schedule 0, 1, 2 and 12 months, first dose with HBIg at separate injection sites. Need for booster not established. IM, anterolateral thigh in neonates, infants, young children; deltoid in older children (thrombocytopenia or bleeding disorders, SC).

Fendrix (from age 15 years and over), *HBVAXPRO 40mcg*, PRIMARY, schedule 0, 1, 2 and 6 months using same product for initiation and completion. Known or presumed exposure, if admin with HBIg, use separate injection sites. BOOSTER, pre-haemodialysis/dialysis patients, consider booster to ensure protective antibody level. IM deltoid. All brands are NOT for intradermal or IV use; avoid gluteal muscle IM admin.

Child: *Engerix 10mcg, HBVAXPRO 5mcg*, up to and including 15 years including neonates, 10mcg *(Engerix)* OR 5mcg *(HBVAXPRO)* dose. Primary schedule as for Adult above. Neonates born of HBV carrier mothers, start immunisation at birth using either schedule; HBIg should be given simultaneously. See Adult above.

Renal Impairment: Primary, adult including dialysis, 4 double doses (*Engerix B*, 2 x 20mcg OR *HBVAXPRO* 40mcg) at 0, 1, 2 and 6 months. Booster, consider if antibody level after vaccination below 10 IU/L. Child, as for Child dose *(Engerix B)*; vaccination with higher dose antigen may improve immune response.

SP: Reduced immune response to Hepatitis B vaccines (older age, males, obesity, smoking, route of admin, some chronic underlying diseases); may need additional. Chronic liver disease, HIV infection, Hepatitis C carriers should not be precluded from Hepatitis B vaccination. Hepatitis B has long incubation; if infected before immunisation, vaccine

Active Immunisation   12.1

may not prevent infection. Caution, thiomersal (sensitisation) *(Fendrix)* and formaldehyde, potassium thiocyanate *(HBVAXPRO)* may cause hypersensitivity. Apnoea risk, see Notes below. Anaphylaxis, allergic reactions (anaphylactoid reactions and mimicking serum sickness).

Pregnancy, Lactation: Pregnancy, if benefit outweighs risk. Lactation, no data; no contraindication established; use if benefit outweighs risk.

ADR: *Common*, injection-site reactions; appetite loss, fatigue, pain, fever, drowsiness, headache, nausea, vomiting, diarrhoea, abdominal pain, irritability.

Notes: See 12.1 Active Immunisation.

Engerix B *(GSK)* A. HSEi(Restricted).
Price, not published by company.
Injection, Hepatitis B surface antigen 10mcg, 20mcg. Adsorbed (aluminium hydroxide); produced in *Saccharomyces cerevisiae* by rDNA technology. 1 dose (0.5mL, 1mL). Susp. PFS. **Store:** See Class Effects.
Fendrix *(GSK)* A. HSEi(Restricted).
Price, not published by company.
Injection, Hepatitis B surface antigen 20mcg. Adsorbed (aluminium phosphate), produced in *Saccharomyces cerevisiae* by rDNA technology. White turbid susp; fine white deposit with clear colourless supernatant upon storage. **Store:** See Class Effects.
HBVAXPRO *(MSD)* A. HSEi(Restricted).
Price, not published by company.
Injection, Hepatitis B virus surface antigen, recombinant (HBsAg) 5mcg (10mcg, 40mcg). Adsorbed. Slightly opaque white susp, PFS. *Dry natural latex rubber.* **Store:** See Class Effects.

Human Papillomavirus Vaccine

ATC Code: J07BM01 *(Gardasil)*. J07BM02 *(Cervarix)*. **Sport:** Permitted.
Driving: ADRs may temporarily affect.

Indications: Prevention, premalignant (genital, anal) lesions, cervical and anal cancers, external genital warts (condyloma acuminata) related to HPV types. Use/efficacy in men, see manufacturers Full Prescribing Information *(Gardasil)*. Prevention, premalignant ano-genital lesions (cervical, vulvar, vaginal, anal), cervical and anal cancers related to certain HPV types *(Cervarix)*.

Dose: Adult, Elderly: *Gardasil*, age 9-13* years, 2-dose schedule of 2x 0.5mL at (0, 6 months) (if admin before 6 months, always admin a third dose) OR 3-dose schedule of 3x 0.5mL at (0, 2 and 6 months) (minimum 1-month between dose 1 and 2; at least 3-months between dose 2 and 3; all 3 within 1-year period). Age 14 years and older, as for 3-dose schedule above. *Admin*, IM deltoid or higher anterolateral thigh; SC, intradermal not recommended. Admin as soon as possible after removing from refrigerator. *Cervarix*, from age 9-14* years, 2x 0.5mL doses; dose 2 between 5 and 13 months after dose 1; from age 15 years and above, 3x 0.5mL doses at (0, 1 and 6 months) (dose 2 between 1 and 2.5 months after dose 1; dose 3 between 5 and 12 months after dose 1). At any age, if dose 2 is admin before the fifth month after dose 1, always admin a third dose. *Admin*, IM injection, deltoid region. Need for booster not established. Not for intravascular or intradermal injection; SC admin, no data. *(including).

Child: Under 9 years, not recommended.

Interactions: Effect of Other Drugs on HPV Vaccine: *Co-admin does not interfere with immune response; inject at different sites*: Hepatitis B (recombinant) vaccine, Hepatitis A and B (HAB) vaccine. *Sequential admin, trend of lower anti-HPV GMTs observed; clinical significance unknown*: dTap-IPV vaccine. *Admin did not appear to affect immune response*: Oral contraceptives.

SP: Psychogenic response to needle injection, see Notes below. Not for treatment or progression prevention of established HPV-related lesions. Not a substitute for routine cervical screening. Protection duration unknown. Does not provide protection against every HPV type; use in adult women, consider HPV type prevalence in different geographical areas. The decision to vaccinate an individual

333

12.1 Active Immunisation

woman should take into account her (risk for previous HPV exposure, potential benefit). No safety, immunogenicity or efficacy data to support interchangeability; use the same vaccine for the whole dose regimen.

Pregnancy, Lactation: Pregnancy, postpone or interrupt vaccination until completion of pregnancy. Lactation, can be used *(Gardasil)*; if benefit outweighs risk *(Cervarix)*.

ADR: *Very common*, headache, injection-site reactions; myalgia *(Cervarix)*. *Common*, nausea; extremity pain, pyrexia; syncope; observe vaccinees (15 minutes post-admin) *(Gardasil)*; vomiting, diarrhoea, abdominal pain, itching/pruritus, rash, urticaria, arthralgia *(Cervarix)*.

Notes: See 12.1 Active Immunisation.

GARDASIL Vaccine *(MSD)* A. HSEi(Used).
Price, not published by company.
Injection, HPV Type 6 20mcg, Type 11 40mcg, Type 16 40mcg, Type 18 20mcg. Adsorbed (aluminium hydroxyphosphate sulfate). Susp in PFS. Clear liquid; white precipitate (before agitation); white cloudy liquid (after agitation). **Store:** See Class Effects.

Cervarix Vaccine *(GSK)* A.
Price, not published by company.
Injection, HPV Type 16, 18 (20mcg). Adsorbed recombinant adjuvanted. Turbid white susp, PFS; upon storage, a fine white deposit; clear colourless supernatant. **Store:** See Class Effects.

Influenza Vaccine

ATC Code: J07BB. **Sport:** Permitted.
Driving: No or negligible effect.

Indications: Prophylaxis of influenza, especially those at increased risk of complications.

Dose: Adult, Elderly: All brands, age over 36 months 1x 0.5mL dose IM or deep SC. Not for intravascular injection.

Child: All brands, age 6-35 months, dosages of 0.25mL or 0.5mL may be used. Previously not vaccinated, admin second dose after 4-weeks *(Influvac).*

CI: Hypersensitivity to egg (chicken protein, ovalbumin), formaldehyde; cetyltrimethylammonium bromide, polysorbate 80, gentamicin *(Influvac)*; neomycin, octoxinal 9 *(Inactivated Influenza Vaccine/Split Virion BP).*

SP: Following influenza vaccination, false positive serology tests detect HIV-1, Hepatitis C, HTLV1 antibodies.

Pregnancy, Lactation: Inactivated influenza vaccines can be used at all stages of pregnancy and during lactation.

ADR: *Common*, headache, sweating, myalgia, arthralgia, fever, malaise, shivering, fatigue, injection-site reactions.

Notes: See 12.1 Active Immunisation.

All brands below comply with WHO recommendation (northern hemisphere), EU decision for year season (2016/2017).

Inactivated Influenza Vaccine (Split Virion) BP Parenteral *(SanofiPasteur)* A. HSEi(Adult).
Price, not published by company.
Injection, inactivated (split) virus. Slightly whitish opalescent susp in PFS (0.5mL). **Store:** See Class Effects.

Influvac Sub-Unit Parenteral *(BGP)* A. HSEi(Adult).
Price, not published by company.
Injection, influenza virus surface antigens. Clear colourless susp. PFS (0.5mL). **Store:** See Class Effects.

Japanese Encephalitis Vaccine

ATC Code: J07BA02. **Sport:** Permitted.
Driving: No studies performed.

Indications: Immunisation against Japanese encephalitis (at risk due to travel or occupation).

Dose: Adult, Elderly: PRIMARY, 0.5mL dose (day 0); second 0.5mL dose 28 days after first dose.

BOOSTER, admin third dose within second year (12-24 months) after primary, prior to potential re-exposure; if at continuous risk of JEV exposure, admin booster 12 months after primary. IM deltoid; exceptionally, SC (thrombocytopenia, bleeding disorders).

Child: PRIMARY, age 3-18 years, as for Adult above. Age 2 months to 3 years, two 0.25mL doses, schedule as for Adult above.

334

BOOSTER, Age 2 months to 18 years, no data. Admin as for Adult (infants, anterolateral thigh may be used).

CI: Hypersensitivity to first dose do not admin second dose. Protamine sulphate hypersensitivity.

SP: Protection against JEV not ensured until second dose received.

Pregnancy, Lactation: Pregnancy, avoid. Lactation, avoid (no effects on breastfed infant anticipated).

ADR: *Very common*, headache, myalgia, injection site reaction.

Notes: See 12.1 Active Immunisation.

IXIARO Parenteral *(Valneva)* A.
Price, not published by company.
Injection, Japanese encephalitis virus strain (0.5mL). Susp; clear liquid; white precipitate. Inactivated, adsorbed. **Store:** See Class Effects.

Measles Mumps Rubella (MMR) Vaccine

ATC Code: J07BD52. **Sport:** Permitted.
Driving: No or negligible influence.

Indications: Immunisation against measles, mumps, rubella (from 12 months). Can be used in infants aged 9-12 months in special circumstances. Measles outbreaks, post-exposure, previously unvaccinated children older than 9 months in contact with pregnant women, persons likely to be susceptible to mumps and rubella *(M-M-RVAXPRO).*

Dose: Adult, Elderly: See Child below.

Child: *M-M-RVAXPRO*, age 12 months and older, 1 dose (elected date); if no response, a second dose may be given at least 4 weeks after first. Age 9-12 months, can be admin if early protection required; revaccinate at 12-15 months.

Priorix, 1x 0.5mL dose. A second dose should be given according to official recommendations. Under 12 months, vaccination may be indicated in some situations (high-risk areas); a second dose should be given in second year of life, preferably within 3 months after first dose.

Under 9 months, no data. SC or IM only. See Notes below.

CI: Not contraindicated in individuals receiving topical or low-dose parenteral corticosteroids (asthma prophylaxis). Neomycin hypersensitivity *(Priorix)*. Active untreated TB, no paediatric data.

M-M-RVAXPRO, vaccination may be considered in patients with selected immune deficiencies where benefit outweighs risk (asymptomatic HIV, IgG subclass deficiencies).

Interactions: Effect of Other Drugs on Measles, Mumps and Rubella Vaccine: *1-month dose interval (unless co-admin):* Other live attenuated vaccines. *Vaccine failure risk (delay for 3 months):* Following human gammaglobulins (immune globulins), blood or plasma transfusion (due to passively acquired antibodies).

Effect of Measles, Mumps and Rubella Vaccine on Other Drugs: Tuberculin testing: *Temporary depression of skin sensitivity; false negative results; test to be done before, with, or 4-6 weeks after vaccination.*

SP: Infants 9-12 months vaccinated with measles-containing vaccine may fail to respond due to presence of circulating antibodies of maternal origin and/or immaturity of immune system. *Severely immunocompromised*, inadvertent vaccination with measles-vaccine, may result in measles inclusion body encephalitis, pneumonitis, and fatal outcome (consequence of disseminated measles vaccine virus infection). Immunocompromised, consider vaccination where benefit outweighs risk (asymptomatic HIV, IgG subclass deficiencies, congenital neutropenia, chronic granulomatous disease, complement deficiency disease). *Vaccine production* is in chick embryo cell culture (measles, mumps); may contain traces of egg protein. History of anaphylactic, anaphylactoid, or other immediate reactions (generalised urticaria, swelling of mouth/throat, difficulty breathing, hypotension, shock) following egg ingestion (enhanced risk of immediate-type hypersensitivity reactions after vaccination); vaccinate with extreme caution. Alcohol (other disinfecting agents) should evaporate fully before injection; can inactivate attenuated viruses in vaccine. Contains traces of recombinant human albumin (rHA). *CNS disorder*, susceptibility to febrile convulsions, convulsions, caution temperature elevation following vaccination. Worsening or recurrence of thrombocytopenia (subjects suffering thrombocytopenia after first dose); consider risk/benefit.

Pregnancy, Lactation: Pregnancy, contraindicated; avoid for 1 month following vaccination. Lactation, caution; if benefit outweighs risk.

ADR: *Very common/common*, fever, injection-site reactions, rash.

Notes: See 12.1 Active Immunisation.

M-M-RVAXPRO Parenteral *(MSD)* A. HSEi(Child).
Price, not published by company.
Injection (PFS), live attenuated measles, mumps, rubella virus strains. Light-yellow crystalline cake; clear colourless solvent. Sorbitol. **Store:** See Class Effects.
Priorix PFS *(GSK)* A. HSEi(Child).
Price, not published by company.
Injection, live attenuated measles, mumps and rubella virus strains. White (slightly pink) powder. Neomycin, sorbitol. Clear colourless diluent. PFS. **Store:** See Class Effects.

Meningococcal Vaccine

ATC Code: J07AH. **Sport:** Permitted.
Driving: Caution.

Indications: Immunisation against disease caused by *Neisseria meningitidis*: Group B, from age 2 months *(Bexsero)*; group C, from age 2 months *(Meningitec, Menjugate)*; group A, C, W-135, Y from age 12 months *(Nimenrix)*; from age 2 years *(Menveo)*.

Dose: Adult: A single 0.5mL dose. *Admin*, deep IM, deltoid (older children, adolescents, adults), anterolateral thigh (infants); not for injection in gluteal area; avoid area near nerves and blood vessels; NOT for IV, intradermal or SC admin. May be given as booster if previously vaccinated with plain polysaccharide meningococcal vaccine *(Nimenrix)*, conjugated or unconjugated *(Menveo)*. Particular risk of exposure to Men A and received *Nimenrix* more than 1 year previously, consider a booster dose; a second dose of *Nimenrix* may be considered.

Bexsero, age 11 years and older, 2x 0.5mL doses at minimum 1-month interval; need for booster not established.

Elderly: Age 56-65 years, limited data; over 65 years, no data *(Menveo, Menjugate)*; over 50 years, no data *(Bexsero)*.

Child: *Meningitec, Menjugate*, primary series (age 2-12 months), 2x 0.5mL doses at 2-month interval; over 12 months*. *Nimenrix*, over 12 months*; under 12 months, not recommended. *Menveo*, age 2 years and older*. Booster recommended after completion of primary immunisation series in infants *(Meningitec, Menjugate)*; need for booster not established *(Nimenrix, Menveo)*.

Bexsero age 2-5 months 3x 0.5mL doses, first at 2 months, then at minimum 1-month intervals; booster of 1x 0.5mL between 12 and 15 months. Unvaccinated infants (6-11 months), children (12 months to 10 years), 2x 0.5mL doses at minimum 2-month interval; infants (6-11 months), booster of 1x 0.5mL in second year of life (minimum 2 months between primary and booster); children (12-23 months), booster of 1x 0.5mL (minimum 12-23 months between primary and booster); children (2-10 years), need for booster not established. Age 11 years and older*. *Admin*, see Adult above. *(as for Adult above).

CI: Hypersensitivity to diphtheria toxoid or non-toxic diphtheria toxin protein *(Meningitec, Menjugate, Menveo)*. Use in kanamycin-sensitive individuals not established *(Bexsero)*.

SP: Petechiae and/or purpura after vaccination, investigate. Symptoms of meningism (neck pain or

stiffness, photophobia), consider co-incidental meningitis. Not a substitute for routine diphtheria admin. *Bexsero*, hypersensitivity to natural latex rubber, kanamycin, caution. Prophylactic paracetamol reduces fever incidence/severity; does not affect immunogenicity.

Pregnancy, Lactation: Pregnancy should not preclude vaccination (exposure risk clearly defined). Lactation, if benefit outweighs risk; *Menveo* may be used.

ADR: *Very common*, loss of appetite/anorexia, irritability, drowsiness, headache, inj-site reaction, GI symptoms, diarrhoea (all brands); *Meningitec*, impaired sleep, vomiting; *Menjugate*, impaired sleep, nausea (adults); myalgia, arthralgia, malaise; *Nimenrix*, fever, fatigue; *Menveo*, nausea, vomiting, malaise, myalgia. *Bexsero*, unusual crying, vomiting, rash, fever, nausea, arthralgia.

Notes: See 12.1 Active Immunisation.

▼ **Bexsero Parenteral** *(GSK)* A.
Price, not published by company.
Injection, N. meningitidis Group B fusion protein. Adsorbed (aluminium hydroxide). White opalescent susp. **Store:** See Class Effects.
Meningitec Parenteral *(Nuron Biotech)* A. HSEi(Child).
Price, not published by company.
Injection, N. meningitidis Group C oligosaccharide, 10mcg conjugated *(Corynebacterium diphtheriae* protein). Adsorbed (aluminium phosphate). Homogenous white susp on shaking. **Store:** See Class Effects.
Menjugate Kit *(GSK)* A. HSEi(Child).
Price, not published by company.
Injection, N. meningitidis (meningococcal) group C 10mcg conjugated *(Corynebacterium diphtheriae* protein). Adsorbed (aluminium hydroxide). White powder; white opalescent solvent (Kit) or white opalescent sus (syringe, vial). **Store:** See Class Effects.
Menveo Vaccine *(GSK)* A.
Price, not published by company.
Injection, N. meningitidis (meningococcal) group A (10mcg), C, W-135, Y polysaccharide (5mcg) conjugated *(Corynebacterium diphtheriae* protein). White powder; clear colourless solvent. **Store:** See Class Effects.
Nimenrix Vaccine *(Pfizer)* A.
Price, not published by company.
Injection, N. meningitidis (meningococcal) group A, C, W-135, Y polysaccharide 5mcg conjugated to tetanus toxoid protein. White powder. Clear colourless solvent for soln. **Store:** See Class Effects.

Pneumococcal Vaccine (PCV)

ATC Code: J07AX. **Sport:** Permitted.
Driving: Unlikely to impair.

Indications: Immunisation against invasive disease (sepsis, meningitis, pneumonia, bacteraemia, acute otitis media) caused by *Streptococcus pneumoniae*, from age 2 years *(PNEUMOVAX 23)*, OR from age 6 weeks to 17 years and against invasive disease and pneumonia in adults from 18 years, elderly *(Prevenar 13)*.

Dose: Adult, Elderly: *PNEUMOVAX 23*, from age 2 years, 1x 0.5mL single dose, IM or SC. Revaccination, 1x 0.5mL dose; interval less than 3 years, increased adverse event risk. *Special dosing*, admin at least 2 weeks before elective splenectomy or initiation of chemo- or radiation therapy; re-admin minimum 3 months after completion if needed; avoid during treatment. HIV infection, vaccinate as soon as possible after diagnosis. Revaccination recommended if at increased risk; healthy adults/children should not be revaccinated routinely.

Prevenar 13, age 18 years and older (including elderly) or individuals with underlying conditions predisposing to pneumococcal disease (sickle cell disease, HIV infection), 1x single dose IM. Haematopoietic stem cell transplant (HSCT), primary 3-dose series with first dose at 3-6 months after HSCT, then at 1-month intervals; fourth (booster) dose recommended 6 months after third dose.

Child: *PNEUMOVAX 23*, see Adult above.

Prevenar 13, age 6 weeks to 6 months as well as preterm infants (under 37 weeks gestation), *3-dose* primary series, 3x 0.5mL doses at 2 months (can be given at 6 weeks) then at 1-month intervals; booster (fourth dose) between

12.1 Active Immunisation

11-15 months. This schedule is also used for pre-term infants (below 37 weeks gestation). Alternatively, *2-dose* primary series, 1x 0.5mL dose at 2 months and second 0.5mL dose 2 months later; booster (third dose) between 11-15 months.

Unvaccinated, age 7-11 months, 2x 0.5mL doses at 1-month intervals; third dose in second year of life; children aged 12-23 months, 2x 0.5mL doses at 2-month intervals; children and adolescents, age 2-17 years, one single 0.5mL dose. *Previous 7-valent vaccination,* may switch to 13-valent at any time in schedule; age 12-59 months completely immunised with 7-valent, or children and adolescents age 5-17 years who have received 1 or more doses of 7-valent, should receive 1 dose (0.5mL) of 13-valent at least 8 weeks after final 7-valent dose IM to elicit immune response to the additional 6 serotypes.

CI: Diphtheria toxoid hypersensitivity.

Interactions: Effect of Other Drugs on Pneumococcal Vaccine (PCV). *Immune response possibly reduced with co-admin (Prevenar)*: Paracetamol (clinical significance unknown).

SP: Pneumococcal polysaccharide vaccine SPMSD and *Zostavax* are not for co-admin (reduced *Zostavax* immunogenicity); separate by at least 4 weeks. Not effective for prevention (acute otitis media, sinusitis, other common upper RTIs). Not a substitute for routine diphtheria immunisation. *Prevenar,* prophylactic antipyretic medication recommended (children with seizure disorders, prior history of febrile seizures, all children receiving simultaneous whole cell pertussis vaccines). Thrombocytopenia, apnoea risk in premature infants, see Notes below.

Pregnancy, Lactation: Pregnancy, avoid. Lactation, unknown if excreted in human milk.

ADR: *Very common,* fever, injection-site reactions; *Prevenar 13, most common,* decreased appetite, irritability, somnolence, increased and/or decreased sleep (age 6 weeks to 5 years).

Notes: See 12.1 Active Immunisation.
PNEUMOVAX 23 *(MSD)* A. HSEi(Adult).
Price, not published by company.
Injection, pneumococcal polysaccharide vaccine. 25mcg/0.5mL of each of 23 serotypes. Clear colourless soln. **Store:** See Class Effects.
Prevenar 13 Vaccine *(Pfizer)* A. HSEi(Child).
Price, not published by company.
Injection, pneumococcal polysaccharide vaccine (13 serotypes). Conjugated to carrier protein, adsorbed onto aluminium phosphate. Homogenous white susp. *Essentially sodium-free.* **Store:** See Class Effects.

Rabies Vaccine

ATC Code: J07BG01. **Sport:** Permitted.
Driving: No adverse effects reported.
Indications: Prophylactic immunisation against rabies. Treatment, following suspected rabies contact.

Dose: Adult, Elderly: PROPHYLAXIS, 3x 1mL injection at schedule 0, 7, 28 days; third dose can be given at day 21 earliest. If at regular and continuing risk, admin a single reinforcing dose 1 year after primary course; admin further doses at 3-5 year intervals.

TREATMENT, adequate prophylaxis, 2 further boosters, schedule day 0 and on day 3; no, or inadequate prophylaxis, first injection to be given as soon as possible after suspected contact (day 0), followed by 5 further doses (days 3, 7, 14, 30); the earliest the fifth dose can be given is day 28. Use of Human Rabies Immunoglobulin on day 0 should be considered only if no adequate prophylaxis. IM deltoid.

Child: As for Adult, Elderly above.

Interactions: Effect of Other Drugs on Rabies Vaccine: *Antibody production altered, vaccine failure*: Corticosteroids, immunosuppressives.

SP: Hypersensitivity to neomycin and betapropiolactone.

Very premature infants, apnoea risk, see Notes below. If rabies immunoglobulin is also indicated, admin at a different anatomical site to the vaccination.

Pregnancy, Lactation: Admin based on clinical decision relating to risk of rabies development; substantial risk of exposure to rabies, pre-exposure prophylaxis may also be indicated during pregnancy.

ADR: *Very common,* lymphadenopathy, headache, nausea, diarrhoea, myalgia, arthralgia, injection-site reactions, malaise, chills. Apnoea in premature infants, see SP above.

Notes: See 12.1 Active Immunisation.
Rabies Vaccine BP *(SanofiPasteur)* A.
Price, not published by company.
Injection, inactivated rabies virus not less than 2.5 IU/1mL. Strain PM/WI 38 1503-3M. Powder; solvent for susp. *Human albumin.*
Store: See Class Effects.

Rotavirus Vaccine

ATC Code: J07BH01. **Sport:** Permitted.
Driving: Not applicable.
Indications: Prevention, gastro-enteritis in infants (age 6-24 weeks), due to rotavirus infection.

Dose: Adult, Elderly: Not for Adult use.

Child: Including preterm infants born at least 27 weeks gestational age, admin first dose from age 6 weeks; second dose preferably before 16 weeks but must be before 24 weeks; minimum 4-week interval between doses. Not for use in children over age 24 weeks. Oral only; NOT for injection.

CI: Intussusception, Severe Combined Immunodeficiency (SCID) disorder. Diarrhoea, vomiting, postpone.

Interactions: Effect of Other Drugs on Rotavirus Vaccine: *Immune response possibly reduced with co-admin*: Oral polio vaccine.

SP: GI illness, growth retardation, use with caution. Follow up symptoms indicative of intussusception (severe abdominal pain, persistent vomiting, bloody stools, abdominal bloating, high fever), advise parents/carers to promptly report. Caution, immunodeficient close contacts (malignancies, immunosuppressive therapy). Contacts with recent vaccinees, observe good personal hygiene (hand washing). See ADR below.

Pregnancy, Lactation: Not for adult use. Breastfeeding may continue during vaccination schedule.

ADR: *Common,* diarrhoea, irritability. *Post-marketing,* apnoea in very premature infants (28 weeks gestation or under), haematochezia, intussusception, gastroenteritis (with vaccine viral shedding in infants with SCID). See SP above.

Notes: See 12.1 Active Immunisation.
Rotarix Oral Susp (Oral Applicator) *(GSK)* A.
Price, not published by company.
Oral susp in pre-filled oral applicator, human rotavirus RIX4414 strain (live attenuated). Clear colourless liquid in pre-filled oral applicator. Sucrose, sorbitol. **Store:** See Class Effects; original pack to protect (light).

Tuberculosis Vaccine

ATC Code: J07AN01. **Sport:** Permitted.
Driving: Unlikely to impair.
Indications: Immunisation against tuberculosis (TB).

Dose: Adult, Elderly: 0.1mL by intradermal injection approx. one third down the upper arm.

Child: Under 12 months, 0.05mL injected intradermally; 12 months and over as for Adult, Elderly above.

CI: Corticosteroid, immunosuppressives (including radiotherapy) treatment, malignancies (lymphoma, leukaemia, Hodgkin's disease, other tumours of reticulo-endothelial system), primary or secondary immunodeficiency, HIV-infected (including infants born to HIV infected mothers); effect of BCG may be exaggerated and a generalised BCG-infection is possible. Patients receiving anti-TB drugs.

SP: Increased lymphadenitis, abscess formation risk (injection too deep); may be given with inactivated live vaccines. Advisable not to give further vaccination in arm used for BCG for 3 months due to regional lymphadenitis risk.

Pregnancy, Lactation: Pregnancy, lactation, not recommended; high risk areas, if benefit outweighs risk.

ADR: Regional lymph node enlargement, ulceration with discharging ulcer at injection site. Disseminated BCG complications, osteitis, osteomyelitis; allergic reactions (anaphylaxis).

Notes: See 12.1 Active Immunisation.

BCG Vaccine SSI *(SSI)* A. HSEi(Used).
Price, not published by company.
Injection, Mycobacterium bovis BCG (Bacillus Calmette-Guerin), Danish strain 1331, live attenuated 1 dose (0.1mL or 0.05mL). White crystalline powder; colourless soln. **Store:** See Class Effects.

Typhoid Vaccine

ATC Code: J07AP. **Sport:** Permitted.
Driving: Caution.

Indications: Immunisation against typhoid fever.

Dose: Adult, Elderly: Age 2 years and older, single dose of 0.5mL admin at least 2 weeks prior to risk of typhoid exposure; remaining at risk, revaccinated with single dose at interval max. 3 years. IM injection only *(Typherix)*; IM or deep SC *(Typhim Vi)*; not for intravascular (IV) use.

Child: Under 2 years, response may be sub-optimal; over 2 years, as for Adult above.

SP: Caution, thrombocytopenia or bleeding disorders *(Typherix)*. Does not protect against paratyphoid.

Pregnancy, Lactation: Pregnancy and lactation, only when there is a high risk of infection.

ADR: General aches, malaise, nausea, itching. Following second dose, increased incidence of redness, soreness.

Notes: See 12.1 Active Immunisation.

Typherix Parenteral *(GSK)* A.
Price, not published by company.
Injection, Vi polysaccharide of Salmonella typhi 25mcg/0.5mL dose. Clear isotonic colourless soln in PFS. *Formaldehyde traces.* **Store:** See Class Effects.

Typhim Vi *(SanofiPasteur)* A.
Price, not published by company.
Injection, Vi polysaccharide of Salmonella typhi 25mcg per 0.5mL dose. Clear colourless soln. **Store:** See Class Effects.

Typhoid, Hepatitis A Vaccine

ATC Code: J07BC20. **Sport:** Permitted.
Driving: Caution.

Indications: Immunisation against hepatitis A virus infection and typhoid fever.

Dose: Adult, Elderly: Single 1mL dose at least 2 weeks prior to exposure risk. Long-term protection against hepatitis A and continued protection against typhoid, see manufacturers Full Prescribing Information. For deltoid IM admin; not for gluteal or intravascular, SC or intradermal use (thrombocytopenia or bleeding disorders, SC).

Child: Under 15 years *(Hepatyrix)*, no safety/efficacy data; under 16 years *(ViATIM)*, not recommended.

CI: Hypersensitivity to neomycin.

Pregnancy, Lactation: If benefit outweighs risk.

ADR: Malaise, general aches, asthenia, nausea, diarrhoea, itching, pruritus, rash, erythema, dizziness, arthralgia, myalgia.

Notes: See 12.1 Active Immunisation.

Hepatyrix Parenteral *(GSK)* A.
Price, not published by company.
Injection, inactivated Hepatitis A virus (HM175 strain) 1440 ELISA units Vi polysaccharide of Salmonella typhi (Ty2 strain) 25mcg. Adsorbed (aluminium hydroxide). Propagated on MRC-5 human diploid cells. Slightly opaque white susp. **Store:** See Class Effects.

ViATIM Parenteral *(SanofiPasteur)* A.
Price, not published by company.
Injection, Hepatitis A virus, GBM strain (inactivated) 160 U*, Salmonella typhi (Ty2 strain) capsular Vi polysaccharide 25mcg. *In-house reference. Produced in human diploid MRC-5 cells; adsorbed (aluminium hydroxide). Susp (cloudy white); soln (clear colourless). **Store:** See Class Effects.

Varicella-Zoster Vaccine

ATC Code: J07BK. **Sport:** Permitted.
Driving: Unlikely to impair.

Indications: *VARIVAX*, primary prevention, varicella age 12 months and older. Susceptible individuals exposed to varicella (vaccination within 3 days of exposure may prevent clinically apparent infection or modify infection course; limited data indicates regarding vaccination up to 5 days after exposure). *ZOSTAVAX*, prevention of herpes zoster (shingles) and herpes-related post-herpetic neuralgia (PHN) (age 50 years and older).

Dose: Adult, Elderly: *VARIVAX**, age 13 years and over, admin 2x 0.5mL doses 4-8 weeks apart; if interval exceeds 8 weeks, admin as soon as possible. SC or IM deltoid or higher anterolateral thigh (younger children). *Elderly*, over 65 years in seronegative persons, no data.
ZOSTAVAX*, age 50 years and older, single 0.65mL dose by SC injection, preferably deltoid. The need for a booster dose is not known. *Admin by SC route in presence of thrombocytopenia or coagulation disorder. NOT for intravascular injection.

Child: *VARIVAX*, from age 9 months, admin 2 doses to ensure optimal protection against varicella. If initiated between age 9-12 months, admin second dose after minimum 3-month interval; initiation from 12 months to 12 years, admin second dose 1 month after first. Age 12 months to 12 years with asymptomatic HIV infection should receive 2 doses 12 weeks apart. Age 13 years and older, as for Adult above.
ZOSTAVAX, not for use in children/adolescents.

CI: Hypersensitivity to neomycin or gelatin. Blood dyscrasias, leukaemia, lymphoma, other malignant neoplasms affecting the haemic and lymphatic systems. Immunosuppressive therapy including corticosteroids, severe humoral or cellular (primary or acquired) immunodeficiency. Family history of congenital or hereditary immunodeficiency. Active untreated TB.

Interactions: Effect of Other Drugs on Varicella Vaccine: *VARIVAX: If not admin at same time, leave 1-month dosing interval:* Other live vaccines (measles, mumps, rubella), varicella zoster virus antibody-containing blood products. *Vaccine failure risk, delay for 5 months:* Following blood or plasma transfusion, normal human immune globulin or varicella zoster immune globulin (VZIg) (due to passively acquired antibodies). *Avoid use:* Salicylates (Reye's syndrome risk for up to 6 weeks post vaccination).
ZOSTAVAX: Co-admin not recommended: 23-valent pneumococcal polysaccharide vaccine (reduced immunogenicity).

SP: Hypersensitivity reactions to active principle, excipients, trace residues. *VARIVAX*, vaccination may be considered with selected immune deficiencies if benefit outweighs risk (asymptomatic HIV, IgG deficiency, congenital neutropenia, chronic granulomatous disease, complement deficiency). Avoid, salicylate use for 6 weeks after vaccination; close contact with susceptible high-risk individuals (immunocompromised, pregnant women/newborns of mother without positive chickenpox history). *ZOSTAVAX*, not indicated for treatment of zoster or PHN. Safety/efficacy not established (HIV infected, with or without immunosuppression).

Pregnancy, Lactation: Do not vaccinate pregnant women with *VARIVAX*; avoid pregnancy for 1 month following vaccination; advise women intending to become pregnant to delay. Lactation, generally not recommended. *ZOSTAVAX*, not intended for use in women of childbearing potential.

337

12.2 Immunoglobulins

ADR: *Very common,* fever *(VARIVAX);* erythema, pain/tenderness, swelling, pruritus *(ZOSTAVAX).*

Notes: See 12.1 Active Immunisation.

VARIVAX Parenteral *(MSD)* A.
Price, not published by company.
Injection, live attenuated varicella virus. Each dose (0.5mL) contains varicella virus (Oka/Merck strain) 1350 PFU (plaque-forming units). White (off-white) powder. Solvent for susp; reconstituted to clear colourless (pale-yellow) liquid. **Store:** See Class Effects.

ZOSTAVAX Parenteral *(MSD)* A.
Price, not published by company.
Injection, live attenuated varicella-zoster virus. Each dose (0.65mL) contains varicella-zoster virus (Oka/Merck strain) 19400 PFU (plaque-forming units). White (off-white) compact crystalline plug; clear colourless solvent in PFS. *Neomycin trace.* **Store:** See Class Effects.

Yellow Fever Vaccine

ATC Code: J07BL. **Sport:** Permitted.
Driving: Unlikely to impair.

Indications: Immunisation against yellow fever required for persons travelling within or living in endemic areas, travellers requiring an International Certificate of Vaccination for entry into a country, laboratory workers.

Dose: Adult: Admin a single dose of 0.5mL of reconstituted vaccine at least 10 days before entering endemic area as protective immunity may not be achieved until at least this time has elapsed. For SC admin; IM (deltoid) may be used with applicable official recommendations; NOT for intravascular use. Duration of protection following a single dose is expected to be at least 10 years and may be life-long.

Elderly: Age 60 years and over, higher risk of yellow fever vaccine-associated severe and potentially fatal disease; use only if unavoidable risk of acquiring yellow fever.

Child: Age 9 months and older, as for Adult above. Age 6-9 months, vaccination against yellow fever is not recommended except in specific circumstances and in accordance with official recommendations; dose is the same as for children 9 months and over. Under 6 months, contraindicated. For SC admin. IM can be used, see Adult above; under 12 months (anterolateral aspect of thigh); 12-35 months (anterolateral aspect of thigh or deltoid if muscle mass is adequate); from 36 months onwards, as for Adult above.

CI: Hypersensitivity to egg, chicken protein; anaphylaxis following previous yellow fever vaccine. Immunosuppression (congenital, idiopathic, systemic steroids, radio- or cytotoxic therapy). Thymus dysfunction (including myasthenia gravis, thymoma, thymectomy), HIV infection. Under 6 months. Moderate or severe febrile illness or acute illness.

Interactions: Effect of Other Drugs on Yellow Fever Vaccine: *Co-admin not recommended, leave 3-month dosing interval:* Injectable cholera vaccine, whole cell paratyphoid vaccine.

SP: Neurotropic, viscerotropic disease. Not for IM admin (bleeding disorders, anticoagulant treatment), use SC route. Can induce false positive results with laboratory and/or diagnostic tests for other flavivirus related diseases (dengue, Japanese encephalitis). NOTE: For compliance with vaccine regulations and for official recognition, vaccine must be admin at an approved WHO vaccination centre and registered on an International Certificate of Vaccination. The validity period of this certificate, established according to International Health Regulations recommendations, starts 10 days after primary vaccination and immediately after re-vaccination.

Pregnancy, Lactation: Pregnancy, only if clearly needed and if benefit outweighs risk. Lactation, not recommended unless cannot be avoided.

ADR: Summary, *most frequent,* headache, asthenia, injection site pain, myalgia; in toddlers, irritability, crying,

appetite loss. Severe hypersensitivity or anaphylactic reactions, neurotropic or viscerotropic disease.

Notes: See 12.1 Active Immunisation.

STAMARIL Parenteral *(SanofiPasteur)* A.
Price, not published by company.
Injection, Yellow fever virus 17 D-204 strain (live, attenuated) not less than 1000 IU/dose (0.5mL). Beige (orange beige) powder and solvent for susp. Produced in pathogen-free chick embryos. **Store:** See Class Effects.

12.2 - Immunoglobulins

Class Effects

Indications: Immunoglobulins are used for passive immunity providing immediate protection against infectious diseases.

CI: Hypersensitivity to any member of the class.

Interactions: Effect of Immunoglobulins on Other Drugs: Live vaccines: *Co-admin not recommended (reduced immune response).*

SP: See manufacturers Full Prescribing Information.

12.2.1 - Normal

In This Chapter: *HNIg.*

Class Effects

CI: Hypersensitivity to any member of the class.

SP: True hypersensitivity reactions rare; can occur with anti-IgA antibodies (caution). HNIg can cause a fall in blood pressure with anaphylactic reaction, even if previous HNIg was tolerated. High risk for allergic reactions, admin only with supportive care available. Inform patients of early signs of anaphylaxis or hypersensitivity. Consider pre-medication. Adverse reactions occur more frequently with high infusion rate; may occur with HNIg for first time or when HNIg product is switched; infuse slowly, monitor. Arterial and venous thromboembolic events (MI, stroke, DVT, pulmonary embolism) with immunoglobulin use, caution with pre-existing risk factors. Ensure adequate hydration. Monitor for haemolysis. Aseptic meningitis with IV and SC immunoglobulins, severe renal failure (reported).

Notes: See 12.2 Immunoglobulins.

Human Normal Ig (HNIg)

ATC Code: J06BA. **Sport:** Permitted.
Driving: Adverse reactions may impair.

Indications: Replacement therapy, primary immunodeficiency syndromes (PID); hypogammaglobulinaemia, agammaglobulinaemia, Wiskott Aldrich syndrome, common variable and severe combined immunodeficiencies; congenital AIDS. Immunomodulation in primary immune thrombocytopenia (ITP) (high bleeding risk), Guillain-Barre syndrome, Kawasaki disease, chronic inflammatory demyelinating polyneuropathy (CIDP), allogeneic bone marrow transplantation.

Dose: Adult, Elderly: *Gammagard, PID,* to achieve trough level of 5-6g/L, admin 0.4-0.8g/kg followed by minimum 0.2g/kg every 3-4 weeks. PID (myeloma or CLL with severe secondary hypogammaglobulinaemia, children with AIDS), 0.2-0.4g/kg every 3-4 weeks. *ITP,* acute episode, 0.8-1g/kg (day 1); repeat on day 3 if needed OR 0.4g/kg/day for 2-5 days; can be repeated. *Kawasaki disease,* 1.6-2g/kg (divided doses) over 2-5 days OR 2g/kg as single dose (with acetylsalicylic acid). *Bone marrow transplant,* 0.2-0.4g/kg every 3-4 weeks (maintain 5g/L trough level). *Guillain-Barre syndrome,* 0.4g/kg/day for 5 days; limited experience in children. *Admin,* IV; individual rate based on tolerability. *Hizentra, PID,* individualise dose to achieve sustained IgG. Loading, 0.2-0.5g/kg divided over several days. Maintenance, at repeated intervals to reach cumulative monthly dose 0.4-0.8g/kg. *Admin,* SC only (abdomen, thigh, upper arm, lateral hip). Doses above 25mL, use multiple sites (up to 4 sites; at least 5cm apart). Infusion rate, initial max. 15mL/hour/site; if tolerated increase gradually to 25mL/hour/site. Not for intravascular injection.

Privigen, replacement, PID, to achieve trough level of 5-6g/L, admin 0.4-0.8g/kg once, then minimum 0.2g/kg every 3-4 weeks. *Hypogammaglobulinaemia*, 0.2-0.4g/kg every 3-4 weeks.

Immunomodulation, ITP, 0.8-1g/kg (day 1); can repeat within 3 days OR 0.4g/kg/day (2-5 days). *Guillain-Barre syndrome*, 0.4g/kg/day over 5 days. *Kawasaki disease*, 1.6-2g/kg (divided doses) over 2-5 days OR 2g/kg as a single dose (with acetylsalicylic acid). *CIDP*, initially 2g/kg divided over 2-5 days then maintenance of 1g/kg over 1-2 days every 3 weeks. *Admin*, IV; initial infusion rate 0.3mL/kg/hour for approx. 30 minutes; if tolerated, gradually increase to max. 4.8mL/kg/hour. In PID, if latter rate is tolerated, may be further increased to max. 7.2mL/kg/hour.

Child: As for Adult above.

CI: Hyperprolinaemia (type I or II) *(Hizentra)*. Patients with IgA antibodies *(Gammagard, Privigen)* or hyperprolinaemia *(Privigen)*.

Interactions: Effect of HNIg on Other Drugs: Live attenuated vaccines (measles, rubella, mumps, varicella). *Efficacy may be impaired.*

SP: IV HNIg admin requires (monitoring of urine output, serum creatinine); avoid loop diuretic co-admin. Aseptic meningitis syndrome reported with IV Ig treatment (correlation with higher doses; higher incidence in women). Diabetics, note glucose in diluent. *Hizentra*, caution, anti-IgA antibodies. *Gammagard*, caution fluid overload. Infusion-related reactions.

Pregnancy, Lactation: Caution.

ADR: Summary, *occasionally*, chills, headache, dizziness, fever, vomiting, allergic reactions, nausea, arthralgia, low BP, moderate low back pain.

Notes: See Immunoglobulins 12.2.1 Normal.

GAMMAGARD S/D Parenteral *(Baxalta)* A.
Price, not published by company.
Infusion, human normal Ig 100mg/mL (10g). Powder and solvent for soln. **Store:** Below 25 deg C; do not freeze.
Hizentra Parenteral *(CSL Behring)* A.
Price, not published by company.
Subcutaneous injection, human normal Ig 200mg/mL. Clear (pale-yellow or light-brown).
Privigen Parenteral *(CSL Behring)* B.
Price, not published by company.
Infusion, human normal Ig 100mg/mL. Clear (slightly opalescent) colourless (pale-yellow) isotonic soln.

Human Normal Ig (HNIg), recombinant human hyaluronidase (rHuPH20)

ATC Code: J06BA. **Sport:** Permitted.
Driving: Adverse reactions may impair.

Indications: Replacement therapy (adults, children 0-18 years) in primary immunodeficiency syndromes; hypogammaglobulinaemia and recurrent bacterial infections in CLL (antibiotics failed or contraindicated) or multiple myeloma; hypogammaglobulinaemia pre- and post- allogeneic haematopoietic stem cell transplant.

Dose: Adult, Elderly: *Replacement therapy, immunoglobulin naïve*, to achieve trough level of 6g/L, admin 0.4-0.8g/kg bodyweight per month; dose interval to achieve steady state levels 2-4 weeks. To reduce infection rate, aim for trough levels above 6g/L; *previous IV treatment*, admin at same (dose, frequency); if previously on a 3-week regimen, increase to 4-week interval by admin of same weekly equivalents; *previous SC treatment*, use same dose; adjust to 3-week or 4-week intervals. Admin first infusion 1 week after last treatment of previous immunoglobulin.

Admin, SC route only. NOT for IV or IM admin. Comprised of 2 vials; do not mix the components. Admin sequentially through same needle; first recombinant hyaluronidase then immunoglobulin. Admin dose in 1 or 2 sites up to every 4 weeks (middle to upper abdomen, thighs). Infusion site leakage can occur with SC admin; consider using longer needles and/or more than 1 infusion site.

Child: Age 0-18 years, as for Adult based on body weight and adjusted to clinical outcome.

CI: Hypersensitivity to human immunoglobulins especially with IgA antibodies.

SP: Accidental admin into a blood vessel may result in shock. Avoid potential complications (slow initial infusion, monitor during and for first hour after infusion, home admin always in presence of another responsible person). Adverse reaction, slow infusion or discontinue; shock, discontinue immediately and treat (applies to both components). Patients to report chronic inflammation, nodules or inflammation at infusion site lasting more than a few days.

Pregnancy, Lactation: Caution.

ADR: Summary, *most frequent*, headache, fatigue, pyrexia, local reactions. Nature, frequency, seriousness, reversibility similar for adults and paediatrics.

Notes: See Immunoglobulins 12.2.1 Normal.
▼ **HyQvia Parenteral** *(Baxalta)* A.
Price, not published by company.
Subcutaneous infusion, human normal Ig 100mg/mL and recombinant human hyaluronidase. Clear (slightly opalescent) colourless (pale-yellow) soln (HNIg); clear colourless soln (hyaluronidase). *Sodium 4.03mg/mL (hyaluronidase)*. **Store:** Refrigerate; do not freeze.

12.2.2 - Specific

In This Chapter: *HBIg, HTIg.*

Class Effects

Notes: See 12.2 Immunoglobulins.

Hepatitis B Ig

ATC Code: J06BB04. **Sport:** Permitted.
Driving: Adverse reactions may impair.

Indications: Prevention, hepatitis B re-infection after liver transplant, hepatitis B induced liver failure. Immunoprophylaxis, accidental post-exposure (non-immunised subjects), haemodialysis patients (until vaccination effective), newborns (HBsAg carrier mother), patients without immune response after vaccination (continuous hepatitis B infection risk).

Dose: Adult, Elderly: Prophylaxis, *accidental post-exposure*, 500 IU as soon as possible preferably within 24-72 hours; *haemodialysed*, 8-12 IU/kg with max. 500 IU every 2 months*; *newborn*, at birth or as soon as possible after, 30-100 IU/kg; repeat*. *No immune response following vaccination*, consider 500 IU (adults) and 8 IU/kg (children) every 2 months. Admin by IV infusion; initial rate 0.1mL/kg/hour for 10 minutes; if tolerated increase slowly to 1mL/kg/hour. Newborns, infusion rate of 2mL in-between 5-15 minutes has been well tolerated. *(until seroconversion following vaccination).

Child: See Adult above.

SP: Caution, thromboembolic risk factors. Monitor for serum anti-HB antibodies. Adverse reactions more frequent (high infusion rate, hypo- or agammaglobinaemia with/without IgA deficiency).

Pregnancy, Lactation: Caution.

ADR: Infusion-related events. See SP above.

Notes: See Immunoglobulins 12.2.2 Specific.
Hepatect CP Parenteral 50 IU *(Biotest)* A.
Price, not published by company.
Infusion, HBIg 50 IU/mL Clear slightly opalescent soln.

12.2.3 Anti-D

Tetanus Ig

ATC Code: J06BB02. **Sport:** Permitted.
Driving: No effects observed.

Indications: Post-exposure prophylaxis, immediate after tetanus prone injuries, patients (not adequately vaccinated, immunisation status not known, severe deficiency in antibody production). Therapy, clinically manifest tetanus (always admin with an active tetanus vaccination unless contraindicated or confirmation of adequate vaccination).

Dose: Adult, Elderly: PROPHYLAXIS, 250 IU unless extremely high risk; increase to 500 IU with infected wounds (surgical treatment not achievable in 24 hours), deep or contaminated wounds or foreign body injury (bites, stings, shots), burns, tissue necrosis, septicaemic abortion, adults weighing more than average. Extensive burns, admin a second injection of 250 IU after the exudative phase of burn has subsided. May be given SC in presence of severe coagulation disorder where IM contraindicated.
TREATMENT, usually 3000-6000 IU in combination with other clinical procedures. *Admin*, IM. In case of simultaneous vaccination, immunoglobulin and vaccine should be admin at contralateral sites of body. NOT for intravascular injection (shock risk).

Child: As for Adult above.

SP: *Tetagam P* contains small quantity of IgA. Observe patient for 20 minutes after admin.

Pregnancy, Lactation: No harmful effects on pregnancy, foetus or neonate anticipated.

ADR: Allergic reactions, chills, fever, headache, malaise, nausea, vomiting, arthralgia, moderate back pain, cardiovascular reactions (intravascular injection), local pain, tenderness, swelling.

Notes: See Immunoglobulins 12.2.2 Specific.

Tetagam P Parenteral *(CSL Behring)* A.
Price, 250 IU/mL (1mL) not published by company.
Injection, antibodies to tetanus toxin 250 IU/mL. Clear (pale-yellow to light-brown) soln.

12.2.3 - Anti-D

In This Chapter: *Anti-D Ig.*

Anti-D Ig

ATC Code: J06BB01. **Sport:** Permitted.
Driving: Not applicable.

Indications: Prevention of Rh(D) immunisation in Rh(D) negative women. Treatment, Rh(D) negative persons after incompatible transfusions of Rh(D) positive blood.

Dose: Adult, Elderly: Base dose on level of exposure. 0.5mL of packed Rh(D) positive RBCs or 1mL or Rh(D) positive blood is neutralised by approx. 10mcg (50 IU) of anti-D immunoglobulin. IV by slow injection.

CI: Hypersensitivity to human immunoglobulins.

Rhophylac *(CSL Behring)* A.
Price, not published by company.
Injection, human anti-D Ig 1500 IU (300mcg) per PFS. Clear or slightly opalescent colourless (pale-yellow) soln.

12.2.4 - Interferons

In This Chapter: *Interferon gamma.*

Interferon Gamma 1-b

ATC Code: L03AB03. **Sport:** Permitted.
Driving: May have minor or moderate influence; may be enhanced by alcohol.

Indications: Reduction of frequency of serious infections in chronic granulomatous disease (CGD); severe, malignant osteopetrosis.

Dose: Adult, Elderly: 50mcg/m2 BSA (BSA above 0.5m2) and 1.5mcg/kg/dose (BSA below or equal to 0.5m2) 3-

times weekly; severe reactions, reduce dose by 50%. SC admin, preferably evening, deltoid or anterior thigh.

Renal Impairment: Severe, caution; possibility of accumulation.

Hepatic Impairment: As for Renal above.

Interactions: Effect of Other Drugs on Interferon Gamma: *Co-admin avoid (amplified immune response):* Other heterologous serum proteins or immunologicals (vaccines). *Clearance altered:* Other nephro- or hepatotoxic drugs. *Effect on acute cellular effects (effect not known):* Anti-inflammatories, NSAIDs, theophylline, immunosuppressives, cytostatics. *Increased toxicity:* Neuro- and/or haemotoxic drugs, myelosuppressives, cardiotoxic drugs.

Effect of Interferon Gamma on Other Drugs: Drugs metabolised by CYP450: *Half-life prolonged.*

SP: Does not exclude need for additional antimicrobial cover in CGD. Exacerbation of cardiac conditions at doses 250mcg/m2/day or higher. Seizures and/or compromised CNS function, caution. AST and/or ALT elevation. Neutropenia and thrombocytopenia, reversible (severe; dose-related). Before and during treatment, monitor haematology (FBC, differential and platelet counts, blood chemistry including renal and LFTs, urinalysis). Interferon gamma-1b may lead to development of antibodies.

Pregnancy, Lactation: Pregnancy, if benefit outweighs risk. Lactation, not recommended.

ADR: *Very common,* nausea, vomiting, diarrhoea, increased hepatic enzymes, rash, abdominal pain, fever, headache, chills, fatigue, injection site pain.

Immukin Parenteral *(Boehringer)* A. HT.
Price, (6) €447.36.
Injection, recombinant human interferon gamma-1b 0.1mg/0.5mL vial. Clear colourless soln. *Natural rubber stopper.*

12.3 - Diagnostic Testing

In This Chapter: *Tuberculin.*

Tuberculin

ATC Code: V04CF01. **Sport:** Permitted.
Driving: Unlikely to impair.

Indications: Tuberculin skin testing (diagnostic use only).

Dose: Adult, Elderly: *Mantoux test,* intradermal injection of 0.1mL tuberculin soln. For medical diagnosis, use 2 T. U. (tuberculin units); if infiltration of injection site is less than 6mm diameter measured at 48-72 hours after injection, repeat with 10 T. U. Admin in middle third of dorsal forearm.
Reaction, white papule 10mm diameter; will remain for about 10 minutes. Read 48-72 hours after injection; positive reaction (flat slightly swollen rough or uneven infiltration; more or less defined area of erythema); must be minimum 6mm diameter (immunosuppressed, induration may be less).

CI: Hypersensitivity to any member of the class.

Interactions: Effect of Other Drugs on Tuberculin: *Sensitivity/reactivity may be reduced:* Viral infection, cancer, sarcoidosis, after vaccination with live virus vaccine, undernourishment, immunosuppressive treatments. *False positive:* Previous BCG vaccination, earlier infection with non-tuberculous mycobacterium which did not cause disease. *Induration less than 6mm:* Immune system severely depressed by TB infection; active TB may be present.

SP: Extreme caution, if previous severe skin reaction to RT23 or a sensitising PPD product.

ADR: See Notes below.

Tuberculin PPD *(SSI)* A. HSEi(Used).
Price, not published by company.
Intradermal injection, tuberculin PPD TR23 2 T.U. (0.4mcg)/0.1mL or 10 T.U. (2mcg)/mL. Soln.

340

Oncology, Immunosuppression

Class Effects

Topical, imiquimod is indicated for treatment of small superficial basal cell carcinomas and actinic keratosis, see Notes below.

Notes: See 10.6 Imiquimod and 10.1.6 Photodamage, Actinic Keratosis.

13.1 - Cytotoxic Drugs

Class Effects

General Principles: Drugs used in treating malignancy and/or conditions requiring immunosuppression are used in specialised units; information provided is less detailed; prescribers should always consult the manufacturers Full Prescribing Information, Scientific Literature and/or local hospital protocols.

CI: Hypersensitivity to any member of the class. See Interactions below.

Interactions: Effect of Other Drugs on Cytotoxics: *Use contraindicated*: Yellow fever vaccine. *Use not recommended*: Live vaccines (measles, mumps, rubella, oral polio, BCG, varicella, typhoid).

Effect of Cytotoxics on Other Drugs: Oral anticoagulants: Monitor INR.

SP: *Admin*, under direction of specialist oncology service with facilities for regular monitoring (biochemistry, haematology) during and after treatment. Individualise dose and treatment duration based on (patient requirement, clinical response, protocol for malignancy type). Monitor haematological parameters for immunosuppression (common in cancer patients either due to disease or treatment; may predispose to opportunistic infections). For full information regarding dose adjustments for toxicity, missed doses, and dosing when used in combination, always consult the manufacturers Full Prescribing Information.

Pregnancy, Lactation: All cytotoxics are potentially teratogenic. *Pregnancy*, use only if considered absolutely essential. Women of childbearing potential and in some cases, males intending to father a child, to ensure adequate contraception during treatment. For contraception duration after treatment, see individual drugs. *Lactation*, generally not recommended due to contraindicated with certain drugs; stop drug or stop breastfeeding.

ADR: Alopecia, common occurring to varying degrees. Immune system depression, opportunistic infection risk (bacterial, fungal, viral). Allergic reactions, anaphylaxis, anaphylactoid. *GI disorders* (diarrhoea, constipation, abdominal pain; mucositis, oral ulceration, stomatitis) may be severe. Nausea, vomiting most common with systemic cytotoxics (may be severe); anti-emetics may alleviate. Anorexia may be severe. Tumour Lysis Syndrome (TLS) due to rapid cell destruction (hyperuricaemia, acute renal

Cytotoxic Drugs   13.1

failure); consider prophylactic allopurinol. Systemic Inflammatory Response Syndrome, capillary leak syndrome and/or organ dysfunction. *Haematological disorders* e.g. dose-related bone marrow depression, leucopenia, neutropenia, thrombocytopenia, pancytopenia, platelet disturbances, anaemia; monitor blood counts regularly; haematological profile may differ for different molecules; myelosuppression may be delayed. Myelodysplastic Syndrome (MDS); antineoplastics, notably alkylating agents, associated with MDS risk, secondary malignancies (leukaemia). *Extravasation* may occur; if irritant, avoid severe soft tissue damage may occur (necrosis). Injection-site reactions are common.

Notes: See manufacturers Full Prescribing Information.

13.1.1 - Alkylating Agents

In This Chapter: *Bendamustine, busulfan, chlorambucil, cyclophosphamide, ifosfamide, melphalan, temozolomide.*

Class Effects

CI: Use in children unless otherwise specified.

SP: Significant increase in acute leukaemia incidence; consider risk/benefit before initiation.

Pregnancy, Lactation: See Notes below.

ADR: Adverse events relate to mode of action; not selective for malignant cells and targets all rapidly dividing cells (bone marrow, lymph tissue, GI mucosa, skin, gonadal and foetal tissue). See Notes below.

Notes: See also 13.1 Cytotoxic Drugs.

Bendamustine

ATC Code: L01AA09. **Sport:** Permitted.

Driving: Ataxia, peripheral neuropathy, somnolence.

Indications: Chronic lymphocytic leukaemia (CLL), non-Hodgkin's lymphomas, multiple myeloma.

Dose: Adult, Elderly: MONOTHERAPY, CLL, 100mg/m2 BSA (days 1 and 2) every 4 weeks. Non-Hodgkin's lymphoma, 120mg/m2 (days 1 and 2) every 3 weeks.

COMBINATION, multiple myeloma, 120-150mg/m2 (days 1 and 2) every 4 weeks with 60mg/m2 prednisone (IV or oral) (days 1 and 4) every 4 weeks. *Admin*, by IV infusion over 30-60 minutes.

Renal Impairment: Severe, limited data.

Hepatic Impairment: Moderate (serum bilirubin 1.2-3mg/dL), 30% dose reduction. Severe (serum bilirubin above 3mg/dL), contraindicated.

CI: Jaundice, severe bone marrow depression, blood count alterations (leucocytes, platelets), major surgery in 30 days before initiation, infection especially with leukocytopenia.

Interactions: Effect of Other Drugs on Bendamustine: *Co-admin caution*: Other myelosuppressives (increased toxicity); ciclosporin, tacrolimus (excessive immunosuppression). *Potential interaction*: CYP1A2 inhibitors (fluvoxamine, ciprofloxacin, aciclovir, cimetidine).

SP: Myelosuppression, monitor leucocytes, platelets. Pneumonia, sepsis; rarely septic shock/death. Rash, toxic reactions, bullous exanthema, withhold or discontinue. Cardiac disorders, monitor potassium. Consider antiemetics for nausea/vomiting. Caution, infusion reactions, extravasation. See Notes below.

ADR: See Notes below.

Notes: See 13.1.1 Alkylating Agents.

Levact Parenteral 25mg, 100mg *(Mundipharma)* A. HOS. *Price*, (5) 25mg, €334.01; 100mg, €1303.51 (PTW). *Infusion*, bendamustine HCl. White powder for conc. **Store:** Protect from light.

Busulfan

ATC Code: L01AB01. **Sport:** Permitted.

Driving: Hospital use.

Indications: Busilvex, conditioning treatment, followed by cyclophosphamide or followed by fludarabine prior to conventional haematopoietic progenitor cell transplantation (HPCT) (adults) or followed by cyclophosphamide or melphalan prior to conventional HPCT (paediatrics). *Myleran*, palliative treatment, chronic phase granulocytic leukaemia. To produce prolonged

13.1.1 Alkylating Agents

remission in polycythaemia vera. Essential thrombocythaemia, myelofibrosis.

Dose: Adult, Elderly: *Busilvex* with cyclophosphamide or melphalan, 0.8mg/kg as 2-hour infusion every 6-hours for 4 consecutive days, total 16 doses; followed by cyclophosphamide at 60mg/kg/day over 2 days starting at least 24 hours after last busulphan dose; with fludarabine, 3.2mg/kg as single daily 3-hour infusion immediately after fludarabine for 2 or 3 consecutive days; fludarabine admin before as single daily 1-hour infusion at 30mg/m2 for 5 consecutive days or 40mg/m2 for 4 consecutive days. *Admin*, by IV infusion via central venous catheter; not for rapid IV bolus or peripheral injection. Premedication, see SP below. Obese, base dose adjusted to ideal body weight. *Elderly*, under 50 years, as for Adult.
Myleran, chronic granulocytic leukaemia, induction, 0.06mg/kg/day; initial max. 4mg as single oral dose; if needed uptitrate after 3 weeks. Polycythaemia vera, 4-6mg/day for 4-6 weeks. Myelofibrosis, essential thrombocytopenia, usually 2-4mg/day. *Admin*, swallow tabs whole; do not divide.

Child: *Busilvex*, age 0-17 years, actual body weight, under 9kg, 1mg/kg; 9-16kg, 1.2mg/kg; 16-23kg, 1.1mg/kg; 23-34kg, 0.95mg/kg; over 34kg, 0.8mg/kg admin as 2-hour infusion, see Adult above; followed by 4 cycles of cyclophosphamide 50mg/kg OR melphalan single dose of 140mg/m2. Combination with fludarabine, safety/efficacy not established. Obese, BMI above 30kg/m2, not recommended.
Myleran, see manufacturers Full Prescribing Information.

Renal Impairment: Caution (*Busilvex*).

Hepatic Impairment: As for Renal above, especially if severe.

CI: Resistance to busulfan.

Interactions: Effect of Other Drugs on Busulfan: *Increased toxicity*: Itraconazole, metronidazole. *Additive effects*: Other pulmonary toxic cytotoxics. *Decreased myeloablative effect (high dose oral but not IV due to increased clearance)*: Phenytoin. *Decreased metabolism*: Paracetamol. *Co-admin caution (plasma levels increased)*: Ketobemidone (analgesic)

Effect of Busulfan on Other Drugs: Cyclophosphamide; melphalan (paeds): *Allow 24-hour dosing interval after last busulphan dose.*

SP: Profound myelosuppression. Classified potentially carcinogenic (IARC). *Busilvex*, premedicate with anticonvulsants (phenytoin, benzodiazepines) to prevent seizures; antiemetics before first dose then on fixed schedule. Children with Fanconi anaemia, caution. Hepatic veno-occlusive disease; increased risk (prior radiation, 3 chemotherapy cycle, progenitor cell transplant). ARDS, respiratory failure, pulmonary toxicity. *Myleran*, respiratory dysfunction, monitor; lung toxicity, discontinue. Do not admin with or soon after radiotherapy. Correct hyperuricaemia and/or hyperuricosuria before starting; ensure adequate hydration, use allopurinol. Seizures, see *Busilvex* above.

Pregnancy, Lactation: Pregnancy, contraindicated; women* to ensure adequate contraception; men* not to father child *(during, up to 6 months after treatment).

ADR: See Notes below.

Notes: See 13.1.1 Alkylating Agents.

Chlorambucil

ATC Code: L01AA02. **Sport:** Permitted.
Driving: Unlikely to impair.

Indications: Hodgkin's disease, non-Hodgkin's lymphoma, chronic lymphocytic leukaemia (CLL); Waldenstrom's macroglobulinaemia (*Leukeran* is one treatment choice for this indication).

Dose: Adult: *Hodgkin's disease, non-Hodgkin's lymphoma*, as monotherapy 0.2mg/kg/day (0.1-0.2mg/kg/day for non-Hodgkin's lymphoma) for 4-8 weeks. *CLL*, initially 0.15mg/kg/day, then resume treatment 4 weeks after end of first course at 0.1mg/kg/day. *Waldenstrom's macroglobulinaemia*, initially 6-12mg/day until leucopenia occurs, then 2-8mg/day indefinitely. Lymphocytic infiltration of bone marrow or hypoplastic bone marrow, max. 0.1mg/kg/day. *Admin*, oral on empty stomach (1 hour before food or 3 hours after); high gastric pH decreases bioavailability.

Elderly: Initiate at low end of dose range; titrate carefully.

Child: Hodgkin's disease, non-Hodgkin's lymphoma, as for Adult above.

Renal Impairment: No adjustment considered necessary.

Hepatic Impairment: Severe, consider dose reduction.

CI: Use in non-malignant disease.

Interactions: Effect of Other Drugs on Chlorambucil: *Admin not recommended*: With current or recent radiotherapy, other recent cytotoxic treatment. *Enhanced toxicity*: Phenylbutazone.

SP: 6.5mg/day associated with irreversible bone marrow damage. Haematology altered; depressed bone marrow, lymphocytic infiltrates, caution. Not for long-term treatment in patients who will have autologous stem cell transplant. Paediatrics with nephrotic syndrome, high pulse dosing regimens, history of seizures, monitor (increased seizure risk). Balance leukaemogenic risk against potential benefit.

Pregnancy, Lactation: Potentially teratogenic.

ADR: See Notes below.

Notes: See 13.1.1 Alkylating Agents.

Cyclophosphamide

ATC Code: L01AA01. **Sport:** Permitted.
Driving: Dizziness, blurred vision, visual impairment.

Indications: Treatment, malignant disease (adults).

Dose: Adult: ORAL, most indications, 100-300mg/day as single or divided doses. Combination use may require dose reduction. *Admin*, ideally in morning with sufficient fluid; do not chew or divide tabs.
PARENTERAL IV, *conventional dose*, 80-300mg/m2/day (single or divided doses) or 300-600mg/m2/week as single weekly dose; *high dose*, 600-1500mg/m2 as single IV dose of short infusion at 10-20 day intervals. Dosage varies depending on malignancy, bone marrow condition, use of radio/chemotherapy. *Admin*, preferably as infusion, caution extravasation.

Elderly: Monitor for toxicity; adjust dose.

Renal Impairment: For optimal admin, consider severity of impairment. Dialysis, use consistent interval between admin and dialysis.

Hepatic Impairment: Severe may be associated with decreased cyclophosphamide activation; may alter effectiveness.

CI: Acute infection, bone marrow aplasia, UTI, acute urothelial toxicity (cytotoxic chemotherapy or radiation), urinary outflow obstruction.

Interactions: Effect of Other Drugs on Cyclophosphamide: *Reduced activation*: Aprepitant, bupropion, busulfan, ciprofloxacin, chloramphenicol, fluconazole, itraconazole, prasugrel, sulfonamides, thiotepa. *Increased conc of cytotoxic metabolites*: Allopurinol, chloral hydrate, cimetidine, disulfiram, glyceraldehyde, CYP450 inducers, protease inhibitors, ondansetron. *Increased toxicities*: ACEIs, natalizumab, paclitaxel, thiazide diuretics, zidovudine, clozapine (haematotoxicity and/or immunosuppression); anthracyclines, cytarabine, pentostatin, radiation, trastuzumab (cardiotoxicity); amiodarone, granulocyte colony-stimulating factor (pulmonary toxicity); amphotericin B, indomethacin (nephrotoxicity); azathioprine, busulfan, protease inhibitors. *Other interactions*: ALCOHOL, etanercept, metronidazole, tamoxifen.

Effect of Cyclophosphamide on Other Drugs: Bupropion, coumarins, ciclosporin, depolarising muscle relaxants, digoxin and analogues, vaccines, verapamil: *Pharmacokinetics affected.*

SP: Consider colony-stimulating factors to reduce myelosuppressive complication risk and/or help facilitate dose delivery. During or immediately after admin, ensure adequate hydration (force diuresis, reduce urinary tract toxicity risk). Anaphylactic reactions, myelosuppression, significant immunosuppression. Urinary tract and renal toxicity. Treatment with mesna and/or strong hydration to force diuresis can reduce bladder toxicity (frequency, severity). Ensure patients empty bladder at regular intervals. Nephrotoxicity, cardiotoxicity, pulmonary toxicity.

Pregnancy, Lactation: Contraindicated.

ADR: See Notes below.

Notes: See 13.1.1 Alkylating Agents.

Endoxana 50mg, Parenteral *(Baxter)* A. GMS.
Price, (100) €52.92. Parenteral, not published by company (non-GMS).
Tablet, cyclophosphamide. White round s/c. *Lactose, sucrose.* **Store:** Below 25 deg C.
Injection, cyclophosphamide 50mg, 1g. Powder for soln. **Store:** As above; outer carton.

Ifosfamide

ATC Code: L01AA06. **Sport:** Permitted.
Driving: Caution.

Indications: Wide range of malignant conditions.

Dose: Adult, Elderly: Guideline 8-12g/m2 BSA IV in equally divided single daily doses over 3-5 days every 2-4 weeks OR 5-6g/m2 (max. 10g) as 24-hour IV infusion every 3-4 weeks. NOT for use WITHOUT Mesna (urothelial toxicity).

Child: Guideline 5g/m2 over 24-hours OR 9g/m2 in equally divided single daily doses over 5 days OR 9g/m2 as continuous IV infusion over 72 hours, repeated at 3-week intervals.

Renal Impairment: Serum creatinine above 1.5mg/100mL, not recommended.

Hepatic Impairment: Bilirubin above 1mg/100mL or serum transaminases or ALP above 2.5xULN, not recommended.

CI: Bone marrow aplasia, myelosuppression, urinary tract obstruction, acute UTI, acute urothelial toxicity from cytotoxic chemo- or radiation therapy. High cumulative doses in presence of renal tubular dysfunction.

Interactions: Effect of Other Drugs on Ifosfamide: *Increased myelotoxicity*: Other cytostatics, intensified skin reaction with irradiation. *Increased bone marrow depression severity*: Allopurinol. *Enhanced toxicity (haematological, nephro-, neuro)*: Other nephrotoxics (cisplatin, aminoglycosides, aciclovir, amphotericin B). *Enhanced neurotoxicity*: Barbiturates. *Metabolism accelerated*: Enzyme inducers.

Effect of Ifosfamide on Other Drugs: Anticoagulants (warfarin): *Increased bleeding risk.* Antidiabetics (sulphonylureas): *Enhanced hypoglycaemic effect.*

SP: Correct electrolyte imbalance before initiation. Debilitated, diabetes, myelosuppression, recent chemo- or radiotherapy, previous platinum treatment, undergone nephrectomy, caution. Drug-induced neoplasia.

ADR: See Notes below.

Notes: See 13.1.1 Alkylating Agents.

Mitoxana Parenteral *(Baxter)* A.
Price, (1) 1g, €23.06. 2g, €42.59.
Injection, ifosfamide 1g, 2g. White powder for conc for soln.

Melphalan

ATC Code: L01AA03. **Sport:** Permitted.
Driving: Effect not studied.

Indications: Neoplastic conditions (malignant melanoma, multiple myelomatosis, breast carcinoma, epithelial ovarian cancer), polycythaemia rubra vera. *Parenteral,* by regional arterial perfusion, localised (malignant melanoma or soft tissue sarcoma of extremities), advanced ovarian carcinoma, multiple myeloma, stage IV neuroblastoma.

Dose: Adult: Before initiating, see SP below.

ORAL, *multiple myeloma,* 0.15mg/kg/day in divided doses (4 days); repeat 6-weekly. *Ovarian adenocarcinoma,* 0.2mg/kg/day in divided doses (5 days); repeat 4-8 weekly. *Advanced breast carcinoma,* 0.15mg/kg/day OR

6mg/m2/day BSA (5 days); repeat 6-weekly. *Polycythaemia rubra vera,* initially 6-10mg/day (5-7 days), then 2-4mg/day until disease control. *Admin,* absorption after oral admin is variable; may need to increase dose until myelosuppression is seen to ensure potentially therapeutic levels achieved.

PARENTERAL (IV), *multiple myeloma,* range 8-30mg/m2 BSA at 2-6 week intervals alone or combination; used alone, 0.4mg/kg (16mg/m2 BSA) at 4-week intervals; high dose, generally 100-240mg/m2 BSA (2.5-6mg/kg) as single IV dose. *Advanced ovarian carcinoma,* monotherapy, 1mg/kg (40mg/m2 BSA) IV every 4 weeks; combination, 0.3-0.4mg/kg (12-16mg/m2 BSA) at 4-6 week intervals.

REGIONAL PERFUSION, malignant melanoma, soft tissue sarcoma, consult scientific literature.

Elderly: High dose, caution.

Child: Stage IV neuroblastoma in childhood, high dose, 100-240mg/m2 BSA sometimes divided equally over 3 consecutive days.

Renal Impairment: Oral, reduce dose. Parenteral, moderate to severe, reduce initial dose by 50% of conventional (IV 8-40mg/m2 BSA); high dose (100-240mg/m2 BSA), reduction depends on degree of impairment; without stem cell rescue in moderate impairment reduce initial dose by 50%.

Interactions: Effect of Other Drugs on Melphalan: *Co-admin not recommended (high dose IV)*: Nalidixic acid. *Impaired renal function (high dose IV)*: Ciclosporin (following bone marrow transplant).

SP: Conduct frequent blood counts; delay dose or adjust. Combination (lenalidomide + prednisone; thalidomide + prednisone or dexamethasone), increased venous thromboembolism risk (VTE, PE); admin thromboprophylaxis (at least first 5 months of treatment, especially with added thrombotic risk factors e.g. smoking, hypertension, hyperlipidaemia, thrombosis history); base decision on careful individual risk factor assessment. Any thromboembolic events, discontinue; start standard anticoagulation.

Caution, recent chemo- or radiotherapy. Chromosomal aberrations. High dose (IV), consider prophylactic anti-infectives, blood products; ensure adequate performance status and organ function before starting. Caution, extravasation (local tissue damage). Possible increased leukaemogenic risk in combination (thalidomide or lenalidomide + prednisone).

Pregnancy, Lactation: Due to increased VTE risk in multiple myeloma patients, combined oral contraceptives are not recommended. Breastfeeding not recommended.

ADR: See Notes below.

Notes: See 13.1.1 Alkylating Agents.

Alkeran 2mg *(Aspen)* A. GMS.
Price, (25) €73.92.
Tablet, melphalan. White (off-white) round f/c. Marked GXEH3; A on reverse. **Store:** Refrigerate.
Alkeran Parenteral 50mg *(Aspen)* A.
Price, 50mg (1) €62.10.
Infusion, melphalan. White (off-white) powder; clear colourless solvent. *46mg sodium, 0.4mg ethanol per vial.* **Store:** Below 30 deg C; do not refrigerate.

Temozolomide

ATC Code: L01AX03. **Sport:** Permitted.
Driving: Caution, fatigue, somnolence.

Indications: Newly diagnosed glioblastoma multiforme (with radiotherapy), then as monotherapy; malignant glioma recurrence or progression after standard therapy.

Dose: Adult: *Glioblastoma multiforme,* 75mg/m2/day BSA for 42 days with focal radiotherapy; after 4 weeks, up to 6 cycles of monotherapy (cycle 1, 150mg/m2 once daily for 5 days then 23 days without treatment; cycle 2 onwards, 200mg/m2 for first 5 days of each subsequent cycle).

Malignant glioma (recurrent, progressive), no previous chemotherapy, 200mg/m2/day for first 5 days, then 23-days rest (28-day cycle); previous chemotherapy, 150mg/m2/day for first cycle increasing to 200mg/m2/day in second cycle if no haematological toxicity. Adjust dose according to neutrophil and thrombocyte counts. *Oral admin,* swallow caps whole with

13.1.2 Cytotoxic Antibiotics

water; do not break or chew; admin in fasting state. Vomiting, a second dose should not be admin that day.
Elderly: Over 70 years, caution; increased neutropenia and thrombocytopenia risk.
Child: *Malignant glioma* (recurrent, progressive), age 3 years and older, as for Adult above; under 3 years, no data.
Renal Impairment: Caution.
Hepatic Impairment: Severe, as for Renal above.
CI: Dacarbazine hypersensitivity, severe myelosuppression.
Interactions: Effect of Other Drugs on Temozolomide: *Clearance decreased*: Valproic acid. *Increased myelosuppression risk*: Other myelosuppressives.
SP: Opportunistic infections (*Pneumocystis jirovecii* pneumonia*), viral infection reactivation (HBV, CMV). Myelodysplasia syndrome, secondary malignancies (myeloid leukaemia); fatal respiratory failure (especially with dexamethasone or other steroids); hepatic injury (including fatal) (perform baseline LFTs before initiation; if abnormal assess benefit/risk). Guidelines for anti-emetic therapy, see manufacturers Full Prescribing Information. *(prophylaxis required).
Pregnancy, Lactation: Contraindicated; women of childbearing potential and males to ensure adequate contraception during and up for to 6 months after treatment.
ADR: See Notes below.
Notes: See 13.1.1 Alkylating Agents.
Interchangeability: Same strengths of all brands of temozolomide caps listed below are deemed interchangeable.
Reference Price: (5) 5mg, €9.46. 20mg, €37.84. 100mg, €189.22. 140mg, €285.97. 180mg, €367.68. 250mg, €473.04.
Temodal Capsules *(MSD)* A. HT.
Price, (5) 5mg, €11.82. 20mg, €47.29. 100mg, €236.49. 140mg, €357.46. 180mg, €459.52. 250mg, €591.20.
Capsule, temozolomide 5mg, 20mg, 100mg, 140mg, 180mg, 250mg. Opaque. Marked Temodal, strength, logo, 2 stripes. 5mg: White/green. 20mg: White/yellow. 100mg: White/pink. 140mg: White/blue. 180mg: White/orange. 250mg: White/white. *Lactose.*
Temozolomide Accord Capsules *(Accord)* A. HT.
Price, see reference price above.
Capsule, temozolomide 5mg, 20mg, 100mg, 140mg, 180mg, 250mg. Marked TMZ and strength. 5mg: Green/white. 20mg: Yellow/white. 100mg: Pink/white. 140mg: Blue/white. 180mg: Maroon/white. 250mg: White/white. *Lactose.*
Temozolomide Clonmel Capsules *(Clonmel)* A. HT.
Price, see reference price above.
Capsule, temozolomide 5mg, 20mg, 100mg, 140mg, 180mg, 250mg. Opaque hard gelatin white/white. Marked T and strength with 2 stripes. *Lactose.*
Temozolomide TEVA Capsules *(TEVA)* A. HT.
Price, see reference price above.
Capsule, temozolomide 5mg, 20mg, 100mg, 140mg, 250mg. Opaque hard gelatin white/white. Marked T and strength (mg) with 2 stripes. *Lactose.*

13.1.2 - Cytotoxic Antibiotics

In This Chapter: *Daunorubicin, doxorubicin, epirubicin, idarubicin, mitomycin, mitoxantrone, pixantrone.*

Class Effects
All in this chapter are anthracyclines; except mitomycin (described under 'other' cytotoxic antibiotics). See Notes below.
CI: Hypersensitivity to any member of the class.
Interactions: Effect of Other Drugs on Anthracyclines: *Use not recommended, avoid*: Live vaccines (use inactivated). *Co-admin caution*: Other cytotoxics (especially myelotoxics). *Increased cardiotoxicity risk (Myocet)*: Other cardiotoxic or cardiologically active drugs. *Generally not recommended*: Admixture with other drugs in same injection or infusion. *Additive myelosuppressive effects*: Other myelosuppressives.
SP: *Anthracyclines*: Toxicity may be early (acute, tachycardia, ECG changes, tachyarrhythmias) or late (delayed, reduced LVEF, CHF, acute arrhythmias, cardiomyopathies). Cardiotoxicity (CHF due to cardiomyopathy); cardiac damage may be irreversible. Risk

increases with total cumulative dose; is higher following radiation (mediastinal-pericardial area), previous anthracycline, anthracenedione treatment or other cardiotoxic agents (5-fluorouracil), clinical disease (anaemia, bone marrow depression, infection, leukaemia pericarditis, myocarditis), drugs suppressing cardiac contractility, pre-existing cardiac disease, children, elderly. Radiation recall (previously irradiated fields). Secondary malignancy (AML, myelodysplastic syndrome). *Acute infusion reactions* with liposomal infusion (flushing, dyspnoea, fever, facial swelling, headache, back pain, chills, chest and/or throat tightness, hypotension). Avoid extravasation (most of class are irritant); severe soft tissue damage may occur (necrosis); some liposomal preparations may be less irritant but avoid paravenous admin. *Bone marrow suppression*, monitor haematology; myelosuppression associated with opportunistic infections. Hyperuricaemia, Tumour Lysis Syndrome (TLS), secondary to rapid lysis of leukaemic cells, monitor blood uric acid; if needed treat (allopurinol); ensure adequate hydration.
Pregnancy, Lactation: Pregnancy, use only if absolutely essential*. Women of child-bearing age and males to ensure adequate contraception during and after treatment. Lactation, contraindicated*. *(unless otherwise specified).
ADR: See Notes below.
Notes: See also 13.1 Cytotoxic Drugs. Always consult manufacturers Full Prescribing Information.

Daunorubicin
ATC Code: L01DB02. **Sport:** Permitted.
Driving: Caution.
Indications: Remission induction, acute lymphocytic (ALL), acute myelogenous (AML) leukaemia.
Dose: Adult: 40-60mg/m2 BSA on alternate days (up to 3 doses); AML, ALL, 45mg/m2/day. Max. cumulative dose (daunorubicin, other cardiotoxic drugs), see manufacturers Full Prescribing Information. *Admin*, IV infusion over 20 minutes; NOT for admin by IM or SC route.
Elderly: Inadequate bone marrow reserve, reduce dose by 50%.
Child: Over 2 years, max. 300mg/m2 BSA; under 2 years or below 0.5m2 BSA, max. 10mg/kg/day.
Renal Impairment: See Notes below.
Hepatic Impairment: As for Renal above.
CI: Non-malignant disease, acute infection, bone marrow suppression, oropharyngeal ulceration, chicken-pox, Herpes zoster.
SP: Cardiotoxicity, see Notes below. Monitor haematology. Red urine discolouration. Caution, extravasation. Dose above 600mg/m2 (adults) or 300mg/m2 (children over 2 years) or 10mg/kg (children under 2 years) increased CHF risk. Acute infusion reactions (too rapid infusion). NOTE: Do not use liposomal daunorubicin interchangeably with conventional daunorubicin.
Pregnancy, Lactation: Women of childbearing potential and males to ensure adequate contraception during and up to 24 weeks following treatment; may cause serious birth defects.
ADR: See Notes below.
Notes: See Class Effects 13.1.2 Cytotoxic Antibiotics.
Cerubidin Parenteral *(SANOFI)* A. HOS.
Price, (1) €14.48 (PTW).
Infusion, daunorubicin HCl 20mg. Orange-red powder for soln.
Store: Below 25 deg C; reconstituted soln in refrigerator (max. 24 hours).

Doxorubicin
ATC Code: L01DB01. **Sport:** Permitted.
Driving: No or negligible effect; dizziness, somnolence reported.
Indications: *Caelyx* (monotherapy) metastatic breast, advanced ovarian cancer; (combination), progressive multiple myeloma, AIDS-related Kaposi's sarcoma (KS). *Doxorubicin (Hospira)*, acute leukaemia, sarcoma (soft tissue, osteogenic), lymphomas, carcinoma (breast, bronchogenic, paediatric malignancy; non-metastatic transitional cell carcinoma, carcinoma *in situ*, papillary bladder tumours. *Myocet*, metastatic breast cancer. *Doxorubicin (Actavis)*, small-cell lung, breast, recurrent ovarian, bladder cancer, soft-tissue and osteosarcoma,

Ewing's sarcoma, lymphoma (Hodgkin's, highly malignant non-Hodgkin's), leukaemia (ALL, AML), advanced (multiple myeloma, endometrial carcinoma), Wilm's tumour, thyroid cancer, neuroblastoma.

Dose: Adult: *Caelyx*, breast/ovarian cancer, 50mg/m2 BSA once every 4 weeks. Multiple myeloma, 30mg/m2 as 1-hour infusion (after bortezomib) on day 4 of bortezomib 3-week regimen. AIDS-Related KS, 20mg/m2 every 2-3 weeks; avoid intervals under 10 days. Not to be used interchangeably with other doxorubicin formulations; IV, not for bolus injection or for use undiluted.

Doxorubicin (Hospira), monotherapy, 60-75mg/m2 BSA as single IV injection at 21-day intervals; combination, 30-40mg/m2 BSA OR 1.2-2.4mg/kg as single dose every 3 weeks.

Myocet, initially 60-75mg/m2 every 3 weeks in combination with cyclophosphamide. *Admin*, by IV infusion over 60 minutes; NOT for IM, SC or IV bolus injection.

Doxorubicin (Actavis), monotherapy, 60-75mg/m2 every 3 weeks. Combination, reduce to 30-60mg/m2 every 3-4 weeks. Full dose not tolerated (immunosuppression, old age), 15-20mg/m2 weekly.

Elderly: *Doxorubicin (Hospira)*, age 70 years and older, restrict to 450mg/m2 BSA total cumulative dose.

Child: *Doxorubicin (Hospira/Actavis)*, as for Adult, consider dose reduction.

Renal Impairment: See Notes below.

Hepatic Impairment: See Notes below.

CI: Not for use in AIDS-KS that can be treated with local therapy or systemic alfa-interferon (*Caelyx*). Bone marrow depression, buccal ulceration or burning sensation which can precede ulceration (do not repeat dose).

Interactions: Effect of Other Drugs on Doxorubicin:
Effect of Doxorubicin on Other Drugs: Other antineoplastic drugs: *Toxicity potentiated*.

SP: Cardiotoxicity, see Notes below. Lethal cardiomyopathy risk, weigh benefit/risk before each admin; max. cumulative total lifetime doxorubicin dose (including related drugs) 450-550mg/m2. Infusion reactions, discontinue; premedicate (antihistamine and/or short-acting corticosteroid); restart at slower rate. Allergic- or anaphylactoid-like reactions.

ADR: See Notes below.

Notes: See Class Effects 13.1.2 Cytotoxic Antibiotics. See manufacturers Full Prescribing Information.

Caelyx Parenteral *(Janssen-Cilag)* A. HOS.
Price, (1) 20mg, €380.29. 50mg, €974.54 (PTW).
Infusion, doxorubicin HCl in pegylated liposomes 2mg/mL. Translucent red susp conc for soln. *Sucrose*. **Store:** Refrigerate; do not freeze.

Doxorubicin (TEVA) Parenteral *(TEVA)* A.
Price, not published by company.
Infusion, doxorubicin HCl 2mg/mL (5mL, 25mL, 50mL). Clear red conc for soln. *Sodium 3.54mg/mL of conc*. **Store:** Refrigerate.

Doxorubicin (Hospira) Parenteral *(Hospira)* A.
Price, (1) 10mg, €19.20. 50mg, €94.71.
Infusion, doxorubicin HCl. Powder for soln.

Myocet Parenteral *(TEVA)* A.
Price, (1) 50mg, €1499.30.
Infusion, doxorubicin-citrate complex liposome-encapsulated 50mg. Red lyophilised powder. *Sodium 108mg/50mg dose*. White (off-white) opaque soln (liposomes). Clear colourless buffer soln. **Store:** Refrigerate.

Epirubicin

ATC Code: L01DB03. **Sport:** Permitted.
Driving: Nausea, vomiting may temporarily impair ability.
Indications: Carcinoma of breast, ovary and lung, superficial bladder carcinoma, gastric cancer.
Dose: Adult: *Conventional dose*, monotherapy, 60-90mg/m2 BSA by IV bolus over 3-30 minutes, repeat at 21-day intervals. *High dose*, monotherapy, small cell lung cancer (NSCLC) (previously untreated), 120mg/m2 single dose (day 1), repeat every 3 weeks; NSCLC (previously untreated), 135mg/m2 (day 1) OR 45mg/m2 (days 1, 2, and 3) every 3 weeks (IV bolus as above or infusion over 30 minutes). For IV admin; NOT for IM or intrathecal use (caution, extravasation).
Intravesical, papillary transition cell carcinoma of bladder, 50mg/50mL instilled weekly for 8 weeks; local toxicity,

reduce to 30mg/50mL. Carcinoma in-situ, increase to 80mg/50mL depending on tolerability. Prophylaxis of recurrences after transurethral resection, 50mg/50mL weekly for 4 weeks then 11 monthly.

Renal Impairment: Serum creatinine above 5mg/dL, consider lower starting doses.

Hepatic Impairment: Dose adjustment required. Severe, contraindicated.

CI: Management, non-malignant disease, current cardiac disorders, acute infection, marked bone marrow depression, already treated with max. cumulative doses of other anthracyclines. Intravesical if (haematuria, UTI, bladder inflammation, invasive tumours penetrating bladder, catheterisation problems, large volume residual urine, contracted bladder).

Interactions: Effect of Other Drugs on Epirubicin: *Plasma levels increased, co-admin not recommended*: Cimetidine. *Stagger co-admin by 24-hours*: Paclitaxel. *Bone marrow depressant effects increased*: Dexverapamil. *Plasma levels (metabolites) increased*: Docetaxel (if admin immediately after epirubicin). *Initial distribution accelerated/red blood cell partitioning influenced*: Quinine. *Terminal elimination half-life, total clearance reduced*: Interferon alpha-2b.

SP: Cardiotoxicity, see Notes below. High CHF risk with prior cumulative dose above 450mg/m2 (doxorubicin, daunorubicin); epirubicin above 900mg/m2 (extreme caution). Intravesical, see CI above. Intra-arterial, localised/regional events e.g. gastro-duodenal ulcers (drug reflux into gastric artery), bile duct narrowing (drug-induced sclerosing cholangitis); can lead to necrosis of perfused tissue. Red colouration of urine.

Pregnancy, Lactation: Males, not to take part in conception during and up to 6 months after treatment. Consider sperm conservation. Amenorrhoea or premature menopause in premenopausal women.

ADR: See Notes below.

Notes: See Class Effects 13.1.2 Cytotoxic Antibiotics.

Epirubicin Parenteral 2mg/mL *(TEVA)* A.
Price, (5mL, 25mL) not published by company.
Soln for injection, epirubicin HCl. Clear red soln.

Idarubicin

ATC Code: L01DB06. **Sport:** Permitted.
Driving: Caution.
Indications: *Oral*, previously untreated AML (elderly) (IV cannot be used). *Parenteral*, (adults) acute non-lymphoblastic leukaemia (ANLL) remission induction, second-line (relapsed ALL); (child) first-line in acute ANLL remission induction (with cytarabine), second-line (relapsed ALL).
Dose: Adult, Elderly: ORAL, AML, monotherapy, 30mg/m2 for 3 days OR combination, 15-30mg/m2 for 3 days. *Admin*, caps to be swallowed whole with some water; not to be sucked, bitten or chewed; may be taken with light meal.
PARENTERAL, acute ANLL, 12mg/m2/day BSA for 3 days with cytarabine OR 8mg/m2/day for 5 days with or without combination. ALL, 12mg/m2/day for 3 days as single agent. Not for intrathecal use.
Child: PARENTERAL, acute ANLL, 10-12mg/m2 IV for 3 days in combination with cytarabine; ALL, 10mg/m2/day for 3 days IV as single agent. Not for intrathecal use.
Renal Impairment: Severe, contraindicated.
Hepatic Impairment: Consider dose reduction. Severe, as for Renal above.
CI: Uncontrolled infection, hypersensitivity (anthracyclines, anthracenediones), severe myocardial insufficiency, recent MI, severe arrhythmias, persistent myelosuppression, previous treatment with max. cumulative doses of idarubicin or other anthracyclines or anthracenediones, profound or persistent bone marrow depression.
Interactions: Effect of Other Drugs on Idarubicin: *Additive myelosuppressive effects*: Other chemotherapy regimen, radiotherapy co-admin or within 2-3 weeks prior to treatment. *Altered metabolism, pharmacokinetics*: Other drugs changing hepatic function. *Monitor cardiac function*: Potentially cardiotoxic drugs, other cardioactive drugs (calcium channel blockers).
SP: Red colouration of urine. Children more susceptible to anthracycline-induced cardiac toxicity.

345

13.1.3 Antimetabolites

ADR: See Notes below.

Notes: See Class Effects 13.1.2 Cytotoxic Antibiotics.

Zavedos 10mg, Parenteral 5mg *(Pfizer)* A. HT.
Price, caps (1) 10mg, €69.84. Injection (1) 5mg, €82.27.
Capsule, idarubicin HCl. Opaque red/white hard gelatine; contains orange powder. Marked IDARUBICIN/strength.
Injection, as above. Orange-red powder for soln. *Lactose.* **NOTE:** Avoid prolonged contact with alkaline solns (drug degradation); do not mix with heparin (precipitation) or other drugs.

Mitomycin

ATC Code: L01DC03. **Sport:** Permitted.
Driving: Generalised weakness, lethargy reported.
Indications: Superficial bladder cancer, adenocarcinoma (breast, stomach, oesophagus, pancreas, biliary tract, colon, rectum). Squamous cell carcinoma (anus), non-small cell lung cancer.

Dose: Adult, Elderly: Usually 4-10mg (0.06-0.15mg/kg) at 1-6 weekly intervals depending on (combination drugs, bone marrow recovery); 10mg/m2 BSA repeated at intervals; 40-80mg (0.58-1.2mg/kg) may be required (alone or combination). Doses above 0.6mg/kg not shown to be more effective or more toxic. *Admin,* IV (care to avoid extravasation); inject as slowly as possible.

Superficial bladder tumours, usually 20-40mg dissolved in 20-40mL diluent; instil into bladder through urethral catheter weekly or 3-times weekly (total 20 doses); retain dose for minimum 1 hour; rotate patient every 15 minutes to ensure contact with all areas of bladder urothelium; recurrence prevention, 20mg in 20mL diluent every 2 weeks or 40mg in 40mL diluent monthly or 3-monthly.

Child: Safety and efficacy not established.

CI: Hepatic/renal disorders, thrombocytopenia, coagulation disorders, increased bleeding tendency.

Interactions: Effect of Other Drugs on Mitomycin: *Potential positive or negative effect:* Drugs altering drug-metabolising enzymes. *Cardiotoxicity potentiated:* Doxorubicin. *Bone marrow depression enhanced:* Antineoplastic agents, irradiation. *Bronchospasm:* Vinca alkaloids.

SP: Caution, extravasation. Intra-arterial admin (induration, pain, redness, erythema, blisters, erosion, ulceration); may lead to skin/muscle necrosis, discontinue. Parenchymatous liver disorder, biloma, cholangitis (also sclerosing), bile duct necrosis after hepatic arterial admin. Bladder wall fibrosis (intravesical use); possible renal failure. Avoid skin contact. Monitor, laboratory testing (bone marrow depression). Leukaemia, myelodysplastic syndrome (combination).

Pregnancy, Lactation: Not for use.

ADR: See Notes below.

Notes: See Class Effects 13.1.2 Cytotoxic Antibiotics.

Mitomycin-C Kyowa Parenteral *(KyowaKirin)* A.
Price, not published by company (10mg, 40mg).
Injection, mitomycin-C. Blue/purple powder for soln. *Sodium* 240mg/10mg vial; 960mg/40mg vial. **Store:** Do not (refrigerate, freeze).

Mitoxantrone

ATC Code: L01DB07. **Sport:** Permitted.
Driving: Not applicable.
Indications: Metastatic breast cancer, non-Hodgkin's lymphoma, adult ANLL, non-resectable primary hepatocellular carcinoma.

Dose: Adult, Elderly: *Breast cancer, non-Hodgkin's lymphoma, hepatoma,* monotherapy, initially 14mg/m2 BSA (single dose); repeat at 21-day intervals; inadequate bone marrow reserves, 12mg/m2 BSA. As a guide, in combination, reduce by 2-4mg/m2 BSA below monotherapy dose.

Adult ANLL, remission induction 12mg/m2/day BSA (single agent dose in relapse) (5 consecutive days); induction in previously untreated, 10-12mg/m2 (3 days) with cytarabine 100mg/m2 (7 days). *Admin,* IV infusion; label for IV use only; not for intrathecal use. Avoid contact with skin, mucous membrane or eyes.

Child: Not recommended.

Hepatic Impairment: Careful supervision.

CI: IV use only. Severe marrow depression.

Interactions: Effect of Other Drugs on Mitoxantrone: *Allergic reactions:* Sulphites (especially with asthma or allergy history). *Increased cardiac toxicity risk:* Cardiotoxic drugs (anthracyclines).

SP: Increased leukaemia risk (use in non-metastatic breast cancer). Dose above 160mg/m2 BSA, increased cardiotoxicity risk (cardiac monitoring). Secondary malignancy with use with other antineoplastics and/or radiotherapy. Blue-green colouration (urine, skin, nails, sclerae).

ADR: See Notes below.

Notes: See Class Effects 13.1.2 Cytotoxic Antibiotics.

Mitoxantrone Parenteral *(Hospira)* A.
Price, 20mg/10mL (1) €150.00.
Injection, mitoxantrone HCl 2mg/mL. Clear dark-blue aqueous soln; pH 3-4.5. *Sodium metabisulphite.* **Store:** Below 25 deg C; do not (refrigerate, freeze).

Pixantrone

ATC Code: L01DB11. **Sport:** Permitted.
Driving: Effect unknown.
Indications: Monotherapy, multiply relapsed or refractory aggressive Non-Hodgkin B-cell lymphoma.

Dose: Adult, Elderly: 50mg/m2 (days 1, 8 and 15) of each 28-day cycle; up to 6 cycles. Caution, obese patients; limited data on BSA dosing. Adjust dose based on haematological toxicity. *Admin,* by slow IV infusion (minimum 60 minutes) using an in-line filter. NOTE: Dose refers to base of active substance (pixantrone); dose calculation based on strength of reconstituted soln containing 5.8mg/mL.

Child: Under 18 years, safety/efficacy not established.

Renal Impairment: Caution.

Hepatic Impairment: Mild/moderate, caution. Severe, contraindicated.

CI: Profound bone marrow suppression.

Interactions: Effect of Other Drugs on Pixantrone: *Monitor (pixantrone side effects):* Repaglinide, rosiglitazone, paclitaxel; ciclosporin, tacrolimus, ritonavir, saquinavir, nelfinavir. *Decreased exposure:* Rifampicin, carbamazepine, glucocorticoids.

Effect of Pixantrone on Other Drugs: Theophylline, warfarin, amitriptyline, haloperidol, ondansetron, clozapine, propranolol: *Plasma levels increased (monitor).*

SP: Benefit not established (used fifth-line or more; refractory to last therapy). Poor performance status, caution. *Prior to initiation,* assess baseline blood counts, total serum (bilirubin, creatinine), cardiac function (LVEF). Severe myelosuppression; neutropenia predominant. *Monitor,* blood counts, leucocytes, red blood cells, platelets, absolute neutrophil counts. Decreased LVEF or fatal CHF may occur; weigh risk/benefit (baseline LVEF below 45%, NYHA III or IV cardiovascular abnormalities, MI within last 6 months, severe arrhythmia, uncontrolled hypertension or angina, prior doxorubicin above 450mg/m2). Secondary malignancy. Extravasation, stop immediately. See Notes below.

Pregnancy, Lactation: Women of childbearing potential and males to ensure adequate contraception during and for up to 6 months following treatment. Lactation, discontinue breastfeeding during treatment.

ADR: See Notes below.

Notes: See Class Effects 13.1.2 Cytotoxic Antibiotics.

▼ Pixuvri Parenteral 29mg *(Servier)* A. HOS.
Price, (1) €674.30 (PTW).
Infusion, pixantrone 5.8mg/mL as pixantrone dimaleate. Dark blue powder for conc for soln. *Sodium 39mg/vial.* **Store:** Refrigerate; outer carton; protect (light).

13.1.3 - Antimetabolites

In This Chapter: *Azacitidine, capecitabine, cytarabine, clofarabine, decitabine, fludarabine, 5-fluorouracil, folinic acid (as calcium folinate), gemcitabine, mercaptopurine, nelarabine, pemetrexed, raltitrexed; tegafur, gimeracil, oteracil combination; tioguanine; trifluridine, tipiracil combination.*

Class Effects

Generally used in specialised units. See Notes below (cytotoxic drugs).

CI: Hypersensitivity to any member of the class. Not for use in children under 18 years unless specified.

Pregnancy, Lactation: Anti-metabolites have potential to cause serious birth defects. Pregnancy, should not be used unless clearly necessary. Women of child-bearing potential to ensure adequate contraception. Lactation, not recommended or contraindicated.

ADR: See Notes below (cytotoxic drugs).

Notes: See also 13.1 Cytotoxic Drugs. See 4.4.1 Drugs Suppressing Rheumatic Disease Process (methotrexate).

Azacitidine

ATC Code: L01BC07. **Sport:** Permitted.
Driving: Minor or moderate influence. Caution, fatigue.

Indications: Treatment, adults not eligible for haematopoietic stem cell transplantation with: Intermediate and high-risk myelodysplastic syndromes (MDS); chronic myelomonocytic leukaemia (CMML), acute myeloid leukaemia (AML).

Dose: Adult, Elderly: 75mg/m2 BSA daily (7 days); then 21-day rest (28-day cycle); minimum 6 cycles. *Admin*, SC injection; rotate sites. *Elderly*, monitor renal function.

Renal Impairment: No adjustment (baseline serum creatinine or BUN above 2xULN; or serum bicarbonate below 20mmoL/L). Unexplained serum bicarbonate below 20mmoL/L, reduce dose by 50% on next cycle; serum creatinine or BUN above 2xULN, delay next cycle until return to normal and reduce dose by 50%. Severe impairment, monitor carefully.

Hepatic Impairment: Severe, monitor carefully. Advanced malignant hepatic tumours, contraindicated.

SP: Anaemia, neutropenia, thrombocytopenia (especially during first 2 cycles), monitor complete blood counts (prior to each treatment). Observe for febrile episodes, signs/symptoms of bleeding. Assess cardiopulmonary function (before, during treatment). Extensive tumour burden due to metastatic disease, progressive hepatic coma, death. *Reported*, renal abnormalities (elevated serum creatinine, renal failure, death), necrotising fasciitis (fatal), tumour lysis syndrome (discontinue). Premedicate (anti-emetics).

Pregnancy, Lactation: Pregnancy, only if clearly necessary (especially first trimester); weigh benefit/risk. Men and women of childbearing potential to ensure adequate contraception during and up to 3 months after treatment. Lactation, contraindicated. Advise men not to father a child during treatment.

ADR: See Notes below.

Notes: See 13.1.3 Anti-Metabolites.

Vidaza Parenteral *(Celgene)* A. HOS.
Price, (1) €364.23 (PTW).
Injection, azacitidine 25mg/mL. White powder for soln.

Capecitabine

ATC Code: L01BC06. **Sport:** Permitted.
Driving: Caution.

Indications: Stage III (Dukes' stage C) colon cancer (after surgery), metastatic colorectal cancer, advanced gastric cancer (with platinum-based regimen). Locally advanced or metastatic breast cancer, monotherapy or combination (docetaxel).

Dose: Adult: MONOTHERAPY, *colon, colorectal, breast* cancer, 1250mg/m2 twice daily morning and evening (14 days), then rest (7 days). Adjuvant, stage III colon cancer, for 6 months.

COMBINATION, *colon, colorectal, gastric* cancer, 800-1000mg/m2 twice daily (14-days), then rest (7 days) OR 625mg/m2 twice daily with cisplatin or oxaliplatin. With irinotecan 200mg/m2 (day 1), 800mg/m2 twice daily (14 days), then rest (7 days). *Breast* cancer, 1250mg/m2 twice daily (14-days), then rest (7 days) with docetaxel. *Admin*, swallow tabs whole with water 30 minutes after food. Disease progression or intolerable toxicity, discontinue.

Elderly: 60 years and over, monitor. Combination (irinotecan), initially 800mg/m2 twice daily.

Renal Impairment: CrCl (mL/min) below 30, not recommended; 30-50, reduce dose to 75% of Adult.

Hepatic Impairment: No dose recommendation.

CI: Reaction to fluoropyrimidine therapy, absence of dihydropyrimidine dehydrogenase (DPD) activity; severe (leucopenia, neutropenia, thrombocytopenia). Combinations, see individual drugs.

Interactions: Effect of Other Drugs on Capecitabine: *Co-admin contraindicated*: Sorivudine, brivudine. *Co-admin avoid*: Allopurinol. *Max. tolerated daily dose reduced*: Folinic acid/folic acid, interferon alpha, radiotherapy.

Effect of Capecitabine on Other Drugs: Warfarin, other coumarins: *Monitor INR or prothrombin time; adjust dose.* Phenytoin: *Plasma levels increased.*

SP: Dose limiting toxicity (diarrhoea, abdominal pain, nausea, stomatitis, hand-foot syndrome). Cardiotoxicity (MI, angina, dysrhythmias, cardiogenic shock, sudden death, ECG changes). *Caution*, hypo- or hypercalcaemia, central or peripheral nervous system disease, diabetes mellitus, electrolyte disturbances; serious renal events (dehydration, hypertension, diabetes); prevent/correct dehydration at onset (may cause acute renal failure, potentially fatal). Known low or absent DPD activity, at highest risk of life-threatening or fatal toxicity (do not treat; *Ecansya*); partial DPD deficiency, caution. Monitor for ophthalmic complications. *Cisplatin combination*, use of Vitamin B6 (pyridoxine) not recommended to treat hand-foot syndrome (may decrease cisplatin efficacy).

Pregnancy, Lactation: Not recommended.

ADR: See Notes below.

Notes: See 13.1.3 Anti-Metabolites, 13.1.4 Plant Alkaloids (docetaxel) and/or 13.1.5 Platinum Compounds.

Interchangeability: Same strengths of all brands of capecitabine f/c tabs listed below are deemed interchangeable.

Reference Price: 150mg (60) €20.74. 500mg (120) €123.12.

Capecitabine Accord 150mg, 300mg, 500mg *(Accord)* A. HT.
Price, see reference price above. 300mg, €47.11.
Tablet, capecitabine. Oblong f/c. Marked with strength. 150mg: Light-peach. 300mg: White (off-white). 500mg: Peach. *Lactose*.

Capecitabine Actavis 150mg, 500mg *(Accord)* A. HT.
Price, see reference price above.
Tablet, capecitabine. Pink cap-shaped f/c. Marked with strength. *Lactose*.

Capecitabine Sandoz 150mg, 500mg *(Rowex)* A. HT.
Price, see reference price above.
Tablet, capecitabine. Modified oval f/c. Marked with strength. 150mg: Light-pink. 500mg: Pink. *Lactose*.

Ecansya 150mg, 500mg *(Krka)* A. HT.
Price, see reference price above.
Tablet, capecitabine. Oblong f/c. Marked with strength. 150mg: Light-peach. 500mg: Peach. *Lactose*.

Clofarabine

ATC Code: L01BB06. **Sport:** Permitted.
Driving: Dizziness, light-headedness, fainting.

Indications: Treatment, ALL in paediatrics (age 21 years or younger at initial diagnosis), relapsed or refractory after at least 2 prior regimens.

Dose: Adult, Elderly: Safety/efficacy not established.

Child: Age 1 year and over, 52mg/m2 BSA by IV infusion over 2 hours daily for 5 consecutive days; repeat every 2-6 weeks for 2 treatment cycles (no improvement, assess risk benefit). Limited experience with more than 3 treatment cycles. Children under 20kg, consider infusion time of longer than 2 hours to reduce symptoms of anxiety and irritability and to avoid unduly high max. clofarabine conc. Under 1 year, no dose recommendation.

Renal Impairment: Caution. CrCl (mL/min) 30-60, reduce dose by 50%. Severe, contraindicated.

Hepatic Impairment: Mild/moderate, caution. Severe, contraindicated.

Interactions: Effect of Other Drugs on Clofarabine: *Increased renal toxicity risk, avoid*: Nephrotoxic drugs or eliminated by tubular excretion (NSAIDs, amphotericin B, methotrexate, aminoglycosides, organoplatines, foscarnet, pentamidine, ciclosporin, tacrolimus, aciclovir,

13.1.3　Antimetabolites

valganciclovir). *Co-admin avoid*: Hepatotoxic drugs. *Co-admin monitor*: Drugs affecting BP or cardiac function.

SP: *Monitor*, blood, platelet counts, renal function, hepatic function (increased creatinine, liver enzymes, bilirubin, discontinue), respiratory status, BP, fluid balance, weight. Bone marrow suppression. Haemorrhage (cerebral, GI, pulmonary) (fatal), hepatitis, hepatic failure (fatal). Enterocolitis. Admin IV fluids to reduce effects of tumour lysis. Prophylactic steroids, 100mg/m2 hydrocortisone (days 1-3) may prevent Systemic Inflammatory Response Syndrome (SIRS) or capillary leak; discontinue if occurs. Hyperuricaemia expected, consider prophylactic allopurinol. Vomiting and/or diarrhoea, avoid dehydration. Renal failure (including acute) as result of infections, sepsis, tumour lysis syndrome; discontinue as needed.

Pregnancy, Lactation: Pregnancy, should not be used (especially first trimester) unless clearly necessary. Inform of possible hazard to foetus. Women of child-bearing potential and sexually active males to ensure adequate contraception. Lactation, contraindicated.

ADR: See Notes below.

Notes: See 13.1.3 Anti-Metabolites.

▼ **Evoltra Parenteral 1mg/mL** *(SANOFI)* A. HOS.
Price, 20mg, €1585.42 (PTW).
Infusion, clofarabine (20mL). Clear practically colourless soln; pH 4.5-7.5. Conc for soln. *Sodium 180mg/vial*.

Cytarabine

ATC Code: L01BC01. **Sport:** Permitted.
Driving: Caution, intrathecal.

Indications: Induction of remission and/or maintenance in leukaemia (AML, ALL, ANLL, CML, erythroleukaemia, blast crises of CML, non-Hodgkin lymphoma) *(Cytarabine Hospira, TEVA)*. Lymphomatous meningitis (intrathecal treatment) *(DepoCyte)*.

Dose: Adult: *Cytarabine (Hospira, TEVA)*, admin IV or SC only; NOT for intrathecal admin. *Remission induction*, continuous dosing, 2mg/kg/day by rapid IV injection (10 days); no response, increase to 4mg/kg/day* OR 0.5-1mg/kg by IV infusion over 1-24 hours (10 days), then 2mg/kg/day*. Intermittent dosing, 3-5mg/kg/day IV (5 consecutive days); repeat at 3-9 day intervals*. Acute leukaemia, 200mg/m2 been given by continuous IV infusion for 5-7 days at 2-4 week intervals. Maintenance, 1-1.5mg/kg IV or SC once or twice weekly. *(until therapeutic response or toxicity observed). *High dose* (Cytarabine TEVA), monotherapy or combination, 2-3g/m2 by IV infusion over 1-3 hours every 12 hours for 2-6 days (12 doses per cycle); max 36g/m2.

DepoCyte Intrathecal, lymphomatous meningitis, *induction*, 50mg every 14 days for 2 doses (weeks 1, 3), then *consolidation*, 50mg (weeks 5, 7, 9) then 50mg (week 13); then *maintenance*, 50mg every 28 days (weeks 17, 21, 25, 29). Neurotoxicity, reduce to 25mg; if persists, discontinue. *Admin*, slow injection (1-5 minutes) directly into CSF; start **all** patients on dexamethasone 4mg twice daily (oral or IV) for 5 days starting on day of first injection.

Child: *Cytarabine (Hospira, TEVA)*, children tolerate higher doses than adults; where dose range is stated, use higher dose; infants, no data. *DepoCyte*, under 18 years, not recommended.

Hepatic Impairment: Caution.

CI: *Cytarabine (Hospira, TEVA)*, drug-induced bone marrow suppression (only if benefit outweighs risk), non-malignant disease (except immunosuppression). *DepoCyte*, meningeal infection.

Interactions: Effect of Other Drugs on Cytarabine: *Increased neurotoxicity risk (DepoCyte)*: Other neurotoxic chemotherapeutics, cranial or spinal irradiation.

Effect of Cytarabine on Other Drugs: Cardiac glycosides: *GI absorption reduced*. Gentamicin, flucytosine: *Effect antagonised*.

SP: *Cytarabine (Hospira, TEVA)*, anaphylaxis; severe (fatal) CNS, GI, pulmonary toxicity; hyperuricaemia. Rapid IV injection, nausea, vomiting may occur for several hours afterwards; less severe with infusion. *DepoCyte*, dexamethasone reduces arachnoiditis symptoms. Neurotoxicity (blindness, myelopathy). Infectious meningitis, hydrocephalus. Blockage or reduced CSF flow, increased neurotoxicity risk. Systemic effects may occur.

DepoCyte particles are similar in size and appearance to WBCs; caution CSF laboratory examination.

Pregnancy, Lactation: Pregnancy, exclude before initiation; use only if benefit outweighs risk (can harm foetus, mainly first trimester). Males and females to ensure adequate contraception. Lactation, not recommended.

ADR: See Notes below.

Notes: See 13.1.3 Anti-Metabolites.

Cytarabine (Hospira) Parenteral *(Hospira)* A.
Price, (1) 100mg/1mL, €14.82. 100mg/5mL, €14.94. 1g/10mL, €32.70.
Injection, cytarabine. Aqueous soln.
Cytarabine TEVA Parenteral *(TEVA)* A.
Price, (1) 1g/10mL, €31.39; 2g/20mL, €62.77 (PTW).
Injection/infusion, cytarabine 100mg/mL. Clear colourless (pale-yellow) soln. **Store:** Below 25 deg C; do not (refrigerate, freeze).
DepoCyte Intrathecal *(Mundipharma)* A. HOS.
Price, 50mg (1) €1643.87 (PTW).
Injection, cytarabine 10mg/mL. White (off-white) susp. **Store:** Refrigerate; do not freeze.

Decitabine

ATC Code: L01BC08. **Sport:** Permitted.
Driving: Moderate influence (anaemia).

Indications: Treatment (adults), newly diagnosed de novo or secondary acute myeloid leukaemia and not candidates for standard induction chemotherapy.

Dose: Adult, Elderly: 20mg/m2 BSA daily (max.) for 5 consecutive days (1 treatment cycle); max 100mg/m2 per cycle. Repeat cycle every 4 weeks; minimum 4 cycles. After 4 cycles if haematological values have not returned to pre-treatment levels or disease progression, consider patient a non-responder; consider alternative. *Admin*, by IV infusion over 1 hour; central venous catheter not needed.

Renal Impairment: Need for dose adjustment not evaluated. CrCl (mL/min), below 30, caution.

Hepatic Impairment: If hepatic function worsens, monitor carefully.

Interactions: Effect of Other Drugs on Decitabine: *Co-admin caution:* Medicinals activated by sequential phosphorylation (cytidine deaminase).

SP: Pre-medication to prevent nausea and vomiting, not routinely recommended; can be used if needed. Manage myelosuppression, related adverse events. Cardiac disease, safety/efficacy not established. Interstitial lung disease reported.

Pregnancy, Lactation: Pregnancy, not recommended. If used during pregnancy counsel patient regarding the potential hazard to the foetus. Lactation, contraindicated.

ADR: See Notes below.

Notes: See 13.1.3 Anti-Metabolites.

Dacogen Parenteral 50mg *(Janssen-Cilag)* A.
Price, not published by company.
Infusion, decitabine 5mg/mL. White (almost) powder for conc for soln. *Potassium 0.5mmoL (39mg/dose; essentially potassium-free), sodium 0.29mmoL per vial*. **Store:** Below 25 deg C.

Fludarabine

ATC Code: L01BB05. **Sport:** Permitted.
Driving: Fatigue, weakness, visual disturbances, confusion, agitation, seizures.

Indications: B-cell chronic lymphocytic leukaemia (CLL). First-line, advanced disease (adults), Rai stages III/IV (Binet stage C), or Rai stages I/II (Binet stage A/B).

Dose: Adult: ORAL, 40mg/m2 BSA daily for 5 consecutive days every 28 days (dose corresponds to 1.6 times the IV dose of fludarabine per day). *Admin*, oral tabs with or without food; swallow whole with water; do not chew or break.
PARENTERAL (IV only), 25mg/m2 BSA daily for 5 consecutive days every 28-days. *Admin*, dilute in 0.9% NaCl by IV bolus OR by IV infusion over approx. 30 minutes. Avoid paravenous admin.

Elderly: Over 75 years, caution; over 65 years, as for Renal below.

Renal Impairment: CrCl (mL/min) 30-70, reduce dose by up to 50% with haematological monitoring; below 30, contraindicated.

Hepatic Impairment: Caution.

CI: Decompensated haemolytic anaemia.

Interactions: Effect of Other Drugs on Fludarabine: *Co-admin not recommended:* Pentostatin (deoxycoformycin) (fatal pulmonary toxicity). *Efficacy reduced:* Dipyridamole, other adenosine uptake inhibitors.

SP: Autoimmune reactions (life-threatening, fatal), monitor (signs of haemolysis, discontinue). High dose IV, associated with severe neurological effects (blindness, coma, death). Leucoencephalopathy (acute toxic or reversible posterior) may be irreversible, life-threatening; if suspected, discontinue. Transfusion-associated graft-versus-host disease, observed after transfusion of non-irradiated blood (fatal); if on or have received treatment, use only irradiated blood. New, worsening or flare up of pre-existing skin cancer lesions. Severe bone marrow impairment, immunodeficiency, opportunistic infection, caution. Nausea/vomiting incidence higher with oral than IV. If resistant to fludarabine, usually resistant to chlorambucil. Tumour lysis syndrome (large tumour burdens); consider hospitalisation for first treatment course.

Pregnancy, Lactation: Pregnancy, use only if clearly necessary; potential to cause foetal harm; avoid becoming pregnant. Women of child-bearing potential and males to ensure adequate contraception during and for 6 months after treatment. Lactation, contraindicated; excreted into breast milk; potential for serious adverse reactions in breast-fed infants.

ADR: See Notes below.

Notes: See 13.1.3 Anti-Metabolites.

Fludara 10mg *(SANOFI)* A. HT.
Price, (15) €384.83. (20) €508.11.
Tablet, fludarabine phosphate. Salmon-pink cap-shaped. Marked LN in regular hexagon. *Lactose. Store:* Original pack to protect (moisture).

Fludara Parenteral 25mg/mL *(SANOFI)* A. HOS.
Price, 50mg (5) €385.75 (PTW).
Injection or infusion, fludarabine phosphate 50mg. Powder for soln.

Fluorouracil

ATC Code: L01BC02. **Sport:** Permitted.
Driving: Unlikely to impair.

Indications: *Topical* treatment, superficial pre-malignant and malignant skin lesions; keratoses (senile, actinic, arsenic); keratoacanthoma, Bowen's disease, superficial basal-cell carcinoma. Palliative treatment, deep, penetrating or nodular basal cell and squamous cell carcinomas. *Parenteral* management of common malignancies (colon, breast).

Dose: Adult, Elderly: TOPICAL, apply cream thinly once or twice daily to lesions; occlusive dressing not essential (malignant lesions use with occlusive dressing where applicable); usually for 3-4 weeks. Severe discomfort, use topical steroid cream. Avoid contact with mucous membranes. Max. treatment area 500cm2 at any one time. PARENTERAL, max. 0.8-1g/day calculated according to body weight. *IV infusion,* 15mg/kg (max. 1g per infusion) over 4 hours OR infuse daily dose over 30-60 minutes or continuous infusion over 24 hours. Total dose 12-15g. *IV injection,* 12mg/kg/day for 3 days; no evidence of toxicity, 6mg/kg on alternate days for further 3 doses OR 15mg/kg as single injection once weekly. *Intra-arterial infusion,* 5-7.5mg/kg/day by 24-hour continuous intra-arterial infusion. Use standard dose in combination with radiation.

Renal Impairment: Parenteral, caution.

Hepatic Impairment: As for Renal above.

CI: Seriously debilitated, bone marrow depression after radiotherapy, treatment with other antineoplastics, non-malignant disease *(parenteral).*

Interactions: Effect of Other Drugs on Fluorouracil: *Co-admin contraindicated:* Brivudine, sorivudine and analogues. *Co-admin caution:* Drugs affecting dihydropyrimidine dehydrogenase activity.

Effect of Fluorouracil on Other Drugs: Warfarin: *Monitor INR or prothrombin time; adjust dose.*

SP: *Topical,* wash hands after application. Systemic absorption with excessive use/area, presence of ulceration. *Normal response,* early and severe inflammatory phases (erythema), a nephrotic phase (skin erosion) then healing (epithelialisation); response may be severe (pain, blistering, ulceration). Increased inflammatory response with occlusion. Avoid exposure to UV-radiation. *Systemic,* initiate in hospital, in isolation to prevent systemic infection. Oral ulceration, GI side effects, discontinue. Jaundice, chest pain during treatment, heart disease, caution.

Pregnancy, Lactation: Contraindicated. *Topical,* pregnancy, not for use; lactation, stop drug or stop breastfeeding.

ADR: *Topical,* erythema, pre-existing lesions may become apparent, exposure to sunlight may increase reaction intensity. *Systemic,* see Notes below.

Notes: See 13.1.3 Anti-Metabolites.

Efudix 5% Cream *(Meda)* A. GMS.
Price, (20g) €20.80. (40g) €41.60.
Topical cream, fluorouracil 5% w/w. Smooth white opaque. *Stearyl alcohol, propylene glycol, parabens.* **Store:** Below 30 deg C.

Fluorouracil (Accord) Parenteral *(Accord)* A.
Price, 50mg/mL (1) 5mL, €3.99. 10mL, €7.99. 20mL, €15.95. 50mL, €39.88. 100mL, €71.99.
Injection or infusion, fluorouracil 50mg/mL. Clear colourless soln. **Store:** Below 25 deg C; do not (refrigerate, freeze).

Fluorouracil (Hospira) Parenteral *(Hospira)* A.
Price, (1) 250mg/10mL, €8.24. 500mg/20mL, €6.59. 2.5g/100mL, €18.08.
Injection, fluorouracil sodium 25mg/mL. Clear colourless (slightly yellow) soln. *Sodium 160mg/1g dose.* **Store:** Below 25 deg C; do not (refrigerate, freeze); outer carton to protect (light).

Folinic Acid (Calcium Folinate, Calcium Leucovorin)

ATC Code: V03AF03. **Sport:** Permitted.
Driving: Unlikely to impair.

Indications: To diminish toxicity and counteract action of folic acid antagonists (methotrexate) (calcium folinate rescue). Megaloblastic anaemia due to folate deficiency.

Dose: Adult, Elderly: PARENTERAL, calcium folinate rescue, methotrexate protocol dictates dosage. First dose usually 15mg (6-12mg/m2) admin 12-24 hours (max. 24 hours) after commencing methotrexate infusion; repeat 6-hourly for 72 hours with maintenance of high urine output, urinary alkalinisation. Calculate additional dose based on residual methotrexate.
Folic acid antagonist antidote, *trimetrexate,* prevention, IV 20mg/m2 for 5-10 minutes 6-hourly OR oral 4 doses of 20mg/m2 at equal time intervals every day during treatment, then for 72 hours after last trimetrexate dose; trimetrexate doses above 90mg/m2 without calcium folinate, after stopping trimetrexate admin 40mg/m2 calcium folinate IV 6-hourly for 3 days. *Trimethoprim,* after stopping trimethoprim, 3-10mg/day calcium folinate until normal blood count. *Pyrimethamine,* high dose or prolonged low-dose, 5-50mg/m2 calcium folinate. IV or IM; IV admin. max. 160mg/min due to calcium content of soln; not for intrathecal use.
ORAL, megaloblastic anaemia, 10-20mg/day.

Child: As for Adult above. Folate deficiency, under 12 years, 0.25mg/kg/day.

CI: Pernicious anaemia, other anaemias due to Vitamin B12 deficiency.

Interactions: Effect of Other Drugs on Folinic Acid: *Not recommended:* Admixture with other drugs in same syringe.

Effect of Folinic Acid on Other Drugs: Anti-epileptics (phenobarbital, phenytoin, primidone, succinimides): *Plasma levels decreased; increased seizure risk.* 5-Fluorouracil: *Toxicity enhanced (reduce dose).* Folic acid antagonists (cotrimoxazole, pyrimethamine): *Efficacy reduced or neutralised.*

SP: May mask pernicious anaemia, other anaemias (as result of Vitamin B12 deficiency). Many cytotoxics lead to macrocytosis; not to be treated with folinic acid. Combination with methotrexate, avoid excessive doses as methotrexate activity may be impaired.

Pregnancy, Lactation: If treated with methotrexate (or other folate antagonists) despite pregnancy or lactation, there are no limitations to use of calcium folinate to diminish toxicity or counteract effects. Lactation, calcium folinate can be used if considered necessary.

ADR: See Notes below.

Notes: See 13.1.3 Anti-Metabolites.

13.1.3　Antimetabolites

Folinic Acid 15mg, Parenteral *(Hospira)* A.
Price, tabs (10) €48.28. Injection 10mg/mL (1) €19.05.
Tablet, folinic acid (as calcium folinate). Yellowish-white round flat u/c scored. Marked CF. *Lactose.*
Injection, as above 10mg/mL. Clear slightly yellow. *Sodium 3.05mg/mL.*

Gemcitabine

ATC Code: L01BC05. **Sport:** Permitted.
Driving: Somnolence especially with alcohol.
Indications: Locally advanced or metastatic, non-small cell lung cancer (NSCLC) (with cisplatin), adenocarcinoma of pancreas, bladder cancer (with cisplatin), epithelial ovarian cancer (with carboplatin), unresectable locally recurrent or relapsed metastatic breast cancer (with paclitaxel).
Dose: Adult, Elderly: *NSCLC* (monotherapy) 1000mg/m2 BSA once weekly for 3 weeks, then 1-week rest (4-week cycle) then repeat; (combination) 1250mg/m2 (days 1 and 8) of each 21-day cycle OR 1000mg/m2 (days 1, 8 and 15) of each 28-day cycle *(Gemcitabine Hospira)* with cisplatin. *Pancreatic cancer,* 1000mg/m2 BSA once weekly for up to 7 weeks followed by 1-week rest; subsequent cycles, once weekly for 3 consecutive weeks out of every 4 weeks. *Bladder cancer,* 1000mg/m2 admin (days 1, 8 and 15) of each 28-day cycle followed by cisplatin. *Ovarian cancer* (combination) 1000mg/m2 (days 1 and 8) of each 21-day cycle followed by carboplatin. *Breast cancer,* paclitaxel followed by gemcitabine 1250mg/m2 (days 1 and 8) of each 21-day cycle.
Renal Impairment: Caution, no data.
Hepatic Impairment: As for Renal above.
Interactions: Effect of Other Drugs on Gemcitabine: *Gemcitabine Hospira: Co-admin not recommended:* Oral anticoagulants, warfarin (potential increased anticoagulant effect; increase INR monitoring), phenytoin (decreased phenytoin GI absorption, increased exacerbation of convulsion risk; toxicity enhancement risk or reduced efficacy of gemcitabine due to increased hepatic metabolism); ciclosporin, tacrolimus (excessive immunosuppression with lymphoproliferation risk).
SP: Radiotherapy co-admin: Concurrent, or 7 or less days apart, optimum regimen not determined for all tumour types; non-concurrent, toxicity not enhanced (radiation recall). Increased toxicity (prolonged infusion time, increased dosing frequency). Exacerbation risk (liver metastases, hepatitis, alcoholism, liver cirrhosis). Microangiopathic haemolytic anaemia, discontinue. Pulmonary oedema, interstitial pneumonitis, ARDS (risk higher with lung cancer, lung metastases). Posterior reversible encephalopathy syndrome, capillary leak syndrome, haemolytic uraemic syndrome.
Pregnancy, Lactation: Pregnancy, avoid; use if benefit outweighs risk. Women of childbearing potential and men to ensure adequate contraception. Lactation, contraindicated.
ADR: See Notes below.
Notes: See 13.1.3 Anti-Metabolites.

Gemcitabine (Accord) Parenteral *(Accord)* A.
Price, 100mg/mL (1) 2mL, €41.99. 10mL, €209.95. 15mL, €314.93. 20mL, €419.99.
Infusion, gemcitabine HCl 100mg/mL. Clear colourless (slightly-yellow) conc for soln.
Gemcitabine Parenteral *(TEVA)* A.
Price, not published by company.
Infusion, gemcitabine HCl 200mg, 1g, 2g. White (off-white) aggregate. *Sodium 3.56mg (17.81mg)/200mg (1g) vial.*
Infusion concentrate, as above 40mg/mL. Clear colourless (pale-yellow) soln. *Sodium 3.95mg/mL, ethanol.*
Gemcitabine (Hospira) Parenteral *(Hospira)* A.
Price, not published by company.
Infusion, gemcitabine HCl 38mg/mL (1g, 2g). White (off-white) powder for soln. *Sodium 3.5mg (17.5mg) (35mg)/200mg (1g) (2g) vial.* Conc 200mg, 1g, 2g. Clear colourless (light straw-coloured). *Sodium up to 0.46mg/mL.*
Gemcitabine TEVA Parenteral *(TEVA)* A.
Price, not published by company.
Infusion, gemcitabine HCl 40mg/mL (200mg, 1g, 2g). Clear colourless (pale-yellow) conc for soln. *Sodium 3.85mg/mL, ethanol anhydrous 395mg/mL.*

Mercaptopurine

ATC Code: L01BB02. **Sport:** Permitted.
Driving: No detrimental effect predicted.
Indications: ALL *(both brands),* AML, chronic granulocytic leukaemia *(Puri-Nethol).*
Dose: Adult: Usually oral 2.5mg/kg/day or 25-75mg/m2/day BSA; reduce with reduced/absent Thiopurine Methyl Transferase enzyme activity. Combination (xanthine oxidase inhibitors), see Interactions below.
Elderly: Monitor renal/hepatic function.
Child: As for Adult above. See manufacturers Full Prescribing Information.
Renal Impairment: Consider dose reduction; monitor for dose-related adverse events.
Hepatic Impairment: Hepatotoxic, monitor LFTs weekly during treatment. Jaundice, discontinue.
CI: No absolute contraindications.
Interactions: Effect of Other Drugs on 6-Mercaptopurine: *Co-admin, reduce dose to one-quarter (does not apply to tioguanine):* Allopurinol, other xanthine oxidase inhibitors. *Cross-resistance:* 6-thioguanine. *Reduce dose:* Other myelosuppressives (primary or secondary). *Co-admin caution:* Drugs inhibiting TPMT enzyme (olsalazine, mesalazine, sulfasalazine).
Effect of 6-Mercaptopurine on Other Drugs: Warfarin: *Inhibition of anticoagulant effect.*
SP: Risk to lymphoproliferative disorders, other malignancies especially skin (melanoma, non-melanoma); multiple immunosuppressants increase risk of Epstein-Barr virus (EBV)-associated lymphoproliferative disorders. Macrophage activation syndrome (life-threatening) may develop with autoimmune conditions. Bone marrow suppression; take full blood counts daily during remission induction and regularly (including platelets) during maintenance. During remission induction (AML), there may be a period of bone marrow aplasia (adequate support facilities important). Renal transplants, consider dose reduction. Chromosomal aberrations, acute leukaemias, Tumour lysis syndrome. Inherited deficiency of TPMT may be unusually sensitive to myelosuppressive effect. Cross resistance usually exists between 6-mercaptopurine and 6-thioguanine. Azathioprine is a pro-drug of 6-mercaptopurine.
Pregnancy, Lactation: Pregnancy, avoid particularly first trimester; use if benefit outweighs risk. Both males and women of childbearing potential to ensure adequate contraception. Lactation, not recommended.
ADR: See Notes below.
Notes: See 13.1.3 Anti-Metabolites.

Puri-Nethol 50mg *(Aspen)* A. GMS.
Price, (25) €70.20.
Tablet, mercaptopurine. Pale-yellow round scored (facilitates breaking). Marked GX and EX2 either side of score. *Lactose.*
Xaluprine Oral Susp *(Nova)* A. GMS.
Price, 20mg/mL (100mL) €232.20.
Oral susp, mercaptopurine monohydrate 20mg/mL. Pink-brown. *Parabens, aspartame, sucrose.* **Store:** Below 25 deg C; tightly closed.

Nelarabine

ATC Code: L01BB07. **Sport:** Permitted.
Driving: Caution.
Indications: T-cell acute lymphoblastic leukaemia (T-ALL) and T-cell lymphoblastic lymphoma (T-LBL) (not responded or relapsed following at least 2 chemotherapy regimen).
Dose: Adult, Elderly: 1500mg/m2 BSA IV over 2 hours (days 1, 3 and 5); repeat every 21 days. See SP below. Nelarabine must not be diluted prior to admin. *Elderly,* 65 years and over, increased neurological events.
Child: Age 21 years and under, 650mg/m2 IV over 1 hour for 5 consecutive days; repeat every 21 days (age 16-21 years may use Adult regimen depending on decision of physician). Under 4 years, limited data. See SP below.
Renal Impairment: CrCl (mL/min) below 50, monitor closely for toxicities.
Hepatic Impairment: Caution.
Interactions: Effect of Other Drugs on Nelarabine: *Co-*

350

admin not recommended: Intrathecal therapy and/or craniospinal irradiation, adenosine deaminase inhibitors (pentostatin).

SP: NOTE: Severe neurological events reported; neurotoxicity is *dose-limiting*; intrathecal chemotherapy or craniospinal irradiation increases risk. Events grade 2 or more, discontinue. Other toxicities (haematological), delay dosing. CNS effects (convulsions, peripheral neuropathy ranging from numbness and paraesthesia to motor weakness and paralysis), demyelinations, ascending peripheral neuropathies similar to Guillain-Barre Syndrome. Monitor complete blood counts regularly. Ensure IV hydration for management of hyperuricaemia (tumour lysis syndrome risk); hyperuricaemia risk, use allopurinol.

Pregnancy, Lactation: Pregnancy, use only if clearly necessary. Inform patient of possible risk to foetus in case of pregnancy. Women of childbearing potential and men to ensure adequate contraception during and for at least 3 months after treatment. Lactation, not recommended; not known if excreted in breast milk.

ADR: See Notes below.

Notes: See 13.1.3 Anti-Metabolites.

▼ **Atriance Parenteral 5mg/mL** *(Novartis)* A. HOS.
Price, (6) €1877.30 (PTW).
Infusion, nelarabine. Clear colourless soln. *Sodium 1.725mg/mL.*

Pemetrexed

ATC Code: L01BA04. **Sport:** Permitted.
Driving: Fatigue.

Indications: Unresectable malignant pleural mesothelioma (chemotherapy-naïve); locally advanced or metastatic non-small cell lung cancer (NSCLC) (monotherapy with cisplatin).

Dose: Adult, Elderly: COMBINATION, 500mg/m2 BSA IV over 10 minutes (day 1) of each 21-day cycle, then cisplatin; ensure adequate anti-emetic treatment, hydration.
MONOTHERAPY, after prior chemotherapy, 500mg/m2 BSA on day 1 of each 21-day cycle. Admin corticosteroid (4mg dexamethasone twice daily) to avoid skin reaction; admin folic acid and Vitamin B12 to reduce toxicity.

Renal Impairment: CrCl (mL/min) below 45, not recommended; 45-79, avoid NSAIDs (ibuprofen) or aspirin (above 1.3g/day) for 2 days before, on day, and 2 days after treatment.

Hepatic Impairment: Bilirubin above 1.5xULN and/or transaminase above 3xULN (hepatic metastases absent) or above 5xULN (hepatic metastases present), no data.

Interactions: Effect of Other Drugs on Pemetrexed: *Co-admin not recommended*: Yellow fever vaccine. *Caution, delayed or decreased clearance*: Nephrotoxic drugs (aminoglycosides, loop diuretics, ciclosporin), substances tubularly excreted (probenecid, penicillin); NSAIDs (monitor for toxicity, myelosuppression, GI toxicity). **Effect of Pemetrexed on Other Drugs:** Oral anticoagulants: *Monitor INR.*

SP: Myelosuppression is a *dose-limiting toxicity*. Avoid NSAIDs with long elimination half-life (piroxicam, rofecoxib) for at least 5 days before, on day, or for 2 days after treatment (with mild/moderate renal insufficiency). Caution, severe dehydration. Serious cardiovascular events (MI) and cerebrovascular events. Genetically damaging. Radiation pneumonitis, caution; radiation recall. Effect of third-space fluid (pleural effusion, ascites) not fully defined.

Pregnancy, Lactation: Women of childbearing potential *and* males to ensure adequate contraception during and for 6 months after treatment. Lactation, contraindicated.

ADR: See Notes below.

Notes: See 13.1.3 Anti-Metabolites.

Alimta Parenteral 500mg *(Lilly)* A.
Price, 500mg (1) €1341.86.
Infusion, pemetrexed disodium 25mg/mL. White (light- or green-yellow) powder for conc for soln. *Sodium 54mg.*

Raltitrexed

ATC Code: L01BA03. **Sport:** Permitted.
Driving: Caution.

Indications: Palliative treatment, advanced colorectal cancer.

Dose: Adult, Elderly: IV as single short infusion 3mg/m2 BSA over 15 minutes; absence of toxicity, repeat every 3 weeks. *Elderly*, caution.

Renal Impairment: CrCl (mL/min) 55-65, 75% of dose every 4 weeks; 25-54, 50% of dose every 4 weeks; below 25, not recommended.

Hepatic Impairment: Mild to moderate, caution. Severe, jaundice or decompensated liver disease, not recommended.

SP: Depressed bone marrow, poor condition, prior radiotherapy, caution. Elderly, monitor (diarrhoea, mucositis).

Pregnancy, Lactation: Pregnancy, avoid. Women of childbearing potential and males to ensure adequate contraception during and for 6 months after treatment. Exclude pregnancy before initiating. Lactation, not recommended.

ADR: See Notes below.

Notes: See 13.1.3 Anti-Metabolites.

Tomudex Parenteral *(Hospira)* A.
Price, 2mg (1) €166.98.
Injection, raltitrexed 2mg. White (cream) solid powder cake.

Tegafur, Gimeracil, Oteracil

ATC Code: L01BC53. **Sport:** Permitted.
Driving: Fatigue, dizziness, blurred vision, nausea.

Indications: Treatment, advanced gastric cancer in combination.

Dose: Adult, Elderly: 25mg/m2 BSA (expressed as tegafur content) twice daily (morning, evening) for 21 consecutive days, then 7 days rest (1 treatment cycle) (with cisplatin). Repeat cycle every 4 weeks. Do not replace doses omitted for toxicity; vomiting, do not replace this dose. *Admin*, with water 1 hour before or 1 hour after a meal.

Child: Under 18 years, not recommended.

Renal Impairment: CrCl (mL/min) 30-50, 20mg/m2 BSA twice daily (expressed as tegafur content); below 30, only if benefit outweighs risk. End-stage renal disease requiring dialysis, contraindicated.

CI: Severe unexpected reactions to fluoropyrimidine therapy, dehydrogenase (DPD) deficiency, severe bone marrow suppression, cisplatin contraindicated.

Interactions: Effect of Other Drugs on Tegafur, Gimeracil, Oteracil Combination: *Co-admin contraindicated*: Fluoropyrimidines (capecitabine, f-fluorouracil, flucytosine), within 4 weeks of other DPD inhibitors (sorivudine, brivudine). *Co-admin avoid*: CYP2A6 inhibitors, allopurinol. *Caution*: Folinate/folinic acid (may enhance 5-fluorouracil activity); nitroimidazoles (metronidazole, misonidazole), methotrexate, cimetidine (may increase toxicity); clozapine (may increase haematological toxicity) **Effect of Tegafur, Gimeracil, Oteracil Combination on Other Drugs:** Oral coumarin-derivative anticoagulants: *Monitor prothrombin time or INR (adjust dose).* Phenytoin: *Increased plasma conc; monitor for phenytoin toxicity.*

SP: Monitor haematology, liver/renal function, serum electrolytes frequently. Combination with cisplatin, ensure pre-treatment hyperhydration. Anti-emetics and anti-diarrhoeals (loperamide) recommended. Dose-limiting toxicities (diarrhoea, dehydration); most reversible and can by managed symptomatically (fluid, electrolytes) or interrupt dose or reduce. Increased lacrimation, dry eye, acquired dacryostenosis, ensure early detection.

Pregnancy, Lactation: Contraindicated.

ADR: See Notes below.

Notes: See 13.1.3 Anti-Metabolites.

Teysuno 15mg, 20mg *(Nordic)* A. HT.
Price, 15mg (126) €389.52.10. 20mg (84) €351.78.
Capsule, tegafur 15(20)mg, gimeracil 4.35(5.8)mg, oteracil 11.8(15.8)mg. Hard opaque. 15mg: White/brown. Marked TC448. 20mg: White/white. Marked TC442. *Lactose.*

Tioguanine

ATC Code: L01BB03. **Sport:** Permitted.
Driving: No detrimental effect predicted.

Indications: Treatment, acute leukaemias (myeloblastic, lymphoblastic).

Dose: Adult, Elderly: Usually 60-200mg/m2 BSA per day. Use at any stage prior to maintenance in short term cycles

13.1.4   Plant Alkaloids, Other Natural Products

(induction, consolidation, intensification); not recommended for use during maintenance or long-term continuous treatment (liver toxicity risk). *Admin*, oral.

Child: As for Adult above with correction for body surface area (BSA).

Renal Impairment: Consider dose reduction.

Hepatic Impairment: As for Renal above.

CI: No absolute contraindications.

Interactions: Effect of Other Drugs on Tioguanine: *Cross-resistance*: Mercaptopurine. *Increased myelosuppression risk*: Other myelotoxic substances, radiation therapy.

SP: Hepatotoxicity (hepatic veno-occlusive disease e.g. hyperbilirubinaemia, tender hepatomegaly, weight gain due to fluid retention, ascites) or signs of portal hypertension (splenomegaly, thrombocytopenia, oesophageal varices), particularly in males, monitor liver function. Patients with TPMT enzyme deficiency or NUDT15 mutation, increased risk of severe tioguanine toxicity (reduce dose); enzyme deficiency (Lesch-Nyhan syndrome), may be drug resistant. Myelosuppressive, monitor frequent full blood counts. Limit exposure to sunlight, UV light. Cross resistance between tioguanine and mercaptopurine.

Pregnancy, Lactation: Pregnancy, avoid particularly first trimester; use if benefit outweighs risk. Both males and women of childbearing potential to ensure adequate contraception. Lactation, not recommended.

ADR: See SP above.

Notes: See 13.1.3 Anti-Metabolites. See Mercaptopurine above.

Lanvis 40mg *(Aspen)* A. GMS.
Price, (25) €162.00.
Tablet, tioguanine. White (off-white) round scored (facilitates breaking). Marked T40. *Lactose*. **Store:** Below 25 deg C; original pack to protect (light, moisture).

Trifluridine, Tipiracil

ATC Code: L01BC59. **Sport:** Permitted.
Driving: Minor influence; fatigue, dizziness, malaise.

Indications: Treatment, metastatic colorectal cancer (previously treated with or not candidates for available therapies).

Dose: Adult: Initially 35mg/m2 BSA* per dose admin twice daily on Days 1-5 and Days 8-12 of each 28-day cycle as long as benefit or until unacceptable toxicity. Max. 80mg/dose. Max. 3 dose reductions permitted to minimum 20mg/m2; dose escalation not permitted after reduction. *(calculated on body surface area; rounded to nearest 5mg). *Admin*, oral with glass of water 1 hour after finishing morning and evening meal.

Elderly: Age over 75 years, limited data.

Child: No relevant use.

Renal Impairment: CrCl (mL/min) 30 and above, no dose adjustment; below 30 or ESRD, not recommended (no data).

Hepatic Impairment: Mild, no adjustment; moderate or severe, not recommended (no data).

Interactions: Effect of Other Drugs on Trifluridine, Tipiracil: *Caution*: Medicinals interacting with transporters (CNT1, ENT1, ENT2), thymidine kinase substrates (zidovudine). *Tipiracil levels may be increased*: OCT2, MAT1 inhibitors.

SP: *Monitor*, complete blood counts prior to (initiation, each treatment cycle), then as needed; proteinuria (dipstick urinalysis) prior to initiation, during treatment. No dose adjustments based on race. Myelosuppression; serious infections reported. GI toxicity (nausea, vomiting, diarrhoea); delay or reduce dose; admin antiemetics, antidiarrhoeals, fluids and electrolytes. Moderate renal impairment, monitor (haematological toxicity).

Pregnancy, Lactation: Pregnancy, only if clinically indicated. Unknown if *Lonsurf* reduces hormonal contraceptive efficacy; use additional barrier contraceptive. Women (and men of partners) of childbearing potential to ensure highly effect contraception during and for 6 months after stopping drug. Lactation, discontinue during treatment.

ADR: See Notes below.

Notes: See 13.1.3 Anti-Metabolites.

352

▼ **Lonsurf Tablets** *(Servier)* A. HT.
Price, 15mg/6.14mg (20), €826.90; (60), €2559.29.
20mg/8.19mg (20), €1061.38; (60), €3263.04.
Tablet, trifluridine 15(20)mg, tipiracil hydrochloride 6.14(8.19)mg. Round f/c. Marked 102 and strength one side. 15/6.14mg: White. Marked 15. 20/8.19: Pale-red. Marked 20. *Lactose*.

13.1.4 - Plant Alkaloids, Other Natural Products

In This Chapter: *Cabazitaxel, docetaxel, etoposide, paclitaxel, trabectedin, vinblastine, vincristine, vinorelbine.*

Class Effects

CI: Hypersensitivity to any member of the class. Use in children under 18 years unless otherwise specified.

ADR: See Notes below. See manufacturers Full Prescribing Information.

Notes: See 13.1 Cytotoxic Drugs.

Cabazitaxel

ATC Code: L01CD04. **Sport:** Permitted.
Driving: Fatigue, dizziness.

Indications: Combination (corticosteroids), castration resistant metastatic prostate cancer (previous docetaxel).

Dose: Adult, Elderly: 25mg/m2 as 1-hour infusion every 3 weeks (with oral prednisone or prednisolone). Premedication, at least 30 minutes prior to each admin to include antihistamine (dexchlorpheniramine or diphenhydramine), corticosteroid (dexamethasone), H2-antagonist (ranitidine), oral or IV antiemetic prophylaxis. Prolonged neutropenia (febrile), diarrhoea, peripheral neuropathy, reduce to 20mg/m2. NOTE: Do not use PVC infusion containers and polyurethane infusion sets.

Child: No relevant use.

Renal Impairment: Impairment not requiring dialysis, no adjustment. ESRD no data, caution.

Hepatic Impairment: Severe (total bilirubin above 3xULN), contraindicated. Mild (total bilirubin between 1-1.5xULN or AST above 1.5xULN), reduce dose.

CI: Taxane hypersensitivity, neutrophils below 1500/mm3. Concomitant yellow fever vaccine.

Interactions: Effect of Other Drugs on Cabazitaxel: *Co-admin avoid (consider dose reduction with CYP3A inhibitors)*: Strong CYP3A inhibitors (ketoconazole, itraconazole, clarithromycin, indinavir, nefazodone, nelfinavir, ritonavir, saquinavir, telithromycin, voriconazole) or inducers (phenytoin, carbamazepine, rifampicin, rifabutin, rifapentine, phenobarbital), St John's Wort. *Co-admin caution*: Moderate CYP3A inhibitors

SP: GI toxicity (serious); diarrhoea more frequent with prior abdomino-pelvic radiation. Ensure adequate hydration; measure serum creatinine at baseline with blood count and if urinary output changes. Renal failure Grade 3, discontinue. Premedicate to reduce risk/severity of hypersensitivity reactions (severe); observe closely during first and second infusion; if it occurs, discontinue. Consider prophylactic G-CSF to reduce neutropenia risk. Monitor complete blood counts weekly (cycle 1), then before each treatment cycle; check Hb and haematocrit if there are signs/symptoms of anaemia or blood loss. Peripheral neuropathy (sensory and motor), consider dose adjustment. Tachycardia, atrial fibrillation risk, interstitial pneumonia or pneumonitis and interstitial lung disease (fatal) reported.

ADR: See Notes below.

Notes: See 13.1.4 Plant Alkaloids.

JEVTANA Parenteral 60mg *(SANOFI)* A. HOS.
Price, (1) €4113.64 (PTW).
Infusion, cabazitaxel 40mg/mL. Clear yellow (brownish-yellow) oily soln (conc); clear colourless solvent. *Ethanol*. **Store:** Below 30 deg C; do not refrigerate.

Docetaxel

ATC Code: L01CD02. **Sport:** Permitted.
Driving: Ethanol content may impair.

Indications: Breast cancer, operable (with doxorubicin + cyclophosphamide); locally advanced or metastatic (with doxorubicin); after cytotoxic therapy failure, monotherapy or (with capecitabine); where tumours overexpress HER2

Plant Alkaloids, Other Natural Products **13.1.4**

(with trastuzumab). Non-small cell lung cancer (NSCLC), locally advanced or metastatic (with cisplatin). Prostate cancer, hormone refractory metastatic (with prednisolone). Gastric adenocarcinoma (metastatic) and locally advanced squamous cell carcinoma of head and neck (with cisplatin + 5-fluorouracil).

Dose: Adult: *Breast cancer*, operable node- (positive, negative), 75mg/m2 after doxorubicin and cyclophosphamide every 3 weeks for 6 cycles; locally advanced or metastatic monotherapy 100mg/m2. Combination, see manufacturers Full Prescribing Information. *NSCLC*, no prior treatment, 75mg/m2 then cisplatin; after treatment failure, 75mg/m2 as single agent. *Prostate cancer*, 75mg/m2 with prednisolone. *Gastric adenocarcinoma*, 75mg/m2 as 1-hour infusion then cisplatin both on day 1 only, followed by 5-fluorouracil for 5 days; repeat every 3 weeks. *Head and neck cancer* as for gastric adenocarcinoma; repeat every 3 weeks for 4 cycles; admin radiotherapy on completion of chemotherapy.

Premedication, breast, NSCLC, gastric cancer, oral dexamethasone 16mg/day in divided doses for 3 days starting 1 day prior to docetaxel. Prostate, oral dexamethasone 8mg admin at 12 hours, 3 hours and 1 hour before infusion.

Renal Impairment: Severe, no data.

Hepatic Impairment: Elevated transaminases (ALT and/or AST) above 1.5xULN *and* ALP above 2.5xULN, reduce 75mg/m2. Serum bilirubin above ULN *and/or* ALT and AST above 3.5xULN *and* ALP above 6xULN, not recommended unless strictly indicated. Severe, contraindicated.

CI: Baseline neutrophils below 1500 cells/mm3.

Interactions: Effect of Other Drugs on Docetaxel: *Co-admin caution (clearance reduced; consider dose adjustment):* Potent CYP3A4 inhibitors (ketoconazole, itraconazole, clarithromycin, indinavir, nefazodone, nelfinavir, ritonavir, saquinavir, telithromycin, voriconazole). *Metabolism modified:* CYP3A4 inducers, inhibitors, substrates (ciclosporin, ketoconazole, erythromycin).

Effect of Docetaxel on Other Drugs: Carboplatin: *Clearance increased.*

SP: Premedication can reduce fluid retention (incidence, severity), hypersensitivity reactions. Neutropenia (most frequent adverse reaction), hypersensitivity especially during first and second infusion (hypotension, bronchospasm). Localised erythema of extremities, desquamation; pleural and pericardial effusion, ascites. Severe peripheral neurotoxicity, reduce dose. HF, monitor function. Cystoid macular oedema (discontinue). Adjuvant use in breast cancer, see manufacturers Full Prescribing Information.

Pregnancy, Lactation: Pregnancy, not recommended. Ensure adequate contraception (men and women) during treatment; men up to 6 months after treatment cessation. Lactation, stop breastfeeding for treatment duration.

ADR: See Notes below.

Notes: See 13.1.4 Plant Alkaloids.

Taxotere Conc Parenteral 20mg/mL *(SANOFI)* A.
Price, not published by company.
Infusion, docetaxel trihydrate (1mL, 4mL). Pale-yellow (brownish-yellow) conc for soln. *Ethanol anhydrous 395mg/1mL or 1.58g/4mL vial.*

Docetaxel Actavis Parenteral 20mg/mL *(Accord)* A.
Price, not published by company.
Infusion, docetaxel (1mL, 4mL, 7mL). Clear pale-yellow conc for soln. *Ethanol 400mg/mL.*

Etoposide

ATC Code: L01CB01. **Sport:** Permitted.
Driving: Fatigue, somnolence.
Indications: Hodgkin's disease, lymphosarcoma, AML, small cell lung cancer, resistant non-seminomatous testicular carcinoma.

Dose: Adult, Elderly: Usually 120-240mg/m2 daily for 5 consecutive days; above 200mg/day to be given in divided doses, twice daily; repeat at minimum 21-day intervals; adjust subsequent doses according to neutrophil count. Caps should be taken on empty stomach.

Renal Impairment: Monitor. CrCl (mL/min) 15-50, admin

75% of usual dose; below 15, consider further dose reduction.

Hepatic Impairment: Monitor. Severe, contraindicated.

Interactions: Effect of Other Drugs on Etoposide: *Increased etoposide exposure:* Ciclosporin. *Reduced clearance:* Cisplatin. *Increased clearance, reduced etoposide efficacy:* Phenytoin. *Possible displacement of etoposide from plasma binding:* Phenylbutazone, sodium salicylate, aspirin. *Cross resistance:* Anthracyclines.

Effect of Etoposide on Other Drugs: Warfarin: *Elevated INR, monitor.* Antiepileptics: *Decreased seizure control.*

SP: Before initiating, allow interval for bone marrow to recover following radio- and/or chemotherapy; control infection. Fatal myelosuppression reported; myelosuppression is *dose-limiting* toxicity. Respiratory dysfunction, caution. Acute leukaemia. Tumour lysis syndrome, cardiac arrhythmias, ischaemia/failure (in combination). Increased etoposide-associated toxicity in patients with low serum albumin. Hypotension (rapid infusion).

Pregnancy, Lactation: Not recommended. Women of child-bearing potential, advise to avoid pregnancy and of potential hazard to foetus.

ADR: See Notes below.

Notes: See 13.1.4 Plant Alkaloids.

Vepesid 50mg, 100mg *(BMS)* A. HT.
Price, 50mg (20) €143.28. 100mg (10) €125.18.
Capsule, etoposide. Soft gelatin opaque pink oval. *Parabens.*

Paclitaxel

ATC Code: L01CD01. **Sport:** Permitted.
Driving: Tiredness, dizziness.
Indications: Ovarian cancer, breast cancer, advanced non-small cell lung cancer (NSCLC), AIDs-related Kaposi's sarcoma (KS).

Dose: Adult, Elderly: *Ovarian cancer* first-line, 175mg/m2 BSA then cisplatin OR 135mg/m2 by IV infusion over 24-hours, then cisplatin; repeat at 3-week intervals; second-line, 175mg/m2 over 3-hours at 3-weekly intervals. *Breast cancer*, 175mg/m2 every 3 weeks for 4 courses following adjuvant therapy; first-line, 220mg/m2 admin 24 hours *after* doxorubicin repeated at 3-weekly intervals OR 175mg/m2 over 3-hours at 3-week intervals with trastuzumab; second-line, 175mg/m2 at 3-weekly intervals. *Advanced NSCLC*, 175mg/m2 then cisplatin at 3-week intervals. *AIDS-related KS*, 100mg/m2 every 2 weeks.

Premedication, corticosteroids (dexamethasone), antihistamines (diphenhydramine), H2-receptor antagonists (cimetidine, ranitidine) to prevent hypersensitivity reactions. *Admin*, using in-line filter; caution, extravasation; usually by 3-hour infusion unless otherwise stated.

Renal Impairment: No dose recommendation.

Hepatic Impairment: Mild to moderate, no dose recommendation. Severe not recommended.

CI: Macrogolglycerol ricinoleate hypersensitivity. Kaposi's sarcoma (concurrent, serious uncontrolled infection). Baseline neutrophils, platelets, see manufacturers Full Prescribing Information.

Interactions: Effect of Other Drugs on Paclitaxel: Ensure co-admin before other cytotoxics: Cisplatin (if admin after, greater myelosuppression). *Caution:* CYP2C8 or CYP3A4 inhibitors (erythromycin, fluoxetine, gemfibrozil, clopidogrel, cimetidine, ritonavir, saquinavir, indinavir, nelfinavir) or inducers (rifampicin, carbamazepine, phenytoin, phenobarbital, efavirenz, nevirapine). *Clearance reduced:* Nelfinavir, ritonavir (not indinavir).

Effect of Paclitaxel on Other Drugs: Doxorubicin: *Elimination reduced, allow 24-hour dosing interval.*

SP: Admin before cisplatin. Hypersensitivity reactions, discontinue; do not rechallenge. Bone marrow suppression, dose-dependent neutropenia. Severe cardiac conduction abnormalities, monitor; hypo-, hypertension, bradycardia. Peripheral sensory neuropathy. Hepatic impairment, increased toxicity risk, caution. Extravasation, severe tissue reactions. Pseudomembranous colitis. Severe mucositis. Possible CNS effects (alcohol content of formulation). Combination (radiation of lung), possible interstitial pneumonitis.

353

13.1.4   Plant Alkaloids, Other Natural Products

Pregnancy, Lactation: Pregnancy and lactation, contraindicated. Sexually active men and women to ensure adequate contraception during and up to 6 months after treatment (men), 1 month (women).
ADR: See Notes below.
Notes: See 13.1.4 Plant Alkaloids.

Cantaxel Parenteral *(Clonmel)* A.
Price, not published by company.
Infusion, paclitaxel 6mg/mL. Clear colourless (slightly yellow) viscous soln. Ethanol.
Paclitaxel (Accord) Parenteral *(Accord)* A.
Price, (1) 5mL, €99.99. 16.7mL, €333.33. 50mL, €999.99.
Infusion, paclitaxel 6mg/mL. Clear colourless (slightly yellow) conc for soln. Polyoxyl castor oil, ethanol 391mg/mL.
Paclitaxel (Actavis) Parenteral *(Accord)* A.
Price, not published by company.
Infusion, paclitaxel 6mg/mL (30mg, 100mg, 300mg). Clear colourless (slightly yellow) viscous conc for soln. Ethanol, macrogolglycerol ricinoleate.
Paclitaxel (Hospira) Parenteral *(Hospira)* A.
Price, not published by company.
Infusion, paclitaxel 6mg/mL. Clear colourless (slightly yellow) viscous soln. Ethanol.

Paclitaxel Albumin

ATC Code: L01CD01. **Sport:** Permitted.
Driving: Tiredness, dizziness.
Indications: Monotherapy, metastatic breast cancer (failed first-line and anthracyclines not indicated). First-line (in combination), metastatic adenocarcinoma of pancreas (with gemcitabine); non-small cell lung cancer (NSCLC) (surgery and/or radiation therapy not suitable; with carboplatin).
Dose: Adult: *Breast cancer* (monotherapy), 260mg/m2 IV every 3 weeks. Severe neutropenia or sensory neuropathy, reduce to 220mg/m2; recurrence, reduce further to 180mg/m2.
Pancreatic adenocarcinoma, 125mg/m2 IV (days 1, 8 and 15) of each 28-day cycle with gemcitabine 1000mg/m2 IV immediately after *Abraxane*.
NSCLC, 100mg/m2 IV (days 1, 8 and 15) of each 21-day cycle with carboplatin. *Admin*, by IV infusion over 30 minutes.
Elderly: Over 75 years, no benefit of combination with gemcitabine demonstrated.
Renal Impairment: Mild/moderate, no adjustment. Severe, no dose recommendation.
Hepatic Impairment: Mild, no dose adjustment (all indications). Moderate/severe impairment, metastatic breast cancer, NSCLC, reduce dose by 20%; metastatic adenocarcinoma, no dose recommendation. Total bilirubin above 5xULN or AST above 10xULN, no dose recommendation (all indications).
CI: Baseline neutrophils below 1500 cells/mm3.
Interactions: Effect of Other Drugs on Paclitaxel Albumin: *Co-admin (paclitaxel albumin + gemcitabine) not recommended*: Erlotinib, other anticancer drugs (except gemcitabine, cisplatin).
SP: Severe hypersensitivity (fatal); discontinue, do not rechallenge. Bone-marrow suppression; neutropenia is dose-dependent and dose-limiting toxicity. Sensory neuropathy, sepsis, pneumonitis (higher incidence in combination). Cardiotoxicity (CHF, LV dysfunction). *Abraxane* is an albumin-bound formulation of paclitaxel; do not substitute with other formulations.
Pregnancy, Lactation: Pregnancy, only if the clinical condition requires paclitaxel treatment; lactation, contraindicated. See Notes below.
ADR: See Notes below.
Notes: See Paclitaxel above.

Abraxane Parenteral 5mg/mL *(Celgene)* A.
Price, not published by company.
Infusion, paclitaxel (albumin bound). White (yellow) powder for susp. Sodium 4.2mg/mL of conc.

Trabectedin

ATC Code: L01CX01. **Sport:** Permitted.
Driving: Fatigue, asthenia.
Indications: Advanced soft tissue sarcoma (anthracycline and ifosfamide failure or contraindicated); combination

(pegylated liposomal doxorubicin) relapsed platinum-sensitive ovarian cancer.
Dose: Adult, Elderly: *Soft tissue sarcoma*, 1.5mg/m2 BSA by IV infusion over 24 hours; 3-week interval between cycles. *Ovarian cancer*, 1.1mg/m2 BSA immediately after doxorubicin by IV infusion over 3 hours every 3 weeks; max. rate 1mg/min initially; no infusion reaction, subsequently infusion over 1 hour. Admin dexamethasone IV to provide anti-emetic, hepatoprotective effect (30 minutes prior to trabectedin). Central venous access recommended; potentially severe injection-site reactions with peripheral line; extravasation (tissue necrosis).
Child: Under 18 years, not recommended, safety concerns.
Renal Impairment: CrCl (mL/min) below 30 (monotherapy), below 60 (combination), not recommended.
Hepatic Impairment: Dose adjustment may be necessary. Elevated bilirubin, not recommended.
CI: Concurrent serious or uncontrolled infection. See Interactions below.
Interactions: Effect of Other Drugs on Trabectedin: *Co-admin contraindicated*: Yellow fever vaccine. *Co-admin not recommended (increased rhabdomyolysis risk)*: Statins. *Co-admin avoid*: Potent CYP3A4 inhibitors (ketoconazole, fluconazole, ritonavir, clarithromycin, aprepitant) (monitor for toxicities, consider trabectedin dose reduction), potent CYP3A4 inducers (rifampicin, phenobarbital, St John's Wort) (may decrease trabectedin systemic exposure), alcohol (hepatotoxicity). *Co-admin caution*: Other hepatotoxic drugs, P-gp inhibitors (ciclosporin, verapamil) (may alter trabectedin distribution or elimination).
SP: CPK above 2.5xULN, ALP below 2.5xULN, not recommended; rhabdomyolysis associated with myelotoxicity, severe LFT abnormalities and/or renal failure; monitor CPK levels. Perform full blood count including differential platelets (baseline, weekly for first two cycles, then once between cycles).
Pregnancy, Lactation: Pregnancy, use only if clearly necessary; inform patient of potential risk to foetus; at end of pregnancy, monitor newborn. Men and women of childbearing potential to use effective contraception during treatment and 3 months after (women) and immediately inform the treating physician if a pregnancy occurs, and 5 months after (men). Lactation, contraindicated.
ADR: See Notes below.
Notes: See 13.1.4 Plant Alkaloids.

Yondelis Parenteral 0.25mg, 1mg *(Pharma Mar)* A.
Price, (1) 0.25mg, €504.87. 1mg, €913.53.
Infusion, trabectedin 0.25mg, 1mg. White (off-white) powder for conc for soln. Potassium 2mg (8mg) per 0.25mg (1mg) vial; sucrose.

Vinblastine

ATC Code: L01CA01. **Sport:** Permitted.
Driving: Unlikely to impair.
Indications: Hodgkin's disease (Stages III, IV), lymphocytic lymphoma, histiocytic lymphoma, advanced (mycosis fungoides, carcinoma of testis), Kaposi's sarcoma, Letterer-Siwe disease (histocytosis X); choriocarcinoma, breast carcinoma.
Dose: Adult, Elderly: IV at weekly intervals, (dose 1) 3.7mg/m2 BSA, (dose 2) 5.5mg/m2, (dose 3) 7.4mg/m2, (dose 4) 9.25mg/m2, (dose 5) 11.1mg/m2. Increase to max. 18.5mg/m2. *Admin*, IV route only (FATAL if given by other routes) directly into vein or into running IV infusion; complete injection in 1 minute (not for IM, SC or intrathecal use).
Child: IV at weekly intervals, initially 2.5mg/m2 BSA (dose 1), then 3.75mg/m2 (dose 2), 5mg/m2 (dose 3), 6.25mg/m2 (dose 4), 7.5mg/m2 (dose 5). Increase dose to max. 12.5mg/m2. *Admin*, see Adult above.
CI: Leucopenia, bacterial infection.
Interactions: Effect of Other Drugs on Vinblastine: *Acute respiratory distress, pulmonary infiltration*: Combinations including mitomycin and/or progesterone (MVP). *Plasma levels increased*: Cisplatin. *Raynaud's phenomenon, gangrene*: Bleomycin. *Vascular events (MI, CVA)*: Bleomycin + cisplatin. *Toxicity increased*: Erythromycin.
Effect of Vinblastine on Other Drugs: Anticonvulsants: *Plasma levels decreased.*

SP: Strictly for IV admin. Extravasation, severe local reaction. Altered elimination with liver disease (increased peripheral nerve toxicity). Monitor for infection. Cachexia, ulcerated areas of skin, avoid use. Avoid eye contamination.

Pregnancy, Lactation: Pregnancy, if benefit outweighs risk. Lactation, not recommended.

ADR: See Notes below.

Notes: See 13.1.4 Plant Alkaloids.

> **Vinblastine Parenteral 1mg/mL** *(Hospira)* A. HOS.
> *Price*, 10mL (5) €99.27 (PTW).
> *Injection*, vinblastine sulfate (10mL). Clear colourless soln.
> *Sodium 35mg/vial*. **Store:** Refrigerate.

Vincristine

ATC Code: L01CA02. **Sport:** Permitted.
Driving: Unlikely to impair.

Indications: Leukaemias (ALL, CLL, AML, blast crisis of chronic myelogenous leukaemia), malignant lymphoma (Hodgkin's disease, non-Hodgkin's lymphoma), multiple myeloma, solid tumours (breast, small cell bronchogenic, head and neck, soft tissue sarcoma), paediatric solid tumours (Ewing's sarcoma, embryonal rhabdomyosarcoma, neuroblastoma, Wilm's tumour, retinoblastoma, medulloblastoma), idiopathic thrombocytopenic purpura.

Dose: Adult, Elderly: 1.4-1.5mg/m2 per week at weekly intervals; max. 2mg. IV only, see Notes below (vinblastine).

Child: 2mg/m2/week; under 10kg, initially 0.05mg/kg.

Hepatic Impairment: Serum bilirubin above 3mg/100mL (51micromoL/L), half dose.

CI: Demyelinating form of Charcot-Marie-Tooth syndrome.

Interactions: Effect of Other Drugs on Vincristine: *Additive neurotoxicity*: Other neurotoxic agents, spinal cord irradiation, neurological disease. *Increased incidence (cytotoxic-induced bone marrow depression)*: Allopurinol, pyridoxine, isoniazid. *Bronchospasm*: Mitomycin-C. *Metabolism inhibited*: Drugs inhibiting CYP3A. *Allow 24-hour dosing interval*: L-asparaginase. *Delay use*: Until radiotherapy completed.

Effect of Vincristine on Other Drugs: Phenytoin: *Plasma levels decreased, increased seizure activity*. Methotrexate: *Increased cellular uptake by malignant cells (high-dose)*.

SP: Strictly for IV admin. Poorly penetrates blood-brain barrier. Secondary malignancies (combination with other mutagenics). Avoid contact with eyes.

Pregnancy, Lactation: Pregnancy, if benefit outweighs risk. Lactation, not recommended.

ADR: See Notes below.

Notes: See Vinblastine above. See 13.1.4 Plant Alkaloids.

> **Vincristine Parenteral** *(Hospira)* A.
> *Price*, (5) 2mg/2mL, €109.98. 5mg/5mL, €173.53.
> *Injection*, vincristine sulfate 1mg/mL (2mL, 5mL). Colourless soln.
> *Benzyl alcohol*. **Store:** Refrigerate; in outer carton; protect (light).

Vinorelbine

ATC Code: L01CA04. **Sport:** Permitted.
Driving: See Adverse Events.

Indications: Treatment, non-small cell lung cancer, advanced breast cancer (stage 3, 4).

Dose: Adult: MONOTHERAPY, 60mg/m2 BSA orally once weekly for first three doses, then 80mg/m2 once weekly depending on neutrophil count.

COMBINATION, 80mg/m2 orally corresponding to 30mg/m2 (IV); max. 160mg/week OR 60mg/m2 orally corresponding to 25mg/m2 IV; max. 120mg/week. Swallow whole with water; do not chew, suck or dissolve cap; admin with food.

Hepatic Impairment: Mild (bilirubin below 1.5xULN and ALT and/or AST 1.5-2.5xULN), 60mg/m2/week. Moderate (bilirubin 1.5-3xULN irrespective of ALT and AST), 50mg/m2/week. Severe, not recommended.

CI: Hypersensitivity to other vinca alkaloids, disease significantly affecting absorption, previous significant surgical resection of stomach or small bowel, neutrophils below 1500/mm3 or severe infection, platelets below 100000mm3, long-term oxygen therapy required.

Interactions: Effect of Other Drugs on Vinorelbine: *Co-admin not recommended*: Phenytoin (convulsions exacerbated), itraconazole (increased vinca-alkaloid neurotoxicity). *Co-admin caution*: Lapatinib. *Monitor bowel mobility*: Morphine, morphinomimetics, laxatives. *Myelosuppression exacerbated*: Bone marrow toxic drugs. *Granulocytopenia incidence (higher in combination)*: Cisplatin. *Pharmacokinetics modified*: Strong CYP3A4 inhibitors (azole antifungals; increased plasma conc); strong inducers (rifampicin, phenytoin; decreased plasma conc). *Increased pulmonary toxicity*: Mitomycin C.

SP: Liquid content of caps irritant; if chewed/sucked in error, rinse mouth with water or normal saline. Vomiting, do not re-admin; 5HT3 antagonists (ondansetron, granisetron) may reduce occurrence. Ischaemic heart disease, poor performance status, caution. Above grade 3 peripheral neuropathy or LFT abnormality, delay admin until recovery. Not for use with radiotherapy if treatment field includes liver. Oral vinorelbine has higher nausea/vomiting incidence than IV (anti-emetic prophylaxis recommended).

Pregnancy, Lactation: Pregnancy, use only if benefit outweighs risk; women of child-bearing potential to ensure adequate contraception during and for up to 3 months after treatment. Lactation, discontinue before initiation. Men should not father a child during and up to 3 months after treatment.

ADR: See Notes below.

Notes: See 13.1.4 Plant Alkaloids.

> **Navelbine 20mg, 30mg** *(Pierre Fabre)* A. HT.
> *Price*, (1) 20mg, €59.76. 30mg, €89.62.
> *Capsule*, vinorelbine tartrate. Soft light brown. Marked N20.
> *Ethanol, sorbitol*. **Store:** Refrigerate; original pack.

13.1.5 - Platinum Compounds

In This Chapter: *Carboplatin, cisplatin, oxaliplatin.*

Class Effects

For use in specialised units under supervision of experienced oncologist. Dose adjustment, missed doses, consult manufacturers Full Prescribing Information.

CI: Hypersensitivity to any member of the class. Not for use in children. Impaired hearing, severe myelosuppression.

SP: Renal, hepatic function, monitor. Allergic reactions (erythematous rash, fever, pruritus; anaphylaxis, angio-oedema, anaphylactoid reactions). See ADR below.

Pregnancy, Lactation: Pregnancy, not recommended. Women of child-bearing age and males to ensure adequate contraception during and for at least 3 months (cisplatin) or 6 months (oxaliplatin) after treatment. Lactation, not recommended.

ADR: Myelosuppression with altered haematology (anaemia, neutropenia, thrombocytopenia, leucopenia, lymphopenia; febrile neutropenia), allergic reaction, nephrotoxicity, ototoxicity (decreased hearing acuity; may be more severe in children), visual disturbances, optic neuritis, papilloedema, cerebral blindness; conjunctivitis, peripheral neuropathies, paraesthesia, decreased deep tendon reflexes, loss of taste, seizures. Injection site reactions. See Notes below.

Notes: See also 13.1 Cytotoxic Drugs.

Carboplatin

ATC Code: L01XA02. **Sport:** Permitted.
Driving: Nausea, vomiting, vision abnormalities, ototoxicity.

Indications: Ovarian carcinoma (epithelial origin) first-line or after other treatment failure, small cell lung carcinoma.

Dose: Adult, Elderly: Previously untreated, 400mg/m2 BSA as single IV infusion over 15-60 minutes. Do not repeat until 4 weeks after previous carboplatin course. With risk factors (previous myelosuppressive therapy, poor performance status), reduce dose by 20-25%. *Admin*, IV only. *Elderly*, adjust dose depending on physical condition.

Renal Impairment: CrCl (mL/min) 41-59, initially 250mg/m2; 16-40, initially 200mg/m2; 15 or less, not recommended. *Admin*, as for Adult above.

Interactions: Effect of Other Drugs on Carboplatin: *Co-admin not recommended*: Aminoglycosides, other nephrotoxic drugs (vancomycin, capreomycin, diuretics), aluminium (do not use aluminium-containing equipment during preparation, admin of carboplatin or cisplatin). *Increased myelosuppression*: Other myelosuppressives (adjust dose).

13.1.6　Protein Kinase Inhibitors

SP: Myelotoxicity related to renal clearance; monitor. Combination therapy, plan dose/timing carefully to minimise additive effects.
ADR: See Notes below.
Notes: See 13.1.5 Platinum Compounds.
　Carboplatin Parenteral 10mg/mL *(Hospira)* A.
　Price, not published by company.
　Infusion, carboplatin. Clear colourless soln.

Cisplatin

ATC Code: L01XA01. **Sport:** Permitted.
Driving: Caution.
Indications: Metastatic, non-seminomatous germ cell carcinoma, advanced stage and refractory (ovarian carcinoma, bladder carcinoma), squamous cell carcinoma of head and neck. Combination, treatment of metastatic testicular tumours.
Dose: Adult, Elderly: Usually 50-100mg/m2 BSA as single dose every 3-4 weeks OR 15-20mg/m2 daily for 5 days every 3-4 weeks by IV infusion over 6-8 hours. Ensure pre-treatment hydration.
Child: As for Adult above.
Renal Impairment: Not recommended.
Interactions: Effect of Other Drugs on Cisplatin: *Co-use not recommended*: Aluminium (aluminium-containing equipment should not be used during preparation and/or admin of carboplatin or cisplatin). *Not recommended*: Admixture with other drugs in same syringe. *Toxicity potentiated*: Aminoglycosides (oto- and nephrotoxicity), other nephrotoxic drugs (nephrotoxicity), other drugs with similar mode of action.
Effect of Cisplatin on Other Drugs: Bleomycin, methotrexate: *Reduced renal excretion; increased toxicity*. Phenytoin: *Plasma levels decreased, adjust dose*.
ADR: See Notes below.
Notes: See 13.1.5 Platinum Compounds.
　Cisplatin Parenteral *(Hospira)* A.
　Price, not published by company.
　Infusion, cisplatin 1mg/mL. Clear colourless soln.

Oxaliplatin

ATC Code: L01XA03. **Sport:** Permitted.
Driving: Dizziness, neurologic symptoms affecting gait/balance; vision abnormalities, transient vision loss.
Indications: Treatment (with 5-fluorouracil), stage III (Duke's C) colon cancer after complete resection of primary tumour *(Eloxatin)*; metastatic colorectal cancer *(Eloxatin, Oxaliplatin Hospira)*.
Dose: Adult, Elderly: Metastatic colorectal cancer, 85mg/m2 by IV infusion over 2-6 hours; repeat every 2 weeks (12 cycles for colon cancer); admin before 5-fluorouracil. Paraesthesia *without* functional impairment persisting until next cycle, reduce dose to 65mg/m2 (metastatic setting) or 75mg/m2 (adjuvant setting); *with* functional impairment, discontinue.
Renal Impairment: Moderate, if benefit outweighs risk; adjust dose according to toxicity. CrCl (mL/min) below 30, not recommended.
CI: Peripheral sensory neuropathy with functional impairment prior to first course.
SP: Extravasation, non-productive cough, dyspnoea, crackles, radiological pulmonary infiltrates, sepsis, neutropenic sepsis, septic shock, discontinue; anaphylactic-type reaction, discontinue (do not re-initiate). Possible peripheral sensory neuropathy after treatment ends. Acute laryngopharyngeal dysaesthesia during or following 2-hour infusion, admin next infusion over 6 hours. Laryngospasm or bronchospasm. Nausea, vomiting, consider anti-emetics; severe may result in (dehydration, paralytic ileus, intestinal obstruction, hypokalaemia, metabolic acidosis, renal impairment). Monitor haematology. Mucositis, stomatitis, delay next treatment until recovery. Drug-induced hepatic vascular disorders. QT-prolongation, Torsade de Pointes (discontinue). Rhabdomyolysis (fatal).
Pregnancy, Lactation: Pregnancy, contraindicated. Male patients advised not to father a child during and up to 6 months after treatment. Women of childbearing potential to ensure adequate contraception.

356

ADR: See Notes below.
Notes: See 13.1.5 Platinum Compounds.
　Eloxatin Parenteral 5mg/mL *(SANOFI)* A. HOS.
　Price, (1) 50mg, €140.56; 100mg (vial) €281.27 (PTW).
　Infusion, oxaliplatin. Clear colourless conc for soln.
　Oxaliplatin (Accord) Parenteral 5mg/mL *(Accord)* A.
　Price, (1) 10mL, €62.00. 20mL, €124.00. 40mL, €248.00.
　Infusion, oxaliplatin. Clear colourless conc for soln.
　Oxaliplatin (Hospira) Parenteral 5mg/mL *(Hospira)* A.
　Price, not published by company.
　Infusion, oxaliplatin. White (off-white) powder for soln.

13.1.6 - Protein Kinase Inhibitors

In This Chapter: *Afatinib, axitinib, bosutinib, ceritinib, crizotinib, dabrafenib, dasatinib, erlotinib, gefitinib, ibrutinib, imatinib, lapatinib, lenvatinib, nilotinib, nintedanib, pazopanib, ponatinib, regorafenib, ruxolitinib, sorafenib, sunitinib, vandetanib, vemurafenib.*

Class Effects
Indications: For individual drugs, Philadelphia chromosome positive is abbreviated as Ph+. Unless otherwise stated, duration of treatment is until disease progression or no longer tolerated.
CI: Hypersensitivity to any member of the class. Not for use in children under 18 years unless specified.
Interactions: Effect of Other Drugs on Protein Kinase Inhibitors: *Decreased plasma levels (reduced efficacy)*: CYP3A4 inducers (phenytoin, carbamazepine, rifampicin, barbiturates, St John's Wort, dexamethasone). *Increased plasma levels*: CYP3A4 inhibitors (itraconazole, ketoconazole, posaconazole, voriconazole, protease inhibitors, clarithromycin, telithromycin, grapefruit juice).
SP: Nintedanib is a triple angiokinase inhibitor blocking vascular endothelial growth factor receptors (VEGFR 1-3), platelet-derived growth factor receptors (PDGFR alpha, beta) and fibroblast growth factor receptors (FGFR 1-3) kinase activity.
Pregnancy, Lactation: Unless otherwise stated, use in pregnancy only if clearly necessary; inform patient of potential risk to foetus; advise to avoid becoming pregnant while being treated; women of childbearing potential to ensure adequate contraception. Lactation, not recommended, discontinue breastfeeding.
ADR: Generally, dose reduction reduces incidence of adverse events. See manufacturers Full Prescribing Information. See Notes below.
Notes: See also 13.1 Cytotoxic Drugs.

Afatinib

ATC Code: L01XE13. **Sport:** Permitted.
Driving: Minor influence; ocular adverse effects reported.
Indications: Monotherapy, treatment of Epidermal Growth Factor Receptor (EGFR) TKI-naive adults with locally advanced or metastatic non-small cell lung cancer (NSCLC); locally advanced or metastatic NSCLC (squamous histology progressing on/after platinum chemotherapy).
Dose: Adult, Elderly: 40mg once daily without food; do not take food for at least (3 hours before and 1 hour after admin). Increase to max. 50mg/day if 40mg/day is tolerated in first cycle (21 days for EGFR positive NSCLC; 28 days for squamous NSCLC) *Admin*, swallow tabs whole with water or disperse in 100mL non-carbonated drinking water (use no other liquids); consume immediately; dispersion can be admin through a gastric tube.
Renal Impairment: eGFR (mL/min/1.73m2) 15-29, monitor, adjust dose if not tolerated; below 15 or on dialysis, not recommended.
Hepatic Impairment: Severe, not recommended.
Interactions: Effect of Other Drugs on Afatinib: *Decreased afatinib exposure*: High-fat meal, strong P-gp inducers (rifampicin, carbamazepine, phenytoin, phenobarbital, St John's Wort). *Increased exposure (stagger dose 6 or 12 hours apart)*: Strong P-gp inhibitors (ritonavir, ciclosporin A, ketoconazole, itraconazole, erythromycin, verapamil, quinidine, tacrolimus, nelfinavir, saquinavir, amiodarone).
Effect of Afatinib on Other Drugs: Rosuvastatin, sulfasalazine: *Increased bioavailability.*

SP: Establish EGFR mutation status before initiating. Diarrhoea (severe); admin anti-diarrhoeal (loperamide); ensure adequate hydration. ILD, see Notes below. Rash, acne may worsen with sun exposure; bullous, blistering, exfoliative skin conditions (Stevens-Johnson syndrome, toxic epidermal necrolysis). Higher afatinib exposure observed (females, lower body weight, underlying renal impairment). Ulcerative keratitis diagnosed, interrupt or discontinue; contact lens use increases risk. Cardiac risk factors, monitor LVEF (baseline, during treatment).

Pregnancy, Lactation: Women of childbearing age to ensure adequate contraception during and for at least 1 month after last dose. See Notes below.

ADR: See Notes below.

Notes: See 13.1.6 Protein Kinase Inhibitors.

▼ **Giotrif Tablets** *(Boehringer)* A. HT.
Price, (28) all strengths, €2115.42.
Tablet, afatinib 20mg, 30mg, 40mg, 50mg. Round f/c. Marked T and strength; logo on reverse. 20mg: White (yellowish). 30mg, 50mg: Dark-blue. 40mg: Light-blue. *Lactose.* **Store:** Original pack to protect (light).

Axitinib

ATC Code: L01XE17. **Sport:** Permitted.
Driving: Minor influence; dizziness, fatigue.
Indications: Treatment (adults), advanced renal cell carcinoma (after failure or prior sunitinib or cytokine).
Dose: Adult, Elderly: Initially 5mg twice daily; if tolerated for 2 weeks*, increase to 7mg twice daily; if tolerated for another 2 weeks*, increase to 10mg twice daily (monitor adverse reactions, BP). Dose reduction, reduce to 3mg twice daily, then 2mg twice daily. *Admin*, 12-hourly with or without food. Vomiting or missed dose, an additional dose should not be taken. *(consecutive).

Renal Impairment: CrCl (mL/min) below 15, no data.
Hepatic Impairment: Moderate, reduce dose to 2mg twice daily. Severe, not recommended.

Interactions: Effect of Other Drugs on Axitinib: *Plasma levels increased:* CYP3A4/5 inhibitors (ketoconazole, itraconazole, clarithromycin, erythromycin, atazanavir, indinavir, nefazodone, nelfinavir, ritonavir, saquinavir, telithromycin), grapefruit juice, strong CYP1A2 and CYP2C19 inhibitors; choose alternative or consider dose reduction. *Plasma levels decreased:* CYP3A4/5 inducers (rifampicin, dexamethasone, phenytoin, carbamazepine, rifabutin, rifapentine, phenobarbital, St John's Wort), possibly CYP1A2 induction by cigarette smoking.
Effect of Axitinib on Other Drugs: CYP1A2 substrates (theophylline): *Plasma levels increased.*
SP: Control hypertension before initiation (monitor); if persistent, reduce dose; severe hypertension, interrupt and restart at lower dose when normotensive. Arterial and venous embolic and thrombotic events, haemorrhagic events. Increased haemoglobin, haematocrit. GI perforation, fistula formation, wound healing complications, posterior reversible encephalopathy syndrome. Thyroid function, proteinuria (monitor before initiation, then periodically); proteinuria if moderate or severe, reduce dose or temporarily interrupt; if nephrotic syndrome develops, discontinue. Liver-related adverse events.

Pregnancy, Lactation: Ensure adequate contraception during and up to 1 week after treatment. See Notes below.
ADR: See Notes below.
Notes: See 13.1.6 Protein Kinase Inhibitors.

▼ **Inlyta 1mg, 5mg** *(Pfizer)* A. HT.
Price, (56) 1mg, €837.52. 5mg, €4186.08.
Tablet, axitinib. Red f/c. Marked Pfizer; strength and XNB on reverse. 1mg: Oval. 5mg: Triangular. *Lactose.*

Bosutinib

ATC Code: L01XE14. **Sport:** Permitted.
Driving: Negligible effect; dizziness, fatigue, visual impairment.
Indications: Treatment, adults with (chronic, accelerated, blast)-phase Ph+ chronic myelogenous leukaemia (Ph+ CML) (previous tyrosine kinase inhibitors).
Dose: Adult, Elderly: 500mg once daily. *Admin*, with food. Dose escalation to 600mg was allowed if no severe or persistent moderate adverse reactions. *Elderly*, caution.
Renal Impairment: CrCl (mL/min) 30-50, 400mg/day with

Protein Kinase Inhibitors   13.1.6

escalation to 500mg; below 30, 300mg/day with escalation to 400mg. See Adult above.
Hepatic Impairment: Contraindicated.

Interactions: Effect of Other Drugs on Bosutinib: *Co-admin avoid:* CYP3A inhibitors, potent (ritonavir, indinavir, nelfinavir, saquinavir, ketoconazole, itraconazole, voriconazole, posaconazole, troleandomycin, clarithromycin, telithromycin, boceprevir, telaprevir, mibefradil, nefazodone, conivaptan, grapefruit) or moderate (fluconazole, darunavir, erythromycin, diltiazem, dronedarone, atazanavir, aprepitant, amprenavir, fosamprenavir, imatinib, verapamil, tofisopam, ciprofloxacin) (increased bosutinib levels); CYP3A inducers, potent (rifampicin, phenytoin, carbamazepine, St John's Wort, rifabutin, phenobarbital) or moderate (bosentan, nafcillin, efavirenz, modafinil, etravirine) (decreased bosutinib levels). *Co-admin caution:* PPIs (use short-acting antacids; separate admin times).
Effect of Bosutinib on Other Drugs: P-gp substrates (digoxin, colchicine, tacrolimus, quinidine, etoposide, doxorubicin, vinblastine, immunosuppressives, protease inhibitors, dexamethasone, NNRTIs): *Plasma levels increased.* Antiarrhythmics (amiodarone, disopyramide, procainamide, quinidine, sotalol), chloroquine, halofantrine, clarithromycin, domperidone, haloperidol, methadone, moxifloxacin: *Caution, QT-prolongation.*
SP: Cardiac disorders (recent MI, CHF, unstable angina), QTc-prolongation, GI disorders, caution. Elevated ALT/AST; monitor LFTs before initiation, then monthly (first 3 months of treatment). Diarrhoea and vomiting. Myelosuppression, perform complete blood counts weekly (month 1), then monthly. Fluid retention, monitor. Treatment may result in decline in renal function; assess prior to initiation, then monitor.

Pregnancy, Lactation: See Notes below.
ADR: See Notes below.
Notes: See 13.1.6 Protein Kinase Inhibitors.

▼ **Bosulif 100mg, 500mg** *(Pfizer)* A. HT.
Price, (28) 100mg, €949.47. 500mg, €4067.30.
Tablet, bosutinib monohydrate. Oval f/c. Marked Pfizer; strength on reverse. 100mg: Yellow. 500mg: Red.

Ceritinib

ATC Code: L01XE28. **Sport:** Pending.
Driving: Minor influence; caution, fatigue, vision disorders.
Indications: Treatment, ALK-positive advance non-small cell lung cancer (NSCLC) (previous crizotinib).
Dose: Adult, Elderly: 750mg/day (max.). Unable to tolerate 300mg/day, discontinue. Temporary interruption or dose reduction may be needed due to adverse events; decrease by 150mg/day. *Elderly*, over 85 years, no data. *Admin*, once daily at same time each day; swallow whole with water; do not crush or chew; take on empty stomach; take no food for 2 hours before and 2 hours after admin.
Child: Under 18 years, safety/efficacy not established.
Renal Impairment: Mild/moderate, no adjustment; severe, caution (no experience).
Hepatic Impairment: Moderate to severe, not recommended.

Interactions: Effect of Other Drugs on Ceritinib: *Plasma levels increased (decrease ceritinib dose by one third):* CYP3A/P-gp inhibitors (ritonavir, saquinavir, telithromycin, ketoconazole, itraconazole, voriconazole, posaconazole, nefazodone). *Plasma levels decreased, avoid co-admin:* CYP3A substrates (astemizole, cisapride, ciclosporin, ergotamine, fentanyl, pimozide, quinidine, tacrolimus, alfentanil, sirolimus), CYP2C9 substrates (phenytoin, warfarin). *Increased bioavailability:* Food, grapefruit juice. *Decreased bioavailability:* Acid-reducing agents (PPIs, H2-antagonists).
Effect of Ceritinib on Other Drugs: BCRP substrates (rosuvastatin, topotecan, sulfasalazine), P-gp substrates (digoxin, dabigatran, colchicine, pravastatin): *Caution, plasms levels increased.* Antiarrhythmics Class I (quinidine, procainamide, disopyramide), Class III (amiodarone, sotalol, dofetilide, ibutilide), other medicinals causing QT prolongation (astemizole, domperidone, droperidol, chloroquine, halofantrine, clarithromycin, haloperidol, methadone, cisapride, moxifloxacin).
SP: Establish ALK-positive status before initiation.

357

13.1.6   Protein Kinase Inhibitors

Hepatotoxicity (dose interruption or reduction). ILD, see Notes below. QT-prolongation (increased ventricular tachyarrhythmias e.g. Torsade de Pointes, sudden death). Bradycardia (below 60bpm), GI toxicity (diarrhoea, nausea, vomiting), hyperglycaemia, lipase/amylase elevations.
Pregnancy, Lactation: See Notes below. Ensure adequate contraception during and for 3 months after treatment.
ADR: See Notes below.
Notes: See 13.1.6 Protein Kinase Inhibitors.
▼ **Zykadia 150mg** *(Novartis)* A. HT.
Price, (150), €6270.64.
Capsule, ceritinib. White/blue; contains white (almost white) powder. Marked LDK 150MG and NVR.

Crizotinib
ATC Code: L01XE16. **Sport:** Pending.
Driving: Caution, symptomatic bradycardia (syncope, dizziness, hypotension), vision disorder, fatigue.
Indications: Treatment (adults), anaplastic lymphoma kinase (ALK)-positive (ALK+) advanced non-small cell lung cancer (NSCLC) (first-line or previously treated); ROS1-positive (ROS1+) advanced NSCLC.
Dose: Adult, Elderly: All indications, 250mg twice daily (500mg/day) taken continuously. Interrupt and/or reduce dose based on individual safety and tolerability. NOTE: Accurate and validated ALK+ or ROS1+ assay is necessary for patient selection for treatment. *Admin*, swallow whole preferably with water; do not crush, dissolve or open; with or without food. Avoid grapefruit or grapefruit juice.
Child: Safety/efficacy not established.
Renal Impairment: CrCl (mL/min) 30 and above; below 30 and not on dialysis (peritoneal or haemodialysis), 250mg once daily; increase after 4 weeks to 200mg twice daily based on safety/tolerability.
Hepatic Impairment: Mild/moderate, caution. Severe, contraindicated.
Interactions: Effect of Other Drugs on Crizotinib: *Co-admin avoid*: Increased crizotinib plasma levels with grapefruit juice, St John's Wort, strong CYP3A4 inhibitors, (ketoconazole, itraconazole, voriconazole, atazanavir, indinavir, nelfinavir, ritonavir, saquinavir, clarithromycin, telithromycin, troleandomycin); decreased plasma levels (CYP3A4 inducers, carbamazepine, phenobarbital, phenytoin, rifabutin, rifampicin, St John's Wort); clinical monitoring (CYP3A4 substrates with narrow therapeutic indices, alfentanil, cisapride, ciclosporin, ergot derivatives, fentanyl, pimozide, quinidine, sirolimus, tacrolimus). *Co-admin caution*: Drugs prolonging QT interval (quinidine, disopyramide, amiodarone, sotalol, dofetilide, ibutilide, methadone, cisapride, moxifloxacin, antipsychotics), bradycardic agents (verapamil, diltiazem, beta-blockers, clonidine, guanfacine, digoxin, mefloquine, anticholinesterases, pilocarpine).
Effect of Crizotinib on Other Drugs: CYP2B6 substrates (bupropion, efavirenz): *Increased plasma levels*. Oral contraceptives: *Effectiveness may be altered*. UGT substrates (UGT1A1) (raltegravir, irinotecan), (UGT2B7) (morphine, naloxone), OCT1 or OCT2 substrates (metformin, procainamide): *May increase plasma levels*. P-gp substrates (digoxin, dabigatran, colchicine, pravastatin): *Caution, therapeutic effect may be increased*.
SP: Drug induced hepatotoxicity, monitor LFTs once weekly (first 2 months) then once monthly. ILD, see Notes below. QT-prolongation (increased ventricular tachyarrhythmias e.g. Torsade de Pointes, sudden death); if diagnosed, discontinue permanently. Patients at risk, monitor (ECG, electrolytes, renal function). Symptomatic bradycardia (syncope, dizziness, hypotension); monitor heart rate, BP. Cardiac failure, GI perforations (fatal). Monitor complete blood counts. Increased blood creatinine and decreased creatinine clearance observed; renal failure, including acute. Visual field defects with vision loss; new onset of severe visual loss (visual acuity below 6/60 in one or both eyes), discontinue; perform ophthalmological evaluation.
Pregnancy, Lactation: Ensure adequate contraception during and for up to 90 days after treatment. See Notes below.
ADR: See Notes below.
Notes: See 13.1.6 Protein Kinase Inhibitors.

▼ **XALKORI 200mg, 250mg** *(Pfizer)* A. HT.
Price, (60) 200mg, €5308.65; 250mg, €5724.00.
Capsule, crizotinib. Hard opaque. Marked Pfizer, CRZ and strength. 200mg: White/pink. 250mg: Pink/pink.

Dabrafenib
ATC Code: L01XE23. **Sport:** Permitted.
Driving: Minor influence; fatigue, eye problems.
Indications: Monotherapy or combination, unresectable or metastatic melanoma with a BRAF V600 mutation.
Dose: Adult, Elderly: Monotherapy or in combination (with trametinib), 150mg (2x 75mg caps) twice daily taken 1 hour before or 2 hours after food; dose interval 12 hours; take at similar time each day. Dose modification or interruption not recommended for adverse reactions of cutaneous squamous cell carcinoma or new primary melanoma; uveitis if ocular inflammation can be controlled. Other dose modifications, see manufacturers Full Prescribing Information. *Admin*, swallow whole with water; do not crush, chew; do not mix with food or liquids.
Renal Impairment: Severe, caution.
Hepatic Impairment: Moderate/severe, caution.
Interactions: Effect of Other Drugs on Dabrafenib: *Dabrafenib plasma levels*: Increased by potent CYP2C8/3A4 inhibitors (azole antifungals, nefazodone, clarithromycin, ritonavir, saquinavir, telithromycin, atazanavir), caution; decreased by potent CYP2C8/3A4 inducers (rifampicin, phenytoin, carbamazepine, phenobarbital, St John's Wort), avoid. *Bioavailability decreased*: Agents increasing gastric pH (PPIs), avoid.
Effect of Dabrafenib on Other Drugs: Warfarin, digoxin: *Decreased exposure*. CYP2B6 and CYP3A4 substrates, OATP1B1/B3 substrates: *Large number of drug classes affected*. See manufacturers Full Prescribing Information.
SP: *Before initiation*, confirm tumour BRAF V600 mutation (not for use with BRAF wild-type melanoma); perform skin examination for cutaneous squamous cell carcinoma (then monthly during treatment and up to 6 months after); perform head and neck examination (then 3-monthly) and chest CT scan (then 6-monthly) (non-cutaneous malignancy risk is increased); perform anal examinations, pelvic examination (women) (then at end of treatment); perform full blood counts, serum creatinine, visual signs/symptoms (then routinely for changed vision, photophobia, eye pain), signs of pancreatitis (serum amylase, lipase); LFTs (then every 4 weeks for 6 months after initiation) when used in combination. *Serious non-infectious febrile events* (typical first month); interrupt or reduce dose; increased pyrexia incidence, severity (combination). New primary melanoma. Colitis and GI perforation (fatal) reported (combination). Combination with trametinib, consult manufacturers Full Prescribing Information (trametinib).
Pregnancy, Lactation: Ensure adequate contraception during and for up to 4 weeks after treatment. See Notes below.
ADR: See Notes below.
Notes: See 13.1.6 Protein Kinase Inhibitors.
▼ **Tafinlar 50mg, 75mg** *(Novartis)* A. HT.
Price, (120) 50mg, €4485.89. 75mg, €6728.40.
Capsule, dabrafenib. Opaque hard. Marked with strength. 50mg: Dark-red. Marked GS TEW. 75mg: Dark-pink. Marked GS LHF.

Dasatinib
ATC Code: L01XE06. **Sport:** Permitted.
Driving: Dizziness, blurred vision.
Indications: Newly diagnosed Ph+ chronic myelogenous leukaemia (Ph+ CML) in (chronic, accelerated or blast)-phase*; Ph+ ALL and lymphoid blast CML*. *(resistant or intolerant to prior therapy).
Dose: Adult, Elderly: *Chronic phase* CML, 100mg once daily at same time of day. *Advanced phase* CML or Ph+ ALL, 140mg once daily. *Admin*, oral with or without food; swallow tabs whole, do not crush or cut.
Hepatic Impairment: Caution.
Interactions: Effect of Other Drugs on Dasatinib: *Co-admin caution, bleeding risk*: Platelet inhibitors, anticoagulants. *Exposure reduced*: Long-term gastric acid suppression with H2-blockers or PPIs (famotidine, omeprazole), antacids (allow 2-hour dosing interval).
Effect of Dasatinib on Other Drugs: CYP3A4 substrates

with narrow therapeutic index (astemizole, terfenadine, cisapride, pimozide, quinidine, bepridil, ergot alkaloids): *Co-admin caution.* Glitazones: *Potential interaction risk.*
SP: Correct hypo- (kalaemia, magnesaemia) before initiation. Myelosuppression. Bleeding (severe CNS, GI), associated with severe thrombocytopenia (fatal). Fluid retention (severe pleural, pericardial effusion, dyspnoea); more likely in elderly. QT-prolongation, PAH.
Pregnancy, Lactation: Suspected to cause congenital malformations (neural tube defects). See Notes below.
ADR: See Notes below.
Notes: See 13.1.6 Protein Kinase Inhibitors.

> **Sprycel 20mg, 50mg, 70mg, 100mg** *(BMS)* A. HT.
> *Price,* (60) 20mg, €1984.04. 50mg, €4010.69. 70mg, €3894.31. 100mg, €4052.11.
> *Tablet,* dasatinib monohydrate. White (off-white) f/c. Marked BMS. 20mg: Round. Marked 527. 50mg: Oval. Marked 528. 70mg: Round. Marked 524. 100mg: Oval. Marked 852. *Lactose.*

Erlotinib

ATC Code: L01XE03. **Sport:** Permitted.
Driving: Unlikely to impair.
Indications: Non-small cell lung cancer (NSCLC) locally advanced or metastatic (first-line or after failure of at least one prior chemotherapy regimen). Treatment, metastatic pancreatic cancer in combination (gemcitabine).
Dose: Adult, Elderly: *NSCLC,* 150mg/day (smokers, max. tolerated dose 300mg); see Interactions below. *Pancreatic cancer,* 100mg/day with gemcitabine. Adjust dose in 50mg steps. *Admin,* oral 1 hour before or 2 hours after food.
Renal Impairment: Severe, not recommended.
Hepatic Impairment: Moderate, caution, reduce dose or interrupt if ADRs occur; severe (AST/SGOT and ALT/SGPT above 5xULN), not recommended.
Interactions: Effect of Other Drugs on Erlotinib: *Co-admin caution:* P-glycoprotein inhibitors (ciclosporin, verapamil). *Co-admin avoid (plasma levels reduced):* Potent CYP3A4 and/or CYP1A2 inducers. *Increased plasma levels/toxicity (consider dose reduction):* Potent CYP3A4 and/or CYP1A2 inhibitors (fluvoxamine, ciprofloxacin). *Plasma levels reduced:* Cigarette smoking (advise current smokers to stop). *Solubility/bioavailability altered (decreased exposure):* Antacids (dose 4 hours before or 2 hours after erlotinib), H2-antagonists (ranitidine; erlotinib to be taken 2 hours before or 10 hours after), PPIs (avoid co-admin). *Plasma levels increased:* Capecitabine (no clinical significance).
Effect of Erlotinib on Other Drugs: Coumarin-derived anticoagulants (warfarin), NSAIDs: *Monitor (prothrombin time, INR).* Statins: *Increased myopathy potential.*
SP: Assess EGFR mutation status before initiation (chemo-naive advanced or metastatic NSCLC). ILD, see Notes below. Diarrhoea, consider dose reduction; caution, dehydration. Monitor LFTs (liver disease, hepatotoxic drugs). GI perforation risk. Severe bullous, blistering or exfoliation conditions, discontinue. Corneal perforation or ulceration; eyelash changes, keratoconjunctivitis sicca, keratitis; interrupt or discontinue.
Pregnancy, Lactation: Adequate contraception during therapy and for minimum 2 weeks upon completion. See Notes below.
ADR: See Notes below.
Notes: See 13.1.6 Protein Kinase Inhibitors.

> **Tarceva 25mg, 100mg, 150mg** *(Roche)* A. HT.
> *Price,* (30) 25mg, €503.02; 100mg, €1743.90; 150mg, €2148.81.
> *Tablet,* erlotinib HCl. White (yellowish) round f/c. Marked T and strength. *Lactose.*

Gefitinib

ATC Code: L01XE02. **Sport:** Permitted.
Driving: Asthenia.
Indications: Monotherapy, locally advanced or metastatic non-small cell lung cancer (NSCLC) with activating mutations (EGFR-TK).
Dose: Adult, Elderly: 250mg once daily. CYP2D6 poor metabolisers, monitor for adverse events. Toxicity (diarrhoea, skin reactions), interrupt for up to 14 days; if not tolerated after interruption, discontinue. *Admin,* with or without food; about same time each day. Swallow whole

---

Protein Kinase Inhibitors   13.1.6

or disperse in non-carbonated water (drink immediately) or admin dispersion by nasogastric or gastrostomy tube.
Renal Impairment: CrCl (mL/min) above 20, no adjustment; 20 and below, caution (limited data).
Hepatic Impairment: Severe, due to cirrhosis, plasma levels elevated; monitor for adverse events.
Interactions: Effect of Other Drugs on Gefitinib: *Increased metabolism, decreased plasma levels (reduced efficacy), avoid co-admin:* CYP3A4 inducers (phenytoin, carbamazepine, rifampicin, barbiturates, St John's Wort). *Increased plasma levels (monitor for adverse events):* Poor CYP2D6 metabolisers, co-admin of CYP3A4 potent inhibitors (ketoconazole, posaconazole, voriconazole, protease inhibitors, clarithromycin, telithromycin). *Reduced bioavailability and plasma conc (possible reduced efficacy):* Medicinals causing sustained gastric pH elevation (PPIs, H2-antagonists), antacids (if taken regularly close to gefitinib admin).
Effect of Gefitinib on Other Drugs: Warfarin: *Monitor prothrombin time or INR.* CYP2D6 substrates with narrow therapeutic window: *Consider dose modification.*
SP: Assess EGFR mutation status. ILD, if confirmed, discontinue, see Notes below. Abnormal LFTs (hepatitis); hepatic failure; recommend periodic LFTs. GI perforation, usually with risk factors (steroids, NSAIDs, GI ulceration history, age, smoking, bowel metastases). Advise patient to seek medical advice if eye symptoms develop, severe or persistent diarrhoea, nausea, vomiting, anorexia.
Pregnancy, Lactation: Lactation, contraindicated. See Notes below.
ADR: See Notes below.
Notes: See 13.1.6 Protein Kinase Inhibitors.

> **IRESSA 250mg** *(AstraZeneca)* A. HT.
> *Price,* (30) €2274.36.
> *Tablet,* gefitinib. Brown round f/c. Marked IRESSA 250. *Lactose.*
> *Store:* Original pack to protect (moisture).

Ibrutinib

ATC Code: L01XE27. **Sport:** Permitted.
Driving: Fatigue, dizziness, asthenia.
Indications: Treatment (adults) monotherapy, relapsed or refractory mantle cell lymphoma (MCL), chronic lymphocytic leukaemia (CLL) (previously untreated), Waldenstrom's macroglobulinaemia (one prior therapy or first-line if chemo-immunotherapy is unsuitable); monotherapy or combination, CLL (one prior therapy).
Dose: Adult, Elderly: *Mantle cell lymphoma,* 560mg/day. *CLL*, Waldenstrom's macroglobulinaemia,* 420mg/day * (as single agent or in combination). *Co-admin* with moderate CYP3A4 inhibitors, reduce dose to 140mg/day; with strong CYP3A4 inhibitors, reduce to 140mg/day or withhold for up to 7 days. Adjust dose for non-haematological toxicity, neutropenia with infection or fever, haematological toxicities. *Admin,* once daily with glass of water; approx. same time each day. Swallow whole; do not open, break or chew. Not for admin with grapefruit juice or Seville oranges.
Renal Impairment: CrCl (mL/min) above 30; no adjustment, maintain hydration; monitor serum creatinine. CrCl (mL/min) below 30, use only if benefit outweighs risk; monitor for toxicity.
Hepatic Impairment: Mild, 280mg/day; moderate, 140mg/day. Monitor for toxicity. Severe, not recommended.
Interactions: Effect of Other Drugs on Ibrutinib: *Co-admin contraindicated:* St John's Wort. *Co-admin not recommended:* Warfarin, other vitamin K antagonists. *Co-admin avoid:* Fish oil, vitamin E supplements, grapefruit juice, Seville oranges, agents increasing plasma levels e.g. strong CYP3A4 inhibitors (ketoconazole, indinavir, nelfinavir, ritonavir, saquinavir, clarithromycin, telithromycin, itraconazole, nefazodone, cobicistat), moderate CYP3A4 inhibitors (voriconazole, erythromycin, amprenavir, aprepitant, atazanavir, ciprofloxacin, crizotinib, darunavir/ritonavir, diltiazem, fluconazole, fosamprenavir, imatinib, verapamil, amiodarone, dronedarone), see Dose; agents decreasing plasma levels e.g. strong or moderate CYP3A4 inducers (carbamazepine, rifampicin, phenytoin). *Ibrutinib exposure may be decreased:* Decreased stomach pH (PPIs).
Effect of Ibrutinib on Other Drugs: P-gp or BCRP substrates

359

13.1.6   Protein Kinase Inhibitors

(digoxin, methotrexate): *Allow 6-hour dosing interval.* Rosuvastatin, CYP3A4 substrates with narrow therapeutic window (oral) (dihydroergotamine, ergotamine, fentanyl, ciclosporin, sirolimus, tacrolimus): *Possible increased exposure, caution.* CYP2B6 substrates (efavirenz, bupropion): *Possible decreased exposure.*

SP: Haemorrhagic events, with and without thrombocytopenia; minor, major, some fatal (GI, intracranial, haematuria). Withhold for 3-7 days pre- and post-surgery depending on surgery type, bleeding risk. Leukostasis; monitor, supportive care (hydration and/or cytoreduction). Atrial fibrillation/flutter with (cardiac risk factors, hypertension, acute infections, atrial fibrillation history); monitor ECG; if anticoagulants required, seek alternative. Tumour lysis syndrome. Monitor for non-melanoma skin cancer. ILD, see Notes below.

Pregnancy, Lactation: Not for use in pregnancy. Women of childbearing potential to use highly effective contraception during treatment and for up to 3 months after; if using hormonal contraceptives, add a barrier method. Stop breastfeeding or stop drug.

ADR: See Notes below.

Notes: See 13.1.6 Protein Kinase Inhibitors.

▼ **Imbruvica 140mg** *(Janssen-Cilag)* A. HT.
Price, (90) €6159.03; (120) €8212.05.
Capsule, ibrutinib. White opaque hard. Marked 'ibr 140 mg'.

Imatinib

ATC Code: L01XE01. **Sport:** Permitted.
Driving: Dizziness, blurred vision.

Indications: Treatment, Ph+ CML, newly diagnosed or chronic phase (interferon-alpha failure) or accelerated phase or blast crisis. Newly diagnosed Ph+ ALL (with chemotherapy). Myelodysplastic or myeloproliferative diseases (MDS/MPD). Advanced hypereosinophilic syndrome (HES) and/or chronic eosinophilic leukaemia (CEL). Kit (CD117) positive unresectable and/or metastatic GI stromal tumours (GIST). Adjuvant, following Kit (CD117)-positive GIST resection. Unresectable dermatofibrosarcoma protuberans (DFSP), recurrent and/or metastatic (not eligible for surgery).

Dose: Adult, Elderly: CML, chronic phase, 400mg/day; can increase to 600mg/day; accelerated phase, blast crisis, 600mg/day; can increase to max. 800mg/day. Ph+ ALL, 600mg/day (with chemotherapy); relapsed or refractory, 600mg/day (monotherapy). *Other indications,* MDS/MPD, 400mg/day; HES/CEL, 100mg/day; consider increase to 400mg/day; GIST, 400mg/day; DFSP, 800mg/day. *Admin,* oral with food and large glass of water to minimise GI irritation. Swallowing difficulty, disperse in glass of mineral water. Doses of 400-600mg, admin once daily; 800mg, admin as 400mg twice daily.

Child: CML, age 2 years and over, chronic and advanced phases, 340mg/m2 BSA; can be increased to 570mg/m2; max. 800mg/day. Admin, in 1 or 2 divided doses, morning and evening. Ph+ ALL, 340mg/m2 daily; max. 600mg/day.

Renal Impairment: Renal dysfunction or on dialysis, initially 400mg/day (caution); not tolerated, reduce dose; if tolerated, can be increased.

Hepatic Impairment: All grades, 400mg/day; unacceptable toxicity, reduce (monitor peripheral blood counts, liver enzymes).

Interactions: Effect of Other Drugs Imatinib: Co-admin caution: Paracetamol (especially high doses). *Hepatotoxicity, myelosuppression increased (caution):* L-asparaginase.

Effect of Imatinib on Other Drugs: Strong CYP3A4 inhibitors (ketoconazole), CYP3A4 substrates with narrow therapeutic window (ciclosporin, pimozide): *Co-admin caution.* Triazolo-benzodiazepines, dihydropyridines, certain statins: *Plasma levels increased.* CYP2C9 substrates with narrow therapeutic window (warfarin, other coumarins): *Not recommended (use heparin or LMWH).* CYP2D6 substrates: *Caution, plasma levels increased.* Levothyroxine: *Plasma levels decreased.*

SP: Serious liver injury (with high-dose chemotherapy). Monitor TSH levels (thyroidectomy with levothyroxine replacement). Severe fluid retention (pleural effusion, oedema, pulmonary oedema, ascites); monitor body weight (increased risk in *elderly* or with prior cardiac risk).

Hypereosinophilic syndrome (HES) and cardiac involvement, cardiogenic shock or LVD. GIST treatment, monitor; gastric antral vascular ectasia (GAVE) reported. Perform complete blood counts. Growth retardation in children, pre-adolescents. Decline in renal function (long-term treatment).

Pregnancy, Lactation: See Notes below.
ADR: See Notes below.
Notes: See 13.1.6 Protein Kinase Inhibitors.

▼ **Glivec 100mg, 400mg** *(Novartis)* A. HT.
Price, 100mg (60) €886.93. 400mg (30) €1772.88.
Tablet, imatinib mesilate. Dark-yellow (brownish-orange) f/c. Marked NVR. 100mg: Round scored. Marked SA. 400mg: Ovaloid. Marked SL. **Store:** Below 30 deg C; protect (moisture).

Imatinib Accord 100mg, 400mg *(Accord)* A. HT.
Price, 100mg (60) €507.03; 400mg (30) €1013.48.
Tablet, imatinib mesilate. Brownish-orange f/c scored (not intended for breaking). 100mg: Round. Marked T1. 400mg: Oval. Marked T2. **Store:** Below 30 deg C.

Imatinib Actavis 400mg *(Accord)* A. HT.
Price, (30) €1017.05.
Tablet, imatinib mesilate. Dark-yellow (brownish) f/c scored (not intended to break tab). Marked with company logo; 37 on reverse. **Store:** Below 25 deg C; protect (moisture).

Imatinib Clonmel 100mg, 400mg *(Clonmel)* A. HT.
Price, 100mg (60) €508.53; 400mg (30) €1017.06.
Tablet, imatinib mesilate. Brownish f/c. Marked with strength one side; NI on reverse. 100mg: Round scored (divisible into equal doses). 400mg: Oval. **Store:** Below 25 deg C. Protect (moisture).

Imatinib Krka 100mg, 400mg *(Krka)* A. HT.
Price, 100mg (60) €508.52; 400mg (30) €1017.05.
Tablet, imatinib mesilate. Orange-brown f/c. 100mg: Round scored (divisible in equal doses). 400mg: Oval. *Lactose.*

Imatinib (Pinewood) 100mg, 400mg *(Pinewood)* A. HT.
Price, 100mg (60) €508.53; 400mg (30) €1017.05.
Tablet, imatinib mesilate. Brownish f/c. Marked with strength one side; NI on reverse. 100mg: Round scored (divisible into equal doses). 400mg: Oval. **Store:** Below 25 deg C.

Imatinib Rowex 100mg, 400mg *(Rowex)* A. HT.
Price, 100mg (60) €508.53; 400mg (30) €1017.05.
Tablet, imatinib mesilate. Very dark-yellow (brownish-orange) f/c scored (divisible into equal halves). 100mg: Round. Marked NVR; SA on reverse. 400mg: Ovaloid. Marked 400 one side; SL on reverse. **Store:** Below 30 deg C; protect (moisture).

Imatinib TEVA 100mg, 400mg *(TEVA)* A. HT.
Price, 100mg (60) €508.53; 400mg (30) €1017.05.
Tablet, imatinib mesilate. Dark-yellow (brownish-orange) f/c scored (divisible into equal doses). 100mg: Round. Marked IT and 1. 400mg: Oblong. Marked IT and 4.

Lapatinib

ATC Code: L01XE07. **Sport:** Permitted.
Driving: Consider adverse event profile.

Indications: Treatment, breast cancer (tumours overexpress ErbB2/HER2) with capecitabine (advanced or metastatic; progression after prior therapy) OR trastuzumab (hormone receptor-negative metastatic) OR aromatase inhibitor (postmenopausal women, hormone receptor positive metastatic; not for chemotherapy).

Dose: Adult, Elderly: 1250mg once daily (with capecitabine) OR 1000mg once daily (with trastuzumab) OR 1500mg once daily (with aromatase inhibitor). *Admin,* 1 hour before or 1 hour after food (always before or always after); to be taken continuously, daily dose not to be divided. *Elderly,* over 65 years, limited data.

Renal Impairment: Severe, caution.

Hepatic Impairment: Moderate/severe, caution (increased exposure). Severe changes in function, discontinue; do not retreat.

Interactions: Effect of Other Drugs on Lapatinib: Co-admin avoid: CYP3A4 strong inhibitors (ritonavir, saquinavir, nefazodone); grapefruit juice; substances increasing gastric pH (esomeprazole; decreased solubility/absorption). *Co-admin caution:* CYP3A4 moderate inhibitors. *Altered exposure and/or distribution:* P-gp and BCRP inhibitors (ketoconazole, itraconazole, quinidine, verapamil, ciclosporin, erythromycin) and inducers (rifampicin, St John's Wort). *Co-admin, severe neutropenia/diarrhoea:* Paclitaxel (175mg/m2 every 3 weeks). *Bioavailability increased:* Food (up to 4 times depending on fat content), grapefruit juice.

Effect of Lapatinib on Other Drugs: Substrates of CYP3A4 (cisapride, pimozide, quinidine) or CYP2C8 (repaglinide) with narrow therapeutic window: *Avoid*. Substrates of P-gp (digoxin), BCRP (topotecan) and OATP1B1 (rosuvastatin): *Pharmacokinetic interaction cannot be excluded.*

SP: Symptoms associated with decreased LVEF, discontinue; restart after minimum 2 weeks at 1000mg/day (with capecitabine) OR 1250mg/day (with aromatase inhibitor) if LVEF returns to normal. Pulmonary symptoms, discontinue. Other toxicities, discontinue; restart when toxicity improves to Grade 1 or less at 1250mg/day (with capecitabine) OR 1500mg/day (with aromatase inhibitor); if toxicity recurs, restart as for LVEF. *Prior to initiation*, evaluate LVEF, monitor for pulmonary toxicity. Monitor liver function prior to initiation, then monthly. Diarrhoea, including severe; manage with anti-diarrhoeals.

Pregnancy, Lactation: See Notes below.

ADR: See Notes below.

Notes: See 13.1.6 Protein Kinase Inhibitors.

Tyverb 250mg *(Novartis)* A. HT.
Price, (70) €1198.76.
Tablet, lapatinib ditosylate monohydrate. Oval yellow f/c. Marked GS XJG. **Store:** Below 30 deg C.

Lenvatinib

ATC Code: L01XE29. **Sport:** Permitted.
Driving: Minor influence; fatigue, dizziness.
Indications: Treatment, progressive, locally advanced or metastatic, differentiated thyroid carcinoma, refractory to radioactive iodine.

Dose: Adult, Elderly: 24mg once daily. Adverse reactions may need dose interruption, adjustment or discontinuation. *Special populations* (75 years and older, Asian race, hypertension, hepatic or renal impairment), initiate with 24mg/day. *Admin*, approx. same time each day; swallow caps whole with water; do not open capsule to avoid repeated exposure to contents.

Child: Age 2-18 years, safety/efficacy not established. Under 2 years, not recommended (safety concerns).

Renal Impairment: See Hepatic below. ESRD, not recommended.

Hepatic Impairment: Mild/moderate, no adjustment. Severe, initially 14mg once daily; adjust based on tolerability.

Interactions: Effect of Other Drugs on Lenvatinib: *Co-admin caution:* CYP3A4 substrates with narrow therapeutic window (astemizole, terfenadine, cisapride, pimozide, quinidine, bepridil, ergot alkaloids). *Lenvatinib immediately after sorafenib:* Ensure 4-week washout.

SP: Control BP prior to initiation; monitor (1 week after initiation, every 2 weeks for 2 months, then monthly). Monitor TSH levels. *Reported* (may need dose modification), proteinuria (monitor), renal failure (dehydration and/or hypovolaemia due to GI toxicity), cardiac failure and decreased LVEF (monitor for cardiac decompensation), posterior reversible encephalopathy syndrome (control BP), serious haemorrhage (fatal intracranial), arterial thromboembolisms (caution, assess risk/benefit), GI perforation, fistulae formation, QT-prolongation (ECG monitoring), diarrhoea.

Pregnancy, Lactation: Women of childbearing potential to use highly effective contraception during and for 1 month after treatment (add barrier method). Lactation, contraindicated. See Notes below.

ADR: See Notes below.

Notes: See 13.1.6 Protein Kinase Inhibitors.

▼ **LENVIMA 4mg, 10mg** *(Eisai)* A. HT.
Price, (30) 4mg, 10mg, €1977.80.
Capsule, lenvatinib mesilate. Marked with E and LENV and strength. 4mg: Yellowish-red. 10mg: Yellow/yellowish-red. **Store:** Below 25 deg C; original blister to protect (moisture).

Nilotinib

ATC Code: L01XE08. **Sport:** Permitted.
Driving: Dizziness, fatigue, visual impairment.
Indications: Treatment, Ph+ CML, newly diagnosed in chronic phase; chronic phase, accelerated phase (resistant or intolerant to prior therapy).

Dose: Adult, Elderly: Newly diagnosed, 300mg twice daily; resistant or intolerant to prior therapy, 400mg twice daily. Haematological toxicity, withhold temporarily and/or

reduce dose. *Admin*, 12-hourly; swallow caps whole with water on empty stomach 2 hours before or 1 hour after food.

Hepatic Impairment: Caution, increased exposure.

Interactions: Effect of Other Drugs on Nilotinib: *Co-admin avoid (if necessary to use, monitor QT-interval):* Grapefruit juice. *Co-admin not recommended (reduced exposure):* Drugs suppressing gastric acid secretion (H2-blockers, PPIs, antacids). *Bioavailability increased:* Admin with food.

Effect of Other Drugs on Nilotinib: CYP (3A4, 2C8, 2C9, 2D6) and UGT1A1 substrates, medicinals with narrow therapeutic index (astemizole, terfenadine, cisapride, pimozide, quinidine, bepridil, ergot alkaloids including ergotamine, dihydroergotamine), warfarin (monitor INR or prothrombin time), certain statins and oral midazolam (increased systemic exposure): *Caution.* Antiarrhythmics (amiodarone, disopyramide, procainamide, quinidine, sotalol), other drugs causing QT-prolongation (chloroquine, halofantrine, clarithromycin, haloperidol, methadone, moxifloxacin): *QT-prolongation risk.*

SP: Myelosuppression. Severe fluid retention (pleural effusion, pulmonary oedema, pericardia effusion); investigate unexpected rapid weight gain. *Cardiovascular events*, evaluate cardiovascular status, monitor risk factors; recent MI, CHF, unstable angina, bradycardia, caution. QT-prolongation, see Interactions above. Sudden death reported (history of cardiac disease or significant risk factors). Elevated serum lipase, increases in serum cholesterol/blood glucose; assess lipid profiles/blood glucose levels prior to initiation and during treatment; hyperlipidaemia treatment, see Interactions above. Pancreatitis (history), caution. Correct dehydration, treat high uric acid levels prior to initiation. Bioavailability reduced with total gastrectomy.

Pregnancy, Lactation: Women of childbearing potential to use highly effective contraception during and up to 2 weeks after treatment. See Notes below.

ADR: See Notes below.

Notes: See 13.1.6 Protein Kinase Inhibitors.

Tasigna 150mg, 200mg *(Novartis)* A. HT.
Price, (112) 150mg, €2852.94. 200mg, €3895.56.
Capsule, nilotinib HCl monohydrate. Hard light-yellow opaque; contains white (slightly yellowish) powder. *Lactose.* **Store:** Below 30 deg C; original pack to protect (moisture).

Nintedanib (oncology)

ATC Code: L01XE31. **Sport:** Permitted.
Driving: Minor influence; caution.
Indications: After first-line chemotherapy, combination (docetaxel), locally advanced metastatic or locally recurrent non-small cell lung cancer (NSCLC) (adenocarcinoma).

Dose: Adult, Elderly: 200mg twice daily (12 hours apart) (days 2-21) of standard 21-day docetaxel cycle; do not admin on same day as docetaxel (day 1). Max. 400mg/day. *Admin*, swallow whole with water; do not chew or crush; preferably with food.

Child: Under 18 years, safety/efficacy not established.

Renal Impairment: Mild/moderate, no adjustment. CrCl (mL/min) under 30, not studied.

Hepatic Impairment: Mild, no adjustment; moderate/severe, not recommended.

CI: Peanut, soya hypersensitivity.

Interactions: Effect of Other Drugs on Nintedanib: *Increased nintedanib exposure:* Potent P-gp inhibitors (ketoconazole, erythromycin). *Decreased nintedanib exposure:* Potent P-gp inducers (rifampicin, carbamazepine, phenytoin, St John's Wort).

Effect of Nintedanib on Other Drugs: Anticoagulants (warfarin, phenprocoumon): *Monitor prothrombin time, INR.*

SP: Diarrhoea (ensure adequate hydration, anti-diarrhoeals e.g. loperamide, reduce dose or discontinue). Nausea, vomiting (interrupt, reduce dose or discontinue). If dehydration occurs (admin fluids, electrolytes). Monitor blood counts, liver enzymes (start of each treatment cycle). Elevated liver enzymes or bilirubin (females at higher risk). Haemorrhage (epistaxis), tumour-associated, see Interactions above. Increased risk of venous thromboembolism (DVT); arterial thromboembolic events; with idiopathic pulmonary fibrosis, GI perforation (caution,

13.1.6 Protein Kinase Inhibitors

abdominal surgery). May impair wound healing. Exposure generally higher in Asian race.

Pregnancy, Lactation: Pregnancy, not for use unless clinically needed. Exclude pregnancy before initiation. Lactation, stop drug or stop breastfeeding.

ADR: See Notes below.

Notes: See 13.1.6 Protein Kinase Inhibitors.

▼ **Vargatef 100mg, 150mg** *(Boehringer)* A. HT.
Price, 100mg (120), 150mg, (60), €2733.17.
Soft capsule, nintedanib esilate. Opaque oblong soft gelatin. Marked with company symbol and strength. 100mg: Peach. 150mg: Brown. Soya lecithin. **Store:** Below 25 deg C; original pack to protect (moisture).

Pazopanib

ATC Code: L01XE11. **Sport:** Permitted.
Driving: Dizziness, tiredness, weakness.

Indications: First-line, advanced renal cell carcinoma (RCC) (prior cytokine therapy); advanced soft tissue sarcoma (STS) (prior chemotherapy for metastatic disease or progressed within 12 months after adjuvant therapy).

Dose: Adult: RCC, STS, 800mg once daily; titrate in 200mg increments to max. 800mg/day. See Hepatic Impairment. Admin on empty stomach 1 hour before or 2 hours after food, whole with water; do not break, chew or crush.

Child: Under 18 years, safety/efficacy not established; under 2 years, safety concerns (organ growth, maturation).

Renal Impairment: CrCl (mL/min) below 30, caution.

Hepatic Impairment: Mild (normal bilirubin and any ALT elevation OR elevated bilirubin up to 1.5xULN*), initially 800mg once daily; moderate (bilirubin above 1.5-3xULN*), 200mg, once daily. Severe (total bilirubin above 3xULN*), not recommended. *(regardless of ALT).

Interactions: Effect of Other Drugs on Pazopanib: *Co-admin avoid (increased plasma levels):* Grapefruit juice. *Co-admin caution:* Other oral BCRP and P-gp substrates. *Co-admin, increased exposure:* CYP3A4 strong inhibitors (ketoconazole, itraconazole, clarithromycin, atazanavir, indinavir, nefazodone, nelfinavir, ritonavir, saquinavir, telithromycin, voriconazole), P-glycoprotein (P-gp) inhibitors (lapatinib), breast cancer resistance protein (BCRP) inhibitors (lapatinib). *Co-admin, decreased exposure:* CYP3A4 inducers (rifampicin). *Co-admin, increased ALT elevation incidence:* Simvastatin.

Effect of Pazopanib on Other Drugs: UGT1A1 substrates (irinotecan): *Caution (pazopanib is a UGT1A1 inhibitor).*

SP: Hepatic failure (fatal), monitor LFTs before initiation, at weeks (3, 5, 7, 9), at months (3, 4), then periodically. Increased ALT elevation risk with HLA-B*5701 allele. Symptomatic hypertensive episodes/crisis, monitor; hypertensive crisis or severe/persistent hypertension, discontinue. QT-prolongation, Torsade de Pointes, monitor ECG (base line, periodic); maintain electrolytes within normal range. Arterial thrombotic events, MI, ischaemic stroke, TIA. *Caution,* haemorrhagic events, haemoptysis, cerebral/GI haemorrhage (past 6 months), GI perforation, fistula. Impaired wound healing (stop pazopanib 7 days prior to surgery). Monitor, CHF, cardiac dysfunction; decreased LVEF, hypothyroidism, proteinuria, Grade 4, discontinue. Serious infection (fatal). Pneumothorax. Posterior reversible encephalopathy syndrome (PRES), reversible posterior leucoencephalopathy syndrome (PPLS) (discontinue). Thrombotic microangiopathy; permanently discontinue.

Pregnancy, Lactation: Women of childbearing age to ensure adequate contraception and males (including those who have had vasectomies) should use condoms during and for at least 2 weeks after last dose. See Notes below.

ADR: See Notes below.

Notes: See 13.1.6 Protein Kinase Inhibitors.

Votrient 200mg, 400mg *(Novartis)* A. HT.
Price, (30) 200mg, €812.30. 400mg, €1611.16.
Tablet, pazopanib HCl. Cap-shaped f/c. Marked GS. 200mg: Pink. Marked JT. 400mg: White. Marked UHL.

Ponatinib

ATC Code: L01XE24. **Sport:** Permitted.
Driving: Lethargy, dizziness, blurred vision.

Indications: Chronic myeloid leukaemia (CML) (chronic, accelerated or blast phase)*. Acute lymphoblastic leukaemia Ph+ (Ph+ ALL)*. *Resistant or intolerant to dasatinib or nilotinib (CML) or dasatinib only (ALL), imatinib not appropriate, T3151 mutation.

Dose: Adult, Elderly: 45mg once daily. Non-haematological adverse reactions, withhold; resume once resolved. Management of toxicities, see manufacturers Full Prescribing Information. *Admin,* swallow whole, do not crush or dissolve; with or without food. Elderly, 65 years and over, more likely to experience adverse events.

Renal Impairment: CrCl (mL/min) below 50 or ESRD, caution.

Hepatic Impairment: Caution.

Interactions: Effect of Other Drugs on Ponatinib: *Co-admin avoid:* Strong CYP3A4 inducers (carbamazepine, phenobarbital, phenytoin, rifabutin, rifampicin, St. John's Wort). *Co-admin, caution (consider reduced ponatinib starting dose):* Strong CYP3A4 inhibitors (clarithromycin, indinavir, itraconazole, ketoconazole, nefazodone, nelfinavir, ritonavir, saquinavir, telithromycin, troleandomycin, voriconazole, grapefruit juice).

Effect of Ponatinib on Other Drugs: P-gp substrates (digoxin, colchicine, dabigatran, pravastatin): *Plasma levels increased.* Methotrexate, rosuvastatin, sulfasalazine: *Increased (therapeutic effect, adverse reactions).*

SP: Vascular occlusion, arterial or venous thrombosis and occlusions; more frequent with (increasing age, history of ischaemia, hypertension, diabetes, hyperlipidaemia); likely to be dose-related. Assess cardiovascular status before initiation; manage risk factors. Fatal and serious CHF, haemorrhage (history of, use only if benefit outweighs risk); consider alternative. *Monitor,* full blood counts every 2 weeks for first 3 months, then monthly (severe myelosuppression); check serum lipase every 2 weeks (first 2 months) then periodically (pancreatitis); consider dose modification. Perform LFTs periodically. Monitor for evidence of thromboembolism and vascular occlusion; decreased vision, perform ophthalmic examination (retinal venous occlusion).

Pregnancy, Lactation: Advise men not to father a child during treatment. See Notes below.

ADR: See Notes below.

Notes: See 13.1.6 Protein Kinase Inhibitors.

▼ **Iclusig 15mg, 45mg** *(Incyte)* A. HT.
Price, (60) both strengths, €6426.00.
Tablet, ponatinib HCl. Round white f/c. 15mg: Marked A5. 45mg: Marked AP4. Lactose. **Store:** Original pack.

Regorafenib

ATC Code: L01XE21. **Sport:** Permitted.
Driving: Caution if ability to concentrate or react is affected.

Indications: Treatment, metastatic colorectal cancer (MCRC) (previously treated, available therapy not suitable); unresectable or metastatic GI stromal tumours (GIST) (progress on or intolerant to prior imatinib and sunitinib).

Dose: Adult, Elderly: Recommended, 160mg once daily for 3 weeks then 1 week off therapy (1-treatment cycle). Dose interruptions or modifications may be required; modifications should be made in 40mg (1 tab) steps; 80mg/day is lowest recommended dose. Admin at same time each day; swallow whole with water after a light meal (less than 30% fat).

Child: MCRC, no relevant use; GIST, under 18 years, safety/efficacy not established.

Renal Impairment: No adjustment.

Hepatic Impairment: Moderate, no dose recommendation (monitor); severe, not recommended.

Interactions: Effect of Other Drugs on Regorafenib: *Avoid co-admin:* Strong UGT1A9 inhibitors (mefenamic acid, diflunisal, niflumic acid). *Regorafenib efficacy may be decreased:* Neomycin.

Effect of Regorafenib on Other Drugs: UGT1A1/9 substrates (irinotecan): *Increased substrate exposure.* BCRP substrates (methotrexate, fluvastatin, atorvastatin): *Plasma levels increased.*

SP: Severe LFT abnormalities, and hepatic dysfunction; perform LFTs before initiation, at least every 2 weeks (first 2 months) then at least monthly; severe LFT abnormalities and hepatic dysfunction*. Impaired wound healing. Hand-foot skin reaction*, rash. *Increased incidence,* haemorrhagic events (fatal), monitor blood counts and coagulation parameters if predisposed to bleeding or on anticoagulants (warfarin, phenprocoumon); severe bleeding, permanently discontinue; myocardial ischaemia and infarction (history of), monitor; if develops, discontinue until resolved. Arterial hypertension, control BP prior to initiation; severe or persistent, temporarily interrupt; hypertensive crisis, discontinue. Electrolyte and metabolic abnormalities. *Reported*, posterior reversible encephalopathy syndrome, GI perforation (fatal), fistulae. *higher incidence reported in Asian (particularly Japanese) patients.

Pregnancy, Lactation: Ensure adequate contraception during and up to 8 weeks after treatment. See Notes below.

ADR: See Notes below.

Notes: See 13.1.6 Protein Kinase Inhibitors.

▼ **Stivarga 40mg** *(Bayer)* A. HT.
Price, (84) €3154.04.
Tablet, regorafenib. Light-pink f/c oval. Marked Bayer; 40 on reverse. *Sodium* 55.8mg/160mg dose; soya lecithin. **Store:** Original pack to protect (moisture); keep desiccant in bottle.

Ruxolitinib

ATC Code: L01XE18. **Sport:** Permitted.
Driving: No or negligible effect; dizziness.
Indications: Treatment (adults), disease-related splenomegaly or symptoms with primary myelofibrosis, post (polycythaemia vera or essential thrombocythaemia myelofibrosis); polycythaemia vera (intolerant or resistant to hydroxyurea).

Dose: Adult, Elderly: Initially, *myelofibrosis (MF)*, 15mg twice daily with platelets between 100-200 (x1000)/mm3 OR 20mg twice daily with platelets 200 (x1000)/mm3 and above; *polycythaemia vera (PV)*, 10mg twice daily; max. 5mg twice daily with platelets 50-100 (x1000)/mm3; titrate cautiously. Do not increase initial dose within first 4 weeks and then at minimum 2-week intervals; max. 25mg twice daily. Oral with or without food. Dose adjustments, combination use with strong CYP3A4 inhibitors and/or CYP2C9 inhibitors, as for Renal below with twice weekly haematological monitoring.

Renal Impairment: CrCl (mL/min) below 30, *MF*, reduce dose by 50% dosed twice daily with careful monitoring; *PV*, 5mg twice daily. ESRD on dialysis, see manufacturers Full Prescribing Information.

Hepatic Impairment: Based on platelet count, reduce by 50% dosed twice daily.

Interactions: Effect of Other Drugs on Ruxolitinib: *Reduce dose by 50%*: Boceprevir, clarithromycin, indinavir, itraconazole, ketoconazole, lopinavir/ritonavir, ritonavir, mibefradil, nefazodone, nelfinavir, posaconazole, saquinavir, telaprevir, telithromycin, voriconazole; fluconazole (avoid at dose 200mg/day or more). *Dose increase may be needed*: CYP3A4 inducers (avasimibe, carbamazepine, phenobarbital, phenytoin, rifabutin, rifampicin, St. John's Wort). *Monitor (cytopenias)*: Erythromycin.

Effect of Ruxolitinib on Other Drugs: CYP3A4 substrates, substances transported by P-glycoprotein and BCRP (dabigatran, ciclosporin, rosuvastatin, 'potentially' digoxin): *Keep admin as far apart as possible.*

SP: Myelosuppression (perform full blood cell count prior initiation); thrombocytopenia; reduce dose or withhold temporarily; anaemia may require blood transfusions. PML reported.

Pregnancy, Lactation: Contraindicated.

ADR: See Notes below.

Notes: See 13.1.6 Protein Kinase Inhibitors.

Jakavi 5mg, 10mg, 15mg, 20mg *(Novartis)* A. HT.
Price, (56) 5mg, €1950.81; 10mg, €3855.23; 15mg, €3880.82; 20mg, €3897.92.
Tablet, ruxolitinib phosphate. White (almost). Marked NVR; L and strength on reverse. 5mg, 10mg: Round. 15mg: Ovaloid. 20mg: Elongated. *Lactose*. **Store:** Below 30 deg C.

Sorafenib

ATC Code: L01XE05. **Sport:** Permitted.
Driving: No evidence that ability affected.
Indications: Treatment, hepatocellular carcinoma; advanced renal cell carcinoma (failed or unsuitable for interferon-alfa or interleukin-2 therapy); progressive, locally advanced or metastatic, differentiated thyroid carcinoma refractory to radioactive iodine.

Dose: Adult, Elderly: 400mg twice daily (800mg/day). If not tolerated reduce to 400mg once daily (hepatocellular, advanced renal cell carcinoma) or 600mg/day in divided doses (thyroid carcinoma). Admin without food or with a low or moderate fat meal; with high fat meal, take 1 hour before or 2 hours after; swallow whole with water. *Elderly*, consider monitoring renal function.

Renal Impairment: At risk, monitor fluid, electrolytes.

Hepatic Impairment: Severe, no data.

Interactions: Effect of Other Drugs on Sorafenib: *Co-admin caution*: Medicinals metabolised/eliminated by UGT1A1 (irinotecan) or UGT1A9 pathways (docetaxel). *Decreased exposure*: Neomycin. *Higher mortality (squamous cell carcinoma) with co-admin*: Platinum-based chemotherapy (carboplatin).

Effect of Sorafenib on Other Drugs: Warfarin, phenprocoumon: *Monitor INR or prothrombin time; adjust dose*. Digoxin: *Possible increased plasma levels*. Docetaxel: *Increased exposure, caution.*

SP: Palmar-plantar erythrodysaesthesia, rash. Hypertension, monitor BP. Increased bleeding risk. Cardiac ischaemia and/or MI, GI perforation, discontinue permanently. Wound healing, caution, major surgery. CHF, prolonged QT/QTc interval; increased ventricular arrhythmia risk. Differentiated thyroid cancer, evaluate prognosis before initiating. Due to potential bleeding risk, tracheal, bronchial, and oesophageal infiltration should be treated with localised therapy prior to initiation. Monitor blood calcium, TSH levels.

ADR: See Notes below.

Notes: See 13.1.6 Protein Kinase Inhibitors.

Nexavar 200mg *(Bayer)* A. HT.
Price, (112) €3799.55.
Tablet, sorafenib tosilate. Red round f/c. Marked with Bayer cross; 200 on reverse. **Store:** Below 25 deg C.

Sunitinib

ATC Code: L01XE04. **Sport:** Permitted.
Driving: Dizziness.
Indications: GI stromal tumour (GIST), unresectable and/or metastatic, after imatinib failure. Metastatic renal cell carcinoma (MRCC) (advanced/metastatic). Pancreatic neuro-endocrine tumours (pNET) (unresectable or metastatic well-differentiated with disease progression).

Dose: Adult, Elderly: *GIST, MRCC*, 6-week cycle, 50mg/day (4 consecutive weeks, then 2-week rest); titrate by 12.5mg steps; max. 75mg/day (87.5mg with CYP3A4 inhibitors); minimum 25mg/day (37.5mg with CYP3A4 inhibitors). *pNET*, 37.5mg daily without rest period; titrate by 12.5mg steps; max. 50mg daily (with CYP3A4 inhibitors, 62.5mg/day; minimum 25mg). *Admin*, oral, with or without food.

Child: Under 18 years, safety/efficacy not established.

Renal Impairment: Nephrotic syndrome, discontinue.

Hepatic Impairment: Severe, no data.

Interactions: Effect of Other Drugs on Sunitinib: *Plasma levels increased*: CYP3A4 inhibitors (grapefruit juice); choose alternative or consider dose reduction.

Effect of Sunitinib on Other Drugs: Warfarin, acenocoumarol: *Monitor (platelets, INR).*

SP: Skin discolouration (active substance is yellow); skin, hair depigmentation may occur; dryness, thickness/cracking, blisters, pyoderma gangrenosum, rash, mouth pain/irritation. Treatment-related haemorrhage; may occur suddenly, severe, life-threatening); epistaxis common. Pulmonary tumour, severe/life-threatening haemoptysis or haemorrhage. Consider anti-emetics, anti-diarrhoeals; may be fatal (perforation). Hypertension, screen (control); reduce dose or temporarily suspend. Perform complete blood counts (each treatment cycle); fatal haemorrhage associated with thrombocytopenia, neutropenic infections. Anaemia. Cardiovascular events (HF, cardiomyopathy, myocardial ischaemia/infarction); evaluate baseline risk factors; CHF, discontinue. QT-prolongation, caution. Thrombolic events, venous (DVT), arterial (DVA, TIA, cerebral infarction); risk

13.1.7   Monoclonal Antibodies

factors (underlying malignancy, age 65 years and older, hypertension, diabetes mellitus, prior thromboembolic disease). Pulmonary events. Hypothyroidism, tumour lysis syndrome (monitor). Pancreatitis, hepatic failure, renal impairment, failure, necrotising fasciitis (fatal); discontinue. Fistula formation, interrupt. Impaired wound healing, osteonecrosis of jaw, dysgeusia. Seizures, temporarily suspend and treat. Hypoglycaemia, temporarily interrupt.

ADR: See Notes below.

Notes: See 13.1.6 Protein Kinase Inhibitors.

SUTENT 12.5mg, 25mg, 50mg *(Pfizer)* A. HT.
Price, (28) 12.5mg, €1252.75. 25mg, €2497.69. 50mg, €4982.73.
Capsule, sunitinib malate. Hard gelatin; contain yellow (orange) granules. Marked Pfizer, STN/strength. 12.5mg: Orange/orange. 25mg: Caramel/orange. 50mg: Caramel/caramel. *Mannitol.*

Vandetanib

ATC Code: L01XE12. **Sport:** Permitted.
Driving: Fatigue, blurred vision.

Indications: Treatment, aggressive and symptomatic medullary thyroid cancer (unresectable locally advanced or metastatic disease).

Dose: Adult, Elderly: 300mg once daily with or without food at about same time each day. Swallowing difficulties, disperse tabs in half a glass of non-carbonated water and swallow or admin through nasogastric or gastrostomy tube; tabs to be dropped whole into water and stirred until dispersed.

Renal Impairment: Moderate, reduce dose; sever, safety/efficacy not established.

Hepatic Impairment: Serum bilirubin above 1.5xULN, not recommended.

CI: Congenital long QTc syndrome, QTc interval above 480 msec, do not initiate.

Interactions: Effect of Other Drugs on Vandetanib: *Co-admin contraindicated:* Drugs prolonging QTc interval or inducing Torsades de Pointes (arsenic, cisapride, IV erythromycin, toremifene, mizolastine, moxifloxacin, Class IA and III antiarrhythmics). *Co-admin not recommended:* Ondansetron, methadone, haloperidol, amisulpride, chlorpromazine, sulpiride, zuclopenthixol, halofantrine, pentamidine, lumefantrine. *Co-admin avoid:* Potent CYP3A4 inducers (rifampicin, St John's Wort, carbamazepine, phenobarbital).

Effect of Vandetanib on Other Drugs: Metformin, P-gp substrates (digoxin, dabigatran): *Lower dose may be required; clinical monitoring.* Vitamin K antagonists: *Increased frequency of INR monitoring.*

SP: Treatment to be initiated by physician experienced in (MTC treatment, use of anticancer medicinals, ECG assessment). Dose of 300mg associated with substantial, concentration-dependent QTc prolongation (first occurred most often in first 3 months); problem due to long half-life (19 days); interval of 500 msec or above, discontinue. Assess QTc interval prior to initiation; toxicity or prolonged QTc interval, reduce dose or temporarily discontinue. Obtain ECG, serum potassium, calcium and magnesium, thyroid stimulating hormone (TSH) at baseline, at weeks 1, 3, 6 and 12, then 3-monthly (minimum 1 year). Posterior reversible encephalopathy syndrome, skin reactions (photosensitivity, palmar-plantar erythrodysaesthesia syndrome); severe (Stevens-Johnson syndrome), seek urgent medical advice. Diarrhoea (routine anti-diarrhoeals), haemorrhage (intracranial), HF (may not be reversible; fatal), hypertension (hypertensive crisis), ILD, see Notes below. Patient to carry a Patient Alert Card.

Pregnancy, Lactation: Lactation, contraindicated.

ADR: See Notes below.

Notes: See 13.1.6 Protein Kinase Inhibitors.

▼ **Caprelsa 100mg, 300mg** *(Genzyme)* A. HT.
Price, (30) 100mg, €2241.51; 300mg, €5142.08.
Tablet, vandetanib. White. Marked Z and strength. 100mg: Round. 300mg: Oval. **Store:** Below 30 deg C.

Vemurafenib

ATC Code: L01XE15. **Sport:** Permitted.
Driving: Minor influence; potential fatigue, eye problems.

Indications: Treatment, melanoma (BRAF V600 mutation-positive unresectable or metastatic).

Dose: Adult, Elderly: 960mg twice daily. *Admin,* with or without food; avoid taking both daily doses on empty stomach. Swallow whole, do not chew or crush. Adverse reactions, QTc prolongation may need dose reduction.

Renal Impairment: Severe, monitor for increased exposure.

Hepatic Impairment: Moderate/severe, as for Renal above.

Interactions: Effect of Other Drugs on Vemurafenib: *Co-admin not recommended:* Ipilimumab. *Co-admin caution:* Potent inhibitors (CYP3A4, glucuronidation and/or transport proteins) (ritonavir, saquinavir, telithromycin, ketoconazole, itraconazole, voriconazole, posaconazole, nefazodone, atazanavir). *Co-admin avoid (suboptimal exposure):* Potent inducers (P-gp), glucuronidation and/or CYP3A4) (rifampicin, rifabutin, carbamazepine, phenytoin, St John's Wort). *Pharmacokinetics may be affected:* Verapamil, clarithromycin, ciclosporin, ritonavir, quinidine, dronedarone, amiodarone, itraconazole, ranolazine.

Effect of Vemurafenib on Other Drugs: Warfarin: *Increased exposure; monitor INR.* CYP1A2 substrates (caffeine): *Increased plasma exposure; consider dose adjustment.* CYP3A4 substrates (midazolam, substrates with narrow therapeutic window), oral contraceptives: *Decreased exposure.* Medicinals transported by P-gp (aliskiren, colchicine, digoxin, everolimus, fexofenadine) or BCRP (methotrexate, mitoxantrone, rosuvastatin): *Exposure may be increased.*

SP: Not for use in wild-type BRAF malignant melanoma. Serious reactions (hypersensitivity, dermatologic); permanently discontinue. Exposure-dependent QT prolongation; monitor before initiation, after (1 month, dose modification). Moderate or severe hepatic impairment; monitor. Pancreatitis. Long half-life (8 days). Renal toxicity; monitor serum creatinine (before initiation, as needed). *Reported (monitor),* serious ophthalmologic reactions; non-cutaneous and cutaneous squamous cell carcinoma; new primary melanoma; other malignancies (RAS-mutation), photosensitivity. Laboratory abnormalities. Dupuytren's contracture and plantar fascial fibromatosis.

Pregnancy, Lactation: Ensure adequate contraception during and up to 6 months after treatment. See Notes below.

ADR: See Notes below.

Notes: See 13.1.6 Protein Kinase Inhibitors.

Zelboraf 240mg *(Roche)* A. HT.
Price, (56) €1849.08.
Tablet, vemurafenib. White (pink/orange) oval f/c. Marked VEM. **Store:** Original pack to protect (moisture).

13.1.7 - Monoclonal Antibodies

In This Chapter: *Bevacizumab, brentuximab, cetuximab, elotuzumab, ipilimumab, nivolumab, obinutuzumab, ofatumumab, panitumumab, pembrolizumab, pertuzumab, ramucirumab, rituximab, trastuzumab, trastuzumab emtansine.*

Class Effects

Store: Before use, all monoclonal antibody parenteral formulations should be stored in the refrigerator i.e. between 2-8 degrees Centigrade (C).

CI: Hypersensitivity to any member of the class. Use in children under 18 years unless specified (generally safety/efficacy not established).

SP: Infusion reactions e.g. anaphylactic or anaphylactoid events, cardiac events (myocardial ischaemia or MI, bradycardia), hypo- and/or hypertension, rigors, fever, shortness of breath, chills, rashes, bronchospasm, cytokine release syndrome; other hypersensitivity reactions (following IV admin of proteins); interrupt or withdraw (premedication may attenuate). Facilities and medication to manage hypersensitivity reactions to be present. Tumour Lysis Syndrome. Acute respiratory failure, with pulmonary interstitial infiltration or oedema, visible on a chest x-ray; death. Transient hypotension, caution (ischaemic heart disease, angina, antihypertensive medication). Monitor, cardiac function (previous treatment with cardiotoxic agents), haematological profile. Decreased LVEF with medicinals blocking HER2 activity. Prior anthracyclines or prior radiotherapy (chest) may increase LVEF decline risk. To improve traceability of biological medicinals, clearly record the brand name AND batch number in the patient file. These drugs are generally initiated and supervised by specialist physicians.

Pregnancy, Lactation: See Notes below.

ADR: See manufacturers Full Prescribing Information. See Notes below.

Notes: See also 13.1 Cytotoxic Drugs.

Bevacizumab

ATC Code: L01XC07. **Sport:** Permitted.
Driving: No or negligible effect; somnolence, syncope.

Indications: Treatment, metastatic carcinoma of colon or rectum (mCRC). First-line, metastatic breast cancer (mBC); unresectable advanced metastatic or recurrent non-small cell lung cancer (NSCLC), including with EGFR mutations; advanced and/or metastatic renal cell cancer (mRCC). Front-line treatment, advanced epithelial ovarian, fallopian tube or primary peritoneal cancer; first recurrence, platinum- (sensitive, resistant) recurrent. Cervical carcinoma, persistent, recurrent, metastatic.

Dose: Adult, Elderly: mCRC, 5mg/kg or 10mg/kg body weight 2-weekly OR 7.5mg/kg or 15mg/kg 3-weekly. mBC, 10mg/kg 2-weekly or 15mg 3-weekly. mRCC, 10mg/kg 2-weekly. NSCLC, 7.5mg/kg or 15mg/kg 3-weelkly (with platinum) for up to 6 cycles, then monotherapy; NSCLC with EGFR mutations, 15mg/kg 3-weekly (with erlotinib).

Other (ovarian, fallopian tube, peritoneal), 15mg/kg 3-weekly (with carboplatin and paclitaxel) for up to 6 cycles, then monotherapy; max. 15 months; platinum-sensitive recurrent, 15mg/kg 3-weekly (with carboplatin and gemcitabine) for 6 cycles up to 10 cycles then monotherapy; platinum-resistant recurrent, 10mg/kg 2-weekly with one of either (paclitaxel or doxorubicin) OR 15mg/kg 3-weekly (with topotecan).

Cervical, 15mg/kg 3-weekly with paclitaxel and (cisplatin or topotecan). Admin, IV infusion over 90 minutes (first dose); if tolerated, infuse over 60 minutes (second dose); if tolerated, infuse over 30 minutes (subsequent infusions). Dose reduction for adverse events not recommended; temporarily suspend or discontinue.

Child: Under 18 years, no dose recommendation.

Hepatic Impairment: As for Renal above.

CI: Hypersensitivity to Chinese hamster ovary (CHO) cell products, other recombinant human antibodies.

Interactions: Effect of Other Drugs on Bevacizumab: Co-admin not recommended: EGFR monoclonal antibodies. Co-admin caution (microangiopathic haemolytic anaemia risk; hypertensive crisis): Sunitinib. Co-admin (increased severe/febrile neutropenia rates, infection): Platinum- or taxane-based therapies. Co-admin, no data: Radiotherapy.

Effect of Bevacizumab On Other Drugs: Irinotecan: Dose modification with co-admin (diarrhoea, leucopenia, neutropenia).

SP: May affect wound healing (serious complications; fatal outcome); withhold elective surgery. Arterial thromboembolism; risk higher in combination (arterial thromboembolism history, diabetes, over 65 years), at greater risk; pulmonary VTE. CNS metastases, monitor (CNS haemorrhage, especially tumour-associated). NSCLC, pulmonary haemorrhage or haemoptysis risk. Increased severe (febrile) neutropenia with infection (combination). Infusion reactions (premedication not warranted). Osteonecrosis of jaw (with prior IV bisphosphonate). NOT for intravitreal use; serious ocular events; degrees of visual loss (permanent blindness).

Discontinue, increased GI, gall bladder perforation risk (prior radiation a risk for GI). Reversible posterior leucoencephalopathy syndrome. Permanently discontinue, GI-vaginal fistulae (increased with prior radiation); non-GI fistulae risk, tracheoesophageal fistula (any grade 4). Uncontrolled hypertension or hypertensive crisis/encephalopathy (control hypertension; diuretics not

advised with cisplatin-based chemotherapy; greater risk for proteinuria development with hypertension, monitor by dipstick urinalysis). Consider discontinuation, internal fistulae (not GI). Caution, congenital bleeding diathesis, acquired coagulopathy, anticoagulant co-admin for thromboembolism. CHF risk (previous anthracyclines, prior radiotherapy to left chest wall, other CHF risk factors); significant CVD.

Pregnancy, Lactation: Pregnancy, contraindicated (crosses placenta; anticipated to inhibit angiogenesis in foetus, serious birth defects suspected). Women of childbearing potential to ensure adequate contraception*. Lactation, not recommended*. *(during and for at least 6 months after treatment).

ADR: See Notes below.

Notes: See 13.1.7 Monoclonal Antibodies.

Avastin Parenteral 25mg/mL (Roche) A. HOS.
Price, (1) 100mg, €309.12; 400mg, €1171.30 (PTW).
Infusion, bevacizumab. Recombinant humanised monoclonal antibody produced by rDNA technology. Clear (slightly opalescent) colourless (pale-brown) conc for soln. **Store:** Refrigerate; do not freeze.

Brentuximab Vedotin

ATC Code: L01XC12. **Sport:** Permitted.
Driving: May have minor influence.

Indications: Treatment (relapsed or refractory), CD30+ Hodgkin's lymphoma (HL), systemic anaplastic large cell lymphoma (sALCL).

Dose: Adult, Elderly: 1.8mg/kg as IV infusion over 30 minutes every 3 weeks; over 100kg, base dose calculation on 100kg. Minimum 8 cycles, max. 16 cycles. Retreatment (relapsed or refractory HL or sALCL) as above or at last tolerated dose. Elderly, age 65 years and older, no data. Not for IV push or bolus; admin through dedicated IV line; not for mixture with other products.

Renal Impairment: Monitor closely. Severe, initially 1.2mg/kg as IV infusion over 30 minutes every 3 weeks.

Hepatic Impairment: As for Renal above.

Interactions: Effect of Other Drugs on Brentuximab Vedotin: Co-admin contraindicated: Bleomycin (pulmonary toxicity). Exposure may be altered: CYP3A4 inhibitors (ketoconazole), CYP3A4 inducers (rifampicin metabolites).

SP: Monitor, complete blood counts prior to each dose; patients during and after infusion (infusion-related reactions, anaphylactic reactions). Neurological, cognitive or behavioural signs/symptoms as progressive multifocal leucoencephalopathy (PML). Possible serious infections and opportunistic infections (Pneumocystis jirovecii pneumonia, oral candidiasis). Liver function (ALT and AST) elevations. Tumour lysis syndrome. Peripheral neuropathy, (sensory and motor). Haematological toxicities, febrile neutropenia. Stevens-Johnson syndrome, toxic epidermal necrolysis*, discontinue. Hyperglycaemia with elevated Body Mass Index with or without diabetes mellitus history. Acute pancreatitis*, monitor. Pulmonary toxicity, GI complications, hepatotoxicity*. *(including fatal).

Pregnancy, Lactation: Pregnancy, if benefit outweighs risk; advise on potential risk to foetus. Women of childbearing potential should be using 2 methods of effective contraception during and for 6 months after treatment. Lactation, stop breastfeeding or stop drug.

ADR: See Notes below.

Notes: See 13.1.7 Monoclonal Antibodies.

▼ **Adcetris Parenteral** (Takeda) A. HOS.
Price, (1) €3191.26 (PTW).
Infusion, brentuximab vedotin 50mg/vial. White (off-white) cake or powder for conc for soln. Sodium 13.2mg/vial. **Store:** Refrigerate; do not freeze.

Cetuximab

ATC Code: L01XC06. **Sport:** Permitted.
Driving: Concentration or reaction altered.

Indications: Treatment, EGFR-expressing, RAS wild-type metastatic colorectal cancer (mCRC), in combination with irinotecan; first-line in combination with FOLFOX; monotherapy following failure of oxaliplatin- and irinotecan-based therapy. Treatment, squamous cell cancer of head and neck in combination with, radiation or platinum-based chemotherapy.

13.1.7 Monoclonal Antibodies

Dose: Adult, Elderly: Initially 400mg/m2 BSA infusion over 120 minutes, then 250mg/m2 once weekly infusion over 60 minutes; max. infusion rate 10mg/min. Colorectal cancer, monotherapy or in combination; squamous cell cancer, in combination with radiation starting cetuximab 1 week before radiation; combination with platinum after cetuximab. *Elderly*, over 75 years, limited data.

Cl: Known severe hypersensitivity reactions. Before initiating combination treatment, consider contraindications for chemotherapy or radiation. Combination with oxaliplatin in mutant-RAS mCRC or if RAS mCRC status unknown.

Interactions: Effect of Other Drugs on Cetuximab: *Increased cardiac ischaemia frequency, Palmar-Plantar erythrodysaesthesia:* Fluoropyrimidine combination. *Frequency increased:* Platinum combination (severe neutropenia/leucopenia), capecitabine and oxaliplatin (severe diarrhoea).

SP: Mild/moderate infusion-related reactions, decrease infusion rate; severe, immediate and permanent discontinuation. Cardio-pulmonary disease and reduced performance status, caution. Interstitial lung disease, discontinue. Skin reactions (severe); interrupt; risk of secondary infections (consider prophylactic oral tetracyclines for 6-8 weeks and topical 1% hydrocortisone cream with moisturiser). Severe hypomagnesaemia, diarrhoea-associated hypokalaemia, hypocalcaemia (platinum combination). Increased frequency of severe/fatal cardiovascular events and treatment emergent deaths. Keratitis, refer to ophthalmologist.

Pregnancy, Lactation: Pregnancy, if benefit outweighs risk; strongly recommended not to use. Women of child-bearing potential to ensure adequate contraception (increased abortion incidence observed). Lactation, not recommended, and for 2 months after last dose.

ADR: See Notes below.

Notes: See 13.1.7 Monoclonal Antibodies.

Erbitux Parenteral (Merck Serono) A. HOS.
Price, (1) 100mg, €198.11 (PTW).
Infusion, cetuximab 5mg/mL. Monoclonal IgG1 antibody produced by rDNA technology. Colourless soln. *Store:* Refrigerate.

Elotuzumab

ATC Code: L01XC23. **Sport:** Permitted.
Driving: Not expected to influence; infusion reactions.

Indications: Treatment (adults), in combination (lenalidomide and dexamethasone), multiple myeloma (received at least one prior treatment).

Dose: Adult: *Premedication* must be admin 45-90 minutes prior to elotuzumab; dexamethasone 8mg IV, diphenhydramine 25-50mg oral or IV (or equiv. H1-blocker), ranitidine 50mg IV or 150mg orally (or equiv. H2-blocker), paracetamol 650-1000mg orally. Management of infusion reactions*.

Recommended, elotuzumab 10mg/kg IV every week on days 1, 8, 15 and 22 (28-day cycle) for first two cycles and then every 2 weeks on days 1 and 15. In combination* with lenalidomide (at least 2 hours after elotuzumab infusion when admin on same day) and dexamethasone (oral before, IV after elotuzumab). *Admin*, by IV infusion; initiate at rate 0.5mL/min; if tolerated increase to max. 5mL/min. *See manufacturers Full Prescribing Information.

Elderly: Age 65 years and over, no adjustment; 85 years and older, limited data.

Child: No relevant use.

Renal Impairment: No adjustment including ESRD requiring dialysis.

Hepatic Impairment: Mild, no adjustment; moderate/severe, not studied.

SP: Monitor patients for second primary malignancies (solid tumours, non-melanoma skin cancer).

Pregnancy, Lactation: Pregnancy, not for use unless needed for clinical condition. Women of child-bearing potential to ensure adequate contraception; male patients to use effective contraception during and for 180 days following treatment if their partner is pregnant or of childbearing potential and not using effective contraception. Lenalidomide, contraindicated. Lactation, stop breastfeeding because of the use of lenalidomide.

ADR: See Notes below.

Notes: See 13.1.7 Monoclonal Antibodies. See 13.2.1 Immunosuppressants (lenalidomide) and 11.1.1 Glucocorticoids (dexamethasone).

▼ *Empliciti Parenteral 300mg, 400mg (BMS)* A.
Price, not published by company.
Infusion, elotuzumab. Produced by rDNA technology. White (off-white) powder cake for conc for soln. *Store:* Refrigerate; do not freeze.

Ipilimumab

ATC Code: L01XC11. **Sport:** Permitted.
Driving: Fatigue.

Indications: Treatment, advanced unresectable or metastatic melanoma in adults.

Dose: Adult, Elderly: 3mg/kg IV over 90 minutes every 3 weeks; total 4 doses. Immune-related adverse reactions, withhold a dose or permanently discontinue; dose reduction not recommended. Not for IV push or bolus injection.

Hepatic Impairment: Transaminases above 5xULN or bilirubin above 3xULN at baseline, caution.

Interactions: Effect of Other Drugs on Ipilimumab: *Co-admin not recommended:* Vemurafenib. *Potential interference with pharmacodynamic activity/efficacy:* Systemic corticosteroids, avoid (at baseline). *Co-admin, monitor:* Anticoagulants (GI haemorrhage).

SP: Immune-related adverse reactions (severe or life-threatening); may need systemic high-dose corticosteroid with or without immunosuppressives. Monitor for immune-related signs and symptoms (GI, liver, skin, neurological, endocrine); cases of Vogt-Koyanagi-Harada syndrome. Evaluate LFTs, thyroid function (baseline, before each dose).

Pregnancy, Lactation: Pregnancy and women of childbearing potential not using effective contraception, use only if benefit outweighs risk. Lactation, stop breastfeeding or stop drug.

ADR: See Notes below.

Notes: See 13.1.7 Monoclonal Antibodies.

▼ *Yervoy Parenteral (BMS)* A. HOS.
Price, (1) 50mg, €3916.62. 200mg, €15615.91 (PTW).
Infusion, ipilimumab 5mg/mL (10mL, 40mL). Clear slightly opalescent colourless (pale-yellow); may contain few particulates. pH 7. *Sodium* 2.3mg/mL. *Store:* Refrigerate; do not freeze.

Nivolumab

ATC Code: L01XC17. **Sport:** Permitted.
Driving: Unlikely to affect; fatigue.

Indications: *Monotherapy or combination (ipilimumab):* Melanoma, advanced (unresectable or metastatic). *Monotherapy:* Non-small cell lung cancer (NSCLC), locally advanced or metastatic*. Renal cell carcinoma (RCC)*. Classical Hodgkin lymphoma (cHL) relapses or refractory (after autologous stem cell transplant and brentuximab vedotin). *(after prior chemotherapy).

Dose: Adult: Recommended, 3mg/kg every 2 weeks. *Combination*, 1mg/kg nivolumab every 3 weeks (first 4 doses) with 3mg/kg ipilimumab IV (over 90 minutes). Then second phase, 3mg/kg nivolumab every 2 weeks. Continue as long as clinical benefit or no longer tolerated. Dose escalation or reduction not recommended; dose delay or discontinuation may be needed. *Admin*, IV infusion over 60 minutes. NOT for IV push or bolus injection. Combination, admin nivolumab first; then ipilimumab on same day; use separate infusion bag and filters.

Elderly: As for Adult. NSCLC, age 75 years and older, limited data.

Renal Impairment: No dose adjustment. Severe, limited data.

Hepatic Impairment: Moderate or severe, caution.

Interactions: Effect of Other Drugs on Nivolumab: *Potential interference with pharmacodynamic activity/efficacy:* Systemic corticosteroids, avoid (at baseline).

SP: Supply patients with patient alert card. Consider delayed nivolumab onset before initiating in rapidly progressing disease (melanoma), poorer prognostic features, aggressive disease (NSCLC, head and neck cancer). Caution, infusion reactions (severe). *Combination*, higher incidence of immune-related adverse reactions (admin corticosteroids; add non-corticosteroid immunosuppressive therapy if worsening or no improvement; prophylactic antibiotics to prevent opportunistic infection); severe, permanently discontinue. Cardiac adverse events, pulmonary embolism (life-threatening, discontinue). *Monitor*, for cardiac and pulmonary events, clinical signs, symptoms, laboratory abnormalities (electrolyte disturbance, dehydration) prior to, then periodically; continuous monitoring (at least up to 5 months after last dose). Pneumonitis (radiographic changes, dyspnoea, hypoxia), diarrhoea, colitis, severe (hepatitis, nephritis, renal dysfunction), severe endocrinopathies e.g. hypo- or hyperthyroidism, adrenal insufficiency (secondary adrenocortical insufficiency), hypophysitis (hypopituitarism), diabetes mellitus, diabetic ketoacidosis), rash, Stevens-Johnson syndrome, toxic epidermal necrolysis, other immune-related reactions (pancreatitis, uveitis, demyelination, autoimmune neuropathy, Guillain-Barre syndrome, myasthenic syndrome, encephalitis). Solid organ transplant rejection reported. Disease-specific precautions, see Full Prescribing Information.

Pregnancy, Lactation: Pregnancy, not recommended unless using effective contraception and if benefit outweighs risk; use effective contraception for at least 5 months after last dose. Lactation, stop breastfeeding or stop drug.

ADR: See Notes below.

Notes: See 13.1.7 Monoclonal Antibodies.

▼ **OPDIVO Parenteral 10mg/mL** *(BMS)* A.
Price, not published by company (4mL, 10mL).
Infusion, nivolumab. Clear (opalescent) colourless (pale-yellow) liquid; might contain few light particles. pH 6.0. *Sodium 2.5mg/mL*. **Store:** Refrigerate; do not freeze.

Obinutuzumab

ATC Code: L01XC15. **Sport:** Permitted.
Driving: No or negligible effect; caution infusion-related symptoms.
Indications: Treatment chronic lymphocytic leukaemia (CLL), (with chlorambucil), previously untreated, unsuitable for fludarabine-based treatment; follicular lymphoma (FL), (with bendamustine), patients who did not responds or progressed during or up to 6 months after rituximab.

Dose: Adult, Elderly: *CLL, cycle 1*, 1000mg over day 1 and day 2 (100mg day 1; 900mg day 2), then 1000mg on day 8 and day 15 of first 28-day cycle. *Cycles 2 to 6*, 1000mg on day 1.
Follicular Lymphoma, cycle 1, 1000mg on days 1, 8 and 15 of first 28-day cycle. *Cycles 2 to 6*, 1000mg on day 1.
Maintenance, 1000mg every 2 months for 2 years or until disease progression.
Admin, by IV infusion (dedicated line after dilution), not for push or bolus. *CLL*, rate 25mg/hour over 4 hours; do not increase infusion rate (day 1); 50mg/hour (can be escalated by 50mg/hour every 30 minutes to max. 400mg/hour) (day 2); 100mg/hour or faster (can be escalated by 100mg/hour every 30 minutes to max. 400mg/hour) (day 8 and 15 of cycle 1; cycles 2-6)*. *FL*, rate 50mg/hour (can be escalated by 50mg/hour every 30 minutes to max. 400mg/hour) (day 1); 100mg/hour or faster (can be escalated by 100mg/hour every 30 minutes to max. 400mg/hour) (day 8 and 15 of cycle 1; cycles 2-6 and maintenance)*. *Manage infusion-related reactions by temporary interruption, rate reduction or discontinue.
Prophylaxis, tumour lysis syndrome, adequate hydration, uricosuric admin (allopurinol, rasburicase) starting 12-24 hours prior to infusion; repeat with each subsequent infusion; *infusion related reactions*, hypotension may occur; consider withholding antihypertensives for 12 hours prior to, throughout, and for first hour after infusion.
Prophylaxis and premedication for tumour lysis syndrome and infusion-related reactions for both indications, IV corticosteroids, oral analgesics or antipyretics and antihistamines, see manufacturers Full Prescribing Information.

Renal Impairment: Mild/moderate, no adjustment; severe, safety/efficacy not established.

Hepatic Impairment: Safety/efficacy not established; no dose recommendation.

Interactions: Effect of Other Drugs on Obinutuzumab: *Possible increased neutropenia*: Chlorambucil.

SP: Infusion-related reactions (predominantly during infusion of first 1000mg). May be related to cytokine release syndrome. Neutropenia, thrombocytopenia (severe, life-threatening). Worsening of pre-existing cardiac conditions. Hepatitis B reactivation. Progressive multifocal leukoencephalopathy.

Pregnancy, Lactation: Pregnancy, if benefit outweighs risk; monitor newborns for B cell depletion; postpone live virus vaccines until infant B cell count has recovered. Women of childbearing potential to use effective contraception*. Lactation, stop breastfeeding*. *during and for 18 months after treatment.

ADR: See Notes below.

Notes: See 13.1.7 Monoclonal Antibodies.

▼ **Gazyvaro Parenteral** *(Roche)* A. HOS.
Price, (1) 1000mg, €3479.37 (PTW).
Infusion, obinutuzumab 25mg/mL (40mL). Clear colourless (slightly brownish). **Store:** Refrigerate; do not freeze.

Ofatumumab

ATC Code: L01XC10. **Sport:** Permitted.
Driving: Unlikely to impair.
Indications: Chronic lymphocytic leukaemia (CLL), refractory to fludarabine and alemtuzumab.

Dose: Adult, Elderly: Always premedicate with analgesic/antipyretic (paracetamol), antihistamine (cetirizine), glucocorticoids (prednisone) 30-120 minutes prior to infusion. Monitor for onset of infusion reactions during admin (cytokine release syndrome, especially with first infusion).
Initially 30mg by IV infusion (first infusion), then 2g for subsequent infusions; schedule 8 consecutive weekly infusions, then 4-5 weeks later, 4 consecutive monthly infusions (4-weekly). Infusions 1 and 2, initial rate 12mL/hour, doubling rate during infusion every 30 minutes to max. 200mL/hour; if no severe infusion reactions, subsequent infusions, initially 25mL/hour doubling every 30 minutes to max. 400mL/hour. Dose (premedication, modification), dilution, see manufacturers Full Prescribing Information.

SP: Infusion reactions; even with premedication, severe reactions (cytokine release syndrome). Tumour lysis syndrome may occur (CLL patients); progressive multifocal leucoencephalopathy (PML) (including death), discontinue if suspected. Avoid live attenuated vaccines; HBV infection and reactivation. History of cardiac disease, monitor; serious or life-threatening arrhythmias, discontinue. Bowel obstruction. Conduct regular complete blood counts and platelets.

Pregnancy, Lactation: Pregnancy, use if benefit outweighs risk. Women of childbearing potential to ensure adequate contraception during and for 12 months after last ofatumumab treatment. Lactation, stop breastfeeding.

ADR: See Notes below.

Notes: See 13.1.7 Monoclonal Antibodies.

Arzerra Parenteral *(Novartis)* A.
Price, not published by company.
Infusion, ofatumumab 100mg/5mL, 1g/50mL (conc). Clear (opalescent) colourless (pale-yellow) conc for soln. *Sodium 34.8mg/300mg*, 232mg/2g dose. **Store:** Store and transport refrigerated; do not freeze.

Panitumumab

ATC Code: L01XC08. **Sport:** Permitted.
Driving: Caution (vision; ability to concentrate).
Indications: Treatment, wild-type RAS metastatic colorectal cancer (mCRC) (adults), first-line (with FOLFOX or FOLFIRI); second-line (with FOLFIRI); monotherapy after (fluoropyrimidine-, oxaliplatin-, irinotecan-containing chemotherapy) failure.

Dose: Adult, Elderly: 6mg/kg once every 2 weeks. Dilute in 0.9% sodium chloride injection to final conc max. 10mg/mL. *Admin*, IV infusion over 60 minutes; dose above 1000mg, infuse over 90 minutes. NOT for IV push or bolus. Establish wild-type RAS (KRAS, NRAS) status before initiation.

CI: Interstitial pneumonitis, pulmonary fibrosis.

Interactions: Effect of Other Drugs on Panitumumab: *Co-admin contraindicated*: Oxaliplatin-containing chemotherapy (mutant KRAS mCRC or status unknown).

13.1.7 Monoclonal Antibodies

Co-admin avoid: IFL (irinotecan, fluorouracil, leucovorin) (severe diarrhoea), bevacizumab-containing chemotherapy (increased toxicity; deaths).

SP: Skin reactions; grade 3 or higher or intolerable, modify dose; skin necrosis, Stevens-Johnson syndrome, toxic epidermal necrolysis. Pulmonary complications (interstitial lung disease, pneumonitis, lung infiltrates), discontinue. Hypo- (magnesaemia, calcaemia); monitor before, during and up to 8 weeks after treatment, hypokalaemia (monitor). Severe or life-threatening infusion-reactions (anaphylactic reactions, bronchospasm, hypotension), stop infusion; if occurs after infusion, discontinue permanently. Severe angioedema post-infusion. Acute renal failure (associated with severe diarrhoea, dehydration). Keratitis, ulcerative keratitis (inflammation, lacrimation, light sensitivity, blurred vision, pain, red eye). Combinations to avoid, see Interactions above.

Pregnancy, Lactation: Pregnancy, not recommended. Women of childbearing potential to ensure adequate contraception*. During pregnancy or if patient becomes pregnant, advise of risk of loss of pregnancy or potential hazard to foetus. Lactation, not recommended*. *(during treatment and minimum 2 months after last dose).

ADR: See Notes below.

Notes: See 13.1.7 Monoclonal Antibodies.

Vectibix Parenteral 20mg/mL *(Amgen)* A. HOS.
Price, (1) 100mg/5mL, €408.72. 400mg/20mL, €1636.29 (PTW).
Infusion, panitumumab. Human monoclonal IgG2 antibody (rDNA). Colourless; may contain translucent (white) visible particles. *Sodium 3.45mg/mL (conc)*. **Store:** Refrigerate; do not freeze.

Pembrolizumab

ATC Code: L01XC18. **Sport:** Permitted.
Driving: Minor influence; fatigue.
Indications: Monotherapy treatment: Advanced (unresectable or metastatic) melanoma; first-line, metastatic non-small cell lung carcinoma (NSCLC) (tumours expressing PD-L1 with 50% or greater TPS*, no EGFR or ALK positive mutations) as well as locally advanced metastatic NSCLS (tumours expressing PD-L1 with 1% or greater TPS*and received 1 prior chemotherapy; EGFR or ALK positive mutations have received targeted therapy); relapsed or refractory classical Hodgkin lymphoma (cHL) (failed autologous stem cell transplant and brentuximab vedotin). *(tumour proportion score).

Dose: Adult, Elderly: 200mg (NSCLC not previously treated with chemotherapy or for cHL) OR 2mg/kg (NSCLC previously treated OR for melanoma) IV every 3 weeks. Immune-related adverse reactions, delay dose or discontinue. See Full Prescribing Information. *Elderly*, no dose adjustment; cHL limited data. *Admin*, IV infusion over 30 minutes; not for IV push or bolus injection.

Child: Under 18 years, efficacy/safety not established.

Renal Impairment: No dose adjustment. Severe, not studied.

Hepatic Impairment: Mild, no dose adjustment. Moderate/severe, not studied.

Interactions: Effect of Other Drugs on Pembrolizumab: *Potential interference with pharmacodynamic activity/efficacy*: Systemic corticosteroids, avoid (before pembrolizumab initiation).

SP: Ocular melanoma, limited data. Immune-related reactions after last dose; based on severity, withhold, admin corticosteroids. Immune-related reactions (monitor), pneumonitis (including fatal), colitis, hepatitis (monitor at start of treatment then periodically), nephritis (observe renal changes), endocrinopathies (hypophysitis, Type 1 diabetes mellitus, diabetic ketoacidosis, hypo/hyperthyroidism). Long-term HRT may be needed for endocrinopathies. Severe infusion-related reactions (permanently discontinue); mild or moderate (monitor); premedicate (antipyretic, antihistamine). Cases of GVHD and hepatic veno-occlusive disease observed with allogeneic haematopoietic stem cell transplantation after previous pembrolizumab exposure; weigh risk/benefit. Patient to carry Patient Alert Card.

Pregnancy, Lactation: Pregnancy, not for use unless clinically needed. Women of childbearing potential to use

368

effective contraception during and for at least 4 months after last dose. Lactation, stop drug or stop breastfeeding.

ADR: See Notes below.

Notes: See 13.1.7 Monoclonal Antibodies.

▼ **KEYTRUDA Parenteral 50mg** *(MSD)* A. HOS.
Price, (1) €1725.50 (PTW).
Infusion, pembrolizumab 25mg/1mL conc. White (off-white) powder for conc for soln. **Store:** Refrigerate.

Pertuzumab

ATC Code: L01XC13. **Sport:** Permitted.
Driving: Unlikely to impair.
Indications: Breast cancer (adults, HER2-positive), with trastuzumab and docetaxel (metastatic or locally recurrent unresectable; no previous anti-HER2 therapy or chemotherapy); with trastuzumab and chemotherapy (neoadjuvant treatment, locally advanced, inflammatory or early stage at high risk of recurrence).

Dose: Adult, Elderly: Recommended initial loading dose 840mg IV (60-minute infusion), then maintenance of 420mg IV over 30-60 minutes every 3-weeks with trastuzumab or docetaxel* admin sequentially. Observation of 30-60 minutes recommended after *Perjeta* infusion and before subsequent trastuzumab or docetaxel. Neoadjuvant treatment, admin for 3-6 cycles.

Renal Impairment: Severe, no dose recommendation.

Hepatic Impairment: No dose recommendation.

SP: Patients must have HER2-positive tumour status. Increased febrile neutropenia risk (with trastuzumab + docetaxel). Anaphylaxis, bronchospasm, acute respiratory distress syndrome, discontinue immediately; severe, discontinue permanently. Assess LVEF prior to initiation, during treatment, every 3 cycles (metastatic setting) or every 2 cycles (neoadjuvant setting). Increased cardiac toxicity risk (with anthracyclines). Severe diarrhoea, initiate anti-diarrhoeal treatment; interrupt if no improvement.

Pregnancy, Lactation: Pregnancy, not recommended. Women of childbearing potential to ensure adequate contraception during treatment and for 6 months following last dose. Lactation, stop breastfeeding or drug.

ADR: See Notes below.

Notes: See 13.1.7 Monoclonal Antibodies.

▼ **Perjeta Parenteral 420mg** *(Roche)* A.
Price, not published by company.
Infusion, pertuzumab 30mg/mL (14mL vial). Humanised IgG1 monoclonal antibody produced by rDNA technology. Clear (slightly opalescent) colourless (pale-yellow) conc for soln. **Store:** Refrigerate; do not freeze.

Ramucirumab

ATC Code: L01XC21. **Sport:** Pending.
Driving: No known influence.
Indications: Treatment (adults), advanced gastric cancer or gastro-oesophageal junction (GEJ) adenocarcinoma with disease progression after platinum and fluoropyrimidine chemotherapy (with paclitaxel or as monotherapy if paclitaxel is not appropriate); metastatic colorectal cancer (mCRC) with disease progression on or after bevacizumab, oxaliplatin and fluoropyrimidine (with FOLFIRI); locally advanced or metastatic non-small cell lung cancer (NSCLC) with disease progression after platinum-based therapy (with docetaxel).

Dose: Adult: *Gastric cancer and GEJ adenocarcinoma, with paclitaxel*, 8mg/kg on days 1 and 15 of a 28-day cycle prior to paclitaxel (paclitaxel admin at 80mg/m2 on days 1, 8 and 15 of a 28-day cycle); *monotherapy*, 8mg/kg every 2 weeks.

Colorectal cancer, recommended 8mg/kg every 2 weeks prior to FOLFIRI.

NSCLC, recommended 10mg/kg on day 1 of 21-day cycle before docetaxel (docetaxel admin at 75mg/m2 over 60 minutes on day 1 of 21-day cycle; East Asian patients, reduce docetaxel initiation to 60mg/m2 on day 1 of 21-day cycle).

Premedicate with a histamine H1-antagonist (e.g. diphenhydramine) prior to ramucirumab infusion; Grade 1 or 2 infusion reaction, admin dexamethasone; second Grade 1 or 2 infusion reaction, admin IV histamine H1 antagonist, paracetamol and dexamethasone. If infusion reactions occur, reduce infusion rate by 50% for duration of infusion and subsequent infusions. Grade 3 or 4 reaction, permanently discontinue. *Admin,* by IV infusion over approx. 60 minutes; max. infusion rate 25mg/minute; NOT for IV bolus or push. Monitor patient for infusion reactions.

Elderly: A trend towards less efficacy with increasing age observed in advanced NSCLC (combination with docetaxel).

Renal Impairment: No dose reductions recommended. Severe, limited data.

Hepatic Impairment: As for Renal above. Severe liver cirrhosis or hepatorenal syndrome, caution; use only if benefit outweighs risk.

CI: In NSCLC where there is tumour cavitation or tumour involvement of major vessels.

SP: *Permanently discontinue* in event of severe arterial thromboembolic events, GI perforation, severe bleeding, spontaneous fistula development, protein levels above 3g/24-hours or event of nephrotic syndrome (monitor for proteinuria). Infusion reactions, see Dose above; majority of events occur during first or second infusion. Discontinue temporarily for 4 weeks prior to elective surgery or with wound healing complications. Conduct complete blood count and blood chemistry before each paclitaxel infusion; complete blood count before FOLFIRI admin. Monitor BP; severe hypertension, discontinue until controlled. NSCLC with squamous histology, higher risk of serious pulmonary bleeding. Increased stomatitis incidence (combination).

Pregnancy, Lactation: Pregnancy, use only if benefit outweighs risk; advise women of childbearing potential to avoid becoming pregnant and to use effective contraception*; stop breastfeeding*. *(during and up to 3 months after last dose).

ADR: See Notes below.

Notes: See 13.1.7 Monoclonal Antibodies.

▼ **Cyramza Parenteral 10mg/mL** *(Lilly)* A.
Price, 100mg, €607.45; 500mg, €3037.24 (PTW).
Infusion, ramucirumab. Human IgG1 monoclonal antibody produced by rDNA technology. Clear (slightly opalescent) colourless (slightly yellow) conc for soln. *Sodium 17(85)mg/10(50)mL* vial. **Store:** Refrigerate; do not freeze.

Rituximab

ATC Code: L01XC02. Sport: Permitted.
Driving: Unlikely to impair.
Indications: Non-Hodgkin's Lymphoma (NHL), Stage III-IV follicular lymphoma, previously untreated (with chemotherapy); follicular lymphoma responding to induction therapy, Stage III-IV chemo-resistant or relapse after chemotherapy; CD20 positive diffuse large B cell NHL combination with CHOP (cyclophosphamide, doxorubicin, vincristine, prednisolone) *(IV and SC).* Chronic Lymphocytic Leukaemia (CLL), first-line (with chemotherapy). Rheumatoid arthritis, severe active (with methotrexate) with inadequate response or intolerance to other DMARDs. Granulomatosis with polyangiitis and microscopic polyangiitis (with glucocorticoids) *(IV).*

Dose: Adult,   Elderly: Premedicate   with analgesic/antipyretic (paracetamol), antihistamine (diphenhydramine), glucocorticoids.

IV INFUSION, *follicular NHL,* (with chemotherapy), previously untreated or relapsed or refractory, 375mg/m2 BSA (up to 8 cycles); maintenance, previously untreated, responded to induction, 375mg/m2 BSA every 2 months (starting 2 months after induction); relapsed or refractory, responded to induction, 375mg/m2 BSA every 3 months (starting 3 months after induction). Monotherapy, relapsed/refractory, 375mg/m2 BSA once every 4 weeks. *Diffuse large B cell NHL,* (with CHOP), 375mg/m2 BSA admin on day 1 of each cycle (8 cycles), after glucocorticoids.

Chronic lymphocytic leukaemia, 375mg/m2 BSA on day 0 of first treatment cycle; then 500mg/m2 BSA on day 1 of each subsequent cycle for 6 cycles before chemotherapy. Ensure adequate hydration/uricosurics starting 48 hours prior to initiation to reduce tumour lysis syndrome risk; admin prednisolone 100mg IV just before infusion.

Rheumatoid arthritis, 1g by IV infusion; followed by 1g after 2 weeks; with methylprednisolone IV 30 minutes prior to infusion. Initial infusion rate (first infusion) 50mg/hour; after first 30 minutes escalate in 50mg/hour increments

every 30 minutes; max. 400mg/hour; second infusion, initially 100mg/hour; increase by 100mg/hour increments every 30 minutes; max. 400mg/hour.

Granulomatosis with polyangiitis and microscopic polyangiitis, 375mg/m2 as IV infusion (rate 50mg/hour) once weekly for 4 weeks; with methylprednisolone 1g IV for 1-3 days prior to infusion; then oral prednisone 1mg/kg/day tapered as rapidly according to clinical need; max. 80mg/day. *Pneumocystis jirovecii* pneumonia prophylaxis recommended.

SC INJECTION, 1.4g is intended for SC use in non-Hodgkin's lymphoma only. Dose of 1.4g irrespective of body surface area; admin over approx. 5 minutes. Before initiating SC injections, all patients must receive a full dose by IV infusion using IV infusion formulation.

CI: Murine protein hypersensitivity, active severe infection, severely immunocompromised state; additional contraindications (rheumatoid arthritis, granulomatosis), severe HF (NYHA Class IV), severe uncontrolled cardiac disease.

Interactions: Effect of Other Drugs on Rituximab: *Co-admin (including sequential),* limited data: Chemotherapy (other than CHOP or CVP), agents liable to cause depletion of normal B cells.

SP: Caution, presence of human antimouse antibody or human antichimeric antibody titres, allergic or hypersensitivity reactions (with other monoclonal antibodies). Posterior reversible encephalopathy syndrome (PRES)/reversible posterior leucoencephalopathy syndrome (RPLS); signs/symptoms include (visual disturbance, headache, seizures, altered mental status, with/without associated hypertension). NHL, CLL, high tumour burden, higher risk of severe Cytokine Release Syndrome (CRS). Infusion-related reactions (CRS, hypotension, bronchospasm). Myelodepression, caution. Hepatitis B reactivation (screen all patients for HBV before initiation); active hepatitis, do not initiate. Cardiac disease, monitor (angina pectoris, arrhythmias, HF and/or MI). Vaccination with live viruses not recommended; may receive non-live vaccines but response rate may be reduced. PML reported. Measure blood neutrophils prior to each course; then regularly up to 6-months after treatment end. Severe skin reactions (toxic epidermal necrolysis, Stevens-Johnson Syndrome), with fatal outcome; permanently discontinue. Rheumatoid arthritis, granulomatosis, infusion reactions, hypersensitivity, moderate HF or severe uncontrolled cardiovascular disease, no data. Serious infections. Risk of solid tumour development. Supply patients with alert card with each admin. Methotrexate-naive patients, not recommended.

Pregnancy, Lactation: Pregnancy, if benefit outweighs risk. Women of childbearing potential to ensure adequate contraception during and for up to 12 months after treatment due to long retention time of rituximab with B cell depletion. Lactation, not recommended during or for up to 12 months after treatment.

ADR: See Notes below.

Notes: See 13.1.7 Monoclonal Antibodies.

MabThera Parenteral *(Roche)* A. HOS.
Price, (10mg/mL) 10mL (2) €499.41; 50mL (1) €1246.64 (PTW).
Infusion (IV), rituximab 10mg/mL (100mg, 500mg) concentrate for soln. Glycosylated immunoglobulin human IgG1. Clear colourless. NOTE: Supply patients with alert card with each infusion. **Store:** Refrigerate.

Trastuzumab

ATC Code: L01XC03. Sport: Permitted.
Driving: No or negligible effect; caution, infusion-related symptoms.
Indications: See Dose below.

Dose: Adult, Elderly: INFUSION, *metastatic breast cancer (MBC),* (weekly), initially 4mg/kg loading dose, then 2mg/kg/week beginning 1 week after loading; (3-weekly), initially 8mg/kg loading dose, then 6mg/kg 3-weeks later, then 6mg/kg repeated at 3-weekly intervals; *early breast cancer (EBC),* (weekly), initially 4mg/kg, then 2mg/kg every week with paclitaxel following chemotherapy with doxorubicin and cyclophosphamide; (3-weekly), initially 8mg/kg loading dose, then 6mg/kg at 3-weekly intervals beginning 3 weeks after loading dose.
Metastatic gastric cancer, (3-weekly), as for EBC. Not for

369

13.1.8   Other Antineoplastics

IV bolus or push; IV infusion over 90 minutes (initial; observe for 2 hours); if tolerated, use 30-minute infusion (subsequent).

SUBCUTANEOUS, *breast cancer*, 600mg irrespective of body weight, SC over 2-5 minutes every 3 weeks.

NOTE: To prevent medication errors, ensure drug administered is *Herceptin* (trastuzumab) and not *Kadcyla* (trastuzumab emtansine).

CI: Hypersensitivity to murine protein, severe dyspnoea at rest (complications of advanced malignancy or requiring oxygen therapy).

SP: HER2 testing mandatory prior to initiation. Caution, HF (NYHA class II-IV) observed (monotherapy or combination), particularly after anthracyclines (doxorubicin, epirubicin); monitor cardiac function 12-weekly; asymptomatic cardiac dysfunction, monitor 6-8 weekly. Caution, with increased cardiac risk (hypertension, CAD, CHF, LVEF below 55%, elderly). *Serious* infusion-related reactions (dyspnoea, hypo-, hypertension, wheezing, bronchospasm, supraventricular tachyarrhythmia, reduced oxygen saturation, anaphylaxis, respiratory distress, urticaria, angioedema). Pulmonary infiltrates, ARDS, pneumonia, pneumonitis, pleural effusion, acute pulmonary oedema, respiratory insufficiency. Interstitial lung disease; risk factors with prior or concomitant antineoplastic therapies (taxanes, gemcitabine, vinorelbine, radiation therapy). Breast cancer (MBC, EBC), do not co-admin anthracyclines; EBC eligible for neoadjuvant-adjuvant treatment, use with anthracyclines in chemotherapy-naive patients with low dose anthracycline regimens. *Check product labels* to ensure correct formulation (intravenous or subcutaneous fixed dose); IV formulation only for IV infusion and not for SC admin.

Pregnancy, Lactation: Pregnancy, avoid unless benefit outweighs risk; cases of foetal renal growth and/or impaired function with oligohydramnios, some with fatal pulmonary hypoplasia of foetus reported in pregnant women receiving *Herceptin*. Women of childbearing potential to use effective contraception*. Lactation, not recommended*. *(during treatment and for 7 months after last dose).

ADR: See Notes below.

Notes: See 13.1.7 Monoclonal Antibodies.

Herceptin Parenteral *(Roche)* A. HOS.
Price, (1) 150mg (infusion), €567.69. 600mg/5mL (SC injection), €1645.24 (PTW).
Infusion, trastuzumab 150mg (21mg/mL reconstituted soln). Humanised IgG1 monoclonal antibody. White (pale-yellow) lyophilised powder for conc for soln. **Store:** Refrigerate.
Injection (SC), as above 600mg/5mL vial. Clear (opalescent) colourless (yellowish) soln. **Store:** Refrigerate; do not freeze. Out of refrigerator, use within 6 hours, store below 30 deg C.

Trastuzumab Emtansine

ATC Code: L01XC14. **Sport:** Permitted.
Driving: No or negligible effect; caution, infusion-related symptoms.
Indications: As single agent, treatment of HER2-positive, unresectable locally advanced or metastatic breast cancer (previous trastuzumab and taxane).
Dose: Adult, Elderly: 3.6mg/kg by IV infusion every 3 weeks (21-day cycle); initial infusion over 90 minutes; observe for infusion-related reactions; monitor infusion site for subcutaneous infiltration. If tolerated, admin following infusions over 30 minutes. Not for IV push or bolus.
NOTE: To prevent medication errors, ensure drug administered is *Kadcyla* (trastuzumab emtansine) and not *Herceptin* (trastuzumab).
Renal Impairment: Mild/moderate, no adjustment. Severe, monitor carefully.
Hepatic Impairment: Mild/moderate, no adjustment. Severe, caution (hepatotoxicity observed).
Interactions: Effect of Other Drugs on Trastuzumab Emtansine: *Co-admin avoid:* Strong CYP3A4 inducers (ketoconazole, itraconazole, clarithromycin, atazanavir, indinavir, nefazodone, nelfinavir, ritonavir, saquinavir, telithromycin, voriconazole).
SP: Interstitial lung disease; signs and symptoms (dyspnoea, cough, fatigue, pulmonary infiltrates); if diagnosed, discontinue permanently. Dyspnoea at rest, all increased risk of pulmonary events. Hepatotoxicity; monitor

liver function (prior to initiation, at each dose). LVD observed; symptomatic CHF a potential risk. Perform standard cardiac function testing (prior to initiation, at regular intervals 3-monthly). Infusion-related reactions due to cytokine release; hypersensitivity reactions may present as infusion-related reactions. Thrombocytopenia, peripheral neuropathy.

Pregnancy, Lactation: Pregnancy, not recommended; inform women of possible harm to foetus. Women of childbearing potential to use effective contraception during and for at least 7 months after treatment. Lactation, not recommended during treatment and for 7 months after last dose.

ADR: See Notes below.

Notes: See 13.1.7 Monoclonal Antibodies.

▼ **Kadcyla Parenteral** *(Roche)* A.
Price, not published by company.
Infusion, trastuzumab emtansine 100mg, 160mg. White (off-white) powder for conc for soln. *Sodium 23mg/dose.* **Store:** Refrigerate.

13.1.8 - Other Antineoplastics

In This Chapter: *Aflibercept, arsenic trioxide, bexarotene, bortezomib, crisantaspase, eribulin, hydroxycarbamide, idelalisib, irinotecan, mitotane, topotecan, tretinoin and mTOR inhibitors* (everolimus, temsirolimus). *mammalian target of rapamycin.*

Class Effects

Advice for missed dose or dose modifications for toxicity, see manufacturers Full Prescribing Information.

CI: Hypersensitivity to any member of the class. Unless stated, not for use in children under 18 years.

SP: *Rapamycin derivatives* (everolimus, temsirolimus), non-infectious pneumonitis (including ILD), impaired wound healing (class effects). Risk factors for interstitial lung disease (ILD) (history of, pulmonary fibrosis, lung cancer, thoracic exposure to radiation, use of pneumotoxic drugs and/or colony stimulating factors); monitor for (cough, fever, dyspnoea and/or hypoxia). See individual drugs.

ADR: See manufacturers Full Prescribing Information. See Notes below.

Notes: See also 13.1 Cytotoxic Drugs. Drugs with immunosuppressant properties, see 13.2 Drugs Affecting Immune Response.

Aflibercept

ATC Code: L01XX44. **Sport:** Permitted.
Driving: No or negligible effect; caution if vision, concentration or ability to react is influenced.
Indications: Treatment, metastatic colorectal cancer in combination (FOLFIRI) (resistant to or progressed after oxaliplatin-containing regimen).
Dose: Adult, Elderly: 4mg/kg by IV infusion over 1 hour followed by FOLFIRI repeated every 2 weeks. *Admin,* not for IV push or bolus; not for intravitreal injection. *Elderly,* increased risk of diarrhoea, dizziness, asthenia, weight loss, dehydration.
Renal Impairment: Severe, caution.
Hepatic Impairment: Severe, no data.
CI: Ophthalmic or intravitreal use.
SP: Increased haemorrhage risk (severe, fatal), monitor for GI, other severe bleeding. Thrombocytopenia, neutropenic complications, monitor complete blood count with platelets at baseline, prior to initiation of each cycle, then as needed. GI perforation, fistula formation (GI, non-GI), thrombolic events (arterial, venous), severe hypersensitivity, discontinue. Control hypertension before initiation. Proteinuria (monitor by urine dipstick analysis or urinary protein creatinine ratio for development or worsening before each admin; 2g or more of proteinuria per 24 hours, suspend; under 2g/24-hours, restart), nephrotic syndrome, thrombotic microangiopathy, severe diarrhoea, compromised wound healing, posterior reversible encephalopathy syndrome. ECOG performance status 2 or below or significant co-morbidities, greater risk of poor clinical outcome. Osteonecrosis of jaw (cancer patients, with prior or concomitant IV bisphosphonates).

Pregnancy, Lactation: Pregnancy, only if benefit outweighs risk; advise women of risk to foetus. Women of childbearing potential and fertile males to use effective contraception during and up to 6 months after last dose of treatment. Lactation, stop breastfeeding or drug.

ADR: See Notes below.

Notes: See 13.1.8 Other Antineoplastics.

▼ **Zaltrap Parenteral** *(SANOFI)* A. HOS.
Price, (1) 100mg, €350.13; 200mg, €700.77 (PTW).
Infusion, aflibercept 25mg/mL. Produced by rDNA technology. Clear colourless (pale yellow) conc for soln. **Store:** Refrigerate; original pack to protect (light).

Arsenic Trioxide

ATC Code: L01XX27. **Sport:** Permitted.
Driving: Not applicable.

Indications: Induction of remission and consolidation, relapsed/refractory acute promyelocytic leukaemia (APL) where previous treatment included a retinoid and chemotherapy.

Dose: Adult, Elderly: *Induction,* fixed daily dose 0.15mg/kg/day until bone marrow remission achieved; no remission at day 50, discontinue. *Consolidation,* commence 3-4 weeks after induction completion at 0.15mg/kg/day for 25 doses; admin 5 days/week followed by 2-day interruption; repeat for 5 weeks. *Admin,* IV over 1-2 hours; extend infusion time up to 4 hours if vasomotor reactions observed. See SP below. *Elderly,* caution.

Child: As for Adult; under 5 years, no data.

Renal Impairment: Caution. Severe, insufficient data to determine if dose adjustment required; dialysis, no data.

Hepatic Impairment: As for Renal above.

Interactions: Effect of Other Drugs on Arsenic Trioxide: *QT-prolongation risk:* Drugs prolonging QT-interval including Class Ia and III antiarrhythmics (quinidine, amiodarone, sotalol, dofetilide), antipsychotics (thioridazine), antidepressants (amitriptyline), macrolides (erythromycin), antihistamines (terfenadine, astemizole), quinolones (sparfloxacin), cisapride, potassium wasting diuretics, amphotericin B.

SP: Clinically unstable APL, more frequent monitoring. Leukocyte Activation Syndrome (APL Differentiation Syndrome) (unexplained fever, dyspnoea and/or weight gain, abnormal chest auscultatory findings, radiographic abnormalities), initiate high dose steroids (dexamethasone 10mg IV twice daily). ECG abnormalities (QT-interval prolongation, AV block); increased QT-prolongation risk with previous anthracyclines; caution (QT-prolongation history, CHF, hypo-, kalaemia or magnesaemia), monitor. Dose modification, interrupt, adjust or discontinue with toxicity (CTC) grade 3 or greater. Laboratory tests, monitor twice weekly (electrolytes, glycaemia levels, haematological, hepatic, renal and coagulation parameters). Hyperleukocytosis.

Pregnancy, Lactation: Pregnancy, not recommended; if used inadvertently, or if pregnancy occurs, inform patient of potential hazard to foetus. Men, and women of child-bearing potential to ensure adequate contraception. Lactation, stop breastfeeding prior to and throughout admin.

ADR: See Notes below.

Notes: See 13.1.8 Other Antineoplastics.

Trisenox Parenteral 1mg/mL *(TEVA)* A.
Price, not published by company.
Infusion, arsenic trioxide. Clear colourless aqueous conc for soln.

Bexarotene

ATC Code: L01XX25. **Sport:** Permitted.
Driving: Caution.

Indications: Treatment, skin manifestations of advanced stage cutaneous T-cell lymphoma (CTCL), refractory to at least 1 systemic treatment.

Dose: Adult, Elderly: Initially 300mg/m2/day BSA; reduce to 200mg/m2/day, then 100mg/m2/day, or temporarily suspend due to toxicity. Doses above 650mg/m2/day not evaluated. *Admin,* single oral dose with food.

Renal Impairment: Monitor.

Hepatic Impairment: Not recommended.

CI: Pancreatitis, uncontrolled (hypercholesterolaemia,

hypertriglyceridaemia, thyroid disease), hypervitaminosis A, ongoing systemic infection.

Interactions: Effect of Other Drugs on Bexarotene: *Co-admin not recommended (plasma levels substantially increased):* Gemfibrozil. *Plasma levels increased:* CYP3A4 substrates (ketoconazole, itraconazole, protease inhibitors, clarithromycin, erythromycin), grapefruit juice. *Plasma levels decreased:* CYP3A4 inducers (rifampicin, phenytoin, dexamethasone, phenobarbital).

Effect of Bexarotene On Other Drugs: Tamoxifen, oral contraceptives: *Plasma levels decreased.*

SP: Retinoid hypersensitivity, caution. Blood donation not recommended during treatment. Hyperlipidaemia, monitor. Pancreatitis (acute, especially with risk factors e.g. prior pancreatitis, uncontrolled hyperlipidaemia, excessive alcohol consumption, uncontrolled diabetes mellitus, biliary tract disease, medications increasing triglycerides or associated with pancreatic toxicity), use only if benefit outweighs risk. LFT elevations, thyroid function test alterations, leucopenia, anaemia, lens opacities. Limit Vitamin A supplements to 15000 IU/day or less. Photosensitivity, minimise sunlight or sun lamp exposure.

Pregnancy, Lactation: Pregnancy, not recommended; if used inadvertently, or if pregnancy occurs while on treatment, inform patient of potential hazard to foetus. Exclude pregnancy before initiating. Women of child-bearing potential to ensure adequate non-hormonal contraception. Lactation, not recommended.

ADR: See Notes below.

Notes: See 13.1.8 Other Antineoplastics.

Targretin 75mg *(Eisai)* A. HT.
Price, (100) €1539.26. HOS: €1132.79 (PTW).
Capsule, bexarotene. Off-white soft containing liquid susp. Marked Targretin.

Bortezomib

ATC Code: L01XX32. **Sport:** Permitted.
Driving: Fatigue, dizziness, orthostatic/postural hypotension, blurred vision, syncope (caution); advise not to drive is these symptoms experienced.

Indications: Treatment (monotherapy or with pegylated liposomal doxorubicin or dexamethasone), progressive multiple myeloma, with 1 prior therapy and undergone or unsuitable for bone marrow transplantation (BMT). Combination (with melphalan and prednisone), previously untreated multiple myeloma not eligible for high-dose chemotherapy or BMT; with (dexamethasone alone or with thalidomide), induction treatment, previously untreated multiple myeloma who are eligible for high-dose chemotherapy or BMT; with (rituximab, cyclophosphamide, doxorubicin and prednisone), previously untreated mantle cell lymphoma unsuitable for haematopoietic stem cell transplantation.

Dose: Adult, Elderly: MONOTHERAPY, initially 1.3mg/m2 BSA twice weekly (days 1, 4, 8, 11) in a 21-day treatment cycle; minimum 72 hours between consecutive doses. Confirmed complete response, admin 2 additional cycles; complete remission not achieved, admin total of 8 cycles. COMBINATION as for monotherapy.
Admin, IV (3-5 second bolus) or SC (thigh, abdomen); rotate sites. Initiate under supervision of physician experienced in cancer treatment; admin by healthcare professional.

Child: Safety/efficacy not established under 18 years; no dose recommendation can be made.

Renal Impairment: CrCl (mL/min) below 20 (not on dialysis), no pharmacokinetic data. Admin after dialysis.

Hepatic Impairment: Moderate/severe, initiate at 0.7mg/m2 per injection (first treatment cycle); based on tolerability escalate to 1mg/m2 or reduce to 0.5mg/m2.

CI: Boron hypersensitivity, acute diffuse infiltrative pulmonary and pericardial disease.

Interactions: Effect of Other Drugs on Bortezomib: *Co-admin not recommended:* Potent CYP3A4-inhibitors (ketoconazole, ritonavir); CYP3A4-inducers (reduced efficacy) (rifampicin, carbamazepine, phenytoin, phenobarbital, St John's Wort); CYP(3A4 or 2C19) substrates.

Effect of Bortezomib on Other Drugs: Oral antiglycaemics: *Confirm normal liver function, caution; monitor glucose levels, consider dose adjustment.*

13.1.8 Other Antineoplastics

SP: Ileus (constipation, monitor), nausea, vomiting, diarrhoea. Thrombocytopenia (platelets lowest, day 11 of cycle). Peripheral neuropathy, predominantly sensory; incidence increases early in treatment, peaks cycle 5; monitor for symptoms (burning sensation, hyper- or hypoaesthesia, discomfort, neuropathic pain or weakness). See Dose above. Seizure risk factors, caution. Orthostatic and/or postural hypotension. CHF, acute development or exacerbation, decreased LVEF. QT-prolongation. *Pulmonary disease*, acute diffuse infiltrative (pneumonitis, interstitial pneumonia, lung infiltration, ARDS); recommend pre-treatment chest X-ray; new or worsening pulmonary symptoms, consider risk/benefit. Hepatic, failure, increased LFTs, hyperbilirubinaemia, hepatitis. Amyloidosis, caution. Potentially immunocomplex-mediated reactions, discontinue (serious). Tumour Lysis Syndrome, Reversible Posterior Leucoencephalopathy Syndrome. Herpes zoster reactivation. JC virus infection resulting in progressive multifocal leucoencephalopathy (very rare). NOT for intrathecal admin.

Pregnancy, Lactation: Pregnancy, inform of potential hazard to foetus. Males and females of childbearing potential to ensure adequate contraception during and for 3 months after treatment. Lactation, not recommended. Caution, thalidomide combination (TERATOGENIC).

ADR: See Notes below.

Notes: See 13.1.8 Other Antineoplastics, 13.1.1 Alkylating Agents (melphalan). See manufacturers Full Prescribing Information.

Velcade Parenteral 3.5mg *(Janssen-Cilag)* A. HOS.
Price, (1) €1079.66 (PTW).
Injection, bortezomib (as mannitol boronic ester) 3.5mg; after reconstitution 2.5mg/1mL (SC injection) or 1mg/1mL (IV injection). White (off-white) cake or powder for soln. **Store:** Below 30 deg C in outer carton (protect from light).

Crisantapase (asparaginase)

ATC Code: L01XX02. **Sport:** Permitted.
Driving: Unlikely to impair.
Indications: Combination, treatment ALL.
Dose: Adult, Elderly: Usually 6000 U/m2 BSA (200 U/kg) 3-times weekly for 3 weeks. IV injection or infusion, IM or SC.
Child: See manufacturers Full Prescribing Information.
Interactions: Effect of Other Drugs on Crisantapase: *Not recommended:* Admixture with other drugs in same syringe.
SP: Admin without interruption; if interrupted, resume at low dose (10 U/kg/day); increase to full dose over 5 days if tolerated. Anaphylaxis. Neurotoxicity, life-threatening sepsis, severe hypersensitivity, fever, CNS depression, biochemical changes.
Pregnancy, Lactation: Not recommended. Women of childbearing potential to ensure adequate contraception.
ADR: See Notes below.
Notes: See 13.1.8 Other Antineoplastics.

Erwinase Parenteral *(Ipsen)* A.
Price, (20) 1000 U, €1206.25.
Injection, crisantapase (asparaginase) 1000 U. From *Erwinia chrysanthemi.* Freeze-dried powder for reconstitution.

Eribulin

ATC Code: L01XX41. **Sport:** Permitted.
Driving: Tiredness, dizziness.
Indications: Treatment (adults), breast cancer (locally advanced or metastatic; progressed after at least one chemotherapy regimen for advanced disease; prior therapy to have included anthracycline and a taxane); unresectable liposarcoma (received prior anthracycline-containing therapy, unless unsuitable, for advanced or metastatic disease).
Dose: Adult, Elderly: Ready to use soln (0.44mg/mL), admin 1.23mg/m2 IV over 2-5 minutes on day 1 and day 8 of every 21-day cycle. Consider antiemetic prophylaxis including corticosteroids. NOTE: Dose is based on active substance (eribulin).
Child: Under 18 years, safety/efficacy not established in soft tissue sarcoma.
Renal Impairment: Mild/moderate, close monitoring; CrCl (mL/min) below 40, dose reduction may be needed.
Hepatic Impairment: Mild, 0.97mg/m2*; moderate, 0.62mg/m2*; severe, not studied, more marked dose reduction expected to be needed. *Admin as for Adult, Elderly above. Cirrhosis, as for mild and moderate but with close monitoring.
Interactions: Effect of Other Drugs on Eribulin: *Caution (monitor):* Substances mainly metabolised by CYP3A4 especially with narrow therapeutic window (alfentanil, ciclosporin, ergotamine, fentanyl, pimozide, quinidine, sirolimus, tacrolimus).
SP: *Monitor,* complete blood counts prior to admin of each dose (myelosuppression is dose-dependent; primarily neutropenia, including febrile); neutropenic sepsis, septic shock (fatal). Signs of peripheral motor or sensory neuropathy (severe peripheral, delay or reduce dose). ECG monitoring with (CHF, bradyarrhythmias, medicines prolonging QT-interval e.g. Class Ia and II antiarrhythmics, electrolyte abnormalities). Correct hypokalaemia or hypomagnesaemia prior to initiation.
Pregnancy, Lactation: Pregnancy, only if clearly necessary. Women of childbearing potential and male partners to use effective contraception during and for up to 3 months after treatment. Lactation, contraindicated.
ADR: See Notes below.
Notes: See 13.1.8 Other Antineoplastics.

HALAVEN Parenteral *(Eisai)* A. HOS.
Price, (1x 2mL) €348.80 (PTW).
Injection, eribulin mesilate equiv. to 0.44mg eribulin. Clear colourless aqueous soln.

Everolimus (oncology)

ATC Code: L01XE10. **Sport:** Permitted.
Driving: Minor or moderate influence; fatigue.
Indications: Treatment, hormone receptor-positive advanced breast cancer (post-menopause, in combination); unresectable or metastatic neuroendocrine tumours of pancreatic (well or moderately differentiated) or GI or lung origin (well differentiated); advanced renal cell carcinoma, disease progression after VEGF-targeted therapy.
Dose: Adult, Elderly: Recommended, 10mg/day as long as benefit or unacceptable toxicity; severe and/or intolerable adverse reactions, reduce to 5mg/day or withhold temporarily; reintroduce at 5mg/day. *Admin,* oral once daily at same time of day with/without food; swallow tabs whole with water; do not crush or chew. See Interactions below.
Hepatic Impairment: Moderate, 5mg daily; severe, if benefit outweighs risk, max. 2.5mg/day.
CI: Hypersensitivity to other rapamycin derivatives.
Interactions: Effect of Other Drugs on Everolimus: *Co-admin not recommended (plasma levels increased):* Potent CYP3A4/P-gp inhibitors (ketoconazole, itraconazole, posaconazole, voriconazole, telithromycin, clarithromycin, nefazodone, ritonavir, atazanavir, saquinavir, darunavir, indinavir, nelfinavir). *Co-admin caution (consider everolimus dose adjustment)*: Moderate CYP3A4/P-gp inhibitors (erythromycin, imatinib, verapamil, ciclosporin oral; fluconazole, diltiazem, dronedarone, amprenavir, fosamprenavir, grapefruit juice, food affecting CYP3A4/P-gp). *Co-admin avoid (consider dose adjustment)*: Potent CYP3A4 inducers (rifampicin, dexamethasone, carbamazepine, phenobarbital, phenytoin, efavirenz, nevirapine, St John's Wort). *Increased angioedema risk with co-admin:* ACEis (ramipril). *See manufacturers Full Prescribing Information.
SP: Non-infectious pneumonitis (including interstitial lung disease) frequently reported (rule out opportunistic infections e.g. *Pneumocystis jirovecii* pneumonia); corticosteroids may be needed (re-initiate at 5mg/day). Hypersensitivity reactions. Oral ulceration, treat topically (alcohol or peroxide-containing mouthwashes may exacerbate). Monitor, blood glucose, lipids prior to initiation then periodically as hyper- (cholesterolaemia, triglyceridaemia) reported, complete blood count.
Pregnancy, Lactation: Not recommended. Women of childbearing age to ensure adequate contraception, otherwise not recommended.
ADR: See Notes below.
Notes: See 13.1.8 Other Antineoplastics.

Afinitor 2.5mg, 5mg, 10mg *(Novartis)* A. HT.
Price, (30) 2.5mg, €1298.43. 5mg, €2596.86. 10mg, €3579.94.
Tablet, everolimus. White (slightly yellow) elongated. Marked NVR. 2.5mg: Marked LCL. 5mg: Marked 5. 10mg: Marked UHE. *Lactose.*

Hydroxycarbamide

ATC Code: L01XX05. **Sport:** Permitted.
Driving: Caution.
Indications: Malignant neoplastic disease including CML; with radiotherapy (cervical cancer, other solid-type tumours).
Dose: Adult, Elderly: Continuous (CML) or intermittent (solid tumours) regimen, start 7 days before concurrent radiation. Continuous, 20-30mg/kg/day* based on actual or ideal weight whichever is less; intermittent, 80mg/kg* every third day. Fall in white cell count or platelets, GI disturbances, mucositis, interrupt treatment. *Elderly,* consider dose reduction, caution. *(as a single dose). Oral admin; contents of capsule may be emptied into a glass of water and taken immediately.
Renal Impairment: Consider dose reduction.
CI: Leucopenia, thrombocytopenia, severe anaemia, non-malignant disease.
Interactions: Effect of Other Drugs on Hydroxycarbamide: *Co-admin caution (avoid):* Antiretrovirals (didanosine with/without stavudine) (fatal and non-fatal pancreatitis, hepatotoxicity, severe peripheral neuropathy in HIV-infected patients). *Myelosuppression potentiated:* Previous or concomitant radiotherapy, cytotoxics.
SP: Full blood counts, bone marrow examination, kidney and liver function test prior to and repeatedly during treatment; do not initiate if bone marrow function depressed. Determine Hb, total leucocytes, platelets at least once weekly. May produce bone marrow suppression and leucopenia (more likely with previous radiotherapy, cytotoxic cancer chemotherapy). Increased serum uric acid (gout, uric acid nephropathy), maintain high fluid intake. Secondary leukaemia (long-term treatment). Cutaneous vasculitic toxicity (vasculitic ulceration, gangrene). Macrocytosis may mask folic acid deficiency; folic acid supplements may be needed. Vaccination with live vaccines may result in severe infection.
Pregnancy, Lactation: Not normally used; women of child-bearing potential and males to ensure adequate contraception. Potential for serious adverse events in nursing infants; stop drug or stop nursing.
ADR: See Notes below.
Notes: See 13.1.8 Other Antineoplastics.

Hydrea 500mg *(BMS)* A. GMS.
Price, (100) €15.02.
Capsule, hydroxycarbamide. Hard gelatin opaque pink/green containing white homogenous powder. Marked BMS 303. *Lactose.*

Idelalisib

ATC Code: L01XX47. **Sport:** Pending.
Driving: No or negligible influence.
Indications: Adults, treatment (with rituximab or ofatumumab), chronic lymphocytic leukaemia (CLL) (received at least 1 prior therapy); first line with 17p deletion or TP53 mutation (not eligible for other treatment); monotherapy, follicular lymphoma (FL) refractory to 2 prior therapies.
Dose: Adult, Elderly: 150mg twice daily. *Admin,* swallow whole with or without food; do not crush or chew.
Hepatic Impairment: Mild/moderate, intensify monitoring for adverse reactions. Severe, insufficient data for dose recommendations.
Interactions: Effect of Idelalisib on Other Drugs: Quetiapine, pimozide, salmeterol: *Co-admin not recommended.* CYP3A inducers (rifampicin, phenytoin, St John's Wort, carbamazepine), reduced plasma levels; CYP3A inhibitors (alfuzosin, amiodarone, cisapride, pimozide, quinidine, ergotamine, dihydroergotamine, quetiapine, lovastatin, simvastatin, sildenafil, midazolam, triazolam), increased plasma levels. *Co-admin avoid; not recommended.* Bosentan, sildenafil: *Co-admin caution.* Fentanyl, alfentanil, methadone, buprenorphine/naloxone (respiratory depression, sedation); bepridil, disopyramide, lidocaine; dasatinib, nilotinib, vincristine, vinblastine,

Other Antineoplastics 13.1.8

amlodipine, diltiazem, felodipine, nifedipine, nicardipine, azole antifungals, rifabutin, boceprevir, telaprevir, telithromycin; clarithromycin (CrCl below 90mL/min), budesonide, fluticasone, atorvastatin, ciclosporin, sirolimus, tacrolimus: *Monitor for adverse events.* Warfarin: *Monitor INR.* Trazodone: *Careful dose titration.* Colchicine, buspirone, clorazepate, diazepam, estazolam, flurazepam, zolpidem: *Dose reduction may be required.*
SP: First-line in CLL with 17p deletion or TP53 mutation, use only if not eligible for other therapies. Inform patient of serious and/or fatal infection risk; do not initiate with ongoing systemic infection (bacterial, fungal, viral). Admin prophylaxis for *Pneumocystis jirovecii* pneumonia throughout treatment. Serious lung events not responding to antimicrobial treatment, assess for drug-induced pneumonitis. Monitor for respiratory signs and symptoms. Screen for cytomegalovirus (CMV) regularly. Elevated transaminases (usually in first 12 weeks), reversible with dose interruption. Severe drug-related colitis (late; months after start of treatment), Stevens-Johnson syndrome, toxic epidermal necrolysis (fatal) (combination use). Caution, admin with active hepatitis. *Monitor,* absolute neutrophil count (ANC) every 2 weeks (first 6 months); weekly if ANC is below 1000/mm3.
Pregnancy, Lactation: Pregnancy, not recommended. Women of childbearing potential to use highly effective contraception during and up to 1 month after ending treatment; add a barrier method to hormonal contraception. Lactation, stop breastfeeding.
ADR: See Notes below.
Notes: See 13.1.8 Other Antineoplastics.

▼ **Zydelig 100mg, 150mg** *(Gilead)* A. HT.
Price, both strengths (60) €4436.35.
Tablet, idelalisib. Oval f/c. Marked GSI; strength on reverse. 100mg: Orange. 150mg: Pink. *Sunset Yellow (100mg).*

Irinotecan

ATC Code: L01XX19. **Sport:** Permitted.
Driving: Dizziness, visual disturbances.
Indications: Treatment, advanced colorectal cancer with (5-fluorouracil AND folinic acid) OR monotherapy (if 5-fluorouracil has failed); with (cetuximab), EGFR-expressing KRAS wild-type metastatic colorectal cancer (no prior treatment for metastatic disease or after irinotecan failure); with (5-fluorouracil, folinic acid, bevacizumab), first-line for metastatic carcinoma of colon or rectum. With (capecitabine) with/without (bevacizumab) first-line for metastatic colorectal carcinoma.
Dose: Adult: MONOTHERAPY, previously treated, 350mg/m2 BSA every 3 weeks.
COMBINATION, previously untreated, 180mg/m2 once every 2 weeks, followed by folinic acid and 5-fluorouracil. Infusion into peripheral or central vein over 30-90 minutes. For dosing in combination with cetuximab, bevacizumab and/or capecitabine, see manufacturers Full Prescribing Information.
Elderly: Intense surveillance.
Renal Impairment: Not recommended.
Hepatic Impairment: Bilirubin up to 1.5xULN, 350mg/m2; bilirubin 1.5-3xULN, 200mg/m2; bilirubin above 3xULN, contraindicated. Combination use, no data.
CI: Chronic inflammatory bowel disease and/or bowel obstruction, severe bone marrow failure, WHO performance status above 2. Combination, see cetuximab, bevacizumab and/or capecitabine.
Interactions: Effect of Other Drugs on Irinotecan: *Co-admin contraindicated (plasma levels decreased):* St John's Wort. *Caution:* Drugs inhibiting CYP3A4 (ketoconazole) or inducing CYP3A4 (rifampicin, carbamazepine, phenobarbital phenytoin). *Potential increased systemic exposure (to SN-38, irinotecan active metabolite):* Atazanavir, a CYP3A4 and UGT1A1 inhibitor.
Effect of Irinotecan on Other Drugs: Suxamethonium: *Prolonged effect.* Non-depolarising neuromuscular blockers: *Effect antagonised.*
SP: Delayed diarrhoea, treat with loperamide, prophylactic broad-spectrum antibiotics, hospitalisation if severe, or fever persists beyond 48 hours; previous abdominal/pelvic radiotherapy, baseline hyperleucocytosis, performance status above 2, females, increased diarrhoea risk;

13.1.8   Other Antineoplastics

diarrhoea can be life-threatening especially with neutropenia. Severe haematological toxicity, reduce dose. Inform patient of neutropenia risk/significance of fever, increased infection risk; monitor complete blood counts weekly. Monitor liver function at baseline, before each cycle. Admin prophylactic antiemetics for nausea and vomiting; if associated with diarrhoea, hospitalise. Acute cholinergic syndrome, admin atropine sulfate (0.25mg SC) unless contraindicated. Interstitial pulmonary disease (fatal). Avoid extravasation; if occurs, flush site/apply ice. Not recommended with bowel obstruction until obstruction resolved. Myocardial ischaemic events; monitor with known risk factors. Thromboembolic events (patients with multiple risk factors). Combination with bevacizumab, severe diarrhoea, leucopenia, neutropenia (modify irinotecan dose).

Pregnancy, Lactation: Pregnancy, use only if clearly necessary. Women of childbearing potential and men to ensure adequate contraception during and up to 1 month (women) and 3 months (men) after treatment. Lactation, not recommended, discontinue for therapy duration.

ADR: See Notes below.

Notes: See 13.1.8 Other Antineoplastics, 13.1.7 Monoclonal Antibodies (cetuximab, bevacizumab).

Campto Parenteral *(Pfizer)* A.
Price, not published by company.
Infusion, irinotecan hydrochloride trihydrate 40mg/2mL, 100mg/5mL. Clear pale-yellow (slightly yellow) conc for soln.

Irinotecan (Accord) Parenteral *(Accord)* A.
Price, 20mg/mL (1) 2mL, €56.36. 5mL, €140.90. 15mL, €421.99. 25mL, €704.49.
Infusion, irinotecan hydrochloride trihydrate 20mg/mL. Pale-yellow clear conc for soln. *Sorbitol, sodium.*

Irinotecan Parenteral *(TEVA)* A.
Price, not published by company.
Infusion, irinotecan hydrochloride trihydrate 40mg/2mL, 100mg/5mL. Clear pale-yellow conc for soln. *Sorbitol.*

Irinotecan (Hospira) Parenteral *(Hospira)* A.
Price, not published by company.
Infusion, irinotecan hydrochloride trihydrate 40mg/2mL, 100mg/5mL. Clear pale-yellow conc for soln. *Sorbitol.*

Mitotane

ATC Code: L01XX23. **Sport:** Permitted.
Driving: Major influence; warn ambulatory patients not to drive.
Indications: Advanced unresectable, metastatic or relapsed adrenal cortical carcinoma.
Dose: Adult, Elderly: Initially 2-3g/day increasing at 2-week intervals until plasma levels reach therapeutic window 14-20mg/L (neurological toxicity above 20mg/L). If urgent to control Cushing's syndrome, initiated at 4-6g/day increasing every week; max. 6g/day. Monitor plasma levels (every 2 weeks) after each dose adjustment (therapeutic window 14-20mg/L); more frequent when high starting dose used (weekly). Admin as 2- divided doses with a glass of water during meals containing fat-rich food. *Elderly,* caution; monitor frequently.
Child: Initiate at 1.5-3.5g/m2/day; with objective of 4g/m2/day. Monitor as for Adult; particular attention when plasma levels 10mg/L reached. Neuro-psychological retardation observed; investigate thyroid function to identify impairment linked to treatment.
Renal Impairment: Mild/moderate, caution; monitor mitotane levels. Severe, not recommended.
Hepatic Impairment: As for Renal above.
Interactions: Effect of Other Drugs on Mitotane: *Co-admin contraindicated:* Spironolactone. *Co-admin caution:* CNS depressants. *Absorption enhanced:* Fat-rich food.
Effect of Mitotane on Other Drugs: Coumarin anticoagulants: *Monitor for change in dose requirements.* Substances metabolised by cytochrome P450 enzymes (anticonvulsants, rifabutin, rifampicin, griseofulvin, St John's Wort): *Plasma conc may be modified.*
SP: Before initiation, surgically remove large metastatic masses to minimise adverse events due to rapid cytotoxic effect. Adrenal insufficiency risk, consider steroid replacement; discontinue immediately following shock, severe trauma or infection. Monitor plasma levels to adjust dose. Fat tissue can act as reservoir (prolonged half-life, potential accumulation). Reversible brain damage/impaired function (long-term treatment).

Prolonged bleeding time; monitor red/white blood cell counts, platelets. Increased plasma levels of hormone-binding proteins. Ovarian macrocysts observed; higher incidence in premenopausal women. Neurotoxicity, consider temporary interruption. Advise caregivers to wear disposable gloves when handling tablets.
Pregnancy, Lactation: Pregnancy, only if clearly needed and benefit outweighs potential risk to foetus (limited number of exposed pregnancies indicated abnormalities on adrenals of foetus). Women of childbearing potential to ensure adequate contraception during treatment. Lactation, contraindicated during and after treatment as long as plasma levels detectable.
ADR: See Notes below.
Notes: See 13.1.8 Other Antineoplastics.

Lysodren 500mg *(HRA)* A.
Price, (100) €705.88.
Tablet, mitotane. White round scored. Marked BL over L1.

Temsirolimus

ATC Code: L01XE09. **Sport:** Permitted.
Driving: IV Torisel, ethanol may affect.
Indications: First-line, advanced renal cell carcinoma (RCC) with at least 3 of 6 prognostic factors. Relapsed and/or refractory mantle cell lymphoma (MCL).
Dose: Adult, Elderly: *RCC,* 25mg once weekly; suspected reactions not managed with dose delays, reduce by 5mg/week. *MCL,* 175mg once weekly for 3 weeks; then 75mg once weekly. Starting dose may be associated with significant adverse events requiring dose reduction/delay in majority of patients. Dilute conc to achieve temsirolimus conc 10mg/mL. 30 minutes before start of infusion, admin 25-50mg diphenhydramine (or similar) IV. Infuse over 30-60 minutes.
Child: Not recommended.
Renal Impairment: Severe, caution.
Hepatic Impairment: Caution. Severe, not recommended. *RCC,* severe, 10mg IV once weekly.
CI: Hypersensitivity to temsirolimus or metabolites (sirolimus), polysorbate 80.
Interactions: Effect of Other Drugs on Temsirolimus: *Dose-limiting toxicity with co-admin:* Sunitinib. *Co-admin caution (angioedema risk):* ACEIs. *Co-admin avoid (reduced exposure):* CYP3A4 strong inducers (carbamazepine, phenobarbital, phenytoin, rifampicin, St John's Wort). *Co-admin avoid:* CYP3A4 inhibitors including protease inhibitors (nelfinavir, ritonavir), antifungals (itraconazole, ketoconazole, voriconazole), nefazodone. *Co-admin caution, especially at temsirolimus doses above 25mg (plasma levels increased):* Moderate CYP3A4 inhibitors (aprepitant, erythromycin, clarithromycin, fluconazole, verapamil, grapefruit juice, diltiazem, amiodarone). *Co-admin caution (amphiphilic pulmonary toxicity):* Other amphiphilic agents (amiodarone, statins).
Effect of Temsirolimus on Other Drugs: P-gp substrates (digoxin, vincristine, colchicine, paclitaxel): *Co-admin, monitor closely.*
SP: CNS tumours (primary, metastases) and/or on anticoagulation therapy, increased intracerebral bleeding risk (including fatal). Thrombocytopenia, neutropenia, anaemia (monitor complete blood counts prior to initiation then periodically). Renal failure. Cataracts (combination with interferon-alpha). Hypersensitivity and/or infusion reactions (including anaphylaxis); stop infusion (observe for 30-60 minutes); resume at physician discretion. Increased blood glucose levels; advise patients to report excessive thirst, increased urination volume/frequency. Increased serum triglycerides, cholesterol (monitor); may predispose to MI. Abnormal wound healing. Caution, alcoholics. Interstitial lung disease. Observe for signs of infection including opportunistic; *Pneumocystis jirovecii* pneumonia.
Pregnancy, Lactation: Pregnancy, not recommended. Women and men with partners of childbearing potential to ensure adequate contraception. Lactation, stop breastfeeding during treatment.
ADR: See Notes below.
Notes: See 13.1.8 Other Antineoplastics.

Torisel Parenteral *(Pfizer)* A. HOS.
Price, (1) €820.73 (PTW).
Infusion, temsirolimus 30mg diluted to 10mg/mL. Clear colourless (light-yellow) conc; clear (slightly turbid) light-yellow (yellow) diluent for soln. *Ethanol 474mg/vial; 358mg/1.8mL diluent.* **Store:** Refrigerate (conc and diluent); do not freeze.

Topotecan

ATC Code: L01XX17. **Sport:** Permitted.
Driving: Caution.
Indications: Monotherapy, relapsed small cell lung cancer (SCLC). Combination with cisplatin, carcinoma of cervix recurrent after radiotherapy; stage IVB disease. Monotherapy, metastatic carcinoma of ovary after failure of first-line or subsequent therapy *(Hycamtin).*
Dose: Adult: ORAL, relapsed SCLC, 2.3mg/m2 BSA/day for 5 consecutive days with 3-week interval between start of each course. Swallow whole with water; do not crush or chew; with or without food.
PARENTERAL, ovarian cancer, relapsed SCLC, initially 1.5mg/m2 BSA/day, schedule as for oral above. Cervical cancer, 0.75mg/m2/day on days 1, 2 and 3 with cisplatin after topotecan on day 1; repeat every 21 days for 6 courses. IV infusion over 30 minutes.
Elderly: Over 65 years, increased incidence drug-related diarrhoea.
Renal Impairment: *Oral,* CrCl (mL/min) 30-49, dose at 1.9mg/m2/day for 5 consecutive days; if well tolerated, increase to 2.3mg/m2/day in subsequent cycles. Korean patients, CrCl (mL/min) below 50, consider further dose reduction. Below 30, no dose recommendation. *Parenteral,* monotherapy, CrCl (mL/min) below 20, no data; 20-39, 0.75mg/m2/day for 5 consecutive days. Combination, see manufacturers Full Prescribing Information.
Hepatic Impairment: No dose recommendation.
CI: Severe bone marrow depression prior to initiation.
Interactions: Effect of Other Drugs on Topotecan: *Oral, Increased exposure:* ABCB1 (p-glycoprotein) (ciclosporin), ABCG2 (BCRP) inhibitors. *Parenteral: Combination therapy:* Reduce dose of each drug. See Notes below (cisplatin, carboplatin).
SP: Platinum admin (day 1 of topotecan dosing), a lower dose of each agent must be admin for improved tolerability, compared to platinum on (day 5 of topotecan dosing). Dose-related haematological toxicity, monitor. Interstitial lung disease. Proactive diarrhoea management with anti-diarrhoeals; severe, may require oral/IV electrolytes and fluids and/or therapy interruption.
Pregnancy, Lactation: Pregnancy, not recommended; can cause foetal harm; advise women of childbearing potential to avoid becoming pregnant during therapy; warn of potential hazard to foetus. Lactation, contraindicated.
ADR: See Notes below.
Notes: See 13.1.8 Other Antineoplastics. See 13.1.5 Platinum Compounds (cisplatin, carboplatin).

Hycamtin 0.25mg, 1mg *(Novartis)* A. HT.
Price, (10) 0.25mg, €136.57. 1mg, €545.27. HOS: (1) 1mg, €58.01; 4mg, €264.37 (PTW).
Capsule, topotecan HCl. Hard opaque. Marked name/strength. 0.25mg: White (yellowish white). 1mg: Pink.
Hycamtin Parenteral *(Novartis)* A.
Price, (1) 1mg, €60.95; 4mg, €393.86 (PTW).
Infusion, topotecan HCl 4mg. Light-yellow (greenish) powder for conc for soln.
Topotecan Hospira Parenteral *(Hospira)* A.
Price, not published by company.
Infusion, topotecan HCl 1mg/mL (4mg). Clear yellow (yellow-green) conc for soln.

Tretinoin (systemic)

ATC Code: L01XX14. **Sport:** Permitted.
Driving: Caution.
Indications: Induction of remission, acute promyelocytic leukaemia previously untreated as well as for relapse after standard chemotherapy with anthracycline and cytosine or refractory to chemotherapy.
Dose: Adult, Elderly: Usually 45mg/m2/day BSA in 2 equal doses until complete remission or max. 90 days. Full dose anthracycline-based chemotherapy should be added. Oral, caps to be taken with or shortly after food swallowed whole with water.

Child: Can be treated as for Adult unless severe toxicity develops. Intractable headache, reduce dose.
Renal Impairment: Decrease to 25mg/m2/day.
Hepatic Impairment: As for Renal above.
CI: Hypersensitivity to retinoids, soya, peanut.
Interactions: Effect of Other Drugs on Tretinoin: *Co-admin not recommended:* Tetracyclines (elevated intracranial pressure risk), Vitamin A (hypervitaminosis A). *Co-admin caution:* Anti-fibrinolytics (tranexamic acid, aminocaproic acid, aprotinin). *Altered pharmacokinetics:* Hepatic enzyme inducers (rifampicin, glucocorticoids, phenobarbital, pentobarbital), inhibitors (ketoconazole, cimetidine, erythromycin, verapamil, diltiazem, ciclosporin).
SP: Hyperleucocytosis associated with Retinoic Acid Syndrome (fever, dyspnoea, acute respiratory distress, pulmonary infiltrates, pleural and pericardial effusions, hypotension, oedema, weight gain, hepatic, renal and multi-organ failure); treat immediately with dexamethasone 10mg 12-hourly for up to 3 days. Pseudotumour cerebri, Sweet's syndrome or acute febrile neutrophilic dermatitis, venous or arterial thrombosis risk, hypercalcaemia.
Pregnancy, Lactation: Micro-dosed progesterone preparations are inadequate method of contraception during tretinoin treatment. Pregnancy and lactation, not recommended.
NOTE: Tretinoin causes serious birth defects and should only be initiated if females meet certain criteria. See Notes below (isotretinoin).
ADR: See Notes below.
Notes: See 13.1.8 Other Antineoplastics. See 10.1.5 Oral Acne Treatments (isotretinoin).

Vesanoid 10mg *(Cheplapharm)* A.
Price, (100) €313.70.
Capsule, tretinoin. Soft orange-yellow/reddish-brown. *Soya-bean oil, sorbitol.*

13.2 - Drugs Affecting Immune Response

Class Effects
General Principles: Immunosuppressants are used to treat a variety of chronic inflammatory and autoimmune diseases. In organ transplantation (rejection prevention), they should be prescribed only by physicians experienced in immunosuppressive use post-transplant. Usually used in specialised units; information provided is less detailed and prescribers should always consult the manufacturers Full Prescribing Information, Scientific Literature and/or local hospital protocols.
Interactions: Effect of Other Drugs on Drugs Affecting Immune Response: *Co-admin not recommended:* Live vaccines (especially BCG, smallpox, yellow fever).
SP: Facilities equipped with adequate laboratory and supportive medical resources (drugs for treating severe hypersensitivity reactions) to be available. Immunosuppression following transplant, increased risk of developing lymphoproliferative disorders, see SP below. *Opportunistic infection* risk increased (bacterial, fungal, viral including latent reactivation and polyomavirus, protozoal); BK virus (nephropathy), John Cunningham (JC) virus (multifocal leucoencephalopathy). Infection relates to high total immunosuppressive burden; consider differential diagnosis if renal function deteriorates, neurological symptoms develop (impaired cognition, visual disturbances, hemiparesis, altered mental state, behavioural changes); increased susceptibility with immunosuppressive combinations.
ADR: Serious life-threatening infections (meningitis, endocarditis, TB, atypical mycobacterial infection). Immunosuppressive combinations increase risk of developing lymphomas, other malignancies (particularly skin). Elderly, generally at increased adverse reaction risk.
Notes: See also 13.1 Cytotoxic Drugs. Use in various chronic diseases, see 4.4.1 Drugs Suppressing Rheumatic Disease Process.

13.2.1 - Immunosuppressants

In This Chapter: *Antithymocyte immunoglobulin, azathioprine, basiliximab, belatacept, everolimus,*

13.2.1 Immunosuppressants

lenalidomide, mycophenolate, pomalidomide, siltuximab, mTOR inhibitors (sirolimus, tacrolimus), thalidomide.

Class Effects

Prednisolone, widely used in treating malignancies, is an immunosuppressant.

CI: Hypersensitivity to any member of the class.

SP: Adjust dose according to (condition treated, response, haematological tolerance, regime used). Advise patients to report signs of immunosuppression (throat ulceration, fever, infection, bruising, bleeding, signs of myelosuppression). Limit exposure to sunlight, UV light (malignancy risk). Tumour lysis syndrome (high tumour burden prior to treatment). Progressive multifocal leucoencephalopathy, opportunistic infection risk, see Notes below (Class Effects, Drugs Affecting Immune Response).

Notes: See Class Effects 13.2 Drugs Affecting Immune Response. See also 11.1.1 Glucocorticoids (prednisolone), 4.4.1 Drugs Suppressing Rheumatic Disease Process (ciclosporin).

Antithymocyte Immunoglobulin

ATC Code: L04AA04. **Sport:** Permitted.
Driving: Cytokine release syndrome.

Indications: Immunosuppression in solid organ transplantation; prevention, graft rejection (renal, heart transplant). Treatment, steroid resistant graft rejection (renal transplant).

Dose: Adult, Elderly: PROPHYLAXIS, graft rejection in kidney transplantation, 1-1.5mg/kg/day for 3-9 days after transplant (cumulative 3-13.5mg/kg); heart, 1-2.5mg/kg/day for 3-5 days (cumulative 3-12.5mg/kg).
TREATMENT, steroid resistant graft rejection in kidney transplant, 1.5mg/kg/day for 7-14 days after transplant (cumulative 10.5-21mg/kg). Base dose on ideal weight. Premedicate (IV corticosteroids, antihistamines, antipyretics) prior to infusion (slowly in high-flow vein; total duration minimum 6 hours).

Child: Do not require a different dose to adults.

CI: Acute chronic infection.

SP: For hospital use only. Monitor during and after infusion until stable (anaphylactic shock). Serious immune-mediated reactions (anaphylaxis, cytokine release syndrome), infection (bacterial, fungal, viral, protozoal), infection reactivation (CMV). Protein composition and conc vary for different antithymocyte globulin products; ensure prescribed dose is for appropriate product. Thrombocytopenia, leucopenia (adjust dose). Human blood components, thymus cells used in manufacturing. Combination with heparin and hydrocortisone in dextrose infusion (precipitation). Live attenuated vaccines not recommended. May interfere with ELISA tests.

Pregnancy, Lactation: Pregnancy, use only if clearly needed. Lactation, stop breastfeeding during treatment. Use in labour/delivery, no data.

ADR: See Notes below.

Notes: See 13.2.1 Immunosuppressants.

> **Thymoglobulin Parenteral** *(SANOFI)* A. HOS.
> *Price,* 25mg/5mL (1) €213.77 (PTW).
> *Infusion,* rabbit anti-human thymocyte immunoglobulin 25mg/vial. Powder for soln.

Azathioprine

ATC Code: L04AX01. **Sport:** Permitted.
Driving: Unlikely to impair.

Indications: *Imuran,* alone or combination (corticosteroids); can have steroid-sparing effect reducing toxicity of (high dose, prolonged) corticosteroid use; combination (corticosteroids, other immunosuppressants), to enhance survival of organ transplants. *Imuger,* prophylaxis, transplant rejection (kidney, liver, heart, lung, pancreas transplants). *Both brands,* alone or combination, severe active rheumatoid arthritis (RA), SLE, dermatomyositis, polymyositis, auto-immune chronic active hepatitis; pemphigus vulgaris, polyarteritis nodosa, auto-immune haemolytic anaemia, chronic refractory thrombocytopenic purpura; *Imuger,* severe or moderately severe inflammatory intestinal disease (Crohn's disease, ulcerative colitis).

Dose: Adult: Transplantation, initially 5mg/kg/day loading dose; maintenance, range 1-4mg/kg/day (oral or IV). Other conditions, generally 1-3mg/kg/day. Chronic active hepatitis, usually 1-1.5mg/kg/day. Maintenance, range 1-3mg/kg/day. *Elderly,* as for Renal below. *Admin,* oral tabs minimum 1 hour before or 3 hours after food or milk *(Imuran);* with at least a glass (200mL) water during meals *(Imuger).* IV by slow injection over minimum 1 minute or IV infusion (if oral route not practical). Avoid perivenous injection (tissue damage).

Child: Under 18 years, not recommended (juvenile chronic arthritis, SLE, dermatomyositis, polyarteritis nodosa). Other indications, as for Adult above.

Renal Impairment: Dose at lower end of normal range.

Hepatic Impairment: *Both brands,* mild to moderate, as for Renal above. Severe, contraindicated *(Imuger).*

CI: 6-mercaptopurine hypersensitivity, severe (infection, impaired bone marrow function), pancreatitis.

Interactions: Effect of Other Drugs on Azathioprine: *Reduce azathioprine dose (25% of original):* Allopurinol, oxipurinol, thiopurinol. *Excessive immunosuppression risk:* Ciclosporin, tacrolimus. *Increased myelosuppressive effect/risk (reduced dose):* Aminosalicylates (olsalazine, mesalazine, sulfasalazine), ACEIs, co-trimoxazole, cimetidine, indomethacin. *Severe myelosuppression:* Ribavirin. *Enhanced myelotoxicity:* Penicillamine. *Adjust dose to maintain adequate WBC count:* Methotrexate (high dose).

Effect of Azathioprine on Other Drugs: Non-depolarising muscle relaxants (curare, d-tubocurarine, pancuronium)*: Effect antagonised.* Succinylcholine: *Blockade potentiated.* Warfarin, phenprocoumon, acenocoumarol: *Anticoagulant effect inhibited.* Killed vaccines (hepatitis B): *Diminished response.*

SP: Withdraw gradually; withdrawal can result in severe worsening of condition. Monitor haematology (high doses, elderly, impaired renal function, mild or moderately impaired hepatic function, hypersplenism). May not be completely metabolised with TMPT deficiency, increased myelotoxic effect. Lesch-Nyhan Syndrome, not recommended (not effective). Acute untreated infection, caution. Mutagenic; potentially carcinogenic (caution, handling). *Varicella zoster* infection may be severe during immunosuppressant therapy. Lymphoproliferative disorders (multiple immunosuppressant regimens); reported fatalities. Macrophage activation syndrome (life-threatening) with autoimmune conditions (inflammatory bowel disease); discontinue. Inherited mutated NUDT15 gene, increased severe thiopurine toxicity risk (early leucopenia, alopecia) from conventional doses; generally require substantial dose reduction. Asian ethnicity at particular risk (increased mutation frequency in this population). Optimal starting dose (heterozygous or homozygous deficient) not established. Consider genotypic and phenotypic testing of NUDT15 variants before initiating in all patients (including paediatric).

Pregnancy, Lactation: Pregnancy, if benefit outweighs risk. Women of childbearing potential and males to ensure adequate contraception during and for at least 3 months after treatment. Lactation, not recommended *(Imuran);* contraindicated *(Imuger).*

ADR: See Notes below.

Notes: See 13.2.1 Immunosuppressants.

> **Imuran 25mg, 50mg, Parenteral** *(Aspen)* A. GMS.
> *Price,* (100) 25mg, €19.13. 50mg, €29.11. Injection 50mg (1) €20.61.
> *Tablet,* azathioprine. Round f/c unscored. 25mg: Orange. Marked GXEL5. 50mg: Yellow. Marked GXCH1. *Lactose.* **Store:** Below 25 deg C.
> *Injection or infusion,* azathioprine sodium 50mg. Yellow (amber) freeze-dried powder for soln. *Sodium 4.5mg.* **Store:** As above; protect (light).

> **Imuger 25mg, 50mg** *(Gerard)* A. GMS.
> *Price,* (100) 25mg, €18.75. 50mg, €28.52.
> *Tablet,* azathioprine. Pale-yellow. Marked AE/strength; G on reverse. 50mg: Round scored (divisible into equal halves). **Store:** Below 25 deg C; original pack.

Basiliximab

ATC Code: L04AC02. **Sport:** Permitted.
Driving: Unlikely to impair.
Indications: Prophylaxis, acute organ rejection in allogeneic renal transplant. Combination with ciclosporin and corticosteroids in patients with panel reactive antibodies below 80%, or triple maintenance immunosuppressive regimen (ciclosporin, corticosteroids and azathioprine or mycophenolate mofetil).
Dose: Adult, Elderly: Standard total dose 40mg (2 equally divided doses). Admin first 20mg within 2 hours prior to transplantation (*must not* be admin unless certain that patient will receive the graft and concomitant immunosuppression); second dose to be given 4 days after transplantation (withhold if severe hypersensitivity reaction to drug or graft occurs). IV bolus or IV infusion over 20-30 minutes. *Elderly*, limited data.
Child: Age 1-17 years, under 35kg, total 20mg (in 2 equally divided doses); 35kg or more, as for Adult above.
SP: Severe, acute hypersensitivity reactions initially and re-exposure (anaphylactoid-type; urticaria, pruritus, sneezing, hypotension, tachycardia, dyspnoea, bronchospasm, pulmonary oedema, respiratory failure); severe, permanently discontinue. Efficacy and safety in recipients of solid organ allografts other than renal not demonstrated; serious cardiac adverse events (cardiac arrest, atrial flutter, palpitation) when used in heart transplant.
Pregnancy, Lactation: Not recommended. Women of childbearing potential to ensure adequate contraception during and for 16 weeks after treatment.
ADR: See Notes below.
Notes: See 13.2.1 Immunosuppressants.

Simulect Parenteral (Novartis) C.
Price, (1) €1130.84.
Injection or infusion, basiliximab 20mg. White powder; solvent; produced by rDNA technology. **Store:** Store and transport refrigerated.

Belatacept

ATC Code: L04AA28. **Sport:** Permitted.
Driving: Fatigue, malaise, nausea.
Indications: Combination (corticosteroids, mycophenolic acid), prophylaxis of graft rejection in renal transplant. Recommended to add interleukin (IL)-2 receptor antagonist for induction regimen.
Dose: Adult, Elderly: Initial phase, 10mg/kg, day 1 (day of transplant, immediate preoperative period or during surgery before completion of transplant vascular anastomoses), day 5, day 14, day 28, end of week 8 and week 12 after transplant. Maintenance phase, every 4 weeks (+/- 3 days) starting end week 16 after transplant. Should be admin in combination with basiliximab induction, mycophenolate mofetil and corticosteroids. *Admin,* diluted solution as IV infusion at relatively constant rate over 30 minutes.
Child: Under 18 years, no data.
Renal Impairment: No dose adjustment.
Hepatic Impairment: Dose modification cannot be recommended.
CI: Epstein-Barr virus (EBV) seronegative or unknown serostatus.
SP: Panel Reactive Antibody titres above 30%, no data. Infusion-related reactions; serious allergic or anaphylactic reaction, discontinue immediately. Graft thrombosis risk. Liver transplant, not recommended. Taper corticosteroids cautiously. Belatacept therapeutic monitoring is not required. NOTE: 8-10 day half-life (when switching to other immunosuppressants).
Pregnancy, Lactation: Pregnancy, use only if clearly necessary. Women of childbearing potential to ensure adequate contraception during and up to 8 weeks after treatment. Lactation, not recommended.
ADR: See Notes below.
Notes: See 13.2.1 Immunosuppressants.

NULOJIX Parenteral (BMS) A.
Price, not published by company (reimbursement-pending).
Infusion, belatacept 25mg/mL. Fusion protein. White (off-white) powder/cake for conc. *Sodium 0.65mmoL/250mg* vial. **Store:** Refrigerate; original pack to protect (light).

Everolimus (immunosuppressant)

ATC Code: L04AA18. **Sport:** Permitted.
Driving: No data available.
Indications: Prophylaxis, organ rejection in renal or cardiac transplant (with ciclosporin microemulsion + corticosteroids) and liver transplant (with tacrolimus + corticosteroids).
Dose: Adult, Elderly: *Renal, cardiac* transplant, initially 0.75mg twice daily (with ciclosporin) as soon as possible after transplant. *Liver transplant,* 1mg twice daily (with tacrolimus); initial dose approx. 4 weeks after transplant. Adjust dose at 4-5 day intervals. Black patients, no efficacy/safety data. Ciclosporin, tacrolimus dose, see manufacturers Full Prescribing Information. *Admin,* oral in 2 divided doses either with or without food and at the same time as ciclosporin or tacrolimus; swallow whole with water; do not crush.
Child: *Renal transplant,* insufficient data; *liver,* not recommended.
Renal Impairment: No dose adjustment.
Hepatic Impairment: Monitor whole blood trough levels; half-life longer with impairment; therapeutic drug monitoring (see SP below) at initiation or adjustment until stable levels reached. Mild, reduce dose to two thirds*; moderate, reduce to one half*; severe, reduce to one third*. *(or normal dose). Reduce dose rounded to nearest tablet strength.
CI: Sirolimus hypersensitivity.
Interactions: Effect of Other Drugs on Everolimus: *Co-admin not recommended unless benefit outweighs risk:* Strong CYP3A4 inhibitors (ketoconazole, itraconazole, voriconazole, clarithromycin, telithromycin, nefazodone, ritonavir, atazanavir, saquinavir, darunavir, indinavir, nelfinavir), strong and moderate CYP3A4 inducers (rifampicin, rifabutin, carbamazepine, phenytoin, phenobarbital, efavirenz, nevirapine). *Co-admin caution:* Moderate CYP3A4/P-gp inhibitors (erythromycin, imatinib, verapamil, oral ciclosporin, fluconazole, diltiazem, nicardipine, dronedarone, amprenavir, fosamprenavir). *Co-admin avoid:* Grapefruit juice. *Co-admin not recommended:* St John's Wort.
Effect of Everolimus on Other Drugs: CYP3A4 substrates with narrow therapeutic index (pimozide, terfenadine, astemizole, cisapride, quinidine, ergot derivatives): *Monitor for adverse effects.* Octreotide, ciclosporin, atorvastatin, pravastatin, oral midazolam: *Plasma levels may be altered.*
SP: *Not studied,* combinations other than ciclosporin (microemulsion), basiliximab, tacrolimus, corticosteroids; use in high immunological risk. Strict caution, thymoglobulin induction and *Certican,* ciclosporin, steroid regimen (serious infections).
Increased lymphoma and other malignancy risk (skin). Increased serum cholesterol and triglycerides, monitor. Angioedema reported with ACEIs. Monitor: Renal function for all patients (caution, other medicinals negatively affecting renal function), proteinuria. Increased kidney arterial and venous thrombosis risk in first 30-days post-transplant (with graft loss). Wound-healing complications; thrombotic (microangiopathy, thrombocytopenic purpura), haemolytic uraemic syndrome (with calcineurin inhibitor). Vaccinations affected. Interstitial lung disease, new onset diabetes. NOTE: Recommend drug assays with adequate performance characteristics for therapeutic drug monitoring when low ciclosporin or tacrolimus conc are targeted; routine everolimus whole blood conc monitoring.
Pregnancy, Lactation: Pregnancy, weigh risk/benefit. Women of childbearing potential to use effective contraception during and up to 8 weeks after treatment. Lactation, not recommended.
ADR: Summary, *most common,* infections, anaemia, hyperlipidaemia, new onset diabetes mellitus, insomnia, headache, hypertension, cough, constipation, nausea, peripheral oedema, impaired healing (including pleural and pericardial effusion).
Notes: See 13.2.1 Immunosuppressants.

13.2.1 Immunosuppressants

Certican Tablets *(Novartis)* A. HOS.
Price, not published by company.
Tablet, everolimus 0.25mg, 0.5mg, 0.75mg, 1mg. White (yellowish) marbled round. Marked NVR. 0.25mg: Marked C. 0.5mg: Marked CH. 0.75mg: Marked CL. 1mg: Marked CU. *Lactose.* **Store:** Original pack to protect (light, moisture).

Lenalidomide

ATC Code: L04AX04. **Sport:** Permitted.
Driving: Caution; fatigue, dizziness, somnolence, blurred vision.
Indications: *Multiple myeloma,* maintenance, newly diagnosed (undergone autologous stem cell transplant) (ASCT)*; previously untreated (not eligible for transplant)**; with dexamethasone (received at least 1 prior therapy)**. *Myelodysplastic syndromes** (transfusion-dependent anaemia). *Mantle cell lymphoma** (relapsed or refractory). **(monotherapy). **(in combination).

Dose: Adult: *Multiple myeloma: Newly diagnosed,* undergone ASCT, 10mg/day continuously (days 1-28)*; after 3 cycles increase to 15mg/day if tolerated. *Combination,* (not eligible for transplant), 25mg/day (days 1-21)* with dexamethasone 40mg/day (days 1, 8, 15 and 22)*; *elderly,* age 75 years and older, use dexamethasone 20mg. *Combination,* 10mg/day (days 1-21)* for 9 cycles, melphalan 0.18mg/kg (days 1-4)*, prednisone 2mg/kg (days 1-4)*. After 9 cycles or if unable to complete 9 cycles (intolerance), monotherapy 10mg/day (days 1-21)*.
Multiple myeloma: Prior therapy, 25mg/day (days 1-21)* with dexamethasone 40mg/day (days 1-4, 9-12, 17-20)* for 4 cycles 40mg/day (days 1-4)*.
Myelodysplastic syndromes, 10mg/day (days 1-21) of repeated 28-day cycles.
Mantle cell lymphoma, 25mg/day (days 1-21)*.
Admin, once daily at the same time on each scheduled day; swallow whole with water with/without food; do not open, break or chew capsules. Recommend to press only one end of capsule to remove from blister to reduce risk of capsule deformation and/or breakage. *(of repeated 28-day cycles).

Elderly: As for Renal.

Child: Under 18 years, not recommended.

Renal Impairment: *Multiple myeloma, mantle cell lymphoma,* CrCl (mL/min) 30-50, 10mg/day; below 30 and not on dialysis, 7.5mg/day or 15mg every other day; ESRD, below 30 and on dialysis, 5mg/day after dialysis on dialysis days. *Myelodysplastic syndromes,* CrCl (mL/min) 30-50, initially 5mg/day; below 30 and not on dialysis, ESRD below 30 and needing dialysis, initially 2.5mg/day. *Admin,* once daily; see Adult above.

Hepatic Impairment: No specific dose recommendations.

Interactions: Effect of Other Drugs on Lenalidomide: *Co-admin caution*: Other myelosuppressives (neutropenia, thrombocytopenia). *Increased thromboembolic risk (combination therapy), caution*: Erythropoietic agents, other agents increasing thrombosis risk (HRT, combined oral contraceptives). *Plasma levels be increased*: P-gp inhibitors (ciclosporin, clarithromycin, itraconazole, ketoconazole, quinidine, verapamil); monitor.
Effect of Lenalidomide on Other Drugs: Oral contraceptives: *Dexamethasone may affect efficacy.* Warfarin: *Close monitoring; effect of dexamethasone unknown.* Digoxin: *Monitor.* Statins: *Increased rhabdomyolysis risk.*

SP: Advise patients NEVER to give this medicine to another person (teratogenic). With dexamethasone, increased DVT and pulmonary embolism risk; shortness of breath, chest pain, arm or leg swelling, seek medical advice. Known risk of MI, monitor; minimise (smoking, hypertension, hyperlipidaemia). Hb above 12g/dL discontinue erythropoietic agents. Neutropenia, thrombocytopenia (consider dose reduction). Monitor thyroid function. Severe peripheral neuropathy. Tumour lysis syndrome. Allergic (severe skin) reactions. Increased incidence of second primary malignancies. Hepatic failure, including fatal (with dexamethasone). Viral reactivation; serious herpes zoster or hepatitis B virus (HBV) reactivation; fatal outcome; establish HBV status before initiation.

Pregnancy, Lactation: Lenalidomide is structurally related to thalidomide; if taken during pregnancy, TERATOGENIC

378

effects are expected. Pregnancy is an ABSOLUTE CONTRAINDICATION; both men and women should understand the teratogenic risk and accept need for effective contraception without interruption commencing 4 weeks before, during, and for 4 weeks after end of treatment (1 week for men). Perform regular pregnancy testing. Women of childbearing potential, contraindicated unless all conditions of the Pregnancy Prevention Programme are met. Lactation, stop breastfeeding.

ADR: See Notes below.

Notes: See 13.2.1 Immunosuppressants.

▼ **Revlimid 5mg, 10mg, 15mg, 25mg** *(Celgene)* A. HT.
Price, (21) 5mg, €5124.28. 10mg, €5355.19. 15mg, €5587.08. 25mg, €6045.51.
Capsule, lenalidomide. Marked REV/strength. 5mg: White. 10mg: Blue-green/pale-yellow. 15mg: Pale-blue/white. 25mg: White. *Lactose.*

Mycophenolate Mofetil

ATC Code: L04AA06. **Sport:** Permitted.
Driving: Unlikely to impair.
Indications: Prophylaxis, acute transplant rejection in allogeneic renal, cardiac or hepatic transplants (with ciclosporin and corticosteroids).

Dose: Adult: ORAL, *renal transplant,* initiate within 72 hours after transplant, 1g twice daily; *cardiac,* initiate within 5 days, 1.5g twice daily; *hepatic,* admin IV for first 4 days then switch to oral as soon as can be tolerated; 1.5g orally twice daily. *Admin,* do not chew or crush tabs/caps; swallow whole. Caps should not be opened to avoid powder inhalation or direct contact with skin or mucous membranes (teratogenic potential).
PARENTERAL, NOT for rapid or bolus IV injection; slow IV infusion over 2 hours is alternative to oral; may be used for up to 14 days.
NOTE: 720mg twice daily (1440mg/day) mycophenolate sodium corresponds to mycophenolate mofetil 1g twice daily in terms of mycophenolic acid (MPA) content. Mycophenolic acid (sodium salt) and mycophenolate mofetil are NOT to be interchanged or directly substituted.

Elderly: 65 years and older, renal transplant, 1g twice daily; cardiac, hepatic, 1.5g twice daily.

Child: ORAL, *renal transplant,* initiate as for Adult; age 2-18 years (BSA at least 1.25m2), 600mg/m2 twice daily; max. 2g/day; (BSA 1.25-1.5m2), 750mg twice daily; max. 1.5g/day; (BSA above 1.5m2), 1g twice daily. Greater adverse event frequency in children; may require temporary dose reduction or interruption. Under 2 years, *renal transplant,* limited data; cardiac and hepatic transplant, no data.

Renal Impairment: Renal transplant with severe chronic impairment, GFR (mL/min/1.73m2) below 25, outside immediate post-transplant period, avoid above 1g twice daily. Cardiac, hepatic transplant, no data.

Hepatic Impairment: Severe, *renal transplant,* no adjustment. Cardiac transplant, no data.

Interactions: Effect of Other Drugs on Mycophenolate Mofetil: *Co-admin not recommended (no data):* Azathioprine. *Potentially increased plasma levels:* Aciclovir, ganciclovir, valaciclovir, other drugs with renal tubular secretion. *Plasma levels increased:* If ciclosporin co-admin stopped, tacrolimus (liver transplant). *Absorption/exposure decreased:* Antacids (magnesium, aluminium hydroxides), PPIs (lansoprazole, pantoprazole), colestyramine, drugs interfering with enterohepatic circulation. See SP below. *Plasma levels decreased:* Rifampicin + ciclosporin co-admin, sevelamer (admin mycophenolate mofetil minimum 1 hour before or 3 hours after sevelamer), norfloxacin + metronidazole, ciprofloxacin, amoxicillin + clavulanic acid (initiation of antibiotic treatment).

SP: Caution, switching combination therapy containing immunosuppressants which interfere with mycophenolic acid (MPA) enterohepatic recirculation (ciclosporin) to one without this effect (sirolimus, belatacept); this may change MPA exposure; active serious digestive system disease. Neutropenia, monitor. Influenza vaccine may be of value. Lesch-Nyhan and Kelley-Seegmiller syndrome, avoid. *Reported,* PML (fatal), usually with risk factors (immunosuppressant therapy, impaired immune function); Pure Red Cell Aplasia (PRCA) (may resolve with dose reduction), hypogammaglobulinaemia in association with recurrent infections, bronchiectasis. Patients not to donate blood during or for six weeks after treatment. Advise patients to report evidence of infection, unexpected bruising, bleeding, other manifestation of bone marrow depression.

Pregnancy, Lactation: Pregnancy, contraindicated unless no suitable alternative available; exclude before initiation. Women of childbearing potential to ensure adequate contraception during and for six weeks after treatment; sexually active men to use condoms during and for at least 90 days after treatment. Congenital malformations including multiple malformations (abnormally formed or absent external/middle ear, external auditory canal atresia, congenital heart disease; malformations of face, fingers, tracheo-oesophageal, CNS; abnormalities of eye and kidney). Spontaneous abortion reported. Ensure women and men understand the risk of harm to the baby and the need for effective contraception. Lactation, contraindicated (not known if excreted in human milk; potential serious adverse events in breast-fed infants).

ADR: See Notes below.

Notes: See 13.2.1 Immunosuppressants.

CellCept 250mg, 500mg, Oral Susp *(Roche)* A. HT.
Price, 250mg (100) and 500mg (50) €69.33. Susp 1g/5mL (175mL) €154.42
Capsule, mycophenolate mofetil. Oblong blue/brown hard. Marked name, strength, Roche.
Tablet, as above. Lavender caplet-shaped f/c. Marked name, strength; Roche on reverse.
Oral susp, as above 1g/5mL. Powder for susp. *Sorbitol, soybean lecithin, aspartame, parabens.*
CellCept Parenteral *(Roche)* A.
Price, 500mg (4) €62.42.
Infusion, mycophenolate mofetil hydrochloride 500mg. Powder for conc for soln. *Sodium chloride.*
Mycolat 250mg, 500mg *(Rowex)* A. HT.
Price, both strengths (50) €55.47.
Capsule, mycophenolate mofetil. Opaque hard gelatin blue/orange.
Tablet, as above. Lavender f/c.
Mycophenolate Mofetil (Accord) Tabs *(Accord)* A. HT.
Price, both strengths (50) €55.47.
Capsule (250mg), mycophenolate mofetil 250mg. Light-blue/peach containing white (off-white) powder. Marked MMF and 250. **Store:** Below 30 deg C.
Tablet (500mg), as above 500mg. Purple cap-shaped f/c. Marked AHI and 500. **Store:** Below 25 deg C; outer carton to protect (light).
Mycophenolate Mofetil Clonmel Caps/Tabs *(Clonmel)* A. HT.
Price, both strengths (50) €55.47.
Capsule, mycophenolate mofetil 250mg, 500mg. Hard containing white (off-white) powder. 250mg: Blue/pink. Marked APO and M250.
Tablet, as above. Lavender cap-shaped f/c. Marked APO; MYC500 on reverse.
Myfenax 250mg, 500mg *(TEVA)* A. HT.
Price, both strengths (50) €55.47.
Capsule, mycophenolate mofetil. Hard opaque caramel/light-blue. Marked M and strength.
Tablet, as above. Pale-purple oval f/c. Marked M500.

Mycophenolate Sodium

ATC Code: L04AA06. **Sport:** Permitted.
Driving: Unlikely to impair.
Indications: Prophylaxis of acute transplant rejection in patients receiving allogeneic renal transplants in combination with ciclosporin and corticosteroids.

Dose: Adult, Elderly: Recommended, 720mg twice daily (1440mg/day) which corresponds to 1g mycophenolate mofetil admin twice daily (2g/day) in terms of mycophenolic acid (MPA) contents. Initiate within 72 hours of transplant. *Admin,* oral with or without food. Do not crush. Where crushing is necessary, avoid inhalation of powder or direct contact with skin or mucous membrane (teratogenic potential). Mycophenolic acid (sodium salt) and mycophenolate mofetil are NOT to be interchanged or directly substituted. See Notes below (mycophenolate mofetil).

Child: Insufficient data; limited data available for paediatric renal transplantation.

Renal Impairment: Delayed renal graft function post-operative, no dose adjustment. Severe impairment, GFR (mL/min/1.73m2) below 25, monitor closely (max. 1440mg/day). Renal transplant rejection, dose modification not required (MPA pharmacokinetics not changed).

Hepatic Impairment: No adjustment.

Interactions: Effect of Other Drugs on Mycophenolate Sodium: *No changes in pharmacokinetics:* PPIs. See Notes below (mycophenolate mofetil).

SP: See Notes below (mycophenolate mofetil).

Pregnancy, Lactation: Powerful human teratogen with increased risk of spontaneous abortions and congenital malformations when exposed during pregnancy. Women of childbearing potential, do not initiate until negative pregnancy test obtained. Contraindicated in women of childbearing potential who are not using highly effective contraception; two reliable from of contraception to be used before initiation, during therapy and for 6 weeks after last dose; sexually active men to use condoms during treatment and for 90 days after cessation (female partners to ensure highly effective contraception for same 90-day period). Men should not donate semen during therapy or for at least 90 days after discontinuation. Pregnancy, contraindicated unless no suitable alternative available to prevent transplant rejection. Lactation, should not be used. See also Notes below (mycophenolate mofetil).

ADR: See Notes below.

Notes: See Mycophenolate Mofetil above. See 13.2.1 Immunosuppressants.

Myfortic 180mg, 360mg *(Novartis)* A. HT.
Price, (120) 180mg, €125.92. 360mg, €252.17.
Tablet, mycophenolate sodium. g/r. 180mg: Lime green round. Marked C. 360mg: Pale-orange/red ovaloid. Marked CT. *Lactose.*

Pomalidomide

ATC Code: L04AX06. **Sport:** Pending.
Driving: Minor or moderate influence; fatigue, depressed consciousness level, confusion, dizziness.
Indications: Treatment (adults), relapsed and refractory multiple myeloma (with dexamethasone).

Dose: Adult: 4mg/day (days 1-21)*; with dexamethasone 40mg/day (days 1, 8, 15, 22)* until disease progression. Haematological toxicity, reduce dose or interrupt. *Admin,* oral once daily at same time each day; do not open caps, break or chew; swallow whole with water, with or without food. *(of repeated 28-day cycles).

Elderly: Age above 75 years, as for Adult above; with dexamethasone 20mg/day.

Child: No relevant use, age 0-17 years.

Renal Impairment: Admin after haemodialysis.

Hepatic Impairment: Monitor carefully.

Interactions: Effect of Other Drugs on Pomalidomide: *Increased exposure:* Strong CYP1A2 inhibitors (fluvoxamine, ciprofloxacin, enoxacin).

Effect of Pomalidomide on Other Drugs: Warfarin: *Monitor closely.*

SP: TERATOGENIC effect expected. Criteria for women to be considered of 'non-childbearing potential', see Notes below. Instruct patients never to give this medicine to another person and not to donate blood, semen or sperm. Monitor haematology at baseline, weekly (8 weeks), then monthly (neutropenia); observe for signs of bleeding. *Caution,* venous thromboembolic events (DVT, pulmonary embolism; especially with risk factors), peripheral neuropathy, caution, cardiac events (CHF, pulmonary oedema) usually with pre-existing cardiac disease (monitor). Tumour lysis syndrome, secondary primary malignancies (non-melanoma skin cancer), allergic reactions (angioedema, severe dermatological), dizziness, confusion, interstitial lung disease, hepatic disorders (elevated ALT, bilirubin; hepatitis). Establish Hepatitis B status before initiation; reactivation reported; monitor for active HBV infection.

Pregnancy, Lactation: Contraindicated in pregnancy or women of childbearing potential (unless all conditions of pregnancy prevention programme are met), males unable to follow or comply with required contraceptive measures (pomalidomide is present in human semen). Counsel regarding teratogenic risk. Effective contraception to be

13.2.1 Immunosuppressants

used for 4 weeks before, during and for 4 weeks after treatment. Combined oral contraceptives not recommended (increased venous thromboembolism risk). Exclude pregnancy before initiation, then every 4 weeks including 4 weeks after end of treatment. Lactation, stop drug or stop breastfeeding.

ADR: See Notes below.

Notes: See 13.2.1 Immunosuppressants.

▼ **Imnovid 1mg, 2mg, 3mg, 4mg** *(Celgene)* A. HT.
Price, (21) 1mg, €9450.70; 2mg, €9567.89; 3mg, €9688.86; 4mg, €9785.34.
Capsule, pomalidomide. Opaque. Marked POML and strength. 1mg: Blue/yellow. 2mg: Dark-blue/orange. 3mg: Dark-blue/green. 4mg: Blue/blue.

Siltuximab

ATC Code: L04AC11. **Sport:** Pending.
Driving: No or negligible influence.

Indications: Treatment, multicentre Castleman's disease in adults negative for HIV and herpesvirus-8.

Dose: Adult, Elderly: Recommended 11mg/kg by IV infusion over 1 hour; admin every 3 weeks until treatment failure.

Child: Age 17 years and younger, no safety/efficacy data.

Hepatic Impairment: Elevated (transaminases, bilirubin), monitor; possible association between treatment and incidence of, and serious adverse events.

Interactions: Effect of Siltuximab on Other Drugs: CYP450 substrates with a narrow therapeutic index (warfarin, ciclosporin, theophylline, oral contraceptives): *Potentially changed therapeutic effect/toxicity with co-admin.*

SP: Perform haematology laboratory tests prior to each dose (first 12 months), then before every third dose cycle. For treatment requirements (absolute neutrophil, platelet count; Hb) see manufacturers Full Prescribing Information. Severe infection or any non-severe haematological toxicity, withhold (treat infections prior to admin); restart at same dose after recovery. Severe infusion reactions (anaphylaxis, severe allergic reactions or cytokine release syndrome), discontinue; mild/moderate reactions may improve with slowed infusion rate or stopping infusion; re-initiate with lower rate and consider (antihistamines, acetaminophen, corticosteroids). Hypoglobulinaemia, decreased (IgG, IgA, IgM) levels, GI perforation. May mask acute inflammation (suppression of fever, acute-phase reactants e.g. C-reactive protein). Elevated triglycerides and cholesterol, monitor.

Pregnancy, Lactation: Pregnancy, not recommended (use only if benefit outweighs risk; infants may be at increased infection risk). Women of childbearing potential to ensure adequate contraception during and for up to 3 months after treatment. Lactation, stop drug or stop breastfeeding.

ADR: See Notes below.

Notes: See 13.2.1 Immunosuppressants.

▼ **Sylvant Parenteral** *(Janssen-Cilag)* A. HOS.
Price, (1) 100mg, €508.70; 400mg, €1986.90 (PTW).
Infusion, siltuximab 20mg/mL (100mg, 400mg). White powder for soln. **Store:** Refrigerate; do not freeze; original pack to protect (light).

Sirolimus

ATC Code: L04AA10. **Sport:** Permitted.
Driving: Unlikely to impair.

Indications: Prophylaxis, organ rejection in renal transplant. Initially, combination with ciclosporin microemulsion + corticosteroids (2-3 months); may be continued as maintenance with corticosteroids only if ciclosporin can be progressively discontinued.

Dose: Adult: Initially (2-3 months post-transplant), 6mg loading dose immediately after transplant, then 2mg once daily; optimise with a tapering regimen of steroids + ciclosporin; individualise (whole blood trough levels 4-12ng/mL). *Maintenance,* progressively discontinue ciclosporin over 4-8 weeks; adjust sirolimus to obtain blood trough levels 12-20ng/mL. Optimal therapy requires therapeutic drug monitoring (all patients). *Admin,* oral consistently with or without food; do not crush, chew or split tabs. Avoid grapefruit juice. See Interactions below.

Elderly: Limited data.

Child: Under 18 years, not recommended.

Hepatic Impairment: Mild to moderate, monitor whole blood trough levels; severe, reduce maintenance dose by one half; loading dose, no modification needed (monitor every 5-7 days until 3 consecutive trough levels have shown stable conc).

Interactions: Effect of Other Drugs on Sirolimus: *Co-admin not recommended:* Strong CYP3A4 inhibitors (ketoconazole, voriconazole, itraconazole, telithromycin, clarithromycin), strong CYP3A4 inducers (rifampicin, rifabutin). *Co-admin caution, possible interaction:* Moderate to weak CYP3A4 inhibitors (nicardipine, clotrimazole, fluconazole, troleandomycin, bromocriptine, cimetidine, danazol, PIs e.g. ritonavir, indinavir, boceprevir, telaprevir), CYP3A4 inducers (St John's Wort, carbamazepine, phenobarbital, phenytoin). *Co-admin caution:* Nephrotoxic drugs. *Co-admin avoid:* Grapefruit juice. Angioedema-type reactions; increased rates of acute rejection: ACEIs. Increased risk (calcineurin inhibitor-induced effects): Calcineurin inhibitors (ciclosporin, tacrolimus). *Admin 4-hours after:* Ciclosporin (microemulsion). *Monitor blood levels, consider dose reduction:* Diltiazem, verapamil.

SP: Liver or lung transplant, not recommended. Increased hepatic artery thrombosis in combination (ciclosporin or tacrolimus). Bronchial anastomotic dehiscence (lung transplants). Peripheral oedema, exfoliative dermatitis, hypersensitivity vasculitis. Anaphylactic/toid reactions, angioedema, hypersensitivity vasculitis. Pneumocystis carinii (jirovecii) pneumonia (antimicrobial prophylaxis for 12 months*); CMV (prophylaxis for 3 months*). Increased serum cholesterol, triglycerides (renal transplants). statin or fibrate admin, monitor (rhabdomyolysis). May delay recovery of renal function. Monitor urinary protein. Combination use (mycophenolate mofetil + corticosteroids) and IL-2 receptor antibody induction, not recommended. Impaired or delayed wound healing. BMI over 30, increased risk. Conversion from calcineurin inhibitor tacrolimus or Rapamune in maintenance renal transplant patients not recommended. *(post-transplant).

Pregnancy, Lactation: Pregnancy, if benefit outweighs risk. Women of childbearing potential to ensure adequate contraception during and for up to 12 weeks after treatment. Lactation, not recommended.

ADR: See Notes below.

Notes: See 13.2.1 Immunosuppressants.

Rapamune 1mg, 2mg, Oral Soln 1mg/mL *(Pfizer)* A. HT.
Price, tabs (30) 1mg, €128.76. 2mg, €259.20. Oral Soln €248.82.
Tablet, sirolimus. Triangular coated. Marked name/strength. 1mg: White. 2mg: Yellow. *Lactose, sucrose.*
Oral soln, as above 1mg/mL. *Soya oil, ethanol.* **Store:** Refrigerate; below 25 degrees C for 24 hours.

Tacrolimus (systemic)

ATC Code: L04AD02. **Sport:** Permitted.
Driving: Visual, neurological disturbances; may be enhanced with ALCOHOL.

Indications: Prophylaxis, transplant rejection in liver, kidney, heart allograft (adults, paediatric recipients) *(all brands);* liver and kidney only (adult only) *(Advagraf, Envarsus).* Treatment, allograft rejection resistant to treatment with other immunosuppressives (adults only) *(Advagraf, Envarsus).*

Dose: Adult, Elderly: STANDARD/R, prophylaxis of transplant rejection. *Liver,* initially 0.1-0.2mg/kg/day orally, commencing approx. 12 hours after surgery OR parenteral 0.01-0.05mg/kg/day IV. *Kidney,* commencing within 24-hours after surgery, 0.2-0.3mg/kg/day orally OR parenteral 0.05-0.1mg/kg/day IV. *Heart,* following antibody induction, 0.075mg/kg/day orally commencing within 5 days post-surgery OR parenteral 0.01-0.02mg/kg/day IV. Admin, oral in 2 divided doses, on empty stomach at least 1 hour before food or 2-3 hours after; admin immediately after removal from blister; swallow with water; cap contents can be suspended in water and admin via nasogastric tube. Parenteral admin as 24-hour continuous IV infusion. Granules, use 2mL water per 1mg tacrolimus to produce susp; max. 50mL depending on body weight.

PROLONGED/R, *Advagraf,* 18 years and over. *Liver,* initially 0.1-0.2mg/kg/day commencing approx. 12-18 hours after surgery. *Kidney*, initially 0.2-0.3mg/kg/day commencing within 24 hours after surgery. Admin as single daily dose in morning; swallow whole on empty stomach.

PROLONGED/R, *Envarsus*, 18 years and over. *Liver*, initially 0.11-0.13mg/kg/day commencing within 24 hours after surgery. *Kidney*, initially 0.17mg/kg/day commencing within 24 hours after surgery. Admin as single daily dose in morning; swallow whole on empty stomach.

Switching: Stable patients should be switched from twice daily Standard/R to once daily Prolonged/R *Advagraf* on a 1:1 (mg:mg) basis; systemic exposure to tacrolimus for *Advagraf* approx. 10% lower than *Prograf*. *Envarsus* should be converted on a 1:0.7 (mg:mg) total daily dose basis; *Envarsus* maintenance dose should be 30% less than *Prograf* or *Advagraf* dose. Tacrolimus Standard/R and Prolonged/R are **NOT** interchangeable without careful blood monitoring and under supervision of a transplant specialist; see SP below. Stable allograft recipients maintained on one Standard/R preparation requiring conversion to another Standard/R preparation should be converted on a 1:1 (mg:mg) total daily basis.

Dose adjustments when co-admin with CYP3A4 inhibitors, see Interactions below.

Child: STANDARD/R, prophylaxis transplant rejection. *Liver*, initially 0.3mg/kg/day orally, starting approx. 12 hours after surgery OR parenteral 0.05mg/kg/day IV infusion. *Kidney*, starting within 24-hours after surgery, 0.3mg/kg/day orally OR parenteral 0.075-0.1mg/kg/day IV infusion. *Heart*, without antibody induction, 0.03-0.05mg/kg/day IV infusion converting to oral soonest at 0.3mg/kg/day starting 8-12 hours after IV discontinuation. Following antibody induction, 0.1-0.3mg/kg/day orally. In general, paediatrics require 1.5-2 times higher than Adult dose. See Adult above.

PROLONGED/R, under 18 years, not recommended.

Renal Impairment: Potentially nephrotoxic, monitor.

Hepatic Impairment: Severe, consider dose reduction.

CI: Macrolide hypersensitivity.

Interactions: Effect of Other Drugs on Tacrolimus: *Co-admin avoid*: Ciclosporin (previously received ciclosporin, caution). *Co-admin avoid (increased hyperkalaemia risk)*: High potassium intake, potassium-sparing diuretics (amiloride, triamterene, spironolactone). *Co-admin avoid (plasma levels decreased)*: St John's Wort, rifampicin, phenytoin, phenobarbital, corticosteroids (maintenance doses), carbamazepine, metamizole, isoniazid. *Plasma levels increased (monitor tacrolimus levels, renal function; consider dose reduction)*: Strong inhibitors of metabolism including azole antifungals (ketoconazole, fluconazole, itraconazole, voriconazole), macrolides (erythromycin), HIV protease inhibitors (nelfinavir, saquinavir, ritonavir) or HCV protease inhibitors (telaprevir, boceprevir), weaker inhibitors (clotrimazole, clarithromycin, josamycin, nifedipine, nicardipine, diltiazem, verapamil, amiodarone, danazol, ethinyloestradiol, omeprazole, nefazodone, Chinese herb extracts containing *Schisandra sphenanthera*), grapefruit juice (avoid), *in vitro* potential inhibitors (bromocriptine, cortisone, dapsone, ergotamine, gestodene, lidocaine, mephenytoin, miconazole, midazolam, nilvadipine, norethisterone, quinidine, tamoxifen, troleandomycin), reported, potentially (lansoprazole, ciclosporin), metoclopramide, cimetidine, magnesium-aluminium hydroxide. *Plasma levels increased or decreased*: Prednisolone, methylprednisolone (high doses). *Visual, neurological disturbances enhanced*: ALCOHOL. *Increased exposure*: Metoclopramide, cisapride, cimetidine, magnesium-aluminium-hydroxide. *Increased nephro/neurotoxic risk*: Aminoglycosides, gyrase inhibitors, vancomycin, sulfamethoxazole + trimethoprim, NSAIDs ganciclovir, aciclovir, other nephro/neurotoxic drugs *Possible interaction*: Other highly protein-bound medicinals (NSAIDs), oral anticoagulants, oral antidiabetics); medicinals increasing systemic exposure include prokinetic agents (metoclopramide, cisapride), cimetidine, magnesium-aluminium-hydroxide.

Effect of Tacrolimus on Other Drugs: Ciclosporin: *Half-life prolonged; synergistic/additive nephrotoxic effects*. Phenytoin: *Increased plasma levels*. Steroid-based contraceptives: *Increased exposure*.

SP: Medication errors, inadvertent, unintentional or unsupervised substitution of immediate- or prolonged-

release formulations; led to serious adverse events (graft rejection, side effects as result of under- or over-exposure to tacrolimus); change formulation only under supervision of transplant specialist. Black patients may require higher doses; limited experience in non-Caucasians; no evidence of gender differences. Initial post-transplant, monitor (BP, ECG, neurological and visual status, fasting blood glucose, electrolytes particularly potassium, liver and renal function, haematology, coagulation values, plasma protein); carefully monitor drug trough levels to ensure adequate exposure. Episodes of diarrhoea, extra monitoring. GI perforation (may be life-threatening). Cardiomyopathies (ventricular hypertrophy, hypertrophy of septum), caution (pre-existing heart disease, corticosteroid usage, hypertension, renal or hepatic dysfunction, infection, fluid overload, oedema), QT-prolongation (Torsades de Pointes). EBV-associated lymphoproliferative disorders; do not co-admin antilymphocyte treatment. Pure Red Cell Aplasia (PRCA).

Pregnancy, Lactation: Pregnancy, if benefit outweighs risk; crosses placenta. *In utero* exposure, monitor newborn (renal). Premature delivery risk, hyperkalaemia risk (newborn). Spontaneous abortion reported. Lactation, not recommended.

ADR: See Notes below.

Notes: See 13.2.1 Immunosuppressants.

Advagraf 0.5mg, 1mg, 5mg *(Astellas)* A. HT.
Price, (50) 0.5mg, €58.00. 1mg, €98.73. 3mg, €294.50. 5mg, €451.84.
Prolonged/R capsule, tacrolimus monohydrate. Hard light yellow/orange. Marked strength. 0.5mg: Marked *647. 1mg, Marked *677. Marked *687. *Lactose, soya lecithin*.

Envarsus 0.75mg, 1mg, 4mg *(Chiesi)* A. HT.
Price, (30) 0.75mg, €47.14; 1mg, €62.86; 4mg, €251.42.
Prolonged/R tablet, tacrolimus monohydrate. U/c oval white (off-white). Marked TCS. Strength on reverse. *Lactose*.

Prograf 0.5mg, 1mg, 5mg, Parenteral *(Astellas)* A. HT.
Price, caps (50) 0.5mg, €59.25. 1mg, €95.27. 5mg, €430.94.
Injection 5mg/mL (10) €675.08.
Standard/R capsule, tacrolimus. Gelatin opaque; contains white powder. Marked with strength. 0.5mg: Light-yellow. Marked [f] 607. 1mg: White. Marked [f] 617. 5mg: Greyish-red. Marked [f] 657. *Lactose; soya lecithin* 0.5mg, 1mg.
Infusion, as above 5mg/mL. Clear colourless conc for soln. *Castor oil, dehydrated alcohol*.

Modigraf 0.2mg, 1mg Sachets *(Astellas)* A. HT.
Price, (50) 0.2mg, €62.95. 1mg, €312.93.
Standard/R granules for oral susp, tacrolimus monohydrate. White. *Lactose*.

Tacrolimus 0.5mg, 1mg *(Accord)* A. HT.
Price, (50) 0.5mg, €50.38. 1mg, €54.46.
Standard/R capsule, tacrolimus. Hard containing white (off-white) granular powder. Marked TCR and strength. 0.5mg: Light-yellow. 1mg: White. *Lactose*.

Thalidomide

ATC Code: L04AX02. **Sport:** Permitted.

Driving: Somnolence, blurred vision.

Indications: First-line (in combination), in untreated multiple myeloma (65 years or over or ineligible for high dose chemotherapy).

Dose: Adult: Age 18 years and over, 200mg/day; max. 12 cycles or 6 weeks (42 days); combination with melphalan and prednisone each dosed once daily on days 1-4 of each 72-day cycle. See SP below. *Admin*, single dose at bedtime (reduce somnolence); with or without food; press only on one end of cap to remove from blister (reduce risk of deforming or breaking cap).

Elderly: Over 75 years, initially 100mg/day; combined with melphalan, use a reduced melphalan starting dose. Risk of higher frequency of serious adverse reactions.

Renal Impairment: No dose recommendations; severe, monitor carefully. Moderate or severe insufficiency, reduce melphalan by 50%.

Hepatic Impairment: No dose recommendation; severe, monitor carefully.

CI: Women who are pregnant or of childbearing potential unless all conditions of the Thalidomide Celgene Pregnancy Prevention Programme are met. Patients unable to follow/comply with required contraception.

Interactions: Effect of Other Drugs on Thalidomide: *Increased bradycardia risk*: Drugs inducing Torsade de

13.2.2   Radiopharmaceuticals

pointes, beta blockers, anticholinesterases. *Increased peripheral neuropathy risk*: Drugs associated with peripheral neuropathy (vincristine, bortezomib). *Increased venous thrombo-embolic disease risk*: Hormonal contraceptives.

Effect of Thalidomide on Other Drugs: Anxiolytics, hypnotics, antipsychotics, H1-antihistamines, opiate derivatives, barbiturates, ALCOHOL: *Enhanced sedation*. Warfarin: *Monitor INR (especially if corticosteroids being used)*.

SP: TERATOGENIC, see CI and Pregnancy. Monitor for thromboembolic events, peripheral neuropathy, rash/skin reactions (may be toxic; Stevens-Johnson Syndrome), bradycardia, syncope, somnolence (possible impairment of mental and/or physical abilities); delay dose, reduce or discontinue, depending on grade. Admin thromboprophylaxis during first 5 months of treatment (especially with other thrombotic risk factors); prophylactic antithrombotics (LMWH, warfarin) recommended. If thromboembolic events occur, manage with anticoagulants; once stabilised restart if benefit outweighs risk. Increased DVT, pulmonary embolism risk. Neutropenia, thrombocytopenia (delay dose, reduce or discontinue). Peripheral neuropathy, Grade 1, monitor, consider dose reduction; Grade 2, reduce dose or interrupt; no improvement or worsening, discontinue; if resolves to Grade 1, restart if benefit outweighs risk. Grade 3, Grade 4, discontinue. Allergic reactions/angioedema, reversible encephalopathy syndrome, reversible posterior leucoencephalopathy syndrome. Viral reactivation (Hepatitis B, herpes zoster); establish HBV status before initiation. Pulmonary hypertension; evaluate for underlying cardiopulmonary disease before initiating.

Pregnancy, Lactation: Thalidomide is TERATOGENIC, inducing a high frequency of severe and life-threatening birth defects; must never be used by women who are pregnant or could become pregnant. The conditions of the Thalidomide Celgene Pregnancy Prevention Programme must be fulfilled for all male and female patients.

Females, pregnancy, use contraindicated. Women of childbearing potential to ensure adequate contraception for 4 weeks before, during, and for 4 weeks after therapy; if pregnancy occurs, therapy must be stopped immediately and patient referred to teratology specialist for evaluation/advice. Lactation, contraindicated.

Males, thalidomide is found in semen; males must use condoms during and for 1 week after treatment when having intercourse with a pregnant woman or woman of childbearing potential not using adequate contraception.

ADR: See Notes below.

Notes: See 13.2.1 Immunosuppressants.

Thalidomide Celgene 50mg *(Celgene)* A. HT.
Price, (28) €391.18.
Capsule, thalidomide. White hard opaque. Marked Thalidomide Celgene 50mg.

13.2.2 - Radiopharmaceuticals

In This Chapter: *Ibritumomab tiuxetan*

Class Effects
CI: Hypersensitivity to any member of the class.
SP: Radiopharmaceuticals should only be used by qualified personnel and admin only by authorised persons in designated settings. Receipt, storage, use, transfer and disposal are subject to regulations and/or appropriate licences of local competent official organisations.
ADR: See manufactures Full Prescribing Information.
Notes: See also 13.2 Drugs Affecting Immune Response.

Ibritumomab tiuxetan

ATC Code: V10XX02. **Sport:** Permitted.
Driving: Caution.
Indications: Consolidation therapy after remission induction in previously untreated follicular lymphoma. Treatment, rituximab-relapsed or -refractory CD20+ follicular B-cell non-Hodgkin's lymphoma (NHL).
Dose: Adult, Elderly: Following rituximab, *monotherapy* platelets 150000/mm3 and more, 15MBq/kg bodyweight;

platelets 100000-150000/mm3, 11 MBq/kg; max. 1200 MBq/kg.
Consolidation remission, platelets 150000/mm3 and above, as for monotherapy; below 150000/mm3, not recommended. *Admin*, slow IV over 10 minutes; not for IV bolus.
Child: Under 18 years, not recommended.
CI: Hypersensitivity to yttrium chloride, rituximab, other murine proteins.
SP: Not recommended with risk of life-threatening haematological toxicity. Caution, bone marrow depletion. Consolidation, admin only after patient has recovered from induction chemotherapy (neutrophils above 1500/mm3, platelets above 150000/mm3). Growth factor treatment (G-CSF) not for admin 2 weeks prior and 2 weeks after ibritumomab tiuxetan (potential sensitivity of rapidly dividing myeloid cells to radiation). Test for hypersensitivity if murine derived protein previously received. Severe infusion reactions related to rituximab (caution, extravasation to avoid radiation-associated tissue damage). Severe mucocutaneous reactions.
Pregnancy, Lactation: Pregnancy, not recommended; exclude before initiating. Women of childbearing potential and males to ensure adequate contraception during and for up to 12 months after treatment. Lactation, not recommended.
ADR: See Notes below.
Notes: See 13.2.2 Radiopharmaceuticals. See Rituximab above.

Zevalin Parenteral 1.6mg/mL *(Thea Pharma)* A.
Price, not published by company.
Infusion, ibritumomab tiuxetan. Genetically engineered. Kit for radiopharmaceutical preparation. *Sodium 28mg/dose*.

13.2.3 - Interferons

In This Chapter: *Interferon alpha-2b.*

Class Effects
Interferon beta is used in treating MS and peginterferon in treating chronic hepatitis B and C. See Notes below.
CI: Hypersensitivity to any member of the class. Severe cardiac disease, severe myeloid dysfunction, uncontrolled seizure disorders and/or compromised CNS function, chronic hepatitis (with advanced decompensated hepatic disease or cirrhosis or treated with immunosuppressives). See also SP below.
SP: *Psychiatric, CNS*, severe CNS effects (depression, suicidal ideation/attempt); during and after treatment (during 6-month follow up); risk higher with children/adolescents. Other CNS effects (aggressive behaviour, bipolar disorder, mania, confusion, altered mental status). Existing or history of severe psychiatric conditions, adults (initiate with adequate therapeutic management), children, adolescents (contraindicated). Substance use or abuse (alcohol, cannabis), increased psychiatric disorder risk. *Infection* risk, including serious (bacterial, fungal, viral). To improve traceability of biologicals, record product brand name in the patient file.
Pregnancy, Lactation: Pregnancy, only if benefit outweighs risk. Women of childbearing age and fertile males to ensure adequate contraception during treatment. Lactation, not recommended; stop drug or stop breast feeding.
ADR: *Very commonly*, *commonly*, leucopenia, thrombocytopenia, anorexia, hypocalcaemia, headache, diarrhoea, nausea, vomiting, alopecia, myalgia, arthralgia, palpitation, tachycardia, fatigue, malaise. See manufacturers Full Prescribing Information.
Notes: See also 13.2 Drugs Affecting Immune Response, 3.6.1 Multiple Sclerosis (MS) and 9.4.2 Viral Hepatitis.

Interferon Alfa-2b

ATC Code: L03AB05. **Sport:** Permitted.
Driving: Caution.
Indications: Chronic hepatitis B and C, hairy cell leukaemia, CML, multiple myeloma, follicular lymphoma, carcinoid tumour, malignant melanoma.
Dose: Adult, Elderly: *Chronic hepatitis B*, range 5-10 million

IU (MIU) 3-times weekly for 4-6 months; chronic hepatitis C, 3 MIU 3-times weekly alone or combination with ribavirin. *Hairy cell leukaemia*, 2 MIU/m2 BSA 3-times weekly; CML, 4-5 MIU/m2/day. *Multiple myeloma*, following induction chemotherapy, 3 MIU/m2 3-times weekly, monotherapy. *Follicular lymphoma*, adjunctive, 5 MIU 3-times weekly for 18 months. *Carcinoid tumour*, 5 MIU (3-9 MIU range) 3-times weekly. *Malignant melanoma*, as induction, 20 MIU/m2 IV for 5 days per week for 4-weeks; maintenance 10 MIU/m2 3-times weekly. For SC admin.

Child: Chronic hepatitis C, 3 million U/m2 SC 3-times weekly in combination with ribavirin.

Renal Impairment: Severe, including caused by metastases, not recommended.

Hepatic Impairment: Decompensated liver cirrhosis, contraindicated. Closely monitor liver enzymes and hepatic function in cirrhotic patients.

CI: See Notes below.

Interactions: Effect of Other Drugs on Interferon Alpha-2b: *Co-admin contraindicated*: Telbivudine. *Co-admin caution*: Narcotics, hypnotics, sedatives, other myelosuppressives. *Increased toxicity*: Ara-C, cyclophosphamide, doxorubicin, teniposide. *Increased frequency/severity cutaneous vasculitis*: Hydroxyurea.

Effect of Interferon Alpha-2b on Other Drugs: Theophylline: *Monitor serum levels, adjust dose.*

SP: Weight loss, growth inhibition that resulted in reduced final adult height (ages 3-17 years) requires risk/benefit assessment. Acute hypersensitivity reactions (urticaria, angioedema, bronchoconstriction, anaphylaxis). Hypotension. Ensure adequate hydration. Investigate persistent fever. Debilitating medical conditions, caution; pulmonary disease (COPD), diabetes mellitus prone to ketoacidosis, coagulation disorders (thrombophlebitis, pulmonary embolism), severe myelosuppression. Pulmonary infiltrates, pneumonitis, pneumonia. Retinal haemorrhages, cotton wool spots, serous retinal detachment, retinal artery or vein obstruction, obtundation and coma (including encephalopathy). CHF, MI and/or previous or current arrhythmic disorders, hypertriglyceridaemia, monitor. Exacerbation of pre-existing psoriatic disease and sarcoidosis, use if benefit outweighs risk. Increased graft rejection risk. Development of auto-antibodies and autoimmune disorders. Vogt-Koyanagi-Harad Syndrome. Monitor thyroid function, especially children, adolescents.

Pregnancy, Lactation: Women of childbearing potential to ensure adequate contraception during and for 4 months after treatment (7 months for males or their female partners).

ADR: See Notes below.

Notes: See 13.2.3 Interferons, 9.4.2 Viral Hepatitis (ribavirin).

IntronA Parenteral *(MSD)* A. HT.
Price, vial 25 MIU/2.5mL (1) €174.64. Pen (1x1.2mL) 18 MIU, €122.45. 30 MIU, €206.07. 60 MIU, €398.63. Infusion 10 MIU/mL, €56.89.
Injection or infusion, interferon alfa-2b. Recombinant genetically engineered. Clear colourless soln (multidose, pen*). *Essentially sodium-free.* *For injection only. **Store**: Refrigerate. Do not freeze.

13.2.4 - Other Immunostimulants

In This Chapter: *Mifamurtide.*

Class Effects
CI: Hypersensitivity to any member of the class.

Mifamurtide
ATC Code: L03AX15. **Sport:** Pending.
Driving: Dizziness, vertigo, fatigue, blurred vision.
Indications: Treatment, high-grade resectable non-metastatic osteosarcoma after surgical resection, in combination with post-op multi-agent chemotherapy.
Dose: Adult: Age 2-30 years, 2mg/m2 BSA by IV infusion (over 1 hour) adjuvant following resection, twice weekly (at least 3 days apart) for 12 weeks, then once weekly for 24 weeks (total 48 infusions in 36 weeks); older than 30 years, no data. Not for bolus injection.
Renal Impairment: Severe, caution.

Hepatic Impairment: Moderate/severe, caution.
Interactions: Effect of Other Drugs on Mifamurtide: *Co-admin contraindicated*: Ciclosporin, other calcineurin inhibitors, high-dose non-steroidal anti-inflammatories (NSAIDS, cyclo-oxygenase inhibitors). *Separate admin times*: Doxorubicin, other lipophilic medicinals. *Avoid chronic co-admin*: Corticosteroids.
SP: History of asthma or other chronic obstructive pulmonary disease, consider prophylactic bronchodilators. Neutropenia, monitor fever. Caution, use with history of autoimmune, inflammatory or other collagen disease (inflammatory response). Monitor, for signs of uncontrolled inflammatory reactions, patients with history of venous thrombosis, vasculitis or unstable cardiovascular disorders. Haemorrhage observed at high doses. Allergic reactions. GI toxicity (nausea, vomiting, loss of appetite).
Pregnancy, Lactation: Not for use in pregnancy or women not using effective contraception. Stop breastfeeding or stop drug.
ADR: See Notes below.
Notes: See 13.2.4 Other Immunostimulants. See manufacturers Full Prescribing Information.

Mepact Parenteral 4mg *(Takeda)* A. HOS.
Price, not published by company.
Infusion, mifamurtide. White (off-white) homogenous cake or powder for conc for dispersion for infusion.

13.3 - Sex Hormones and Hormone Antagonists In Malignancy

13.3.1 - Breast Cancer

In This Chapter: *Anastrozole, exemestane, letrozole (aromatase inhibitors); megestrol; fulvestrant, tamoxifen, toremifene (oestrogen-receptor antagonists).*

Class Effects
Also used as progestogens, goserelin and triptorelin. See Notes below.
CI: Hypersensitivity to any member of the class. Not for use in children or premenopause.
SP: Aromatase inhibitors are potent oestrogen-lowering agents (loss of bone mineral density, osteoporosis, increased fracture risk); assess baseline bone density (high osteoporosis risk assess individually). Initiate osteoporosis prophylaxis. Routine vitamin D assessment (high prevalence of severe deficiency in women with early breast cancer); consider Vitamin D supplementation.
Pregnancy, Lactation: Pregnancy and lactation, contraindicated. Women of childbearing potential to ensure adequate contraception.
ADR: Hot flushes occur with all drugs in this class. See manufacturers Full Prescribing Information and Notes below (cytotoxic drugs).
Notes: See Class Effects 13.1 Cytotoxic Drugs, 11.7.3 Female Sex Hormones, Progestogens (medroxyprogesterone), and 13.3.2 Prostate Cancer (goserelin, triptorelin).

Anastrozole
ATC Code: L02BG03. **Sport:** Prohibited.
Driving: Unlikely to impair.
Indications: Treatment, advanced breast cancer (postmenopause); hormone-receptor positive early breast cancer (following 2-3 years of tamoxifen).
Dose: Adult, Elderly: 1mg orally once daily.
Renal Impairment: Severe, contraindicated (consider risk/benefit).
Hepatic Impairment: Moderate/severe, contraindicated.
Interactions: Effect of Other Drugs on Anastrozole: *Co-admin not recommended*: Tamoxifen, other oestrogen-containing therapy.
SP: Growth hormone deficiency in addition to growth hormone treatment (boys, girls), use not recommended. Early disease, recommend 5-year duration.
ADR: See Notes below.
Notes: See 13.3.1 Breast Cancer.

383

13.3.1 Breast Cancer

Interchangeability: Same strengths of all brands of anastrozole f/c tabs listed below are deemed interchangeable.
Reference Price: 1mg (28) €21.00.

Arimidex 1mg *(AstraZeneca)* A. GMS.
Price, (28) €48.09.
Tablet, anastrozole. White round f/c. Marked with A; Adx1 on reverse. *Lactose.*
Agerdex 1mg *(Gerard)* A. GMS.
Price, (28) €16.80.
Tablet, anastrozole. White round f/c. Marked ANA and 1. *Lactose.*
Amidex 1mg *(Clonmel)* A. GMS.
Price, (28) €16.80.
Tablet, anastrozole. White round f/c. Marked A1. *Lactose.*
Anastrozole (Accord) 1mg *(Accord)* A. GMS.
Price, (28) €16.80.
Tablet, anastrozole. White (off-white) round f/c. Marked AHI. *Lactose.*
Anastrozole (Actavis) 1mg *(Accord)* A. GMS.
Price, (28) €16.80.
Tablet, anastrozole. White round f/c. Marked ANA and 1. *Lactose.*
Anastrozole Bluefish 1mg *(Bluefish)* A. GMS.
Price, (28) €16.80.
Tablet, anastrozole. White round f/c. *Lactose.*
Anastrozole (Rowex) 1mg *(Rowex)* A. GMS.
Price, (28) €16.80.
Tablet, anastrozole. White round f/c. Marked 1. *Lactose.*
Anastrozole TEVA 1mg *(TEVA)* A. GMS.
Price, (28) €16.80.
Tablet, anastrozole. White (off-white) round f/c. Marked 93; A10 on reverse. *Lactose.*

Exemestane

ATC Code: L02BC06. **Sport:** Prohibited.
Driving: Caution.
Indications: Adjuvant treatment, invasive early breast cancer (postmenopause), oestrogen receptor positive (following 2-3 years of tamoxifen); advanced breast cancer (postmenopause, natural or induced with disease progression after anti-oestrogen therapy).
Dose: Adult, Elderly: 25mg once daily after food.
Renal Impairment: Caution.
Hepatic Impairment: As for Renal above.
Interactions: Effect of Other Drugs on Exemestane: *Co-admin not recommended*: Oestrogen-containing drugs. *Efficacy may be reduced*: Potent CYP3A4 inducers (rifampicin, phenytoin, carbamazepine, St John's Wort). *Caution*: Drugs metabolised by CYP3A4 with narrow therapeutic window. *Co-admin (no experience)*: Other anticancer drugs.
SP: Confirm postmenopausal status (LH, FSH, oestradiol levels).
ADR: See Notes below.
Notes: See 13.3.1 Breast Cancer.

Aromasin 25mg *(Pfizer)* A. GMS.
Price, (30) €72.89.
Tablet, exemestane. White (off-white) round s/c. Marked 7663. *Sucrose, parabens.*
Exemestane Accord 25mg *(Accord)* A. GMS.
Price, (30) €58.33.
Tablet, exemestane. White (off-white). Marked E25. *Mannitol.*
Exemestane Actavis 25mg *(Accord)* A. GMS.
Price, (30) €58.33.
Tablet, exemestane. White round lenticular f/c.

Fulvestrant

ATC Code: L02BA03. **Sport:** Prohibited.
Driving: Asthenia.
Indications: Treatment, locally advanced or metastatic breast cancer (postmenopause, oestrogen-receptor positive), for disease relapse (on or after anti-oestrogens) OR disease progression (on anti-oestrogens)
Dose: Adult, Elderly: 500mg at 1-monthly intervals; additional 500mg dose given 2 weeks after initial dose. *Admin*, as 2 consecutive 5mL injections; slow IM (1-2 minutes per injection) in each buttock (gluteal area).
Renal Impairment: CrCl (mL/min) below 30, no data.
Hepatic Impairment: Mild to moderate, caution. Severe, not recommended.
SP: Bleeding diatheses, thrombocytopenia, anticoagulant treatment, caution (IM route). Thromboembolic events.

Osteoporosis risk. Injection site events, caution with dorsogluteal admin (underlying sciatic nerve).
ADR: See Notes below.
Notes: See 13.3.1 Breast Cancer.

Faslodex Parenteral 250mg *(AstraZeneca)* A. HT.
Price, 250mg/5mL PFS (2) €655.14.
Injection, fulvestrant 250mg/5mL. Clear colourless (yellow) viscous soln. *Benzyl alcohol.* **Store:** Refrigerate (store and transport).

Letrozole

ATC Code: L02BG04. **Sport:** Prohibited.
Driving: Caution.
Indications: Postmenopause. Adjuvant, early breast cancer hormone receptor positive; extended adjuvant treatment, hormone-dependent (following 5 years of tamoxifen). Advanced breast cancer, first-line (hormone dependant); post natural or induced menopause after relapse or disease progression with previous anti-oestrogens.
Dose: Adult, Elderly: 2.5mg once daily as monotherapy for 5 years or until recurrence. Adjuvant, consider sequential letrozole 2 years, then tamoxifen 3 years; neoadjuvant setting continue treatment for 4-8 months to establish optimal tumour reduction. *Admin*, oral with or without food.
Renal Impairment: CrCl (mL/min) below 30, no data.
Hepatic Impairment: Severe, no data.
Interactions: Effect of Other Drugs on Letrozole: *Co-admin (no data)*: Other anticancer drugs. *Caution*: Drugs metabolised by CYP (2A6, 2C19) with narrow therapeutic index.
SP: Confirm postmenopausal status (LH, FSH, oestradiol levels). Caution, osteoporosis risk.
ADR: See Notes below.
Notes: See 13.3.1 Breast Cancer.

Femara 2.5mg *(Novartis)* A. GMS.
Price, (30) €50.36.
Tablet, letrozole. Dark yellow round slightly. Marked FV; CG on reverse. *Lactose.*
EirFem 2.5mg *(Niche)* A. GMS.
Price, (30) €24.17.
Tablet, letrozole. Yellow round f/c. Marked 2.5. *Sunset Yellow.*
Letrozole (Accord) 2.5mg *(Accord)* A. GMS.
Price, (30) €24.17.
Tablet, letrozole. Round yellow. *Lactose.*
Letrozole (Clonmel) 2.5mg *(Clonmel)* A. GMS.
Price, (30) €24.17.
Tablet, letrozole. Yellow round f/c. *Lactose.*
Letrozole Actavis 2.5mg *(Accord)* A. GMS.
Price, (30) €24.17.
Tablet, letrozole. Yellow round lenticular f/c. *Lactose.*
Letrozole Bluefish 2.5mg *(Bluefish)* A. GMS.
Price, (30) €24.17.
Tablet, letrozole. Yellow round f/c. *Lactose.*
Letrozole Mylan 2.5mg *(Gerard)* A. GMS.
Price, (30) €24.17.
Tablet, letrozole. Dark-yellow cap-shaped f/c. Marked LZ2.5; G on reverse. *Lactose.*
Letrozole TEVA 2.5mg *(TEVA)* A. GMS.
Price, (30) €24.17.
Tablet, letrozole. Dark-yellow round f/c. Marked 93; B1 on reverse. *Lactose, tartrazine aluminium lake.*
Letzo 2.5mg *(Rowex)* A. GMS.
Price, (30) €24.17.
Tablet, letrozole. Dark-yellow round f/c. Marked FV; CG on reverse. *Lactose.*

Megestrol

ATC Code: L02AB01. **Sport:** Permitted.
Driving: Unlikely to impair.
Indications: Treatment, certain hormone dependent neoplasms including breast cancer (tabs); anorexia or weight loss secondary to cancer or AIDS (males, females) (oral susp).
Dose: Adult: *Breast cancer*, 160mg once daily. *Anorexia, weight loss*, 400-800mg as single daily dose. At least 2 months continuous treatment to determine efficacy.
Elderly: Caution; greater frequency of decreased hepatic, renal*, cardiac function, concomitant disease or drug therapy. *Monitor.
Hepatic Impairment: Caution. Severe, not recommended.

CI: Thromboembolic disorders.

SP: Thrombophlebitis, caution. Can exert adrenocortical effects. Weight gain.

Pregnancy, Lactation: Certain progesterones produce reversible virilisation in some female offspring of women treated during pregnancy. See Notes below.

ADR: See Notes below.

Notes: See 13.3.1 Breast Cancer.

Megace 160mg, Oral Susp (SOBI) A. GMS.
Price, 160mg (30) €36.83. Susp (240mL) €78.76.
Tablet, megestrol acetate. Off-white oval scored (facilitates breaking). Marked 160. Lactose.
Oral susp, as above 40mg/mL. White (cream) milky. Sucrose.

Tamoxifen

ATC Code: L02BA01. Sport: Prohibited.
Driving: Fatigue.

Indications: Treatment, breast cancer.

Dose: Adult, Elderly: 20-40mg/day in 1 or 2 divided doses (duration 5 years in early disease).

Interactions: Effect of Other Drugs on Tamoxifen: Co-admin avoid (plasma levels of active metabolite, endoxifen lowered): Potent CYP2D6 inhibitors (paroxetine, fluoxetine, quinidine, cinacalcet, bupropion). Increased thromboembolic risk: Combination with cytotoxics.

Effect of Tamoxifen on Other Drugs: Coumarin anticoagulants: Anticoagulant effect increased.

SP: Pre-menopause, suppressed menstruation. Increased incidence of endometrial (hyperplasia, polyps, cancer), uterine sarcoma (malignant mixed Mullerian tumours); abnormal gynaecological symptoms (vaginal bleeding, menstrual irregularities, post-menopausal bleeding, vaginal discharge), investigate. Endometrial neoplasia. Second primary tumours in sites other than endometrium, opposite breast. Combination (anastrozole), not shown improved efficacy. Increased risk of microvascular flap complications.

ADR: See Notes below.

Notes: See 13.3.1 Breast Cancer.

Nolvadex D 20mg (AstraZeneca) B. GMS.
Price, (30) €4.68.
Tablet, tamoxifen citrate. Octagonal white f/c. Marked Nolvadex D. Lactose. Store: Below 30 deg C; original pack.

Soltamox Oral Soln (Fannin) B. GMS.
Price, 10mg/5mL (150mL) €33.70.
Oral soln, tamoxifen citrate 10mg/5mL. Clear colourless. Ethanol, sorbitol.

Tamox 10mg, 20mg (Rowex) B. GMS.
Price, (30) 10mg, €6.39. 20mg, €4.58.
Tablet, tamoxifen citrate. White round f/c. 20mg: Scored (facilitates breaking). Lactose.

Tamoxifen (Gerard) 20mg (Gerard) B. GMS.
Price, (30) 20mg, €4.58.
Tablet, tamoxifen citrate. White round scored. Marked TN over strength and G on reverse. Mannitol.

Toremifene

ATC Code: L02BA02. Sport: Prohibited.
Driving: Unlikely to impair.

Indications: First-line, hormone-dependent metastatic breast cancer (postmenopause).

Dose: Adult, Elderly: 60mg once daily with or without food.

Hepatic Impairment: Caution. Severe, contraindicated.

CI: Pre-existing endometrial hyperplasia; QT-prolongation, electrolyte disturbances (uncorrected hypokalaemia), clinically relevant (bradycardia, HF with reduced LVEF), symptomatic (history of) arrhythmias.

Interactions: Effect of Other Drugs on Toremifene: Co-admin contraindicated: Drugs prolonging QT-interval e.g. antiarrhythmics Class IA (quinidine, hydroquinidine, disopyramide), Class III (amiodarone, sotalol, dofetilide, ibutilide), neuroleptics (phenothiazines, pimozide, sertindole, haloperidol, sultopride), antimicrobials (moxifloxacin, erythromycin IV, pentamidine, halofantrine), antihistamines (terfenadine, astemizole, mizolastine), cisapride, vincamine IV, bepridil, diphemanil. Increased hypercalcaemia risk: Thiazides. Plasma levels decreased

Prostate Cancer 13.3.2

(consider double daily dose): Phenobarbital, phenytoin, carbamazepine. Carefully consider co-admin: CYP3A inhibitors (azole antifungals, ritonavir, nelfinavir, clarithromycin, erythromycin, telithromycin).

Effect of Toremifene on Other Drugs: Warfarin-type anticoagulants: Increased bleeding time; avoid.

SP: Before initiation, gynaecologic examination (ascertain pre-existing endometrial abnormality); repeat yearly; increased endometrial cancer risk (hypertension, diabetes, BMI over 30, history of HRT therapy), monitor. Severe thromboembolic disease (history of), not recommended. Changes in cardiac electrophysiology observed; caution, ongoing proarrhythmic conditions (especially elderly) (acute myocardial ischaemia, QT prolongation); may lead to increased risk for ventricular arrhythmias (Torsade de pointes), cardiac arrest. Non-compensated cardiac insufficiency, severe angina pectoris, monitor. QTC above 500ms, not recommended. Presence of bone metastases, hypercalcaemia may occur at initiation. Anaemia, leucopenia, thrombocytopenia; monitor RBCs, leucocytes, platelets. Cases of liver injury (liver enzymes above 10xULN), hepatitis, jaundice.

ADR: See Notes below.

Notes: See 13.3.1 Breast Cancer.

Fareston 60mg (Orion) B. GMS.
Price, (30) €35.89.
Tablet, toremifene citrate. White round flat. Marked TO/strength. Lactose.

13.3.2 - Prostate Cancer

In This Chapter: Abiraterone, bicalutamide, buserelin, degarelix, enzalutamide, goserelin, leuprorelin, triptorelin.

Class Effects

Diethylstilboestrol is used in both breast and prostate cancer. Buserelin (LHRH-analogue) is also used in treatment of endometriosis and pituitary desensitisation in preparation for ovulation induction, see Notes below.

CI: Hypersensitivity to any member of the class. No relevant use in children.

Interactions: Effect of Other Drugs on Anti-Androgens: Carefully evaluate co-admin: Drugs prolonging QT interval or inducing Torsade de Pointes e.g. antiarrhythmics Class Ia (quinidine, disopyramide), Class III (amiodarone, sotalol, dofetilide, ibutilide), methadone, moxifloxacin, antipsychotics. See SP below.

SP: LHRH-analogues (buserelin, goserelin, histrelin, leuprorelin, triptorelin): Males, reduced glucose tolerance; in prostate cancer, disease or tumour flare, bone pain exacerbation (with bone metastases), neurological signs due to tumour compression/spinal compression (muscle weakness in legs), impaired micturition, hydronephrosis or lymphostasis, thrombosis with pulmonary embolism; prophylactic anti-androgens e.g. cyproterone. Females, loss of bone mineral density (some recovery after cessation); endometriosis, HRT may reduce bone mineral density loss), vasomotor symptoms. Ovulation induction, exclude pregnancy. Risks specific to ART (increased miscarriages, ectopic and multiple pregnancies), unaltered with adjuvant buserelin. Follicle recruitment may be increased. Combination (gonadotrophins), higher OHSS risk. Pedicle torsion or ovary rupture may lead to acute abdomen. Severe thromboembolic events (fatal). Ovarian cysts. Increased risk of depression (may be severe) with GnRH agonist treatment; inform patients. Known depression, monitor. Caution, co-admin with medicinals prolonging QT-interval; androgen-deprivation therapy may prolong QT-interval (consider all cardiovascular risk factors; weigh benefit/risk); Torsade de Pointes risk. Cardiovascular disease (stroke, MI, prolonged QT interval).

Pregnancy, Lactation: Unless otherwise stated, not indicated for use in women.

ADR: See manufactures Full Prescribing Information. See Notes below (cytotoxic drugs).

Notes: See also 13.1 Cytotoxic Drugs, 13.3.1 Breast Cancer (stilboestrol), 11.9 Other Endocrine Drugs (buserelin) and 11.7.2 Male Sex Hormones, Anti-Androgens (cyproterone).

13.3.2   Prostate Cancer

Abiraterone

ATC Code: L02BX03. **Sport:** Permitted.
Driving: No or negligible effect.

Indications: Treatment, metastatic castration-resistant prostate cancer (asymptomatic or mildly symptomatic; after androgen-deprivation therapy failure, chemotherapy not indicated); with disease progression on or after docetaxel.

Dose: Adult, Elderly: 1000mg as single daily dose with prednisolone 10mg/day. Hepatotoxicity (ALT above 5xULN), withhold immediately. Retreat after LFTs return to normal, 500mg once daily. Hepatotoxicity at reduced dose, discontinue. *Admin*, swallow whole with water. NOTE: Must NOT be taken with food (admin at least 2 hours after food; take no food for 1 hour after admin); food increases systemic exposure.

Renal Impairment: Severe, caution.

Hepatic Impairment: Mild, no adjustment. Moderate, if benefit outweighs risk. Severe, not for use.

Interactions: Effect of Other Drugs on Abiraterone: Co-admin not recommended: Spironolactone, food. *Co-admin avoid (unless no alternative), reduced exposure:* CYP3A4 strong inhibitors or strong inducers (phenytoin, carbamazepine, rifampicin, rifabutin, rifapentine, phenobarbital, St John's Wort).

Effect of Abiraterone on Other Drugs: CYP2D6 substrates* (metoprolol, propranolol, desipramine, venlafaxine, haloperidol, risperidone, propafenone, flecainide, codeine, oxycodone, tramadol): *Caution, consider dose reduction.* CYP2C8 substrates* (pioglitazone): *Monitor for toxicity.* *(with narrow therapeutic index).

SP: Monitor serum transaminases prior to initiation, every 2 weeks (first 3 months), then monthly; signs of hepatotoxicity, measure immediately; ALT or AST above 5xULN, interrupt; ALT or AST 20xULN, discontinue; do not re-treat. Acute liver failure, fulminant hepatitis (fatal). Monitor, BP, serum potassium, fluid retention, monthly. Cardiovascular disease, caution; control hypertension, hypokalaemia before initiation. QT-prolongation (with hypokalaemia). If continued after corticosteroids withdrawn, monitor for mineralocorticosteroid excess. Decreased bone density. Lower response rates with previous ketoconazole treatment. Myopathy.

Pregnancy, Lactation: Males and females to ensure adequate contraception.

ADR: See Notes below.

Notes: See 13.3.2 Prostate Cancer.

ZYTIGA 500mg *(Janssen-Cilag)* A. HT.
Price, (56) €3302.21.
Tablet, abiraterone acetate. Oval purple. Marked AA and strength. *Lactose; sodium 13.5mg.*

Bicalutamide

ATC Code: L02BB03. **Sport:** Permitted.
Driving: Somnolence.

Indications: Treatment, prostate cancer, advanced in combination with luteinising-hormone releasing hormone(LHRH) analogue or surgical castration; locally advanced, monotherapy or with radical prostatectomy or radiotherapy (at high disease progression risk) *(Casomide).*

Dose: Adult, Elderly: Prostate cancer: *Advanced,* 50mg/day (same time of day). Start: *Casodex* at same time; *Bicalutamide Teva* 1 week prior to; *Biluta, Casomide* 3 days before LHRH analogue; all at same time as surgical castration; *Locally advanced,* 150mg/day (continuously); minimum 2 years or until disease progression) *(Casomide).* *once daily.

Renal Impairment: CrCl (mL/min) below 30, no data.

Hepatic Impairment: Moderate to severe, increased accumulation may occur. Severe, contraindicated.

CI: Use in females.

Interactions: Effect of Other Drugs on Bicalutamide: Co-admin contraindicated *(Casodex, Bicalutamide Teva, Biluta, Casomide):* Terfenadine, astemizole, cisapride. Co-

386

admin caution *(Bicalutamide Teva, Biluta):* CYP3A4 substrates, substances inhibiting oxidation (ketoconazole, cimetidine).

Effect of Bicalutamide on Other Drugs: Coumarin anticoagulants, warfarin: *Monitor prothrombin time.* Ciclosporin, calcium channel blockers: *Consider dose reduction (Bicalutamide Teva, Casomide, Casodex).*

SP: Perform periodic LFTs; severe hepatic changes, failure (fatal). Severe changes, discontinue.

Pregnancy, Lactation: Contraindicated in females; must not be given to pregnant or nursing mothers.

ADR: See Notes below.

Notes: See 13.3.2 Prostate Cancer.

Casodex 50mg *(AstraZeneca)* A. HT.
Price, (28) €58.15.
Tablet, bicalutamide. Round white f/c. Marked CDX50; logo on reverse. *Lactose.*

Bicalutamide (Accord) 50mg *(Accord)* A. HT.
Price, (28) €44.99.
Tablet, bicalutamide. White (off-white) f/c. Marked B50. *Lactose.*

Bicalutamide TEVA 50mg *(TEVA)* A. HT.
Price, (28) €56.98.
Tablet, bicalutamide. White (off-white) f/c. Marked 93; 220 on reverse. *Lactose.*

Biluta 50mg *(Rowex)* A. HT.
Price, (28) €56.98.
Tablet, bicalutamide. White round f/c. *Lactose.*

Casomide 50mg *(Clonmel)* A. HT.
Price, (28) €41.31.
Tablet, bicalutamide. White round. *Lactose.*

Buserelin (prostate cancer)

ATC Code: L02AE01. **Sport:** Prohibited (in men).
Driving: Caution.

Indications: Treatment, advanced prostate cancer (testosterone suppression indicated). Pituitary desensitisation prior to ovulation induction regimens using gonadotrophins.

Dose: Adult, Elderly: *Prostate cancer,* initiate in hospital; 0.5mg *Suprefact* injection 8-hourly (7 days). *Depot,* 1 dose (2 rods) containing 6.3mg (buserelin), injected in abdominal wall every 2 calendar months. *Ovulation induction,* 0.5mg in 1 injection starting in early follicular phase (day 1) or in mid-luteal phase (day 21) (if early pregnancy excluded). Admin at approx. equal intervals. *Admin*, SC.

CI: Hormone insensitive tumours, after orchiectomy.

Interactions: Effect of Other Drugs on Buserelin: Co-admin: Sex hormones (adjust dose).

Effect of Buserelin on Other Drugs: Antidiabetic agents: *Effect attenuated.*

SP: Depression, caution (recurrence or worsening). Monitor BP, blood glucose (deterioration of metabolic control), testosterone levels (3-monthly).

Pregnancy, Lactation: Exclude pregnancy before initiating.

ADR: Ovulation induction, see Notes below (other endocrine drugs), see Notes below (prostate cancer).

Notes: See Class Effects 13.3.2 Prostate Cancer. See 11.9 Other Endocrine Drugs (buserelin).

Suprefact Parenteral *(SANOFI)* A. HT.
Price, depot 6.3mg (1) €271.52; injection 1mg/mL (5.5mLx2) €38.55.
Injection, buserelin acetate 1mg/mL, Depot 6.3mg. Depot: Syringe containing implant of 2 cream-coloured rods. *Benzyl alcohol.* Inj: Clear colourless soln.

Degarelix

ATC Code: L02BX02. **Sport:** Permitted.
Driving: No or negligible effect.

Indications: Treatment, advanced hormone-dependent prostate cancer.

Dose: Adult, Elderly: Initially 240mg admin as 2 injections of 120mg each; maintenance, 80mg starting 1 month after initial dose. *Admin*, SC in abdominal region rotating site; NOT for IV admin.

Renal Impairment: Severe, caution.

Hepatic Impairment: As for Renal above.

Interactions: Effect of Other Drugs on Degarelix: *Carefully evaluate co-admin*: Medicinals prolonging QTc interval or inducing Torsades de Pointes e.g. antiarrhythmics Class Ia (quinidine, disopyramide), Class III (amiodarone, sotalol, dofetilide, ibutilide), methadone, cisapride, moxifloxacin, antipsychotics.

SP: Prolonged QT-interval, consider benefit/risk. Decreased bone density. Reduced glucose tolerance.

ADR: See Notes below.

Notes: See 13.3.2 Prostate Cancer.

> **Firmagon Parenteral 80mg, 120mg** *(Ferring)* A. HT.
> *Price,* 80mg, €155.35. 120mg, €297.00.
> *Injection,* degarelix 40mg/mL. White (off-white) powder; clear colourless solvent for soln. Do not shake vials.

Enzalutamide

ATC Code: Pending. **Sport:** Permitted.

Driving: Moderate influence; psychiatric, neurologic events (seizures).

Indications: Treatment, metastatic castration-resistant prostate cancer, after androgen deprivation therapy failure; chemotherapy not indicated or where disease has progressed (on or after docetaxel).

Dose: Adult, Elderly: 160mg as single oral daily dose. Continue medical castration with LHRH analogue during treatment if not surgically castrated. *Admin,* swallow whole with water, with or without food. Co-admin, see Interactions below.

Renal Impairment: Severe or ESRD, caution.

Hepatic Impairment: No dose adjustment; increased drug half-life with severe impairment.

Interactions: Effect of Other Drugs on Enzalutamide: *Co-admin avoid or caution*: Strong CYP2C8 inhibitors (gemfibrozil), reduce enzalutamide to 80mg once daily; moderate CYP2C8, strong CYP3A4 inducers (rifampicin). *Co-admin caution*: Drugs lowering seizure threshold; drugs prolonging QT-interval (Torsades de Pointes risk).

Effect of Enzalutamide on Other Drugs: Warfarin, coumarin-like anticoagulants, acenocoumarol: *Avoid or additional INR monitoring.* Cytotoxic chemotherapy: *Co-admin (safety/efficacy not established).* Colchicine, dabigatran, digoxin: *Caution, consider dose adjustment.* Fentanyl, tramadol, clarithromycin, doxycycline, cabazitaxel, carbamazepine, clonazepam, phenytoin, primidone, valproic acid, haloperidol, bisoprolol, propranolol, diltiazem, felodipine, nicardipine, nifedipine, verapamil, digoxin, dexamethasone, prednisolone, indinavir, ritonavir, diazepam, midazolam, zolpidem, statins metabolised by CYP3A4 (atorvastatin, simvastatin), levothyroxine: *Possible interactions.*

SP: Caution, seizures (history of, predisposing factors) e.g. underlying brain injury, stroke, primary brain tumours or metastases, alcoholism, medicinals lowering seizure threshold. Excluded from clinical trials (recent MI, unstable angina, CHF NYHA Class III/IV, long QT interval, bradycardia, uncontrolled hypertension). Posterior reversible encephalopathy syndrome, hypersensitivity reactions, oedema (tongue, lip, pharyngeal).

Pregnancy, Lactation: Contraindicated for use in women who are or may become pregnant; may harm unborn child. Men to ensure adequate contraception during and for 3 months after treatment.

ADR: See Notes below.

Notes: See 13.3.2 Prostate Cancer.

> ▼ **Xtandi 40mg** *(Astellas)* A. HT.
> *Price,* (112), €3245.49.
> *Soft capsule,* enzalutamide. White (off-white) oblong. Marked ENZ. *Sorbitol.*

Goserelin

ATC Code: L02AE03. **Sport:** Prohibited (in men).

Driving: Unlikely to impair.

Indications: Prostate cancer, endometriosis, uterine fibroids, endometrial thinning, assisted reproduction.

Dose: Adult, Elderly: 1x depot 3.6mg every 28 days OR 1x depot LA 10.8mg every 3 months. With assisted reproduction, once pituitary down-regulation achieved, superovulation and oocyte retrieval should be carried out. *Admin,* SC into anterior abdominal wall with caution (proximity of underlying inferior epigastric artery and branches) especially with low BMI (vascular injury risk) and/or on full anticoagulant medication.

SP: Reduced bone mineral density. Mood changes e.g. depression. Hypertension, monitor. *Males,* risk of ureteric obstruction, spinal cord compression; serum acid phosphatase levels may rise, consider anti-androgen use. *Females,* vaginal bleeding (early treatment); probably oestrogen withdrawal. May increase cervical resistance, care when dilating cervix.

Pregnancy, Lactation: Exclude pregnancy before initiating.

ADR: See Notes below.

Notes: See 13.3.2 Prostate Cancer.

> **Zoladex Implant 3.6mg, LA 10.8mg** *(AstraZeneca)* A. HT.
> *Price,* 3.6mg, €118.88. LA 10.8mg, €351.78.
> *Implant,* goserelin 3.6mg, (LA) 10.8mg. White (cream-coloured) cylindrical. **Store:** Below 25 deg C.

Leuprorelin

ATC Code: L02AE02. **Sport:** Prohibited (in men).

Driving: Fatigue, visual disturbances, dizziness.

Indications: Prostate cancer: *Eligard, Leuprex,* hormone-dependent advanced; *Eligard,* high-risk localisation and locally advanced hormone-dependent (with radiotherapy); *Prostap,* testosterone suppression indicated *(3 DCS, SR DCS)*; metastatic, locally advanced (alternative to surgical castration), high-risk localised or locally advanced (with radiotherapy), locally advanced at high risk of disease progression (adjuvent to radical prostatectomy) *(6 DCS)*. Other indications: *Prostap,* oestrogen-dependent gynaecological disorders e.g. pain and lesions (endometriosis); pre-operative management, uterine fibroids *(3 DCS, SR DCS)*, endometrial preparation before intrauterine surgery *(SR DCS)*. Children, central precocious puberty (girls under 9 years, boys under 10 years) *(3 DCS, SR DCS)*.

Dose: Adult, Elderly: *Eligard,* 7.5mg as single SC depot injection every month OR 22.5mg as single SC injection every 3 months; avoid intra-arterial or IV injection. May be used with radiotherapy (high-risk, locally advanced). Do not discontinue when remission or improvement occurs.

Prostap, males, 3.75mg as single SC injection every month (SR) OR 11.25mg as 3-month depot injection SC or IM every 3 months (3 DCS) OR 30mg as 6-month depot injection SC (6 DCS, not to be used IM). *Females,* initiate during first 5 days of menstrual cycle, 3.75mg (SR) every month OR 11.25mg every 3 months (3 DCS).

Leuprex, single-dose 5mg implant injected SC once every 3 months; local anaesthetic may be given before injection. Start anti-androgen adjunctive about 5 days before initiation.

Child: *Prostap (3 DCS, SR DCS),* weight 20kg and above, 3.75mg once monthly* OR 11.25mg (sustained release) every 3 months**; under 20kg, 1.88mg once monthly* OR 5.625mg (sustained release) every 3 months**. *Admin,* as single cutaneous injection. Use minimum effective dose; adapt individually. Sterile abscesses at injection site with IM admin at higher than recommended dose; in such cases, admin SC. *(30 +/- 2 days). ** (90 +/- 2 days).

Contraindicated *(Leuprex).* Safety and efficacy not established *(Eligard).*

CI: Spinal cord compression or evidence of spinal metastases *(Eligard),* post orchiectomy, use in women

13.3.2   Prostate Cancer

(Eligard, Leuprex). Use in men (endocrine therapy insensitive, post orchiectomy), women and girls with central precocious puberty (undiagnosed vaginal bleeding) *(Prostap).* Confirmed hormone independent carcinoma *(Leuprex).*

Interactions: Effect of Other Drugs on Leuprorelin: *QT-interval prolongation risk*: Drugs prolonging QT interval or inducing Torsade de Pointes e.g. antiarrhythmics, Class IA (quinidine, disopyramide), Class III (amiodarone, sotalol, dofetilide, ibutilide), methadone, moxifloxacin, antipsychotics.

SP: Androgen deprivation therapy and QT interval, see Notes below. Bone pain, neuropathy, haematuria, ureteral or bladder outlet obstruction. Following surgical castration, serum testosterone levels are not further decreased. *Monitor,* vertebral or brain metastases, urinary tract obstruction; those at high risk for metabolic or cardiovascular disease, decreased bone density, see Notes below; osteoporosis and/or increased fracture risk (caution). Spinal fracture, paralysis, hypotension, worsening depression. Pituitary adenomas. Advise women to report if regular menstruation persists. Uterine fibroids, confirm diagnosis prior to initiation. May cause increased uterine cervical resistance, caution dilating cervix for intrauterine surgical procedures. Abscess at injection site, may have inadequate leuprorelin absorption from depot formulation (monitor testosterone levels).

Brands, *Eligard,* incorrect preparation may result in lack of efficacy; evaluate testosterone levels if handling errors have occurred. *Prostap, Eligard,* reports of seizures/convulsions (adults, children; with/without history of or at risk of seizures).

Pregnancy, Lactation: Not for use in women *(Eligard, Leuprex, Prostap 6 DCS).* Contraindicated *(Prostap SR, 3 DCS).*

ADR: See Notes below.

Notes: See 13.3.2 Prostate Cancer.

  ELIGARD Parenteral 7.5mg, 22.5mg, 45mg *(Astellas)* A. HT.
  Price, 7.5mg, €118.01. 22.5mg, €3289.97. 45mg, €550.03.
  Injection, leuprorelin acetate 7.5mg, 22.5mg, 45mg. White (off-white) powder (syringe B); clear colourless (pale-yellow) soln (syringe A) (7.5mg) or colourless (pale-yellow) (22.5mg, 45mg) solvent. Store: Refrigerate; outside refrigerator below 25 deg C (max. 4 weeks).

  Leuprex 5mg (3) Implant *(Rowex)* A. HT.
  Price, (1) €312.12.
  Implant, leuprorelin acetate 5mg. Biodegradable white (slightly yellowish) cylinder-shaped stick in PFS.

  Prostap 3, 6 DCS, SR DCS Parenteral *(Takeda)* A. HT.
  Price, per vial 3-DCS (11.25mg) €310.81. 6-DCS (30mg) €659.92. SR DCS (3.75mg) €114.04.
  Injection Prolonged/R, leuprorelin acetate 11.25mg, 30mg, SR 3.75mg. Lyophilised white odourless microsphere powder; clear colourless slightly viscous solvent for susp. Dual Chamber Syringe (DCS). *Sodium approx. 0.4mg/PFS (SR 3.75mg).*

Triptorelin (acetate, pamoate)

ATC Code: L02AE04. **Sport:** Prohibited (in men).

Driving: Dizziness, somnolence, visual disturbances.

Indications: Advanced prostatic carcinoma *(Decapeptyl 3, 6, SR; Gonapeptyl).* Genital, extragenital endometriosis *(Decapeptyl 3, SR; Gonapeptyl).* Female infertility *(Decapeptyl SR).* Breast cancer (endocrine responsive, early, high recurrence risk or pre-menopausal) in combination (tamoxifen or aromatase inhibitor) *(Decapeptyl SR).* Pre-operative reduction of myoma size in women with symptomatic uterine myomas *(Gonapeptyl).* Treatment, central precocious puberty (girls under 9 years, boys under 10 years) *(Gonapeptyl)* OR (girls under 8 years, boys under 9 years) *(Decapeptyl 3)* OR (girls before 8 years, boys under 10 years) *(Decapeptyl 6).*

Dose: Adult, Elderly: Prostate cancer*, *Decapeptyl 3 (IM or SC),* 6 *(IM),* males only, 1 injection every 3 months (11.25mg) OR every 6 months (24 weeks) (22.5mg); *Decapeptyl SR, Gonapeptyl,* 1 injection every 28 days.

*(metastatic castration-resistant not surgically castrated receiving triptorelin and eligible for androgen biosynthesis inhibitor; triptorelin needs to be continued).

Endometriosis, *Decapeptyl 3 (IM),* females only, 1 injection every 3 months starting in first 5 days of cycle; *Decapeptyl SR, Gonapeptyl,* 1 injection every 28 days.

Female infertility, 1x *Decapeptyl SR* injection IM on second day of cycle with gonadotrophin stimulation around day 15.

Breast cancer, 1x *Decapeptyl SR* injection IM every 4 weeks with (tamoxifen or aromatase inhibitor). Commence triptorelin after chemotherapy completion and pre-menopausal status confirmed and 6-8 weeks (minimum 2 triptorelin injections; 4-week interval between) before aromatase inhibitor initiation.

Admin, IM only *Decapeptyl SR, 6-month (3-month* can be used SC in men with prostate cancer); NOT for intravascular injection. Admin SC or deep IM *(Gonapeptyl).*

Child: Precocious puberty: *Gonapeptyl,* 30kg and over (full dose), 1 injection SC or deep IM, with 1 syringe (days 0, 14, 28), then 1 injection every 4 weeks; insufficient effect, injection may be given every 3 weeks; 20-30kg, two-thirds of dose; under 20kg, half dose.

Decapeptyl 3, 1 injection IM repeated 3-monthly OR *Decapeptyl 6,* 1 injection IM repeated 6-monthly; stop around physiological puberty age (bone maturation age 13-14 years) (boys), and with bone maturation or more than 12-13 years (girls). Treatment under specialist supervision.

Renal Impairment: No dose adjustment.

Hepatic Impairment: As for Renal above.

CI: *Gonapeptyl,* men (hormone independent prostate carcinoma, sole treatment in prostate cancer with spinal compression or evidence of spinal metastases, after orchiectomy); women (osteoporosis); children (progressive brain tumours). *Decapeptyl,* initiation of aromatase inhibitor before adequate ovarian suppression with triptorelin.

Interactions: Effect of Other Drugs on Triptorelin: *Carefully evaluate co-admin*: Medicinals prolonging QT-interval (quinidine, disopyramide, amiodarone, sotalol, dofetilide, ibutilide, methadone, moxifloxacin, antipsychotics. *Interaction cannot be ruled out*: Commonly used medicinals, including histamine liberating products *(Gonapeptyl).*

SP: *Prostate cancer,* initial transient increased serum testosterone, worsening of symptoms (increased pain, activity of vertebral lesions, tumours causing urinary tract obstruction); consider anti-androgen to counteract initial rise in serum testosterone.

Female infertility, ovulation induction requires strict monitoring; excessive ovarian response, stop gonadotropin to interrupt stimulation cycle. *Endometriosis,* admin of 1 vial (3-month) or regular 28-day admin (SR) results in constant hypo-gonadotrophic amenorrhoea (month 1, use non-hormonal contraceptive; may need contraception 3 months after last injection; Decapeptyl 3). *Breast cancer,* admin triptorelin on schedule and without interruption throughout aromatase inhibitor treatment. Confirm ovarian suppression prior to aromatase inhibitor initiation; repeat every 3 months (FSH, oestradiol levels). Combination in breast cancer (osteoporosis risk). Hypertension, hyperglycaemia, depression reported.

Children, preclude pseudo-precocious puberty (gonadal or adrenal tumour or hyperplasia) and gonadotropin-independent precocious puberty (testicular toxicosis, familial Leydig cell hyperplasia). Progressive brain tumours, weigh risk/benefit.

Pregnancy, Lactation: Contraindicated *(Decapeptyl).* Pregnancy, exclude prior to treatment. Lactation, not to be used during breastfeeding.

ADR: See Notes below.

Notes: See 13.3.2 Prostate Cancer.

Decapeptyl 3-Month, 6-Month, SR Parenteral *(Ipsen)* A. HT.
Price, per vial 3-month (11.25mg) €306.06. 6-month (22.5mg) €604.95. SR 3mg, €105.52.
Injection, triptorelin pamoate 11.25, 22.5mg, SR 3mg. 3-Month: Slightly yellow lyophilised cake; clear colourless solvent for susp. 6-month: White (off-white powder); clear soln for Prolonged/R susp. SR 3mg: White (off-white) powder reconstituted to clear colourless liquid. *Sodium 23mg/11.25(22.5)mg vial.* **Store:** Below 25 deg C (all formulations).

Gonapeptyl Depot Parenteral *(Ferring)* A. HT.
Price, (1) PFS €141.36.
Injection, triptorelin acetate 3.75mg. Powder and solvent for susp prolonged release. *Sodium 3.69mg/mL.*

13.3.3 - Somatostatin Analogues

In This Chapter: *Lanreotide, octreotide.*

Class Effects

CI: Hypersensitivity to any member of the class.
SP: Transient inhibition of insulin and glucagon secretion, monitor blood glucose. Thyroid function may be reduced. Reduced gall bladder motility (gall bladder echography advisable). Monitor hepatic function.
ADR: See manufactures Full Prescribing Information. See Notes below (cytotoxic drugs).
Notes: See also 13.1 Cytotoxic Drugs, 11.6.3 Anterior Pituitary Hormones, Growth Hormone Antagonists.

Lanreotide

ATC Code: H01CB03. **Sport:** Permitted.
Driving: Dizziness.
Indications: Acromegaly, circulating levels of growth hormone and insulin-like growth factor remain abnormal after surgery and/or radiotherapy, or require medical treatment. Relief of symptoms associated with acromegaly, carcinoid tumours. Treatment, gastroenteropancreatic neuroendocrine tumours (GEP-NETs) (midgut, pancreatic, unknown origin) in adults with unresectable locally advanced or metastatic disease.
Dose: Adult, Elderly: *LA 30mg* (IM injection only), acromegaly, neuroendocrine tumours, adenomas, 30mg every 14 days varying site; digestive fistulae, 30mg to assess response. With fistulae volume drainage reduction of minimum 50% after 72-hours, admin 30mg every 10 days until fistula closure OR max. 3x 30mg additional IM injections.
Autogel, acromegaly, neuroendocrine tumour (symptoms), 60-120mg every 28 days; if controlled on a somatostatin analogue, *Somatuline Autogel* 120mg every 45-56 days can be used. GEP-NETs (see Indications above) (unresectable locally advanced or metastatic disease), 120mg injection every 28 days as long as needed for tumour control. *Admin*, deep SC into buttock; self-injection in upper outer thigh; alternate between left and right side.
Child: Not recommended.
Renal Impairment: No dose adjustment.
Hepatic Impairment: As for Renal above.
Interactions: Effect of Lanreotide on Other Drugs: Ciclosporin: *Levels decreased, monitor; may require adjustment*. Insulin, oral hypoglycaemics: *Requirement may be reduced*. Bromocriptine: *Bioavailability may be increased*. Bradycardia inducing drugs (beta-blockers): *May require dose adjustment*. Drugs metabolised by CYP3A4 with low therapeutic index (quinidine, terfenadine): *Caution; potential decreased metabolic clearance*.
SP: Bradycardia, caution.
Pregnancy, Lactation: Pregnancy, only if clearly needed. Lactation, caution.
ADR: See Notes below.
Notes: See 13.3.3 Somatostatin Analogues.

Somatostatin Analogues   13.3.3

Somatuline Autogel, LA Parenteral *(Ipsen)* A. HT.
Price, injection (1) 60mg, €826.64. 90mg, €1101.18. 120mg, €1400.91. LA vial (1) 30mg, €436.39.
Injection (IM), lanreotide acetate (LA 30mg Prolonged/R; Autogel 60, 90, 120mg). *Autogel:* White (off-white) translucent and viscous super saturated soln in PFS. *LA:* Practically white friable powder (cake); clear colourless soln. **Store:** Refrigerate; original pack. Do not freeze (LA).

Octreotide

ATC Code: H01CB02. **Sport:** Permitted.
Driving: Unlikely to impair.
Indications: See Dose below. Acromegaly, TSH-secreting pituitary adenoma (surgery inappropriate or until interim radiotherapy becomes effective).
Dose: Adult, Elderly: *Acromegaly*, 0.05-0.1mg SC every 8-12 hours (max. 1.5mg/day) OR LAR 20mg IM 4-weekly (3 months); may be increased to 30mg LAR or 40mg LAR 4-weekly.
Functional gastro-entero-pancreatic endocrine tumours, initially 0.05mg SC once or twice daily; titrate gradually to 0.1-0.2mg 3-times daily; if controlled with SC treatment, consider LAR 20mg IM 4-weekly; well controlled after 3 months reduce to 10mg LAR 4-weekly; partially controlled, increase to 30mg LAR 4-weekly. *Advanced neuroendocrine tumours* (midgut or unknown primary origin), 30mg LAR 4-weekly.
TSH-secreting pituitary adenoma, 100mcg 3-times daily SC for at least 5 days to assess efficacy before dose adjustment OR 20mg LAR IM 4-weekly for 3 months then consider dose adjustment.
Pancreatic surgery, prevention of complications, 0.1mg 3-times daily SC for 7 consecutive days starting day of surgery minimum 1 hour before laparotomy.
Bleeding gastro-oesophageal varices, 25mcg/hour for 5 days by continuous IV infusion; cirrhotic patients, up to 50mcg/hour has been tolerated.
NOTE: Standard/R is for SC injection or IV infusion after dilution. Prolonged/R (LAR) admin by deep intragluteal injection, alternating left and right gluteal muscle.
Child: Limited data.
Hepatic Impairment: Elimination may be reduced; consider dose adjustment.
Interactions: Effect of Other Drugs on Octreotide: *Caution (limited data, cannot exclude interaction)*: Drugs metabolised by CYP3A4 with narrow therapeutic window (quinidine, terfenadine).
Effect of Octreotide on Other Drugs: Ciclosporin: *Reduced intestinal absorption*. Insulin, oral hypoglycaemics: *Requirement may be changed*. Cimetidine: *Delayed intestinal absorption*. Bromocriptine: *Increased bioavailability*. Beta-blockers, calcium channel blockers, agents to control fluid/electrolyte balance: *Dose adjustment may be required (bradycardia)*.
SP: *Monitor*, GH-secreting pituitary tumours may expand causing serious complications (visual field defects); thyroid function (with prolonged treatment); gall bladder ultrasonic examination (before, then 6 monthly during treatment), gallstones reported; glucose tolerance and antidiabetic treatment; vitamin B12 levels. Bradycardia. May alter dietary fat absorption.
Pregnancy, Lactation: Pregnancy, avoid. Females of childbearing potential to ensure adequate contraception. Lactation, not recommended.
ADR: See Notes below.
Notes: See 13.3.3 Somatostatin Analogues.

Sandostatin, LAR Parenteral *(Novartis)* A. HT.
Price, injection (5) 50mcg, €3.81. 100mcg, €7.18. 500mcg, €34.80. LAR injection (1) 10mg, €751.93. 20mg, €1005.10. 30mg, €1306.58.
Injection (SC) or infusion (IV), octreotide acetate. Amps: 50, 100, 500mcg. Clear colourless soln. *Essentially sodium free.* **Store:** Refrigerate; do not freeze. May be stored below 30 deg C (2 weeks).
Injection (IM) Prolonged/R, as above. LAR 10, 20, 30mg: White (yellowish) powder; clear colourless (slightly yellow-brown) solvent for soln *Essentially sodium-free.* **Store:** Refrigerate; do not freeze; can remain below 25 degrees C on day of injection.

14

Anaesthesia

14.1 - General Anaesthesia

Class Effects

These medicinals are used under specialist supervision in specialised units. Always consult manufacturers Full Prescribing Information.

SP: *General anaesthetics* should be used under supervision of an experienced anaesthetist with adequate facilities for endotracheal intubation and artificial ventilation. Inform anaesthetist of all patient medication. *Local anaesthetic*, perform procedures in facilities where equipment and drugs necessary for monitoring and emergency resuscitation are available.

14.1.1 - Muscle Relaxants

In This Chapter: *Atracurium, cisatracurium, mivacurium, rocuronium, suxamethonium.*

Class Effects

All are non-depolarising muscle relaxants (neuromuscular blockers) with the exception of suxamethonium which is depolarising.

Driving: Advise not to drive until effects of anaesthetic, and the immediate effects of surgery have passed. Advise not to drink alcohol for 24 hours after anaesthesia.

CI: Hypersensitivity to any member of the class.

Interactions: Effect of Other Drugs on Non-Depolarising Neuromuscular Blockers: *Co-admin not recommended*: Depolarising muscle relaxants used to prolong effects of non-depolarising neuromuscular blockers (may result in prolonged and complex block, difficult to reverse with anticholinesterases). *Magnitude and/or duration of blockade increased*: Anaesthetics (enflurane, isoflurane, halothane), ketamine, other non-depolarising neuromuscular blockers, antibiotics (aminoglycosides, polymyxins, spectinomycin, tetracycline, lincomycin, clindamycin), antiarrhythmics (propranolol, calcium channel blockers, lidocaine, procainamide, quinidine), diuretics (frusemide, possibly mannitol, thiazides, acetazolamide), magnesium and lithium salts, ganglion blockers (trimetaphan, hexamethonium). *Onset of blockade lengthened, duration shortened (effect decreased)*: Prior chronic anticonvulsant therapy (phenytoin, carbamazepine). *Increased drug sensitivity*: Drugs aggravating or unmasking latent myasthenia gravis or inducing myasthenic syndrome including various antibiotics, beta-blockers (propranolol, oxprenolol), antiarrhythmics (procainamide, quinidine), antirheumatics (chloroquine, D-penicillamine), trimetaphan, chlorpromazine, steroids, phenytoin, lithium.

SP: These drugs paralyse respiratory and other skeletal muscles; have no effect on consciousness; always admin with adequate anaesthesia, ventilatory support, analgesia. Monitor neuromuscular function to individualise dose (method, duration, interaction with other drugs, condition of patient). Residual curarisation reported. *Anaphylactic reaction risk*, caution (previous anaphylactic reactions to neuromuscular blockers; allergic cross-

reactivity greater than 50% reported). Combination with corticosteroids, limit duration of neuromuscular blocker (myopathy risk). Potential for histamine release in susceptible patients, caution (history of increased histamine sensitivity). Increased (sensitivity and effect) with myasthenia gravis (other neuromuscular disease, after poliomyelitis), severe electrolyte imbalance. Resistance (burns patients); consider increased dose and shortened duration of action. No effect on heart rate; will not counteract bradycardia. Hypotonic, not for admin into infusion line of blood transfusion. *Hypothermia*, neuromuscular block increased; decreases with rewarming. Malignant hyperthermia-susceptible patients, no data (except suxamethonium). Observe for evidence of spontaneous recovery prior to admin of reversal (neostigmine). *Obese patients*, base initial dose on ideal body weight (not actual). *Reduced plasma cholinesterase activity* e.g. pregnancy and puerperium, genetic plasma cholinesterase abnormality, TB, severe (generalised tetanus, chronic infections, burns), chronic (debilitating disease, anaemia), malignancy, malnutrition, autoimmune disease, myxoedema, collagen disease, end-stage hepatic failure, acute or chronic renal failure (prolonged and intensified neuromuscular blockade; reduce dose).

ADR: Flushing, hypotension. Injection site reactions. In some cases, anaphylactic or anaphylactoid reactions. See manufacturers Full Prescribing Information.

Notes: See 14.1 General Anaesthesia.

Atracurium

ATC Code: M03AC04. **Sport:** Permitted.
Driving: Not applicable.

Indications: Adjunct to general anaesthesia to enable tracheal intubation; relax skeletal muscles during surgery or controlled ventilation.

Dose: Adult, Elderly: IV INJECTION, range 0.3-0.6mg/kg (depending on duration of full block required) provides relaxation for 15-35 minutes. Endotracheal intubation within 90 seconds from IV injection of 0.5-0.6mg/kg; prolong full block with supplementary 0.1-0.2mg/kg as required. C-section, 0.3-0.6mg/kg; does not cross the placenta; spontaneous recovery in about 35 minutes.

CONTINUOUS INFUSION, normothermia, initial bolus 0.3-0.6mg/kg; maintain block during long surgical procedures with continuous infusion 0.3-0.6mg/kg/hour. Induced hypothermia reduces rate of atracurium inactivation; full neuromuscular block may be maintained by approx. half original infusion rate at low temp. *Elderly*, use lower end of dose range; slow admin. *Cardiovascular disease*, admin initial dose over 60 seconds.

Child: Over 1 month, as for Adult above. Neonates, not recommended (no data).

CI: Use before, or with depolarising agent.

Interactions: Effect of Other Drugs on Atracurium: *Not recommended*: Admixture with thiopentone or any alkaline agent in same syringe. *Duration/magnitude of blockade diminished*: Anticholinesterases (donepezil).

SP: Unusual sensitivity to fall in arterial BP (hypovolaemic), admin over 60 seconds. Carcinomatosis (especially bronchial carcinoma), may show marked sensitivity; neuromuscular block may respond poorly to neostigmine. Severe cardiovascular disease, more susceptible to transient hypotension; slow IV (divided doses).

Pregnancy, Lactation: Pregnancy, if benefit outweighs risk. May be used in C-section (does not cross placenta in significant amounts). Lactation, not known if excreted in human milk.

ADR: See Notes below.

Notes: See 14.1.1 Muscle Relaxants.

    Tracrium Parenteral 10mg/mL (GSK) A. HOS.
    Price, 50mg/5mL (5) €17.21 (PTW).
    Injection or infusion, atracurium besilate. Clear slightly yellow soln.

Cisatracurium

ATC Code: M03AC11. **Sport:** Permitted.
Driving: Not applicable.

Indications: Surgical, other procedures (adults, children 1 month and over) and in ICU (adults). Adjunctive, general anaesthesia, or sedation in ICU to relax skeletal muscles, and to facilitate tracheal intubation and mechanical ventilation.

Dose: Adult, Elderly: IV BOLUS, for tracheal intubation, 0.15mg/kg for intubation 120 seconds after admin; maintenance 0.03mg/kg provides approx. 20 minutes additional neuromuscular block. Reversible with anticholinesterases.

IV INFUSION, initially 3mcg/kg/min; after initial stabilisation, 1-2mcg/kg/min; reduce infusion rate by up to 40% during isoflurane or enflurane anaesthesia.

Child: IV BOLUS, tracheal intubation (age 1 month to 12 years), 0.15mg/kg over 5-10 seconds; maintenance (2-12 years), 0.02mg/kg provides approx. 9 minutes additional neuromuscular block.

Renal Impairment: May have slightly slower onset.

Hepatic Impairment: May have slightly faster onset.

CI: Hypersensitivity to atracurium, benzenesulfonic acid.

Interactions: Effect of Other Drugs on Cisatracurium: *Not recommended*: Admixture with thiopentone or any alkaline agent, or propofol emulsion in same syringe. *Duration shortened, blockade magnitude diminished*: Anticholinesterases used in Alzheimer's (donepezil). *Decreased effect*: Phenytoin, carbamazepine (chronic admin).

SP: Seizures (ICU).

Pregnancy, Lactation: Not recommended.

ADR: See Notes below.

Notes: See 14.1.1 Muscle Relaxants.

 Nimbex Parenteral 2mg/mL *(GSK)* A.
 Price, not published by company.
 Injection or infusion, cisatracurium besilate. Colourless (pale-yellow, greenish yellow) soln practically free from visible particles.

Mivacurium

ATC Code: M03AC10. **Sport:** Permitted.
Driving: Not applicable.

Indications: Adjunct to general anaesthesia to relax skeletal muscles and facilitate tracheal intubation and mechanical ventilation.

Dose: Adult: IV INJECTION, tracheal intubation, 0.2mg/kg over 30 seconds for intubation within 2-2.5 minutes OR 0.15mg/kg followed 30 seconds later by 0.1mg/kg for intubation within 1.5-2 minutes; bolus range 0.07-0.25mg/kg; maintenance, 0.1mg/kg provides approx. 15 minutes additional block.

CONTINUOUS INFUSION, 8-10mcg/kg/min; increase infusion rate by 1mcg/kg/min; maintenance, 6-7mcg/kg/min for narcotic anaesthesia; reduce by up to 40% during isoflurane or enflurane anaesthesia.

Elderly: Onset time, duration, recovery rate may be extended. Use slower infusion rates or smaller or less frequent maintenance bolus doses.

Child: Age 7 months to 12 years, IV INJECTION, 0.1-0.2mg/kg over 5-15 seconds; with narcotic or halothane anaesthesia, 0.2mg/kg produces average of 9 minutes block; for tracheal intubation, 0.2mg/kg with max. block within 2 minutes; maintenance, 0.1mg/kg providing 6-9 minutes block.

CONTINUOUS INFUSION, age 7-23 months, during halothane anaesthesia 11mcg/kg/min; range 3-26mcg/kg/min; age 2-12 years, during halothane or narcotic anaesthesia, 13-14mcg/kg/min; range 5-31mcg/kg/min.

Age 2-6 months, IV INJECTION, 0.1-0.15mg/kg over 5-15 seconds; with halothane anaesthesia, 0.15mg/kg produces 9 minutes block; for tracheal intubation, 0.15mg/kg with max. block within 1.4 minutes; maintenance, 0.1mg/kg providing approx. 7 minutes block.

CONTINUOUS INFUSION, during halothane anaesthesia, 11mcg/kg/min; range 4-24mcg/kg/min.

Renal Impairment: Prolonged, intensified neuromuscular blockade with acute or chronic failure due to reduced plasma cholinesterase levels.

Hepatic Impairment: End-stage, duration of block produced by 0.15mg/kg is approx. 3-times longer than in normal function; adjust dose.

CI: Patients known to be homozygous for the atypical plasma cholinesterase gene.

Interactions: Effect of Other Drugs on Mivacurium: *Not recommended*: Admixture with highly alkaline solns (barbiturate solns) in same syringe. *Prolonged blockade*: Drugs reducing plasma cholinesterase activity (anti-mitotic drugs, MAOIs, ecothiopate iodide, pancuronium, certain hormones, anticholinesterases, organophosphates, bambuterol, SSRIs).

SP: Reduced cholinesterase activity with genetic abnormalities of cholinesterase (extremely sensitive to neuromuscular blocking effect of mivacurium; antagonised by conventional doses of neostigmine). See Notes below. Increased histamine sensitivity (asthma), caution. Patients unusually sensitive to fall in arterial BP (hypovolaemic), admin over 60 seconds.

Pregnancy, Lactation: If benefit outweighs risk. Can be used in C-section.

ADR: See Notes below.

Notes: See 14.1.1 Muscle Relaxants.

 Mivacron Parenteral 2mg/mL *(GSK)* A.
 Price, (1) 10mg/5mL, €17.65. 20mg/10mL, €28.70.
 Injection, mivacurium chloride. Clear pale-yellow soln.

Rocuronium

ATC Code: M03AC09. **Sport:** Permitted.
Driving: Not applicable.

Indications: Adjunct, in adults and paediatric patients, to general anaesthesia to facilitate tracheal intubation and to provide skeletal muscle relaxation, during surgery. Adjunct, in adults, in ICU to facilitate intubation and mechanical ventilation.

Dose: Adult: Tracheal intubation for surgery, 0.6mg/kg for intubation within 60 seconds; during rapid sequence induction, 1mg/kg. *C-section*, 0.6mg/kg; maintenance, 0.15mg/kg; long-term inhalational anaesthesia, reduce to 0.075-0.1mg/kg.

Continuous infusion, loading dose 0.6mg/kg and when neuromuscular block starts to recover, start infusion (rate adjusted to maintain twitch response at 10% of control twitch height); range 0.3-0.6mg/kg (IV anaesthesia) OR 0.3-0.4mg/kg (inhalation anaesthesia).

ICU, tracheal intubation, as for surgery above; maintenance, initial loading dose 0.6mg/kg followed by continuous infusion 0.3-0.6mg/kg/hour (first hour), decreasing during next 6-12 hours depending on response.

Elderly: Over 65 years, routine anaesthesia/rapid sequence induction, 0.6mg/kg; maintenance, 0.075-0.1mg/kg at infusion rate of 0.3-0.4mg/kg/hour. Facilitation of mechanical ventilation (ICU), not recommended.

Child: Neonates (0-27 days), infants (28 days-2 months), toddlers (3-23 months), children (2-11 years), adolescents (12-17 years), intubation dose during routine anaesthesia, maintenance dose, as for Adult above. Duration of action of single dose will be longer in neonates and infants.

Continuous infusion as for Adult except children (2-11 years) may need higher infusion rates.

Rapid sequence induction, facilitation of mechanical ventilation (ICU), not recommended.

Renal Impairment: As for Elderly above.

Hepatic Impairment: As for Elderly above.

Interactions: Effect of Other Drugs on Rocuronium: *Effect increased*: Halogenated volatile anaesthetics (effect apparent with maintenance dosing), suxamethonium (after intubation with), concomitant corticosteroids (long-term), antibiotics (aminoglycosides, lincosamide and polypeptide

14.1.2 Opioids In Anaesthesia

antibiotics, acylaminopenicillins), diuretics, quinidine, quinine, magnesium salts, calcium channel blockers, lithium salts, local anaesthetics (lidocaine IV, bupivacaine epidural). *Effect decreased*: Phenytoin or carbamazepine (prior chronic admin), protease inhibitors (gabexate, ulinastatin), neostigmine, edrophonium, pyridostigmine. *Variable effect*: Non-depolarising neuromuscular blockers, suxamethonium.

Effect of Rocuronium on Other Drugs: Lidocaine: *Quicker onset of action*.

SP: Ventilatory support mandatory; anticipate intubation difficulties, need for immediate reversal of rocuronium-induced neuromuscular block; if immediate reversal is needed, consider reversal agent. Residual curarisation, caution (geriatrics). Doses over 0.9mg/kg may increase heart rate. Slower onset of action with prolonged circulation time (cardiovascular disease, old age, oedematous state). Hypothermic conditions (blocking effect increased; duration prolonged). Effect increased with hypo- (kalaemia, calcaemia, proteinaemia), dehydration, acidosis, hyper- (capnia, magnesaemia), cachexia; correct severe electrolyte disturbances.

Pregnancy, Lactation: Pregnancy, caution. Can be used in C-section as part of rapid sequence induction. Does not affect Apgar score, foetal muscle tone or cardiorespiratory adaptation; limited placental transfer. Lactation, if benefit outweighs risk.

Notes: See 14.1.1 Muscle Relaxants.

Esmeron Parenteral *(MSD)* A. HOS.
Price, (10) 100mg/10mL, €76.19; 50mg/5mL, €38.09 (PTW).
Injection or infusion, rocuronium bromide 10mg/mL. Clear colourless (slightly yellow/brown) aqueous soln. *Sodium 1.64mg/mL.*

Suxamethonium

ATC Code: M03AB01. **Sport:** Permitted.
Driving: Not applicable.

Indications: Skeletal muscle relaxant to facilitate tracheal intubation, mechanical ventilation in surgical procedures. Reduction of intensity of muscular contractions associated with convulsions.

Dose: Adult, Elderly: *Anectine*, 1mg/kg by bolus IV injection for intubation within 30-60 seconds (duration 2-6 minutes); maintenance, supplementary doses of 50-100% of initial dose at 5-10 minute intervals.

Suxamethonium (Concordia), usually 20-100mg IV, repeat if needed; electro-convulsive therapy, usually 0.5-0.75mg/kg; continuous IV infusion, 500mg in 500mL sterile isotonic saline; admin rate 2.5-5mg/min.

Child: *Anectine*, IV injection, neonates and infants, 2mg/kg; older children, 1mg/kg. IM bolus of 4-5mg/kg (infants) up to 4mg/kg (older children). Onset of useful neuromuscular relaxation, within 3 minutes; max. 150mg. IV infusion, initially 36-57mcg/kg/min; max. 500mg/hour.

Suxamethonium (Concordia) IV, children, 1-2mg/kg; neonates, 1-2mg, followed by 0.25-0.5mg/kg supplements; max. 50mg. IM, infants and children, 2mg/kg; max. 150mg.

Renal Impairment: See SP below.

Hepatic Impairment: See SP below.

CI: Reduced plasma cholinesterase activity (see SP). Malignant hyperthermia, previous prolonged apnoea after suxamethonium, caution. Rise in serum potassium following admin, not for use when recovering from major trauma or severe burns, neurological deficits involving spinal cord injury, peripheral nerve injury, acute major muscle wasting (motor neurone lesions), prolonged immobilisation, pre-existing hyperkalaemia. Open eye injuries or if increased IOP is undesirable (unless benefit outweighs risk). Congenital myotonic diseases, severe myotonic spasms and rigidity. Skeletal myopathies e.g. Duchenne muscular dystrophy (malignant hyperthermia, ventricular dysrhythmias and cardiac arrest secondary to acute rhabdomyolysis with hyperkalaemia).

Interactions: Effect of Other Drugs on Suxamethonium: *Reduce plasma cholinesterase, prolonged neuromuscular*

blockade: Organophosphate insecticides and metriphonate, ecothiopate eye drops, specific anticholinesterases (neostigmine, pyridostigmine, physostigmine, edrophonium, tacrine), cytotoxics (cyclophosphamide, mechlorethamine, triethylene-melamine, thiotepa), trimetaphan, psychiatric drugs (phenelzine, promazine, chlorpromazine), anaesthetics (ketamine, morphine and morphine antagonists, pethidine, pancuronium), selective serotonin reuptake inhibitors (SSRIs), other drugs with deleterious effects on plasma cholinesterase (aprotinin, diphenhydramine, promethazine, oestrogens, high-dose steroids, oral contraceptives, terbutaline, metoclopramide). *Enhanced or prolonged neuromuscular effect*: Volatile inhalational anaesthetics (halothane, enflurane, desflurane, isoflurane, diethylether, methoxyflurane; little effect on Phase I block; accelerate onset and enhance the intensity of Phase II suxamethonium-induced block), antibiotics (aminoglycosides, clindamycin, polymyxins), antiarrhythmics (quinidine, procainamide, verapamil, beta-blockers, lidocaine, procaine), magnesium salts, lithium carbonate, azathioprine.

Effect of Suxamethonium on Other Drugs: Digitalis-like drugs: *Increased susceptibility to suxamethonium-exacerbated hyperkalaemia.*

SP: Reduced plasma cholinesterase activity reduce dose (see Interactions). Repeated or continued admin, Phase II block may develop. May cause or potentiate bradycardia. Continuous infusion, tachycardia, rise in BP. Caution, cachectic and ill patients, acid-base disturbances, electrolyte imbalance, parenchymatous liver disease, obstructive jaundice, carcinomatosis, contact with certain insecticides (organophosphates), receiving therapeutic radiation, fractures or muscle spasms (initial muscle fasciculations). Muscarinic effects (increased bronchial and salivary secretions), prevented by atropine. May cause cardiac rhythm change (arrest).

Pregnancy, Lactation: Pregnancy, if benefit outweighs risk. Lactation, not known if excreted in breast milk.

ADR: *Common*, IOP, bradycardia, tachycardia. See Notes below.

Notes: See 14.1.1 Muscle Relaxants.

Anectine Parenteral 50mg/mL *(GSK)* A.
Price, 50mg/mL (5x2mL) €4.28.
Injection or infusion, suxamethonium chloride. Clear colourless soln.

Suxamethonium Parenteral 50mg/mL *(Concordia)* A.
Price, 50mg/mL (5x2mL) €6.05 (PTW).
Injection or infusion, suxamethonium chloride. Clear colourless soln.

14.1.2 - Opioids In Anaesthesia

In This Chapter: *Alfentanil, fentanyl, remifentanil.*

Class Effects

Driving: Where early discharge is envisaged, advise patients not to drive or operate machinery for 24 hours following admin. Cognitive function can be impaired; with some members of the class it may be an offence to drive under the influence of these medicines.

CI: Hypersensitivity to any member of the class.

Interactions: Effect of Other Drugs on Opioids: *Respiratory depression potentiated*: Barbiturates, benzodiazepines, neuroleptics, halogenated gases, ALCOHOL. *Co-admin not recommended*: MAOIs (or within 2 weeks). *Metabolism inhibited, prolonged or delayed respiratory depression risk*: Azole antifungals (fluconazole, ketoconazole, itraconazole, voriconazole), erythromycin, diltiazem, cimetidine (alfentanil), ritonavir (alfentanil, fentanyl). *Bradycardia, hypotension risk*: Drugs depressing heart or increasing vagal tone (beta-blockers, anaesthetics, suxamethonium). *Enhanced or prolonged respiratory depression*: Opioid premedication.

SP: Hospital use only by trained anaesthetists in environment where airway can be controlled by trained personnel and resuscitation equipment available. Potent opioids, respiratory depression is dose-related; can be reversed by specific opioid antagonist (naloxone); additional doses of antagonist may be needed as respiratory depression may last longer than duration of action of antagonist. Profound analgesia is accompanied by respiratory depression, which can persist or recur in post-operative period; patients should remain under surveillance. Hyperventilation during anaesthesia may alter response to CO2 (affecting respiration post-operative). Hypotension, especially with hypovolaemia. Compromised intracerebral compliance, avoid rapid bolus injection. Chronic opioid therapy or abuse may require increased dose. Increased intracranial pressure; caution head injuries. Muscle rigidity, non-epileptic (myo)clonic movements. Cardiovascular monitoring (bradycardia, cardiac arrest). Titrate with caution (uncontrolled hypothyroidism, pulmonary disease, decreased respiratory reserve, alcoholism, impaired hepatic or renal function); require prolonged post-op monitoring. Techniques involving analgesia in a spontaneously breathing child only to be used as part of anaesthetic or sedation analgesia technique; with experienced personnel in environment to manage sudden chest wall rigidity requiring intubation, or apnoea requiring airway support.

Pregnancy, Lactation: Pregnancy, if benefit outweighs risk. Use during childbirth including C-section, not recommended (can cross placenta; foetal respiratory centre particularly sensitive to opioids). If used, an opioid antagonist for the child must be available. Lactation, not recommended for 24 hours following admin.

ADR: See manufacturers Full Prescribing Information.

Notes: See 14.1 General Anaesthesia. Opioids used primarily for analgesia, see 4.2.2 Opioid Analgesics.

Alfentanil

ATC Code: N01AH02. **Sport:** Prohibited (in-competition).
Driving: See Notes below.

Indications: *Adults*, induction general anaesthesia (GA), adjunctive, maintenance of general anaesthesia and analgesia. Sole IV anaesthetic agent for short minor surgical procedures. Provision of analgesia and suppression of respiratory activity in mechanically ventilated ICU patients and providing analgesic cover for painful procedures. *Paediatrics* (neonates, infants, children, adolescents), as opioid analgesic with a hypnotic to induce anaesthesia; opioid analgesic with GA (short and long surgical procedures).

Dose: Adult: Induction, 120mcg/kg by slow IV bolus. *Sole IV anaesthetic*, initially 7mcg/kg (up to 500mcg) by slow IV bolus (over 30 seconds) with supplemental doses of 3.5mcg/kg (or 250mcg); longer procedures with controlled ventilation, single IV bolus 30-50mcg/kg with supplemental 15mcg/kg bolus doses OR by infusion, initial loading 50-100mcg/kg over 10-15 minutes and then 0.5-1mcg/kg/min. ICU, 2mg/hour or 30mcg/kg/hour; more rapid control, 5mg loading dose in divided doses over 10 minutes by IV bolus or continuous infusion. *Admin*, with cardiovascular monitoring (bradycardia, hypotension); to avoid bradycardia, admin of small IV dose anticholinergic just before induction recommended. Obese, calculate dose according to lean body mass.

Elderly: Age 65 years and older and debilitated, reduce dose and dosing frequency due to reduced clearance and prolonged elimination half-life. Reduce dose and speed of injection to avoid hypotension.

Child: Neonates (0-27 days), titrate dose according to response (clearance lower; lower dose requirement). Infants/toddlers (28 days to 23 months), maintenance analgesia, infusion rate may need increasing (clearance higher than adults). Children (2-11 years), increase infusion rate (clearance higher in children). Adolescents, as for Adult above.

Older children, bolus 10-20mcg/kg for anaesthesia induction with supplemental boluses of 5-10mcg/kg. Analgesia maintenance, use infusion rate of 0.5-2mcg/kg/min. Combined with IV anaesthetic, 1mcg/kg/min.

Renal Impairment: Consider dose reduction.

Hepatic Impairment: As for Renal above.

CI: Obstructive airways disease or respiratory depression if not ventilated. During labour or C-section prior to clamping of cord.

Interactions: Effect of Alfentanil on Other Drugs: Propofol: *Lower dose of alfentanil may be needed with co-admin.*

SP: Respiratory arrests have occurred within 90 minutes of infusion cessation. Lacks sedative or hypnotic activity. Reserve rapid reversal (using antagonist) for when benefit outweighs disadvantage (opioid withdrawal, exaggerated responses to painful stimuli).

Pregnancy, Lactation: Not of IV admin during childbirth; crosses placenta and may suppress spontaneous respiration in the newborn period. If admin, ventilation equipment to be available for mother and infant; opioid antagonist must be available for child. Lactation, not recommended for 24 hours following admin.

ADR: *Most frequent*, nausea, vomiting. See Notes below.

Notes: See 14.1.2 Opioids In Anaesthesia.

Rapifen Parenteral *(Janssen-Cilag)* CD. HOS.
Price, 500mcg/mL: 2mL x 10, €6.04; 10mL x 5, €14.20 (PTW).
Injection or infusion, alfentanil HCl 500mcg/mL. Clear aqueous soln. *Sodium 3.54mg/mL.*

Fentanyl (anaesthesia)

ATC Code: N01AH01. **Sport:** Prohibited (in-competition).
Driving: See Notes below.

Indications: Adjunct, maintenance of general anaesthesia (GA) and analgesia. Conjunction with neuroleptics in neuroleptanalgesia. Respiratory depressant/analgesic in patients requiring prolonged assisted ventilation. Sole IV analgesic in surgical procedures.

Dose: Adult: *Sublimaze (IV),* general anaesthetic, 0.05mg supplements*. Neuroleptanalgesia, initially 0.1mg; maintenance 0.05mg*. Assisted ventilation, prolonged, initially up to 0.6mg, then 0.05-0.2mg supplements*. Sole IV analgesic in surgery, usually 0.1-0.8mg; maintenance 0.05mg*. Obese patients, calculate dose on estimated lean body mass. Debilitated, as for Elderly below. For IV admin. *(as needed).

Fentanyl (Concordia) (IV), sole IV analgesic in surgery, initially 100-800mcg; maintenance 50mcg/kg*. GA, adjunctive, 50mcg supplements*. Neuroleptanalgesia, initially 100mcg; maintenance 50mcg*. Assisted ventilation, prolonged, initially up to 600mcg with supplemental 50-200mcg doses. Obese, calculate according to lean body mass. *(as needed).

Elderly: *Sublimaze (IV),* reduce initial dose.

Fentanyl (Concordia) (IV), assisted ventilation, prolonged, reduce dose.

Child: *Sublimaze (IV),* GA, 0.001mg/kg supplements as needed. Neuroleptanalgesia, initially 0.01mg/kg; maintenance 0.001mg/kg as needed. Assisted ventilation, prolonged, 0.001mg/kg as needed. Sole IV analgesic in surgery, usually 0.01mg/kg; maintenance 0.001mg/kg as needed.

Fentanyl (Concordia) (IV), sole IV analgesic in surgery, initially 10mcg/kg; maintenance 50mcg/kg as needed. GA, adjunctive, 1mcg/kg supplements as needed. Neuroleptanalgesia, initially 100mcg; maintenance 50mcg as needed. Assisted ventilation, prolonged, initially 10mcg with supplemental 1mcg/kg doses.

Renal Impairment: *Sublimaze (IV),* consider dose reduction; monitor for fentanyl toxicity.

CI: Respiratory depression, cyanosis, excessive bronchial exudation, bronchoconstriction, chronic pulmonary disease, post-op biliary tract interventions.

Interactions: Effect of Other Drugs on Fentanyl: Co-admin caution: Neuroleptics (hypotension risk; extrapyramidal symptoms).

SP: Tolerance (repeated use). Use slow IV (premedicate with benzodiazepines), muscle relaxants (to avoid muscle rigidity induction).

ADR: *Most common*, nausea, vomiting, muscle rigidity,

14.1.3   Other Anaesthetic Adjuncts

hypotension, hypertension, bradycardia, sedation. See Notes below.

Notes: See 14.1.2 Opioids In Anaesthesia.

Sublimaze Parenteral *(Janssen-Cilag)* CD.
Price, (10) 50mcg/mL, 2mL, €23.46. 10mL, €11.95.
Injection, fentanyl citrate 50mcg/mL. Clear colourless soln. *Sodium 3.5mg/mL.*

Fentanyl (Concordia) Parenteral *(Concordia)* CD.
Price, (10) 100mcg/2mL, €2.09. 500mcg/10mL, €10.16 (PTW).
Injection, fentanyl citrate 50(100)mcg/mL. Clear colourless soln. *Sodium 3.542mg/mL.* Store: Below 25 deg C; outer carton to protect (light).

Remifentanil

ATC Code: N01AH06. **Sport:** Prohibited (in-competition).
Driving: See Notes below.

Indications: Adjunctive, as analgesic agent during induction and/or maintenance of general anaesthesia (GA) in conjunction with controlled ventilation. Provision of analgesia in mechanical ventilation in ICU.

Dose: Adult: GA induction, continuous infusion rate 0.5-1mcg/kg/min with or without initial bolus 1mcg/kg; maintenance, during anaesthesia, increase infusion rate by 25-100% or decrease by 25-50% every 2-5 minutes. IV only; not for epidural or intrathecal injection. Consider anticholinergic premedication. Cardiac anaesthesia, use in ICU, see manufacturers Full Prescribing Information.

Elderly: Over 65 years, initially half Adult dose.

Child: Age 1-12 years, GA maintenance, bolus over minimum 30 seconds. 0.4mcg/kg/min infusion rate. Co-admin with IV anaesthetic for induction of anaesthesia not recommended. Total intravenous anaesthesia (TIVA), no dosage recommendations.

Renal Impairment: Severe, might be slightly more sensitive to respiratory depressant effects.

Hepatic Impairment: As for Renal above.

CI: Epidural, intrathecal use (contains glycine). Sole agent for induction of anaesthesia.

Interactions: Effect of Remifentanil on Other Drugs: Inhaled and IV anaesthetics, benzodiazepines (required during anaesthesia): *Co-admin caution, reduce dose.*

SP: May produce dependency. Due to very rapid offset, no residual opioid activity will be present 5-10 minutes after discontinuation; surgery (post-operative pain expected), prior to discontinuation admin analgesics and/or sedatives.

ADR: *Very common,* skeletal muscle rigidity, hypotension, nausea, vomiting. See Notes below.

Notes: See 14.1.2 Opioids In Anaesthesia.

Ultiva Parenteral *(GSK)* A. HOS.
Price, (5) 1mg, €31.93; 2mg, €63.58; 5mg, €122.78 (PTW).
Infusion, remifentanil 1mg, 2mg, 5mg. White (off-white) powder for conc for soln.

Remifentanil Parenteral *(TEVA)* A.
Price, not published by company.
Injection or infusion, remifentanil 1mg, 2mg, 5mg per vial. White (slightly yellow) cake or powdery mass for conc for soln. *Sodium 1.15mg/mL.*

Remifentanil TEVA Parenteral *(TEVA)* A.
Price, not published by company.
Injection or infusion, remifentanil 1mg/vial. White (off-white or yellowish) compact powder for conc for soln. *Essentially sodium-free.*

14.1.3 - Other Anaesthetic Adjuncts

In This Chapter: *Atropine, dexmedetomidine, glycopyrronium (neostigmine combination), midazolam, neostigmine, sugammadex.*

Class Effects

CI: Hypersensitivity to any member of the class.

SP: Elderly are more sensitive to effects of benzodiazepines, caution. Hypersensitivity reactions (anaphylaxis) possible.

ADR: See manufactures Full Prescribing Information.

394

Notes: See 14.1 General Anaesthesia. See 3.4.1 Anxiolytics (lorazepam) and 3.4.1 Hypnotics (temazepam).

Atropine (systemic)

ATC Code: A03BA01. **Sport:** Permitted.
Driving: Not applicable.

Indications: See Dose below.

Dose: Adult: *Atropine Sulphate (Concordia, Aguettant),* anaesthesia (as parasympatholytic agent) 0.3-0.6mg IM or IV. With neostigmine to limit muscarinic effects, 0.6-1.2mg by slow IV injection; admin atropine before neostigmine. Cardiopulmonary resuscitation, 0.2-0.5mg IV (repeat if needed). Sinus bradycardia, 0.5mg IV every 3-5 minutes (until desired heart rate). AV block, 0.5mg every 3-5 minutes (max. 3mg). Antidote, cholinesterase inhibitors, organo-phosphates, range 0.5-2mg; repeat after 5 minutes according to patient response. *Admin,* IV, IM or SC.
Atropine Sulphate (Concordia), treatment, cholinergic crisis of myasthenia gravis, 0.4-2mg IV (increase based on patient response).
Atropine Minijet, bradyarrhythmias, 0.3-0.6mg IM or IV every 4-6 hours (total 2mg). Cardiac resuscitation, 0.5mg IV every 5 minutes (until desired heart rate); asystole, 3mg IV as a single dose. Premedication, 0.3-0.6mg IM or SC before surgery or IV immediately before surgery. With neostigmine to limit muscarinic effects, 0.6-1.2mg by slow IV injection. Anticholinesterase poisoning, 1-2mg IV or IM every 5-60 minutes until signs and symptoms disappear (max. 100mg in first 24 hours).

Elderly: Caution, more susceptible to adverse effects.

Child: *Atropine Sulphate (Aguettant),* pre-anaesthesia, 0.01-0.02mg/kg (max. 0.6mg/dose). With neostigmine to limit muscarinic effects, 0.02mg/kg IV. Bradycardia, AV block, cardiopulmonary resuscitation, 0.02mg/kg IV as single dose (max. 0.6mg). Antidote (organophosphates, cholinesterase inhibitors), 0.02mg/kg*.
Atropine Sulphate (Concordia), anaesthesia IM or IV, premature infants, 65mcg; full-term infants, 100mcg; age 6-12 months, 200mcg; over 1 year, 10-20mcg/kg bodyweight.
Atropine Minijet, under 30kg (IM, IV or SC) usually 0.01mg/kg; max. 0.4mg repeated 4-6-hourly. Advanced life support, 20mcg/kg (0.02mg/kg) IV; minimum 10mcg (0.01mg) repeated at 5 minute intervals; max. 100mcg (0.1mg). Premedication, IM or SC 30-60 minutes before surgery; up to 3kg, 100mcg (0.1mg); 7-9kg, 200mcg (0.2mg); 12-16kg, 300mcg (0.3mg); over 20kg, as for Adult above. With neostigmine to limit muscarinic effects (neonates, infants, children), 20mcg/kg (0.02mg/kg). Anticholinesterase poisoning, 50mcg/kg (0.05mg) IM or IV every 10-30 minutes*. *(repeated until symptoms disappear).

Renal Impairment: Caution.

Hepatic Impairment: As for Renal above.

CI: Not applicable in life-threatening emergencies (asystole). Obstruction of bladder neck (prostatic hypertrophy), reflux oesophagitis, closed angle glaucoma, myasthenia gravis (unless used to treat anticholinesterase adverse effects), paralytic ileus, severe ulcerative colitis, obstructive GI tract disease.

Interactions: Effect of Other Drugs on Atropine: *Effect enhanced:* Drugs with anticholinergic activity (TCADs, antispasmodics, anti-Parkinson drugs, some antihistamines, phenothiazines, disopyramide, quinidine). *Heart rate responsiveness (to IV atropine) decreased (possible) during anaesthesia:* Propofol. *Extreme caution:* Dobutamine-atropine stress ECG, catecholamine co-admin.

Effect of Atropine on Other Drugs: Other oral drugs: *Absorption altered (delayed gastric emptying).*

SP: Caution, hyperthyroidism, hypertension, febrile or high ambient temperature (may increase temperature especially in pyrexial children), tachyarrhythmias, CHF, CHD, gastric ulcer, oesophageal reflux, hiatus hernia (associated with reflux oesophagitis), diarrhoea, GI infection. *Parenteral,* caution (chronic pulmonary disease;

reduced bronchial secretions, bronchial plug formation). Autonomic neuropathy, extreme caution. Cholinergic crisis in myasthenia gravis, withdraw all anti-cholinesterase medication. Dose up to 1mg mild CNS stimulant; higher doses induce mental disturbance, CNS depression.

Pregnancy, Lactation: Pregnancy, if benefit outweighs risk; crosses placenta; during pregnancy or at term, tachycardia risk in foetus. Lactation, trace amounts appear in breast milk may cause antimuscarinic effects in infant; may inhibit lactation.

ADR: See Notes below.

Notes: See 14.1.3 Anaesthetic Adjuncts.

Atropine Sulfate Aguettant Parenteral *(Aguettant)* A.
Price, not published by company.
Injection, atropine sulfate 0.1mg/mL. Clear colourless soln in PFS. *Sodium 3.5mg/mL, 17.7mg/5mL.*

Atropine Sulphate (Concordia) Parenteral *(Concordia)* A.
Price, (10) €4.90 (PTW).
Injection, atropine sulfate. Clear colourless aqueous soln.

Atropine Sulfate Minijet 100mcg/mL *(IMS)* A.
Price, not published by company.
Injection, atropine sulfate 0.1mg/mL. Clear colourless soln. For use with Minijet Injector supplied. *Sodium, max. 0.22mmoL/1mL.*

Glycopyrronium (anaesthesia)

ATC Code: A03AB02. **Sport:** Permitted.
Driving: Not applicable.

Indications: To protect against peripheral muscarinic actions of anticholinesterases (neostigmine, pyridostigmine), used to reverse residual neuromuscular blockade due to non-depolarising muscle relaxants. Pre-operative to reduce (salivary tracheobronchial and pharyngeal secretion, acidity of gastric contents). Pre- or intra-operative to attenuate or prevent intra-operative bradycardia (due to suxamethonium or cardiac vagal reflexes).

Dose: Adult, Elderly: *Premedication* and *intra-operative*, 200-400mcg IV or IM before anaesthesia induction OR 4-5mcg/kg up to max. 400mcg (use IV intra-operatively). *Reversal (residual non-depolarising neuromuscular block)*, 200mcg IV per 1mg neostigmine or equiv. pyridostigmine dose OR 10-15mcg/kg IV with 50mcg/kg neostigmine or equiv. pyridostigmine dose.

Child: *Premedication* and *intra-operative*, IM or IV, 4-8mcg/kg; max. 200mcg. *Reversal (residual non-depolarising neuromuscular block)*, 10mcg/kg IV with 50mcg/kg neostigmine or equiv. pyridostigmine dose.

Interactions: Effect of Other Drugs on Glycopyrronium: *Increased muscarinic side effect risk*: TCADs, some antihistamines, clozapine, disopyramide, MAOIs, phenothiazines. *Caution*: Belladonna alkaloids, other synthetic anticholinergic agents, procainamide, quinidine, narcotic analgesics (meperidine), corticosteroids (IOP).

SP: *Caution*, CAD, CHF, cardiac dysrhythmias, hypertension, thyrotoxicosis, cardiac insufficiency, GORD, diarrhoea, ulcerative colitis, acute MI. Angle-closure glaucoma, myasthenia gravis, paralytic ileus, pyloric stenosis, prostatic enlargement. Prolonged QT-interval (avoid). Pyrexial patients, caution (sweating inhibited).

ADR: See Notes below.

Notes: See Atropine above. See 14.1.3 Anaesthetic Adjuncts.

Glycopyrronium Bromide Parenteral *(Concordia)* A. GMS.
Price, 200mcg/1mL, 1mL (10) €9.34. 3mL (3) €4.70.
Injection, glycopyrronium bromide 200mcg/mL. Clear colourless aqueous soln. *Sodium 3.5mg/mL.*

Glycopyrronium, Neostigmine

ATC Code: N07AA01. **Sport:** Permitted.
Driving: Not applicable.

Indications: Reversal of residual non-depolarising neuromuscular block.

Dose: Adult, Elderly: IV injection 1-2mL* OR 0.02mL/kg IV*; max. 2mL (dose in excess of 2mL not recommended; neostigmine may produce depolarising neuromuscular block). 1mL equiv. to glycopyrronium bromide 0.5mg, neostigmine metilsulfate 2.5mg. *(over 10-30 seconds).

Child: 0.02mL/kg IV over 10-30 seconds (equiv. to neostigmine methylsulfate 0.05mg + glycopyrrolate 0.01mg per kg).

Cl: Mechanical obstruction of GI, urinary tract.

Interactions: Effect of Other Drugs on Glycopyrronium, Neostigmine Combination: *Co-admin not recommended (depolarising blocking effect potentiated)*: Suxamethonium. *Increased muscarinic side-effect risk*: MAOIs, amantadine, clozapine, TCADs, nefopam.

SP: Caution, bronchospasm or severe bradycardia, glaucoma, CAD, CHF, cardiac dysrhythmia, hypertension, thyrotoxicosis and cardiac insufficiency, epilepsy, Parkinson's disease. Intestinal anastomoses, anticholinesterase may produce rupture or leakage of intestinal contents. Caution, in presence of pyrexia (sweating inhibited; especially children).

Pregnancy, Lactation: Safety not established.

ADR: See Notes below.

Notes: See 14.1.3 Anaesthetic Adjuncts. See Glycopyrronium above, Neostigmine below.

Glycopyrronium, Neostigmine Parenteral *(Concordia)* A.
Price, 0.5mg/2.5mg, 1mL (10) €14.55 (PTW).
Injection, glycopyrronium bromide 0.5mg, neostigmine metilsulfate 2.5mg per 1mL. Colourless soln. *Sodium 3mg/mL.*

Dexmedetomidine

ATC Code: N05CM18. **Sport:** Permitted.
Driving: Not relevant.

Indications: Adult sedation in ICU (sedation level not deeper than arousal in response to verbal stimulation).

Dose: Adult, Elderly: Already intubated and sedated, switch to dexmedetomidine, initially 0.7mcg/kg/HOUR; adjust stepwise within range 0.2mcg/kg/hour to max. 1.4mcg/kg/HOUR to achieve desired level of sedation. Frail, lower starting infusion. Loading dose not recommended. *Admin,* as diluted IV infusion using controlled infusion device.

Child: Under 18 years, no dosing recommendation.

Hepatic Impairment: Consider reduced maintenance dose. Severe, caution (reduced clearance, over sedation).

Cl: Advanced heart block unless paced, uncontrolled hypotension, cerebrovascular conditions.

Interactions: Effect of Other Drugs on Dexmedetomidine: *Enhanced effects (sedative, anaesthetic, cardiorespiratory) with co-admin*: Anaesthetics, sedatives, hypnotics, opioids, isoflurane, propofol, alfentanil, midazolam.

Effect of Dexmedetomidine on Other Drugs: Drugs causing hypotension or bradycardia (beta blockers): *Effect possibly enhanced*.

SP: DO NOT, use as induction agent for intubation or sedation during muscle relaxant use (does not cause deep sedation); admin by loading or bolus dose; use for sole treatment of status epilepticus (does not suppress seizure activity). Caution, bradycardia, impaired peripheral autonomic activity, hypertension (reduce infusion rate), myocardial or cerebral ischaemia (reduce dose). Agitation, hypertension after discontinuation, consider withdrawal reaction. Malignant hyperthermia-sensitive individuals, not recommended. Sustained unexplained fever, discontinue. Non-intubated patients, respiratory depression risk, apnoea (monitor respiration).

Pregnancy, Lactation: Pregnancy or women of childbearing potential not using contraception, not recommended. Lactation, stop breastfeeding or stop drug.

ADR: See Notes below.

Notes: See 14.1.3 Anaesthetic Adjuncts.

Dexdor Parenteral 100mcg/mL *(Orion)* A. HOS.
Price, (4) 4mL, €160.00; 10mL, €360.00 (PTW).
Infusion, dexmedetomidine HCl. Clear colourless conc for soln. pH 4.5-7.0.

14.1.3 Other Anaesthetic Adjuncts

Midazolam (anaesthesia)

ATC Code: N05CD08. **Sport:** Permitted.
Driving: Not recommended.

Indications: Conscious sedation before and during diagnostic or therapeutic procedures with or without local anaesthesia. Premedication before induction of anaesthesia. Sedation in ICU; induction of anaesthesia *(Hypnovel, Midazolam Concordia)*; induction agent or sedative component in combined anaesthesia *(Hypnovel)*.

Dose: Adult: Conscious sedation, initially 2-2.5mg IV over 30 seconds; titrate by 0.5-1mg increments; usual range 2.5-7.5mg.
Anaesthesia induction, IV 0.15-0.2mg/kg (0.3-0.35mg/kg without premedication); sedative in combined anaesthesia, intermittent 0.03-0.1mg/kg doses OR continuous IV infusion 0.03-0.1mg/kg/hour.
ICU sedation, loading dose, 0.03-0.3mg/kg in 1-2.5mg increments; maintenance 0.03-0.2mg/kg/hour.
Premedication, 0.07-0.1mg/kg admin IM.
Elderly: Conscious sedation, initially 0.5-1mg IV; titrate by 0.5-1mg increments; total max. dose less than 3.5mg.
Anaesthesia induction, 0.1-0.5mg/kg (0.15-0.3mg/kg without premedication); sedative in combined anaesthesia, lower doses than for Adults under 60 years.
Premedication, 0.025-0.05mg/kg admin IM; over 60 years, debilitated or chronically ill (caution). ICU, as for Adult.
Child: Conscious sedation, *IV*, under 6 months, only for ICU use. Age 6 months to 5 years, initially 0.05-0.1mg/kg; total max. dose less than 6mg; age 6-12 years, initially 0.025-0.05mg/kg; total max. dose less than 10mg. *IM*, age 1-15 years, 0.05-0.15mg/kg (IM route only for exceptional cases). *Rectal*, range 0.3-0.5mg/kg.
Premedication, age 1-15 years, 0.08-0.2mg/kg; use under 6 months, caution; IV or IM deep into large muscle mass.
Midazolam (Concordia), anaesthesia induction, over 7 years, 0.15mg/kg IV.
Renal Impairment: Prolonged infusion (ICU), mean duration of sedative effect increased.
Hepatic Impairment: Clearance reduced; effect may be prolonged; adjust dose.
CI: Use for conscious sedation with severe respiratory failure or acute respiratory depression.
Interactions: Effect of Other Drugs on Midazolam IV: *Caution:* Azole antifungals (itraconazole, fluconazole, ketoconazole), macrolides (erythromycin, clarithromycin), saquinavir, other protease inhibitors (ritonavir, indinavir, nelfinavir, amprenavir), verapamil, diltiazem. *Effect potentiated:* Other CNS depressants (opiates, antipsychotics, other benzodiazepines, phenobarbital, sedative antidepressants, antihistamines, centrally acting antihypertensives, alcohol).
Effect of Midazolam IV on Other Drugs: Inhalation anaesthetics: *Minimum alveolar conc required for anaesthesia decreased (IV midazolam).*
SP: Only for use if age- and size-appropriate resuscitation facilities available; IV admin may depress myocardial contractility, cause apnoea. Respiratory depression, apnoea, respiratory arrest, and/or cardiac arrest (more likely if injected too rapidly or high dose). Use for premedication, adequate observation mandatory. *Special caution*, high risk (over 60 years, chronically ill, debilitated, chronic respiratory insufficiency, impaired cardiac function, chronic renal failure, impaired hepatic function, paediatrics with cardiovascular instability); lower doses, continuous monitoring. Caution, alcohol or drug abuse, myasthenia gravis. Long-term ICU sedation (tolerance, dependence, withdrawal risk). Anterograde amnesia, paradoxical reactions (agitation, involuntary movements, hyperactivity, hostility, rage, aggressiveness, paroxysmal excitement, assault). Delayed elimination (liver dysfunction, low cardiac output). Preterm infants and neonates, increased apnoea risk. Cardiovascular changes (decreased mean arterial pressure, cardiac output, stroke volume, systemic vascular

396

resistance); caution with impaired myocardial oxygen delivery capacity, hypovolaemia.
Pregnancy, Lactation: Pregnancy, only if clearly necessary; if admin during late phase of pregnancy or during labour at high doses, effects on neonate to be expected (hypothermia, hypotonia, moderate respiratory depression); avoid during C-section. Lactation, not recommended for 24 hours following admin.
ADR: See Notes below (benzodiazepines).
Notes: See 14.1.3 Anaesthetic Adjuncts. See 3.3.5 Benzodiazepine Anxiolytics.

> **Hypnovel Parenteral** *(Roche)* A. GMS.
> Price, (10) 10mg/2mL, €9.68. 10mg/5mL, €11.49.
> Injection, midazolam HCl 10mg/2mL (5mL). Clear colourless soln.
> Sodium 2.2mg/mL (10mg/2mL amp), 3.48mg/mL (10mg/5mL amp).

> **Midazolam (Accord) Parenteral** *(Accord)* A.
> Price, 1mg/mL (10) 5mL, €7.99. 5mg/mL (1) 10mL, €28.99.
> Injection or infusion, midazolam 1(5)mg/mL. Clear colourless (pale-yellow) soln. Sodium 3.53mg/mL (1mg/mL), 1.96mg/mL (5mg/mL).

> **Midazolam (Concordia) Parenteral** *(Concordia)* A.
> Price, (10) 10mg/2mL, €7.16. 10mg/5mL, €8.50 (PTW).
> Injection or infusion, midazolam 2(5)mg/mL. Clear colourless (slightly yellow) soln. Essentially sodium-free.

Neostigmine

ATC Code: N07AA01. **Sport:** Permitted.
Driving: Caution.

Indications: Symptomatic treatment, myasthenia gravis. Reversal of effects of non-depolarising neuromuscular blockers. Management, post-op distension, paralytic ileus, urinary retention.
Dose: Adult: Myasthenia gravis, 1-2.5mg IM or SC at intervals during day when strength most needed; range 5-20mg/day.
Reversal non-depolarising neuromuscular blockers, 0.05-0.07mg/kg with or after atropine sulfate by slow IV injection over 60 seconds; max. 5mg.
Post-op distension, 0.5-2.5mg SC or IM.
Elderly: May be more susceptible to dysrhythmias.
Child: Neonatal myasthenia gravis, initially 0.1mg IM; then titrate in range 0.05-0.25mg; duration rarely beyond 8 weeks.
Reversal non-depolarising neuromuscular blockers, as for Adult; max. 2.5mg.
Post-op distension, 0.125-1mg SC or IM.
CI: Mechanical obstruction (GI, urinary tract), peritonitis, doubtful bowel viability.
Interactions: Effect of Other Drugs on Neostigmine: *Co-admin not recommended (depolarising blocking effect potentiated):* Suxamethonium. *Co-admin not recommended (vagotonic effects potentiated):* Cyclopropane, halothane, thiopentone (may be used after withdrawal of these agents). *Muscarinic effect antagonised:* Atropine. *Bradycardia, hypotension risk:* Beta-blockers.
SP: Atropine sulfate (0.6-1.2mg) should always be available to counteract excessive muscarinic effects. Caution, bradycardia, cardiac arrhythmia, bronchial asthma, recent coronary occlusion, epilepsy, hypotension, Parkinsonism, hyperthyroidism, peptic ulcer.
Pregnancy, Lactation: Only if considered essential.
ADR: See Notes below.
Notes: See 14.1.3 Anaesthetic Adjuncts.

> **Neostigmine Parenteral 2.5mg/mL** *(Concordia)* A.
> Price, 2.5mg/1mL (10) €9.17 (PTW).
> Injection, neostigmine metilsuphate. Clear colourless soln.

Sugammadex

ATC Code: V03AB35. **Sport:** Permitted.
Driving: Hospital use.

Indications: Reversal, neuromuscular blockade induced by rocuronium or vecuronium; paediatrics, only routine reversal of rocuronium blockade.
Dose: Adult, Elderly: *Routine reversal*, 4mg/kg if recovery

has reached at least 1-2 post-tetanic counts; dose depends on level of neuromuscular blockade required; 2mg/kg if spontaneous recovery has occurred.

Immediate reversal following rocuronium, 16mg/kg. Exceptional situation of re-occurrence of neuromuscular blockade, after initial 2-4mg/kg a repeat dose of 4mg/kg is recommended. Wait 24 hours before rocuronium or vecuronium re-admin; if blockade required before 24 hours, use nonsteroidal neuromuscular blocker. Obese, base dose on actual body weight. *Elderly*, recovery tends to be slower. Admin IV as single bolus injection given rapidly (within 10 seconds) into an existing IV line.

Child: Routine reversal, age 2-17 years, 2mg/kg (rocuronium-induced blockade). Immediate reversal, not recommended.

Dilute to 10mg/mL to increase accuracy of dosing in children.

Renal Impairment: CrCl (mL/min) below 30, not recommended.

Hepatic Impairment: Severe or accompanied by coagulopathy, caution.

Interactions: Effect of Other Drugs on Sugammadex: *Delayed recovery*: Toremifene, IV (fusidic acid, high dose flucloxacillin). *Caution*: Anticoagulants (see SP).

Effect of Sugammadex on Other Drugs: Hormonal contraceptives: *Reduced efficacy*.

SP: Ventilatory support mandatory. Recurrence of neuromuscular blockade usually with sub-optimal dosing. Caution, with therapeutic anticoagulation for pre-existing or co-morbid condition; cannot exclude increased bleeding risk with (hereditary Vitamin K dependent clotting factor deficiencies, pre-existing coagulopathies, on coumarin derivatives and INR above 3.5, using anticoagulants and receiving 16mg/kg sugammadex). Intentional neuromuscular blockade reversal during anaesthesia, signs of light anaesthesia noted (movement, coughing, grimacing, sucking of tracheal tube). Marked bradycardia observed within minutes of admin. ICU use, not investigated. *NOT for use* to reverse block induced by nonsteroidals or steroidals other than rocuronium or vecuronium. Longer recovery time associated with conditions of prolonged circulation (cardiovascular disease, old age, oedematous state, severe hepatic impairment). Allergic reactions, QTc prolongation.

Pregnancy, Lactation: Pregnancy, caution. Lactation, can be used.

ADR: See Notes below.

Notes: See 14.1.3 Anaesthetic Adjuncts.

Bridion Parenteral *(MSD)* A. HOS.
Price, (10) 2mL, €770.19; 5mL, €1930.20 (PTW).
Injection, sugammadex sodium 100mg/mL (1mL, 2mL, 5mL). Clear colourless (slightly yellow) soln pH 7-8. *Sodium up to 9.7mg/mL*. **Store:** Do not freeze.

14.1.4 - Inhalation Anaesthetics

In This Chapter: *Isoflurane, sevoflurane.*

Class Effects
Driving: General anaesthetics may cause a slight decrease in intellectual function for 2-3 days following anaesthesia; small mood changes and symptoms may persist for up to 6 days; caution when resuming normal daily activities, including driving or operating machinery.

Used in specialised units. Always consult the manufacturers Full Prescribing Information.

Indications: General anaesthesia (GA), induction and maintenance. Restrict use in dental anaesthesia to hospitals or day care units. For Elderly and Child dose, see manufacturers Full Prescribing Information.

CI: Hypersensitivity to any member of the class (history of hepatotoxicity, fever, leucocytosis and/or eosinophilia related to anaesthesia). Known or suspected genetic susceptibility to malignant hyperthermia. Where general anaesthesia is contraindicated.

Interactions: Effect of Halogenated Anaesthetics on Other Drugs: All muscle relaxants (especially non-depolarising): *Effect potentiated, reduce dose.* Adrenaline: *Myocardium sensitised to arrhythmogenic effect of exogenously admin adrenaline*

SP: Patients should be constantly monitored (ECG, BP, oxygen saturation, end tidal CO_2); full resuscitative equipment and trained staff to be available. All general anaesthetics, admin without airway care may result in fatal respiratory complications. For delivery via a specifically calibrated vaporiser. Hypotension and respiratory depression increase as anaesthesia is deepened. Repeated exposure to halogenated hydrocarbons in relatively short interval, increased hepatic injury risk (mild transient increased liver enzymes to fatal hepatic necrosis, rare). Potent inhalation anaesthetics may trigger skeletal muscle hypermetabolic state leading to high O_2 demand and clinical syndrome malignant hyperthermia (discontinue triggering agent, IV dantrolene, supportive therapy). *Caution*, cardiac arrhythmias due to increased serum potassium; caution, latent or overt neuromuscular disease, paediatrics. Renal insufficiency. Patients with mitochondrial disorders.

Pregnancy, Lactation: For use in pregnancy only if clearly necessary. Inhalation agents have a relaxant effect on the uterus with potential risk for uterine bleeding; exercise clinical judgement during obstetric anaesthesia; use lowest possible conc. Lactation, caution.

ADR: Adverse reactions are generally dose dependent and extensions of the pharmacophysiolgic effects (cardio-respiratory depression, hypotension, arrhythmias) see manufacturers Full Prescribing Information.

Notes: See 14.1 General Anaesthesia.

Isoflurane

ATC Code: N01AB06. **Sport:** Permitted.
Driving: See Notes below.
Dose: Adult, Elderly: *Premedication*, individualise with consideration for respiratory depressant effect of isoflurane; anticholinergics may be advisable in paediatrics. *Induction*, IV induction agent (to avoid excitement) followed by inhalation initiated at 0.5% conc (range 1.5-3% usually produce surgical anaesthesia in 7-10 minutes); maintenance, surgical anaesthesia, 1-2.5% in oxygen/nitrous oxide mixtures; additional 0.5-1% may be needed if oxygen is used alone; C-section, 0.5-0.75% in oxygen/nitrous oxide mixture. *Elderly*, usually require lesser concentrations to maintain surgical anaesthesia.

Child: Not recommended (cough, breath-holding, desaturation, increased secretions, laryngospasm).

Hepatic Impairment: Pre-existing disease, caution.

CI: Liver dysfunction, jaundice, unexplained fever, leucocytosis, eosinophilia after previous halogenated anaesthetics. Use in dental procedures outside a hospital or day care unit.

Interactions: Effect of Other Drugs on Isoflurane: *Co-admin not advised*: Succinylcholine with inhaled anaesthetics (increased serum potassium); cardiac arrhythmias and death in paediatric patients). *Co-admin caution*: Aminoglycosides, beta-blockers (may be used with propranolol). *MAC decreased*: Nitrous oxide. *Increased isoflurane metabolism*; *increased plasma fluoride*: Isoniazid (increased hepatotoxicity), ALCOHOL.

Effect of Isoflurane on Other Drugs: Adrenaline: *Prevent overdosage or unduly rapid absorption*. Non-depolarising muscle relaxants: *Action markedly potentiated*.

SP: Profound respiratory depressant effect, caution premedication choice (accentuated by narcotics). Myocardial depression related to depth of anaesthesia. Increased intracranial pressure, caution; may cause rise in CSF pressure and cerebral blood flow. Hepatic injury (mild transient increased liver enzymes to fatal hepatic necrosis). Neostigmine does not antagonise muscle relaxant effect of isoflurane. Malignant hyperthermia (fatal).

ADR: See Notes below.

14.1.5   Other General Anaesthetics

Notes: See 14.1.4 Inhalation Anaesthetics.

Forane Inhalation *(AbbVie)* A.
Price, not published by company.
Inhalation vapour liquid, isoflurane 99.9% w/w. Slightly musty odour for vaporisation and admin as inhalation gas.

Sevoflurane

ATC Code: N01AB08. **Sport:** Permitted.
Driving: See Notes below.

Dose: Adult: Individualise dose; titrate to desired effect according to patient age, clinical status. A short acting barbiturate or other IV induction agent may be admin followed by sevoflurane inhalation.

Induction, inspired concentrations of up to max. 8% sevorane usually produces surgical anaesthesia in less than 2 minutes (adults, children). *Maintenance,* 0.5-3% with or without nitrous oxide. Emergence times usually shorter, patient may require post-operative pain relief earlier. Select premedication according to individual patient need.

Elderly: Minimum alveolar conc (MAC) values decrease with increasing age; average conc sevoflurane required to achieve MAC at age 80 years, approx. 50% of that required age 20 years.

Child: See manufacturers Full Prescribing Information.

Renal Impairment: Caution.

Hepatic Impairment: Underlying conditions or drugs causing hepatic dysfunction, exercise clinical judgement.

Interactions: Effect of Other Drugs on Sevoflurane: *Caution*: Isoprenaline, adrenaline, noradrenaline (ventricular arrhythmia risk), non-selective MAOIs (stop 2 weeks prior to surgery), calcium antagonists (additive negative inotropic effect), succinylcholine (increased serum potassium; arrhythmias, death (paediatrics). *Synergistic fall (heart rate, BP, respiratory rate)*: Opioids (alfentanil, sufentanil). *Acute hypertensive episode*: Amphetamines, ephedrine. *Increased sevoflurane metabolism; increased plasma fluoride conc*: Isoniazid, ALCOHOL. *Severe hypotension, delayed emergence*: St John's Wort (long-term treatment). *Sevoflurane MAC reduced*: Nitrous oxide.

Effect of Sevoflurane on Other Drugs: Beta-blockers: *Increased negative inotropic, chronotropic, dromotropic effects.* Verapamil: *Atrioventricular conduction impairment.* Isoniazid: *Increased hepatotoxic effects.*

SP: Dose-dependent BP decrease. May cause respiratory depression (augmented by narcotic premedication, other agents causing respiratory depression). Maintain haemodynamic stability to avoid myocardial ischaemia (CAD patients). Seizures reported. *Paediatrics,* agitation with rapid emergence; Pompe's disease, ventricular arrhythmia. Higher degree of bradycardia (Down's syndrome).

Pregnancy, Lactation: Not known if excreted in breast milk.

ADR: See Notes below.

Notes: See 14.1.4 Inhalation Anaesthetics.

Sevorane (AbbVie) Inhalation *(AbbVie)* A. HOS.
Price, 250mL, €80.67 (PTW).
Inhalation gas, sevoflurane 100% v/v. Non-flammable, volatile liquid or admin as inhalation anaesthetic.
Sevoflurane Baxter Inhalation *(Baxter)* A.
Price, not published by company.
Inhalation vapour, liquid, sevoflurane 100% v/v. Clear colourless.

14.1.5 - Other General Anaesthetics

In This Chapter: *Ketamine, propofol, thiopental.*

Class Effects
Driving: See Notes below.

Used in specialised units. Always consult the manufacturers Full Prescribing Information.

CI: Hypersensitivity to any member of the class.

SP: Only for use in hospital by anaesthetists, except under emergency conditions (ketamine). Outpatient use, do not release patient until recovery from anaesthesia is complete; should be accompanied by a responsible adult. Caution, cardiac, respiratory, renal or hepatic impairment, hypovolaemic or debilitated patients.

ADR: See manufacturers Full Prescribing Information.

Notes: See 14.1 General Anaesthesia. See 14.1.4 Inhalation Anaesthetics (driving)

Ketamine

ATC Code: N01AX03. **Sport:** Permitted.
Driving: See Notes below.

Indications: Anaesthetic, short diagnostic and surgical procedures (no skeletal muscle relaxation needed). Anaesthesia induction, prior to other general anaesthetics. Anaesthetic supplementation. Specific areas of application or types of procedures e.g. IM route more convenient; debridement, painful dressings, skin grafting (burns); superficial surgical procedures; neurological, radiodiagnostic, therapeutic procedures in children (to abolish movement), airway control difficult.

Dose: Adult, Elderly: Onset and duration, 1-2mg/kg IV produces anaesthesia within 30-60 seconds lasting 5-10 minutes; 10mg/kg IM produces anaesthesia within 3-4 minutes lasting 12-25 minutes. All doses expressed as ketamine *base.*

Sole anaesthetic agent, IV infusion, induction, 0.5-2mg/kg as total dose; maintenance, 10-40mcg/kg/min (approx. 1-3mg/min) by microdrip infusion OR intermittent injection, 1-4.5mg/kg IV (slowly over 60-120 sec) OR 6.5-13mg/kg IM (usually 10mg/kg); maintenance by additional IV or IM doses. Induction, prior to general anaesthetic full IV or IM dose as for sole agent above; supplement, to other anaesthetic, usually as for sole agent; may be able to reduce dose.

Obstetrics, vaginal delivery or C-section 0.2-1mg/kg IV recommended.

Child: As for Adult above.

CI: Where elevated BP would be a serious hazard. Eclampsia or pre-eclampsia, severe coronary or myocardial disease, CVA, cerebral trauma, psychiatric disorders (history).

Interactions: Effect of Other Drugs on Ketamine: *Admixture not recommended*: Barbiturates, diazepam. *Co-admin not recommended*: Gallamine (tachycardia). *Co-admin caution*: Thyroid hormones (hypertension, tachycardia). Pancuronium (hypertension, tachycardia). *Co-admin caution*: Thyroid hormones (hypertension, tachycardia). *Prolonged recovery time*: Barbiturates, narcotics, benzodiazepines (premedication). *Elimination half-life lengthened, delayed recovery; cardiovascular depression (bradycardia, hypotension, decreased cardiac output risk)*: Halogenated anaesthetics (halothane, enflurane). *Hepatic metabolism inhibited*: Halothane. *Plasma levels increased, clearance reduced*: Diazepam, other benzodiazepines, CYP3A4 enzyme inhibitors. *Dose reduction*: Nitrous oxide. *CNS depression potentiated*: Other CNS depressants (ethanol, phenothiazines, sedating H1-blockers, skeletal muscle relaxants). *Increased hypotension risk*: Antihypertensives.

Effect of Ketamine on Other Drugs: Atracurium, tubocurarine: *Neuromuscular blocking effects enhanced.* Thiopental: *Hypnotic effect antagonised.* Theophylline: *Seizure threshold reduced.*

SP: NOTE: Caution, surgical procedures involving pharynx, larynx or trachea (increases salivary and tracheo-bronchial secretions); does not reliably suppress pharyngeal or laryngeal reflexes. Avoid mechanical stimulation of pharynx. Use atropine, hyoscine or other drying agent before use. Emergence delirium, reduced if verbal and tactile stimulation minimised; monitor vital signs. Following IV admin, high plasma concentrations depress respiration, pharyngo-laryngeal reflexes; minimised by slow injection of dilute soln. Increased myocardial oxygen consumption, caution (hypovolaemia, dehydration, cardiac disease especially CHF, myocardial ischaemia, MI, mild/moderate hypertension, tachyarrhythmias). Pulmonary or upper RTI (gag reflex sensitised, potential laryngospasm). Hypertension, cardiac decompensation, monitor.

398

Increased CSF pressure. Rapid admin, transient respiratory depression or apnoea, enhanced pressor response. Procedures involving visceral pain pathways, supplement with agent for visceral pain. Caution, use in chronic alcoholics or acutely intoxicated, increased IOP, neurotic traits or psychiatric illness, acute intermittent porphyria, seizures, hyperthyroidism/thyroid replacement, intracranial mass lesion or head injury. Dependence, tolerance if used daily for few weeks especially with history of drug abuse/dependence; been reported as a drug of abuse. Not indicated or recommended for long-term use. Hepatotoxicity with extended use (3 days or more).

Pregnancy, Lactation: Not recommended except for C-section or vaginal delivery. Neonates exposed to ketamine during delivery have experience respiratory depression and low Apgar scores. Lactation, not recommended.

ADR: See Notes below.

Notes: See 14.1.5 General Anaesthetics.

Ketalar Parenteral *(Pfizer)* A. HOS.
Price, (12) 10mg/mL (20mL) €57.65. (1) 50mg/mL (10mL) €7.98 (PTW).
Injection (IV or IM) or IV infusion, ketamine HCl 10mg(50mg)/mL. Clear colourless aqueous soln. *Sodium 2.6mg/mL (only 10mg/mL injection)*. Store: Below 25 deg C; do not freeze.

Propofol

ATC Code: N01AX10. **Sport:** Permitted.
Driving: See Notes below.
Indications: Short-acting IV general anaesthetic (GA) for induction and maintenance; sedation of ventilated patients in ICU; conscious sedation for surgical and diagnostic procedures.

Dose: Adult: *General anaesthetic*, induction, titrate against response, 40mg every 10 seconds; usually 1.5-2.5mg/kg; maintenance, continuous infusion 4-12mg/kg/hour. Repeat bolus in increments of 25-50mg.

ICU sedation, continuous infusion 0.3-4mg/kg/hour (not recommended under 16 years). Conscious sedation, initiate with 0.5-1mg/kg over 1-5 minutes; single infusion max. 12 hours.

The Diprifusor TCI system may be used for induction and maintenance of general anaesthetic. Not recommended for ICU use or use in children.

Elderly: Reduce dose.

Child: *General anaesthesia*, induction, over 1 month, titrate slowly until clinical signs of anaesthesia; over 8 years, usually 2.5mg/kg; under 8 (especially 1 month to 3 years) may need higher dose; maintenance, range 9-15mg/kg/hour; age 1 month to 3 years as above. 1 month, not recommended. *Conscious sedation*, usually 1-2mg/kg for onset; maintenance usually 1.5-9mg/kg/hour. *ICU sedation*, use contraindicated in patients 16 years and younger as safety/efficacy not established. Admin by a Diprifusor TCI system not recommended for any indication in children.

CI: ICU sedation, 16 years and younger.

Interactions: Effect of Other Drugs on Propofol: *Consider propofol dose reduction*: Valproate. *Hypotensive effect potentiated*: Opiate analgesics; rifampicin (profound hypotension).

SP: Supplementary analgesia required. Monitor, conscious sedation, hypotension, airway obstruction, O2 desaturation; involuntary movements may occur. Post-operative unconsciousness. Bradycardia, asystole (consider anticholinergic before induction). Convulsion risk. Disorders of fat metabolism, other conditions requiring cautious use of lipid emulsions; monitor lipid levels (if risk of fat overload). Metabolic acidosis, rhabdomyolysis, hyperkalaemia and/or rapidly progressive cardiac failure (high doses). EDTA is a chelator of metal ions, including zinc; prolonged admin, consider zinc supplements (burns, diarrhoea and/or major sepsis). Abuse of, and dependence on, predominantly by healthcare professionals. *Caution*, mitochondrial disease, peanut/soya allergy. *ICU management*, use for sedation associated with a constellation of metabolic derangements and organ system

failures that may result in death (Propofol Infusion Syndrome). Risk factors (decreased oxygen delivery to tissues, serious neurological injury and/or sepsis, high dosages of vasoconstrictors, steroids, inotropes and or propofol).

Pregnancy, Lactation: Pregnancy, only if clearly necessary; crosses placenta, caution, neonatal depression. Anaesthesia, avoid doses above 2.5mg/kg (induction) or 6mg/kg/h (maintenance). Lactation, stop breastfeeding; discard breast milk for 24 hours after admin.

ADR: See Notes below.

Notes: See 14.1.5 General Anaesthetics.

Diprivan 1% Parenteral *(Aspen)* A. HOS.
Price, (1) 50mL, €12.54 (PTW).
Injection or infusion, propofol 10mg/mL PFS. White (almost) homogenous emulsion. *Soya-bean oil, sodium 0.0018mmoL/mL; preservative free*. Store: Below 25 deg C; do not freeze.

Thiopental

ATC Code: N01AF03. **Sport:** Permitted.
Driving: Vertigo, disorientation, sedation may be prolonged; do not drive within 24-36 hours.

Indications: Induction, short-duration general anaesthesia; control of convulsive disorders. May be used rectally to produce basal anaesthesia. Reduction of intracranial pressure in patients with increase intracranial pressure if controlled ventilation is provided.

Dose: Adult, Elderly: PARENTERAL (IV), anaesthesia induction, 100-150mg injection over 10-15 seconds; if needed a repeat dose of 100-150mg can be given over 1 minute; anaesthesia usually produced 1 minute after IV admin. Average adult dose (70kg adult) roughly 200-300mg; max. 500mg. Admin atropine (or similar) prior to thiopental to depress vagal reflexes, mucous secretions; also narcotic analgesics (thiopental poor analgesic).

Convulsive states, 75-125mg as soon as possible after convulsion begins.

Neurological patients with raised intracranial pressure, intermittent bolus injection of 1.5-3mg/kg to reduce intracranial pressure if controlled ventilation provided.

RECTAL, 25-45mg/kg dissolved in 25mL water; anaesthetic effect within 10 minutes of admin. See SP below.

Child: Range 2-7mg/kg. See Adult above.

Renal Impairment: Severe, caution.

Hepatic Impairment: Consider dose reduction.

CI: Respiratory obstruction, acute asthma, severe shock, dystrophia myotonica. Porphyria (any barbiturate). Hypersensitivity or idiosyncratic reactions to barbiturates.

Interactions: Effect of Other Drugs on Thiopental: *Consider dose reduction*: Sulphafurazole, narcotic analgesic premedication.

Effect of Thiopental on Other Drugs: Beta-blockers, calcium channel blockers: *Enhanced hypotensive effect*. Antipsychotics, anxiolytics: *Enhanced sedative effect*.

SP: Rapid injection produces more rapid anaesthesia and recovery. May be used non-ventilated undergoing short duration procedure. Respiratory depression (apnoea, reduced cardiac output, fall in BP); may precipitate acute circulatory failure with cardiovascular disease (constrictive pericarditis). Associated with severe or refractory hypokalaemia during infusion; severe rebound hyperkalaemia may occur after infusion cessation (neurological patients with raised intracranial pressure). Shock, dehydration, severe anaemia, toxaemia, myxoedema, other metabolic disorders, reduce dose. Alcohol habituation/addiction, drug abuse, increase dose, use supplementary analgesia. Accidental intra-arterial injection, severe arterial spasm, intense burning injection site pain; if occurs, use antispasmodic (papaverine) or prilocaine; anticoagulant to reduce haematoma risk. Adrenocortical insufficiency or raised intracranial pressure, caution. See ADR below.

Pregnancy, Lactation: Can be used without adverse effects during pregnancy; max. dose 250mg. Crosses

14.1.6   Malignant Hyperthermia

placental barrier, appears in breast milk; use if benefit outweighs risk.

ADR: See Notes below.

Notes: See 14.1.5 General Anaesthetics.

Thiopental Parenteral *(KyowaKirin)* A.
Price, 500mg (25) €136.49.
Injection, thiopental sodium 500mg. Yellow (white) freeze-dried powder for soln.

14.1.6 - Malignant Hyperthermia

Class Effects

Dantrolene (IV) is used for the treatment of malignant hyperthermia.

Notes: See 4.3.1 Skeletal Muscle Relaxants (dantrolene).

14.2 - Local Anaesthesia

In This Chapter: *Bupivacaine (adrenaline, glucose combinations), levobupivacaine, lidocaine (adrenaline, chlorhexidine; prilocaine combinations), ropivacaine, tetracaine.*

Class Effects

Lidocaine is also used in emergency management of ventricular arrhythmias, see Notes below (lidocaine). Adrenaline is used in combination with local anaesthetics when a vasoconstrictor effect is required.

CI: Hypersensitivity to any member of the group.

Intrathecal anaesthesia, active CNS disease (meningitis, poliomyelitis, intracranial haemorrhage, sub-acute combined degeneration of the cord due to pernicious anaemia, cerebral and spinal tumours; raised intracranial pressure; spinal stenosis; spondylitis, tumour, TB of spine), recent trauma in vertebral column; septicaemia; pyogenic infection (skin, adjacent lumbar puncture site); cardiogenic or hypovolaemic shock; coagulation (disorders or treatment).

Adrenaline co-admin, anaesthesia in areas supplied by end arteries or with compromised blood supply (digits, nose, external ear, penis), spinal anaesthesia.

Interactions: Effect of Other Drugs on Local Anaesthetics (including with Adrenaline): *Additive cardiac effects:* Class III Antiarrhythmics (amiodarone). *Adrenaline, avoid co-admin:* MAOIs, TCADs (prolonged hypertension), ergot oxytocics (severe hypertension; CVA or cardiac accidents), phenothiazines, butyrophenones (may oppose vasoconstrictor effects), anaesthesia (halothane, enflurane) (cardiac arrhythmia risk), non-cardioselective beta-blockers (propranolol) (enhanced pressor effects). *Lidocaine clearance reduced (high, repeated doses):* Cimetidine, beta-blockers (no clinical importance with short-term lidocaine at recommended dose).

SP: Monitor cardiovascular and respiratory vital signs, state of consciousness after local anaesthetic injection (sympathetic blockage during spinal anaesthesia may cause peripheral vasodilatation and hypotension). Monitor, level of anaesthesia (not always predictable in spinal techniques). High/total spinal blockade can cause cardiovascular and respiratory depression (increased risk, elderly, late stages of pregnancy); reduce dose. Exacerbation of CNS disease with local anaesthetic admin via intrathecal or epidural route. Use with caution (epilepsy; impaired cardiac conduction, respiratory and hepatic function; severe renal dysfunction, elderly, poor general condition). Partial or complete heart block, caution. Adrenaline co-admin, caution, hypertension, arteriosclerotic heart disease, cerebrovascular insufficiency, heart block, thyrotoxicosis, diabetes. NOTE: Adjust dose according to patient response, area to be anaesthetised, vascularity of tissue, number of neuronal segments to be blocked; use lowest conc and smallest dose to produce effect. Intrathecal anaesthesia only under supervision of clinicians with necessary knowledge and experience.

Pregnancy, Lactation: Generally only if benefit outweighs

risk. Adrenaline may decrease uterine blood flow and contractility especially if inadvertently injected into maternal blood vessels.

ADR: Acute systemic toxicity (CNS, cardiovascular) due to high blood conc with (accidental intravascular injection, overdose, rapid absorption from highly vascularised areas). Hypotension, bradycardia, hypertension, cardiac conduction depression, arrhythmias, nausea, vomiting, urinary retention, paraesthesia, dizziness, headache. Local application site reactions. See manufacturers Full Prescribing Information.

Notes: See 14.1 General Anaesthesia. See 2.5.2 Class Ib Antiarrhythmics (lidocaine).

Bupivacaine

ATC Code: N01BB01. **Sport:** Permitted.

Driving: Direct anaesthetic effect; also mild effect on mental function and co-ordination.

Indications: Surgical anaesthesia (adults, children from age 12 years), acute pain management (adults, children from age 1 year).

Dose: Adult: Lumbar epidural, surgery or C-section, (conc 5mg/mL) 15-30mL (75-150mg), onset 15-30 minutes, duration 2-3 hours; thoracic epidural, surgery (conc 2.5mg/mL), 5-15mL (12.5-37.5mg) onset 10-15 minutes, duration 1.5-2 hours OR (conc 5mg/mL) 5-10mL (25-50mg), onset 10-15 minutes, duration 2-3 hours; caudal epidural block (conc 2.5mg/mL), 20-30mL (50-75mg) onset 20-30 minutes, duration 1-2 hours OR (conc 5mg/mL) 20-30mL (100-150mg), onset 15-30 minutes, duration 2-3 hours.

Major nerve block (brachial plexus, femoral, sciatic), (conc 5mg/mL) 10-35 mL (50-175mg), onset 15-30 minutes, duration 4-8 hours; field block (minor nerve blocks and infiltration), (conc 2.5mg/mL) less than 60mL (less than 150mg) onset 1-3 minutes, duration 3-4 hours OR (conc 5mg/mL) less than 30mL (less than 150mg), onset 1-10 minutes, duration 3-8 hours.

Acute pain management (use only conc 2.5mg/mL), lumbar epidural, intermittent injection (post-operative pain), 6-15mL (minimum interval 30 minutes) (15-37.5mg), onset 2-5 minutes, duration 1-2 hours OR continuous infusion, 5-7.5mL/hour (12.5-18.8mg/hour); thoracic epidural, continuous infusion, 4-7.5mL/hour (10-18.8mg/hour).

Intra-articular block (following knee arthroscopy), 40mL or less (100mg or less), onset 5-10 minutes, duration 2-4 hours after wash-out. Field block (minor nerve blocks and infiltration), 60mL or less (150mg or less), onset 1-3 minutes, duration 3-4 hours.

Elderly: Including debilitated, reduce dose.

Child: Age 1-12 years, acute pain management (caudal, lumbar, thoracic epidural) (conc 2.5mg/mL) 0.6-0.8mL/kg (1.5-2mg/kg), onset 20-30 minutes, duration 2-6 hours. Field block (minor nerve blocks and infiltration) and peripheral nerve blocks (conc 2.5mg/mL or 5mg/mL), 0.5-2mg/kg. Max. 2mg/kg. Peripheral nerve block onset/duration depends on type of block and dose.

Renal Impairment: See SP below.

Hepatic Impairment: As for Renal above.

CI: Hypersensitivity (amide type local anaesthetics). Not for injection into inflamed or infected areas. IV regional anaesthesia (Bier's-block) *(Marcain).* Not for IV use, obstetrical paracervical block *(Bupivacaine Concordia).*

Interactions: Effect of Other Drugs on Bupivacaine: *Systemic additive toxic effects:* Other amide anaesthesics (lidocaine, mexiletine). *Metabolism affected:* Highly protein-bound drugs (anticonvulsants, anticoagulants), drugs metabolised in liver (cimetidine). *Caution:* Class III antiarrhythmics (amiodarone).

SP: Ensure IV infusion in place before starting intrathecal anaesthesia. High systemic conc (ventricular arrhythmia and/or fibrillation, sudden cardiovascular collapse, death). Elderly, late stages of pregnancy, increased risk (high or total spinal blockade). Intercostal paralysis. Hypotension, bradycardia. Increased intraspinal abscess formation (septicaemia). Retrobulbar injection (may reach cranial subarachnoid space; temporary blindness, cardiovascular collapse, apnoea, convulsions). Retro- and peribulbar injection of local anaesthetics; persistent ocular muscle dysfunction risk. Injection in head and neck region (inadvertently into an artery), immediate cerebral symptoms. Paracervical block, foetal (bradycardia, tachycardia); monitor foetal heart rate. Horner's syndrome, alert anaesthetist (excessive cranial spread of local anaesthetic, possibility of autonomic and motor complications). Caution, epilepsy, impaired cardiac conduction, hepatic impairment (including reduced hepatic blood flow), renal damage.

Pregnancy, Lactation: Not for use in early pregnancy unless benefit outweighs risk. Enters human milk in small quantities; generally no risk to child at therapeutic doses. Obstetric epidural analgesia, essential to place mother on her side or tilted laterally to avoid caval occlusion (maternal hypotension, foetal acidosis).

ADR: See Notes below.

Notes: See 14.2 Local Anaesthesia.

> **Marcain Polyamp Steripack** *(AstraZeneca)* A. HOS.
> *Price,* 10mL (10) 0.25%, €13.13. 0.5%, €15.08.
> *Injection,* bupivacaine HCl equiv. to bupivacaine HCl anhydrous 2.5mg (5mg)/mL. Clear colourless aqueous soln. *Sodium* 3.2mg/L.
> **Bupivacaine Parenteral** *(Concordia)* A. HOS.
> *Price,* 10mL (10) 0.25%, €9.51. 0.5%, €10.95 (PTW).
> *Injection,* bupivacaine HCl equiv. to 0.25% or 0.5% w/v anhydrous bupivacaine HCl. Clear colourless soln.

Bupivacaine, Adrenaline

ATC Code: N01BB51. **Sport:** Permitted.
Driving: Caution.

Indications: See Notes below (bupivacaine).

Dose: Adult: See Notes below (bupivacaine). See Pregnancy, Lactation below.

Child: Strength 0.25%, age 1-12 years, acute pain management (caudal, lumbar, thoracic* epidural) (conc 2.5mg/mL) 0.6-0.8mL/kg (1.5-2mg/kg), onset 20-30 minutes, duration 2-6 hours. Strength 0.5%, under 12 years, safety/efficacy not established. *Thoracic blocks need to be given incrementally until desired anaesthesia level achieved.

CI: Paracervical block (obstetrics). Thyrotoxicosis, severe heart disease especially with tachycardia.

Interactions: Effect of Other Drugs on Bupivacaine, Adrenalin Combination: *Vasoconstrictor effects of adrenaline opposed (hypotensive response, tachycardia):* Neuroleptics (phenothiazines).

SP: Cardiac arrhythmia during or following admin of chloroform, halothane, cyclopropane, trichloroethylene. Caudal, epidural or paracervical block during labour, may reduce uterine and spinal blood flow and uterine contractility; serious systemic effects in pre-eclampsia or where an oxytocic drug is used post-partum.

Pregnancy, Lactation: Not for use for epidural block in labour analgesia (except test dose) as benefit of addition of adrenaline not shown to outweigh risk. Not known if adrenaline enters breast milk; unlikely to affect. See Notes below.

ADR: See Notes below.

Notes: See Bupivacaine above. See Bupivacaine, Dextrose below.

> **Marcain with Adrenaline** *(AstraZeneca)* A.
> *Price,* 20mL (5) 0.25%, €14.68. 0.5%, €16.56.
> *Injection,* bupivacaine HCl 2.5mg, 5mg (0.25%, 0.5% w/v), adrenaline tartrate equiv. to adrenaline 5mcg/mL. Clear colourless aqueous soln. *Sodium metabisulphite.* **Store:** Refrigerate; do not freeze.

Bupivacaine, Dextrose

ATC Code: N01BB51. **Sport:** Permitted.
Driving: Caution.

Indications: Intrathecal spinal anaesthesia in adults, children (all ages).

Dose: Adult, Elderly: Urological (conc 5mg/mL), 1.5-3mL (7.5-15mg), onset 5-8 minutes, duration 2-3 hours. Lower abdominal surgery (conc 5mg/mL), 2-4mL (10-20mg), onset 5-8 minutes, duration 1.5-3 hours. Pregnant women, 2-2.5mL (10-12.5mg). Late stages of pregnancy and elderly, reduce dose.

Child: Neonates, infants and children, under 5kg (0.4-0.5mg/kg), 5-15kg (0.3-0.4mg/kg), 15-40kg (0.25-0.3mg/kg). Age 12 years and older, as for Adult above. Recommended injection site below L3.

Pregnancy, Lactation: Obstetric analgesia, see Notes below (bupivacaine).

ADR: See Notes below.

Notes: See Bupivacaine above. See 14.2 Local Anaesthesia.

> **Marcain Heavy Steripack** *(Aspen)* A.
> *Price,* 20mg/4mL (5) €5.80.
> *Injection,* bupivacaine HCl equiv. to 5mg/mL (20mg/4mL) anhydrous bupivacaine HCl, dextrose anhydrous equiv. to 80mg/mL dextrose monohydrate. Clear colourless aqueous soln.
> **Store:** Below 25 deg C; amps in outer carton.

Levobupivacaine

ATC Code: N01BB10. **Sport:** Permitted.
Driving: Caution. Can have major influence.

Indications: Surgical anaesthesia, management of post-operative pain and labour analgesia, ilioinguinal/iliohypogastric blocks in children, see Dose below.

Dose: Adult, Elderly: Motor block (moderate to complete), surgical anaesthesia, epidural, (conc 5-7.5mg/mL), (slow) bolus for surgery, 10-20mL (50-150mg); (conc 5mg/mL), slow injection for C-section, 15-30mL (75-150mg). Intrathecal, (conc 5mg/mL), 3mL (15mg). Peripheral nerve block, (conc 2.5-5mg/mL), 1-40mL (2.5-150mg max); ilioinguinal block (conc 2.5mg/mL), 0.5mL (1.25mg)/kg/side; Iliohypogastric blocks, children under 12 years, (conc 5mg/mL), 0.25mL(1.25mg)/kg/side. Ophthalmic (peribulbar block), (conc 7.5mg/mL), 5-15mL (37.5-112.5mg). Local infiltration, (conc 2.5mg/mL), 1-60mL (2.5-150mg max.).

Motor block (minimal to moderate), pain management, labour analgesia, epidural bolus (conc 2.5mg/mL), 6-10mL (15-25mg); epidural infusion (conc 0.625mg/mL), 8-20mL (5-12.5mg) OR (conc 1.25mg/mL), 4-10mL/hour (5-12.5mg/hour).

Post-operative pain, (conc 0.625mg/mL), 20-30mL/hour (12.5-18.75mg/hour) OR (conc 1.25mg/mL), 10-15mL/hour (12.5-18.75mg/hour) OR (conc 2.5mg/mL), 5-7mL/hour (12.5-18.75mg/hour). Therapy exceeding 24 hours, limited safety data (monitor patient/duration).

Child: Ilioinguinal/iliohypogastric blocks, see Adult above. Other indications, not for use.

Hepatic Impairment: Caution, hepatic disease or reduced blood flow (alcoholics, cirrhosis).

CI: Amide type local anaesthetic hypersensitivity. IV regional anaesthesia (Bier's-block). Severe hypotension (cardiogenic or hypovolaemic shock), paracervical block in obstetrics.

Interactions: Effect of Other Drugs on Levobupivacaine: *Metabolism may be affected:* CYP3A4 inhibitors (ketoconazole), CYP1A2 inhibitors (methylxanthines).

SP: Can cause acute allergic reactions, cardiovascular effects, neurological damage. Chondrolysis (shoulder most reported) with intra-articular continuous infusion* of local anaesthetics. Caution, debilitated, elderly or acutely ill patients. *Epidural anaesthesia,* caution unintentional intravascular or intrathecal injection; may cause hypotension, bradycardia. Cauda equina syndrome indicative of neurotoxicity. *(not an approved indication).

Pregnancy, Lactation: Contraindicated for paracervical block in obstetrics. Not for use during pregnancy unless clearly necessary. Lactation, possible after local anaesthesia.

ADR: See Notes below.

Notes: See Bupivacaine above.

14.2　Local Anaesthesia

Chirocaine Parenteral (AbbVie) A. HOS.
Price, 200mL (bag): 1.25mg/mL (1), €26.54. 10 Amps
Overwrap: 2.5mg/mL, €24.70; 5mg/mL, €34.54; 7.5mg/mL, €41.46 (PTW).
Injection or infusion, levobupivacaine HCl. 1.25mg/mL: Clear colourless soln for inj/inf. 2.5mg, 5mg, 7.5mg per mL (10mL vials): Soln for injection or conc for infusion. Sodium 3.6mg/mL per bag/vial.

Lidocaine (anaesthesia)

ATC Code: N01BB02. **Sport:** Permitted.
Driving: Caution.
Indications: Local anaesthetic.
Dose: Adult: Max. 3mg/kg or 200mg whichever is lower. Infiltration by injection (IV, epidural).
Elderly: Lower doses depending on age, physical status.
Child: As for Elderly above.
CI: Hypersensitivity to amide anaesthetics.
Interactions: Effect of Other Drugs on Lidocaine: Increased ventricular arrhythmia risk, avoid co-admin: Quinupristin + dalfopristin. Plasma levels increased: Propranolol, cimetidine. Effect antagonised: Acetazolamide, loop diuretics, thiazides (hypokalaemia). Additive cardiac depressant effect: Other antiarrhythmics.
Effect of Lidocaine on Other Drugs: Suxamethonium: Action prolonged.
SP: Not for intravascular injection (rapid toxicity onset, marked restlessness, twitching, convulsions; coma, apnoea, cardiovascular collapse); caution when anaesthetising mucous membranes/highly vascular areas (especially if inflamed, traumatised); systemic absorption. Repeated admin, possible cumulative toxicity/tachyphylaxis. Hypersensitivity.
Pregnancy, Lactation: Pregnancy, crosses placenta (neonatal toxicity includes decreased muscle strength and tone, bradycardia, apnoea, convulsions); consider when used for obstetric analgesia. Early pregnancy, only if considered essential.
ADR: See Notes below.
Notes: See 14.2 Local Anaesthesia.

Lidocaine, Adrenaline

ATC Code: N01BB52. **Sport:** Permitted.
Driving: Caution.
Indications: Local anaesthesia (age above 12 years).
Dose: Adult: Max. single dose, 7mg/kg or 500mg total (whichever lower).
Field block, infiltration, surgery using 1% soln, max. 300mg/dose; intercostals (per nerve), surgery, post-operative pain, fractured ribs, using 1% soln, 20-50mg; max. 300mg/dose. Pudendal, instrument delivery, using 1% soln, max. 100mg/dose.
Major nerve block, paracervical (each side), surgery, cervical dilatation, obstetric pain, using 1% soln, max. 100mg/dose. Sciatic, surgery using 2% soln, max. 300mg/dose. 3-in-1 (femoral, obturator, lateral cutaneous), surgery, using 1% soln, max 300mg/dose.
Elderly: Lower doses depending on age, physical status.
Child: Over 12 years, as for Adult above.
Renal Impairment: Severe, caution.
Hepatic Impairment: Advanced disease, caution.
CI: Amide-type local anaesthetic hypersensitivity, IV or intrathecal use, end-organ anaesthesia (fingers, toes, ear lobe, penis) or spinal anaesthesia (adrenaline content).
SP: Solns containing adrenaline, caution (hypertension, cardiac disease, cerebrovascular insufficiency, hyperthyroidosis, advanced diabetes, conditions aggravated by adrenaline). Porphyriacs, caution; use only in urgent indications. Not for use by intrathecal, intracisternal or intra- or retro-bulbar routes.
ADR: See Notes below.
Notes: See Lidocaine above.

Xylocaine 2% with Adrenaline Parenteral (AstraZeneca) A.
Price, (5) 20mL, €2.69.
Infiltration by injection, lidocaine HCl 20mg, adrenaline tartrate 5mcg. Clear colourless aqueous soln. Metabisulphite, parabens, sodium 2.49mg/mL.

Lidocaine, Chlorhexidine

ATC Code: N01BB52. **Sport:** Permitted.
Driving: Unlikely to impair.
Indications: Catheterisation, cystoscopy, exploratory and intra-operative investigations, exchange of fistula catheters.
Dose: Adult, Elderly: Urethral sounding, catheterisation, instil 6-11mL into urethra. Cystoscopy, coat entire urethra including external sphincter with film of lubricant, usually 11mL; an additional 6-11mL can be used; effect begins after 3-5 minutes.
CI: Damaged or bleeding mucous membranes.
SP: Oropharyngeal use (difficulty in swallowing; increased aspiration risk; biting trauma due to tongue numbness).
Pregnancy, Lactation: first trimester, only if absolutely necessary.
ADR: See Notes below.
Notes: See 14.2 Local Anaesthesia.

Instillagel (Farco) OTC. GMS.
Price, 6mL, €1.06. 11mL, €1.33.
Lubrication gel, lidocaine HCl 2%, chlorhexidine digluconate 0.05%, methylhydroxybenzoate 0.06%, propylhydroxybenzoate 0.025%.

Lidocaine, Prilocaine

ATC Code: N01BB54. **Sport:** Permitted.
Driving: No influence at recommended dose.
Indications: Topical anaesthesia: Skin (needle insertion, superficial surgical procedures) (adults, children); leg ulcers to facilitate cleansing or debridement (adults); genital mucosa prior surgical procedures or infiltration anaesthesia (age 12 years and over).
Dose: Adult, Elderly: Topical skin anaesthesia (from 12 years)*: Minor procedures (needle insertion, superficial surgery), apply 2g or 1.5g/10cm2 for 1-5 hours; dermal surgical procedures (hospital setting e.g. split skin grafting), 1.5-2g/10cm2 for 2-5 hours; dermal procedures (self-application) on newly shaven skin of large body areas, max. 60g; max. area 600cm2 for minimum 1 hour, max. 5 hours. Skin of genital organs, prior to local anaesthetic injection*, males, 1g/10cm2 for 15 minutes; females, 1-2g/10cm2 for 60 minutes.
Genital mucosa, prior to (surgical treatment of localised lesions, local anaesthetic injection), 5-10g of cream for 5-10 minutes; prior to cervical curettage, 10g of cream in lateral vaginal fornices for 10 minutes.
Leg ulcer*, cleansing/debridement, apply 1-2g/10cm2 up to 10g to leg ulcer for 30-60 minutes. *(use with occlusive dressing).
Child: Age 0-11 years, minor procedures (needle insertion, surgery for localised lesions), neonates (0-2 months), up to 1g and 10cm2 for 1hour; infants (3-11 months), up to 2g and 20cm2 for 1 hour; children (1-5 years), up to 10g and 100cm2 for 1-5 hours; (6-11 years), up to 20g and 200cm2 for 1-5 hours. Age 12 years and over, as for Adult above. Prior to removal of mollusca, apply for 30 minutes. Use with occlusive dressing.
CI: Hypersensitivity to amide local anaesthetics, lidocaine and/or prilocaine.
Interactions: Effect of Other Drugs on Lidocaine, Prilocaine Combination: Increased methaemoglobin levels: Sulfonamides, nitrofurantoin, phenytoin, phenobarbital. Additive systemic toxic effects: Other local anaesthetics (structurally related). Caution: Anti-arrhythmics Class III (amiodarone). Potentially toxic lidocaine plasma concentrations: Drugs reducing lidocaine clearance (cimetidine, beta-blockers).
SP: Defective G6PD methaemoglobinaemia is more

susceptible to active-substance induced methaemoglobinaemia; methylene blue is ineffective (cannot be given). Not for application to open wounds (excluding leg ulcers). In atopic dermatitis, application over 30 minutes, increased incidence of local vascular reactions. Avoid contact with eyes. Do not apply to impaired tympanic membrane. Not for use, newborn infants/infants (up to 12 months) if co-admin with methaemoglobin-inducing agents; preterm newborn infants, gestational age under 37 weeks, risk of increased methaemoglobin levels. Use on genital (skin, mucosa) in children under 12 years, safety and efficacy not established. Adequate efficacy for circumcision not demonstrated.

Pregnancy, Lactation: Pregnancy, caution. Lactation, can be used if needed.

ADR: See Notes below.

Notes: See 14.2 Local Anaesthesia.

> **Emla 5% Cream** *(AstraZeneca)* A.
> *Price*, 5g (5) €11.31.
> *Cream*, lidocaine 25mg, prilocaine 25mg per 1g. White homogenous. *Macrogolglycerol hydroxystearate.*

Lidocaine, Tetracaine

ATC Code: N01BB52. **Sport:** Permitted.
Driving: No or negligible effect.

Indications: Local dermal anaesthesia on intact skin prior to dermatological procedures.

Dose: Adult, Elderly: Apply to skin at thickness of 1mm (1.3g per 10cm2) for 30 minutes (pulsed-dye laser therapy, laser-assisted hair removal, non-ablative laser facial resurfacing, dermal filler injection, vascular access) OR for 60 minutes (laser-assisted tattoo removal, laser leg vein ablation). After the required time, the peel must be removed from skin prior to procedure. Max. application area 400cm2.

Child: Under 18 years, not recommended.

Renal Impairment: Caution.

Hepatic Impairment: As for Renal above.

Interactions: Effect of Other Drugs on Lidocaine, Tetracaine Combination: *Additional systemic toxicity:* Class I antiarrhythmics (quinidine, disopyramide, tocainide, mexiletine), Class III antiarrhythmics (amiodarone), other local anaesthetics. *Increased methaemoglobinaemia risk:* Sulphonamides, naphthalene, nitrates, nitrites, nitrofurantoin, nitroglycerin, nitroprusside, pamaquine, quinine.

SP: Cardiac impairment, caution. Do not apply to broken or irritated skin. Avoid contact with eyes.

Pregnancy, Lactation: Pregnancy, caution. Lactation, can be used as long as not applied to breast.

ADR: See Notes below.

Notes: See 14.2 Local Anaesthesia.

> **Pliaglis 70mg/70mg** *(Galderma)* A.
> *Price*, 15g, €27.00.
> *Cutaneous cream*, lidocaine 70mg, tetracaine 70mg. White (off-white). *Parabens.* **Store:** Refrigerate; do not freeze; below 25 deg C (max. 3 months) and do not refrigerate again.

Ropivacaine

ATC Code: N01BB09. **Sport:** Permitted.
Driving: Dose-dependent; may have a minor influence (mental function, co-ordination); may impair locomotion and alertness.

Indications: 7.5mg/mL, 10mg/mL: Epidural anaesthesia (surgery including C-section, major nerve blocks, field blocks). 2mg/mL: Acute pain management (intermittent bolus post-operative or labour pain, field blocks, continuous peripheral nerve block via intermittent bolus injection e.g. post-operative pain); pre- and post-operative, age 1-12 years, single and continuous peripheral nerve block; in neonates and up to 12 years, caudal epidural block.

Dose: Adult, Elderly: *Surgical anaesthesia:* Lumbar epidural, for surgery (7.5mg/mL conc), 15-25mL (113-188mg) OR (10mg/mL conc), 15-20mL (150-200mg); C-

section (7.5mg/mL conc), 15-20mL (113-150mg). Thoracic epidural: Post-operative pain relief, (7.5mg/mL conc), 5-15mL (38-113mg). Major nerve block: Brachial plexus block, (7.5mg/mL conc), 30-40mL (225-300mg). Field block: Minor nerve block infiltration, (7.5mg/mL conc), 1-30mL (7.5-225mg).

Acute pain management (2mg/mL conc): Lumbar epidural, bolus, 10-20mL (20-40mg); intermittent injection (top up) 10-15mL (20-30mg) (labour pain management, minimum 30-minute interval); post-operative pain 6-14mL/hour (12-28mg/hour).

Field block (2mg/mL conc): Minor nerve block, infiltration, 1-100mL (2-200mg); peripheral nerve block (femoral or interscalene block), intermittent injection, 5-10mL/hour (10-20mg/hour).

Admin, caution, intravascular injection. Large dose for injection, recommend test dose of 3-5mL lidocaine with adrenaline.

Child: *Acute pain management* (2mg/mL conc): Age 0-12 years, single caudal epidural block, 1mL/kg (2mg/kg). Age 1-12 years, single injections for peripheral nerve block e.g. ilioinguinal nerve block, brachial plexus block, fascia iliaca compartment block, 0.5-0.75mL/kg (1-1.5mg/kg); multiple blocks, 0.5-1.5mL/kg (1-3mg/kg).

Renal Impairment: No adjustment. Chronic renal failure may increase systemic toxicity risk.

Hepatic Impairment: Severe, caution; repeated doses may need reduction (delayed elimination).

CI: Amide type local anaesthetic hypersensitivity. Anaesthesia (IV regional, obstetric paracervical), hypovolaemia.

Interactions: Effect of Other Drugs on Ropivacaine: *Systemic toxic effects additive:* Other amide-type anaesthetics (mexiletine). *Mutual potentiation:* General anaesthetics, opioids. *Avoid prolonged admin:* Strong CYP1A2 inhibitors.

SP: Chronic renal failure, acidosis, reduced plasma proteins. Acute porphyria, use only if no alternative.

Pregnancy, Lactation: Obstetric use only. Lactation, no data.

ADR: *Very common*, hypotension, nausea.

Notes: See 14.2 Local Anaesthesia.

> **Naropin Parenteral** *(Aspen)* A.
> *Price*, (5 x 10mL) 2mg/mL, €10.09; 7.5mg/mL, €19.58 (trade).
> *Soln for injection*, ropivacaine hydrochloride monohydrate 2mg, 7.5mg (10mL). Clear colourless. *Sodium.* **Store:** Below 30 deg C; do not freeze.

Tetracaine (anaesthesia)

ATC Code: N01BA03. **Sport:** Permitted.
Driving: Unlikely to impair.

Indications: Local anaesthesia of skin prior to venipuncture or venous cannulation.

Dose: Adult, Elderly: Apply contents of tube (approx. 1g) to centre of area to be anaesthetised and occlude; sufficient to anaesthetise up to 30cm2 usually achieved following 30-minute application time (venipuncture) and 45 minute application time (venous cannulation); after which gel should be removed and site prepared. Anaesthesia remains for 4-6 hours.

Child: Premature babies, full term infants under 1 month, not recommended.

CI: Broken skin, mucous membranes, eyes, ears.

SP: Apply to intact skin. May be ototoxic (instilled into middle ear, used for procedures penetrating into middle ear). Increased sensitisation reactions (repeated exposure). Not for oral use.

Pregnancy, Lactation: Pregnancy, no data; been widely used without problem. Lactation, not recommended.

ADR: See Notes below.

Notes: See 14.2 Local Anaesthesia.

> **Ametop Gel** *(Smith&Nephew)* OTC.
> *Price*, 1.5g (12) single tube, €22.86; dispensing pack, €33.24.
> *Topical gel*, tetracaine base 4% w/w. White opalescent. *Parabens.*

15

Toxicology

15.1 - Specific Substance Antagonists

Class Effects

National Poisons Information Centre of Ireland: Tel: +353 (0)1 8092566. Where a brand is not licensed in Ireland, contact the National Poisons Information Centre for advice. Always consult the manufacturers Full Prescribing Information.

Parenteral atropine is an antidote for cardiovascular collapse following anticholinesterase overdose; also used to treat poisoning from organophosphorus insecticides, chemical warfare 'nerve' gases and mushrooms.

CI: Hypersensitivity to any member of the class.

SP: All antidotes to be used in conjunction with decontamination and supportive measures.

ADR: See manufacturers Full Prescribing Information.

15.1.1 - Benzodiazepines

In This Chapter: *Flumazenil.*

Flumazenil

ATC Code: V03AB25. **Sport:** Permitted.
Driving: Do not drive during first 24-hours as effect of earlier benzodiazepine may recur.

Indications: Complete or partial reversal of central sedative effects of benzodiazepines in termination of general anaesthesia; reversal of sedation/conscious sedation in diagnostic and therapeutic procedures; paradoxical reactions due to benzodiazepines; return to spontaneous respiration and consciousness in ICU patients. Diagnosis and/or management of benzodiazepine overdosage.

Dose: Adult: Anaesthesia, initially 200mcg; if desired degree of consciousness not obtained within 60 seconds, admin second 100mcg dose; repeat at 60 second intervals; max. total 1mg; usually 300-600mcg.

ICU, initially 300mcg; if desired degree of consciousness not obtained, then as for Anaesthesia above; max. total 2mg. Adjust dose and/or infusion rate to desired sedation level; IV; either undiluted or diluted; can be admin with other reanimation measures.

Elderly: Caution, more sensitive to benzodiazepine effects.

Child: Reversal, conscious sedation, benzodiazepine induced, age over 1 year, initially 10mcg/kg (up to 200mcg) IV over 15 seconds; if desired level of conscious not obtained after additional 45 seconds, further 10mcg/kg may be admin (up to 200mcg), repeated at 60-sec intervals if needed (max. 4 times; max. total dose 50mcg/kg OR 1mg whichever is lower). Under 1 year, if benefit outweighs risk.

Hepatic Impairment: Primary metabolised in liver, titrate carefully; elimination may be delayed (effects delayed; extended observation period required).

CI: When benzodiazepines are used for control of potentially life-threatening conditions (intracranial pressure, status epilepticus).

SP: Short duration of action. Caution, convulsion risk (epileptics receiving benzodiazepines for prolonged periods, head injury); rapid reversal may lead to raised intracranial pressure with severe head injury; long-term treatment, caution withdrawal. Should not be injected until neuromuscular blockade fully reversed. Anxious patients (especially with CHD), considerable pain; maintain a degree of sedation post-op. Not for treatment of benzodiazepine dependence or protracted abstinence syndromes. Mixed intoxications (benzodiazepines + antidepressants), antidepressant toxicity can be masked by protective benzodiazepine effects. Should not be used with autonomic, motor neurological or cardiovascular symptoms of severe tri and/or tetracyclic intoxication. Slow injection/infusion should not produce withdrawal symptoms, even with high benzodiazepine doses and/or for prolonged time; if signs of stimulation occur, admin diazepam or midazolam by slow IV injection. At end of surgery anaesthesia, effect of peripheral muscle relaxants must first have disappeared.

Pregnancy, Lactation: Pregnancy, caution. Lactation, not contraindicated in emergency situations.

ADR: See Notes below.

Notes: See 15.1 Specific Substance Antagonists.

Anexate Parenteral *(Cheplapharm)* A. HOS.
Price, 5mL (5) 100mcg/mL, €77.09 (PTW).
Injection or infusion, flumazenil 100mcg/mL. Clear almost colourless soln. *Sodium 3.7mg/mL.*

15.1.2 - Cyanide

In This Chapter: *Hydroxocobalamin.*

Hydroxocobalamin (cyanide poisoning)

ATC Code: V03AB33. **Sport:** Permitted.
Driving: No studies performed.

Indications: Treatment, cyanide poisoning.

Dose: Adult, Elderly: Initially 5g by IV infusion over 15 minutes; based on severity/clinical response, admin second dose of 5g over 15-120 minutes; max. 10g.

Child: Initially 70mg/kg; max. 5g; second dose of 70mg/kg (max. 5g) if needed, see Adult above. Max. 140mg/kg not exceeding 10g.

Renal Impairment: Emergency therapy, no adjustment.

Hepatic Impairment: As for Renal above.

SP: Treatment must include airway patency, adequate (oxygenation, hydration), cardiovascular support, seizure management. *Cyanokit* is not a substitute oxygen therapy; must not delay setup of above measures. Base treatment on history and/or signs/symptoms of cyanide intoxication. *Poisoning may result from*, smoke exposure (closed space fires), inhalation, ingestion, dermal exposure. Common signs/symptoms e.g. nausea, vomiting, headache, altered mental status (confusion, disorientation), chest tightness, dyspnoea, tachypnoea or hyperpnoea (early), bradypnoea or apnoea (late), hypertension (early) or hypotension (late), cardiovascular collapse, seizures/coma, mydriasis, plasma lactate conc above 8mmoL/L. Hypersensitivity, consider risk/benefit. May induce red colouration of skin; may interfere with burn assessment. Interference with laboratory tests.

Pregnancy, Lactation: Pregnancy, may be admin; no more than 2 injections in potentially life-threatening condition with no alternative treatment. In case of pregnancy at time or becomes known after treatment, contact the pharmaceutical company. Lactation, not contraindicated for use.

ADR: See Notes below.

Notes: See 15.1 Specific Substance Antagonists.

Cyanokit Parenteral *(SOBI)* A.
Price, 5g, €876.07.
Infusion, hydroxocobalamin 2.5g. Dark red crystalline powder for soln.

15.1.3 - Iron

In This Chapter: *Deferiprone, deferoxamine, deferasirox.*

Deferiprone

ATC Code: V03AC02. **Sport:** Permitted.
Driving: No studies performed.

Indications: Iron overload in thalassaemia major, monotherapy where current chelation therapy contraindicated or inadequate; combination (another chelator), monotherapy is ineffective or prevention or treatment of life-threatening consequences of iron overload (mainly cardiac overload) requires rapid or intensive correction.

Dose: Adult, Elderly: *Monotherapy,* 25mg/kg oral 3-times daily (calculated to nearest half tab); total dose 75mg/kg/day; above 100mg/kg not recommended (increased adverse reaction risk). *Combination* with deferoxamine, use standard dose as above; iron-induced heart failure, 75-100mg/kg/day should be added to deferoxamine. Concurrent use of iron chelators not recommended if serum ferritin falls below 500mcg/L (excessive iron removal risk).

Child: Age 6-10 years, limited data; under 6 years, no data.

Renal Impairment: Caution, monitor function.

Hepatic Impairment: As for Renal above.

CI: Recurrent neutropenia, agranulocytosis.

Interactions: Effect of Other Drugs on Deferiprone: *Co-admin contraindicated:* Medicinals associated with neutropenia or causing agranulocytosis. *Co-admin not recommended:* Aluminium-based antacids. *Co-admin caution:* Vitamin C.

SP: Deferiprone may cause neutropenia, including agranulocytosis; monitor neutrophil counts every week; do not initiate if neutropenic. Cannot exclude carcinogenicity. Monitor, serum ferritin every 2-3 months, plasma zinc. HIV positive, other immunocompromised, weight risk/benefit. Reddish/brown discolouration of urine. Neurological disorders with chronic overdose (more than 2.5 times max. for several years; also observed with standard dose); if observed, discontinue. *Combination use,* consider on case-by-case basis; fatalities and life-threatening situations (agranulocytosis) reported. See Dose above (ferritin levels).

Pregnancy, Lactation: Pregnancy, lactation, contraindicated.

ADR: Summary, *most common,* nausea, abdominal pain, vomiting, chromaturia; *most serious,* agranulocytosis.

Notes: See 15.1 Specific Substance Antagonists.

Ferriprox 500mg, Oral Soln *(SOBI)* A. HT.
Price, tabs (100) €213.11. Soln 100mg/mL (500mL) €219.54.
Tablet, deferiprone. White (off-white) cap-shaped f/c scored (divisible into equal halves). Marked APO 500. **Store:** Below 30 deg C; bottle tightly closed to protect (moisture).
Oral soln, as above 100mg/mL. Clear reddish orange. *Sunset Yellow, sucralose.* **Store:** Below 30 deg C; original pack to protect (light).

Deferoxamine

ATC Code: V03AC01. **Sport:** Permitted.
Driving: Dizziness, other CNS disturbances, vision/hearing impairment.

Indications: Iron chelation treatment of chronic iron overload (primary, secondary haemochromatosis including thalassaemia); transfusional haemosiderosis (concomitant disorders preclude phlebotomy). Treatment, acute iron poisoning. Diagnosis, iron storage disease, certain anaemias. Maintenance dialysis for ESRD with aluminium-related bone disease and/or anaemia, dialysis encephalopathy, diagnosis of aluminium overload.

Dose: Adult: Chelation, generally, serum ferritin below 2000ng/mL requires 25mg/kg/day; ferritin 2000-3000ng/mL requires 35mg/kg/day; higher ferritin up to 55mg/kg/day; inadvisable to regularly exceed 50mg/kg/day except if intensive chelation needed; if ferritin falls below 1000ng/mL, increased toxicity risk. *Admin,* by slow SC infusion over 8-12 hours; may be given over 24-hours; 5-7 times/week. Not for SC bolus; use continuous IV infusion for intensive chelation; IM only if SC not feasible. Admin Vitamin C, adjuvant.

Acute iron poisoning, 15mg/kg/hour by continuous IV infusion; reduce after 4-6 hours; total IV dose is max. 80mg/kg in any 24-hour period.

Diagnostic (iron storage disease, anaemia), 500mg IM and 400mL water only; collect all urine over next 6 hours; excretion of 1-1.5mg of iron during 6-hour period suggests of iron-storage disease; values above 1.5mg pathological.

Aluminium overload in ESRD, maintenance haemodialysis, 5mg/kg once-weekly; peritoneal dialysis, 5mg/kg once-weekly prior to final exchange of day. Diagnostic (aluminium overload), see manufacturers Full Prescribing Information.

Elderly: Use lowest end of dose range; consider renal function.

Child: As for Adult above. Chelation begun before age 3 years, max. mean daily dose 40mg/kg.

Renal Impairment: Caution as metal complexes are excreted mainly via kidneys. Dialysis increases chelated iron and aluminium elimination. Monitor function (serum creatinine).

Interactions: Effect of Other Drugs on Deferoxamine: *Co-admin not recommended:* Prochlorperazine (prolonged unconsciousness). *Co-admin not recommended (within 1 month of starting deferoxamine):* Vitamin C (initiate only after initial month of *regular* deferoxamine treatment; max. 200mg/day). *Vitamin C co-admin (severe chronic iron-storage):* Monitor cardiac function.

Effect of Deferoxamine on Other Drugs: Erythropoietin: *Adjust dose.*

SP: May exacerbate neurological dysfunction in aluminium-related encephalopathy; precipitate dialysis dementia; pretreat (clonazepam). Aluminium overload treatment may result in decreased serum calcium. Always admin by slow infusion; rapid IV infusion (hypotension, shock); IM accidentally given IV (circulatory collapse); high doses by SC admin (local irritation). Iron overload, increased susceptibility to infection; if occurs, discontinue. *High doses,* disturbed vision and hearing (prolonged use; low serum ferritin levels; monitor; low ferritin or young children (under 3 years), growth retardation (rare if dose kept below 40mg/kg); ARDS, do not exceed recommended dose. Reddish-brown discolouration of urine. Monitor 24-hour urinary iron excretion daily.

Pregnancy, Lactation: Use only if benefit to mother outweighs risk to child.

ADR: *Very common,* injection-site reactions, arthralgia, myalgia.

Notes: See 15.1 Specific Substance Antagonists.

Desferal Parenteral *(Novartis)* A. GMS.
Price, 500mg (10) €39.40.
Injection or infusion, deferoxamine mesilate 500mg. White (practically white) lyophilised powder for soln.

Deferasirox

ATC Code: V03AC03. **Sport:** Permitted.
Driving: Minor influence; dizziness.

Indications: Treatment, chronic iron overload due to frequent blood transfusions: In beta thalassaemia major (from 6 years); when deferoxamine contraindicated or inadequate i.e. paediatric receiving frequent transfusion (2-5 years) or infrequent transfusions (from 2 years) in beta thalassaemia major or other anaemias (from 2 years). Non-transfusion-dependent thalassaemia syndromes (deferoxamine not indicated or inadequate) (from 10 years).

Dose: Adult, Elderly: NOTE: *Exjade f/c tabs (f/c) have higher bioavailability compared to dispersible formulation (disp); when switching, f/c tab dose to be 30% lower than disp dose (rounded to nearest tab).*

Transfusional iron overload, initially (mg/kg/day) 14 (f/c) OR 20 (disp) after transfusion or 20 units packed red blood cells (PRBC). Alternatively (mg/kg/day), 21 (f/c) OR 30 (disp) with transfusion of under 14mL/kg/month PRBC. Second alternative (mg/kg/day), 7 (f/c) OR 10 (disp) with transfusions under 7mL/kg/month PRBC. Patients well managed on deferoxamine, one-third of deferoxamine dose (f/c) OR half of deferoxamine dose (disp).

Adjustment steps, increase every 3-6 months (mg/kg/day) by 3.5-7 (f/c) OR 5-10 (disp); max. 28 (f/c) OR 40 (disp); if ferritin falls below 500mcg/L, consider interruption. Increased serum creatinine (33% or more), consider dose reduction (see SP below). NOTE: Initiate after transfusion of approx. 20 units (approx. 100mL/kg) PRBC OR if serum ferritin above 1000mcg/L.

Non-transfusional-dependent thalassaemia syndromes, initially (mg/kg/day) 7 (f/c) OR 10mg (disp). Consider increasing every 3-6 months by (mg/kg/day) 3.5-7 (f/c) OR 5-10mg/kg (disp) according to liver iron concentration (LIC) or ferritin levels; max. 14 (f/c) OR 20 (disp). If ferritin falls below 300mcg/L, consider interruption Retreatment not recommended.

Admin, once daily, preferably same time of day, on empty stomach or with a light meal. F/c tabs, swallow whole; may be crushed and full dose sprinkled on soft food e.g. yogurt, apple sauce and taken immediately. Disp tabs, disperse by stirring in glass of water, orange or apple juice (100-200mL); do not chew tablets or swallow whole.

Child: *Transfusional iron overload,* age 2-17 years, as for Adult above. Age 2-5 years, exposure may be lower and higher doses may be needed; initiate as for Adult and titrate. Rise in serum creatinine above age-appropriate ULN, reduce dose.
Non-transfusional-dependent thalassaemia syndromes (mg/kg/day), max. 7 (f/c) OR 10 (disp). Monitor LIC and serum ferritin to avoid over-chelation. Birth to 23 months, safety/efficacy not established.

Renal Impairment: CrCl (mL/min) below 60, contraindicated. See SP below.

Hepatic Impairment: Moderate, decrease dose up to 50%. Severe, not recommended.

Interactions: Effect of Other Drugs on Deferasirox: *Co-admin not recommended:* Other iron chelators, aluminium-containing preparations (antacids), CYP2C8 substrates (paclitaxel, repaglinide), CYP1A2 substrates (theophylline, clozapine, tizanidine). *Bioavailability increased:* Food. *Possible decreased (plasma levels, efficacy):* UGT inducers (rifampicin, phenobarbital, phenytoin, carbamazepine, ritonavir). *Co-admin caution (GI toxicity risk):* Ulcerogenics (NSAIDs, high dose acetylsalicylic acid, corticosteroids, oral bisphosphonates), anticoagulants. *Decreased exposure:* Colestyramine.

Effect of Deferasirox on Other Drugs: CYP3A4 substrates (ciclosporin, simvastatin, hormonal contraceptives, bepridil, ergotamine, midazolam): *Possible decreased efficacy.* Anticoagulants: *Increased GI haemorrhage risk.*

SP: Increased serum creatinine observed; dose-dependent. Before initiation, assess serum creatinine (in duplicate), creatinine clearance and/or plasma cystatin C levels; monitor weekly (month 1), then monthly (co-admin, medication depressing renal function at greater complication risk; maintain adequate hydration with diarrhoea or vomiting). *Monitor* proteinuria (monthly), other renal tubular function markers (as needed); hepatic function before initiation, every 2 weeks (month 1), then monthly; persistently elevated serum transaminases interrupt; when LFTs return to normal, re-initiate (caution). Upper GI (ulceration, haemorrhage). Rash. Serious hypersensitivity, discontinue (do not reintroduce; anaphylactic shock risk). Decreased hearing, lens opacities, monitor (before initiation, 12-monthly). Cardiac dysfunction (iron overload complication). Body weight, height, sexual development, monitor (paediatrics). Leucopenia, thrombocytopenia, pancytopenia. Metabolic acidosis.

Pregnancy, Lactation: Pregnancy, only if clearly necessary. Women of childbearing potential to use additional or alternative non-hormonal contraception. Lactation, not recommended.

ADR: Summary, *most frequent,* nausea, vomiting, diarrhoea (more common in paediatrics), abdominal pain, skin rash.

Notes: See 15.1 Specific Substance Antagonists.

▼ **Exjade Tablets, Dispersible** *(Novartis)* A. HT.
Price, (30) f/c tabs 90mg, €194.40; 180mg, €388.80; 360mg, €755.66. (28) Disp tabs 125mg, €181.73. 250mg, €363.14. 500mg, €723.96.
F/c tablet, deferasirox 90mg, 180mg, 360mg. Ovaloid. Marked NVR; strength on reverse. 90mg: Light-blue. 180mg: Medium-blue. 360mg: Dark-blue.
Dispersible tablet, as above 125mg, 250mg, 500mg. Off-white round flat. Marked NVR; J/strength on reverse. *Lactose.* **Store:** Original pack to protect (moisture).

15.1.4 - Lead

Class Effects

Contact the Poisons Information Centre of Ireland for advice regarding treatment of lead and other heavy metal poisoning.

Notes: See 15.1 Specific Substance Antagonists.
Price,

15.1.5 - Opiates

In This Chapter: *Naloxone, naltrexone.*

Naloxone

ATC Code: V03AB15. **Sport:** Permitted.
Driving: Not applicable. When used to reverse opioids, effect of opioids may return; driving not recommended for 24 hours.

Indications: Reversal of opioid-induced respiratory depression (dextropropoxyphene, methadone, mixed agonist/antagonist including nalbuphine, pentazocine). Diagnosis, suspected acute opioid overdosage. To counteract respiratory and other CNS depression in newborn (from analgesics admin to mother during childbirth) *(Naloxone Paed, Naloxone 400mcg Concordia).*

Dose: Adult, Elderly: Overdose, initially 0.4-2mg IV repeated at 2-3 minute intervals if needed; no response after 10mg, reconsider diagnosis. If duration of action of opioid exceeds naloxone IV bolus, use continuous infusion. Post-operative, usually 0.1-0.2mg, approx. 1.5-3mcg/kg IV with 2-minute interval between 100mcg increments. *Admin,* IV (injection, infusion), IM or SC.

Child: Overdose, usually 0.01mg/kg IV; a second dose of

100mcg/kg may be admin. Neonatal opioid induced depression, 10mcg/kg IV, IM or SC; repeat at 2-3 minute intervals if needed OR 200mcg as single dose (60mcg/kg) IM at birth.

Post-operative, initially in 5-10mcg increments IV at 2-3 minute intervals.

Renal Impairment: Caution. Dialysis with increased elimination of chelated iron and aluminium.

Hepatic Impairment: Caution.

SP: High opioid doses or physical opioid dependence; too rapid reversal may precipitate withdrawal (hypertension, cardiac arrhythmias, pulmonary oedema, cardiac arrest); also applies to newborn. Repeated doses may be needed (long-acting opioids). Reversal of buprenorphine-induced respiratory depression may be incomplete. Caution, cardiac disease or cardiotoxic drugs (hypo/hypertension, ventricular tachycardia, fibrillation, pulmonary oedema). Severe hypertension with naloxone admin in coma due to clonidine overdose.

Pregnancy, Lactation: Pregnancy, if benefit outweighs risk; can be used in second stage labour; can cause withdrawal in newborn. Lactation, not recommended; avoid for 24 hours after admin.

ADR: See Notes below.

Notes: See 15.1 Specific Substance Antagonists.

Naloxone Parenteral *(Concordia)* A.
Price, 1mL (10) 400mcg/mL, €51.66 (PTW).
Injection or infusion, naloxone hydrochloride dihydrate 400mcg/mL. Clear colourless soln. *Sodium 3.55mg/mL.*
Naloxone, Paed Minijet *(IMS)* A.
Price, (5) 400mcg/mL, €24.51. Paed 40mcg/mL, €20.81.
Injection, naloxone HCl 400mcg/mL. Paed 40mcg/mL. Clear colourless soln in syringe.

Naltrexone

ATC Code: N07BB04. **Sport:** Permitted.
Driving: Caution.

Indications: Maintenance, detoxified formerly opioid-dependant patients (adjunctive).

Dose: Adult: Initially 25mg, then 50mg daily OR 100mg 3-times weekly (Mon, Wed, Fri). Above 150mg/day, not recommended; single doses above 50mg, higher hepatocellular injury risk. NOTE: Do not initiate before naloxone challenge test performed and negative result obtained.

Child: Under 18 years, not recommended.

Renal Impairment: Caution; failure, contraindicated.

Hepatic Impairment: Mild, moderate, caution; failure, acute hepatitis, contraindicated.

CI: Currently opioid-dependence (acute withdrawal risk), positive opioid screen or failed naloxone challenge, acute opioid withdrawal.

Interactions: Effect of Other Drugs on Naltrexone: *Co-admin contraindicated*: Methadone. *Co-admin not recommended, avoid*: Opioid-containing medicines (analgesics, antitussives, substitution treatments), high dose opioids (acute intoxication, see SP below), agonist-antagonist opioids, central antihypertensives (alpha-methyldopa). *Caution*: Barbiturates, benzodiazepines, anxiolytics, meprobamate, hypnotics, sedative antidepressants (amitriptyline, doxepin, mianserin, trimipramine), sedative antihistamines, droperidol. *Co-admin, lethargy, somnolence*: Thioridazine.

SP: Consider treatment only if opioid-free for minimum 7-10 days, not showing signs of withdrawal; recommend naloxone challenge to screen for opioid use. Warn patients of risk of attempting to overcome blockade with large opioid dose (can lead to life-threatening opioid poisoning; respiratory, circulatory impairment). Monitor LFTs (before, during treatment). Emergency opioid analgesia (higher dose required; respiratory depression deeper); non-receptor mediated actions (facial swelling, itching, generalised erythema). Increased suicide risk (substance abusers with/without depression); naltrexone does not eliminate risk.

Pregnancy, Lactation: Pregnancy, use only if benefit outweighs risk. Lactation, not recommended.

ADR: See Notes below.

Notes: See 15.1 Specific Substance Antagonists.

Nalorex **50mg** *(BMS)* A. GMS.
Price, (28) €51.41.
Tablet, naltrexone HCl. Pale-yellow cap-shaped f/c scored. Marked R11; 50 on reverse. *Lactose.*
Naltrexone **50mg** *(Accord)* A. GMS.
Price, (28) €60.36.
Tablet, naltrexone HCl. Yellow oval f/c scored (divisible into equal halves). *Lactose.*

15.1.6 - Paracetamol

In This Chapter: *Acetylcysteine.*

Acetylcysteine (toxicology)

ATC Code: V03AB23. **Sport:** Permitted.
Driving: Unlikely to impair.

Indications: Paracetamol overdose in staggered overdose; where there is any doubt over time of overdose; plasma paracetamol level on or above line joining points 100mg/L (4 hours) and 15mg/L (15 hours).

Dose: Adult, Elderly: Initially 150mg/kg body weight in 200mL infusion fluid over 15 minutes; then 50mg/kg in 500mL infusion fluid over next 4 hours; then 100mg/kg in 1L infusion fluid over next 16 hours; total 300mg/kg over 21 hours. Dose calculation for obese patients, ceiling weight 110kg using actual weight.

Child: As for Adult, reduce infusion volume. Initially 150mg/kg infusion over 1 hour as 50mg/mL soln (rate 3mL/kg/hour); then 50mg/kg infused over 4 hours as 6.25mg/mL soln (rate 2mL/kg/hour); then 100mg/kg infused over 16 hours as 6.25mg/mL soln (rate 1mL/kg/hour).

Interactions: Effect of Acetylcysteine on Other Drugs: Carbamazepine: *Increased clearance (seizure risk).*

SP: IV acetylcysteine admin within 24 hours of ingestion of potentially hepatotoxic paracetamol overdose is indicated to reduce severity of liver damage. Most effective if admin within 8-10 hours of overdose; efficacy diminished between 10-24 hours post overdose (still can benefit). May be admin after 24 hours if at risk for severe liver damage. Increased hepatotoxicity risk, drugs inducing liver enzymes, routine excess alcohol consumption, malnutrition (anorexia, HIV; risk of hepatotoxicity at lower paracetamol plasma conc due to depleted glutathione reserves). Anaphylactoid hypersensitivity reactions (especially initial dose). Asthma, history of bronchospasm, caution. Changes in haemostatic parameters. Fluid overload risk/hyponatraemia, seizures, death (children, fluid-restricted patients, under 40kg weight).

Pregnancy, Lactation: If benefit outweighs risk.

ADR: *Most common,* nausea, vomiting, flushing, skin rash. Adverse reactions usually occur 15-60 minutes after start of infusion.

Notes: See 15.1 Specific Substance Antagonists.

Parvolex Parenteral *(Phoenix)* A.
Price, 10mL (10) 200mg/mL, €36.10.
Infusion, acetylcysteine 200mg/mL. Clear colourless conc for soln. *Sodium 322.6mg/10mL.*

15.1.7 - Potassium

In This Chapter: *Calcium polystyrene sulfonate.*

15.2   Detoxifying Agents Used For Antineoplastic Treatment

Calcium Polystyrene Sulphonate

ATC Code: VO3AE01. **Sport:** Permitted.
Driving: None stated.

Indications: Hyperkalaemia, associated with anuria or severe oliguria (patients requiring acute dialysis, regular haemodialysis, prolonged peritoneal dialysis).

Dose: Adult, Elderly: ORAL, 15g 3-4 times daily.

RECTAL, 30g resin in susp daily as retention enema; retain for at least 9 hours, then colonic irrigation to remove.

Child: ORAL, acute, 1g/kg in divided doses; maintenance 0.5g/kg.
RECTAL, dose at least as great as oral, in susp. Neonates, 0.5-1g/kg. See SP below.

CI: Plasma potassium below 5mmoL/L, hypercalcaemia, obstructive bowel disease, neonates with reduced gut motility. See Child above.

Interactions: Effect of Other Drugs on Calcium Polystyrene Sulphonate: *Co-admin not recommended:* Sorbitol (oral or rectal) due to cases of intestinal necrosis and other serious GI adverse events which may be fatal (see SP). *Co-admin caution:* Cation-donating agents, non-absorbable cation-donating antacids and laxatives, aluminium hydroxide, digitalis-like drugs.

Effect of Calcium Polystyrene Sulphonate on Other Drugs: Lithium, levothyroxine: *Absorption reduced (possible).* Fat soluble vitamins: *Absorption inhibited.*

SP: GI stenosis, intestinal ischaemia (necrosis, perforation) may occur especially in patients using sorbitol. Hypokalaemia (severe; caution with digitalis co-admin), hypomagnesaemia, hypercalcaemia, monitor. Acute hyperkalaemia not due to excess potassium (IV glucose infusion with soluble insulin recommended in conjunction with calcium polystyrene sulphonate). Constipation, magnesium-containing laxatives not recommended. Position patient carefully when ingesting resin, to avoid aspiration. Neonates/children, oral route not recommended; rectal, impaction risk (excessive dosage/inadequate dilution). Premature infants, low birth weight (digestive haemorrhage or colonic necrosis).

Pregnancy, Lactation: If benefit outweighs risk.

ADR: GI irritation, anorexia, nausea, vomiting, constipation, diarrhoea. Rectal admin, faecal impaction (children).

Notes: See 15.1 Specific Substance Antagonists.

Calcium Resonium Powder *(SANOFI)* OTC. GMS.
Price, (30g) €43.04.
Powder for oral or rectal susp, calcium polystyrene sulfonate 99.934% w/w. Buff-coloured fine.

15.2 - Detoxifying Agents Used For Antineoplastic Treatment

In This Chapter: *Mesna.*

Class Effects

Calcium folinate is used to diminish toxicity and counteract action of folic acid antagonists (methotrexate) in cytotoxic therapy (calcium folinate rescue) and overdose. See Notes below.

CI: Hypersensitivity to any member of the class. Hypersensitivity to thiol *(Mesna).*

Notes: See 13.1.3 Antimetabolites (calcium folinate).
Price,

Mesna

ATC Code: VO3AF01. **Sport:** Permitted.
Driving: Syncope, light-headedness, lethargy, drowsiness, dizziness, blurred vision.

Indications: Prophylaxis, urothelial toxicity (haemorrhagic

cystitis, micro/macrohaematuria) with ifosfamide and cyclophosphamide (oxazaphosphorines) at urotoxic doses.

Dose: Adult, Elderly: ORAL, intermittent oxazaphosphorine, mesna 40% of oxazaphorine dose weight for weight (w/w) rounded down to nearest whole tablet. *Admin,* 2 hours before then 2 hours and 6 hours after oxazaphorine i.e. -2, +2, +6 hours. High risk patients, dose at shorter than 4-hour intervals and/or increase number of doses. Intermittent oxazaphosphorine, if IV is used at start, replace -2 hours (oral) with 0 hours IV. Ifosfamide 24-hour infusion, admin oral mesna as ifosfamide-mesna infusion finishes, then at +2 and +6 hours. Ifosphamide long-term continuous infusion, admin as for 24-hour infusion but all oral mesna doses should be 40% of final 24-hour ifosfamide dose rounded as above.

PARENTERAL, oxazaphosphorine as IV bolus, admin mesna 20% w/w of co-admin oxazaphosphorine by IV injection over 15-30 minutes (0 hours); repeat at +4 and +8 hours. If needed increase to 40% w/w 4-times daily at 3-hourly intervals (0, 3, 6 and 9 hours) (total dose = 160% w/w oxazaphosphorine dose). Ifosfamide 24-hour infusion, initially 20% w/w of ifosfamide dose admin as IV bolus, then infusion of 100% w/w over 24 hours, then 60% w/w over 12 hours. Ifosfamide long-term infusion, initially 20% w/w as IV bolus as ifosfamide infusion starts, then co-admin 24-hour mesna 100% w/w infusion with each 24-hour ifosfamide, then 60% w/w for 12 hours as ifosfamide-mesna infusion finishes. *Admin,* mesna can be mixed in same infusion bag as ifosfamide.

PARENTERAL USED AS ORAL (ampoules), compared with IV admin, overall availability of mesna in urine after oral admin, approx. 50%. Dosage 40% w/w as for oral above. *Admin,* add contents of ampoule to flavoured soft drink (orange juice, cola).

Child: Under 16 years, safety/efficacy not established. See Adult, high risk patients. See medical literature.

SP: High risk patients (damaged urothelium from previous treatment, pelvic irradiation, not protected by standard mesna dose e.g. with urinary tract disease). Hypersensitivity reactions (various skin reactions, other reactions, anaphylaxis); may worsen with re-exposure (life-threatening). Maintain sufficient urinary output.

Pregnancy, Lactation: If benefit outweighs risk.

ADR: Summary, *most frequent,* headache, abdominal pain/colic, light-headedness, lethargy, drowsiness, pyrexia, rash, diarrhoea, nausea, flushing, influenza-like illness; *most severe,* toxic epidermal necrolysis, Stevens-Johnson syndrome, anaphylaxis, DRESS.

Notes: See 15.2 Detoxifying Agents Used For Antineoplastic Treatment.

Uromitexan 400mg, 600mg, Parenteral *(Baxter)* A.
Price, (10) 400mg, €23.13. 600mg, €30.05. Parenteral 100mg/mL (15) 4mL, €32.62. 10mL, €73.21.
Tablet, mesna. White oblong f/c scored (facilitates breaking). 400mg: Marked M4. 600mg: Marked M6. *Lactose.*
Injection or infusion, as above 100mg/mL. Clear colourless soln.

15.3 - Dependence

15.3.1 - Alcohol Dependence

In This Chapter: *Acamprosate, disulfiram, nalmefene.*

Class Effects

CI: Hypersensitivity to any member of the class. Use in children.

SP: Use in conjunction with psychiatric treatment and/or support programmes. Due to the complex interrelationship between alcohol dependence, depression and suicidality, monitor.

Pregnancy, Lactation: Not recommended.

Acamprosate

ATC Code: N07BB03. **Sport:** Permitted.
Driving: Unlikely to impair.
Indications: Maintenance of abstinence in alcohol-dependent patients.
Dose: Adult: Over 60kg, 2 tabs 3-times daily; below 60kg, 2 tabs in morning, 1 at midday, 1 at night. Oral, with food.
Elderly: Over 65 years, not recommended.
Renal Impairment: Serum creatinine above 120micromoL/L, not recommended.
Hepatic Impairment: Severe, not recommended.
SP: Specialist supervision. Does not constitute treatment for withdrawal period.
ADR: Nausea, vomiting, diarrhoea, abdominal pain, pruritus, maculo-papular rash, bullous reactions, hypersensitivity, frigidity, impotence, decreased or increased libido.
Notes: See 15.3.1 Alcohol Dependence.

> **Campral EC 333mg** *(Merck Serono)* B. GMS.
> *Price,* (84) €21.24.
> *Tablet,* acamprosate calcium. White e/c.

Disulfiram

ATC Code: N07BB01. **Sport:** Permitted.
Driving: Caution.
Indications: Adjunctive, treatment of co-operative chronic alcohol dependents.
Dose: Adult, Elderly: 800mg (day) 1 in 1 dose (strict instruction NOT to take any alcohol); 600mg (day 2), 400mg (day 3), 200mg (day 4, 5), then 100-200mg daily or 2-3 times weekly. *Admin,* disperse tabs in water, stir and take immediately; may be swallowed whole.
CI: Decompensated cardiac disease, severe hypertension, psychoses.
Interactions: Effect of Other Drugs on Disulfiram: *Co-admin not recommended*: Alcohol (reaction can occur within 10 minutes; intensity may be increased by amitriptyline and decreased by diazepam; overall intensity may be increased by chlorpromazine). *Synergistic action, toxicity*: Metronidazole, isoniazid.
Effect of Disulfiram on Other Drugs: Paraldehyde, phenytoin, barbiturates, amphetamines, morphine, diazepam, rifampicin, chlordiazepoxide, oral hypoglycaemics: *Metabolism altered.* Coumarin anti-coagulants: *Activity enhanced.* Pimozide: *Potentiation of organic brain syndrome.*
SP: Initial treatment (fatigue, drowsiness, headache, nausea, vomiting, halitosis, taste disorders, reduced libido), if marked reduce dose. Caution (renal, hepatic or respiratory disease, diabetes, epilepsy, peripheral neuropathy, hypothyroidism, irreversible brain damage). Do not admin until minimum 24 hours after last alcohol ingestion. NOTE: Inform patient and relatives that the patient must not take alcohol during treatment; should not be given without full knowledge; caution, certain food sauces, some medicines contain alcohol. Never admin with state of alcoholic intoxication. Alcohol should not be taken for 1 week after discontinuation.
ADR: Elevated LFTs. See SP above.
Notes: See 15.3.1 Alcohol Dependence.

> **Antabuse 400mg** *(TEVA)* B. GMS.
> *Price,* (50) €24.04.
> *Effervescent tab,* disulfiram. White flat round scored. Marked CJ.

Nalmefene

ATC Code: N07BB05. **Sport:** Pending.
Driving: Nausea, dizziness, insomnia, headache.
Indications: Reduction, alcohol consumption, adults with alcohol dependence who have a high drinking risk level

(DRL), without withdrawal symptoms not requiring immediate detoxification.
Dose: Adult, Elderly: Initiate only if a high DRL continues after initial assessment. Take as-needed on each day the patient perceives a risk of drinking alcohol; take 1 tab preferably 1-2 hours prior to anticipated time of drinking. If the patient has started drinking without dosing, take 1 tab as soon as possible. Max. 1 tab/day; swallow whole with or without food; do not divide or crush. *Elderly*, limited data, caution.
Renal Impairment: Mild/moderate, caution (frequent monitoring). Severe, contraindicated.
Hepatic Impairment: As for Renal above.
CI: Opioids (currently taking, addiction, acute withdrawal, suspected use); acute alcohol withdrawal syndrome (hallucinations, seizures, delirium tremens). See Interactions and SP below.
Interactions: Effect of Other Drugs on Nalmefene: *Co-admin contraindicated*: Opioid agonists (opioid analgesics), for substitution therapy (methadone) or partial agonists (buprenorphine). *Co-admin caution*: Medicinals containing opioids (cough medications, opioid analgesics). *Increased nalmefene exposure*: UGT2B7 potent inhibitors (diclofenac, fluconazole, medroxyprogesterone, meclofenamic acid). *Sub-therapeutic nalmefene plasma levels*: UGT inducers (dexamethasone, phenobarbital, rifampicin, omeprazole).
SP: *Selincro* is not for patients where the goal is abstinence; reduction of alcohol consumption is intermediate goal. In emergency if opioids must be admin, the amount of opioid required may be greater to have desired effect; monitor for respiratory depression. Elective surgery, discontinue one week prior to anticipated opioid use. Psychiatric effects; caution with current psychiatric conditions (major depression). Seizure disorders, caution. Simultaneous intake of alcohol with nalmefene does not prevent intoxicating effects of alcohol.
ADR: Summary, *most common*, nausea, dizziness, insomnia, headache.
Notes: See 15.3.1 Alcohol Dependence.

> ▼ **Selincro 18mg** *(Lundbeck)* A. GMS.
> *Price,* (14), €49.97. (28), €101.90.
> *Tablet,* nalmefene hydrochloride dihydrate. White oval f/c. Marked S. *Lactose.*

15.3.2 - Smoking Cessation

In This Chapter: *Bupropion, nicotine, varenicline.*

Class Effects
CI: Hypersensitivity to any member of the class. Use in children.
Interactions: Effect of Drugs Used For Smoking Cessation on Other Drugs: Due to smoking cessation: Drugs with narrow therapeutic window, metabolised by CYP1A2 (theophylline, tacrine, clozapine), possibly (imipramine, olanzapine, clomipramine, fluvoxamine), may require dose reduction (caffeine, pentazocine, phenacetin, phenylbutazone, flecainide): *Reduced clearance, plasma levels increased.* Insulin: *Increased SC absorption.* Isoprenaline, salbutamol: *Consider dose increase.* Propoxyphene, frusemide, H2-antagonists: *Adjust dose (smoking reduces effect).*
SP: *Neuropsychiatric symptoms,* depressed mood associated with nicotine withdrawal; rarely suicidal ideation and suicide attempt with smoking cessation. Smoking cessation may also cause exacerbation of underlying psychiatric illness (depression); history of psychiatric illness (caution). Possible emergence of significant depressive symptomatology in patients undergoing a smoking cessation attempt; advise patients accordingly.

15.3.2 Smoking Cessation

Dose may require adjustment of some co-admin drugs. Drug therapy should be in combination with motivation support, in accordance with smoking cessation guidelines. More likely to succeed where there is motivation to quit, with motivational support.

ADR: Transdermal, local skin reactions. Chronic dermatological disorders (psoriasis, chronic dermatitis, urticaria); do not apply patch to affected areas. Erythema; severe or persistent, discontinue.

Bupropion

ATC Code: N07BC01. **Sport:** Permitted (included in monitoring programme).

Driving: Caution.

Indications: Aid to smoking cessation.

Dose: Adult: Initially 150mg/day (6 days); increase on day 7 to 150mg twice daily (at 8 hour intervals); max. single dose 150mg; max. daily dose, 300mg. *Admin*, swallow tabs whole; do not cut, crush or chew; with or without food.

Elderly: Possible greater sensitivity; 150mg once daily.

Child: Under 18 years, not recommended.

Renal Impairment: As for Elderly above.

Hepatic Impairment: Mild to moderate, as for Elderly above.

CI: Current seizure disorder, CNS tumour, undergoing abrupt withdrawal associated with seizures (alcohol, benzodiazepines), bulimia or anorexia nervosa, severe hepatic cirrhosis, bipolar disorder (may precipitate manic episode during depressed phase).

Interactions: Effect of Other Drugs on Bupropion: *Co-admin contraindicated:* Other bupropion-containing products (incidence of seizures, dose dependent; to avoid overdosage). *Co-admin not recommended:* MAOIs (allow 14-day dosing interval; reversible MAOIs, 24-hour interval). *Increased plasma levels, lower active metabolite levels:* CYP2B6 substrates (cyclophosphamide, ifosfamide), CYP2B6 inhibitors (orphenadrine, ticlopidine, clopidogrel). *Metabolism induced (consider dose increase; not to exceed max. dose):* Carbamazepine, phenytoin, ritonavir, efavirenz. *Metabolism inhibited:* Valproate. *Avoid:* Alcohol. *Increased exposure:* High fat meal.

Effect of Bupropion on Other Drugs: Drugs with narrow therapeutic window, metabolised by CYP2D6 including antidepressants (desipramine, imipramine, paroxetine), antipsychotics (risperidone, thioridazine), beta-blockers (metoprolol), Type 1c antiarrhythmics (propafenone, flecainide): *Reduce dose.* Citalopram: *Plasma levels increased.* Tamoxifen: *Reduced endoxifen metabolite conc (reduced efficacy); avoid co-admin. Plasma levels decreased:* Digoxin (may rise with bupropion discontinuation).

SP: Risk of dose-related seizures increased with predisposing risk factors (medicinals lowering seizure threshold, alcohol abuse, head trauma, diabetes treated with oral hypoglycaemics or insulin, stimulants or anorectic products), use only if benefit outweighs risk (max. 150mg/day). Seizures, discontinue. Dry mouth, insomnia. Neuropsychiatric reactions. Psychotic and manic symptomatology (patients with psychiatric illness history); depression, suicidal ideation/behaviour. Hypersensitivity; discontinue, treat (antihistamines or corticosteroids). Hypertension (severe), monitor. Hepatic impairment, monitor (insomnia, dry mouth, seizures) indicating high drug or metabolite levels. Interference with some rapid urine drug screening tests.

Pregnancy, Lactation: Pregnancy, not recommended. Lactation, stop breastfeeding or stop drug.

ADR: *Very common,* insomnia.

Notes: See 15.3.2 Smoking Cessation.

Zyban 150mg *(GSK)* A. GMS.
Price, (100) €98.96.
Prolonged/R tablet, bupropion HCl. White f/round. Marked GXCH7.
Store: Below 25 deg C; original pack.

Nicotine

ATC Code: N07BA01. **Sport:** Permitted.

Driving: Smoking cessation can cause behavioural changes

Indications: Relief of nicotine craving and withdrawal symptoms, to facilitate smoking cessation, to assist temporary abstinence, to reduce smoking prior to stopping (gradual cessation).

Dose: Adult, Elderly: Smoking cessation: ORAL, low/moderate dependence (under 20 cigarettes/day), use 2mg (gum or tab) per hour OR 1mg (lozenge) every 1-2 hours; strong dependence (20-30 cigarettes/day), use gum 2mg or 4mg depending on patient characteristics OR 1-2mg (lozenge); very strong dependence (over 30 cigarettes/day) use 4mg (gum or tab) per hour OR 2-4mg (lozenge) every 1-2 hours.

INHALER, up to 8 weeks, 3-6 cartridges/day; reduce over following 2 weeks to zero; max. 6 cartridges in 24 hours. May be used with transdermal.

OROMUCOSAL SPRAY, up to 4 sprays per hour; max. 2 sprays per dosing episode and 64 sprays in any 24-hour period. Weeks 1-6, most smokers will need 1-2 sprays every 30-60 minutes; weeks 7-9, reduce number of sprays to half used in weeks 1-6; weeks 10-12, continue reducing to max. 4 sprays/day in week 12. At 2-4 sprays per day, discontinue.

TRANSDERMAL, 1 patch delivering 15mg, 10mg, 5mg released over 16 hours, as needed; max. application time 16 hours in any 24-hour period *(Nicorette)* OR 1 patch delivering 21mg (TTS 30), 14mg (TTS 20), 7mg (TTS 10) per 24 hours; using each size/strength for 3-4 weeks *(Nicotinell)* OR 1 patch delivering 21mg/24 hours (first six weeks), then 14mg/24 hours (next 2 weeks), then 7mg/24 hours (last 2 weeks) *(NiQuitin)*.

Temporary abstinence, use when required. Gradual cessation, if unwilling to quit abruptly, use gum when strong urge to smoke to reduce number of cigarettes; max. 15 pieces per day. It may be beneficial to utilise more than one form of nicotine replacement therapy (NRT) concurrently (heavy smokers; relapsed on monotherapy), see manufacturers Full Prescribing Information.

Child: Under 18 years, not recommended. *Nicorette* (lozenges), use with medical advice (age 12-17 years); under 12 years not recommended.

Renal Impairment: Moderate, caution; severe, not recommended.

Hepatic Impairment: Moderate to severe, as for Renal above.

CI: Non-smokers. Phenylketonuria *(NiQuitin lozenges).* Acute MI, unstable or worsening angina pectoris, severe cardiac arrhythmias, recent CVA, diseases of skin which may complicate patch *(Nicotinell TTS).*

Interactions: Effect of Other Drugs on Nicotine: *Buccal absorption decreased (gum, lozenges):* Acidic beverages (coffee, soda).

Effect of Nicotine on Other Drugs: Adenosine: *Haemodynamic effects may be enhanced.*

SP: Benefits of quitting smoking outweigh risks of nicotine replace therapy (NRT). Assess risk/benefit: Dependent smokers with recent MI, unstable or worsening angina (including Prinzmetal's), severe cardiac arrhythmias, recent CVA, uncontrolled hypertension (initiate under close supervision); diabetes mellitus (monitor blood sugar); renal and hepatic impairment (caution decreased clearance); phaeochromocytoma, uncontrolled hyperthyroidism (caution, nicotine causes catecholamine release); GI disease (oesophagitis, gastric or peptic ulcers) (caution, symptom exacerbation). Do not apply patches to affected skin (chronic psoriasis, dermatitis). Nicotine may cause dependence syndrome (chronic use); highly toxic (acute use); dependence with pharmaceutical forms is less harmful and easier to break than smoking dependence. Keep out of reach of children (suspected nicotine poisoning in a child is a medical emergency); if excessive amount of nicotine is swallowed, activated charcoal reduces GI absorption.

Pregnancy, Lactation: Pregnancy, only on medical advice especially third trimester; haemodynamic effects on foetus. Lactation, nicotine is excreted in breast milk in quantities that may affect the child; not recommended; if smoking withdrawal not achieved, use only on medical advice.

ADR: *Common,* headache, nausea, GI discomfort/pain, hiccups, mouth or throat irritation, jaw muscle ache with gum; sore mouth or throat, dry mouth, burning sensation with sublingual tab; nasal congestion with inhaler; itch or contact sensitisation/application site reaction with patch; dysgeusia with oromucosal spray.

Notes: See 15.3.2 Smoking Cessation.

Nicorette Gum, Spray *(McNeil)* OTC. GMS.
Price, gum (210) 2mg, €26.90. 4mg, €33.19. QuickMist Oromucosal Spray 1-pack (2x150-dose) €25.16.
Chewing gum, nicotine 2mg, 4mg. Resin complex. Plain. *Sorbitol.* Fresh fruit. *Butylhydroxytoluene.* **Store:** Below 25 deg C; original pack.
Oromucosal spray (QuickMist), nicotine 13.6mg/1mL. Clear (opalescent) colourless (light-yellow) soln. *Ethanol.* **Store:** Below 25 deg C.

Nicorette Inhaler, Transdermal *(McNeil)* OTC. GMS.
Price, inhaler 15mg (20) €17.11. Patch (per 16 hours): Invisi 10mg, 15mg (7) €11.63; Extra Strength 25mg (7) €11.63, (14) €23.26.
Inhalation cartridge, nicotine 15mg. White (slightly coloured) porous plugs sealed in transparent plastic cartridge.
Transdermal patch (Invisi), nicotine 10mg, 15mg, Extra Strength 25mg per 16 hours. Pre-coated backing layer, nicotine source layer, skin contact adhesive layer. Printed Nicorette. **Store:** Below 25 deg C.

Nicotinell Gum, Lozenge *(Novartis Consumer)* OTC. GMS.
Price, gum (12) €2.05; (24) €3.61. 4mg (12) €2.19; (96) €14.39. Lozenge 1mg (12) €2.44; (36) €5.99; (96) €12.73.
Medicated chewing gum, nicotine polacrilin 2mg, 4mg. Off-white rectangular. *Sodium 11.5mg (Fruit) or 11.44mg (Cool Mint) per piece; sorbitol, butylhydroxytoluene.*
Compressed lozenge, nicotine bitartrate dihydrate 1mg. White round compressed; mint. *Aspartame, maltitol; sodium 9.5mg/lozenge (Nicotinell Mint).*

Nicotinell TTS Transdermal *(Novartis Consumer)* OTC. GMS.
Price, (7) 7mg, €11.38. 14mg, €11.89. 21mg, €12.39.
Transdermal patch, nicotine TTS 10 (7mg), 20 (14mg), 30 (21mg). Round flat matrix-type self-adhesive patch.

NiQuitin Lozenge 2mg, 4mg, Transdermal *(Chefaro)* OTC. GMS.
Price, lozenge (72) 2mg, 4mg, €15.91. Patch CQ, (7) 7mg, 14mg, 21mg, €12.81; 21mg (14) €23.09.
Lozenge 2mg, 4mg, nicotine resinate. White round. Marked NL/strength, and S. *Aspartame, mannitol, sodium 17mg, mint flavour.*
Transdermal patch, nicotine 7mg, 14mg, 21mg. Rectangular, matt pinkish tan-coloured/clear.

Varenicline

ATC Code: N07BA03. **Sport:** Permitted.
Driving: Minor/moderate effect (dizziness, somnolence).
Indications: Smoking cessation (adults).
Dose: Adult: Initiate 1-2 weeks before date on which patient has decided to stop smoking. Initially 0.5mg once daily (days 1-3), then 0.5mg twice daily (days 4-7), then 1mg twice daily (day 8 to end of treatment). Duration 12 weeks. If smoking cessation achieved, consider second 12-week course at 1mg daily. If adverse reactions are not tolerated, lower dose temporarily or permanently to 0.5mg twice daily. *Admin,* oral; swallow whole with water, with or without food.
Elderly: Consider renal status.
Child: Under 18 years, safety/efficacy not established.
Renal Impairment: Mild, no adjustment. Moderate impairment and not tolerated, reduce to 1mg once daily.

CrCl (mL/min) below 30, initially 0.5mg once daily (3 days), then 1mg once daily. ESRD, not recommended.
Hepatic Impairment: No adjustment.
Interactions: Effect of Other Drugs on Varenicline: *Co-admin avoid (severe renal impairment)*: Cimetidine.
Effect of Varenicline on Other Drugs: ALCOHOL: *Increased intoxicating effects reported.*
SP: New or worsening cardiovascular symptoms. Seizures reported (post-marketing). Discontinuation associated with increased irritability, urge to smoke, depression and/or insomnia; taper dose. Patients with or without history of psychiatric disorder (use not associated with increased risk of serious neuropsychiatric adverse events).
Pregnancy, Lactation: Pregnancy, not recommended; women of childbearing potential should avoid becoming pregnant during treatment. Lactation, not known if excreted in breast milk; stop breastfeeding or stop drug.
ADR: Summary, *most common,* nausea. Smoking cessation is associated with various symptoms (dysphoric or depressed mood, insomnia, irritability, frustration or anger, anxiety, difficulty concentrating, restlessness, decreased heart rate, increased appetite, weight gain).
Notes: See 15.3.2 Smoking Cessation.

CHAMPIX 0.5mg, 1mg *(Pfizer)* A. GMS.
Price, (56) 0.5mg, €81.69. 1mg, €79.06. Initiation pack (4-week), €75.69.
Tablet, varenicline tartrate. Cap-shaped f/c. Marked Pfizer; CHX/strength on reverse. 0.5mg: White. 1mg: Light blue.

15.3.3 - Opiate Dependence

In This Chapter: *Buprenorphine, buprenorphine/naloxone combination, methadone.*

Class Effects
Buprenorphine and methadone are also indicated for pain management. See Notes below.
CI: Hypersensitivity to any member of the class. Under 15 years, not recommended *(buprenorphine and combination)*; under 18 years, not recommended *(methadone)* as children more sensitive to respiratory and CNS depressant effects.
SP: Treatment by physicians with specialist training (consultants, and/or Level I or Level II GPs); all treated patients must be on central register according to Drug Misuse Programme guidelines. Potential for morphine type dependence. Discontinue gradually to avoid withdrawal.
ADR: See manufacturers Full Prescribing Information.

Buprenorphine (opiate dependence)

ATC Code: N07BC01. **Sport:** Prohibited (in-competition).
Driving: Caution.
Indications: Substitution treatment in major opioid dependence within comprehensive programme.
Dose: Adult, Elderly: Initially 0.8-4mg as single daily dose; titrate as needed to max. single daily dose 32mg. Opioid-dependents (not undergone withdrawal), admin 1 dose at least 6 hours after last opioid use or when signs of craving appear. Methadone treated, reduce methadone to max. 30mg/day before commencing; may precipitate withdrawal symptoms in opioid or methadone dependants. Sublingual, do not chew or swallow tabs whole; keep tab under tongue until dissolved (5-10 minutes).
Child: Age 15-18 years, caution.
Renal Impairment: Titrate slower to allow for stabilisation.
Hepatic Impairment: As for Renal above.
SP: Determine (baseline LFTs, viral hepatitis status) before initiation; monitor if at risk of accelerated liver injury (viral hepatitis positive, medication co-admin and/or existing liver dysfunction). Marked dependence, initial admin can

15.3.3 Opiate Dependence

produce withdrawal effect similar to naloxone (has partial agonist profile; can precipitate withdrawal especially if admin less than 6 hours after last heroin dose or 24 hours after last methadone dose). Chronic admin produces dependence of the opiate type. Respiratory depression (fatal) reported (combination with benzodiazepines, alcohol, other opioids); in some non-opioid dependent individuals not tolerant to effects of opioids and/or children (especially with accidental ingestion). Caution, asthma or respiratory insufficiency (COPD, cor pulmonale, decreased respiratory reserve, hypoxia, hypercapnia, pre-existing respiratory depression, kyphoscoliosis).

ADR: See Notes below.

Notes: See 15.3.3 Opiate Dependence.

> **Subutex Sublingual** *(Indivior)* CD.
> Price, not published by company.
> *Sublingual tablet*, buprenorphine HCl 0.4mg, 2mg, 8mg. White flat oval. Marked with logo; B and strength on reverse. *Lactose.*

Buprenorphine, Naloxone

ATC Code: N07BC51. **Sport:** Prohibited (in-competition).
Driving: Drowsiness, dizziness, impaired thinking.
Indications: As for buprenorphine (naloxone component is to deter IV misuse).

Dose: Adult: 2mg/0.5mg (or 8mg/2mg) as single dose or 2 divided doses taken directly after each other. Initially 1 or 2 tablets (2mg/0.5mg); an additional 1 or 2 tables may be admin on day 1 depending on requirement. Opioid-dependent addicts not undergone withdrawal, methadone treated, see Notes below (buprenorphine); initiate not less than 24 hours after last methadone usage. Titrate in 2-8mg increments to max. 24mg/day as needed. Sublingual is only effective and safe admin route; place under tongue until dissolved (5-10 minutes).

Elderly: Over 65 years, no data.

Child: Under 15 years, no data.

Renal Impairment: CrCl (mL/min) below 30, caution.

Hepatic Impairment: Lower initial doses, titrate carefully. Severe, contraindicated.

SP: See Notes below (buprenorphine). No notable interaction with cocaine.

Pregnancy, Lactation: Pregnancy, if benefit outweighs risk; towards end of pregnancy, buprenorphine may induce respiratory depression in the newborn; long-term admin in last trimester may cause neonatal withdrawal. Lactation, stop breastfeeding.

ADR: See Notes below.

Notes: See Buprenorphine above. See 15.3.3 Opiate Dependence.

> **Suboxone Sublingual** *(Indivior)* CD.
> Price, not published by company.
> *Sublingual tablet*, buprenorphine HCl 2mg (8mg), naloxone HCl dihydrate 0.5mg (2mg). White hexagonal. Marked with logo; N and strength on reverse. *Lactose.*

Methadone

ATC Code: N07BC02. **Sport:** Prohibited (in-competition).
Driving: Moderate influence (orthostatic hypotension, drowsiness).
Indications: Treatment, opioid drug addiction (narcotic abstinence syndrome suppressant). Analgesic, relief of severe pain where morphine may be reasonable alternative (severe cancer pain) *(Phymet, Pinadone).*

Dose: Adult: Opioid addiction, initially a daily dose of 10-40mg orally; titrate by max. 10mg in one day; max. 30mg weekly increase up to total daily dose 60-120mg until no signs of withdrawal or intoxication. After stabilisation, gradually decrease dose until total withdrawal achieved.

Analgesia, initially 5-10mg orally; subsequent doses according to individual patient response; if admin more frequently than 6-8 hourly, accumulation may occur (increased sedation and respiratory depression).

Elderly: Long half-live may cause accumulation especially with impaired renal function.

Child: Under 18 years, not recommended.

Renal Impairment: GFR (mL/min) 10-50, dose interval minimum 8-hourly; below 10, minimum 12-hourly.

Hepatic Impairment: Reduce dose (metabolised more slowly). Severe, contraindicated (may precipitate hepatic encephalopathy).

CI: Respiratory depression (with cyanosis, excessive bronchial secretions), during bronchial asthma attack, acute alcoholism, head injury, raised intracranial pressure, ulcerative colitis (toxic dilatation, colonic spasm).

Interactions: Effect of Other Drugs on Methadone: *Co-admin not recommended:* MAOIs. *Co-admin caution:* Drugs prolonging QT-interval (Class I and III antiarrhythmics, some neuroleptics, TCADs, calcium channel blockers), drugs causing electrolyte disturbances (diuretics, laxatives, mineralocorticoid hormones). *Metabolism increased:* Rifampicin, phenytoin, carbamazepine, St John's Wort, antiretrovirals (nevirapine, efavirenz, some protease inhibitors). *Metabolism decreased (increased methadone toxicity):* Fluconazole, some SSRIs (fluvoxamine). *Decreased clearance:* CYP3A4 inhibitors (some anti-HIV agents, macrolides, cimetidine, azole antifungals). *Urinary clearance increased:* Acid urine. *Urinary clearance decreased:* Alkaline urine (common in vegetarians).

Effect of Methadone on Other Drugs: Nelfinavir, zidovudine, fluconazole, desipramine: *Plasma levels increased.* Abacavir, amprenavir: *Plasma levels decreased.*

SP: *Extreme caution,* phaeochromocytoma (aggravated hypertension). *Caution,* hypothyroidism, adrenocortical insufficiency, hypopituitarism, prostatic hypertrophy, shock. Respiratory depression is the major hazard associated with methadone treatment (peak depressive effect persists longer than peak analgesic effect, especially during initiation; during dose initiation and adjustment, caution advisable). QT-interval prolongation and serious arrhythmia (Torsade de Pointes) observed (especially above 100mg/day); caution, QT-interval prolongation risk (cardiac hypertrophy, concomitant diuretic use, hypokalaemia, hypomagnesaemia), history of cardiac repolarisation prolongation, medications affecting cardiac repolarisation or methadone metabolism, increased arrhythmia risk. NOTE: Deaths due to cardiac arrhythmias and respiratory depression may occur, (especially when used for analgesia during treatment initiation or conversion from other opioids).

Pregnancy, Lactation: Pregnancy, if benefit outweighs risk; crosses placenta; neonatal (respiratory depression, abstinence syndrome). Not for use during labour (long duration of action, neonatal respiratory depression risk). Lactation, permitted (monitor baby for sedation).

ADR: Very common, dizziness, drowsiness, light-headedness, nausea, vomiting, dry mouth, constipation, sweating. See SP above.

Notes: See 15.3.3 Opiate Dependence. Reimbursed under Methadone Treatment Scheme.

> **Phymet DTF 1mg/mL** *(GSK)* CD.
> Price, not published by company.
> *Oral syrup*, methadone HCl. Clear viscous green. *Parabens, Sunset Yellow, maltitol, sorbitol.*
>
> **Methadone 1mg/mL Sugar Free** *(Rosemont)* CD.
> Price, 500mL, €11.66.
> *Oral soln*, methadone HCl 1mg/mL. Green. *Maltitol, benzoate, propylene glycol.*
>
> **Methadone TEVA 1mg/mL** *(TEVA)* CD.
> Price, not published by company.
> *Oral soln*, methadone HCl 1mg/mL. Clear green. *Parabens, maltitol.*
>
> **Pinadone DTF 1mg/mL** *(Pinewood)* CD.
> Price, not published by company.
> *Oral soln*, methadone HCl 1mg/mL. Clear viscous green sugar-free. *Sunset Yellow, Green S.*

16

Haematology, Obesity, Nutritionals

16.1 - Haematology

Class Effects
Iron/folic acid combinations are used during pregnancy; iron overload, see Notes below. Most of these drugs are used in specialised units. Always consult the manufacturers Full Prescribing Information.
Notes: See 15.1.3 Iron.

16.1.1 - Hypoplastic, Haemolytic, Renal Anaemias

In This Chapter: *Darbepoetin alfa, eculizumab, epoetin alfa, epoetin beta, epoetin theta, epoetin zeta.*

Class Effects
Sport: EPO is prohibited for use in sport, see WADA Prohibited List 2017.
CI: Hypersensitivity to any member of the class.
Interactions: Effect of Erythropoietin (EPO) on Other Drugs: Drugs highly bound to red cells (ciclosporin, tacrolimus): *Monitor serum levels, adjust dose.*
SP: Monitor, ensure lowest effective dose used to provide adequate anaemia symptom control but maintaining Hb conc below or at 12g/dL (7.5mmoL/L). Caution, dose escalation in CRF (**target Hb range 10-12g/dL (child, 9.5-11g/dL**); avoid sustained Hb above 12g/dL; increased risk of mortality, serious cardiovascular or cerebrovascular events (stroke) observed when ESA targets Hb above 12g/dL (7.5mmoL/L) or with high cumulative doses (CRF). Supplementary iron recommended (serum ferritin below 100mcg/L or transferrin saturation below 20%). Poor Hb response, consider alternative diagnosis. Paradoxical Hb decrease, severe anaemia associated with low reticulocyte counts, discontinue epoetin (perform antibody testing). Not for anaemia associated with hepatitis C. *CRF*, BP increased or existing hypertension aggravated, monitor; acute complications (hypertensive encephalopathy), related complications (seizure, stroke). Caution, sharp migraine-like headaches. *Non-response to EPO*, iron, folic acid or vitamin B12 deficiency may reduce ESA effectiveness; intercurrent infection, inflammatory or traumatic episodes, occult blood loss, haemolysis, severe aluminium toxicity, iron deficiency, underlying haematological diseases, bone marrow fibrosis. Monitor Hb, BP, platelets. *Caution*, porphyria exacerbation, epilepsy, chronic liver failure. Misuse in healthy persons, excessive increase in packed cell volume may have life-threatening cardiovascular complications. All growth factors, including epoetin, risk of

stimulation of tumour growth; cannot exclude tumour progression or reduced progression-free survival. With active malignant disease (untreated), ESAs are not indicated (blood transfusions preferred). PRCA, see CI above. To improve traceability of ESAs, record brand name in patient file. Preterm infants, potential risk of erythropoietin to cause retinopathy (caution); risk/benefit.
ADR: Expect approx. 8% of patients treated with EPO to experience adverse events especially (CRF, underlying malignancy). *Most common*, headache, hypertension (dose-dependent); hypertensive crisis. 'Flu-like' symptoms (headache, joint pain, weakness, dizziness, tiredness). Thrombotic/vascular events (access-related, shunt thrombosis), hypersensitivity (anaphylaxis, antibody-mediated erythroblastopenia). See SP above. Consult manufacturers Full Prescribing Information.
Notes: See 16.1 Haematology.

Darbepoetin Alfa

ATC Code: B03XA02. **Sport:** Prohibited.
Driving: Unlikely to impair.
Indications: Treatment, symptomatic anaemia, CRF-associated; non-myeloid malignancies on chemotherapy.
Dose: Adult, Elderly: Anaemia (CRF), target Hb max. 12g/dL (7.5mmoL/L), correction phase, initially 0.45mcg/kg as single injection once weekly; not on dialysis, initially 0.75mcg/kg once every 2 weeks SC or in adults only, 1.5mcg/kg once monthly. Hb increase inadequate (below 1g/dL) in 4 weeks, increase dose by 25%; Hb increase over 2g/dL in 4 weeks, reduce by 25%. Maintenance, single injection once weekly or once every 2 weeks; to achieve target, adjust dose by 25%.
Cancer, initially 6.75mcg/kg once every 3 weeks OR 2.25mcg/kg once weekly SC or IV.
Child: Anaemia (CRF), age 11 years and older, as for Adult above. Age 1-18 years, receiving r-HuEPO 2-3 times weekly, convert to *Aranesp* once weekly; r-HuEPO once weekly, convert to *Aranesp* once every other week.
Hepatic Impairment: Caution.
CI: Poorly controlled hypertension.
SP: Sickle cell anaemia, caution.
Pregnancy, Lactation: Pregnancy, caution. Lactation, not recommended.
ADR: *Very common*, hypersensitivity, oedema.
Notes: See 16.1.1 Anaemias.
   Aranesp SureClick PFS *(Amgen)* A. H.T.
   Price, (1) PFP SureClick (mcg) 20, €38.58; 40, €80.19; 60, €120.24; 80, €159.65; 100mcg, €198.73; 150mcg, €299.84. 300mcg, €582.40, 500mcg, €959.13; PFS (mcg) 300, €573.76; 500, €944.30. (4) (mcg) 10, €80.19; PFS (mcg) 20, €159.65; 30, €240.57; 40, €318.17; 50, €400.77; 60, €481.15; 80, €640.56; 100, €794.61; 150, €1178.22. *Injection*, darbepoetin alfa (PFS) (mcg) 10, 20 and 30-100 (in multiples of ten); 150, 300, 500. Clear colourless soln. *Sodium* 3.79mg/mL. **Store:** Refrigerate; do not freeze.

Eculizumab

ATC Code: L04AA25. **Sport:** Pending.
Driving: No or negligible effect.
Indications: Treatment, paroxysmal nocturnal haemoglobinuria (PNH) (high disease activity regardless of transfusion history); atypical haemolytic uraemic syndrome (aHUS).
Dose: Adult, Elderly: PNH, initial phase, 600mg every week (4 weeks); maintenance, 900mg (week 5), then 900mg every 14 days (+/- 2 days).
aHUS, initial phase, 900mg (4 weeks); maintenance, 1200mg (week 5), then 1200mg every 14 days (+/- 2 days).
Admin, by 25-45 minute IV infusion; not for IV push or bolus injection; monitor patients for 1 hour after infusion.
Child: PNH, aHUS, 40kg and above, as for Adult above. Under 40kg, body weight 30-40kg, initially 600mg/week (2 weeks); maintenance, 900mg (week 3), then 900mg every 2 weeks; 20-30kg as for 30-40kg; maintenance 600mg (week 3), then 600mg every 2 weeks. Weight 10-20kg, initially 600mg/week (1 week), 300mg (week 2), then 300mg every 2 weeks. Weight 5-10kg,

16.1.1 Hypoplastic, Haemolytic, Renal Anaemias

300mg/week (1 week), 300mg (week 2), then 300mg every 3 weeks. *Admin*, as for Adult above.

Hepatic Impairment: No data.

CI: Do not initiate in patients with unresolved *Neisseria meningitidis* infection or are not currently vaccinated against *Neisseria meningitidis* (unless receiving prophylactic antibiotics until 2 weeks after vaccination).

SP: *Soliris* increases susceptibility to meningococcal infection (serious or fatal reported); vaccinate all patients 2 weeks before initiation; if treated with *Soliris* under 2 weeks after vaccination, admin prophylactic antibiotics until 2 weeks after vaccination. Vaccines against serotypes A, C, Y, W135 and B recommended. Patients with complement-mediated diseases may have increased signs/symptoms of underlying disease (PNH, aHUS). Caution, presence of other active infections. Under 18 years, vaccinate against *Haemophilus influenzae*. Infusion reactions or immunogenicity (allergic or hypersensitivity reactions). Discontinuation, monitor for, intravascular haemolysis (PNH), thrombotic microangiopathy (aHUS). Treatment should not alter anticoagulant management.

Pregnancy, Lactation: Pregnancy, only if clearly needed. Women of childbearing potential to ensure adequate contraception during and for 5 months after treatment. Lactation, stop breastfeeding during and for up to 5 months after treatment.

ADR: Summary, *most common*, headache; *most serious*, meningococcal sepsis.

Notes: See 16.1.1 Anaemias.

Soliris Parenteral *(Alexion)* A.
Price, 300mg (1) €4557.50.
Infusion, eculizumab 10mg/mL (30mL). Clear colourless conc for soln. *Sodium 5mmoL/vial.* **Store:** Refrigerate; do not freeze; original pack to protect (light). Unrefrigerated max. 3 days (once).

---

5 days between doses. Dose increase max. 1050 IU/kg (80 thousand IU) per week at minimum 4-week intervals.

Admin, where IV access is readily available use IV route; if not readily available, use SC. Not for IV infusion or mixed with other drugs. Admin iron supplement prior to initiation to achieve adequate iron stores.

Child: Anaemia in CRF (age 1-18 years), recommended Hb conc range 9.5-11g/dL. Correction phase, initially 50 IU/kg IV 3-times weekly; maintenance, children under 30kg generally require higher dose than children under 30kg adjusted to maintain Hb at recommended levels. Other indications, adult use only.

CI: Patients developing Pure Red Cell Aplasia (PRCA) following erythropoietin treatment. Uncontrolled hypertension. Major elective orthopaedic surgery (not participating in autologous blood predonation), patients with (severe coronary, peripheral arterial, carotid or cerebral vascular diseases; recent MI or CVA). Surgery patients who cannot receive adequate antithrombotic prophylaxis.

SP: Elective surgery, ensure adequate antithrombotic prophylaxis. Measure Hb regularly.

Pregnancy, Lactation: CRF, use in pregnancy only if benefit outweighs risk. Pregnant or lactating surgical patients using autologous blood predonation, not recommended.

ADR: Summary, *most frequent*, increased BP; diarrhoea, nausea, vomiting, pyrexia, headache, flu-like illness.

Notes: See 16.1.1 Anaemias.

Eprex Parenteral *(Janssen-Cilag)* A. HT.
Price, (IU x 1000) (6), 1, €45.45; 2, €89.54; 3, €134.32; 4, €181.76; 5, €217.19; 6, €260.61; 8, €363.52; 10, €454.41. (1), 20, €151.34; 30, €229.68; 40, €292.25.
Injection, epoetinum alfa 20, 30, 40 thousand units (U). PFS (U thousand) 1, 2, 3, 4, 5, 6, 8, 10. Clear colourless soln. PFS *Essentially sodium-free.* **Store:** Refrigerate; do not freeze or shake; original pack to protect (light). Below 25 deg C (max. 3 days), discard.

Epoetin Alfa

ATC Code: B03XA01. **Sport:** Prohibited.
Driving: Unlikely to impair.

Indications: Treatment, anaemia associated with chronic renal failure (CRF) (adults, children, age 1-18 years) on haemodialysis, (adults) on peritoneal dialysis; severe anaemia of renal origin (adults) not on dialysis. Treatment, anaemia and reduction of transfusions (adults) on chemotherapy (solid tumours, malignant lymphoma, multiple myeloma). Predonation programmes to increase yield of autologous blood. Non-iron deficient adults prior to major elective orthopaedic surgery to reduce exposure to allogeneic blood transfusions. Treatment, symptomatic anaemia (adults) with low or intermediate-1-risk primary myelodysplastic syndromes (MDS) with low serum erythropoietin.

Dose: Adult, Elderly: Anaemia (CRF), recommended Hb conc range 10-12g/dL.
Haemodialysis correction phase, 50 IU/kg IV 3-times weekly, adjust at 4-week intervals by 25 IU/kg 3-times weekly; maintenance, 75-300 IU/kg/week. *Not on dialysis*, correction phase 50 IU 3-times weekly IV or SC; increase by 25 IU/kg 3-times weekly until goal achieved; maintenance, 150 IU 3-times weekly or 240 IU (up to max. 20 thousand IU) once weekly or 480 IU (up to max. 40 thousand IU) once every 2 weeks. *Peritoneal dialysis*, correction phase, 50 IU/kg IV twice weekly IV or SC; maintenance, 25-50 IU/kg twice weekly in 2 equal injections.
Anaemia (chemotherapy), initially 150 IU SC 3-times weekly OR 450 IU SC once weekly; continue until 1 month after the end of chemotherapy.
Autologous predonation, mildly anaemic (haematocrit 33-39%), 600 IU/kg IV twice weekly for 3 weeks prior to surgery; elective orthopaedic, 600 IU/kg weekly on days 21, 14 and 7 prior to surgery and on day of surgery (day 0); lead time under 3 weeks, 300 IU/kg daily for 10 consecutive days prior to surgery, on day of surgery, and for 4 days after.
Symptomatic anaemia, (Hb below 10g/dL), 450 IU/kg (max. total 40 thousand IU) SC once every week; minimum

Epoetin Beta

ATC Code: B03XA01. **Sport:** Prohibited.
Driving: Unlikely to impair.

Indications: Treatment, symptomatic anaemia in chronic renal failure (CRF) *(both brands)*; prevention of anaemia of prematurity in infants with birth weight 750-1500g and gestational age below 34 weeks; non-myeloid malignancies receiving chemotherapy; increase yield of autologous blood pre-donation *(NeoRecormon)*.

Dose: Adult, Elderly: *NeoRecormon*, anaemia (CRF) correction phase, initially 3x 20 IU/kg/week SC; increase every 4 weeks by 3x 20 IU/kg/week if Hb increase below 0.25g/dL/week. Maintenance (to maintain Hb at 10-12g/dL), usually half of previous dose*.
Symptomatic anaemia (malignancy), 450 IU/kg/week*; max. 60000 IU/week. Autologous blood, individualise dose; admin twice weekly over 4 weeks SC or IV over 2 minutes. Do not exceed PCV of 48%.
Mircera, anaemia in CRF, NOT currently ESA-treated, initially 0.6mcg/kg every 2 weeks as single IV or SC injection OR 1.2mcg/kg once monthly (to increase Hb to above 10g/dL)**. Currently ESA-treated, starting dose based on previous weekly darbepoetin alfa (mcg/week) or epoetin (IU/seek). Previous darbepoetin alfa below 40 (40-80) (above 80) or epoetin below 8000 (8000-16000) (above 16000), admin *Mircera* 120mcg once monthly (200) (360)**.
*(admin as single injection per week or divided doses 3 or 7 times/week). **If Hb rise is below 1g/dL, increase by 25%; if Hb rise is above 2g/dL, decrease by 25%.

Child: *NeoRecormon*, 3x 250 IU/kg/week; transfused premature infants not likely to benefit as much as untransfused infants; duration 6 weeks. *Mircera*, under 18 years not recommended.

CI: Uncontrolled hypertension. To increase yield of autologous blood in patients with (MI or stroke in month preceding treatment, unstable angina pectoris, increased venous thrombosis risk e.g. DVT history) *(NeoRecormon)*.

SP: Refractory anaemia with excess blasts in

transformation, thrombocytosis, caution. Severe aluminium overload may reduce efficacy. Failure to respond, investigate. Some cases blood transfusions preferred for anaemia of cancer, assess risk/benefit. *NeoRecormon*, increased heparin during haemodialysis often needed (increased packed cell volume), hypertension. *Mircera*, PRCA, do not switch to *Mircera*. PRCA with Hepatitis C, paradoxical Hb decrease, development of severe anaemia associated with low reticulocyte counts (discontinue; perform anti-erythropoietin antibody testing). Not approved in management of associated anaemia (hepatitis C or cancer).

Pregnancy, Lactation: Pregnancy, caution. Lactation, if benefit outweighs risk; stop drug or stop breastfeeding.

ADR: Summary, *most frequent*, increased blood pressure or aggravation of existing hypertension.

Notes: See 16.1.1 Anaemias.

> **Mircera Parenteral** *(Roche)* A. HT.
> *Price*, (0.3mL PFS) 30mcg, €60.71. 50mcg, €102.70. 75mcg, €152.57. 100mcg, €204.99. 120mcg, €248.37. 150mcg, €307.37. 200mcg, €407.19. 250mcg, €500.08.
> *Soln for injection (PFS)*, methoxy polyethylene glycol-epoetin beta (mcg) 30, 50, 75, 100, 120, 150, 200, 250. Recombinant. Clear colourless (slightly yellow). PFS. *Essentially sodium-free*.
> **NeoRecormon Parenteral** *(Roche)* A. HT.
> *Price*, 500 IU, €24.08. IU x 1000 (6): 2, €105.31; 3, €157.74; 4, €208.61; 5, €255.58; 6, €313.09; 10, €486.25; 20, €1018.26. IU x 1000 (4): 30, €977.19.
> *Injection*, epoetin beta PFS 500, 2000-6000 IU (in 1 thousand IU increments); 10, 20, 30 (thousand) IU. Recombinant human erythropoietin. Multidose: White lyophilisate; clear colourless solvent for soln. *Sodium below 1mmoL/dose, benzyl alcohol*. PFS: Colourless clear (slightly opalescent) soln. *Sodium as for multidose, phenylalanine*.

Epoetin Theta

ATC Code: B03XA01. **Sport:** Prohibited.
Driving: No or negligible effect.
Indications: Treatment, symptomatic anaemia associated with CRF; non-myeloid malignancies (on chemotherapy).

Dose: Adult, Elderly: Anaemia in CRF, correction phase, initially 20 IU/kg body weight SC 3-times weekly; titrate to 40 IU/kg 3-times weekly if Hb increase inadequate OR initially 40 IU/kg 3-times weekly IV titrating to 80 IU/kg 3-times weekly. Max. 700 IU/kg/week (SC and IV). Maintenance, adjust to maintain Hb range 10g/dL-12g/dL. Cancer, initially 20000 IU independent of body weight; after 4 weeks Hb increased by minimum 1g/dL, continue current dose; if Hb not increased minimum 1g/dL, consider doubling weekly dose. If after another 4 weeks, Hb still insufficient, consider increase to max. 60000 IU per week.

Child: No experience.

CI: Uncontrolled hypertension.

ADR: See Notes below.

Notes: See 16.1.1 Anaemias.

> **Eporatio Parenteral** *(Ratiopharm)* A. HT.
> *Price*, (IU x 1000) (6), 1, €32.40; 2, €64.80; 3, €97.20; 4, €129.60; 5, €162; 10, €324; 20, €921.94; (4) 30, €907.69.
> *Injection*, epoetin theta 1000-5000 IU (1000 IU increments); 10, 20, 30 thousand IU. Recombinant human erythropoietin. Clear colourless soln in PFS. *Essentially sodium-free*.

Epoetin Zeta

ATC Code: B03XA01. **Sport:** Prohibited.
Driving: Unlikely to impair.
Indications: Treatment, anaemia associated with CRF on haemodialysis, peritoneal dialysis; severe anaemia in renal insufficiency not on dialysis. Anaemia and reduction of transfusions with chemotherapy for solid tumours, malignant lymphoma, multiple myeloma. Increase yield of autologous blood predonation.

Dose: Adult, Elderly: CRF, haemodialysis, correction phase, 50 IU/kg IV 3-times weekly; adjust by 25 IU/kg 3-times weekly at 4-week intervals; maintenance, adjust dose to maintain Hb between 10-12g/dL; recommended, 75-300 IU/kg IV per week. Peritoneal dialysis, correction phase, 50 IU/kg IV twice weekly; maintenance, 25-50 IU/kg twice weekly in 2 equal doses. Not on dialysis, correction phase,

Megaloblastic Anaemias   16.1.2

as for haemodialysis; maintenance, 17-33 IU/kg 3-times weekly; max. 200 IU/kg 3-times per week.

Anaemia of chemotherapy, initially 150 IU/kg SC 3-times weekly OR 450 IU/kg SC once weekly; if Hb increases by 1g/dL after 4 weeks, maintain initial dose; if Hb increase below 1g/dL increase to 300 IU/kg 3-times weekly; if after 4 additional weeks at this dose, Hb increase above 1g/dL maintain dose; if Hb increase below 1g/dL, response unlikely, discontinue.

Autologous predonation, IV admin at completion of blood donation; haematocrit 33-39%, requiring pre-deposit of more than 4 units blood, 600 IU/kg twice weekly for 3 weeks prior to surgery; supplement with 200mg/day oral elemental iron. *Admin*, IV over 1-5 minutes; SC, max. 1mL at 1 injection site.

Child: *CRF*, on haemodialysis, as for Adult to maintain Hb 9.5-11g/dL.

CI: See Epoetin Alfa (both brands).

Notes: See 16.1.1 Anaemias.

> **Retacrit Parenteral** *(Hospira)* A. HT.
> *Price*, PFS (IU x 1000) (6) 1, €25.92; 2, €48.84; 3, €73.32; 4, €97.74; 5, €122.22; 6, €146.64; 8, €195.48. 10, €244.38. (1) 20, €81.46. 30, €122.19; 40, €162.92.
> *Injection*, epoetin zeta 20000 IU, 30000 IU. Clear colourless soln (PFS). *Phenylalanine; essentially 'sodium-free'*.

16.1.2 - Megaloblastic Anaemias

In This Chapter: *Folic acid, hydroxocobalamin.*

Class Effects
CI: Hypersensitivity to any member of the class.

Macrocytic anaemia associated with Vitamin B12 deficiency may be due to gastrectomy, some malabsorption syndromes, strict vegetarianism. A rise in the reticulocyte count induced by folic acid may mask Vitamin B12 deficiency.

Notes: See 16.1 Haematology.

Folic acid

ATC Code: B03BB01. **Sport:** Permitted.
Driving: Unlikely to impair.
Indications: Treatment, folate-deficient megaloblastic anaemia (infancy, pregnancy), nutritional macrocytic anaemia, pellagra, sprue, post-gastrectomy anaemia, pernicious anaemia (adjunctive), deficiency refractory to dietary measures. Prevention, neural tube defects.

Dose: Adult, Elderly: *Clonfolic*, megaloblastic anaemias, 5mg/day for 4 months; maintenance, 5mg every 1-7 days as needed. Prevention of neural tube defects, 0.4mg/day commencing before conception; continue for first 12 weeks of pregnancy.
Folic Acid (Clonmel), usually 10-20mg/day; maintenance 2.5-10mg/day.

Child: *Clonfolic*, megaloblastic anaemias, over 1 year, as for Adult; under 1 year, 500mcg/kg/day. *Folic acid (Clonmel)*, usually 5-15mg/day.

CI: Folic acid monotherapy should not be used to treat pernicious anaemia or other Vitamin B12 deficiencies.

Interactions: Effect of Folic Acid on Other Drugs: *Mutual inhibition (high dose folic acid)*: Folic acid antagonists (trimethoprim, proguanil, pyrimethamine, methotrexate). *Severe diarrhoea (high dose folic acid)*: Fluorouracil. *Response hindered*: Chloramphenicol (not for admin if severe folic acid deficiency).

Effect of Folic Acid on Other Drugs: Phenytoin, barbiturate antiepileptics: *Serum level decreased; increased seizure risk.*

SP: Caution, use with folate dependent tumours. Megaloblastic anaemia, exclude Vitamin B12 deficiency before initiating.

Pregnancy, Lactation: Used for the prevention of neural tube defects, treatment of megaloblastic anaemia during pregnancy. No known risks for use during pregnancy and lactation.

415

16.1.3   Neutropenia

ADR: GI disturbance, rarely hypersensitivity. High doses (sleep disturbances, agitation, depression).

Notes: See 16.1.2 Megaloblastic Anaemias.

Cionfolic 0.4mg *(Clonmel)* OTC. GMS.
Price, (98) €3.79.
Tablet, folic acid. Pale-yellow.

Folic Acid 5mg *(Clonmel)* A. GMS.
Price, (56) €1.58.
Tablet, folic acid. Mottled round orange. Lactose.

Hydroxocobalamin (anaemia)

ATC Code: B03BA03. **Sport:** Permitted.
Driving: None stated.

Indications: Addisonian pernicious anaemia. Prophylaxis and treatment, macrocytic anaemias associated with vitamin B12 deficiency. Tobacco amblyopia, Leber's optic atrophy.

Dose: Adult, Elderly: *Pernicious, macrocytic anaemias,* without neurological involvement, 250-1000mcg IM (alternate days for 1-2 weeks); then 250mcg/week until blood count normal; maintenance, 1000mcg every 2-3 months. With neurological complications, initially 1000mcg on alternate days*; maintenance, 1000mcg every 2 months. Prophylaxis, macrocytic anaemia, 1000mcg every 2-3 months.

Tobacco amblyopia, Leber's optic atrophy, 1000mcg or more IM daily for 2 weeks, then twice weekly*; maintenance, 1000mcg/month. *(for as long as improvement occurs).

Child: As for Adult above.

CI: Not for treatment of megaloblastic anaemia of pregnancy unless vitamin B12 deficient.

Interactions: Effect of Other Drugs on Cyanocobalamin: *Poor response:* Chloramphenicol treated patients. *Plasma levels decreased:* Oral contraceptives.

SP: Monitor blood profile; failure to respond, investigate folate metabolism. Above 10mcg/day may produce incomplete response in patients with folate deficiency. Cardiac arrhythmias secondary to hypokalaemia; monitor plasma potassium.

Pregnancy, Lactation: Is secreted into breast milk; unlikely to harm infant. See CI above.

ADR: Reactive thrombocytosis, arrhythmia (see SP above), hypersensitivity, nausea, vomiting, diarrhoea, headache, paraesthesia, tremor, chromaturia, acneiform and bullous eruptions, fever, chills, hot flushing, dizziness, malaise, pain, injection-site reactions.

Notes: See 16.1.2 Megaloblastic Anaemias.

Neo-Cytamen Parenteral *(Recipharm)* A. GMS.
Price, (5) 1000mcg/1mL, €13.25.
Injection, hydroxocobalamin chloride 1000mcg/mL. Clear red-brown soln.

16.1.3 - Neutropenia

In This Chapter: Filgrastim, lenograstim, lipegfilgrastim, pegfilgrastim.

Class Effects

They drugs are used under specialist supervision. Always consult the manufacturers Full Prescribing Information.

CI: Hypersensitivity to any member of the class. Use to increase intensity of cytotoxic chemotherapy beyond established dose and dosage regimens. Concurrent admin with cytotoxic chemotherapy.

Interactions: Effect of Other Drugs on Granulocyte Colony-Stimulating Factors: *Co-admin not recommended:* Cytotoxic chemotherapy (24-hours before; 24-hours after chemotherapy). *Co-admin (neutropenia severity exacerbated):* 5-fluorouracil.

SP: With G-CSF admin, possible cross-reactivity regarding hypersensitivity to G-CSF or derivatives. With all therapeutic proteins, potential for immunogenicity; antibody response may lead to undesirable effects or loss of efficacy. Pulmonary adverse events (interstitial lung disease, capillary leak syndrome) may be life-threatening). Admin

only in collaboration with oncology centre experienced in G-CSF treatment and haematology; perform mobilisation and apheresis under specialist supervision. Possibility of intensified chemotherapy doses being used, caution increased toxicity (cardiac, pulmonary, neurologic, dermatologic); thrombocytopenia, anaemia. Admin at least 24 hours after last chemotherapy dose. *PBPC mobilisation,* very extensive prior myelosuppressive therapy, may not show sufficient mobilisation to reach minimum yield or acceleration of platelet recovery; some cytotoxics may reduce progenitor yield. Normal donors, no data under 16 years, over 60 years. Allogeneic PBPC graft and recipient, possible increased risk of acute and chronic GvHD compared with bone marrow transplantation. Severe chronic neutropenia, perform complete blood counts (differential, platelets), and evaluate bone marrow before treatment. Exclude causes of transient neutropenia. Glomerulonephritis reported (filgrastim, pegfilgrastim).

Pregnancy, Lactation: Pregnancy, if benefit outweighs risk (avoid if possible) unless otherwise stated. Lactation, not recommended.

Notes: See 16.1 Haematology.

Filgrastim

ATC Code: L03AA02. **Sport:** Permitted.
Driving: Fatigue.

Indications: Neutropenia, reduction in duration, incidence (febrile) with cytotoxic chemotherapy (except CML, myelodysplastic syndromes) or undergoing myeloablative therapy followed by bone marrow transplant (BMT). Mobilisation of peripheral blood progenitor cells (PBPC). Severe congenital, cyclic, or idiopathic neutropenia and history of infections (severe or recurrent). Persistent neutropenia (HIV infection).

Dose: Adult, Elderly: *Chemotherapy,* 0.5 MU/kg/day at least 24 hours after chemotherapy (usually for 14 days) by SC injection or IV infusion over 30 minutes. Myeloablative therapy followed by BMT, 1 MU/kg/day at least (24 hours after chemotherapy and 24 hours after bone marrow infusion) by IV infusion (30 minute or 24-hour) OR 24-hour continuous SC infusion. *PBPC mobilisation,* myelosuppressive or myeloablative therapy followed by autologous PBPC transplantation: Used alone, 1 MU/kg/day as 24-hour SC continuous infusion or single daily SC injection (5-7 consecutive days); following myelosuppressive chemotherapy, 0.5 MU/kg/day; normal donors prior to allogeneic PBPC transplantation, 1 MU/kg/day SC (4-5 consecutive days). *Neutropenia,* congenital, initially 1.2 MU/kg/day; idiopathic or cyclic, initially 0.5 MU/kg/day SC (single or divided doses); reversal in HIV, 0.1 MU/kg/day SC titrating to max. 0.4 MU/kg/day until normal neutrophil count reached; maintenance, adjust dose by 30 MU/day.

NOTE: 1 MU (million units)=10mcg filgrastim=1 MIU (million international units).

Child: Cytotoxic chemotherapy, as for Adult above.

SP: Use not recommended (severe congenital neutropenia with leukaemia, myelodysplastic syndrome, CML); caution, secondary AML. Monitor bone density with underlying osteoporotic bone disease (use longer than 6 months). Cancer patients, splenomegaly, splenic rupture; leucocytosis, monitor (WBC counts); high dose chemotherapy, monitor (platelets, haematocrit).

Pregnancy, Lactation: Pregnancy, not recommended; if becoming pregnant or breastfeeding during treatment, encourage patient to enrol in the Amgen Pregnancy Surveillance Programme. Lactation, stop breastfeeding or stop drug.

ADR: See Notes below.

Notes: See 16.1.3 Neutropenia.

Neupogen Parenteral, Singleject *(Amgen)* A. HT.
Price, injection 30 MIU/1mL vial (5) €335.30. Singleject 30 MIU (1) €76.82. (5) €384.12. 48 MIU (1) €122.52. (5) €612.52.
Injection, filgrastim. Clear colourless soln. Sodium 0.023-0.051mg/mL; sorbitol; natural dry rubber (needle cover). **Store:** Refrigerate; accidental freezing does not affect stability.

416

Nivestim Parenteral *(Hospira)* A. HT.
Price, (5) PFS 12 MIU/0.2mL, €188.84. 30 MIU/0.5mL, €285.34. 48 MIU/0.5mL, €454.98.
Injection or infusion, filgrastim (MU) 12, 30, 48. Clear colourless soln. **Store:** Refrigerate; do not freeze (accidental freezing, up to 24 hours does not affect stability); room temp. (max. 7 days).
Ratiograstim Parenteral *(Ratiopharm)* A. HT.
Price, (5) PFS 30 MIU/0.5mL, €411.56. 48 MIU/0.8mL, €656.26.
Injection or infusion, filgrastim (MU) 30, 48. Clear colourless soln. *Sorbitol.* **Store:** Refrigerate.
Tevagrastim Parenteral *(TEVA)* A. HT.
Price, (5) PFS 30 MIU/0.5mL, €373.09. 48 MIU/0.8mL, €594.97.
Injection or infusion, filgrastim (MU/0.5mL) 30, 48. Clear colourless soln. *Sorbitol.* **Store:** Refrigerate.

Lenograstim

ATC Code: L03AA10. **Sport:** Permitted.
Driving: Unlikely to impair.
Indications: Reduction in neutropenia duration in non-myeloid malignancy undergoing myeloablative therapy followed by bone marrow transplantation (BMT) (increased prolonged severe neutropenia risk); severe neutropenia undergoing cytotoxic chemotherapy (with febrile neutropenia incidence). Mobilisation, peripheral blood progenitor cells (PBPC).
Dose: Adult, Elderly: BMT, chemotherapy, PBPC mobilisation after chemotherapy, 150mcg (19.2 MIU)/m2/day BSA by SC injection (equiv. to 5mcg OR 0.64 MIU/kg/day) starting on day after chemotherapy completed or day after transplant.
PBPC mobilisation, 10mcg (1.28 MIU)/kg/day; monotherapy, SC injection for 4-6 days.
Child: Over 2 years, as for Adult (all indications except PBPC).
Renal Impairment: Severe, no data.
Hepatic Impairment: As for Renal above.
CI: Myeloid malignancy other than AML, acute AML (age below 55 years and/or with good cytogenetics).
SP: Normal donors, pulmonary (haemoptysis, haemorrhage, lung infiltrates, dyspnoea, hypoxia). Caution, patients with sickle cell trait or sickle cell disease (sickle cell crisis).
ADR: See Notes below.
Notes: See 16.1.3 Neutropenia.
Granocyte Parenteral *(Chugai)* A. HT.
Price, (5) injection 13.4 MIU, €191.02. 33.6 MIU, €478.97.
Injection or infusion, lenograstim (rHuG-CSF) 33.6 MIU (263MU)/mL after reconstitution. White lyophilised powder; clear colourless solvent for soln. *Phenylalanine, latex rubber tip cap.* **Store:** Below 30 deg C; do not freeze.

Lipegfilgrastim

ATC Code: L03AA14. **Sport:** Permitted.
Driving: No or negligible effect.
Indications: Reduction in duration of neutropenia and incidence of febrile neutropenia associated with cytotoxic chemotherapy for malignancy (adults), except CML and myelodysplastic syndromes.
Dose: Adult, Elderly: 6mg SC for each chemotherapy cycle given approx. 24-hours after cytotoxic chemotherapy.
Child: Under 17 years, no data.
Renal Impairment: No dose recommendation.
Hepatic Impairment: As for Renal above.
SP: Leucocytosis, elevated white blood cells (monitor regularly). Splenomegaly, interstitial pneumonia, sickle cell anaemia, hypokalaemia.
ADR: See Notes below.
Notes: See 16.1.3 Neutropenia.
▼ **Lonquex Parenteral** *(TEVA)* A. HT.
Price, (1) 6mg, €890.09.
Injection, lipegfilgrastim (conjugate of filgrastim with methoxy polyethylene glycol) 6mg (0.6mL PFS). Clear colourless soln. *Sorbitol, sodium 23mg/PFS.* **Store:** Refrigerate; do not freeze. Below 25 deg C (max. 3 days), discard.

Pegfilgrastim

ATC Code: L03AA13. **Sport:** Permitted.
Driving: Unlikely to impair.
Indications: See Notes below.
Dose: Adult, Elderly: One 6mg dose SC for each chemotherapy cycle given at least 24 hours after cytotoxic chemotherapy.
Child: Safety/efficacy not established.
CI: Hypersensitivity to *E. coli*-derived proteins.
SP: Acute myeloid leukaemia (AML), caution. Not for use in myelodysplastic syndrome, CML, secondary AML. Splenomegaly (fatal). Sickle cell disease, caution. Serious hypersensitivity reactions, anaphylaxis with initial or subsequent treatment, permanently discontinue.
Pregnancy, Lactation: Pregnancy, not recommended. Women of childbearing potential to ensure adequate contraception. Lactation, stop breastfeeding or stop drug.
ADR: See Notes below.
Notes: See Lipegfilgrastim above. See 16.1.3 Neutropenia.
Neulasta Parenteral *(Amgen)* A. HT.
Price, PFS 6 MIU/0.6mL (1) €1043.79.
Injection, pegfilgrastim 6mg/0.6mL. Clear colourless soln. *Sorbitol, sodium acetate; dry natural rubber (needle cover).*

16.1.4 - Platelet Disorders

In This Chapter: *Anagrelide.*

Class Effects
Treatment to be initiated by clinicians experienced in essential thrombocythaemia management.
CI: Hypersensitivity to any member of the class.
Notes: See 16.1 Haematology.

Anagrelide

ATC Code: L01XX35. **Sport:** Permitted.
Driving: Dizziness.
Indications: Reduction of elevated platelet counts in at risk essential thrombocythaemia patients.
Dose: Adult, Elderly: Initially 1mg/day in 2 equally divided doses, for at least 1 week; then titrate by max. 0.5mg/day in any 1-week; max. single dose 2.5mg. *Admin,* swallow caps whole; do not crush or dilute contents in liquid.
Child: Safety/efficacy not established. Caution; no dose recommendation available.
Renal Impairment: Mild, assess risk/benefit; CrCl (mL/min) below 50, not recommended.
Hepatic Impairment: Mild, as for Renal; moderate to severe (transaminases above 5xULN), not recommended.
Interactions: Effect of Other Drugs on Anagrelide: *Co-admin not recommended:* Other phosphodiesterase (PDE III) inhibitors (milrinone, amrinone, enoximone, olprinone, cilostazol). *Co-admin caution (anti-aggregatory effects additive):* Acetylsalicylic acid (associated with major haemorrhagic events). *Clearance adversely affected:* CYP1A2 inhibitors (fluvoxamine, enoxacin). *Decreased exposure:* CYP1A2 inducers (omeprazole) (biological monitoring).
Effect of Anagrelide on Other Substances: CYP1A2 substrates (theophylline): *Potential interaction.* Oral contraceptives: *Absorption may be compromised.*
SP: Monitor FBC, liver, renal function. Platelets will increase within 4 days of stopping treatment; return to pre-treatment levels within 10-14 days. Serious cardiovascular adverse events (Torsades de Pointes, ventricular tachycardia, cardiomyopathy, cardiomegaly, CHF). Caution, known risk factors for QT-prolongation (monitor QTc-interval).
Pregnancy, Lactation: Not recommended. Women of childbearing potential to ensure adequate contraception. Stop breastfeeding during treatment.
ADR: Summary, *most common,* headache, palpitations, fluid retention, nausea, diarrhoea.
Notes: See 16.1.4 Platelet Disorders.

16.1.5 Drugs Used To Mobilise Stem Cells

▼ **Xagrid 0.5mg** *(Shire)* A. HT.
Price, (100) €462.38.
Capsule, anagrelide HCl. Hard gelatin opaque white. Marked S 063. *Lactose.*

16.1.5 - Drugs Used To Mobilise Stem Cells

In This Chapter: *Plerixafor.*

Class Effects
To be initiated and supervised by physician experienced in oncology and/or haematology. Mobilisation and apheresis to be performed only where haematopoietic progenitor cell monitoring can be performed.
CI: Hypersensitivity to any member of the class.
Notes: See 16.1 Haematology.

Plerixafor
ATC Code: L03AX16. **Sport:** Pending.
Driving: Dizziness, fatigue, vasovagal reactions.
Indications: In combination with G-CSF to enhance haematopoietic stem cells mobilisation to peripheral blood for collection and subsequent autologous transplantation (patients with lymphoma and multiple myeloma whose cells mobilise poorly).
Dose: Adult, Elderly: 0.24mg/kg/day; commonly used for 2-4 (and up to 7) consecutive days. *Admin,* by SC injection 6-11 hours prior to apheresis initiation following G-CSF pre-treatment. *Elderly,* according to renal function. Over 60 years and/or (prior myelosuppressive chemotherapy; extensive prior chemotherapy; peak circulating stem cell count below 20 stem cells/microlitre) predictors of poor mobilisation.
Child: Limited data.
Renal Impairment: CrCl (mL/min) 20-50, reduce dose by one third to 0.16mg/kg/day (max. 27mg/day); below 20 or on dialysis, no dose recommendation.
SP: Potential for tumour cell mobilisation in lymphoma, multiple myeloma. Leukaemia, not recommended; may cause mobilisation of leukaemic cells, contamination of apheresis product. Hyperleukocytosis (monitor WBC counts), thrombocytopenia (monitor platelets). Allergic reactions including systemic. Vasovagal reactions, orthostatic hypotension and/or syncope following injection. Cannot exclude splenic enlargement.
Pregnancy, Lactation: Pregnancy, only if necessary. Women of childbearing potential to ensure adequate contraception. Stop breastfeeding.
ADR: *Very common,* diarrhoea, nausea, injection and infusion site reactions.
Notes: See 16.1.5 Drugs Used To Mobilise Stem Cells.

Mozobil Parenteral *(SANOFI)* A.
Price, not published by company.
SC injection, plerixafor 20mg/mL. Clear colourless (pale-yellow) soln; pH 6-7.5. *Essentially sodium-free.*

16.1.6 - Plasma Substitutes, Protein Fractions

In This Chapter: *Human albumin.*

Class Effects
Under normal conditions the total exchangeable albumin pool is 4-5g/kg bodyweight of which 40-45% is present intravascularly and 55-60% in the extravascular space.
CI: Hypersensitivity to any member of the class.
SP: Suspicion of allergic or anaphylactic reaction, discontinue immediately. Shock, implement standard medical treatment.

Human Albumin
ATC Code: B05AA01. **Sport:** Pending.
Driving: No influence.
Indications: Restoration and maintenance of circulating blood volume (volume deficiency demonstrated; use of colloid appropriate).

Dose: Adult, Elderly: Individualise concentration of albumin preparation, dose and infusion rate. Dose depends on (patient size, severity of trauma or illness, continuing fluid and protein losses). Use measures of adequacy of circulating volume and not plasma albumin levels to determine required dose. In plasma exchange adjust infusion rate to removal rate. *Admin,* directly IV or diluted in an isotonic soln (0.5% glucose or 0.9% sodium chloride).
SP: *If human albumin is admin,* monitor haemodynamic performance regularly (arterial BP and pulse rate, central venous pressure, pulmonary artery wedge pressure, urine output, electrolytes, haematocrit, haemoglobin, cardiac or respiratory failure e.g. dyspnoea, increasing intra-cranial pressure e.g. headache). *Use with caution,* if hypervolaemia or haemodilution could be a risk (decompensated cardiac insufficiency, hypertension, oesophageal varices, pulmonary oedema, haemorrhagic diathesis, severe anaemia, renal and post-renal anuria). The colloid-osmotic effect of human albumin 200g/L or 250g/L is approx. 4-times that of blood plasma; ensure adequate hydration; monitor (circulatory overload, hyperhydration). Monitor electrolytes. Do not dilute with water for injection (may cause haemolysis). Ensure adequate substitution of other blood constituents (coagulation factors, electrolytes, platelets, erythrocytes). Signs of cardiovascular overload, or increased BP, raised venous pressure and pulmonary oedema, stop infusion immediately. Record name and batch number of product.
Pregnancy, Lactation: Clinical experience with albumin suggest no harmful effects to be expected.
ADR: *Rare,* nausea, flushing, skin rash, fever.
Notes: See 16.1.6 Plasma Substitutes, Protein Fractions.

Flexbumin Parenteral *(Baxalta)* A.
Price, not published by company.
Infusion, human albumin 200g/L (50mL, 100mL). Clear slightly viscous; almost colourless (yellow, amber or green) soln. *Sodium 130-160mmol/L.*

Human Albumin Baxalta Parenteral *(Baxalta)* A.
Price, not published by company.
Infusion, human albumin 50g/L (250mL, 500mL). Clear slightly viscous; almost colourless (yellow, amber or green) soln. *Sodium 130-160mmol/L.* **Store:** Below 25 deg C; do not freeze.

16.2 - Obesity

In This Chapter: *Orlistat, naltrexone, bupropion combination.*

Class Effects
CI: Hypersensitivity to any member of the class.
SP: Patients should be on a nutritionally balanced mildly hypocaloric diet with dietary and behavioural modification and increased physical activity.

Orlistat
ATC Code: A08AB01. **Sport:** Permitted.
Driving: Unlikely to impair.
Indications: Treatment, adjunctive (diet, exercise), of obese patients (BMI 30kg/m2 or more) or overweight patients (BMI 28kg/m2 or more) with associated risk factors (type 2 diabetes, dyslipidaemia).
Dose: Adult: 120mg admin with water immediately before, during or up to 1 hour after each main meal; if meal missed or contains no fat, omit dose.
Child: Not recommended.
CI: Chronic malabsorption syndrome, cholestasis.
Interactions: Effect of Other Drugs on Orlistat: *Co-admin avoid:* Acarbose.
Effect of Orlistat on Other Drugs: Antidiabetics: *Monitor.* Ciclosporin: *Plasma levels decreased.* Warfarin, oral anticoagulants: *Monitor INR.* Fat soluble vitamins (ADEK), anti-epileptics, levothyroxine (cannot be ruled out), HIV antiretrovirals: *Absorption impaired.* Amiodarone: *Slightly decreased plasma levels; monitor ECG.* Antidepressants, antipsychotics: *Reduced efficacy, caution.*
SP: Faecal fat increases 24-48 hours after dose; returns to pre-treatment levels within 48-72 hours after

discontinuation. GI adverse events increase with increased fat intake. Rectal bleeding. Hyperoxaluria/oxalate nephropathy with underlying kidney disease and/or volume depletion (renal failure). Hypothyroidism. Decreased anti-epileptic medication absorption (convulsions). Anticoagulants, see Interactions above.

Pregnancy, Lactation: Pregnancy, caution. Lactation, contraindicated. Severe diarrhoea, use additional contraceptive methods to prevent oral contraceptive failure.

ADR: *Very common,* headache, upper RTI, abdominal pain/discomfort, oily spotting from rectum, flatus with discharge, faecal urgency, fatty/oily stools, flatulence, liquid stools, oily evacuation, increased defecation, hypoglycaemia, influenza.

Notes: OTC available as *alli 60mg.* See 16.2 Obesity.

Xenical 120mg *(Cheplapharm)* A.
Price, (84) €49.35.
Capsule, orlistat. Hard turquoise. Marked Roche Xenical 120.

Naltrexone, Bupropion (obesity)

ATC Code: A08AA62. **Sport:** Permitted.
Driving: Minor influence; dizziness.

Indications: Treatment, adjunctive (diet, exercise), of obese patients (BMI 30kh/m2 or more) or overweight patients (BMI 27-30kg/m2) with associated risk factors (type 2 diabetes, dyslipidaemia, or controlled hypertension). Discontinue after 16 weeks if at least 5% of initial body weight has not been lost.

Dose: Adult: Initially, 1 tab in morning (week 1), 1 tab morning and evening (week 2), 2 tabs in morning and 1 tab evening (week 3) then 2 tabs morning and evening (week 4 onwards); max. 32mg naltrexone, 360mg bupropion per day. Re-evaluate after 16 weeks. *Admin,* swallow whole with some water preferably with food; do not cut, chew or crush tablets.

Elderly: Over 65 years, caution; over 75 years, not recommended.

Child: Under 18 years, safety/efficacy not established; not for use.

Renal Impairment: Mild, no adjustment. Moderate, not recommended. Severe or end stage renal failure, contraindicated.

Hepatic Impairment: Mild/moderate, not recommended. Severe, contraindicated.

CI: Uncontrolled hypertension, seizures*, CNS tumour, undergoing acute alcohol or benzodiazepine withdrawal, bipolar disorder (history), bulimia or anorexia nervosa*, acute opiate withdrawal. *(current, history of).

Interactions: Effect of Other Drugs on Naltrexone, Bupropion: *Co-admin contraindicated*: Chronic opioids or opioid agonists, (methadone), MAOIs (or within 14 days of), other naltrexone or bupropion containing drugs. *Caution, efficacy may be affected*: Decreased plasma levels, CYP2B6 inducers (carbamazepine, phenytoin, ritonavir, efavirenz); increased plasma levels, CYP2B6 inhibitors (orphenadrine, ticlopidine, clopidogrel), CYP2B6 substrates (cyclophosphamide, ifosfamide). *Caution:* Drugs which may increase seizure risk e.g. insulin, oral antidiabetics (assess dose to avoid hypoglycaemia), drugs lowering seizure threshold (antipsychotics, antidepressants, antimalarials, tramadol, theophylline, systemic steroids, quinolones, sedating antihistamines); levodopa, amantadine (increased adverse events), valproate (metabolism inhibited).

Effect of Naltrexone, Bupropion on Other Drugs: Drugs metabolised by CYP2D6 e.g. antidepressants (SSRIs, TCAD including desipramine, imipramine, paroxetine), antipsychotics (haloperidol, risperidone, thioridazine), beta-blockers (metoprolol) and Type 1C antiarrhythmics (propafenone, flecainide), citalopram: *Caution, dose at lower end of dose range.* Tamoxifen: *Efficacy may be reduced.* ALCOHOL: *Minimise or avoid.*

SP: Assess safety/tolerability are regular intervals. Suicidality reported (all ages) post-marketing; closely supervise high risk patients. Seizures (bupropion, dose-related); increased risk (head trauma, excessive alcohol, stimulant/cocaine addiction, hypoglycaemia, drugs lowering seizure threshold). Minimise/avoid alcohol. For admin with chronic opiate therapy.

Attempt to overcome naltrexone opioid blockade with large amounts of exogenous opioids is dangerous (fatal overdose or life endangering opioid toxicity). Hypersensitivity, hypertension, hepatotoxicity. Caution, active CAD (angina, recent MI), cerebrovascular disease (history). Activation of mania, hypomania reported.

Pregnancy, Lactation: Not for use.

ADR: Summary, *most frequent,* nausea, constipation, vomiting, dizziness, dry mouth.

Notes: See 15.1.5 Specific Substance Antagonists (naltrexone), 15.3.2 Dependence (bupropion) and 16.2 Obesity.

▼ **Mysimba 8/90 Tablets** *(Consilient)* A.
Price, (112) €83.00 (PTW). GMS-pending.
Prolonged/R tablet, naltrexone hydrochloride, bupropion hydrochloride 8mg/90mg. Blue round. Marked NB-890. *Lactose.*
Store: Below 30 deg C.

16.3 - Minerals, Vitamins, Dietary Supplements

In This Chapter: *Minerals (calcium, iron, magnesium, potassium, zinc), vitamins (B, C, D, K), multivitamins.*

Class Effects
CI: Hypersensitivity to any member of the class.

16.3.1 - Calcium

In This Chapter: *Calcium (and combinations).*

Class Effects
CI: *Calcium, vitamin combinations,* severe renal impairment (GFR below 30mL/min), except when used as phosphate binder in CRF. Severe hypercalcaemia, hypercalciuria (hyperparathyroidism, Vitamin D overdose or hypervitaminosis D, decalcifying tumours including plasmocytoma, myeloma, skeletal metastases), immobilisation (osteoporosis or prolonged) accompanied by hypercalcaemia and/or hypercalciuria, nephrolithiasis, nephrocalcinosis, myeloma, renal calculi (nephrolithiasis). *Calcium, magnesium combinations,* as for above and elevated serum magnesium (above 2mmoL/L) and/or hypermagnesaemia symptoms, myasthenia gravis.

Interactions: Effect of Other Drugs on Calcium: *Urinary excretion reduced:* Thiazides. *Absorption reduced:* Systemic corticosteroids. *Absorption inhibited:* Oxalic acid (found in spinach, rhubarb), phytic acid (whole cereals) (allow 2-hour interval between dosing and eating these foods). *Absorption enhanced:* Vitamin D3, oestrogens.

Effect of Calcium on Other Drugs: Tetracyclines, doxycycline, some (quinolones, cephalosporins, azole antifungals), anticholinergics, urso- and chenodesoxychol acid, halofantrine, levothyroxine: *Absorption altered (admin 2 hours before or 4-6 hours after oral calcium).* Bisphosphonates, sodium fluoride, iron, zinc, strontium ranelate, colestyramine, estramustine: *Decreased absorption (allow 1-2 hour dosing interval before or after).* Cardiac glycosides: *Increased toxicity/arrhythmia risk.*

SP: High dose treatment, especially Vitamin D and in immobilised patients with osteoporosis, increased hypercalcaemia risk. Monitor renal function, especially elderly. Renal impairment, caution Vitamin D use, monitor calcium, phosphate; severe impairment, colecalciferol is not metabolised normally, use other Vitamin D forms. Sarcoidosis, risk of increased Vitamin D metabolism to active metabolite. Calculate total Vitamin D intake when other Vitamin D-containing drugs are co-admin. Long-term treatment, max. urinary calcium 300-360mg/24 hours. Orlistat may impair fat-soluble vitamin absorption.

Pregnancy, Lactation: Adequate calcium intake (food, supplements) in normal pregnant and lactating women, 1000-1300mg/day; max. 1500mg and colecalciferol max. 600 IU/day (*Calcichew,* calcium max. 2500mg/day and

16.3.1 Calcium

Vitamin D max. 4000 IU/day). Calcium is secreted in breast milk. Can be used in pregnancy if calcium deficient.

ADR: Hypercalcaemia, hypercalciuria, hypophosphataemia, GI disorders (constipation, flatulence, nausea, abdominal pain, diarrhoea), hypersensitivity reactions (pruritus, rash, urticaria). Symptoms of hypercalcaemia (anorexia, nausea, vomiting, headache, weakness, apathy, drowsiness); more severe (thirst, dehydration, polyuria, nocturia, abdominal pain, paralytic ileus, cardiac arrhythmia).

Notes: See 8.4.5 Dialysis (calcium phosphate binders).

Calcium Carbonate

ATC Code: A12AA04. **Sport:** Permitted.
Driving: Unlikely to impair.

Indications: To correct calcium deficiency states and maintain appropriate balance (osteoporosis, osteomalacia, rickets, tetany, malabsorption states, pregnancy and lactation); as a phosphate binder in renal failure (patients on dialysis).

Dose: Adult, Elderly: Osteoporosis, dietary deficiency, 2-3 tabs/day; osteomalacia, 2-6 tabs/day. As phosphate binder, dose is dependent on serum phosphate level. Suck or chew tabs just before, during, or just after food.

Child: Dietary deficiency, 2-3 tabs/day.

Renal Impairment: Admin under controlled conditions for hyperphosphataemia. Caution, history of renal calculi. Potential risk (hyperphosphataemia, nephrolithiasis, nephrocalcinosis).

Notes: See 16.3.1 Calcium.

Calcichew 500mg *(Takeda)* OTC. GMS.
Price, (100) €10.64.
Chewable tablet, calcium carbonate equiv. to 500mg calcium. Round white u/c. *Sorbitol, isomalt, aspartame.*

Calcium Carbonate, Colecalciferol

ATC Code: A12AX. **Sport:** Permitted.
Driving: No or negligible effect.

Indications: Prevention and treatment, combined Vitamin D and calcium deficiency (elderly). Vitamin D and calcium supplement, adjunctive to specific osteoporosis treatment; therapeutic supplement (established osteomalacia, pregnancy, malnutrition).

Dose: Adult, Elderly: 1 tab morning and evening *(Calcichew Forte)* or 1 tablet daily *(Calciup, Kalcipos, Calcichew Double Strength)*. Pregnancy, 1 tab/day *(Caltrate)* OR half tab/day *(Calciup)*. Swallow f/c tabs whole with water; chew or suck chewable tabs and then swallow.

Child: Not for use in children and adolescents.

Renal Impairment: Potential risk (hyperphosphataemia, nephrolithiasis, nephrocalcinosis). Severe, contraindicated.

CI: Soya or peanut hypersensitivity *(Calcichew Double Strength)*.

Interactions: Effect of Other Drugs on Calcium, Colecalciferol: *Reduced Vitamin D absorption:* Colestyramine, laxatives, orlistat. *Increased Vitamin D3 metabolism, reduced activity:* Rifampicin, phenytoin, barbiturates.

Notes: See Calcium Carbonate above.

Calcichew D3 Forte, Double Strength *(Takeda)* OTC. GMS.
Price, Forte (60) €5.49; (100) €9.15. Forte DS (30) €5.49.
Chewable tablet, calcium carbonate equiv. to 500mg calcium, colecalciferol 400 IU (Forte); 1000mg/800 IU (Forte Double Strength). Round white u/c; may have small specks. *Isomalt, sucrose (both formulations), aspartame, sorbitol (Forte), soya-bean oil (Double Strength).*

Calciup D3 Forte *(Rowex)* OTC. GMS.
Price, (30) €5.12.
Chewable tablet, calcium carbonate 2500mg equiv. to 1000mg calcium, colecalciferol 880 IU. Round white scored (divisible into equal halves). *Aspartame, sorbitol, isomalt, sucrose.*

Caltrate 600/400 *(Pfizer Consumer)* OTC. GMS.
Price, (90) €8.47.
Tablet, calcium carbonate 600mg, cholecalciferol 400 IU. Cap-shaped grey/beige f/c scored (facilitates breaking). Marked D, 600 either side of score; Caltrate on reverse. *Soya bean oil, sucrose.*

Calvidin 600mg/400 IU *(Meda)* OTC. GMS.
Price, (60) €9.19.
Chewable tablet, calcium carbonate 1500mg (600mg calcium), colecalciferol 400 IU. White with snap groove. Marked C/D. *Sucrose.* Tabs contain 0.47g digestible carbohydrate; 2 tabs equiv. to 0.08 carbohydrate units.

Ideos Chewable *(Fannin)* OTC. GMS.
Price, (60) €8.01.
Chewable tablet, calcium carbonate 1250mg equiv. to 500mg calcium, colecalciferol 400 IU. Greyish-white square. *Sorbitol, soya bean oil.*

Kalcipos-D Forte *(Meda)* B. GMS.
Price, tabs and chewable (30) €7.72 (60) €10.48.
Tablets, calcium carbonate equiv. to 500mg calcium, colecalciferol 800 IU (20mcg). White oval f/c. Marked R150. *Sucrose.*
Chewable tablet, as above. White (off-white) round. Marked R152. *Glucose, sucrose.*

Calcium Chloride

ATC Code: A12AA07. **Sport:** Permitted.
Driving: Not applicable.

Indications: Immediate treatment, hypocalcaemic tetany. Cardiac resuscitation, especially after open heart surgery (adrenaline failed to improve weak or ineffective myocardial contractions). Adjunctive, severe hyperkalaemia, aid in treatment of depression due to magnesium sulfate overdosage (calcium antagonises magnesium toxicity).

Dose: Adult, Elderly: INTRACARDIAC, into ventricular cavity 200-400mg (2-4mL). INTRAVENOUS, slow IV, hypocalcaemic disorders, 500mg-1g at 1-3 day intervals; magnesium toxicity, 500mg admin promptly; hyperkalaemic ECG disturbances, use constant ECG monitoring to adjust dose during admin.

Child: INTRACARDIAC, into ventricular cavity. 0.2mL/kg bodyweight. INTRAVENOUS, slow IV, hypocalcaemic disorders, 0.2mL/kg; max. 1-10mL/day. Infants, not for oral admin (GI irritation); not for admin through scalp.

CI: Cardiac resuscitation (with ventricular fibrillation). Treatment, asystole and electromechanical dissociation. See Interactions below.

Interactions: Effect of Other Drugs on Calcium Chloride: *Co-admin or admixture contraindicated:* Ceftriaxone IV in premature and full-term newborns (risk of ceftriaxone-calcium precipitation). *Co-admin not recommended:* Digitalis group. *Not for parenteral admixture:* Carbonates, phosphates, sulphates, tartrate. *Increased hypercalcaemia risk with co-admin:* Thiazide diuretics.

Effect of Calcium Chloride on Other Drugs: Calcium channel blockers: *Effectiveness may be reduced.*

SP: Ceftriaxone, see Interactions above. Moderate BP fall. Not for treatment of hypocalcaemia of renal insufficiency, respiratory acidosis, respiratory failure. Caution, venous irritation; severe necrosis, sloughing if injected into tissue; avoid extravasation or injection into perivascular or myocardial tissue. If perivascular infiltration occurs, discontinue immediately (local 1% procaine HCl infiltration with hyaluronidase may reduce venospasm and dilute remaining calcium in tissue).

Pregnancy, Lactation: Pregnancy, if benefit outweighs risk. Lactation, is excreted in breast milk.

ADR: Tingling sensation, calcium taste, sense of oppression ('heat wave') (rapid IV injection). Peripheral vasodilation, local burning sensation. Necrosis, sloughing (SC or IM admin, or extravasation). Soft tissue calcification, bradycardia, arrhythmia, hypertension, venous thrombosis, hypercalcaemia.

Notes: See 16.3.1 Calcium.

Calcium Chloride Minijet *(IMS)* A.
Price, not published by company.
Injection, calcium chloride dihydrate 10% w/v (100mg/mL) (10mL). Soln. 0.68mmol/mL calcium ions.

Calcium Phosphate, Colecalciferol

ATC Code: A12AX. **Sport:** Permitted.
Driving: Unlikely to impair.

Indications: Correction, calcium and Vitamin D deficiency (elderly). Adjunctive, in osteoporosis, with Vitamin D and calcium combined or needing supplements.

Dose: Adult, Elderly: 1 sachet/day during evening meal; pour into non-carbonated water, stir and drink.
Child: Not recommended.
Pregnancy, Lactation: Not recommended.
Notes: See Calcium Carbonate, Cholecalciferol above.

Osteofos D3 (*A.Menarini*) B. GMS.
Price, 30 sachets, €5.39.
Powder for oral susp, calcium phosphate equiv. to 1200mg calcium, colecalciferol 800 IU per sachet. White (slightly orange) granular. *Mannitol, sucrose, Sunset Yellow E110.* **Store:** Below 25 deg C.

16.3.2 - Iron, Folic Acid Combinations

In This Chapter: *Ferric carboxymaltose, ferrous (fumarate, sulfate), iron (dextran, sucrose).*

Class Effects
Individualised dose of these drugs according to Hb and body weight. Use Ganzoni formula to calculate cumulative iron dose: Total iron deficit [mg] = BW (body weight) [kg] x (target Hb-actual Hb) [g/dL] x 2.4* + depot storage iron [mg].

NOTE: Recommend using ideal body weight or pre-pregnancy weight. Other laboratory tests include Hb, serum ferritin, transferrin saturation (TSAT, serum iron. *Factor 2.4 = 0.0034 (iron content of Hb = 0.34%) x 0.07 (blood volume = 7% of BW) x 1000 (conversion of [g] to [mg] x 10).

CI: Hypersensitivity to any member of the class. Caution, history of asthma, eczema, other atopic or known allergies (may be more susceptible to allergic reactions). *Parenteral,* serious hypersensitivity to other parenteral iron products; non-iron deficiency anaemia (haemolytic anaemia), iron overload or disturbed iron utilisation (haemochromatosis, haemosiderosis), decompensated liver cirrhosis, hepatitis.

Interactions: Effect of Other Drugs on Oral Iron: *Co-admin avoid:* Dimercaprol. *Absorption mutually reduced:* Tetracyclines, zinc, trientine. *Absorption reduced:* Calcium, magnesium (caution antacids).

Effect of Oral Iron on Other Drugs: Bisphosphonates, fluoroquinolones (ciprofloxacin, norfloxacin, levofloxacin, ofloxacin), penicillamine, levodopa, entacapone: *Absorption reduced.*

SP: Use iron supplements with caution (haemochromatosis, haemolytic anaemia). May cause tooth discolouration (oral solns), black-coloured faeces. Children, avoid prolonged or excessive use (toxic accumulation).

Parenteral, hypersensitivity reactions (potentially fatal allergic or anaphylactic or anaphylactoid reactions; cardiac arrest, respiratory arrest, hypotension, syncope, unresponsiveness; ensure resuscitation facilities available; monitor during and after admin for hypersensitivity. Increased risk with known allergies (drug or atopic allergies, severe asthma, eczema); immune or inflammatory conditions (SLE, rheumatoid arthritis). Hypersensitivity after previously uneventful doses. Bacteraemia, discontinue; chronic infection, weigh risk/benefit. Paravenous leakage, brown discolouration and irritation of skin.

Pregnancy, Lactation: Not for use in first trimester; if iron-containing products considered essential, use only with medical supervision. *Parenteral,* use only if clearly necessary; confine to second and third trimesters (risk/benefit). Lactation, not recommended.

ADR: *Oral,* GI irritation, nausea, epigastric pain, constipation. *Parenteral,* hypotension (rapid IV admin), injection-site reactions, hypersensivity (may be acute, severe, life-threatening), see SP above.

Ferric Carboxymaltose
ATC Code: B03AC01. **Sport:** Permitted.
Driving: Unlikely to impair.
Indications: Iron deficiency (parenteral indicated).
Dose: Adult, Elderly: Max. single dose 1000mg/day; max. once weekly. *Admin,* IV bolus injection or IV infusion.

Iron, Folic Acid Combinations   16.3.2
Child: Under 14 years, not recommended.
Hepatic Impairment: Risk/benefit.
CI: See Notes below.
ADR: *Common,* headache, dizziness, hypertension, nausea, injection-site reactions, increased ALT, hypophosphataemia.
Notes: See 16.3.2 Iron.

▼ **Ferinject Parenteral** (*Vifor*) A.
Price, (5) 2mL, €142.50. 10mL, €712.50. 20mL, €270.75.
Injection or infusion, ferric carboxymaltose 50mg/mL. Dark-brown non-transparent aqueous. *Sodium 5.5mg/mL.*

Ferrous Fumarate
ATC Code: B03AA02. **Sport:** Permitted.
Driving: Unlikely to impair.
Indications: Treatment and prophylaxis, iron deficiency anaemia.
Dose: Adult, Elderly: Treatment, 1 cap (or 10mL) twice daily. Prophylaxis, once daily.
Child: Syrup, 2.5-5mL once or twice daily.
Notes: See 16.3.2 Iron.

Galfer 305mg, Syrup (*Thornton&Ross*) OTC. GMS.
Price, caps €8.81. Syr 100mL, €2.86.
Capsule, ferrous fumarate. Red/green. Marked Galfer.
Oral susp, as above 140mg/5mL. Brown; chocolate/mint odour.

Ferrous Fumarate, Folic Acid
ATC Code: B03AD02. **Sport:** Permitted.
Driving: Unlikely to impair.
Indications: Prophylaxis, iron and folic acid deficiency in pregnancy.
Dose: Adult: 1 cap daily before meals.
Notes: See 16.3.2 Iron.

Galfer FA (*Thornton&Ross*) OTC. GMS.
Price, (28) €1.37.
Capsule, ferrous fumarate 305mg, folic acid 305mg. Red/yellow. Marked Galfer FA.

Ferrous Sulfate
ATC Code: B03AA07. **Sport:** Permitted.
Driving: Unlikely to impair.
Indications: Prevention and treatment, iron deficiency anaemia.
Dose: Adult, Elderly: 1 daily before food (*Ferrograd*).
CI: Haemochromatosis, iron overload.
Interactions: Effect of Ferrous Sulfate on Other Drugs: Methyldopa: *Hypotensive effect reduced.*
SP: Caution, undiagnosed haemochromatosis, iron overload (overdose may be fatal in children).
Pregnancy, Lactation: *Ferrograd* may be used in pregnancy after 13 weeks.
Notes: See 16.3.2 Iron.

Ferrograd 325mg (*Teofarma*) OTC. GMS.
Price, (150) €11.61.
Prolonged/R tablet, ferrous sulfate equiv. to 105mg iron. Red. Marked with iron.

Ferrous Sulfate, Folic Acid
ATC Code: B03AD03. **Sport:** Permitted.
Driving: Unlikely to impair.
Indications: Prophylaxis, iron and folic acid deficiency in pregnancy after 13 weeks; second and third trimesters.
Dose: Adult: 1 tab daily before food.
CI: Active peptic ulcer, regional enteritis, ulcerative colitis, diverticular disease, intestinal obstruction, Vitamin B12 deficiency, paroxysmal nocturnal haematuria, haemosiderosis, repeated blood transfusion.
Interactions: Effect of Other Drugs on Ferrous Sulfate, Folic Acid Combination: *Co-admin caution:* Co-trimoxazole, anticonvulsants, penicillamine, chloramphenicol, sulfasalazine, colestyramine.
SP: History of peptic ulcer, folate dependent tumours, caution. Delayed intestinal transit.
Notes: See 16.3.2 Iron.

16.3.3 Magnesium

Ferrograd Folic *(Teofarma)* OTC. GMS.
Price, (150) €15.43.
Prolonged/R tablet, ferrous sulfate 325mg, folic acid 350mg. Red f/c. Marked with logo.

Iron (III)-Dextran

ATC Code: BO3AC. **Sport:** Permitted.
Driving: Unlikely to impair.
Indications: Iron deficiency (intolerance or lack of effect of oral iron); need for rapid delivery of iron to iron stores.
Dose: Adult, Elderly: 100-200mg 2-3 times weekly. Rapid delivery to iron stores, 20mg/kg iron as total replacement dose. Slow IV injection or infusion or IM.
Child: Under 14 years, not recommended.
Renal Impairment: Acute, contraindicated.
CI: Acute or chronic infection, rheumatoid arthritis. See Notes below.
Interactions: Effect of Iron (III)-Dextran on Other Drugs: *Co-admin not recommended:* Other iron-carbohydrate complexes.
Notes: See 16.3.2 Iron.

▼ **Cosmofer Parenteral** *(Pharmacosmos)* A. GMS.
Price, 50mg/mL, 2mL (5) €59.34.
Injection, iron (III)-hydroxide dextran complex 50mg/mL. Dark brown soln.

Iron (III)-Isomaltoside

ATC Code: BO3AC. **Sport:** Permitted.
Driving: No data.
Indications: Iron deficiency anaemia when rapid delivery of iron is needed, when oral iron is ineffective of cannot be used.
Dose: Adult: Individualise dose based Ganzoni formula* (see Notes below) or Hb (g/dL) 10 or below 1000mg (bodyweight 50-70kg) or 1500mg (70kg and above); Hb below 10, 1500mg (50-70kg) or 2000mg (70kg and above). Max. total single dose 200mg, admin max. 3-times weekly as slow IV injection or IV infusion. NOT for IM injection. *Recommended where individual adjustments needed (anorexia nervosa, cachexia, obesity, pregnancy, anaemia due to bleeding). Admin by IV bolus injection, IV drip infusion or direct into venous limb of dialyser.
Child: Under 18 years, not recommended.
Interactions: Effect of Iron (III)-Isomaltoside on Other Drugs: Oral iron: *Absorption reduced; commence 5 days after last parenteral dose.*
SP: Caution, presence of acute or chronic infection; ongoing bacteraemia, not recommended
Notes: See 16.3.2 Iron.

▼ **Monover Parenteral** *(Pharmacosmos)* A.
Price, not published by company.
Injection or infusion, iron (III)-isomaltoside 100mg/mL. Dark brown non-transparent soln.

Iron (III)-Sucrose

ATC Code: BO3AC. **Sport:** Permitted.
Driving: Dizziness, confusion, light-headedness following admin.
Indications: Iron deficiency, rapid iron supply needed; oral not tolerated; active inflammatory bowel disease (oral iron ineffective), chronic kidney disease (oral iron less effective than *Venofer*).
Dose: Adult: Use Ganzoni formula to individualise dose (see Notes below). 5-10mL *Venofer* (100-200mg iron) 1-3 times weekly. *Admin,* IV (slow injection or infusion or directly into venous line of dialysis machine); NOT for IM injection. Dilute only in 0.9% sodium chloride soln.
Child: Not recommended.
Hepatic Impairment: Careful risk/benefit assessment.
CI: History of asthma, eczema, other atopic allergy. See Notes below.
Interactions: Effect of Other Drugs on Iron (III)-Sucrose: *Co-admin not recommended:* Oral iron (absorption reduced).
Pregnancy, Lactation: Pregnancy, first trimester, contraindicated; then weigh risk/benefit; use only if oral iron ineffective. Lactation, non-metabolised iron sucrose unlikely to pass into breast milk.
ADR: Summary, *most common,* dysgeusia; *most important serious,* hypersensitivity reactions.
Notes: See 16.3.2 Iron.

▼ **Venofer Parenteral 20mg/mL** *(Vifor)* A.
Price, (5) 5mL, €51.70.
Injection or infusion, iron (III)-hydroxide sucrose complex. Dark-brown non-transparent aqueous. **Store:** Do not freeze.

16.3.3 - Magnesium

In This Chapter: *Magnesium.*

Class Effects
Magnesium salts are also used in the symptomatic relief of dyspepsia and GORD. See 1.1.1 Metallic Salts.

SP: Symptoms of hypermagnesaemia (thirst, nausea, vomiting, flushing of the skin, hypotension, drowsiness, confusion, loss of tendon reflexes, muscle weakness, respiratory depression, cardiac arrhythmias, coma, cardiac arrest).

Magnesium

ATC Code: A12CC. **Sport:** Permitted.
Driving: Unlikely to impair.
Indications: Magnesium deficiency in hypomagnesaemia; prevention, recurrent seizure in eclampsia.
Dose: Adult, Elderly: Magnesium deficiency, up to 160mmoL magnesium by slow IV infusion of diluted soln for up to 5 days.
Seizure prevention in eclampsia, initial IV loading dose 16mmoL magnesium over 5-15 minutes then 4mmoL magnesium (1g) every hour by IV infusion for at least 24-hours after last seizure OR 5g by deep IM injection into upper quadrant of each buttock, then a further 5g IM 4-hourly; duration 24 hours after last seizure provided (respiratory rate above 16/min, urine output above 25mL/min, knee jerks present). Recurrent convulsions, both IV and IM regimens, further 2-4g depending on body weight IV over 5 minutes.
Child: Magnesium deficiency, dilute appropriately and admin IM.
Renal Impairment: Severe, reduce dose.
Hepatic Impairment: Hepatic (encephalopathy, failure, coma) with renal function risk, not recommended.
Interactions: Effect of Other Drugs on Magnesium: Caution: Digitalis glycosides. *Respiratory depression risk:* Barbiturates, opioids, hypnotics (high doses).
Effect of Magnesium on Other Drugs: Neuromuscular blocking agents: *Effect enhanced (parenteral magnesium).* Nifedipine: *Profound hypotension.* Tubocurarine: *Effect potentiated, prolonged.*
SP: *Parenteral* soln MUST be diluted before IV use (up to 20% w/v soln); IM (25% or 50% w/v soln).
Pregnancy, Lactation: As eclampsia may be life-threatening to mother and baby, magnesium sulfate (parenteral) may be used. Lactation, if essential.
ADR: High dose oral (diarrhoea, loose stools). Hypermagnesaemia (impaired renal function, high dose parenteral).
Notes: See 16.3.3 Magnesium.

Magnesium Sulphate Parenteral *(Pinewood)* A.
Price, (10) 2mL, €27.00. 10mL, €52.00.
Injection, magnesium sulfate heptahydrate 50%. Soln.

16.3.4 - Potassium

In This Chapter: *Potassium.*

Potassium

ATC Code: A12BA. **Sport:** Permitted.
Driving: Unlikely to impair.
Indications: Patients requiring supplemental potassium e.g. potassium depleting diuretics, hypokalaemia

(corticosteroid, ACTH, carbenoxolone therapy), inadequate dietary intake, increased potassium loss (GI e.g. vomiting, diarrhoea; renal, stress-related), Cushing's syndrome, renal tubular disease, altered transcellular potassium shifts, hypochloraemic alkalosis, alcoholism.

Dose: Adult: ORAL, *Kay-Cee-L* 10-50mL/day (divided doses) *Admin*, after food.

PARENTERAL, 50-100mmoL/day with normal dietary intake; slow IV infusion max. 20mmoL/hour; monitor ECG.

Elderly: Consider renal status; increased hyperkalaemia risk (monitor).

Child: *Kay-Cee-L*, with medical supervision; up to 1 year, 0.5-0.75mL/kg/day in divided doses after food; age 1-12 years, 0.5-1mL/kg/day.

Renal Impairment: *Oral*, mild/moderate, caution; advanced/severe, contraindicated. *Parenteral*, inadequate urinary excretion or defective cellular uptake of potassium, life-threatening hyperkalaemia at standard dose.

Hepatic Impairment: Caution, increased likelihood of electrolyte disturbances (monitor).

CI: All forms of hyperkalaemia. *Oral*, untreated Addison's disease, hyporeninaemic hypoaldosteronism, acute dehydration, extensive cell destruction (severe burns). Hyperkalaemic periodic paralysis (potassium precipitated), congenital paramyotonia. GI obstruction (all solid forms). Metabolic acidosis, use alkaline potassium salt (bicarbonate). *Parenteral*, conc (15%) never use undiluted.

Interactions: Effect of Other Drugs on Potassium: *Co-admin not recommended*: Potassium-sparing diuretics (spironolactone, triamterene, amiloride) *(Kay-C-Lee)*, ACEIs, AIIAs, other drugs containing potassium, ciclosporin, NSAIDs, beta-blockers, heparin, digoxin. *Co-admin caution*: Direct renin inhibitors (aliskiren), PPIs. *Caution (solid forms, high doses)*: Anticholinergics (reduce GI motility).

SP: *Oral*, peptic ulcer, renal or hepatic dysfunction (hyperkalaemia); caution. May induce ulceration, haemorrhage or GI stricture; risk increased with (GI disorders, cardiovascular disease, prolonged therapy, anticholinergic admin). Diuretic induced magnesium deficiency will prevent restoration of intracellular deficits of potassium. *Parenteral*, admin slowly (high conc may cause serious cardiac toxicity); renal or adrenal insufficiency, cardiac disease, extensive tissue destruction (severe burns), caution. See CI above.

Pregnancy, Lactation: With medical supervision; pregnancy, solid forms only if essential; parenteral, if considered essential. Lactation, if benefit outweighs risk.

ADR: Nausea, vomiting, abdominal pains, diarrhoea, GI (obstruction, haemorrhage, ulceration with/without perforation). Pruritus, rash, urticaria, hyperkalaemia. Injection-site reactions.

Notes: See 16.3.4 Potassium.

Kay-Cee-L *(Geistlich)* OTC. GMS.
Price, 500mL, €6.27.
Oral syrup, potassium chloride 7.5% w/v. Clear red slightly viscous liquid. *Sorbitol, parabens.*

Potassium Chloride Conc Parenteral *(Concordia)* A. GMS.
Price, (10) 1.5g/10mL, €3.51.
Infusion, potassium chloride 1.5g/10mL. Clear colourless conc for soln.

16.3.5 - Zinc

In This Chapter: *Zinc acetate.*

Class Effects
Indications: Zinc deficiency (nutritional deficiency, wound healing, infection), genetic disorders of zinc metabolism, copper absorption inhibitors in Wilson's disease (slow onset of action). Also used topically to promote wound healing.

SP: Wilson's disease, initiate treatment under physician experienced in this disease. Life-long therapy.

Zinc Acetate
ATC Code: A16AX05. **Sport:** Permitted.
Driving: No studies performed.

Indications: Treatment, Wilson's Disease.

Dose: Adult, Elderly: 50mg 3-times daily; max. 50mg 5-times daily.

Child: Under 6 years, consider prophylactic treatment as early as possible; age 1-6 years, 25mg twice daily; age 6-16 years, under 57kg, 25mg 3-times daily; over 57 kg, 50mg 3-times daily. Admin on empty stomach, 1 hour before or 2-3 hours after food. Switch from chelating agents, maintain and co-admin for 2-3 weeks; admin 1 hour apart.

Interactions: Effect of Other Drugs on Zinc: *Mutually decreased effect*: Chelators (penicillamine, trientine); ensure dosing 1 hour apart. *Absorption decreased*: Iron, calcium supplements, tetracyclines, phosphorus-containing compounds, food (bread, hard boiled eggs, coffee, milk; phytates and fibres bind zinc and prevent entry to intestinal cells); protein appears to interfere least.

Effect of Zinc on Other Drugs: Iron, tetracyclines, fluoroquinolones: *Absorption decreased*.

SP: If symptomatic treat initially with chelating agent. Once copper levels below toxic, consider maintenance treatment with *Wilzin*; switch from chelating agent to *Wilzin*, caution portal hypertension.

Pregnancy, Lactation: Pregnancy, extremely important to continue therapy; physician to decide treatment choice. Adjust dose to guarantee foetus will not be copper deficient; mandatory monitoring. Lactation, avoid; zinc-induced copper deficiency in baby may occur.

ADR: *Common*, gastric irritation, blood amylase, lipase, ALP increased.

Notes: See 16.3.5 Zinc.

Wilzin 25mg, 50mg *(Orphan Europe)* A. HT.
Price, (250) 25mg, €215.14. 50mg, €395.39.
Capsule, zinc acetate dihydrate. Opaque. 25mg: Aqua blue. Marked 93-376. 50mg: Orange. Marked 93-377.

16.3.6 - Vitamin B Group

In This Chapter: *Vitamin B complex and ascorbic acid combination.*

Class Effects
The Vitamin B group comprises a number of water soluble vitamins, including thiamine (B1), riboflavin (B2), niacin or nicotinamide (B3), pantothenic acid (B5), pyridoxine and pyridoxamine (B6), biotin (B7) and cyanocobalamin (B12). Cyanocobalamin, used in the treatment of megaloblastic anaemia, see Notes below.

CI: Hypersensitivity to any member of the class.

Interactions: Effect of Other Drugs on Vitamin B Group: (B1) *Effect neutralised*: Thiosemicarbazone, 5-fluorouracil. *Resorption inhibited*: Antacids. (B12) *GI absorption reduced*: Neomycin, aminosalicylic acid, H2-blockers. (B12 and Pyridoxine) *Serum levels lowered*: Oral contraceptives.

Effect of Vitamin B Group on Other Drugs: (Pyridoxine) Levodopa: *Effect reduced (if given without dopa-decarboxylase inhibitor)*.

Notes: See 16.1.2 Drugs Used In Megaloblastic Anaemia (cyanocobalamin).

Vitamin B1, B2, B3, B6 and combinations
ATC Code: A11EB. **Sport:** Permitted.
Driving: Unlikely to impair.

Indications: Rapid therapy of severe depletion or malabsorption of water soluble vitamins (B, C) especially in alcoholism where severe thiamine depletion can lead to Wernicke's encephalopathy.

Dose: Adult, Elderly: Contents of 2-3 pairs of amps (amp 1 + amp 2) diluted with 50-100mL infusion soln (infuse over 30 minutes) 8-hourly. Drip infusion preferred. NOTE: For IV admin only; unintentional IM admin reported; not associated with serious adverse reactions.

16.3.7 Vitamin C

Interactions: Effect of Vitamin B Combination on Other Drugs: Levodopa: *Pyridoxine may interfere with effect.*

SP: Facilities to manage anaphylactic reactions to be available; initial warning signs (sneezing, mild asthma); further injections may result in anaphylactic shock. Use only if parenteral treatment essential. NOTE: This medicine is for injection into a vein only; not for admin by any other route.

Pregnancy, Lactation: No adverse effects at recommended dose. Pregnancy, caution.

ADR: *Incidence unknown,* hypersensitivity, paraesthesia, hypotension, bronchospasm, nausea, vomiting, sweating, injection-site reactions.

Notes: See 16.3.6 Vitamin B Group.

> **Pabrinex IV High Potency Parenteral** *(KyowaKirin)* A.
> *Price,* 10 pairs, €49.73 (high potency).
> *Infusion (1 and 2),* No 1: Thiamine HCl 250mg, riboflavin phosphate sodium 4mg, pyridoxine HCl 50mg. No 2: Ascorbic acid 500mg, nicotinamide 160mg, glucose (monohydrate) 1000mg. *Sodium 79mg/dose (1 pair of amps).* **Store:** Below 25 deg C; do not freeze; protect (light).

16.3.7 - Vitamin C

In This Chapter: Ascorbic acid.

Class Effects

Indications: Prophylaxis and treatment, ascorbic acid deficiency.

CI: Hypersensitivity to any member of the class. Hyperoxaluria (max. 1g/day; may be increased urinary oxalate excretion).

Interactions: Effect of Other Drugs on Ascorbic Acid: *Deterioration in LV function (ascorbic acid 500mg):* Deferoxamine.

Effect of Ascorbic Acid on Other Drugs: Fluphenazine: *Decreased plasma levels.*

SP: Hyperoxaluria, G-6-PD deficiency (haemolytic anaemia), prolonged use, increased renal clearance (deficiency if withdrawn rapidly). Do not exceed stated dose. Caution, increased plasma iron. May interfere with some tests for glucose in urine.

Pregnancy, Lactation: Max. dose 1g/day.

ADR: GI disturbances, rarely allergic reactions. G-6-PD deficiency patients, haemolytic anaemia. Nausea, vomiting, abdominal cramping, headaches, diarrhoea, renal calcium calculi.

Notes: See 16.3.7 Zinc.

16.3.8 - Vitamin D, Analogues

In This Chapter: Alfacalcidol, colecalciferol, paricalcitol.

Class Effects

Vitamin D analogues include ergocalciferol (Vitamin D2), dihydrotachysterol (DHT), alfacalcidol, calcitriol, colecalciferol (Vitamin D3), calcifediol, paricalcitol.

CI: Hypersensitivity to any member of the class. Hypercalcaemia, Vitamin D toxicity.

Interactions: Effect of Other Drugs on Vitamin D Analogues: *Increased dose requirement (increased metabolism):* Anticonvulsants (barbiturates, phenytoin, carbamazepine, primidone), corticosteroids. *Impaired absorption:* Bile acid sequestrants (colestyramine, colestipol), orlistat, paraffin oil laxatives. *Hypercalcaemia risk:* Thiazides, calcium-containing preparations (high dose), preparations containing (Vitamin D, phosphate). *Hypermagnesaemia risk:* Magnesium-containing drugs (antacids). *Aluminium-related toxicity:* Aluminium-containing preparations. *Interfered Vitamin D activity:* Actinomycin, imidazole antifungals.

Effect of Vitamin D Analogues on Other Drugs: Cardioactive glycosides, digitalis: *Hypercalcaemia (arrhythmias).*

SP: *Monitor,* serum (calcium, phosphate) regularly; PTH, alkaline phosphatase, calcium and phosphate as needed. *Hypercalcaemia,* individualise dose according to response. Ensure adequate daily calcium intake; caution, abrupt increased calcium intake (hypercalcaemia); early signs, (anorexia, fatigue, nausea, vomiting, constipation or diarrhoea, polyuria, sweating, headache, polydipsia, hypertension, somnolence, vertigo); chronic manifestations (fever, dehydration, nocturia, abdominal pain, paralytic ileus, cardiac arrhythmias, dystrophy, arrested growth, sensory disturbances, UTI; rarely overt psychosis, metastatic calcification). *Caution,* chronic renal failure (ectopic calcification); maintain plasma phosphate at normal (2-5mg/100mL) using oral phosphate binders; prolonged hypercalcaemia may aggravate decline of renal function. These drugs increase serum inorganic phosphate levels; desirable in hypophosphataemia. *Caution,* granulomatous disease (sarcoidosis) (Vitamin D sensitivity increased due to increased hydroxylation activity).

Pregnancy, Lactation: Pregnancy, if benefit outweighs risk (with Vitamin D deficiency). Hypercalcaemia during pregnancy may produce congenital disorder in offspring. Lactation, avoid or stop breastfeeding or stop drug; otherwise monitor infants for hypercalcaemia.

ADR: Hyper- (calcaemia, phosphataemia).

Notes: Other drugs used in dialysis, see 8.4.5 Dialysis.

Alfacalcidol

ATC Code: A11CC03. **Sport:** Permitted.
Driving: Dizziness.

Indications: Disturbed calcium metabolism due to impaired 1-alpha-hydroxylation of vitamin D3 (reduced renal function). Uraemic bone disease, hyperparathyroidism (with bone disease), hypoparathyroidism; osteoporosis (post-menopause, senile, steroid-induced); nutritional and malabsorptive rickets and osteomalacia; pseudo-deficiency (D-dependent) rickets; hypophosphataemic vitamin D resistant rickets and osteomalacia. Prophylaxis, therapy, neonatal hypocalcaemia.

Dose: Adult: All indications, adults, children over 20kg, 1mcg/day.

Elderly: All indications, 0.5mcg/day may be sufficient.

Child: All indications, neonates, premature infants, 0.05-0.1mcg/kg/day; children under 20kg, 0.05mcg/kg/day; over 20kg, as for Adult above.

SP: Nephrolithiasis, caution.

ADR: *Common,* abdominal pain/discomfort, rash, pruritus, hypercalciuria.

Notes: See 16.3.8 Vitamin D.

> **One-Alpha 0.25mcg, 1mcg, Drops** *(LEO)* B. GMS.
> *Price,* (30) 0.25mcg, €4.57. 1mcg, €13.14. Drops (10mL) €13.11.
> *Capsule,* alfacalcidol. Soft gelatin ellipsoid (egg-shaped); contains oily soln. 0.25mcg: Cream-coloured. 1mcg: Brown. *Sesame oil.* **Store:** Below 25 deg C.
> *Oral drops,* as above 2mcg/mL. Clear aqueous soln. *Ethanol, sorbitol, parabens, macrogolglycerol hydroxystearate.* **Store:** Refrigerate.

Colecalciferol

ATC Code: A11CC05. **Sport:** Permitted.
Driving: Unlikely to impair.

Indications: Prevention and treatment, Vitamin D deficiency*; adjunctive, to specific osteoporosis treatment with Vitamin D deficiency risk *(Desunin 800 IU, altavitaD3 25000 IU).* Treatment, Vitamin D deficiency* *(Desunin 4000 IU),* in pregnant and breastfeeding women* *(altavitaD3 1000 IU).* Prophylaxis, vitamin D deficiency* (malabsorption), rickets in preterm newborn; prophylaxis and treatment, rickets and osteomalacia *(Thorens).* *(identified risk).

Dose: Adult, Elderly: *Desunin* (800 IU, 4000 IU), 1 tab (800 IU)/day; max. 5 tabs/day OR max. 1 tab (4000 IU)/day. *Admin,* swallow whole or can be crushed; can be taken with food.

Thorens, Vitamin D deficiency, prevention, 600-800 IU/day

424

(3-4 drops) or 25000 IU/month (1 bottle); treatment, 50000 IU/week (6-8 weeks); maintenance, 1400-2000 IU/day). Osteoporosis, adjunctive, 800 IU/day (4 drops) or 25000 IU/month. Pregnancy and breastfeeding, deficiency prevention, 400 IU/day (2 drops); up to 2000 IU/day may be needed; even higher doses during breastfeeding. *Admin*, preferably with food; admin as is or mix with a small amount of cold or lukewarm food.

altavitaD3, Vitamin D deficiency, prevention, 25000 IU/month OR 1000 IU/day; treatment, oral soln 50000 IU/week (2 single-dose oral solns) (6-8 weeks) OR caps 1000-4000 IU/day (12 weeks); maintenance, 1400-2000 IU/day. Osteoporosis, adjunctive, 25000 IU/month OR 1000 IU/day. Pregnancy and breastfeeding, deficiency prevention, caps 1000-2000 IU/day (25000 IU strength not recommended). NOTE: 1000 IU/day is considered equiv. to 7000 IU/week. *Admin*, swallow caps whole with water; empty contents of single-dose oral soln into mouth or onto a spoon; can mix with small amount of cold or lukewarm food. Preferably with food.

Child: *Desunin*, under 12 years, safety/efficacy not established.

Thorens, Vitamin D deficiency, prevention, (0-1 year) 400 IU/day (2 drops) OR 25000 IU every 8 weeks (1 bottle), (1-18 years) 600 IU/day (3 drops) OR 25000 IU every 6 weeks; up to 1000 IU/day (5 drops) may be needed; treatment, (0-18 years), 2000 IU/day (10 drops) OR 25000 IU once every 2 weeks (6 weeks); maintenance, 400-1000 IU/day (2-5 drops). *Admin*, see Adult above.

altavitaD3, Vitamin D deficiency: CAPS, up to 1000 IU/day may be needed. ORAL SOLN, (0-1 year), 25000 IU (1 single dose soln) every 8 weeks; (1-18 years), 25000 IU every 6 weeks. Treatment: (0-18 years) 25000 IU (1 single dose soln) every 2 weeks OR (10-18 years) caps 2000 IU/day (6 weeks); maintenance, 400-1000 IU/day. NOTE: Caps, 1000 IU/day is considered equiv. to 7000 IU/week. *Admin*, see Adult above.

Renal Impairment: Caution, monitor (calcium, phosphate). Severe, not recommended; colecalciferol not metabolised normally (use other forms of Vitamin D; do not use with calcium).

CI: Hypercalcaemia (calciuria), nephrolithiasis (calcinosis), hypervitaminosis D, serious renal impairment.

SP: Sarcoidosis, caution. Monitor (elderly, co-admin of cardiac glycosides or diuretics), if high tendency to calculus formation. *High risk populations for Vitamin D3 deficiency*: Institutionalised or hospitalised, dark skin, limited sun exposure, obese, possible osteoporosis, concomitant medication (anticonvulsants, glucocorticoids), malabsorption (inflammatory bowel disease, coeliac disease), pregnancy, recently treated for Vitamin D3 deficiency (requiring maintenance therapy). Recommended Tolerable Upper Intake Levels of Vitamin D3, adults, including (pregnant, lactating) women, 4000 IU/day; children, adolescents (11-17 years) 4000 IU/day; children (1-10 years) 2000 IU/day; infants (0-1 year) 1000 IU/day.

Pregnancy, Lactation: Prevention of deficiency during pregnancy or breastfeeding, see Dose above. High strength formulations not recommended.

ADR: Uncommon, hypercalcaemia, hypercalciuria.

Notes: See 16.3.8 Vitamin D.

altavitaD3 Capsules, Oral Soln *(Consilient)* B. GMS.
Price, caps 1000 IU (28) and 7000 IU (4), €3.28; 25000 IU (3), €6.00. Oral soln 25000 IU (3) 1mL, €6.00.
Soft capsules, colecalciferol. Oval; contain slightly yellow oily liquid. 1000 IU: Dark-red. Marked 1. *Allura Red*. 7000 IU: Yellow. Marked 7. *Sunset Yellow*. 25000 IU: Light-red. Marked 25. *Allura Red*. **Store:** Below 30 deg C.
Oral soln, as above 25000 IU/1mL single dose soln. Clear slightly-yellow oily liquid; orange odour. **Store:** As above.

Desunin 800 IU, 4000 IU *(Meda)* B. GMS.
Price, 800 IU (90) €10.58. 4000 IU (70) €21.33.
Tablet, colecalciferol. White (light-yellow). 800 IU: Round. 4000 IU: Oblong scored (facilitates breaking). *Isomalt, sucrose*. **Store:** Below 30 deg C; original pack to protect (light, moisture).

Thorens Oral Drops, Soln *(Galen)* B. GMS.
Price, oral drops (10000 IU/mL) 10mL, €8.05. Oral soln (25000 IU/2.5mL) 2.5mL (4) €9.71.
Oral drops (soln), cholecalciferol oral drops 200 IU/drop OR oral soln 10000 IU/mL (25000 IU/2.5mL single dose bottle). Clear colourless (greenish-yellow) oily soln. **Store:** Below 30 deg C; do not (refrigerate, freeze); outer carton to protect (light).

Paricalcitol

ATC Code: H05BX02. **Sport:** Permitted.
Driving: Unlikely to impair.

Indications: Prevention and treatment, secondary hyperparathyroidism (with chronic renal insufficiency and chronic renal failure on haemodialysis or peritoneal dialysis).

Dose: Adult, Elderly: ORAL, chronic kidney disease (Stages 3, 4), iPTH level (pg/mL) 500 or below, 1mcg daily or 2mcg 3-times weekly; above 500, 2mcg daily or 4mcg 3-times weekly. Titrate dose based on iPTH levels. CKD (Stage 5), admin 3-times weekly every other day. Initially based on iPTH level (pg/mL)/60 [(pmOL/L)/7] up to initial max. of 32mcg. Oral can be taken with food.
PARENTERAL, initial dose calculation is based on baseline PTH levels as follows: Initial dose (mcg) = baseline intact PTH level (pmOL*/L) divided by 8. Max. 40mcg safely admin in clinical studies. Soln for injection is admin via haemodialysis access. *(picomole)*. *Elderly*, greater sensitivity cannot be ruled out. Dose titration, see manufacturers Full Prescribing Information.

Child: Under 18 years, safety/efficacy not established. No dose recommendation.

Renal Impairment: Renal transplant, see manufacturers Full Prescribing Information.

Hepatic Impairment: Mild/moderate, no adjustment. Severe, no data.

Interactions: Effect of Other Drugs on Paricalcitol: *Co-admin not recommended (hypercalcaemia risk)*: Other Vitamin D or phosphate-containing medications. *Co-admin caution*: Ketoconazole, digitalis (toxicity potentiated by hypercalcaemia), calcium-containing preparations, thiazide diuretic (hypercalcaemia risk), magnesium-containing preparations (antacids) (hypermagnesaemia risk). *Chronic co-admin not recommended (increased aluminium levels/bone toxicity)*: Aluminium-containing preparations (antacids, phosphate-binders). *Impaired absorption*: Drugs impairing intestinal fat-soluble vitamin absorption (colestyramine).

SP: Over PTH suppression, may result in elevated serum calcium. Significant hypercalcaemia and receiving calcium-based phosphate binder, reduce dose or interrupt phosphate binder. Chronic hypercalcaemia (generalised vascular calcification, other soft tissue calcification). Ethanol content, caution alcoholics, epilepsy, liver disease.

ADR: *Common*, hypoparathyroidism, hyper-(phosphataemia, calcaemia), dysgeusia, rash, pruritus, headache, stomach discomfort.

Notes: See 16.3.8 Vitamin D.

Zemplar Capsules, Parenteral *(AbbVie)* A. HT.
Price, caps (28) 1mcg, €89.32; 2mcg, €171.02. HOS (PTW): Parenteral (5) 5mcg/mL (1mL) €93.00.
Injection, paricalcitol 5mcg/mL. Clear colourless aqueous soln. *Propylene glycol, ethanol*.
Capsules, as above 1mcg, 2mcg. Oval soft. Marked with logo. 1mcg: Gray. Marked ZA. 2mcg: Orange-brown. Marked ZF. **Store:** As above.

16.3.9 - Vitamin K

In This Chapter: *Phytomenadione*.

Class Effects
CI: Hypersensitivity to any member of the class.

Phytomenadione

ATC Code: B02BA01. **Sport:** Permitted.
Driving: None known.

Indications: Prophylaxis and treatment, Vitamin K deficiency bleeding (VKDB) in neonates and infants.

16.4 Multivitamin Preparations

Treatment, of overdose with coumarin anticoagulants where small quantities of Vitamin K are required including haemorrhage (threatened) associated with low prothrombin or Factor VII levels.

Dose: Adult: Asymptomatic high INR with or without mild haemorrhage: *Warfarin* INR 5-9, Vitamin K oral 1-2.5mg (initial reversal) OR 2-5mg (rapid reversal) OR 0.5-1mg IV; add 1-2mg orally if INR remains high after 24 hours. INR above 9, Vitamin K oral 2.5-5mg (up to 10mg) OR 1mg IV. *Acenocoumarol*, INR 5-8, Vitamin K 1-2mg oral or IV. INR above 8, Vitamin K oral 3-5mg OR 1-2mg IV. *Phenprocoumon*, INR 5-9, Vitamin K 2-5mg oral or IV. INR above 9, as for INR 5-9. INR above 10, Vitamin K oral not recommended; individually adapt IV doses.

Anticoagulant antidote (severe or life-threatening haemorrhage): Withdraw anticoagulant, admin 5-10mg Vitamin K by slow IV with fresh frozen plasma (FFP) or prothrombin complex conc (PCC). *Warfarin*, major bleeding, Vitamin K 5-10mg IV (with FFP or PCC); life-threatening bleeding, Vitamin K 10mg IV (with FFP, PCC or rFactor VIIa). *Acenocoumarol*, major bleeding, Vitamin K 5mg IV with (FFP, PCC or rFactor VIIa). *Phenprocoumon*, major bleeding (INR below 5), Vitamin K 5mg IV (with PCC); major bleeding (INR above 5), Vitamin K 10mg IV (with PCC).

Admin, amp for IV injection or oral use. Do not mix with other parenteral medicines.

Elderly: More sensitive to anticoagulation reversal; use lower end of dose ranges. High INR, with or without mild haemorrhage (INR 5-9), 0.5-1mg IV or oral effective to reduce INR to below 5 within 24 hours.

Child: Prophylaxis Vitamin K deficiency bleeding, *neonates*, 36 weeks gestation and older, 1mg IM at birth* OR 2mg orally at birth (follow oral dose with 2mg orally at 4-7 days and a further 2mg at 1 month after birth (this third dose can be omitted in exclusively formula fed infants; *preterm neonates*, under 36 weeks gestation (2.5kg or more) or term neonates at special risk (prematurity, birth asphyxia, obstructive jaundice, inability to swallow, maternal anticoagulant or antiepileptic use), admin 1mg IM or IV at birth*; (under 2.5kg), 0.4mg/kg IM or IV at birth*. Base further doses on coagulation status. Further oral doses advised for breast-fed infants.

Asymptomatic high INR, with/without mild haemorrhage, 30mcg/kg IV. Infants under 1 year, use paediatric formulation which can be admin by IV injection or orally. IM route only suitable for VKDB indication in babies. *or soon after birth.

Major life-threatening bleeding, Vitamin K 5mg IV suggested (with FPP or PCC).

Hepatic Impairment: Severe, carefully monitor INR (1x 10mL amp contains 54.6mg glycocholic acid).

CI: Admin by IM route (depot characteristics; haematoma risk).

Interactions: Effect of Phytomenadione on Other Drugs: Coumarin-type anticoagulants: *Effect antagonised.*

SP: Potentially fatal/severe haemorrhage (coumarin overdose), admin by slow IV; max. 40mg during 24-hour period; with whole blood or clotting factors (immediate treatment). Presence of prosthetic heart valves, use FFP. Dose selection, caution that sub-therapeutic infusion not produced (thrombosis or subsequent resistance to re-initiation of anticoagulant therapy); smaller doses (1mg) found to reduce INR effectively. Severe haemorrhage, fresh whole blood may be needed while waiting for Vitamin K effect. NOT ANTIDOTE FOR HEPARIN. Admin to premature babies (under 2.5kg) may increase kernicterus (bilirubin encephalopathy) risk. Cholestatic disease, admin IM or IV (oral absorption impaired).

Pregnancy, Lactation: If benefit outweighs risk. Not recommended for pregnant women as prophylaxis of Vitamin K deficiency bleeding in the newborn.

ADR: Too rapid IV (facial flushing, sweating, chest constriction, cyanosis, peripheral vascular collapse). Anaphylactoid* reactions after IV admin. Venous irritation or phlebitis. *Paediatric*, anaphylactoid* reactions (IV); local irritation, injection-site reactions (may be severe; inflammation, atrophy, necrosis). *Possible.

Notes: See 16.3.9 Vitamin K.

Konakion MM, Paed Parenteral, Oral Soln *(Roche)* A. GMS.
Price, injection 10mg/1mL (10) €5.14. Paed injection 2mg/0.2mL (5) €4.85. HOS: Paed injection, €4.49.
Injection or oral soln, phytomenadione (Vitamin K1) 10mg/mL (IV), paed 2mg/0.2mL (IV or IM) or admin as oral soln. Clear (slightly opalescent) pale-yellow soln. Glycocholic acid 54.6mg, essentially sodium-free. **Store:** Below 25 deg C; do not freeze; original pack to protect (light).

16.4 - Multivitamin Preparations

Class Effects

CI: Hypersensitivity to any member of the class.

Pregnancy, Lactation: Large doses of Vitamin A have been found to be teratogenic especially during first trimester. Vitamin D given during last trimester or while breastfeeding may cause hypercalcaemia in infants.

Multivitamins

ATC Code: A11A. **Sport:** Permitted.
Driving: None known.

Indications: Vitamin supplement for prevention of vitamin deficiency (galactosaemia, disaccharide intolerance, phenylketonuria, other disorders of carbohydrate or amino acid metabolism, restricted, specialised or synthetic diets).

Dose: Adult, Elderly: Age 4 years and over, 1 tab 3-times daily OR 5mL oral soln daily.

Child: As for Adult above.

CI: Hypercalcaemia *(Liquid)*.

Interactions: Effect of Other Drugs on Multivitamins: *Serum B12 levels may be decreased*: Oral contraceptives. *Vitamin absorption may be reduced*: Conditions of fat malabsorption, co-admin (neomycin, colestyramine, liquid paraffin, aminoglycosides, aminosalicylic acid, anticonvulsants, biguanides, chloramphenicol, cimetidine, colchicine, potassium salts, methyldopa).

Effect of Multivitamins on Other Drug: Levodopa: *Peripheral metabolism may be increased by pyridoxine; reduced efficacy.*

SP: Do not exceed dose without medical supervision. Hypervitaminosis (prolonged Vitamin A and D ingestion).

Pregnancy, Lactation: Use only if considered essential by physician.

ADR: None known at recommended dose.

Notes: See 16.4 Multivitamin Preparations.

Ketovite Tabs *(Essential Pharma)* OTC. GMS.
Price, tabs (100), €10.86. Liquid 150mL, €22.53.
Tablet, thiamine* 1mg, riboflavin 1mg, pyridoxine* 0.33mg, nicotinamide 3.3mg, calcium pantothenate 1.16mg, ascorbic acid 16.6mg, alpha-tocopheryl acetate 5mg, inositol 50mg, biotin 0.17mg, folic acid 0.25mg, acetomenaphthone 0.5mg per tab (*hydrochloride). Yellow.
Oral soln (liquid), Vitamin A 2500 IU, ergocalciferol (Vitamin D2) 400 IU, cyanocobalamin 12.5mcg, choline chloride 150mg. Pale-pinkish clear opalescent. Parabens.

16.5 - Metabolic Disorders

In This Chapter: *Agalsidase alfa, alglucosidase alfa, imiglucerase, laronidase, miglustat, nitisinone, sapropterin, sodium phenylbutyrate.*

Class Effects

These drugs are used with specialist supervision. Always see manufacturers Full Prescribing Information.

Pharmacology: These drugs are used for long-term enzyme replacement therapy (ERT) in enzyme deficiency disorders.

CI: Hypersensitivity to any member of the class.

ADR: Serious and life-threatening hypersensitivity reactions. Infusion-related reactions.

Agalsidase Alfa

ATC Code: A16AB03. **Sport:** Permitted.
Driving: Unlikely to impair.

Indications: Long-term ERT in Fabry Disease (alfa-galactosidase A deficiency).

Dose: Adult: 0.2mg/kg every other week; IV over 40 minutes.

Elderly: Over 65 years, no data.

Child: Age 0-6 years, no data; 7-18 years, who received 0.2mg/kg every other week, no unexpected safety issues encountered.

Renal Impairment: eGFR (mL/min) below 60 may limit renal response to ERT.

Hepatic Impairment: No data.

Interactions: Effect of Other Drugs on Agalsidase Alfa: *Co-admin not recommended*: Chloroquine, amiodarone, benoquin, gentamicin (potentially inhibit intra-cellular alfa-galactosidase activity).

SP: Infusion-related reactions within first 2-4 months; *serious* reactions (haemodynamic stress triggering cardiac events; with pre-existing cardiac manifestations of Fabry disease). Mild/moderate reactions, temporarily interrupt infusion; restart when symptoms subside. Pre-treat with antihistamines and/or corticosteroids (oral or IV) prior (1-24 hours) to infusion. Hypersensitivity (IV proteins); severe, discontinue. Antibodies to protein may develop (IgG, IgE).

Pregnancy, Lactation: Caution; very limited data; not known if excreted in breast milk.

ADR: See Notes below.

Notes: See 16.5 Metabolic Disorders.

Replagal Parenteral *(Shire Genetics)* A. HOS.
Price, (1) €1710.09.
Infusion, agalsidase alfa 1mg/mL (3.5mL). Clear colourless soln. *Preservative-free.* **Store:** Refrigerate.

Agalsidase Beta

ATC Code: A16AB04. **Sport:** Permitted.
Driving: No specific studies.

Indications: As for agalsidase alfa above.

Dose: Adult: 1mg/kg once every 2 weeks by IV infusion; initially max. 0.25mg/min (15mg/hour) to minimise infusion-related reactions; if tolerated, increase rate gradually.

Elderly: Over 65 years, no data.

Child: Age 0-7 years, no dose recommendation.

Hepatic Impairment: No data.

SP: Antibodies to agalsidase beta, greater IAR risk. Premedicate (antihistamines, paracetamol, ibuprofen and/or corticosteroids).

Pregnancy, Lactation: Pregnancy, use only if clearly necessary. Lactation, stop breastfeeding; may be excreted in milk.

ADR: See Notes below.

Notes: See Agalsidase Alfa above. See 16.5 Metabolic Disorders.

Fabrazyme Parenteral *(Genzyme)* A. HOS.
Price, (1) 5mg, €484.88; 35mg, €3247.64 (PTW).
Infusion, agalsidase beta 5mg, 35mg. Recombinant. White (off-white) lyophilised cake or powder for conc for soln. **Store:** Refrigerate.

Alglucosidase Alfa

ATC Code: A16AB07. **Sport:** Permitted.
Driving: Dizziness.

Indications: Long-term ERT in confirmed Pompe disease (acid alfa-glucosidase deficiency).

Dose: Adult, Elderly: 20mg/kg by IV infusion every 2-weeks. Initial rate 1mg/kg/hour; increase gradually by 2mg/kg/hour every 30 minutes if no sign of infusion-reaction; max. 7mg/kg/hour.

Child: As for Adult above.

CI: Life-threatening hypersensivity reaction when rechallenge unsuccessful.

SP: Infantile onset with high antibody titres at higher risk for infusion-associated reaction (IAR) (severe or delayed); with acute illness (pneumonia, sepsis) greater IAR risk. Re-admin, caution. Advanced disease (compromised cardiac, respiratory function) possible higher risk of severe IAR complications, monitor. Antibodies develop within 3 months (majority of patients). Nephrotic syndrome, severe cutaneous reactions. Respiratory infections (progressive effects of disease on respiratory muscles); risk increased with immunosuppressives.

Pregnancy, Lactation: Pregnancy, use only if clearly necessary. Lactation, stop breastfeeding.

ADR: See Notes below.

Notes: See 16.5 Metabolic Disorders.

Myozyme Parenteral *(Genzyme)* A. HOS.
Price, (1) €507.43 (PTW).
Infusion, alglucosidase alfa 50mg. White (off-white) powder for soln. **Store:** Refrigerate.

Imiglucerase

ATC Code: A16AB02. **Sport:** Permitted.
Driving: No or negligible effect.

Indications: Long-term ERT in Gaucher disease, non-neuronopathic (Type 1), chronic neuronopathic (Type 3).

Dose: Adult, Elderly: Initially 60 U/kg once every 2 weeks (improvement in haematological, visceral parameters) OR 15 U/kg once every 2 weeks (improved haematological parameters, organomegaly; no bone parameters). *Admin,* IV infusion, initial rate 0.5 U/kg/min; subsequent, increase to max. 1 U/kg/min.

Child: As for Adult above.

SP: Decreased response, monitor (IgG antibodies); if present, higher hypersensitivity reaction risk; severe reactions, discontinue. Chronic disease, consider registration in ICGG Gaucher Registry.

Pregnancy, Lactation: Pregnancy, risk/benefit (for each pregnancy). Lactation, not known if excreted in human milk; unlikely to be digested in GI tract of child.

ADR: See Notes below.

Notes: See 16.5 Metabolic Disorders.

Cerezyme Parenteral 400 IU *(Genzyme)* A. HOS.
Price, (1) €1497.19 (PTW).
Infusion, imiglucerase 40 U/mL. White (off-white) powder for conc for soln. *Sodium.* *Enzyme unit (U): Amount of enzyme catalysing hydrolysis of 1 micromole of synthetic substrate (pNP-Glc) per minute. *Sodium 1.24mmoL (400 U/10mL) after reconstitution.* **Store:** Refrigerate.

Laronidase

ATC Code: A16AB05. **Sport:** Permitted.
Driving: No studies performed.

Indications: Long-term ERT with confirmed Mucopolysaccharidosis I (MPS I) (alfa-L-iduronidase deficiency) to treat non-neurological disease manifestations.

Dose: Adult: 100 U/kg by IV infusion over 3-4 hours once every week; initial rate 2 U/kg/hour; if tolerated, increase every 15 minutes to max. 43 U/kg/hour.

Elderly: Over 65 years, no dose recommendation.

Interactions: Effect of Other Drugs on Laronidase: *Co-admin not recommended (interfered intracellular uptake)*: Chloroquine, procaine.

SP: Pre-existent severe underlying upper airway involvement, caution. Acute underlying illness, greater IAR risk. Premedicate with antihistamines and/or antipyretics (paracetamol or ibuprofen) 60 minutes prior to infusion.

Pregnancy, Lactation: Pregnancy, only if clearly necessary. Lactation, stop breastfeeding.

ADR: See Notes below.

Notes: See 16.5 Metabolic Disorders.

Aldurazyme Parenteral *(Genzyme)* A. HOS.
Price, (1) 5mL, €639.07 (PTW).
Infusion, laronidase 100 U/mL. Recombinant alfa-L-iduronidase. Clear (slightly opalescent) colourless (pale-yellow) soln. *Sodium 1.29mmoL/vial.* **Store:** Refrigerate.

Miglustat

ATC Code: A16AX06. **Sport:** Permitted.
Driving: Caution.

Indications: Mild/moderate Type 1 Gaucher Disease (ERT unsuitable); progressive neurological manifestations of Niemann-Pick Type C disease.

Dose: Adult: Type 1 Gaucher, initially 100mg 3-times daily; diarrhoea, reduce temporarily to 100mg once or twice daily. *Admin*, with or without food. *Elderly*, over 70 years, no data. Niemann-Pick, age 12 years and over, 200mg 3-times daily; diarrhoea, consider dose reduction.

Child: Type 1 Gaucher, under 18 years, no data. Niemann-Pick, under 12 years, BSA above 1.25m2 (200mg 3-times/day), above 0.88-1.25m2/ (200mg twice daily), above 0.73-0.88m2 (100mg 3-times daily), above 0.47-0.73m2 (100mg twice daily), 0.47m2 and under (100mg once daily); under 4 years, limited data.

Renal Impairment: CrCl (mL/min/1.73m2) 50-70, initially 100mg twice daily (Gaucher), 200mg twice daily (Niemann-Pick); 30-50, initially 100mg/day (Gaucher), 100mg twice daily (Niemann-Pick); below 30, not recommended.

Hepatic Impairment: Caution.

Interactions: Effect of Other Drugs on Miglustat: *Decreased exposure:* Cerezyme (imiglucerase).

SP: *Gaucher,* hand tremor, reduce dose or discontinue. Monitor Vitamin B12. Peripheral neuropathy; baseline and repeat neurological evaluation; numbness and tingling (re-assess risk-benefit). GI events (diarrhoea). *Niemann-Pick,* assess treatment benefit 6-monthly. Monitor, reduced growth reported (paed); mild platelet reduction without bleeding.

Pregnancy, Lactation: Pregnancy, not recommended. Females of childbearing potential to ensure adequate contraception. Males to ensure reliable contraception during and for 3 months after treatment. Lactation, not recommended.

ADR: See Notes below.

Notes: See 16.5 Metabolic Disorders.

Zavesca 100mg *(Actelion)* A. HT.
Price, (84) €6009.90.
Capsule, miglustat. White hard. Marked OGT918 and 100.

Nitisinone

ATC Code: A16AX04. **Sport:** Pending.
Driving: Vision may be affected.

Indications: Treatment, hereditary tyrosinemia type 1 (HT-1) with dietary tyrosine/phenylalanine restriction.

Dose: Adult, Elderly: Initially 1mg/kg/day. *Admin*, once daily; under 20kg body weight, admin in two divided doses; if initiated with food, continue with food. Admin oral susp using oral syringe without dilution; shake vigorously before use.

Child: As for Adult above.

Interactions: Effect of Other Drugs on Nitisinone: *Consider dose adjustment:* CYP3A4 inhibitor/inducers.

SP: Visual disorders (restrict dietary tyrosine/phenylalanine). Monitor, liver function; increasing alpha-fetoprotein, signs of liver nodules (evaluate for malignancy); platelets, white cell counts.

Pregnancy, Lactation: Pregnancy, use if only clearly necessary. Lactation, contraindicated.

ADR: See Notes below.

Notes: See 16.5 Metabolic Disorders.

Orfadin Capsules, Oral Susp *(SOBI)* A. HT.
Price, (60) 2mg, €909.79. 5mg, €1828.93. 10mg, €3221.41. 20mg, €6442.83. Oral susp 90mL, €2725.35.
Capsule, nitisinone. White opaque. Marked NTBC/strength. **Store:** Refrigerate.
Oral susp, as above 4mg/1mL. White slightly viscous opaque. *Sodium 0.7mg/mL; glycerol, benzoate.* **Store:** Upright; refrigerate; do not freeze.

Sapropterin

ATC Code: A16AX07. **Sport:** Permitted.
Driving: No or negligible effect.

Indications: Treatment, hyperphenylalaninaemia (HPA) with phenylketonuria (PKU) or tetrahydrobiopterin (BH4) deficiency.

Dose: Adult: HPA/PKU, initially 10mg/kg/day; titrate at 5-20mg/kg/day to achieve adequate phenylalanine levels. BH4, initially 2-5mg/kg/day; titrate by up to 20mg/kg/day (may need admin as 2-3 divided doses). *Admin*, with food to increase absorption; single daily dose at same time each day (preferably morning). Dissolve tabs in water; drink within 15-20 minutes.

Elderly: Over 65 years, caution.

Child: As for Adult above. Above 20kg, dissolve tabs in 120mL water; below 20kg, dissolve tabs in a graduated medicine cup or use a graduated syringe.

Renal Impairment: Caution, no data.

Hepatic Impairment: As for Renal above.

Interactions: Effect of Other Drugs on Sapropterin: Co-admin caution: Levodopa (increased excitability/irritability, convulsions), dihydrofolate reductase inhibitors (methotrexate, trimethoprim) (may interfere with BH4 metabolism), vasodilators (glyceryl trinitrate, isosorbide dinitrate, sodium nitroprusside, molsidomin) (may affect nitric acid metabolism), PDE-5 inhibitors, minoxidil.

SP: Continue restricted phenylalanine diet; monitor (phenylalanine, tyrosine) levels, nutrient intake, psychomotor development. Consult medical advice during illness (blood phenylalanine levels may increase). Convulsions, see Interactions above.

Pregnancy, Lactation: Pregnancy, strictly control maternal blood phenylalanine* levels before and during pregnancy. *(uncontrolled levels associated with very high incidence of neurological, cardiac, facial dysmorphism, growth anomalies). Lactation, not for use.

ADR: See Notes below.

Notes: See 16.5 Metabolic Disorders.

Kuvan 100mg *(BioMarin)* A.
Price, not published by company.
Soluble tablet, sapropterin dihydrochloride equiv. to sapropterin 77mg. Off-white (light-yellow). Marked 177. *Essentially sodium-free.*

Sodium Phenylbutyrate

ATC Code: A16AX03. **Sport:** Pending.
Driving: No studies performed.

Indications: Adjunctive, chronic management of urea cycle disorders (neonatal/late-onset).

Dose: Adult, Elderly: See Child below.

Child: Neonates, infants (under 20kg), 450-600mg/kg/day; children (above 20kg), adolescents, adults, 9.9-13g/m2/day (BSA). *Admin*, in divided doses with food.

Renal Impairment: Caution.

Hepatic Impairment: Caution.

Interactions: Effect of Other Drugs on Sodium Phenylbutyrate: *Co-admin may affect renal excretion:* Probenecid. *Frequent monitoring (plasma ammonia) with co-admin:* Haloperidol, valproate, corticosteroids.

SP: Caution, CHF, renal insufficiency (sodium content). Monitor serum potassium. Acute hyperammonaemic encephalopathy may occur. Acute hyperammonaemia management, not recommended.

Pregnancy, Lactation: Pregnancy, lactation, contraindicated.

ADR: See Notes below.

Notes: See 16.5 Metabolic Disorders.

AMMONAPS 500mg, Granules *(SOBI)* B. HT.
Price, tabs 500mg (250) €809.02. Grans 940mg/g (266) €1446.03.
Tablets, sodium phenylbutyrate. Off-white oval. Marked UCY 500. *Sodium 62mg/tab.*
Granules, as above 940mg/g. Off-white. *Sodium 149mg/5mL.*

Routine Childhood Immunisation Schedule, Ireland[1] (babies born before 01 October 2016)

Age	Immunisations	Comment
Birth	BCG	1 injection
2 months	DTaP/Hib/IPV/Hep B + PCV	2 injections
4 months	DTaP/Hib/IPV/Hep B + MenC	2 injections
6 months	DTaP/Hib/IPV/Hep B + PCV	2 injections
12 months	MMR + PCV	2 injections
13 months	MenC + Hib	2 injections
4 to 5 years	DTaP/IPV + MMR	2 injections
12 to 13 years (girls only)	HPV x 2 doses over 6 months	2 injections
12 to 13 years	Tdap	1 injection
12 to 13 years	MenC	1 injection

BCG	Bacille Calmette Guerin vaccine
DTaP	Diphtheria, Tetanus and acellular Pertussis vaccine
Hib	Haemophilius influenzae b vaccine
IPV	Inactivated Polio Virus vaccine
Hep B	Hepatitis B vaccine
HPV	Human Papillomavirus vaccine
MenB	Meningococcal B vaccine
MenC	Meningococcal C vaccine
MMR	Measles, Mumps and Rubella vaccine
PCV	Pneumococcal Conjugate vaccine
Rotavirus	Rotavirus oral vaccine (2 or 3 dose schedule)
Tdap	Tetanus, low-dose diphtheria and low-dose acellular pertussis vaccine

Routine Childhood Immunisation Schedule 2016, Ireland[2] (babies born on or after 01 October 2016)

Age	Immunisations		Comment
Birth	BCG*		1 injection
2 months	DTaP/Hib/IPV/Hep B + MenB + PCV + Rotavirus		3 injections + oral vaccine
4 months	DTaP/Hib/IPV/Hep B + MenB		2 injections + oral vaccine
6 months	DTaP/Hib/IPV/Hep B + PCV + MenC (+ Rotavirus)		3 injections (+ oral vaccine)
12 months	MMR + MenB		2 injections
13 months	Hib/MenC + PCV		2 injections
4 to 5 years	DTaP/IPV** + MMR		2 injections
12-13 years	Girls	HPV (2 doses 6 months apart), Tdap, MenC	4 injections
	Boys	Tdap, MenC	2 injections

*BCG not available since May 2015.
**dTap/IPV can be given if DTaP/IPV is not available

Adrenaline (epinephrine) should be available at all times when vaccines are administered.
Unless the Summary of Product Characteristics (SmPC) requires mixing of vaccines in one syringe (e.g. DTaP/IPV/HepB with Hib), multiple vaccines given at the same visit must be given at different sites.

Reference 1: Routine Childhood Immunisation Schedule 2014. See http://www.hse.ie/eng/health/immunisation/hcpinfo/guidelines/ Changes Chap 2, General Immunisation Guidelines (17 Sep 2015).
Reference 2: As for Reference 1, New Immunisation Schedule 2016, Chap 2, General Immunisation Guidelines (06 Sep 2016).

Adult Enteral Nutrition

Indication(s): A. Disease-related malnutrition. **B.** Short bowel syndrome. **C.** Intractable malabsorption. **D.** Pre-operative and post-operative management of undernourished patients. **E.** Inflammatory bowel disease. **F.** Total gastrectomy. **G.** Bowel fistulae. **H.** Dysphagia. **I.** Anorexia, poor appetite. **J.** Cystic fibrosis. **K.** Malignant disease. **L.** Increased nutritional needs due to various conditions (with clarification). **M.** Other conditions (with clarification).

Contraindication(s): All sip feeds are indicated for enteral nutrition. Sip feeds intended for enteral nutrition are NOT for parenteral (IV) use. Enteral supplements are not suitable when enteral nutrition is not permitted or contraindicated.

Special Precaution(s): All nutritional supplements should be used with medical/healthcare professional (HCP) supervision. ADDITIONAL contraindication(s) and/or Precaution(s) are listed under individual brands. Use in children may be contraindicated in infants (under 1 year) and/or in children (under 3 years) and may have a cautionary note for children (under 5 and 6 years). Nutritional information below is for adult use (unless specified). When using in children always consult the full Prescribing Information provided by the manufacturer.

Note: Energy is expressed as g/100mL or g/100g (unless otherwise specified) and/or % of total energy.

Abbreviations: CI (contraindications); GMS (reimbursed under the GMS Scheme); Euro price (price reimbursed by GMS); CAPD (continuous ambulatory peritoneal dialysis); RTH (ready to hang); SIRS (systemic inflammatory response syndrome); ARDS (adult respiratory distress syndrome).

Sip Feeds: Non-Disease Specific
Class Effects: See Adult Enteral Nutrition above.

Product	Indication(s)	Contraindications (not suitable for use):	Nutritionally Complete or Supplement only	Energy (kcal/mL)	Protein	Fat	Carbohy-drate	Fibre	Special Note	Pack size(s), Options	Price (Euro)
Energy 1cal/mL											
Ensure *(Abbott Nutrition)*	A. D. I. J. K.	Children. Galactosaemia. Diabetes (unless routine monitoring).	Complete	1kcal/mL	10g per 250mL (15.9%)	30.1%	54.0%		Gluten, lactose free	Liquid (3 flavours)	250mL (1), €2.00 (GMS)
Fresubin Original Drink *(Fresenius Kabi)*	A–H.	Children.	Complete or supplement	1kcal/mL	3.8g (15%)	3.4g (30%)	13.8g (55%)	0g (0.35g*)	Gluten, lactose free	Liquid (6 flavours) *chocolate	200mL (1), €1.90 (GMS)

Energy 1.5–1.9kcal/mL

Product	Indication	Type	Energy	Protein	Fat	Carbohydrate	Fibre	Free-from	Style (flavours)	Presentation
Altraplen Protein (Nuatra)	A. L (chronic wounds, post surgery).	Complete	1.5kcal/mL	10g	5.6g	15g	0g	Gluten-free	Milkshake style (1 flavour)	200mL (1), €1.60 (GMS)
Diben Drink (Fresenius Kabi)	A (with diabetes and/or glucose intolerance).	Complete	1.5kcal/mL	7.5g	7g	13.1g	2g	Gluten, lactose free	Liquid (3 flavours)	(1) 200mL, €2.50 (GMS)
Enshake (Abbott Nutrition)	A. I. J.	Supplement	1.9kcal/mL	11.20%	36.5%	52.3%		Gluten-free	Powder (4 flavours)	96.5g sachet (6), €15.05 (GMS)
Ensure Plus (Abbott Nutrition)	A. D. I. M (neurological disorders).	Complete	1.5kcal/mL	12.5g per 200mL (16.7%)	29.5%	53.8%		Gluten, lactose free	Milkshake style (6 flavours)	200mL (1), €1.70 (GMS)
Ensure Plus Crème (Abbott Nutrition)	A. D. H. I. M (taste fatigue).	Complete	1.4kcal/g	7.1g per 125g (16.8%)	28.8%	54.4%		Gluten, lactose free	Pudding style (3 flavours, neutral)	125g (1), €1.60 (GMS)
Ensure Plus Fibre (Abbott Nutrition)	A. D. I. M (constipation or diarrhoea, neurological disorders).	Complete	1.6kcal/mL	13g per 200mL (16.1%)	28.6%	52.1%	3.22% (FOS)	Gluten, lactose free	Liquid (5 flavours)	200mL (1), €1.80 (GMS)
Ensure Plus Juce (Abbott Nutrition)	A. I. K. M (fat malabsorption or steatorrhoea, fat restriction, taste fatigue, aversion to milky drinks).	Supplement	1.5kcal/mL	10.6g per 220mL (12.8%)	0.0%	87.2%		Gluten, lactose free	Fat-free juice style (6 flavours)	220mL (1), €1.80 (GMS)
Ensure Plus Savoury (Abbott Nutrition)	A. D. I. K. M (neurological disorders).	Complete	1.5kcal/mL	14g per 220mL (16.7%)	29.5%	53.8%		Gluten, lactose free	Savoury style (chicken)	220mL (1), €1.70 (GMS)
Ensure Plus Yoghurt (Abbott Nutrition)	A. D. I. M (neurological disorders).	Complete	1.5kcal/mL	13.8g per 220mL (16.7%)	29.5%	53.8%			Yoghurt style (1 flavour)	220mL (1), €1.70 (GMS)
Forticreme Complete (Nutricia)	M (patients unable to meet requirements from other foods).	Complete	1.6kcal/mL	11.9g per 125g (23.8%)	28.2%	47.8%	0.13g	Gluten free	Dessert style (4 flavours)	125g (1), €1.60 (GMS)
Fortijuce (Nutricia)	A-H.	Supplement	1.5kcal/mL	4g (11%)	0g (0%)	33.5g (89%)	0g	Gluten, lactose free	Juice tasting (non-milk) (6 flavours)	200mL (1) €1.80 (GMS)
Fortisip (Nutricia)	A-H.	Complete	1.5kcal/mL	6g (16%)	5.8g (35%)	18.4g (49%)	0g (0.3g*)	Gluten, lactose free	Milk style (7 flavours, neutral) *chocolate	200mL (1), €1.70 (GMS)

Product	Indication(s)	Contraindications (not suitable for use):	Nutritionally Complete or Supplement only	Energy (kcal/mL)	Protein	Fat	Carbohydrate	Fibre	Special Note	Pack size(s), Options	Price (Euro)
Fortisip Multi Fibre *(Nutricia)*	A-H. M (unable to meet requirements from other foods).	Children. Galactosaemia. Fibre-free diet required.	Complete	1.5kcal/mL	6g (16%)	5.8g (35%)	18.4g (49%)	2.3g (0.9%)	Gluten, lactose free	Milk style (5 flavours)	200mL (1), €1.80 (GMS)
Fortisip Yoghurt Style *(Nutricia)*	A-H.	Children.	Complete	1.5kcal/mL	6g (16%)	5.8g (35%)	18.7g (49%)	0.2g	Gluten free	Yoghurt style (3 flavours)	200mL (1), €1.70 (GMS)
Fresubin Crème *(Fresenius Kabi)*	A-H. M (continuous peritoneal dialysis, haemodialysis).	Children.	Supplement	1.8kcal/mL	10g per 100g (22%)	7.2g (36%)	19g (42%)	2g	Gluten, lactose free	Dessert style (5 flavours)	125g (1), €1.60 (GMS)
Fresubin Energy Drink *(Fresenius Kabi)*	A-H.	Children.	Complete	1.5kcal/mL	5.6g (15%)	5.8g (35%)	18.8g (50%)	0g	Gluten, lactose free	Liquid (8 flavours, neutral)	200mL (1), €1.70 (GMS)
Fresubin Energy Fibre Drink *(Fresenius Kabi)*	A-H.	Children.	Complete	1.5kcal/mL	5.6g (15%)	5.8g (35%)	18.8g (50%)	2g	Gluten, lactose free	Liquid (6 flavours)	200mL (1), €1.80 (GMS)
Fresubin Protein Energy Drink *(Fresenius Kabi)*	A-H. M (continuous peritoneal dialysis, haemodialysis).	Children.	Supplement	1.5kcal/mL	10g (27%)	6.7g (40%)	12.4g (33%)	0g (0.5g chocolate)	Gluten, lactose free	Protein drink (5 flavours)	200mL (1), €1.60 (GMS)
Fresubin Thickened *(Fresenius Kabi)*	A. H.	Children.	Supplement	1.5kcal/mL	10g (27%)	6.7g (40%)	12g*, 12.2g** (32.1%)	0.48g*, 0.7g** (0.9%)	Gluten, lactose free	Modified texture liquid. Stage 1, syrup texture; stage 2, custard texture (*vanilla, **wild strawberry)	200mL (1), €2.40 (GMS)
Fresubin Yocreme *(Fresenius Kabi)*	A-H. M (continuous peritoneal dialysis, haemodialysis).	Children.	Supplement	1.5kcal	7.5g per 100g (20%)	4.7g (28%)	19.5g (52%)	0g	Gluten free	Yoghurt style 125g (4 flavours, neutral)	Non-GMS
Nutricrem *(Nualtra)*	L (secondary to illness or unable to meet their nutritional requirements from other foods). H.	Children. Galactosaemia. Soya intolerance.	Complete	1.8kcal/g	10g per 100g	7.2g	18.8g	0g	Gluten, lactose free	Dessert style (3 flavours)	125g (1) €1.60 (GMS)

Product				Energy	Protein	Fat	Carbohydrate	Fibre	Dietary	Format (flavours)	Pack size & cost
Altraplen Compact (Nualtra)	A.	Children. Galactosaemia. Soya intolerance.	Complete	2.4kcal/mL	9.6g	9.6g	28.8g	0g	Gluten-free	Milkshake style (5 flavours)	125mL (1), €1.38 (GMS)
Calshake Powder (Fresenius Kabi)	A. C. J. K. L (HIV/AIDS). M (fat/carbohydrate supplement required).	Children.	Supplement	2kcal/mL	4.7g	25.3g	68.4g	0g	Gluten-free	Powder (4 flavours, neutral) *(reconstituted)	(7) 87g sachet, €15.83 (GMS)
Ensure Compact (Abbott Nutrition)	A. M (fluid restriction, volume intolerance).	Children. Galactosaemia.	Complete	2.4kcal/mL	12.8g per 125mL (17%)	35.1%	47.9%		Gluten free	Low volume feed (3 flavours)	125mL (1), €1.38 (GMS)
Ensure TwoCal (Abbott Nutrition)	A. D. K. M (liver disease, moderate burns, CHF, fluid restriction or volume intolerance, bolus feeding).	Children. Galactosaemia.	Complete	2kcal/mL	16.8g per 200mL (16.8%)	40.0%	42.1%		Gluten, lactose free	Nutrition and hydration (3 flavours, neutral)	200mL (1), €2.20 (GMS)
Foodlink Complete (Nualtra)	I (secondary to illness or unable to meet their nutritional requirements from other foods).	Children. Galactosaemia. Soya or milk protein intolerance.	Supplement	3.78-4.35kcal per g*	18.7-20.9g per 100g*	11.8-13g*	55.1-59.8g*	0g-7.3g*	Gluten free	Powder 57g sachet (4 flavours, natural *(flavour dependent)	Non-GMS
Fortisip Compact (Nutricia)	A.	Children. Galactosaemia.	Complete	2.4kcal/mL	12g per 125mL (16%)	11.6g (35%)	37.1g (37.1%)	0g	Gluten free	Milkshake style (7 flavours, neutral)	125mL (1), €1.38 (GMS)
Fortisip Compact Fibre (Nutricia)	A.	Children.	Complete	2.4kcal/mL	12g per 125mL (15.7%)	13g (39.3%)	31.5g (42%)	4.5g	Gluten free	Milkshake style (2 flavours)	125mL (1), €1.38 (GMS)
Fortisip Compact Protein (Nutricia)	A.	Children.	Supplement	2.4kcal/mL	14.4g (24%)	9.4g (35.3%)	24.4g (40.7%)	0g		Milkshake style. 125mL (5 flavours)	Non-GMS
Fresubin 2kcal Drink (Fresenius Kabi)	A-G. M (continuous ambulatory peritoneal dialysis, haemodialysis).	Children.	Supplement	2kcal/mL	10g (20%)	7.8g (35%)	22.5g (45%)	0g	Gluten, lactose free	Liquid (5 flavours)	200mL (1), €2.20 (GMS)
Fresubin 2kcal Fibre Drink (Fresenius Kabi)	As for Fresubin 2kcal above.	Children.	Supplement	2kcal/mL	10g (20%)	7.8g (35%)	22.5g (45%)	1.5g (1.6g*)	Gluten, lactose free	Liquid (4 flavours)	200mL (1), €2.20 (GMS)
Fresubin 5kcal SHOT (Fresenius Kabi)	A. C. M (high fat supplement with/ or without fluid and electrolyte restriction required).	Children.	Supplement	5kcal/mL	0g (0%)	53.8g (96.8%)	4g (3.2%)	0.4g (0%)	Gluten, lactose free	Fat emulsion (1 flavour, neutral)	120mL (1), €2.97 (GMS)

Tube Feeds: Non-Disease Specific

Class Effects: See Adult Enteral Nutrition above.

Product	Indication(s)	Contraindications (not suitable for use):	Nutritionally Complete or Supplement only	Energy (kcal/mL)	Protein	Fat	Carbohy-drate	Fibre	Special Note	Pack size(s), Options	Price (Euro)
Energy 1kcal/mL											
Diben *(Fresenius Kabi)*	A. M (diabetes and/or glucose intolerance).	Children.	Complete	1kcal/mL	4g	4.5g	8.3g	2g	Gluten, lactose free Low sodium	Liquid. EasyBag	(1) 500mL, €5.00 (GMS)
Fresubin 1000 Complete *(Fresenius Kabi)*	A-H. M (low energy intake required).	Children. Galactosaemia.	Complete	1kcal/mL	5.5g (22%)	2.7g (24%)	12.5g (50%)	2g (4%)	Gluten, lactose free	Liquid. EasyBag	(1) 1L, €10.00 (GMS)
Fresubin 1500 Complete *(Fresenius Kabi)*	A-H. M (low energy intake required).	Children.	Complete	1kcal/mL	3.8g (15%)	3.4g (30%)	13g (52%)	1.5g (3%)	Gluten, lactose free	Liquid. EasyBag	(1) 1.5L, €13.50 (GMS)
Fresubin Original *(Fresenius Kabi)*	A-G.	Children.	Complete	1kcal/mL	3.8g (15%)	3.4g/100mL (30%)	13.8g/100mL (55%)	0g	Gluten, lactose free	Liquid. EasyBag	500mL, €4.00; 1L, €8.00; 1.5L, €12.00 (GMS)
Fresubin Soya Fibre *(Fresenius Kabi)*	A-H. M (mild protein intolerance/objection, lactose intolerance).	Children.	Complete	1kcal/mL	3.8g (15%)	3.6g (32%)	12.1g (49%)	2g (4%)	Gluten, lactose free	Liquid. EasyBag	500mL, €4.50. 1L, €9.00 (GMS)
Jevity Promote *(Abbott Nutrition)*	A-H.	Children. Galactosaemia.	Complete	1kcal/mL	21.50%	28.90%	46.30%	3.29%		Liquid. RTH bottle	1L, €10.00 (GMS)
Osmolite *(Abbott Nutrition)*	A-G.	Children. Galactosaemia.	Complete	1kcal/mL	15.90%	30.30%	53.80%			Liquid. RTH bottle	500mL, €4.00. 1L, €8.00. 1.5L, €12.00.
Osmolite HP *(Abbott Nutrition)*	A. Post surgery. M (critically ill, catabolic, poor wound healing, metabolically stressed, liver disease, GI intolerance, neurological disorders).	Children. Galactosaemia.	Complete	1kcal/mL	24.90%	23.30%	51.80%		Gluten, lactose free	Liquid. RTH 500mL bottle	Non-GMS

Product	Indication	Contraindication		Energy	Protein	Fat	Carbohydrate	Fibre	Free from	Form	Non-GMS
Reconvan (Fresenius Kabi)	M (increased infection risk e.g. post-operative/ trauma particularly burns), severely malnourished. Not indicated (critically ill with severe SIRS, sepsis).	Children. Gluten sensitive enteropathy.	Complete	1kcal/mL	5.5g (22%)	3.3g (30%)	12g (48%)	0g (0%)	Lactose free	Liquid. EasyBag	(1) 500mL, €6.98; 1L, €13.61 (GMS)
Survimed OPD (Fresenius Kabi)	A-G.	Children. Galactosaemia.	Complete	1kcal/mL	4.5g (18%)	2.8g (25%)	14.3g (57%)	0.1g (0%)	Gluten, lactose free	Liquid. EasyBag	(1) 500mL, €4.50. 1L, €9.00 (GMS)
Fresubin Original Fibre (Fresenius Kabi)	A-G.	Children.	Complete	1kcal/mL	3.8g	3.4g	13g	1.5g	Gluten, lactose free	Liquid. EasyBag	(1) 500mL, €4.50. 1L, €9.00 (GMS)
Energy 1.1-1.5kcal/mL											
Jevity (Abbott Nutrition)	A-G.	Children. Galactosaemia.	Complete	1.1 kcal/mL					Gluten Free	Liquid. RTH bottle	500mL, €4.50. 1L, €9.00 (GMS)
Fresubin 1200 Complete (Fresenius Kabi)	A-H. M (low energy intake required).	Children.	Complete	1.2kcal/mL	6g (20%)	4.1g (30%)	14g (47%)	2g (3%)	Gluten, lactose free	Liquid. EasyBag	(1) 1L, €10.00 (GMS)
Fresubin 1800 Complete (Fresenius Kabi)	A-G.	Children. Galactosaemia.	Complete	1.2kcal/mL	6g (20%)	4.1g (30%)	14g (47%)	2g (3%)	Gluten, lactose free	Liquid. EasyBag	(1) 1.5L, €15.00 (GMS)
Jevity Plus (Abbott Nutrition)	A-G.	Children. Galactosaemia.	Complete	1.2 kcal/mL	18.20%	28.90%	49.30%	3.60%		Liquid. RTH bottle	500mL, €6.00. 1L, €12.00. 1.5L, €18.00 (GMS)
Osmolite Plus (Abbott Nutrition)	A-G.	Children. Galactosaemia.	Complete	1.2 kcal/mL	18.40%	29.30%	52.30%		Gluten, lactose free	Liquid. RTH bottle	500mL, €5.00. 1L, €10.00. 1.5L, €15.00 (GMS)
Jevity Plus HP (Abbott Nutrition)	A-H. M (CAPD, haemodialysis)	Children. Galactosaemia.	Complete	1.3 kcal/mL	24.80%	29.70%	43.20%	2.29%		Liquid. RTH bottle	500mL, €5.00 (GMS)
Fresubin 2250 Complete (Fresenius Kabi)	A-G. M (malnutrition risk; high energy requirement and/or fluid restriction).	Children. Galactosaemia.	Complete	1.5kcal/mL	5.6g (15%)	5.8g (35%)	18g/100mL (48%)	1.5g (2%)	Gluten, lactose free	Liquid. EasyBag	(1) 1.5L, €15.00 (GMS)
Fresubin Energy (Fresenius Kabi)	A-H.	Children.	Complete	1.5kcal/mL	5.6g (15%)	5.8g (35%)	18.8g (50%)	0g	Gluten, lactose free	Liquid. EasyBag	500mL, €5.00; 1L, €10.00; 1.5L, €15.00 (GMS)

Product	Indication(s)	Contraindications (not suitable for use):	Nutritionally Complete or Supplement only	Energy (kcal/mL)	Protein	Fat	Carbohydrate	Fibre	Special Note	Pack size(s), Options	Price (Euro)
Fresubin Energy Fibre (Fresenius Kabi)	A-H.	Children. Galactosaemia.	Complete	1.5kcal/mL	5.6g (15%)	5.8g (35%)	18g (48%)	1.5g (2%)	Gluten, lactose free	Liquid. EasyBag	500mL, €5.00. 1L, €10.00 (GMS)
Fresubin HP Energy (Fresenius Kabi)	A-H.	Children. Galactosaemia.	Complete	1.5kcal/mL	7.5g (20%)	5.8g (35%)	17g (45%)	0g	Gluten, lactose free	Liquid. EasyBag	500mL, €5.00. 1L, €10.00 (GMS)
Fresubin HP Energy Fibre (Fresenius Kabi)	A-H. M (CAPD, haemodialysis).	Children. Galactosaemia.	Complete	1.5kcal/mL	7.5g (20%)	5.8g (35%)	16.2g (43%)	1.5g (2%)	Gluten, lactose free	Liquid. EasyBag	500mL, €5.00. 1L, €10.00 (GMS)
Jevity 1.5kcal (Abbott Nutrition)	A-G.	Children. Galactosaemia.	Complete	1.5 kcal/mL	16.50%	28.60%	52.10%	2.85%		Liquid. RTH bottle	500mL, €5.00. 1L, €10.00. 1.5L, €15.00 (GMS)
Osmolite 1.5kcal (Abbott Nutrition)	A-H. M (CAPD, haemodialysis).	Children. Galactosaemia.	Complete	1.5 kcal/mL	16.60%	29.30%	54.00%		Gluten, lactose free	Liquid. RTH bottle	500mL, €5.00. 1L, €10.00. 1.5L, €15.00 (GMS)
Energy 2kcal/mL											
TwoCal (Abbott Nutrition)	A. D. J. M (liver disease and ascites, fluid restriction or volume intolerance, burns, multiple trauma, catabolic e.g. sepsis, infection, CHF neurological disorders).	Children. Galactosaemia.	Complete	2kcal/mL	16.80%	40.10%	42.10%	1.00%	Gluten, lactose free	Liquid. RTH bottle	1L, €15.00 (GMS)

Disease-Specific Feeds

Class Effects: See Adult Enteral Nutrition above.

Product	Indication(s)	Contraindications (not suitable for use):	Nutritionally Complete or Supplement only	Energy (kcal/mL)	Protein	Fat	Carbohy-drate	Fibre	Special Note	Pack size(s), Options	Price (Euro)
Energy 1kcal/mL and under											
preOp *(Nutricia)*	Pre-operative (up to 2 hours before surgery).	Infants. Emergency surgery. Delayed gastric emptying.	Supplement	0.5kcal/mL	0g	0g	12.6g	0g	Gluten, lactose, fat, protein, fibre free	Drink 200mL (1 flavour)	Non-GMS
Ketocal 3:1 Powder *(Nutricia)*	Intractable epilepsy (from birth).		Complete	0.66kcal/mL	1.5g	6.4g	0.68g			Powder (plain)	300g (1), €29.86 (GMS)
Elemental 028 Extra Liquid *(Nutricia)*	B. C. E. G.	Infants.	Complete	0.86kcal/mL	2.5g	3.5g	11g	0g		Liquid drink (3 flavours)	250mL (1), €3.72 (GMS)
Glucerna SR *(Abbott Nutrition)*	Diabetes mellitus. Hyperglycaemia (stress induced). Impaired glucose tolerance.	Galactosaemia.	Complete	0.93kcal/mL	18.40%	33.80%	37.40%	4.83%		Drink (2 flavours)	200mL (1), €2.50 (GMS)
Diasip *(Nutricia)*	M (diabetes, impaired glucose tolerance).	Children. Galactosaemia.	Complete	1kcal/mL	4.9g	3.8g	11.7g	2g	Gluten free	Milkshake style (3 flavours)	(1) 200mL, €2.50 (GMS)
Ketocal 4:1 Powder *(Nutricia)*	Intractable epilepsy.		Complete or supplement	1kcal/mL	2.05g	9.9g	0.41g	0.75g		Powder (neutral, 1 flavour)	300g (1), €29.86 (GMS)
Souvenaid *(Nutricia)*	Early Alzheimer's disease.	Galactosaemia.	Supplement	1kcal/mL	3g	3.9g	13.2g	0g	Gluten, lactose free	Milk-based drink 125mL	Non-GMS
Nutrison Advanced Diason *(Nutricia)*	Diabetes, impaired glucose tolerance.	Infants. Galactosaemia.	Complete	1kcal/mL	4.3g	4.2g	11.3g	1.5g	Gluten free	RTH Bag tube feed	1L(1), €10.00 (GMS)
Nutrison Advanced Peptisorb *(Nutricia)*	A-C. E. G.	Infants. Galactosaemia.	Complete	1kcal/mL	4.0g	1.7g	17.6g	0g	Gluten free	Tube feed	1L(1), €13.80 (GMS)
Peptamen *(Nestle Nutrition)*	B. C. E. G.	Cows' milk protein allergy. Children.	Complete	1kcal/mL	4g	3.7g	12.7g	0g	Gluten free	Liquid tube feed	500mL (1), €6.99; 1L (1), €12.58 (GMS)

Energy above 1kcal/mL to 2kcal/mL

Product	Indication(s)	Contraindications (not suitable for use):	Nutritionally Complete or Supplement only	Energy (kcal/mL)	Protein	Fat	Carbohydrate	Fibre	Special Note	Pack size(s), Options	Price (Euro)
Nutrison Soya Multi Fibre (Nutricia)	A.	Infants. Soy protein allergy. Fibre-free diet.	Complete	1.03kcal/mL	4.0g	3.9g	12.3g	1.5g	Gluten, lactose, milk protein free	Tube feed	Non-GMS
Cubitan (Nutricia)	L (chronic wounds).	Children. Galactosaemia.	Supplement	1.25kcal/mL	10g (30%)	3.5g (25%)	11.7g (45%)	0g*	Gluten free	Milkshake style (3 flavours); *trace (chocolate)	(1) 200mL, €1.60 (GMS)
Ensure Plus HP (Abbott Nutrition)	A. D. M (poor wound healing, moderate burns, general surgery, acute and chronic infections).	Children. Galactosaemia.	Complete	1.25kcal/mL	15.8g per 200mL (25.3%)	23.80%	50.90%	0%		Drink (2 flavours)	200mL (1), €1.60 (GMS)
Perative (Abbott Nutrition)	B. E. F. G. J. S. M (gastroenteritis, GI injury, malabsorption, pancreatic insufficiency, surgical resection).	Children. Galactosaemia.	Complete	1.3kcal/mL	20.50%	25.40%	54.10%		Gluten, lactose free	Liquid (plain)	500mL (1), €7.41: 1L (1), €14.83 (GMS)
ProSure (Abbott Nutrition)	Weight loss (oncology).	Children. Galactosaemia.	Supplement	1.3kcal/mL	20.90%	18.10%	57.70%	3.26%	Gluten, lactose free	Liquid (1 flavour)	220mL (1), €3.12 (GMS)
Nutilis Fruit Stage 3 (Nutricia)	A-F. H. Dialysis.	Children. Galactosaemia. Fibre-free diet.	Complete	1.33kcal/g	7g per 100g (21%)	4g (27%)	17g (51%)	2.6g	Lactose free	Pudding style (2 flavours)	150g (1), €1.60 (GMS)
Fortini Smoothie Multi Fibre (Nutricia)	A (in children from 1 year of age).	Infants (under 1 year). Galactosaemia. Fibre free diet.	Complete	1.5kcal/mL	3.4g (9.1%)	6.4g (38.5%)	19g (50.67%)	1.4g (1.8%)	Gluten, lactose free	Smoothie style (2 flavours)	200mL (1), €3.00 (GMS)
Ketocal 4:1 LQ (Nutricia)	Intractable epilepsy.		Complete or supplement	1.5kcal/mL	3.09g (8.2%).	14.8g (88.7%).	0.61g (1.6%).	1.12g		Liquid (plain)	200mL (1), €4.48 (GMS)
Oxepa (Abbott Nutrition)	SIRS. ARDS. Multiple organ failure. Acute lung injury. Mechanical ventilation.	Children. Galactosaemia.	Complete	1.5kcal/mL	16.50%	55.60%	27.90%		Gluten, lactose free	Liquid 500mL (plain)	Non-GMS
Pulmocare (Abbott Nutrition)	Bronchitis. COPD. Emphysema. Weaning ventilated patients. Respiratory failure. Oxygen therapy.	Children. Galactosaemia.	Complete	1.5kcal/mL	16.50%	55.50%	28.00%		Gluten, lactose free	Liquid (1 flavour)	500mL (1), €5.94 (GMS)

Product	Indications	Cautions	Type	Energy					Free from	Presentation	Pack size, price
Vital 1.5kcal (Abbott Nutrition)	B. E. G. J. Gastroenteritis. Surgical resection. Pancreatic insufficiency. Transition from elemental feeding. GI injury.	Galactosaemia.	Complete	1.5kcal/mL	18%	33%	49%	0g	Gluten, lactose free	Liquid 200mL, 1 L RTH (1 flavour)	Non-GMS
Respifor (Nutricia)	COPD.	Children. Galactosaemia.	Supplement	1.5kcal/mL	7.5g	3.3g	22.5g	0g	Gluten free	Milk-tasting drink (3 flavours)	125mL (1), €2.16 (GMS)
Forticare (Nutricia)	Cachexia (oncology), cancer (pancreatic, lung) on chemotherapy.	Children (caution, age 3-6 years with bleeding disorders). Anticoagulants. Galactosaemia. Fibre-free diets.	Complete	1.6kcal/mL	9g (22.5%)	5.3g (29.8%)	19.1g (47.7%)	2.1g		Milkshake style (3 flavours)	125ml (1), €1.63 (GMS)
Nepro HP (Abbott Nutrition)	Chronic renal failure (on dialysis). Cirrhosis. Conditions requiring high-energy, low (fluid, electrolyte) diet.	Galactosaemia.	Complete or supplement	1.8kcal/mL	18%	48.80%	31.80%	0.93%	Gluten, lactose free	Liquid (2 flavours)	220ml (1), €2.60: 500mL (1), €6.64 (GMS)
Renilon 7.5 (Nutricia)	Renal disease.	Children. Galactosaemia.	Supplement	2kcal/mL	7.5g	10g	20g	0g	Gluten, fibre free	Milk-tasting drink (2 flavours)	125mL (1), €1.63 (GMS)
Energy above 2kcal/mL to 5kcal/mL											
Nutilis Complete (Nutricia)	H.	Children. Galactosaemia. Fibre-free, lactose-free diets.	Complete or supplement	2.45kcal/mL	9.6g	9.3g	29.1g	3.2g	Gluten free	Milkshake style (2 flavours)	125ml (1), €1.50 (GMS)
Polycal Liquid (Nutricia)	A. Conditions requiring high or readily available carbohydrate supplement.	Children.	Supplement	2.47kcal/g	0g	0g	61.9g	0g		Drink (carbohydrate)	200mL (1), €1.75 (GMS)
Nutilis Clear (Nutricia)	H.	Children under 3 years of age.	No contribution to energy intake	2.9kcal/g	0.8g per 100g	0g	57.6g per 100g	28g per 100g		Powder. Fluid thickener only.	175g (1), €8.19 (GMS)
Phlexy-Vits Sachets (Nutricia)	Mineral and trace element supplement (from 11 years).	Infants.	Supplement	3kcal/g	0.3g per 100g	0	0.5g	5.8g		Powder 210g (30 x 7g sachets)	Non-GMS
Pro-Cal Shot (Vitaflo)	A. C. M (conditions requiring fat/carbohydrate supplement with protein).	Lactose or milk protein intolerance. Children.	Supplement	3.34kcal/mL	6.7g	28.2g	13.4g		Gluten free	Liquid (2 flavours, plain)	120mL (1), €2.52; 250mL (1), €5.26 (GMS)
Protifar (Nutricia)	Hypoproteinaemia. Increased protein requirement (burns, wound healing). Unable to meet protein requirements from normal food/drink.	Protein restricted diet.	Supplement	3.68kcal/g	87.2g per 100g	1.6g	1.2g	0g	Gluten free	Powder (protein)	225g (1), €8.10 (GMS)

Product	Indication(s)	Contraindications (not suitable for use):	Nutritionally Complete or Supplement only	Energy (kcal/mL)	Protein	Fat	Carbohydrate	Fibre	Special Note	Pack size(s), Options	Price (Euro)
Maxijul Super Soluble (Nutricia)	Energy enhancer (infant formula, tube and sip feeds). Energy intake enhancer (high energy, low fluid required).	Caution, diabetes.	Supplement	3.8kcal/g	0g per 100g	0g	95g	0g		Powder	200g (1), €2.55 (GMS)
Polycal Powder (Nutricia)	Conditions requiring high or readily available carbohydrate supplement.	Infants.	Supplement	3.84kcal/g	0g per 100g	0g	96g	0g		Powder (carbohydrate)	Non-GMS
Calogen Extra (Nutricia)	M (energy not met from normal food). Energy enhancer (sip/ tube feeds).	Children. Galactosaemia. Fibre-free diets.	Supplement	4kcal/mL	5g (5%)	40.3 (90.8%)	4.5g (4.2%)	0g	Gluten, lactose free	Emulsion (1 flavour, neutral)	Non-GMS
Calogen Extra Shots (Nutricia)	High energy supplement.	Children. Galactosaemia.	Supplement	4kcal/mL	5g (5%)	40.3g (90.8%)	4.5g (4.2%)	0g		Emulsion (1 flavour, neutral)	Non-GMS
Dialamine (Nutricia)	Advanced chronic renal failure. Certain urea cycle disorders (essential amino acid supplement required).		Supplement	3.78-4.35 kcal/g*	18.7g-20.9g per 100g*	11.8g-13g*	55.1-59.8g*	0-7.3g*	Gluten free	Powder *(flavour dependent)	400g (1), €68.66 (GMS)
Emsogen (Nutricia)	Severe malabsorption (LCT poorly tolerated). Overnight feeding (CF, pancreatic enzyme need reduced).	Infants.	Supplement	4.18-4.38 kcal/g*.	12.5g per 100g	16.4g	55-60g*			Powder (1 flavour, plain) *(flavour dependent)	100g (1), €7.20 (GMS)
Elemental 028 Extra Powder (Nutricia)	B. C. E. G.	Infants.	Complete	4.27-4.43 kcal/g*	12.5g per 100g	17.45g	55-59g*			Powder (3 flavours, plain) *(flavour dependent)	100g (1), €7.00 (GMS)
Calogen (Nutricia)	M (energy not met from normal food). Milk-replacement (protein-restriction), energy enhancer (sip/tube feeds); suitable with electrolyte restrictions.		Supplement	4.5kcal/mL	0g	50g	0.1g	0g	Gluten, lactose free	Emulsion (2 flavours, neutral)	(1) 200mL, €4.66; 500mL, €11.65 (GMS)

Product	Indication	Type	Energy					Form	Pack size (no.), price
Liquigen *(Nutricia)*	High energy required (with impaired fat absorption; high MCT intake indicated). Part of MCT ketogenic diet.	Supplement	4.5kcal/mL	0g	50g	0g	0g	Emulsion	250mL (1), €9.53 (GMS)
MCT Duocal *(Nutricia)*	Need for extra calories from combined fat + carbohydrate source (LCT fat malabsorption, MCT required).	Supplement	4.97kcal/g	0g per 100g	23.2g	72g	0g	Powder	400g (1), €20.09 (GMS)
Energy 5kcal/mL and above									
Scandishake Mix *(Nutricia)*	A. J. L (malabsorption).	Supplement	5kcal/g	4.7g per 100g	24.7g	65g	0g	Powder	85g (6), €13.26 (GMS)
Locasol *(Nutricia)*	Use only in hypercalcaemia.	Supplement	5.08kcal/g	14.6g per 100g	26.1g	53.7g		Powder	400g (1), €22.88 (GMS)
Pro-Cal Powder *(Vitaflo)*	A. C. M (conditions requiring fat/carbohydrate supplement with protein). Lactose or milk protein intolerance. Children.	Supplement	6.67kcal/g	13.6g per 100g	55.5g	28.2g	Gluten free	Powder	15g (25), €15.91; 510g (1), €14.74 (GMS)
MCT Oil *(Nutricia)*	Intractable epilepsy (ketogenic diet). Fat malabsorption (cystic fibrosis, chronic liver disease). Flavouring is not recommended for infants less than six months.	Supplement	8.55kcal/mL	0g	95g	0g	0g	Liquid	500mL (1), €15.10 (GMS)

Commonly Used Herbals and Possible Effects on Prescribed Medicines[1]

Herb: Common Name or Synonym	Most Common Indication(s) (Other Uses)	Potential Herbal-Drug Interaction(s)
Acai: Assai palm	Weight loss. *Other Uses:* Osteoarthritis, high cholesterol, erectile dysfunction, "detoxification", improving general health.	Possible interference with cholesterol-lowering and anti-diabetic drugs.
Alfalfa: Lucerne	Kidney, bladder conditions (diuresis). *Other Uses:* Prostate problems. High cholesterol, diabetes, upset stomach. Asthma, arthritis.	Contains large amounts of vitamin K; may decrease efficacy (warfarin, contraceptives, immune suppressants). May cause increased sensitivity to sunlight.
Bilberry: Huckleberry, Blaeberry, Whortleberry	Eye problems. *Other Uses:* Varicose veins, venous insufficiency. Urinary tract infections, gout, kidney disease.	May cause hypoglycaemia (used with anti-diabetic drugs). May slow blood clotting (used with anti-coagulants).
Black Cohosh: Black snakeroot	Menopause symptoms. *Other Uses:* Pre-menstrual syndrome. Osteo- (arthritis, porosis). Acne, mole removal, cough, sore throat.	May cause liver damage. With atorvastatin, increased risk of liver damage. Cisplatin, decreased efficacy. Antidepressants, antihypertensives, other CYP2D6 substrates, risk of increased (potency, side-effects).
Black Psyllium: Fleaseed, Plantago	Constipation. *Other Uses:* Diarrhoea, irritable bowel syndrome (IBS). High cholesterol.	May decrease efficacy (carbamazepine, digoxin, lithium). Might enhance effects (antidiabetic drugs).
Bladderwrack: Atlantic Kelp, Rock Weed, Sea (Oak, Kelp)	Thyroid disorders (underactive and goitre). *Other Uses:* Obesity, digestive problems. Arthritis. Blood cleansing.	Large iodine content; may enhance effects of anti-thyroid drugs. May slow blood clotting (used with anticoagulants, increased risk of bleeding, bruising).
Calendula: Marigold (garden marigold, pot marigold)	Skin problems (anal fissure, nappy rash, wound healing) (topical). *Other Uses:* Leg ulcers, varicose veins. Nose bleeds. Cancer.	Use with sedatives, enhanced effect; can cause drowsiness or sleepiness.
Cranberry: Mossberry	Cystitis. *Other Uses:* UTI.	May increase effects of warfarin.
Clover (Red): Clover (Wild, Meadow, Cow)	Menopause symptoms. *Other Uses:* Cancer prevention. High cholesterol.	Might increase effects (anticoagulants, antiplatelets). May decrease efficacy (contraceptives, HRT drugs, tamoxifen).
Dandelion: Blowball, Lion's tooth, wild endive	A "tonic for liver and kidney". *Other Uses:* Mild diuresis. Minor GI complaints. Cure for warts.	Use with antibiotics (quinolones); may decrease absorption. Use with lithium, may increase levels (diuretic effect); with diuretics, may cause increased serum potassium.
Devil's Claw: Harpagophytum, Wood spider, Grapple plant	Arthritis/Back pain. *Other Uses:* High cholesterol. Gout.	Might reduce effectiveness of Cytochrome P450 (and enhance effects of drugs that utilise that system); might enhance effects of warfarin.
Echinacea: Cone flower. Snakeroot	Cold and flu. *Other Uses:* To ward off infections (UTIs, thrush, herpes, AIDS/HIV, septicaemia).	May decrease efficacy of immunosuppressants, chemotherapy drugs (tamoxifen), some antivirals.
Evening Primrose Oil: EPO, Primrose Oil	Premenstrual syndrome, menopause symptoms. *Other Uses:* Eczema, psoriasis, acne. Rheumatoid arthritis. Osteoporosis.	May cause increased effects of anticoagulants and antiplatelets. Use with phenothiazines; reduced efficacy, increased risk of seizures.
Fenugreek: Greek clover, Bird's foot	To lower cholesterol. *Other Uses:* Loss of appetite, upset stomach, constipation, gastritis. Painful menstruation. Atherosclerosis. Diabetes.	May decrease blood sugar levels. May increase effect of anticoagulants and antiplatelets.
Feverfew: Batchelor's buttons	Headache/Migraine. *Other Uses:* Reduce fever. Arthritis.	Can impair blood clotting; avoid use with (anticoagulants, antiplatelets).
Flaxseed: Linseed	Constipation, diverticulitis, IBS. *Other Uses:* Anti-inflammatory (arthritis). High (cholesterol, BP). Menopause symptoms.	Use with antidiabetic drugs; risk of hypoglycaemia. Use with anticoagulants and antiplatelets; increased risk of bleeding.
Garlic: Allium sativum	Circulatory disorders, lower (cholesterol, triglycerides), inhibit platelet aggregation, high BP. *Other Uses:* Prevent cancer (stomach, prostate). Treat/prevent, common cold.	May cause reduced absorption of isoniazid. May enhance anticoagulant and antiplatelet effect; may decrease efficacy HIV/AIDS drugs. May enhance hypoglycaemic effect; decrease efficacy of some contraceptives, cyclosporin.
Ginger: Ginger root	Relief (indigestion, nausea). *Other Uses:* Osteoarthritis, vertigo.	May enhance effects (anticoagulants, antiplatelets, antidiabetic) drugs. Antihypertensives; ginger can lower BP; may (in combination) cause hypotension and/or irregular heartbeat.

Commonly Used Herbals and Possible Effects on Prescribed Medicines[1]

Herbal	Uses	Possible Effects on Prescribed Medicines
Ginkgo: Ginkgo biloba, Maidenhair tree	Dementia, improved memory. *Other Uses:* Improved blood circulation, intermittent claudication. Vertigo, tinnitus. Improved sexual performance.	Use with Ibuprofen; increased clotting risk. May enhance effects (anticoagulants, antiplatelets, antidiabetic) drugs. May reduce efficacy (diuretics, anticonvulsants); may dangerously enhance MAOI (effects, side-effects).
Ginseng, Panax: Ginseng, Asian ginseng	Improved stamina and energy levels. *Other Uses:* Alzheimer's disease. Erectile dysfunction (ED). Flu prevention.	May increase BP. May decrease blood sugar levels. May reduce efficacy of anti-rejection drugs, warfarin. May over-stimulate (used with antidepressants).
Green Tea: Camellia sinensis, Japanese tea, Green tea extract	To help with weight loss. *Other Uses:* Cancer risk reduction. Gingivitis. High cholesterol/triglycerides, hypertension. Prevention of Parkinson's disease.	Majority of potential interactions are due to green tea caffeine content. Vitamin K content may slow blood clotting. May decrease efficacy of hypoglycaemics.
Hawthorn: Haw, May, Maybush	To prevent heart disease. *Other Uses:* Heart failure, arrhythmias, hypertension, high cholesterol, angina, anxiety.	May cause increased efficacy, increased side-effects (beta-blockers, calcium channel blockers, digoxin, nitrates). Taken with PDE-5 inhibitors, may cause hypotension.
Horse Chestnut: Chestnut	Varicose veins, other circulatory problems. *Other Uses:* Joint pain, cough, haemorrhoids, eczema, menstrual pain, arthritis.	May decrease blood sugar levels. May slow blood clotting.
Lavender: Common, English, French Lavender	Sedative. *Other Uses:* Anxiety, depression, insomnia, migraine, toothache, nerve pain, spasms, hair loss.	May enhance effect of sedatives.
Liquorice: Liquorice, Sweet root, Can cao, Glycyrrhizic Acid	Dyspepsia. *Other Uses:* Gastritis, ulcers. Laxative. Bronchitis, cough, sore throat.	May cause salt and water retention (increasing BP). Increased potassium loss may increase side-effects (digoxin); use with diuretics may cause serious hypokalaemia. May cause decreased efficacy (warfarin).
Milk Thistle: Holy Thistle, St. Mary's Thistle, Silymarin	Liver tonic. *Other Uses:* Gallstones. Dyspepsia. Diabetes. Kidney disease.	May increase effects (hypoglycaemics, some NSAIDs). May decrease effects (oral contraceptives). Extract may affect liver function (may underlie any herbal-drug interactions).
Nettle: Stinging Nettle, Urtica dioica	Urinary problems. *Other Uses:* BPH. Aid to digestion.	Larger amounts may decrease (blood sugar levels, BP), induce drowsiness. Vitamin K content may increase blood clotting reducing efficacy of warfarin.
Peppermint: Peppermint Oil	Irritable Bowel Syndrome. *Other Uses:* Anti-spasmodic. Upset stomach. Muscle and nerve pain (topical).	May affect metabolism of ciclosporin (increased side-effects). May cause dyspepsia and nausea if taken with antacids.
Pumpkin: Pumpkin Seed	Bladder problems. *Other Uses:* Kidney infections, BPH. Intestinal worms.	The key effect is diuretic; caution (drugs with a narrow therapeutic window).
Saw Palmetto: Cabbage palm	Benign prostatic hyperplasia. *Other Uses:* Diuretic. To increase libido.	May reduce efficacy (oral contraceptives, HRT). May increase effect (blood thinners).
Soy: Soya, Soya Bean, Soy Milk	To help lower cholesterol. *Other Uses:* Hypertension, heart disease, diabetes, asthma, cancer, osteoporosis, kidney disease, menopause.	Fermented products of soybean contain significant levels of tyramine (involved in BP control). MAOIs can decrease the rate of breakdown of tyramine (causing elevated BP). May decrease efficacy (HRT, tamoxifen, warfarin).
St. John's Wort: Goatweed, Roisin Rose, Tipton Weed	Depression. *Other Uses:* Anxiety. Menopause. Wound healing (topical).	This list is not exhaustive, further caution advised. Alprazolam, amitriptyline, contraceptives, ciclosporin, digoxin, imatinib, HIV/AIDS drugs, dyspepsia and ulcer treatments, anti-epileptics, tacrolimus, warfarin (decreased efficacy). Antidepressants (increased side-effects). Narcotic analgesics, increased (efficacy, side-effects). Increased sensitivity to sunlight.
Tea Tree Oil (Topical): Australian Tea Tree Oil	Skin problems. *Other Uses:* Acne, fungal nail infections, Athlete's Foot, bacterial vaginosis, dandruff, antiseptic.	No specific interactions documented. Toxic if ingested; should not be used in or around the mouth. May cause skin irritation if used topically in high concentrations.
Turmeric: Curcumin, Indian Saffron	To help maintain bowel health. *Other Uses:* Digestive, respiratory conditions. Arthritis, fibromyalgia, inflammatory conditions. Protect against cancer. Ringworm, acne (topical).	Use with anticoagulants and antiplatelets, may increase efficacy.
Valerian: Common Valerian, Garden Heliotrope	Insomnia. *Other Uses:* Anxiety, depression. migraine. Dysmenorrhea.	Use with benzodiazepines (may increase efficacy), with antifungals (may increase side-effects).

1. References available on request.

443

Prescription Writing[1]

Prescriptions must[2]

- Be in ink
- Be dated
- Be signed by the prescriber with his usual signature
- Clearly indicate the prescriber's name and the prescriber's address (except for a GMS prescription)
- State whether the prescriber is a registered doctor, registered dentist or registered nurse
- Specify the name and address of the patient
- State the patient's age if under 12 years

Prescriptions should also include the prescriber's Medical Council Registration Number (MCRN). In the case of nurse prescribers the registration number must be included.

A GMS prescription should have the patient's GMS number

Name of Drug

- Preferably the generic approved name (International Non-Proprietary Name INN)
- Should never be abbreviated

Strength of Drug

Directions for Use

- Dose and frequency
- Duration
- Any additional information e.g. with food
- Avoid the term 'as directed' - if you write the directions on the prescription the label will provide a reminder to the patient of how to take the medicine safely

The prescription can only be dispensed if it is **'an original'** as issued by the prescriber. This means that faxes, emails etc. are not considered legal prescriptions. The only exception is a GMS three-monthly repeat prescription where three months are prescribed at once by creating two carbon copies of the original prescription. (Note: Repeat by 2 must be written on the top copy in order for the prescription to be legally repeated). Dentists cannot issue repeat prescriptions except for sodium fluoride tablets.

Dr A. Kashan
123 High Street
Dublin 2
Tel: 01 234 5678
Fax: 01 234 5679

1/8/17
Mr Joe Black
456 Main Street
Beaumont, D9

Rx Aspirin 75mg daily po x 28 days

A B Kashan (MCN 12345)

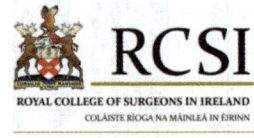

RCSI
ROYAL COLLEGE OF SURGEONS IN IRELAND
COLÁISTE RÍOGA NA MÁINLEÁ IN ÉIRINN

Department of General Practice

Requirements for prescriptions written for Controlled Drugs in Schedules 2 and 3[3]

- Be in ink
- Be dated
- Be signed by the prescriber with his/her usual signature
- Clearly indicate the prescriber's address (except for a GMS prescription). The address must be within the State
- Indicate whether the prescriber is a registered doctor, registered dentist or registered nurse
- Specify a telephone number at which the prescriber may be contacted
- Name and address of the patient (no longer required to be handwritten)
- For controlled drugs in Schedule 2 and 3, the following information **must continue to be handwritten by the prescriber:**
  - **name** of the controlled drug (either generic name/INN or proprietary/brand name)
  - dose
  - pharmaceutical **form** of the drug (e.g. tablets or capsules)
  - **strength** of the drug (where appropriate)
  - the **total quantity** to be dispensed written in both words and figures

If the prescription is for instalments it should additionally state the quantity to be dispensed in each instalment, number of instalments and the intervals between them.
There are a number of other schemes, aside

from the GMS. Please consult http://www.hse.ie/eng/Staff/PCRS/Contractor_Handbooks/PCRS_Handbook_for_Pharmacists.pdf for further information.

Dr A. Kashan

123 High Street

Dublin 2

Tel: 01 234 5678

Fax: 01 234 5679

1/8/17

Joe Barnes

45 Main Street

Beaumont, D9

Morphine Sulphate tablets (MST®) 10mg

ONE twice a day

Mitte 14 (fourteen) tablets

A B Kashan (MCN 12345)

The Medicinal Products (Prescription and Control of Supply) (Amendment) (No.2) Regulations 2014 add further requirements for the writing of prescriptions which are to be dispensed in another EEA member state and for the dispensing of prescriptions in Ireland which have been issued in another EEA member state. Practitioners should familiarise themselves with the requirements as appropriate.

References:
1. Prescription Writing. Dr Sumi Dunne, Professor Tom Fahey, Department of General Practice, Royal College of Surgeons in Ireland. Dr Judith Strawbridge, Mr Matthew Lynch, School of Pharmacy, Royal College of Surgeons in Ireland.
2. S.I. No. 540/2003 — Medicinal Products (Prescription and Control of Supply) Regulations 2003, as amended.
   See **http://www.irishstatutebook.ie/2003/en/si/0540.html**
3. S.I. No. 172 of 2017 – Misuse of Drugs (Amendment) Act 2016 (No. 9 pf 2016).
   See **http://www.irishstatutebook.ie/eli/2016/act/9/enacted/en/print.html**

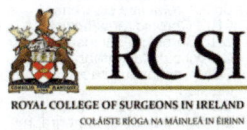

RCSI

ROYAL COLLEGE OF SURGEONS IN IRELAND
COLÁISTE RÍOGA NA MÁINLEÁ IN ÉIRINN

Department of General Practice

Abbreviations and Excipients

Term: Explanation

5-HT: 5-hydroxytryptamine (serotonin)

A

ACEI: Angiotensin Converting Enzyme Inhibitor
ACS: Acute coronary syndrome
ADH: Antidiuretic hormone
ADHD: Attention Deficit Hyperactivity Disorder
Admin: Administer
ADP: Adenosine diphosphate
ADR: Adverse Drug Reaction
AGEP: Acute generalised exanthematous pustulosis
AIDS: Acquired immunodeficiency syndrome
AIIas: Angiotensin II inhibitors
ALAT (ALT) (SGPT): Serum alanine aminotransferase
ALL: Acute lymphoblastic leukaemia
ALS: Amyotrophic lateral sclerosis
AMD: Age-related macular degeneration
AMI: Acute myocardial infarction
AML: Acute myeloid leukaemia
AMPA: alpha-amino-3-hdroxy-5-methyl-4-isoxazoleproprionic acid
ANLL: Acute non-lymphoblastic leukaemia
Approx.: Approximately
aPTT: Activated partial thromboplastin time
ARB: Angiotensin II receptor blocker
ARDS: Acute respiratory distress syndrome
ART: Assisted reproductive technologies
ASAT (AST): Aspartate transaminases
ATP: Adenosine triphosphate
ATPase: Adenosine triphosphatase
AUR: Acute urinary retention

B

BAN: British Approved Name
BMD: Bone mineral density
BMI: Body mass index
BMT: Bone marrow transplantation
BP: Blood pressure
BPH: Benign prostatic hyperplasia
BSA: Body surface area

C

CABG: Coronary artery bypass graft
CAD: Coronary artery disease
Cap: Capsule
CAPD: Continuous ambulatory peritoneal dialysis
CBG: Corticosteroid binding globulin
CEE: Conjugated equine oEstrogens
CF: Cystic fibrosis
CFTR: Cystic Fibrosis Transmembrane Conductance Regulator
CGD: Chronic granulomatous disease
CHD: Coronary heart disease
CHF: Congestive heart failure
CI: Contraindicated
CML: Chronic myeloid leukemia
CNS: Central nervous system
COC: Combined oral contraceptive
CHC: Combined hormonal contraceptive
COMT: Catecholamine O-methyl transferase Inhibitor
Conc: Concentrate, concentration
COX-2: Cyclo-oxygenase-2
CPK: Creatinine phosphokinase
CPT: Child-Pugh-Turcotte
CrCl: Creatinine clearance
CRF: Chronic renal failure
CRI: Chronic renal insufficiency
C-Section: Caesarean section
CSII: Continuous subcutaneous insulin infusion
CSF: Cerebrospinal fluid
CT: Computerised tomography
CTCAE: Common Terminology Criteria for Adverse Events
CVA: Cerebrovascular accident

D

DDC: Dopa decarboxylase
DHA: Docosahexaenoic acid
DHT: Dihydrotestosterone
DIC: Disseminated intravascular coagulation
DMARD: Disease-modifying anti-rheumatic drug
DPP-4: Dipeptidyl peptidase-4
DRESS: Drug Reaction with Eosinophilia and Systemic Symptoms. Also called multiorgan hypersensitivity reactions
DRI: Direct renin inhibitor
DSA: Digital subtraction angiography
DVT: Deep vein thrombosis

E

e/c: Enteric coated
ECT: Electroconvulsive therapy
ED: Erectile dysfunction
EDTA: Disodium edetate
EGFR: Epidermal growth factor receptor
EOD: Every other day
EPA: Eicosapentaenoic acid
EPO: Erythropoietin
Equiv.: Equivalent
ERT: Enzyme replacement therapy
ESA: Erythropoietin stimulating agent
ESR: Erythrocyte sedimentation rate
ESRD: End-stage renal disease

F

f/c: Film-coated
FBC: Full blood count
FDP: Fibrin degradation products
FHR: Foetal heart rate
FOLFIRI: Folinic acid, fluorouracil, irinotecan
FOLFOX: Folinic acid, fluorouracil, oxaliplatin
FSH: Follicle-stimulation hormone
FVC: Forced vital capacity

G

g/r: Gastro-resistant
G-6-PD: Glucose-6-phosphate dehydrogenase
GAD: General anaesthetic
GAD: Generalised anxiety disorder
GFR: Glomerular filtration rate
GHD: Growth hormone deficiency
GI: Gastrointestinal
GIFT: Gamete intra-fallopian transfer
GIST: GI stromal tumour
GnRH: Gonadotrophin releasing hormone
GORD: Gastro-oesophageal reflux disease
GU: Genito-urinary
GVHD: Graft versus host disease

H

HAART: Highly active antiretroviral therapy
Hb: Haemoglobin
HbIg: Hepatitis B immunoglobulin
HBV: Hepatitis B virus
hCG: Human chorionic gonadotrophin
HCl: Hydrochloride
HCTZ: Hydrochlorothiazide
HDL: High density lipoproteins
HER2 (ErbB2): Human epidermal growth factor receptor 2
HF: Heart failure
Hg: Mercury
HHV: Human herpes virus
Hib: Haemophilus influenzae type b
5-HIAA: 5-hydroxyindoleacetic acid
HIV: Human immunodeficiency virus
hMG: Human menopausal gonadotrophin
HNIG: Human normal immunoglobulin
HOCM: Hypertrophic obstructive cardiomyopathy
HoFH: Homozygous familial hypercholesterolaemia
HPA: Hypothalamic-pituitary-adrenal
HRT: Hormone replacement therapy

HSV: Herpes simplex virus
HTIg: Human tetanus immunoglobulin

I

IARC: International Agency for Research in Cancer
IARs: Infusion associated reactions
IBD: Inflammatory bowel disease
IBS: Irritable bowel syndrome
ICH: Intracranial haemorrhage
ICU: Intensive care unit
IDDM: Insulin dependent diabetes mellitus
Iga: Immunoglobulin A
IGF: Insulin-like growth factor
IM: Intramuscular
Immediate/R: Immediate release
Inf: Infusion
Inj: Injection
INN: International Non-Proprietary Name
INR: International normalised ratio
IOP: Intraocular pressure
IU: International units
IUI: Intrauterine insemination
IV: Intravenous
IVF: In vitro fertilisation

K

K: Potassium
KGF: Keratinocyte growth factor
KP: Kaposi sarcoma

L

LDL: Low density lipoproteins
LH: Luteinising hormone
LHRH: Luteinising hormone releasing hormone
LMWH: Low molecular weight heparins
LT: Leukotriene
LUTS: Lower urinary tract symptoms
LVD: Left ventricular dysfunction
LVEF: Left ventricular ejection fraction
LVF: Left ventricular failure
LVH: Left ventricular hypertrophy

M

m2: Square metres (metres squared)
MAC: Minimum alveolar concentration
MAOIs: Monamine oxidase inhibitors
MATE: Multidrug and toxin extrusion transporter
Max.: Maximum
mcg: Microgram
MDS: Myelodysplastic syndrome
mg: Milligram
mg/kg: Milligram per kilogram bodyweight
MI: Myocardial infarction
min: Minute
min.: Minimum
mmHg: Millimetres of mercury
MND: Motor neuron disease
Modified/R: Modified release
MOH: Medication overuse headache
MS: Multiple sclerosis
MTIR: Maximum tolerated infusion rate
mTOR: Mammalian target of rapamycin

N

Na: Sodium
NAION: Non-arteritic anterior ischaemic optic neuropathy
NCICTCAE: National Cancer Institute Common Terminology Criteria for Adverse Events
NGMN: Norelgestromin
NIDDM: Non-insulin dependent diabetes mellitus
NIHSS: National Institutes of Health Stroke Scale
NMDA: N-methyl-D-aspartate
NMR: Nuclear magnetic resonance scanning
NMS: Neuroleptic Malignant Syndrome
NNRTIs: Non-nucleoside reverse transcriptase inhibitors
non-STEMI: non-ST segment elevation myocardial infarction

NRTIs: Nucleoside reverse transcriptase inhibitors
NSAIDs: Non-steroidal anti-inflammatory drugs
NSCLC: Non-small cell lung cancer
NYHA: New York Heart Association

O
OA: Osteoarthritis
OAB: Overactive bladder
OATP: Organic anion transporting polypeptide
OC: Oral contraceptives
OCAS: Oral controlled absorption system
OCD: Obsessive compulsive disorder
OCT: Organic cation transporter
ODT: Orodispersible tablet
OGTT: Oral glucose tolerance testing
OHSS: Ovarian hyperstimulation syndrome
ONJ: Osteonecrosis of the jaw

P
PABA: Para-amino benzoic acid
PBPC: Peripheral blood progenitor cells
PCI: Percutaneous coronary intervention
PCOD: Polycystic ovarian disease
PCRS: Primary Care Reimbursement Service
PE: Pulmonary embolism
PEEP ventilation: Positive end expiratory pressure ventilation
PFMT: Pelvic floor muscle training
PFP: Prefilled pen
PFS: Prefilled syringe
Ph'-: Philadelphia chromosome negative
Ph'+: Philadelphia chromosome positive
PI: Protease inhibitors
PID: Pelvic inflammatory disease
PIL: Patient information leaflet
PML: Progressive Multifocal Leucoencephalopathy
PMS: Premenstrual syndrome
Polyene: Containing many double bonds
PONV: Post-operative nausea and vomiting
PPAR: Peroxisome proliferator activated receptors
PRCA: Pure red cell aplasia
Prolonged/R: Prolonged release
PSA: Prostate specific antigen
PSE: Portosystemic encephalopathy
PTH: Parathyroid hormone
PUBs: Perforations, ulcers and bleeds
PUVA: Combination of psoralen (P) and long-wave ultraviolet radiation (UVA)
PVCs: Premature ventricular contractions
PVD: Peripheral vascular disease
PWS: Prader-Willi syndrome

R
RA: Rheumatoid arthritis
RAAS: Renin-angiotensin-aldosterone system
RAST: RadioAllergoSorbent Test
RBC: Red blood cell/count
RCC: Renal cell carcinoma
RDS: Respiratory distress syndrome
RIMAs: Reversible MAO-A inhibitors
rINN: Recommended International Non-Proprietary Name
RLS: Restless Leg Syndrome
RLMD: Rapid Limb Movement Disorder
RO: Reflux oesophagitis
RTI: Respiratory tract infection

S
s/c: Sugar-coated
SBECD: Sulphobutylether beta cyclodextrin sodium
SC: Subcutaneous
SCC: Squamous cell carcinoma
SCLC: Small cell lung cancer
SGA: Short for gestational age
SHBG: Sex-hormone binding globulin
SIADH: Syndrome of Inappropriate Antidiuretic Hormone Secretion
SLE: Systemic lupus erythematosis
SNRIs: Selective noradrenaline reuptake inhibitors

SP: Special precautions
SPF: Sun protection factor
SQ-T: Standardised quality units
SSRIs: Selective serotonin reuptake inhibitors
Standard/R: Standard release
STD: Sexually transmitted disease
STEMI: ST segment elevation myocardial infarction
SUI: Stress Urinary Incontinence

T
Tab: Tablet
TB: Tuberculosis
TCADs: Tricyclic antidepressants
TIA: Transient ischaemic attack
TIH: Tumour-induced hypercalcaemia
TIVAD: Totally implantable venous access line
TNF: Tumour necrosis factor
TPMT: Thiopurine methyl transferase
TPP: Thrombotic thrombocytopenic purpura
TSH: Thyroid stimulating hormone
TT: Thrombin time
TURP: Transurethral prostatectomy

U
u/c: Uncoated
UGT: Uridine diphosphate-glucuronosyltransferase
ULN: Upper limit of normal
UV: Ultraviolet

V
VEGF: Vascular endothelial growth factor
Vit A: Retinol
Vit E: Tocopherol
VLDL: Very low density lipoprotein
VMA: Vanillylmandelic acid
VMT: Vitreomacular traction
VTE: Venous thromboembolism
VZIG: Varicella zoster immunoglobulin

W
WBC: White blood cells/count
WFI: Water for injection
WHA: World Health Association
WPW: Wolff (Wolfe)-Parkinson-White Syndrome

Z
ZIFT: Zygote intra-fallopian transfer

Excipients:
Excipient: Note, Caution (where applicable)

A
Alcohol: See Ethanol
Arachis (Peanut) oil: Caution, peanut and soya allergics
Ascorbate, sodium (E301), calcium (E302): Glucose-6-phosphate dehydrogenase deficiency, not recommended
Ascorbic acid (E300): See Ascorbate
Aspartame (E951): Phenylalanine source, caution phenylketonuria

B
Benzalkonium chloride: May cause irritation, punctate keratopathy, toxic ulcerative keratopathy. Not recommended for use with soft contact lenses
Benzyl alcohol: Premature babies or neonates (up to 3 years), not recommended; may cause toxic or anaphylactoid reactions
Butylhydroxyanisole (BHA) (E320): Irritant to eyes, skin (contact dermatitis) and mucous membranes
Butylated hydroxytoluene (BHT) (E321): As for butylhydroxyanisole

C
Castor oil (hydrogenated): Stomach upset, diarrhoea
Cetostearyl alcohol: Local skin reactions (contact dermatitis)

Cetyl alcohol: As for Cetostearyl alcohol
Chlorocresol: Allergic reactions

E
Ethanol: Consider possible CNS effects, drug interactions

G
Glucose: Rare glucose-galactose malabsorption, not recommended

L
Lactose: Rare hereditary problems of galactose intolerance, Lapp lactase deficiency or glucose-galactose malabsorption, not recommended
Lanolin (wool fat): Allergic skin reactions, contact dermatitis

M
Macrogolglycerol hydroxystearate: Diarrhoea, stomach upset
Maltitol, maltitol syrup (hydrogenated glucose syrup) (E965): Rare hereditary problems of fructose intolerance, not recommended
Maltose: May interfere with readings of blood glucose monitors (test strips with glucose dehydrogenase pyrroloquinolinequinone) (GDH-PQQ)
Mannitol (E421): Rare hereditary problems of fructose intolerance, glucose-galactose malabsorption, sucrose-isomaltase insufficiency, not recommended
Metabisulphite sodium (E223): Allergic reactions (anaphylactic symptoms, life threatening or less severe asthmatic episodes; more frequent in asthmatics)
Metacresol: Allergic reactions
Methyl-parahydroxybenzoate (E218): Allergic reactions (possibly delayed), exceptionally bronchospasm

P
Ponceau 4R (E124): Allergic reactions
Propyl-parahydroxybenzoate (E216): Allergic reactions (possibly delayed)
Parabens: See methyl, ethyl, propyl p-hydroxybenzoate
Phenylalanine: Caution, phenylketonuria
Potassium Sorbate: Allergic skin reactions, contact dermatitis
Propylene glycol: Skin irritation
Purified egg phosphatide: Allergic reactions

S
Saccharose: Saccharose-isomaltase insufficiency, not recommended. See Sucrose
Sesame Oil: Severe allergic reactions
Sodium: Caution, sodium restricted diets
Sodium benzoate (E211): Mild irritant to eyes, nose, mucous membranes May increase jaundice risk in newborns
Sodium Metabisulphite: See Metabisulphite
Sorbic acid: Local skin reactions (contact dermatitis)
Sorbitol (E420): Flatulence, abdominal distension, diarrhoea if admin in large quantities to adults. Rare hereditary problems of fructose intolerance, glucose-galactose malabsorption, sucrose-isomaltase insufficiency, not recommended
Soya lecithin: Caution, soya or peanut allergics
Stearyl alcohol: See Cetostearyl alcohol
Sucrose: Diabetes mellitus, caution. Rare hereditary problems of fructose intolerance, glucose-galactose malabsorption, sucrose-isomaltase insufficiency, not recommended
Sulphite sodium (E221): Anaphylaxis
Sulphur dioxide (E220): Allergic reactions
Sunset Yellow FCF; Orange Yellow S (E110): Allergic reactions including asthma

Pharmaceutical Companies and Agents

A. Menarini Pharma (Ire) Ltd
T: (0)1 2846744

Abbott AMO (Ophthalmics)
See WMO H/Care

Abbott Nutrition Ireland
T: (01) 4691500

AbbVie Ltd
T: (0)1 4287900

Accord H/Care Ltd
T: +44 (0)1271 385257

Actavis PCL
See Accord H/Care

Actelion Pharma Ltd
T: +44 (0)8450 750555

Aguettant Ltd
T: (0)1 431 1350

Alcon Laboratories UK Ltd
T: +44 (0)845 2669363

Alexion Pharma UK
T: +44 (0)1932 359220

ALK-Abello Ltd
T: +44 (0)118 9037940

Allergan Ltd
T: +44 (0)1628 494026

Alliance Pharma (Ire)
T: +44 (0)1249 466966

Allphar Services/Uniphar
T: (0)1 428 7777

Almirall Ltd
T: +44 (0)2071 602500

Amgen Ltd
T: 1800 535 160

Aribamed
T: (0)1 4688202

Aspen
T: 00800 004 04142

Astellas Pharma Co. Ltd
T: (0)1 4671555

AstraZeneca Pharma (Ire) DAC
T: 1800 800 899

Athlone Laboratories
T: (0)90 6661109

Atnahs Pharma UK
T: +44 (0)1268 535200

Auden McKenzie Ltd
T: +44 (0)1895 627420

Ayrton Saunders
T: +44 (0)151 7092074

Bausch & Lomb UK Ltd
T: +44 (0)1748 828849

Baxalta UK Ltd
T: +44 (0)1635 798777

Baxter H/Care (Ire)
T: (0)1 2065500

Baxter Oncology
T: +44 (0)1635 206345

Bayer Ltd
T: (0)1 2999313

Besins International H/Care
T: +33 (0)1 53015301

BGP Products (Ire) Ltd
T: +44 (0)1628 773355

Biogen Idec Ltd
T: 1800 812 719

Biotest (UK) Ltd
T: +44 (0)121 7448444

Bluefish Pharmaceuticals
T: +46 (0)8 51911600

Boehringer Ingelheim (Ire) Ltd
T: (0)1 2959620

Bristol-Myers Squibb (BMS)
T: 1800 749 749

Bristol-Myers Squibb/Pfizer
T: 1800 749 749

Caragen Ltd
T: (0)1 5552609

Cardiome Canada
T: 1800 330 9928

Carysfort H/Care Ltd
T: (0)1 2882332

CD Pharma AB
T: +46 (0)8 68436800

Celgene Ltd
T: 1800 333 111

Chefaro/Omega Pharma
T: +44 (0)207 5548888

Chemidex Pharma Ltd
T: +44 (0)1784 477444

Cheplapharm Arzneimittel GmbH
T: 0800 145 5034

Chiesi Ltd
T: 1800 817 459

Chugai Pharma Europe Ltd
T: +44 (0)208 9875680

Cipla Ltd
T: +91 (0)22 23082891

Clonmel H/Care Ltd
T: (0)52 77777

Concordia/AMCo Ltd
T: 1890 252 473

Consilient Health Ltd
T: +44 (0)203 7511888

Co-pharma Ltd
T: +44 (0)1923 255580

Creo Pharma
T: +44 (0)1371 822022

CSL Behring UK Ltd
T: +44 (0)1444 447400

Daiichi Sankyo
T: (0)1 4893000

Daiichi Sankyo/Eli Lilly
See Individual Companies

Dermal Laboratories Ltd
T: +44 (0)1462 458866

Dexcel Pharma UK Ltd
T: +44 (0)1748 828784

Dr Falk Pharma UK Ltd
T: +44 (0)1628 536616

Eisai Ltd
T: +44 (0)845 6761400

Essential Generics
T: +44 (0)1784 477167

Essential Pharmaceuticals
T: +44 (0)1784 477167

Fannin Pharma
T: (0)1 2907000

Farco Pharma
See Allphar

Ferring (Ire) Ltd
T: (0)1 4637355

Fidia Farmaceutici s.p.a.
T: +39 (0)49 8232111

Flynn Pharma Ltd
T: +44 (0)1438 727822

Forest Labs
T: (0)21 4619040

Fresenius Kabi Ltd
T: (01) 8413030

Fresenius Medical Care (UK)
T: 1800 902286

Galderma (UK) Ltd
T: +44 (0)1923 208950

Galen Ltd
T: 0483 8334974

Gedeon Richter (UK) Ltd
T: +44 (0)207 6048806

Geistlich Pharma AG
See Allphar

Genentech Roche
See Roche

Genus Pharmaceuticals Ltd
T: +44 (0)870 8510207

Genzyme Therapeutics Ltd
T: +44 (0)1865 405283

Gerard Laboratories
T: (0)1 8393788

Gilead Sciences Int. Ltd
T: +44 (0)1223 897555

GlaxoSmithKline (GSK) Consumer
T: 1800 441 442

GlaxoSmithKline (Ire) Ltd (GSK)
T: (0)1 4955000

Grunenthal Pharma Ltd
T: +44 (0)8703 518960

Hospira (Ire) Ltd
T: (0)1 2962102

HRA Pharma
T: 1800 812 984

Incyte Biosciences UK Ltd
T: 00800 000 27423

Indivior UK Ltd
T: +44 (0)1753 217800

International Medication Systems (IMS)
T: +44 (0)1753 447690

Intrapharm Laboratories Ltd
T: +44 (0)800 1455031

Ipsen Pharma Ltd
T: (0)1 8098200

Janssen-Cilag Ltd
T: 1800 709 122

Johnson & Johnson (Ire) Ltd (J&J)
T: 1800 220 044

KoRa Pharmaceuticals
T: 1890 0406

KrKa Pharma Dublin
T: (0)1 293 9180

Kyowa Kirin
T: +44 (0)1896 664045

Laboratorio Farma SIT (LAB)
T: +39 (0)384 820416

LEO Pharma
T: (0)1 4908924

Lilly (Eli Lilly) & Co (Ire) Ltd
T: +44 (0)1256 315000

Lincoln Medical Ltd
T: +44 (0)1722 742900

Lundbeck (Ire) Ltd
T: (0)1 4689800

Martindale Pharma
T: +44 (0)1277 266600

McNeil H/Care
T: (0)1 4665200

Meda Health Sales (Ire) Ltd
T: (0)1 8026627

Merck Serono
T: +44 (0)208 8187261

Merck Sharp & Dohme (Ire) (MSD)
T: (0)1 2998700

Merit Pharma
T: (0)1 8131010

Merus Labs
T: +31 20 350 2350

Moorfields Pharma
T: +44 (0)20 7684 9090

Mundipharma Pharma
T: (0)1 2063800

Myogen GmbH
See Allphar

Nestle UK
T: +44 (0)20 82824318

Niche Generics
T: (0)1 8167300

Nicox Pharma SNC
T: +44 (0)1483 549211

Nordic Pharma Ltd
T: (0)1 4004141

Norgine Ltd
T: +44 (0)1895 826600

Nova Laboratories Ltd
T: +44 (0)8707 120655

Novartis (Ire) Ltd
T: (0)1 2601255

Novartis Consumer Health
T: +44 (0)1276 687202

Novartis Vaccines
T: +44 (0)8457 451 500

Novo Nordisk Ltd
T: (0)1 678 5989

NPS Pharma
T: 1 855 215 5550

Nualtra (Ire)
T: (061) 518413

Nuron Biotech
T: 1800 948 878

Nutricia Ireland
T: (01) 2890283

Orion Pharma (Ire) Ltd
See Allphar

Orphan Europe (UK)
T: +44 (0)149 1414333

Otsuka Pharma Europe
T: 1800 936 539

Ovelle Ltd
T: (0)42 9332305

Pamex Ltd
T: (0)94 9024000

Pfizer H/Care (Ire)
T: (0)1 4676500

Pharma Mar S.A
T: +44 (0)1932 824026

Pharma Nord Ltd
T: (0)1 6305470

Pharmacosmos UK Ltd
T: +44 (0)1844 269007

Pharmadel (Ire)
T: (0)21 4217470

PharmaSwiss Ceska rep s.r.
T: +42 (0)234 719600

Phoenix Labs (Ire)
T: (0)1 4688917

Pierre Fabre Ltd
T: +44 (0)1962 874435

Pinewood H/Care
T: (0)1 4569123

Pliva Pharma Ltd
T: +44 (0)1730 710900

Ratiopharm Direct UK Ltd
T: +44 (0)239 2386330

Recipharm
T: +46 8 6025200

Reckitt Benckiser Ire Ltd
T: (0)1 4689200

Recordati (Ire) Ltd
T: 1800 303 351

Ricesteele Manufacturing Ltd
T: (0)1 4510144

Roche Products (Ire) Ltd
T: (0)1 4690700

Rosemont Pharmaceuticals
See Fannin Pharma

Rottapharm Ltd
T: (0)1 8852700

Rowa/Rowex Pharma Ltd
T: (0)27 50077

RPH Pharmaceuticals AB
See Recipharm

SANOFI
T: (0)1 4035600

Sanofi Pasteur
T: (0)1 4035600

Santen UK Ltd
T: +44 (0)8450 754863

Servier Laboratories Ltd
T: (0)1 6638110

Shire Human Genetic Therapies
T: 1800 818 016

Shire Pharma (Ire) Ltd
T: 1800 818 016

Sigma-tau Pharma Ltd UK
T: +44 (0)8000 431268

Sinclair IS Pharma Ltd
T: (0)1 8225417

Smith & Nephew Ltd
T: (0)1 2170444

SpePharm UK Ltd
T: +44 (0)1748 828890

SSL H/Care (Ire) Ltd
T: (0)1 4601925

Stallergenes (UK) Ltd
T: +44 (0)207 9606753

Statens Serum Institut (SSI)
See United Drug

Stiefel Laboratories
See GlaxoSmithKline

Swedish Orphan Biovitrum (SOBI)
T: +44 (0)1638 722380

Takeda UK Ltd
T: 1800 937 970

Talecris Biotherapeutics
T: +44 (0)2089 776118

Teofarma S.r.l.
T: +44 (0)1748 828857

TEVA Pharma (Ire)
T: (0)51 331331

The Medicines Company
T: 1800 812 065

Thea Pharma Ltd
T: +44 (0)870 1923283. See Pamex

Thornton & Ross Ltd
See Allphar

Tillomed
T: +44 (0)1480 402400

Tillotts Pharma Ltd
T: +44 (0)8450 344476

TMC Pharma Services Ltd
T: +44 (0)1252 842255

UCB (Pharma) (Ire) Ltd
T: +44 (0)1753 447690

Uniphar
See Allphar

United Drug PLC
T: (0)1 4632300

Valneva SE
T: +44 (0)1506 446608

Vertex Pharma Inc
T: +44 (0)1923 437672

Vifor Pharma UK Ltd
T: +44 (0)1276 853633

ViiV H/Care UK Ltd
See GlaxoSmithKline

Vitaflo
See Nestle

Warner Chilcott UK Ltd
T: +44 (0)800 0328701

WMO H/Care Ltd
T: (0)1 4291200

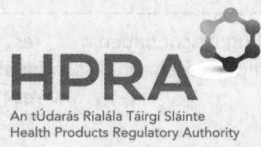

HPRA
An tÚdarás Rialála Táirgí Sláinte
Health Products Regulatory Authority

Adverse Reaction Report Form for Human Medicines

IN CONFIDENCE
Please complete this form in confidence and return to Freepost, Pharmacovigilance Section, Health Products Regulatory Authority, Earlsfort Centre, Earlsfort Terrace, Dublin 2. Telephone 353-1-6764971, Fax 353-1-6762517, e-mail medsafety@hpra.ie.

Reporter name:
Address:
E-mail:
Telephone number:
If healthcare professional, state profession and area of speciality:
Profession:
Area of speciality:

Patient Initials/Record Number	Sex Male ☐ Female ☐	Age:

Reason for treatment:

Suspect Drug(s)/Vaccine(s)[1]	Daily Dose	Route	Batch No.	Dates/Duration of treatment

Suspected reaction: *(Brief description of the effects/side effects/interactions, including any information relevant to the circumstances of this reaction, such as in use conditions, medication error, occupational exposure etc.)*

Time to onset (hours/days)	Onset of reaction (date)	Duration of reaction

Treatment given / Action taken

Outcome of reaction   ☐ Recovered   ☐ Recovering   ☐ Continuing   ☐ Fatal

---

[1] *Please use brand names where possible. Please note that for biological products, including vaccines, it is essential to include the brand name and batch number of the product.*

Drug Discontinued: Yes ☐ No ☐	Do you consider the reaction serious?
Improvement on discontinuation	Yes ☐ No ☐
Yes ☐ No ☐	If yes, please indicate the basis for this, ticking all the criteria that apply:
	☐ Fatal
Patient rechallenged Yes ☐ No ☐	☐ Life threatening (immediately)
If yes, state outcome	☐ Patient hospitalised / hospitalisation prolonged
	☐ Persistent or significant disability/incapacity
	☐ Congenital anomaly or birth defect
	☐ Medically significant - provide details:

Any other drugs used over this period? *(Please state below)*   None ☐   Unknown ☐

Drug/Vaccine	Daily dose:	Route:	Dates/ Duration of Treatment:	Reason for treatment:

Relevant medical history *(including significant concomitant illness/previous drug reaction)*:

Description	Start Date	End Date	Continuing

Additional information

| Supply of report cards required Yes ☐ No ☐ | Manufacturer notified: Yes ☐ No ☐ |

Signature _____   Date:

Thank you for taking the time to complete this form

Pre-Paid HPRA Quality Defect Report Card
HPRA TEL: 01-676 4971   FAX: 01-676 4061

Please complete (in BLOCK LETTERS) with as much information as possible.

EXACT NAME OF PRODUCT

PHARMACEUTICAL FORM

STRENGTH

TYPE OF CONTAINER

BATCH NUMBER

EXPIRY DATE

NAME OF PA / VPA / EU or other MA <u>HOLDER</u>

PA / VPA / EU or other MA <u>NUMBER</u> (Important)

Please state where you obtained the product from. (Please give name and address in box below)

FROM WHOLESALER (Wholesaler Name)

FROM MANUFACTURER (Manufacturer Name)

Please describe in detail the Defect, giving as much information as possible:

WERE ALL UNITS IN THE PACK AFFECTED (If applicable)?   YES ☐   NO ☐

DEFECT NOTICED BY: PHARMACIST ☐   PATIENT ☐   OTHER (please specify)

ARE SAMPLES AVAILABLE FOR SENDING TO HPRA?   YES ☐   NO ☐
If YES, please retain samples for 14 days. If we require a sample for inspection, we will contact you within 14 days.

If a wholesaler, marketing authorisation holder or manufacturer was notified of the defect, please state the name and company of the person you notified:

YOUR NAME & ADDRESS:

Do you agree to HPRA providing your name / your pharmacy name to the Investigating Company for their own follow-up with you?

YES ☐   NO ☐

DATE _____

Tel:

INN/Brand Index

A

456

458

461

464

468

47